DIAGNOSTIC STRATEGIES FOR INTERNAL MEDICINE: A CASE-BASED APPROACH

DIAGNOSTIC STRATEGIES FOR INTERNAL MEDICINE: A CASE-BASED APPROACH

CHARLES J. GRODZIN, M.D.
Fellow, Section of Pulmonary and Critical Care Medicine
Adjunct Attending-Housestaff
Department of Internal Medicine
Rush Presbyterian-St. Luke's Medical Center
Chicago, Illinois

STEPHEN C. SCHWARTZ, M.D.
Assistant Professor of Medicine
Section of Medical Oncology and Hematology
Department of Internal Medicine
Wayne State University
School of Medicine
Detroit, Michigan

ROGER C. BONE, M.D.
Professor of Medicine
President and Chief Executive Officer
The Medical College of Ohio, Toledo
Toledo, Ohio

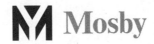

St. Louis Baltimore Boston Carlsbad Chicago Naples New York Philadelphia Portland
London Madrid Mexico City Singapore Sydney Tokyo Toronto Wiesbaden

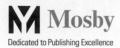

Mosby
Dedicated to Publishing Excellence

A Times Mirror Company

Editor: Stephanie Manning
Developmental Editor: Carolyn Malik, Laura Berendson
Project Manager: Linda Clarke
Senior Production Editor: Allan S. Kleinberg
Editing and Production: Graphic World Publishing Services
Designer: Carolyn O'Brien
Illustrations: Martens & Kiefer Illustration

Printed in the United States of America
Composition by Graphic World, Inc.
Printing/binding by R. R. Donnelley

Mosby–Year Book, Inc.
11830 Westline Industrial Drive
St. Louis, Missouri 63146

Library of Congress Cataloging-in-Publication Data

Grodzin, Charles J.
  Diagnostic strategies for internal medicine: a case-based approach / Charles J. Grodzin, Stephen C. Schwartz, Roger C. Bone.
      p.   cm.
  Includes bibliographical references and index.
  ISBN 0-8151-0642-4
  1. Internal medicine—Case studies. I. Schwartz, Stephen C., 1961–. II. Bone, Roger C. III. Title.
  [DNLM: 1. Internal Medicine—case studies. WB 115 G873c 1995]
  RC66.G76 1995
  616'.09—dc20
  DNLM/DLC
  for Library of Congress   95-32579
                                                                   CIP

96 97 98 99 00 / 9 8 7 6 5 4 3 2 1

CONTRIBUTORS

Robert Balk, M.D.
Section Director
Pulmonary and Critical Care Medicine
Department of Internal Medicine
Rush Presbyterian-St. Luke's Medical Center
Chicago, Illinois

M. Jeffrey Barkoviak, M.D.
Fellow
Section of Pulmonary and Critical Care Medicine
Department of Internal Medicine
Rush Presbyterian-St. Luke's Medical Center
Chicago, Illinois

John Barron, M.D.
Assistant Professor of Medicine
Section of Cardiology
Department of Internal Medicine
Rush Presbyterian-St. Luke's Medical Center
Chicago, Illinois

Yasmeen Bilimoria, M.D.
Fellow
Section of Allergy/Immunology
Department of Internal Medicine
Rush Presbyterian-St. Luke's Medical Center
Chicago, Illinois

Calvin R. Brown, M.D.
Assistant Professor of Medicine
Section of Rheumatology
Department of Internal Medicine
Rush Presbyterian-St. Luke's Medical Center
Chicago, Illinois

Michael Brown, M.D.
Assistant Professor of Medicine
Section of Digestive Diseases
Department of Internal Medicine
Rush Presbyterian-St. Luke's Medical Center
Chicago, Illinois

Godofredo Carandang, M.D.
Attending Physician
Infectious Disease
Cook County Hospital
Chicago, Illinois

Vishnu Chundi, M.D.
Fellow
Section of Infectious Disease
Department of Internal Medicine
Cook County Hospital
Chicago, Illinois

Scott Cotler, M.D.
Fellow
Section of Digestive Diseases
Department of Internal Medicine
Rush Presbyterian-St. Luke's Medical Center
Chicago, Illinois

Peter G. Curran, M.D.
Chief
Section Endocrinology
Columbus Hospital
Clinical Instructor, Northwestern Medical School
Department of Internal Medicine
Chicago, Illinois

Paul R. Delbusto, M.D.
Attending Physician
Section of Rheumatology
Department of Internal Medicine
Rush Presbyterian-St. Luke's Medical Center
Chicago, Illinois

Catherine Dimou, M.D.
Attending Physician
Internal Medicine
Rush Presbyterian-St. Luke's Medical Center
Chicago, Illinois

William J. Elliott, M.D.
Attending Physician
Section of Preventive Medicine
Department of Internal Medicine
Rush Presbyterian-St. Luke's Medical Center
Chicago, Illinois

Conrad Fischer, M.D.
Fellow
Section of Infectious Disease
Department of Internal Medicine
Sloan Kettering Memorial Cancer Center
New York, New York

Staci Fischer, M.D.
Fellow
Section of Infectious Disease
Department of Internal Medicine
Rush Presbyterian-St. Luke's Medical Center
Chicago, Illinois

Walter Fried, M.D.
Attending Physician
Department of Hematology/Oncology
Lutheran General Hospital
Park Ridge, Illinois

Philip Gorelick, M.D., MPH, FACP
Professor and Director
Stroke and Neuroepidemiology Unit
Department of Neurological Sciences
Chicago, Illinois

Charles J. Grodzin, M.D.
Fellow
Section of Pulmonary and Critical Care Medicine
Adjunct Attending-Housestaff
Department of Internal Medicine
Rush Presbyterian-St. Luke's Medical Center
Chicago, Illinois

Charlotte A. Harris, M.D.
Attending Physician
Section of Rheumatology
Department of Internal Medicine
Rush Presbyterian-St. Luke's Medical Center
Chicago, Illinois

James J. Herdegen, M.D.
Assistant Professor of Medicine
Section of Pulmonary and Critical Care Medicine
Department of Internal Medicine
Rush Presbyterian-St. Luke's Medical Center
Chicago, Illinois

Patricia Herrera, M.D.
Attending Physician
Section of Infectious Disease
Department of Internal Medicine
Cook County Hospital
Chicago, Illinois

Christopher Hughes, M.D.
Fellow
Section of Neurology
Department of Internal Medicine
Rush Presbyterian-St. Luke's Medical Center
Chicago, Illinois

Francis P. A. Jamilla
Fellow
Section of Pulmonary and Critical Care Medicine
Department of Internal Medicine
Rush Presbyterian-St. Luke's Medical Center
Chicago, Illinois

Amy Jenkins-Mangrum, M.D.
Resident
Department of Internal Medicine
Rush Presbyterian-St. Luke's Medical Center
Chicago, Illinois

Donald Jensen, M.D.
Attending Physician
Section of Digestive Diseases
Department of Internal Medicine
Rush Presbyterian-St. Luke's Medical Center
Chicago, Illinois

Jeffrey D. Kent, M.D.
Fellow
Section of Digestive Diseases
Department of Internal Medicine
Rush Presbyterian-St. Luke's Medical Center
Chicago, Illinois

Peter Kures, M.D.
Fellow
Section of Cardiology
Department of Internal Medicine
Rush Presbyterian-St. Luke's Medical Center
Chicago, Illinois

Jeffrey Lisowski, M.D.
Attending Physician
Section of Infectious Disease
Department of Internal Medicine
Grant Hospital
Chicago, Illinois

Kevin Maquiling, M.D.
Fellow
Section of Cardiology
Department of Internal Medicine
Rush Presbyterian-St. Luke's Medical Center
Chicago, Illinois

Theodore Mazzone, M.D.
Section Director
Endocrinology
Department of Internal Medicine
Rush Presbyterian-St. Luke's Medical Center
Chicago, Illinois

Kyoko Misawa, M.D.
Fellow
Section of Digestive Diseases
Department of Internal Medicine
Rush Presbyterian-St. Luke's Medical Center
Chicago, Illinois

John C. Pottage, Jr., M.D.
Attending Physician
Section of Infectious Disease
Department of Internal Medicine
Rush Presbyterian-St. Luke's Medical Center
Chicago, Illinois

David Rabin, M.D.
Fellow
Section of Cardiology
Department of Internal Medicine
Rush Presbyterian-St. Luke's Medical Center
Chicago, Illinois

G. Wendell Richmond, M.D.
Assistant Professor of Medicine
Section of Immunology/Microbiology and Internal
  Medicine
Department of Internal Medicine
Rush Presbyterian-St. Luke's Medical Center
Chicago, Illinois

Roger A. Rodby, M.D.
Assistant Professor of Medicine
Section of Nephrology
Department of Internal Medicine
Rush Presbyterian-St. Luke's Medical Center
Chicago, Illinois

Karen S. Sable, M.D.
Assistant Professor
Section of Digestive Disease/Internal Medicine
Rush Presbyterian-St. Luke's Medical Center
Chicago, Illinois

Jessica Santiago, M.D.
Fellow
Section of Infectious Disease
Department of Internal Medicine
Cook County Hospital
Chicago, Illinois

Deborah Schiappa, M.D.
Fellow
Section of Infectious Disease
Department of Internal Medicine
Rush Presbyterian-St. Luke's Medical Center
Chicago, Illinois

David Schwartz, M.D.
Attending Physician
Section of Infectious Disease
Department of Internal Medicine
Cook County Hospital
Chicago, Illinois

Gary Schwartz, M.D.
Assistant Attending
Department of Medicine
Division of Solid Tumor Oncology
Memorial Sloan-Kettering Cancer Center
New York, New York

Stephen C. Schwartz, M.D.
Assistant Professor of Medicine
Section of Medical Oncology and Hematology
Department of Internal Medicine
Wayne State University
School of Medicine
Detroit, Michigan

Panos Sechopoulos, M.D.
Chief Resident
Department of Internal Medicine
Rush Presbyterian-St. Luke's Medical Center
Chicago, Illinois

Kent Sepkowitz, M.D.
Attending Physician
Infectious Disease
Sloan-Kettering Memorial Cancer Center
New York, New York

Winston Sequiera, M.D., FACP
Chairman
Division of Rheumatology
Cook County Hospital—Chicago
Associate Professor of Medicine
Rush Presbyterian-St. Luke's Medical Center
Chicago, Illinois

Susannah E. Spiess, M.D.
Gastroenterology Fellow
Section of Digestive Diseases
Department of Internal Medicine
Rush Presbyterian-St. Luke's Medical Center
Chicago, Illinois

James H. Stein, M.D.
Fellow
Section of Cardiology
Department of Medicine
Rush Presbyterian-St. Luke's Medical Center
Chicago, Illinois

Paul Tamburro, M.D.
Fellow
Section of Cardiology
Department of Internal Medicine
Rush Presbyterian-St. Luke's Medical Center
Chicago, Illinois

Gordon Trenholme, M.D.
Professor of Medicine
Director
Section of Infectious Disease
Rush Presbyterian-St. Luke's Medical Center
Chicago, Illinois

C. William Wester, M.D.
Chief Resident
Department of Internal Medicine
Rush Presbyterian-St. Luke's Medical Center
Chicago, Illinois

Robert Winn, M.D.
Resident
Department of Internal Medicine
Rush Presbyterian-St. Luke's Medical Center
Chicago, Illinois

Rebecca Wurtz, M.D.
Attending Physician
Section of Infectious Disease
Cook County Hospital
Chicago, Illinois

Jong-Yoon Yi, M.D.
Fellow in Hypertension/Clinical Research
Department of Preventive Medicine
Rush Presbyterian-St. Luke's Medical Center
Chicago, Illinois

Neringa Zadeikis, M.D.
Fellow
Section of Infectious Disease
Department of Internal Medicine
Rush Presbyterian-St. Luke's Medical Center
Chicago, Illinois

IN MEMORIAM

"When something is working, keep doing it.
When something isn't working, do something different.
When all else fails, call a pediatrician."

"Deeds speak louder than words."

Harvey H. Grodzin, M.D.

DEDICATION

To my son Aaron:
Let your dreams be your guide through this life.

Stephen C. Schwartz, M.D.

PREFACE

Medical teaching is a challenge and a responsibility. In medicine's infancy teaching was rooted at the bedside. Early physicians demonstrated the subtleties of history taking, physical examination, and the natural history of disease as exemplified in patients. From this paradigm emerged educational tradition such as Osler's famous "Chairman's Rounds." To many young physicians the infirmed patient is a black box. Osler and others realized that answers to the mystery of disease lie within the patient before them. It was their commitment to patient care and the exhaustive search for medical knowledge acquired therein that serve as a benchmark by which excellence in medicine is measured.

It became apparent that textbooks of medicine would be required in order to impart this knowledge to future generations of physicians. Through time major textbooks have strayed from the patient as the focus. Works containing extensive information on separate disease entities are now the rule. These texts have become larger and all encompassing beyond the practical. The charge of the physician in training has become the digestion of long lists of facts. Learning theory would suggest that this is an inefficient method for knowledge acquisition and the formulation of interpretive thought. Formal medical education has itself witnessed a shift to a problem-solving format.

From experience, each hospital admission begins with an introduction, the formulation of a relationship, and an interpretive process from which the following questions will be answered: "Who is this patient?", "What is the chief complaint?", "What information can be gleaned from the history and physical examination?", "How will a diagnosis be established?" and "What is the correct therapeutic intervention?" Clearly, a patient-focused approach will make answering these questions less difficult.

Diagnostic Strategies for Internal Medicine: A Case-Based Approach provides the reader with a patient-directed framework from which sound clinical reasoning is explored. The individual cases and their respective clinical problems have been selected with the intent of improving clinical reasoning and strengthening the reader's knowledge base. This work has been written for the house officer, young attending, and senior medical student. It is this cohort that struggles to link patient complaints to disease and therapy. The material found within is representative of the seminal problems encountered in each discipline of internal medicine.

Charles J. Grodzin, M.D.
Stephen C. Schwartz, M.D.
Roger C. Bone, M.D.

INTRODUCTION

MEDICAL DECISION MAKING

Medical decision making requires a thorough understanding of the seminal manifestations of disease, acquisition, and organization of relevant data and an orderly and logical interpretative process. Data acquisition develops from a complex interaction between patient and physician known as the clinical interview. The success of the clinical interview rests in the development of a rapport between doctor and patient. This facilitates the collection of factual, complete, and sometimes sensitive personal information. A sense of trust must be established such that the patient acknowledges the physician as an advocate for his or her well-being.

ASPECTS OF DISEASE

Essential to the formulation of medical diagnoses is a cogent understanding of the *seminal manifestations* of disease. These include the temporal aspects of symptom presentation, patterns of pain, homeostatic changes including alterations in temperature, mental status, cardiorespiratory function, and autonomic reflexes.

Essential to providing insight into possible diagnoses is an understanding of "time frames" and their interplay in various disease processes. *Acute phenomena* have abrupt presentations with no antecedent signs or symptoms. This time frame lasts moments to hours. Testicular torsion may present acutely, producing an abrupt onset of excruciating testicular pain. Acute presentations may arise from thromboembolic disease, a ruptured viscus, or trauma. For every acute presentation, a review of each event leading up to the onset of symptoms is necessary. It is often easier to begin with the question, "When was the last time you were without this symptom?" and move serially through time with attention to every event. *Subacute presentations* have evidence of premonitory signs and symptoms, and a more insidious course ranging from days to weeks is the rule. This is best exemplified by epididymitis, which

presents with crescendo testicular pain. *Chronic disease* denotes an extended course with stable symptomatology. Often, patients present late in the course of their illness as symptoms may not impair daily function. This time course ranges from months to years. Chronic epididymitis is seen classically as a painful unremitting chronic inflammatory state lasting months.

Nociception, the perception of pain, is separated into somatic and neuropathic categories. Somatic pain emanates from damage to tissue, ultimately activating afferent sensory pathways. It is easily describable in exact terms by the patient (sharp, crampy, stabbing, etc.). Fracture, crush injury, and laceration represent sources of somatic pain. Pain arising from a visceral organ may, however, be vague and poorly localizable. Perception of visceral pain is often mediated by pain referral to a superficial dermatome.

Neuropathic pain results from damage to peripheral or central somatosensory pathways. This pain is less well-defined in location and description. The patient often describes the sensation in broad terms without specificity. Postherpetic neuralgia is a common form of neuropathic pain. Somatic pain is often treatable with analgesic agents. Neuropathic pain, in contradistinction, is poorly controlled by standard measures and often requires modification of ascending neural pathways (i.e., tricyclic antidepressants and TENS units have been known to benefit subsets of patients).

Fever is a product of cellular cytokine production, central hypothalamic regulation, and hypermetabolic states. Clinical settings in which fever is seen include infection (via secretion of the endogenous pyrogen IL-1), neoplasms (via production of tumor necrosis factor), hypermetabolic states (i.e., hyperthyroidism less commonly), metabolic aberrations (i.e., hypoglycemia), and generalized inflammatory diseases (i.e., active SLE or RA, inflammatory bowel disease). Fever patterns often serve as clues to specific disease entities.

Examples include the tertian and quartan fevers seen in malaria, the high spiking fever of Adult Onset Still's disease, and the Pel-Ebstein fever of Hodgkin's disease.

Changes of mental status accompany a multitude of systemic diseases. The level of mental status is determined by an assessment of the patient's response to environmental stimuli. *Acute confusional states* consist of changes of mental status, which include depressed cognitive capability, a decreased ability to attend, and abnormal responses to stimuli. *Delirium* encompasses these elements and a concomitant heightened level of arousal. The term *stupor* describes a depressed mental status from which a patient may be aroused only with the aid of physical stimuli. In contrast, the term *coma* refers to a level of consciousness from which a patient cannot be aroused. Presentation with any of these mental status profiles may provide insight into the etiology of disease. The patient who has used cocaine may appear delirious, whereas the patient with symptomatic hypoglycemia from insulin use may present stuporous or comatose.

The cardiopulmonary system subserves the function of supplying oxygen and nutrients to tissues. Perturbations in cardiovascular parameters are often manifestations of systemic illness. Tachycardia with increased cardiac output accompanies diseases requiring increased organ perfusion. Such entities include infection, fever, thyrotoxicosis, pain, etc. Paradoxically, cardiac ischemia may produce tachycardia secondary to stimulation of the autonomic nervous system. Bradycardia is a finding in severe hepatic dysfunction with significant hyperbilirubinemia and in cases of traumatic brain injury. Alterations in arterial blood pressure may result from such systemic illnesses as endocrinopathy, cardiovascular disease, severe head trauma, or infection. The respiratory system reacts by increasing the respiratory rate in response to metabolic demands in disease (acidosis, hypermetabolism, hypoxemia, etc.) for the purpose of enhancing oxygen delivery or excretion of carbon dioxide. The autonomic nervous system (ANS) func-

tions to support all homeostatic mechanisms. It is responsible for such diverse processes as the stimulation of counter-regulatory hormones in hypoglycemia and the production of fever by stimulation of tachycardia and tachypnea. It also serves to shunt perfusion to selected vascular beds under appropriate circumstances (i.e., peripheral vasoconstriction in septic shock). Additionally, the autonomic nervous system mediates the sensation of nausea that accompanies visceral injury.

THE CHIEF COMPLAINT: HOW TO GET THE INFORMATION YOU WANT

The first important piece of information obtained is the chief complaint. This statement reveals the patient's reason for seeking medical attention. The physician focuses on this point while acquiring facts extracted from the history of present illness. The history of present illness affords the physician the opportunity to methodically examine the chief complaint. Examination of such issues as the onset, duration, and course of the symptoms (fever, chills, nausea, vomiting, diarrhea, pain location, and patterns of radiation), successful or unsuccessful interventions (pain medicines, antibiotics, home remedies, herbal preparations, etc.), exacerbating or ameliorating factors (eating, position changes), and prior hospitalizations must be explored exhaustively. From this point the physician must allow the patient to relate the events of his or her illness, while carefully directing the conversation so that relevant issues are highlighted. Open-ended questions are preferable to "yes/no" format. The physician should maintain a degree of skepticism when evaluating information gleaned from the history. Often, patients will not be able to deliver objective information either because of lack of understanding the interviewer's questions or as the result of fear engendered by those same questions. Therefore, the interviewer should learn to ask questions that approach particular topics from a different direction. An example is a patient with an extensive history of smoking who presents to the hospital with productive cough and fever. Upon questioning she states that her breathing had not been limiting until her current problem began. However, upon investigation of her daily activity, it is clear that her son now does all her grocery shopping, her daughter must clean her home for her, and, although the weather has been warm, she has not gone outside for the preceding 2 months. In some cases, other sources of historical data should be sought. For example, an alcoholic patient with obvious massive weight loss may deny such a history out of fear of being diagnosed with hepatocellular carcinoma. In such a case the doctor should attempt to confirm suspicions from an additional source.

Other required information should include the patient's comorbid conditions and medications, as well as the patient's age, sex, race, and other identifying information. The patient profile remains the cornerstone on which the differential diagnosis is erected. For example, the complaint of chest pain in a 25-year-old man without significant past medical history generates an alternate differential diagnosis than does the same complaint in a 65-year-old hypertensive patient with known coronary artery disease. Defining the extent of existing disease is also critical. Thus, the evaluation should not only be tailored to the chief complaint, but to the possible manifestations of existing diseases. This may be important in the contrast between a patient recently identified as HIV positive versus an HIV positive patient with a CD4 count of 25, current candidal esophagitis, and three known episodes of *Pneumocystis pneumonia*. Assuredly, these patients must be approached differently.

Similarly, the ascertainment of lifestyle risk factors have a great impact on the patient profile and the approach to the differential diagnosis. Important diseases that have significant risk factors include coronary heart disease (cigarette smoking, hypercholesterolemia, Diabetes Mellitus, hypertension, etc.) and HIV infection (intravenous drug abuse, sexual promiscuity, unprotected intercourse, exposure to others with the infection, or history of recurrent infection). An example of how this may be important is the evaluation of an infiltrate on chest radiograph.

The approach taken is markedly different for patients on chronic corticosteroids for Systemic Lupus Erythematosus when compared to those with known HIV positivity or patients who are otherwise healthy.

Commonly, patients are unable to provide historical information concerning medical problems and medications. This may result from language barriers, altered mental status, or lack of familiarity with medical terms. These situations require contact with family members/interpreters or pertinent caregivers (i.e., primary physician, home health nurse, or dialysis center, etc.). The importance of acquiring past medical records cannot be overstated. Not only are they the source of important information regarding medical issues, but they may also be the source of baseline studies including chest x-rays and electrocardiograms. Inquiries made with health care providers in the field (paramedics) regarding the initial presentation, mechanism of injury, personal belongings at the scene, and eyewitness accounts of the event all provide the necessary information to formulate a firm understanding of the patient's presentation. Only with the above information is the physician capable of interpreting the patient's chief complaint in the appropriate context.

In various situations the level of acuity becomes an overriding issue. Included in this initial evaluation is the rapid assessment of hemodynamic, respiratory, and central nervous system stability. Thus, it follows that hemodynamic stability is of immediate concern in a patient with unstable angina due to the potential for impending morbidity and mortality.

THE PHYSICAL EXAMINATION: WHAT THE PATIENT DOESN'T SAY

The physical examination commences prior to the doctor actually entering the room. It is imperative that the physician avail all senses for information-gathering. This includes sounds, smells, visual clues regarding the patient's position, keptness, and such subtleties as skin pigmentation, breathing rhythm, and facial expression. This may help order thinking as fully as verbal history. As an example, patients often assume positions of comfort. A patient with chronic obstructive lung disease may manifest his dyspnea by sitting upright on the edge of the bed, hands on knees, leaning forward. He or she may not otherwise be able to tell you that he or she is extremely short of breath. Patients with sickle cell occlusive crisis writhe in an effort to find a position of comfort. Positional pain may also be seen with pericarditis, pancreatitis, or sinusitis.

Assessment of the vital signs is critical. While simple, these parameters are of the utmost importance. Indeed, in the emergency room setting, hospital admission may rest on interpretation of vital signs. As an example, fever in a neutropenic patient warrants immediate hospital admission for evaluation. From this point on, the physical examination, while thorough, is directed at the spectrum of physical manifestations of the disease processes that may be implicated by the chief complaint. While there may not seem reason to investigate all organ systems for a very specific complaint, it is not possible to predict what information may be collected. Often, an unsuspected finding may suggest or clinch a diagnosis. For example, in a patient who presents with shortness of breath and no history of smoking or lung disease, it remains important to examine the anterior and posterior chambers of the eyes and to palpate the angle of the jaw. When uveitis is present and the angle of the jaw is obscured in such a patient, the diagnosis of uveo-parotid fever or sarcoidosis may be entertained. In a similar situation, a febrile patient in whom endocarditis is suspected may be found to have conjunctival splinter hemorrhages observed on eversion of the left lower lid in the absence of a cardiac murmur.

THE DIFFERENTIAL DIAGNOSIS: A WIDE ANGLE LENS

With the chief complaint established, identifying data gathered, lifestyle risk factors delineated, and the physical examination completed, a differential diagnosis is generated. The construction of a differential diagnosis is essential in planning the course of diagnostic evaluation. Possible diseases should be ranked in order of likelihood and according to prevalence in the population. The impact of this rank order list is determined by the physician's fund of knowledge, patient age, origins, and lifestyle risk factors. The axiom, common diseases present commonly, and its converse, uncommon diseases present uncommonly, should serve to focus the physician's attention on the importance of disease prevalence when formulating a differential diagnosis. In the same vein, the physician must also realize that he or she is more likely to see an uncommon presentation of a common illness than a common presentation of an uncommon illness. Additionally, no matter how contrary to the presentation, there should be serious consideration given to those conditions that are potentially life-threatening. Discarding a diagnosis too early may ultimately jeopardize patient care. An example is the consideration of meningococcemia in patients presenting with fever and skin rash. Although it may rarely be present, the process is lethal unless diagnosed and treated early.

The depth of the differential is determined by the fund of knowledge of the physician. A disease cannot be diagnosed and treated unless known and understood by the physician. While this may seem obvious, it requires a sense of chronic dissatisfaction with one's own knowledge base that stimulates investigation and learning. One scheme that exists to help order diagnostic considerations is the mnemonic INDOCIN, which stands for **I**nfection, **N**eoplasia, **D**rug effect, **O**ccupational, **C**onnective tissue or **C**ardiovascular, **I**diopathic, and **N**oninfectious granulomatous/ other diseases. For a given specific complaint, each category is mentally perused for possible etiologies.

In construction of the differential, the first question to be answered is whether the current presenting complaint is an extension of a preexisting disease or a manifestation of a new syndrome. Therefore, consideration toward implicating a new aspect of a known comorbidity that may have not been previously active takes primacy over the diagnosis of a new disease. Extensive knowledge as to the potential complications of disease is necessary so that new disease processes are not falsely identified and the patient is not mistakenly exposed to additional testing or therapy.

The differential diagnosis should be built off a presumptive or working diagnosis that stands as the entity to be proven or disproven by the workup. This need not be a specific disease but should narrow the disease to an "infectious" versus "neurologic" versus "musculoskeletal" or other processes. *Settling on a specific diagnosis too early is often hazardous.* It is often useful to interpret the patient's complaints in symptom complexes, rather than as disparate findings, to maximize one's diagnostic power. For example, the pentad of renal insufficiency, mental status changes, fever, microangiopathic hemolytic anemia, and thrombocytopenia when taken together confirm the diagnosis of thrombotic thrombocytopenic purpura. However, the differential diagnosis for each symptom when taken separately is unmanageable. This does not negate the possibility of multiple diagnoses coexisting in the same patient to explain presenting symptoms.

FROM DIFFERENTIAL TO SPECIFIC DIAGNOSES: THE POWER OF MEDICAL TESTING

Once constructed, the most likely and most threatening diseases identified should be evaluated with the applicable tests. Methodically, each diagnosis should be ruled in or out. Diagnostic testing should be aimed at determining the presence or absence of a feature of a disease that would assuredly be present should the diagnosis be correct. If one was considering a diagnosis of a community-acquired pneumonia caused by *Streptococcus pneumoniae*, a gram stain of the sputum would be expected to contain leukocytes and Gram-positive diplococci in pairs in the majority of cases. Their presence in a noncontaminated sputum sample confirms the diagnosis. Another example is the consideration of meningitis in a patient with fever and disorientation. If this diagnosis were present, a pleocytosis in the cerebrospinal fluid should be present. Therefore, acquiring a sample of the CSF is the diagnostic test of choice. Diagnostic testing follows the "go where the money is" approach in many cases.

Often young physicians cling to a diagnosis when data is contrary. This is known as the *intern syndrome:* the wish to confirm exotic diagnoses when the evidence is not supportive. When one's clinical suspicion is high, one should not be dissuaded by the collection of unsupportive data. In such a case, the physician must actively seek alternate confirmatory data. The use of laboratory tests to yield information that does not impact on patient treatment or diagnosis is unwarranted. Multiple confirmatory tests that yield redundant information are not necessary.

When the leading diagnosis is less well-defined initially, several tests may be carried out at once. An example of this situation is the nursing home resident with fever and lethargy. A working diagnosis of mental status changes is made. The patient cannot provide a full history and the nursing home staff or family is unavailable. In this case, it may be necessary to carry out a urinalysis, chest radiograph, electrolyte panel, serum chemistries, CBC, blood cultures, head CT, and lumbar puncture before a diagnosis is reached. In this manner, all possibilities that may prove life-threatening are addressed in a timely fashion and empiric therapy is initiated when warranted.

THE TRANSITION FROM DIAGNOSIS TO THERAPEUTICS

Treatment is initiated in either of two situations: the diagnosis is well-established and requires therapy, or there is concern that the patient is so tenuous that empiric treatment is necessary based on clinical grounds to avoid morbidity and mortality. For example, a patient in the emergency room is complaining of acute dyspnea, worsening bilateral lower extremity edema, and is well-known to have an ejection fraction of 15%. Pulse oximetry found his saturation to be 84% on room air. He also complained that he had developed a productive cough of green sputum and had night sweats recently. While being evaluated he stated that he felt more short of breath. Because of the severity of his symptoms, he was given antibiotics to treat pneumonia, diuretics and topical nitroglycerin to treat heart failure, and exogenous nasal cannula oxygen to improve presumed hypoxemia. In this case, treatment was necessary before his specific pathophysiology was known due to impending cardiorespiratory failure.

When a patient is stable, one should not overlook the power of conservative therapy. This provides the physician with the opportunity to look for evolving aspects of disease, evaluate the need for therapy, and intervene before the onset of significant morbidity. In such circumstances the doctor must show the restraint to follow the credo: "Don't just do something, stand there!" When an infection is being considered, it is important to isolate a source and the specific organism. Cultures of all sites are always necessary prior to starting antibiotics. While observing a patient, antibiotic therapy may be started should the clinical situation change. Treatment should be directed due to the emergence of drug-resistant strains of organisms such as *Mycobacterium tuberculosis, Streptococcus pneumoniae,* and vancomycin-resistant *Enterococcus faecalis.* When treatment is started empirically, it should be kept in mind that the decision to treat is not binding once a definitive diagnosis is made. For example, if a patient is begun on heparin empirically for deep venous thrombosis, but further evaluation by ultrasound reveals a Baker's cyst, the heparin is appropriately stopped in the face of a new diagnosis. The same applies to a choice of antibiotic therapy. As new information about a patient is collected, antibiotic coverage may be altered in an effort to take advantage of an organism's susceptibility pattern, positive blood cultures, or development of other localizing signs or symptoms.

If the patient evaluation was thoughtful and complete, the physician may adhere to the original plan with confidence even though the day-to-day complaints and/or condition of the patient may change. Reasons for early failure of a treatment regimen include inadequate drug level for optimum effect, adverse effects that may impair tolerance, inadequate delivery, or absorption of medication and a lengthier time frame required for greatest efficacy. Physicians are often concerned about a patient who presents with a febrile illness who fails to defervesce immediately after starting therapy. A practical example is the AIDS patient with extensive cellulitis who presents with a febrile episode to 40°C shortly after his 11 PM vancomycin dose after a 4-day course. Cultures of blood, urine, and stool were obtained, along with a chest x-ray, CBC, and sputum induction for culture and AFB. A Gallium scan was also ordered to evaluate the new fever. Discussion with the housestaff the next morning did not suggest a deterioration in the patient's clinical picture consistent with worsening infection. Thus, a drug reaction was now considered a potential source of the fever. As his infection was not considered life-threatening, the vancomycin was held. Over the next several days his fever dissipated and his cellulitis was treated successfully with ampicillin. The clinical diagnosis secure, the patient's clinical status was interpreted correctly, and he responded to another antibiotic promptly with resolution of his infection.

As an adjunct to medical therapy, surgical consultation may be imperative. It may be necessary to evacuate purulent material from superficial or deep tissue in order to clear infection. An extreme example is necrotizing Group-A streptococcal fasciitis, which requires wide surgical debridement as a life-saving intervention. On a smaller scale, skin abscesses benefit from incision and drainage in the outpatient setting or the emergency room.

PUTTING THE RIGHT FOOT FORWARD

The importance of the initial patient evaluation should not be underestimated. Arrival at a working and differential diagnosis in conjunction with a plan to evaluate all potential diagnoses should determine whether an inpatient or outpatient evaluation is necessary. Often, discussion with the patient's primary physician can help determine a course of action. If an outpatient mode is chosen, information about the current problem is essential to the practitioner in arranging tests or subsequent therapy. Hospital admission is necessitated when there is concern that the medical condition is tenuous and that it would be unlikely that those assisting the patient at home would be able to recognize or treat the onset of symptoms prior to significant morbidity. Admission is also required when the therapeutic needs of the patient outstrip home care limits (i.e., intravenous antibiotics, surgical intervention). In this case, the initial evaluation orders subsequent thought processes, diagnostic testing, goals of hospitalization, and understanding on the part of the patient concerning his or her condition.

THE PHYSICIAN-TEAM CARE GROUP

An important element of the learning process is the understanding of personal limits. The ultimate goal of the doctor-patient relationship is the rapid treatment of premorbid processes. If the examining physician has reached a diagnostic limit, it is important to ask for help. In most teaching institutions, each admitting team is made up of a hierarchy of medical students→interns→senior residents→attending physicians. In addition, there may be intensive care unit fellows, specialty services on call, and medical chief residents available for consultation, patient evaluation, and placement of the patient in the correct care unit. These resources are adjunctive sources of information and should be utilized to broaden the differential diagnosis, to make light of subtle clues that reorganize the differential diagnosis, to help choose more specific diagnostic tests, and to bring a greater clinical experience to the patient care team. Attendant to this care team is the responsibility at each level to impart teaching to the levels below. In this way, each patient interaction becomes a learning experience; each physician expands the power of his or her diagnostic and therapeutic armamentarium.

An example of this system working well is the patient with rheumatoid arthritis on corticosteroid therapy presenting with a fever and a dense infiltrate on the initial chest radiograph. The patient is markedly diaphoretic and becomes more dyspneic to the point of respiratory failure. The patient is subsequently intubated and transferred to the intensive care unit for ventilatory support. The patient remains persistently hyperkalemic, hyponatremic, and hypotensive. She is felt to be adrenally insufficient. "Stress" doses of corticosteroids are administered, and the patient is rendered stable. In this scenario, there are several levels of complexity: the identification of a patient with a long-standing illness, the identification of a severely immunosuppressive therapy, recognition of a new acute problem, serious metabolic or endocrinologic problems, the skill to perform endotracheal intubation, and the subtlety of identifying the risk of atlantoaxial subluxation when extending the cervical spine to open the airway. Additional choices concerning fluid management, antibiotic therapy, need for invasive hemodynamic monitoring, and use of pressor agents when required are made by the patient care team. A complicated case such as this may require the additive input of different levels of the health care team to come to a complete evaluation of the patient. Again, the limitation to serving the patient is based on how well the team works together, sums their collective knowledge, and turns every effort toward patient advocacy.

THE NEXT STEP

Each of the following cases describes a patient's initial presentation, pertinent history, and findings from the physical examination. Each exercise is organized in a question-and-answer format. This provides the reader with a knowledge base and access to a line of reasoning with which to approach each patient.

For maximum yield, it is suggested the physician read each case, taking time to consider the questions individually and putting forth an answer before that provided in the text. It is hoped that this approach will yield not only pertinent information but a process of thought that is useful in all areas of medical decision making.

CONTENTS

ALLERGY/
IMMUNOLOGY

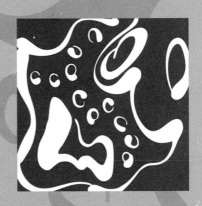

....

G. WENDELL RICHMOND
SECTION EDITOR

CASE

I

Yasmeen Bilimoria
G. Wendell Richmond
· · · · · · · · ·

The patient is a 67-year-old retired woman who presented with complaints of postnasal drip initially noted 2 years ago after she had Legionella pneumonia. She associates exacerbations of her symptoms with humid or windy weather conditions. She also correlates an increase in her symptoms with a recent change in eye drops used to treat glaucoma. A trial of intranasal corticosteroids and cromolyn did not improve her condition. She has found that one half tablet of terfenadine transiently decreases her postnasal drip. However, her symptoms have worsened since moving from Palm Springs to Chicago.

QUESTION 1 You believe that the patient's symptoms are consistent with rhinitis. What are the important historical and examination points you should now pursue?

Evaluation of a patient with symptoms of rhinitis is based on a thorough history. The most important information includes the circumstances of onset, duration and severity of symptoms, and precipitating factors. Information about environmental exposures the patient has throughout the day, both in the home and at work, can add vital insight into possible potentiating factors. Other important factors in the evaluation include a family history of allergic rhinitis, urticaria, or asthma. Many patients will attempt self-medication for this problem so that responses to trials of therapy can be useful pieces of information. One should be careful not to label any home trial a failure until it is clear that the patient administered the medication correctly and used adequate doses for an acceptable period of time.

Allergic rhinitis may be diagnosed by history alone if classic seasonal symptoms predominate. However, in many patients, symptoms do not fall into a distinct seasonal pattern and further work-up is necessary.

The physical examination can also yield important information. Attention should be directed at target end organs to assess severity of the disease process. Common findings are nasal mucosal edema with pale turbinates. Secretions, if present, are clear and watery. Atopic patients may display the classic findings of allergic shiners, an allergic nasal crease, or the accentuated fold of the lower eyelid known as *Dennie's line*.

QUESTION 2 The patient's past medical history was significant for urticaria at age 30 without signs of atopic disease. She also has been treated with isoptocarpine for desquamative glaucoma. Her family history revealed a son with asthma and severe allergies and a maternal grandmother with asthma. Physical examination found systolic hypertension and bilateral miosis. Skin testing was positive to *Dermatophagoides farinae, D. pteronyssinus,* and *Aspergillus.* What is rhinitis, what is your differential diagnosis based on the provided information, and what are the key elements of each entity?

Rhinitis is a common disorder affecting up to 20% of the North American population. It may be classified according to the scheme outlined in Fig. 1-1-1 on p. 6. Rhinitis may be experienced as a component of an upper respiratory tract infection or an allergic syndrome. Physicians should construct a differential diagnosis of rhinitis and recognize that in some patients an "overlap" of rhinitides may explain their disease.

Allergic rhinitis has an estimated prevalence ranging from 5% to 22% with onset between 5 and 20 years of age. Disease is due to the relationship between allergens and associated antigen-specific IgE antibodies that bind to both high- and low-affinity IgE receptors on mast cells and basophils. The immediate response to the allergen is the result of mast cell activation and subsequent release of inflammatory mediators including histamine, prostaglandin D2, leukotrienes, and neutral proteases. In some patients who have been challenged with retronasal allergen, a late phase response occurs 6 to 8 hours after the immediate response and is dominated by an influx of basophils, eosinophils, lymphocytes, and neutrophils with release of similar inflammatory mediators. It is postulated that the late-phase response explains the chronicity of symptoms.

The disease process may range from paroxysmal sneezing to stridorous breathing secondary to severe posterior nasal obstruction. Most commonly, patients complain of nasal congestion/obstruction, rhinorrhea, pruritus, and sneezing. The excessive, clear, watery mucous secretion results in chronic sniffling, rhinorrhea, postnasal drip, or coughing. Pruritus commonly involves the eyes, ears, palate, and nasopharynx. Sequelae include chronic or recurrent rhinosinusitis and otitis media.

Vasomotor rhinitis is a noninflammatory rhinitis characterized by marked nasal congestion, rhinorrhea, and posterior nasopharyngeal drainage. Although the etiology of disease is poorly understood, it appears that patients have a relative accentuation of parasympathetic stimulation in the nasal mucosa. Nasal mucosal responses to stimuli appear to be hyperactive (e.g., responses to perfumes, smoke, cold air, emotional arousal). Skin tests are routinely negative.

Rhinitis medicamentosa is defined as rhinitis due to the administration either locally or systemically, of medications that potentiate nasal congestion. The classic example is prolonged administration of topical alpha adrenergic agonists (e.g., oxymetazoline). Other systemic agents known to increase nasal congestion include oral contraceptives and reserpine.

Polypoid rhinitis is due to the presence of nonmalignant nasal polyps often originating in the ethmoid sinuses. Symptoms include marked nasal congestion, rhinorrhea, postnasal drainage, and occasionally anosmia. Polyps may be noted bilaterally but often may produce persistent unilateral obstruction. An evaluation of nasal secretions reveals the presence of eosinophils. Skin tests are negative in pure polypoid rhinitis.

Nonallergic rhinitis with eosinophilia (NARES) is a non-allergic rhinitis considered by some investigators a "pre-polypoid" rhinitis. Symptoms are similar to those noted in allergic rhinitis.

Less common causes of diseases resembling allergic or nonallergic rhinitis occasionally need to be considered. *Cerebrospinal rhinorrhea* should be thought of in a patient with symptoms of clear, watery, unilateral rhinorrhea that may or may not be preceded by head trauma. Immediate neurosurgical evaluation is necessary in such cases. Children presenting with purulent, foul smelling, and often unilateral nasal discharge must be evaluated for *foreign body rhinitis. Sarcoidosis, Wegener's granulomatosis,* and *nasopharyngeal tumors* must be considered in those cases where the clinical presentation or lack of response to appropriate medications suggests that the differential diagnosis of rhinitis needs to be expanded.

QUESTION 3 After you have constructed the preceding differential diagnosis, what are the means of establishing a definitive diagnosis?

Skin testing with appropriate allergens forms the cornerstone for diagnosis of allergic disease. Application of allergens by puncture technique and intradermal testing, if indicated, provides rapid sensitive results that must be correlated clinically. In patients who have severe cutaneous disease, or those who cannot discontinue antihistamines before skin testing, in vitro testing is indicated. *Radioallergosorbent testing (RAST)* measures levels of antigen-specific IgE. An advantage of RAST technology is that results are not affected by the ingestion of antihistamines. Although good correlation exists for high titers of antigen-specific IgE as identified by RAST and skin tests, RAST is generally not as sensitive as skin testing in defining clinically pertinent allergens. Additional disadvantages of RAST include added cost and delays in providing results.

A nasal smear can be extremely valuable. The patient blows his or her nose into a piece of waxed paper; secretions are transferred to a microscope slide, dried, and stained with the Hansel's stain. Eosinophil clearing or eosinophil counts greater than 10% of the total white blood cell count are highly suggestive of allergic disease. Severe eosinophilia may be suggestive of atopy; however, the usefulness is limited because many patients with severe allergic rhinitis do not have a significant eosinophilia, and eosinophilia is not specific for atopic disease. Other diseases with increased nasal eosinophils include nonallergic rhinitis with eosinophilia syndrome (NARES) and nasal polyposis. Elevated numbers of neutrophils seen on nasal smear is indicative of infectious rhinitis. Total serum IgE is generally not useful in differentiating allergic from nonallergic rhinitis. However, in young patients elevated IgE levels are very suggestive of allergic disease.

A direct approach, although not routinely used, is the nasal provocation test. The allergen is aerosolized into the nasal cavity in an attempt to reproduce any or all symptoms of that patient's rhinitis. Diagnosis of allergic disease by other controversial methods including sublingual testing has failed to satisfy scientific scrutiny. Careful observation is essential when testing for IgE-mediated reactions since systemic effects, although uncommon, may occur.

QUESTION 4 Further history revealed that the patient had moved into a furnished apartment wherein the initial owner had owned a cat. Although the apartment had been thoroughly cleaned, she is adamant that there is a lot of dust from the furniture. You have decided that the diagnosis is allergic rhinitis. What is the correct treatment for this patient?

Once the type of rhinitis has been identified, a therapeutic scheme may be constructed. If the patient has allergic rhinitis, the initial therapeutic measure is environmental control. This is often difficult, particularly with airborne allergens. Exposure to outdoor allergens may be modified by closing windows and using an air conditioner during the summer. Careful, frequent cleaning will decrease the exposure to indoor allergens. Electronic air filtration systems are also useful in decreasing allergen exposure.

The mainstay of treatment for allergic rhinitis remains antihistamines. A wide variety of preparations allows the physician to individualize the therapy based on potency and clinical response. Continuous therapy provides control of chronic symptoms. Antihistamines act competitively at H_1 receptor sites ameliorating symptoms of sneezing, rhinorrhea, and pruritus. Combination medications including antihistamines and alpha-adrenergic agonists effectively also relieve nasal congestion. Of all the side effects, including anticholinergic properties, sedation is the most limiting. Newer products such as astemizole, terfenadine, and loratidine are examples of nonsedating antihistamines.

Allergic rhinitis, uncontrolled by the therapies outlined above, may be controlled by the initiation of allergen immunotherapy. Patients receive injections of appropriate allergens in an incremental dose protocol. Improvement in symptoms may be noted within 3 months in some patients. The goal of allergen immunotherapy is to decrease the severity of symptoms so that previously ineffective therapies will be more effective or aggressive multi-drug regimens may be tapered. Although increasing titers of antigen-specific IgG blocking antibodies have been correlated with clinical improvement, induction of antigen-specific cellular tolerance is critical for long-term effects.

Intranasal (IN) corticosteroids can be used for effective management of rhinitis. Beclomethasone, triamcinolone flunisolide, fluticasone, and budesonide are commonly used intranasal steroid preparations. These agents, in prescribed doses,

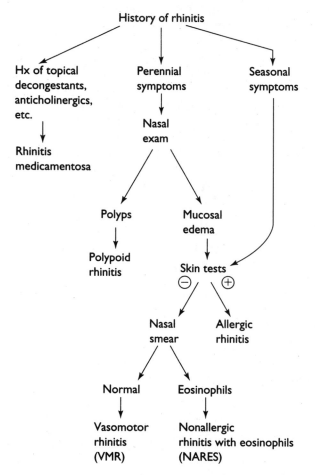

I-I-I Diagnostic algorithm for rhinorrhea.
(From Greene HL, Johnson WP, Maricic MJ: *Decision making in medicine*, St Louis, 1993, Mosby.)

do not cause adrenal suppression. The anti-inflammatory effects of IN corticosteroids have been effective in blocking the late phase of allergic rhinitis, although recent data suggest that even the early phase is diminished by these agents.

Intranasal cromolyn has been shown to be effective in both the early and late phases of allergic rhinitis by inhibiting the degranulation of mast cells. The medication is generally well tolerated and is not systemically absorbed.

Topical alpha-adrenergic agonists cause nasal vasoconstriction and reduction of mucosal edema. Therapy for periods of greater than three to five days can result in rebound congestion (rhinitis medicamentosa). Oral administration of alpha adrenergic agonists relieves nasal congestion without the rebound effect. However, concerns have arisen that phenylpropanolamine may elevate blood pressure.

Management of NARES usually requires intranasal corticosteroids occasionally in combination with decongestants. Patients with severe symptoms may need systemic corticosteroids.

Rhinitis medicamentosa is relieved and best treated by discontinuation of therapy with systemic medications or topical decongestants. Intranasal corticosteroids are used with oral decongestants as the initial regimen is tapered with two days overlap to allow the IN preparation to take effect. Occasionally, oral corticosteroids are required during initial therapy.

BIBLIOGRAPHY

Badhwar AK, Druce HM: Allergic rhinitis, *Med Clin North Am* 76:789-803, 1992.

Druce HM: Allergic and non-allergic rhinitis. In Middleton E Jr, Reed CE, Ellis EF, et al, eds: *Allergy; principles and practice,* ed 4, vol 2, St Louis, 1993, Mosby.

Naclerio RM: Allergic rhinitis, *N Engl J Med* 325:860-869, 1991.

Naclerio RM, Proud D, Togias AG, et al: Inflammatory mediators in late antigen-induced rhinitis, *N Engl J Med* 313:65-70, 1985.

Simons FER, Simons KJ: The pharmacology and use of HI-receptor-antagonist drugs, *N Engl J Med* 330:1663-1670, 1994.

CASE

2

Yasmeen Bilimoria
G. Wendell Richmond

A 35-year-old male presented to the emergency room complaining of the onset of a generalized pruritic rash. He also complained of throat tightness. The symptoms developed within minutes after eating an orange. He had previously noted a mild rash after drinking orange juice. On physical examination, the patient was very anxious and in mild respiratory distress. Vital signs revealed a BP of 85/50 mm Hg, a regular pulse of 120 bpm, a respiratory rate of 30/min, and a temperature of 98° F. Periorbital edema was present. The lung examination revealed diffuse wheezing without stridor. The skin over the trunk and extremities exhibited diffuse erythema and an urticarial eruption.

QUESTION I What elements of this presentation support a presumptive diagnosis of acute anaphylaxis? What other disorders may have a similar presentation?

This patient presented with a spectrum of complaints that occurred acutely after the ingestion of an orange. His history includes a mild cutaneous reaction after eating an orange in the past. The present episode, however, had multisystem involvement with potential life-threatening consequences.

Clinically, cutaneous reactions are the most common finding. These include the symptoms of generalized warmth and tingling and the signs of flushing, erythema, and urticaria with or without angioedema. Pruritus and tingling of the mucous membranes, axillae, and perineum may be the initial signs of an impending reaction.

The respiratory system is the second most commonly involved. Upper airway symptoms are due to edema of the larynx and surrounding tissue. Extensive edema of the larynx may result in stridor. Patients may also complain of chest tightness with dyspnea and wheezing. Poor gas exchange because of ventilation and perfusion mismatching leads to hypoxia and hypercapnia if airway obstruction is prolonged.

Cardiovascular collapse is an important prognostic factor in anaphylaxis. Peripheral vasodilatation and increased vascular permeability cause hypotension. The increased vascular permeability results in a shift of plasma extravascularly with a resultant decrease in intravascular volume. Dysrhythmias are usually sinus tachycardias, although rarely ventricular tachycardias occur. Cases of reversible myocardial ischemia have been reported. Central nervous system manifestations such as confusion, dizziness, syncope, or seizures are less commonly described. Gastrointestinal symptoms including nausea, crampy abdominal pain, vomiting, and diarrhea may be experienced.

The differential diagnosis of anaphylaxis would include systemic mastocytosis, hereditary angioedema, and carcinoid syndrome; all of which can present with flushing, wheezing, abdominal pain, and diarrhea. Central nervous system manifestations should be differentiated from vasovagal episodes, arrhythmias, and seizures. The bronchoconstriction of anaphylaxis may be confused with status asthmaticus, foreign body aspiration, or pulmonary embolus.

QUESTION 2 What is the pathophysiological mechanism for anaphylaxis and what differentiates an anaphylactoid response?

Although the term *anaphylaxis* is generally used to describe immediate, life-threatening reactions to foreign substances, anaphylaxis classically dictates that an IgE-mediated reaction has occurred. Prior exposure to the antigen in a genetically predisposed individual results in the synthesis of a specific IgE antibody. On subsequent reexposure, the antigen binds to cell surface-associated-specific IgE. Cross-linking of contiguous IgE molecules triggers the release of preformed mediators (histamine, heparin, tryptase, chymase) and, as a result of cell activation, newly synthesized, membrane-derived lipid mediators. These include members of the prostaglandin and leukotriene families and platelet activating factor (PAF). All may increase vascular permeability, cause vasodilatation, or both.

Mediator release may be achieved by non–IgE-dependent mechanisms. Symptomatically, these reactions are identical to IgE-mediated anaphylaxis but are termed *anaphylactoid* reactions. Immune complex-mediated activation of the complement cascade with the generation of the complement anaphylatoxins C3a and C5a is an example. Infusions of blood products, especially packed red blood cells, and immunoglobulins may rarely result in immune complex-mediated reactions. An example is the activation of complement by ethylene oxide-sterilized cupriammonium cellulose membranes that has resulted in anaphylactoid reactions in patients on hemodialysis.

Direct activation of mast cells by radiocontrast media, opiates, and plasma expanders such as dextran may cause anaphylactoid reactions. Likewise, nonsteroidal antiinflammatory drugs (NSAID) including aspirin are believed to inhibit cyclo-oxygenase metabolism, thereby shunting arachidonic acid precursors into the leukotriene pathway with the subsequent synthesis of leukotrienes. Leukotrienes C_4, D_4, and E_4, originally termed *slow reacting substance of anaphylaxis (SRSA)*, increase vascular permeability and cause bronchoconstriction. Everyone who takes these compounds inhibits the cyclo-oxygenase enzyme, which suggests that other mediators must be involved to explain these adverse reactions.

The most common causes of anaphylaxis include antibiotics (beta-lactams or penicillin), venomous bites of Hymenoptera, foods (shellfish, nuts, legumes), drugs, and heterosera. Exercise-induced anaphylaxis may occur with or without the previous ingestion of foods including shrimp or celery. Avoidance of the alleged food would allow for normal function during exercise in those patients with food-associated exercise-induced anaphylaxis. Finally, some patients have recurrent anaphylaxis despite aggressive attempts to define an etiology. Idiopathic anaphylaxis is therefore a troublesome diagnosis and should ensure repeated evaluations with each episode.

QUESTION 3 What is the method of treatment this patient requires acutely in the emergency department and over the next 12 to 24 hours?

Acute management of anaphylaxis relies on the maintenance of a patent airway and cardiovascular stability. Administration of epinephrine is the initial therapy for anaphylaxis. The usual dose is 0.1 ml/kg of a 1:1000 solution given intramuscularly or subcutaneously (0.3 to 0.5 ml in adults, 0.15 to 0.3 ml in children). Pharmacological effects of epinephrine include relaxation of bronchial smooth muscle constriction, support of vascular tone, and inhibition of mediator release. Although the initial dose may be effective, subsequent doses may be necessary to maintain that improvement. Careful observation is of paramount importance immediately after intervention. Progressive deterioration requires aggressive measures to maintain an adequate airway and cardiac output. Administration of oxygen and potential intubation, or in cases of severe laryngeal edema, cricothyrotomy, may be necessary. Intensive cardiac support measures including intravascular volume replacement and administration of cardiac pressors are necessary in severe episodes. Bronchoconstriction may require therapy with inhalational β_2 adrenergic agonists, intravenous methylxanthenes, and corticosteroids. All patients should be closely monitored for 8 to 12 hours after presentation. Patients on

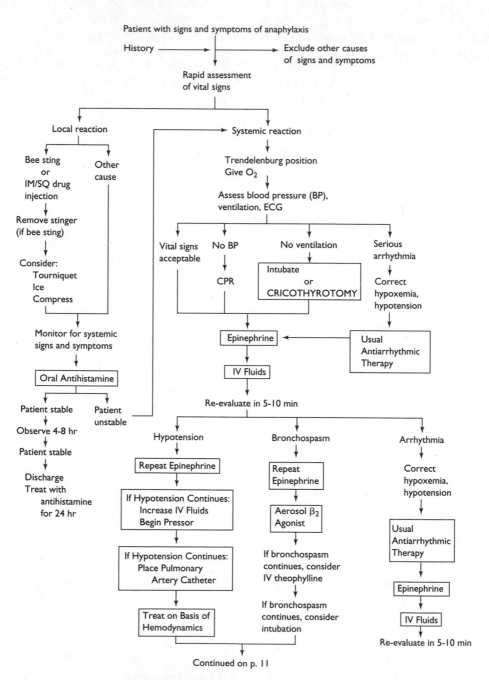

1-2-1   Diagnostic algorithm for anaphylaxis.
(From Greene HL, Johnson WP, Maricic MJ: *Decision making in medicine,* St. Louis, 1993, Mosby.)

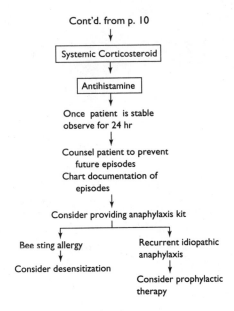

Cont'd. from p. 10

Systemic Corticosteroid

Antihistamine

Once patient is stable
observe for 24 hr

Counsel patient to prevent
future episodes
Chart documentation of
episodes

Consider providing anaphylaxis kit

Bee sting allergy

Consider desensitization

Recurrent idiopathic
anaphylaxis

Consider prophylactic
therapy

1-2-1   Cont'd.

beta-adrenergic agonists may be refractory to therapy and may require prolonged intervention, representing a subgroup of patients with protracted anaphylaxis. If routine measures are inadequate, the administration of glucagon (1 mg in 1 liter D_5W) at 5 to 15 ml/min may be life-saving. A small number of patients may experience biphasic anaphylaxis. The second episode occurs hours after relief of the initial symptoms. Therapy in these cases would be identical to those measures undertaken initially. A diagnostic algorithm for anaphylaxis is shown in Fig. 1-2-1.

BIBLIOGRAPHY

Bochner BS, Lichtenstein LM: Anaphylaxis, *N Engl J Med* 324:1785-1790, 1991.

Boxer M, Greenberger PA, Patterson R: Clinical summary and course of idiopathic anaphylaxis in 73 patients, *Arch Intern Med* 147:269-272, 1987.

Patterson R, et al: Malignant idiopathic anaphylaxis, *J Allergy Clin Immunol* 85:86-88, 1990.

Raper RF, Fisher M: MCD, Profound reversible myocardial depression after anaphylaxis, *Lancet* 1(8582):386-388, Feb. 20, 1988.

Sheffer AL: Anaphylaxis, *J Allergy Clin Immunol* 75:227-233, 1985.

Slater JE, Rubber anaphylaxis, *N Engl J Med* 320:1126-1130, 1989.

Sonin L, et al: Idiopathic anaphylaxis, *Ann Intern Med* 99:634-635, 1983.

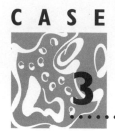

3

Yasmeen Bilimoria
G. Wendell Richmond

A 20-year-old woman presents with a history of recurrent pneumonia. Her history includes chronic diarrhea between the ages of 9 and 18 months. She also was hospitalized at age 11 with complaints of headache and found to have pneumonia. The patient was treated for pneumonia four times between the ages of 12 and 14 years— twice as an inpatient. During those admissions, she had blood cultures with the growth of Streptococcus pneumoniae, *and on a third occasion sputum cultures were positive for* Haemophilus influenzae B (H.I.B). *Her medical history was significant for asthma and rhinitis.*

On physical examination she is a young female in no acute distress; afebrile, P 80 bpm, RR 14/min, BP 110/60 mm Hg.

  Skin: No rashes
  HEENT: Tympanic membranes were negative, oropharynx clear, no sinus tenderness
  Neck: Supple
  Lymph nodes: Mildly increased anterior cervical nodes, nontender and mobile; no other adenopathy
  Lungs: Clear to auscultation and percussion
  Heart: Regular rate and rhythm: S_1 S_2 normal; no murmur
  Abdomen: Soft, nontender, normal abdominal bowel sounds with no hepatosplenomegaly
  Extremities: Normal
  Neurological: Nonfocal
  LABORATORY DATA
  Chem panel = WNL
  CBC: H/H 11.5/34
  WBC: 12.6 $69^S/21^B/8^L/2^E$
  Anti-tetanus and diphtheria normal
  Anti-H.I.B. undetectable

Anti-pneumococcus undetectable
Quantitative immunoglobulins
IgG: 113 (600-1000) mg/dl
IgA: 0 (80-350) mg/dl
IgM: 22 (50-250) mg/dl
Lymphocyte phenotyping

1.	Absolute lymphocyte count:		1368
2.	T lymphocytes:	CD3	72% NL
		CD4	35% NL
		CD8	21% NL
	CD4/CD8 T helper/suppressor ratio:		1.7
3.	Absolute T lymphocytes:		985
4.	Natural killer (HNK-1/CD56):		6% NL
5.	B lymphocytes (CD19):		3% NL
6.	Absolute B lymphocytes:		41

QUESTION I What is the significance of recurrent bacterial infections?

Recurrent bacterial infections may result from multiple etiologies of which immunologic disorders are of key importance. Primary immune deficiencies involve T cells and/or B cells if the immune deficiency is not due to a viral etiology, malignancy, chronic disease (renal failure, hepatic failure), chemotherapy, trauma, drug effects (cyclosporine, corticosteroids, azathioprine, etc.) or a variety of other immunocompromising factors. Patients with antibody deficiency may have select immunoglobulin deficiencies (e.g., IgA) or have a deficiency in all immunoglobulin classes. The lack of these immunoglobulins clinically presents as recurrent infections in most patients.

Diagnostic clues may be gleaned from the type and site of infection (Fig. 1-3-1). Defects of leukocyte function often present with either cellulitis or more importantly, deep tissue bacterial infections. Complement deficiencies of terminal components (C5—C8) present with recurrent Neisserial infections of the urogenital tract or meninges; while a deficiency of C3 often presents with recurrent infection with encapsulated bacteria. Defects of T-cell number or function result in infections with opportunist organisms. B cell defects present with infections of the upper and lower respiratory tract caused by encapsulated bacterial pathogens. The most common pathogens include *Haemophilus influenzae B* and *Streptococcus pneumoniae*, although *Streptococcus pyogenes* and *Staphylococcus aureus* are occasionally isolated.

Chronic diarrhea is a common finding and may be caused by *giardia, salmonella, rotavirus, and campylobacter*. Unfortunately, stool cultures for *giardia*, the most common pathogen, are frequently negative, requiring a more extensive evaluation.

Isolated *IgA deficiency* is the most common of the antibody deficiencies with a prevalence of approximately 1:750. Patients most frequently have no symptoms of recurrent infections. Some patients have severe recurrent sinus and pulmonary infections that are associated with concurrent IgG 2 and 4 sub class deficiencies. Chronic GI infections are not typical of IgA deficiency.

Patients diagnosed with *common variable immunodeficiency (CVID)* are found to have IgG levels often <250 mg/dl, with undetectable IgA and low IgM levels. These patients have recurrent infections including bacterial pneumonia, sinusitis, and otitis, presenting at any age.

X-linked Agammaglobulinemia (XLA) is another primary humoral immunodeficiency which clinically presents as recurrent bacterial infections in males usually after 6 months of age (after maternal IgG has been metabolized) and routinely before 2 years of age. Production of all immunoglobulin is defective, resulting in serum IgG levels <200 mg/dl as well as undetectable IgM and IgA isotypes. Classically, *XLA* is thought to be due to a genetic defect affecting the B cell lineage including plasma cells, sparing T-cells. Like CVID, upper and lower respiratory bacterial infections and malabsorption are the most common complica-

tions. Untreated, patients rarely live into the fourth decade.

QUESTION 2 What steps should be taken to make the diagnosis of a primary immune deficiency syndrome?

A patient presenting with frequent infections should have a thorough history of all known infections since childhood. Specific pathogens should be documented if known. Special attention should be paid to sinus, pulmonary, and gastrointestinal symptoms. Family history is an essential factor in diagnosing the genetically transmitted disorders. In adult onset disease, a list of all drugs ingested by the patient should be recorded, since medications such as phenytoin have been known to cause an IgA deficiency that is reversible.

On physical examination, special attention should be paid to evidence of persistent lymphadenopathy or hepatosplenomegaly, as this may be present in 60% of patients with CVID. Identifications of digital clubbing suggest that recurrent infections of the airways have resulted in bronchiectasis. Autoimmune diseases associated with CVID that may be detected on examination include a rheumatoid-like polyarthritis, thyroiditis, and polymyositis.

After one has conducted a complete history and physical, laboratory data, including a complete blood count, is necessary in the evaluation of a patient with recurrent infections. Quantitative serum immunoglobulin levels including IgE are essential when hypogammaglobulinemia is considered. Antibody responses to specific antigens provide additional insight into the humoral defects. Antitetanus, diphtheria, pneumococcus, and *Haemophilus influenzae* B titers are now available from reference laboratories. Isohemagglutinin titers provide information on functional IgM antibody responses.

Phenotyping for surface immunoglobulin or the detection of specific B cell surface markers (e.g., CD19 or CD20) is performed. Patients with CVID often have normal peripheral blood B cell

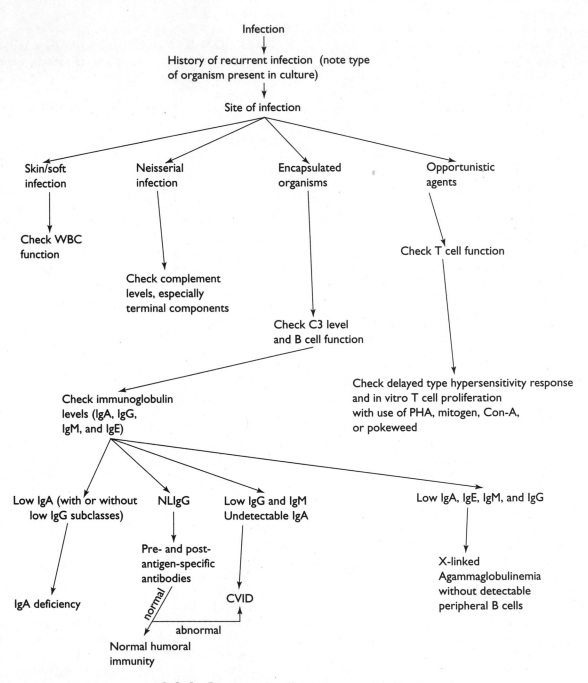

I-3-I Diagnostic algorithm for agammaglobulinemia.

numbers, whereas XLA patients have no detectable peripheral blood B cells. T cell phenotype is important in the evaluation of genetic T cell disorders, although the important clue of marked lymphopenia is evident in a complete blood count. T cell response can be measured by delayed hypersensitivity skin testing or in vitro T-cell proliferative responses to a variety of mitogens including phytohemagglutinin (PHA), concanavalin A (con A), or anti-CD3.

QUESTION 3 What role does immunization play, if any, in these patients?

Patients with severe forms of agammaglobulinemia should not receive live vaccines such as the polio vaccine. These patients have been known to develop post vaccination complications (i.e., poliomyelitis). Patients with deficiencies of specific immunoglobulin isotypes may have an inadequate response to immunizations. IgG_2-deficient patients have a poor antibody response to carbohydrate antigens such as the capsular polysaccharide of *H. influenzae*, predisposing them to recurrent infections by polysaccharide encapsulated bacteria. These patients must be immunized by conjugates of carbohydrates coupled to protein antigens like the diphtheria/*H. influenzae* type B vaccine. This approach results in a switch of the predominant antibody response from IgG_2 to IgG_1 subclass, thereby providing effective prophylaxis.

Immunoglobulin response to vaccines may be quantified for diagnostic purposes as well. Antigen specific titers drawn before and after protein and carbohydrate vaccinations provide valuable information on one's ability to appropriately respond to antigens.

QUESTION 4 What therapy is available for patients suffering from primary immune deficiency syndromes?

Most of the management of these patients revolves around their recurrent infections. Patients should be treated with antibiotics at the first suspicion of an infection. Prompt therapy can avoid more severe, disseminated infections. Some patients may be candidates for chronic prophylactic antimicrobial therapy.

Immunoglobulin therapy is also crucial therapy for patients with panhypogammaglobulinemia. One hundred to 400 mg/kg of immunoglobulin is administered each month with doses customized to keep preinfusion IgG levels at >500 mg/dl. Mild symptoms such as fever, chills, and nausea have been noted during the first few infusions. This may resolve with further doses or by premedicating with acetaminophen and antihistamines. The most catastrophic reaction is anaphylaxis, which can occur in patients with no detectable IgA. Although very uncommon, preparations with very low titers of IgA must be administered to such people. As in any infusion, careful monitoring is essential.

CASE FOLLOW-UP The patient has successfully received monthly immunoglobulin therapy for CVID, without any further systemic infections. Additional treatment with antimicrobial agents has been necessary for recurrent sinusitis.

• •

BIBLIOGRAPHY

Herrod HG: Management of the patient with IgG subclass deficiency and/or selective antibody deficiency, *Ann Allergy* 70:3-8, 1993.

Huston DP, Kavanaugh AF, Rohane PW, Huston MM: Immunoglobulin deficiency syndromes and therapy, *J Allergy Clin Immunol* 87:1-17, 1991.

Rosen FS, Cooper MD, Wedgewood RJP: The primary immunodeficiencies, *N Engl J Med* 311:235-242, 1984.

Sneller MC, Strober W, Eisenstein E, et al: New insights into common variable immunodeficiency, *Ann Intern Med* 118: 720-730, 1993.

C A S E

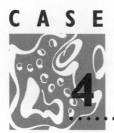

4

Yasmeen Bilimoria
G. Wendell Richmond

A 25-year-old man with a history of asthma since childhood presented to the outpatient clinic with complaints of worsening dyspnea and wheezing. He has had similar intermittent symptoms over the past 3 months, usually requiring emergency room visits. His last visit to an emergency room was 2 weeks earlier, at which time he was discharged on inhaled bronchodilators and a 10-day course of steroids. He has received oral glucocorticosteroids intermittently, and required high-dose therapy approximately once a month for the past year. The patient claims that he has been compliant with his medications but still has multiple episodes of wheezing and shortness of breath.

His medications include timed-release theophylline 300 mg bid and albuterol metered-dose inhaler 2 puffs every hour. Previous pulmonary function tests had revealed that lung volumes were normal with the exception of an increase in residual volume. DLCO was normal.

QUESTION I This patient has required multiple emergency room visits because of dyspnea and wheezing. What are the potential reasons for this patient's difficulty controlling his asthma?

This patient has a form of asthma known as chronic-persistent or recalcitrant asthma. Multiple factors may account for the difficulty these patients have in attempts to control their symptoms.

Adverse reactions to medications and additives may exacerbate asthma. Rhinitis, nasal polyps, and asthma are the classic findings of the aspirin sensitivity triad described by Samter. Sinusitis is frequently seen in the aspirin-sensitive patients as well. Nonsteroidal antiinflammatory agents may also stimulate bronchospasm. Sulfite-sensitive patients have chronic corticosteroid-dependent asthma, but usually they are nonatopic or have incidentally positive skin tests.

Sinusitis alone can be a factor in poorly controlled asthma. The exact mechanism of how sinus disease affects the lower airways is not known. Leakage of secretions to the lungs from the sinuses is unlikely as was tested by radionuclide study. The presence of a nasal-sinus bronchial reflex has also been speculated as another possible explanation relating the upper to the lower respiratory tract.

Another relationship exists between recalcitrant asthma and gastroesophageal reflux disease (GERD). The mechanism of how GERD is associated with asthma is unclear. Possible theories include microaspiration of refluxed gastric contents into the lungs or a vagal reflex initiated by reflux of gastric contents into the upper gastrointestinal tract resulting in bronchoconstriction. Both of these possible mechanisms have been tested in animals and humans with varying results. Despite these results, there is a subset of asthmatics with reflux disease who have an improvement in their respiratory symptoms and pulmonary function after institution of H2-blockers or surgical treatment for GERD.

Allergic bronchopulmonary aspergillosis (ABPA) may be the cause of recalcitrant asthma in some patients. These patients typically have poorly controlled asthma for many years. As opposed to treatment with bronchodilators, these patients usually require steroid therapy to control their asthma.

Many patients with asthma are atopic, and often environmental triggers may exacerbate their asthma. A complete environmental history including details of living and sleeping areas, presence of pets, differential symptoms on weekdays-weekends, travel history, and occupational exposures is integral when evaluating a patient with asthma. Based on the history and physical examination, these patients should be skin-tested to potential allergens.

Patient noncompliance is also a frustrating and too common cause. Because bronchospasm may become established subacutely, these patients disregard physician instructions for maintenance therapy, or wait until overtly symptomatic at which time they present for acute care. Patients are prescribed a short course of corticosteroids that results in rapid improvement; unfortunately, proper outpatient care and home therapy is not sought, and the cycle is again repeated. This cycle can only be arrested with improved patient education, home peak expiratory flow monitoring, and establishment of a patient-physician relationship that fosters communication about presence of symptoms early.

QUESTION 2 Physical examination revealed a well-nourished, well-developed male in mild respiratory distress: T 98.9°F; P 112/min; RR 40/min; BP 136/86 mm Hg; no pulsus paradoxicus. Head examination revealed bilateral inferior turbinate edema without polyps, normal oropharynx, and no sinus tenderness. There were no cervical or supraclavicular nodes palpable. Lung examination revealed diffuse inspiratory and expiratory wheezing. The cardiac, abdominal, and extremity examinations were normal. Laboratory values from his emergency room visit 2 weeks ago are as follows:

Arterial blood gas	pH 7.42
(on room air)	P_{O_2} 95 mm Hg
	P_{CO_2} 35 mm Hg
Electrolytes, BUN, creatinine	normal
CBC	Hb 13.1 g/dl
	Hct 39.3%
	plt 305 K/μL
	WBC 11,000/μl
	seg 87 band 3
	mono 1 eos 9
EKG	normal

How do you approach the evaluation and treatment of patients with recalcitrant asthma?

It is first necessary to document objectively that the patient has reversible airway disease. It is then important to review all the historical facts that can help identify the possible exacerbating factors in the asthmatic patient (Fig. 1-4-1).

Pulmonary function testing that shows an improvement of flow rates when compared before and after bronchodilator therapy is the best way to prove a reversible component to the patient's bronchospasm. Patients may also note a rapid temporal improvement when using inhaled bronchodilators.

In our index patient, possible diagnoses include allergic disease and ABPA. Eosinophilia and elevated IgE can be seen in any of these three processes; however, positive skin test to Aspergillus is an important clue for the syndrome of ABPA. Diagnostic criteria necessary for ABPA include asthma, immediate cutaneous reactivity to *Aspergillus fumigatus* (Af), total serum IgE > 1000 ng/ml, precipitating antibodies to Af, and elevated serum IgE-Af and IgG-Af. Chest roentgenographic infiltrates, central bronchiectasis, and eosinophilia are also seen in ABPA; however, they are not essential for the diagnosis. Patients with recalcitrant asthma secondary to ABPA should be treated with systemic corticosteroids on a daily or alternate day schedule in addition to their other asthma medications.

Chronic persistent asthma secondary to GERD can be treated medically or surgically with improvement of respiratory symptoms. Avoidance of foods that decrease lower esophageal sphincter tone (caffeine, chocolate, garlic, fatty foods), mechanical maneuvers (i.e., elevating the head of the bed, wearing loose-fitting clothes), or a trial of H2-blocker therapy that relieves symptoms of reflux and wheezing and suggests the diagnosis.

If sinusitis is suspected, the patients should undergo imaging of the sinuses to evaluate for acute or chronic inflammatory changes. Some patients may require prolonged antibiotic therapy, while others may suffice with topical nasal steroids. Patients identified as possibly sensitive to ingestants should eliminate these products and monitor their respiratory symptoms. Medications including nonsteroidal anti-inflammatory agents and beta-adrenergic antagonists must be considered potential exacerbating factors in patients with persistent asthma. Aspirin-sensitive patients should also avoid other NSAIDs that inhibit the cyclooxygenase pathway, since "crossreactivity" with aspirin has been well documented. Environmental allergies can also be controlled through avoidance (such as pets), medications (as outlined in the Allergy/Immunology Case 1), and immunotherapy.

QUESTION 3   Additional outpatient evaluation included a total IgE level of 2047 ng/ml (nl < 1000 ng/ml). Additionally, IgE skin testing was positive for reactions to cat, dust mite, Af, Alternaria, and cockroach antigens. What is the significance of an elevated eosinophil count in this asthmatic patient?

The mild elevation of eosinophils may be attributable to multiple etiologies. Wheezing may be an additional component of diseases that have associated eosinophilia. Asthma with or without an allergic component, acute or prolonged exposure to an allergen, and ABPA are all associated with eosinophilia. This also includes aspirin-induced asthma, Churg-Strauss angiitis (allergic granulomatosis), chronic eosinophilic pneumonia, and tropical eosinophilia related to filarial infection (*Strongyloides stercoralis* or *Ascaris lumbricoides*). However, it is not specific for any of these diseases. Before a diagnosis of refractory asthma is decided upon, one should consider the exclusion of these alternative diagnoses first.

QUESTION 4   A chest radiograph revealed a RML infiltrate not present 3 months ago. What is the significance of an infiltrate on a chest radiograph in a patient with an exacerbation of asthma?

Although viral or mycoplasm infections can be the inciting factors in an asthma exacerbation, more commonly an infiltrate represents areas of atelectasis and/or mucus plugging. Without other

information to support the diagnosis of infection such as fever, chills, productive cough, or leukocytosis, patients should be treated for asthma exacerbation without the use of antibiotics. Fleeting infiltrates because of mucoid impaction or atelectasis have also been identified in patients with ABPA. Additionally, central bronchiectasis seen in ABPA predisposes to recurrent infection in that area because of alteration of normal airway clearance mechanisms from ciliary destruction. If the infiltrates persist beyond the asthma exacerbation, other considerations should include bacterial or viral pneumonias, tuberculosis, vasculitis, or neoplasm. Eosinophilic pneumonia can be seen in ABPA patients as well. This disease presents with a characteristic infiltrate pattern known as the "reverse pulmonary edema" or "bat-wing" pattern.

QUESTION 5   Pulmonary function testing revealed an improvement of the $FEV_{1.0}$ from 55% to 72% and of the $FEF_{25-75\%}$ from 29% to 45%. Precipitating antibodies to Af and elevated IgE-Af and IgG-Af were present. How do you interpret these laboratory findings in light of the patient's refractory symptoms?

The above evaluation represents a full workup for recalcitrant asthma. The pulmonary function tests support the diagnosis of reversible airway disease after challenge with a bronchodilator. The presence of an elevated IgE titer, positive precipitins, and IgM and IgG antibodies to Af supports a diagnosis of ABPA. The infiltrate on CXR resolved within 2 weeks on steroids. A positive Aspergillus skin test is an important marker for the diagnosis of ABPA.

After this thorough evaluation for possible causes of recalcitrant asthma, the patient was diagnosed with ABPA. The need for close monitoring and regular physician evaluations were discussed with the patient in attempts to develop reliable communication between doctor and patient. The patient was started on Prednisone 40 mg po daily for 3 weeks, then eventually tapered to alternate day therapy with control of the patient's symptoms.

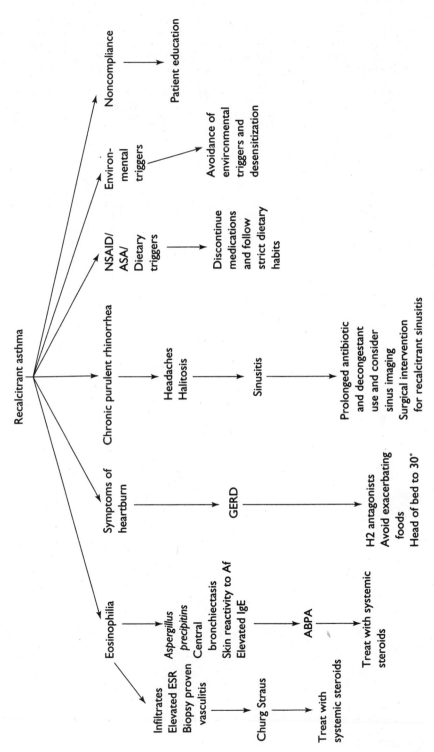

1-4-1   Diagnostic algorithm for recalcitrant asthma.

BIBLIOGRAPHY

Bardin PG, Van Heerden BB, Joubert JR: Absence of pulmonary aspiration of sinus contents in patients with asthma and sinusitis, *J Allergy Clin Immunol* 86:82-88, 1990.

Greenberger PA, Patterson R: Allergic bronchopulmonary aspergillosis and the evaluation of the patient with asthma, *J Allergy Clin Immunol* 81:646-649, 1988.

Irwin RS, Curley FJ, French CL: Difficult to control asthma, *Chest* 103:1662-1669, 1993.

Mansfield LE: Gastroesophageal reflux and diseases of the respiratory tract: a review, *J Asthma* 26(5):271-278, 1989.

Samter M, Beers RF Jr: Intolerance to aspirin, *Ann Intern Med* 68:975, 1968.

Slavin RS: Asthma and sinusitis, *J Allergy Clin Immunol* 90:534-537, 1992.

Stevenson DD, Simon RA: Sensitivity to ingested metabisulfites in asthmatic subjects, *J Allergy Immunol* 68(1):26, 1981.

CASE

5

Yasmeen Bilimoria
G. Wendell Richmond

....

A 23-year-old woman presents to your office with complaints of fever to 101°F, green nasal discharge, and facial pressure for the past 4 days. Previous to these symptoms she had experienced sore throat and nasal congestion with clear rhinorrhea for 1 week. The patient's past medical history included seasonal allergic rhinitis and bronchitis. She had a tonsillectomy as a child. She was currently taking terfenadine 60 mg po bid and pseudoephedrine 60 mg po q 4-6 hours prn.

QUESTION I What are the important elements of normal sinus function? Which clinical considerations would you have in a patient presenting with this picture?

Normal sinus function is dependent on normal ciliary function, intact mucous membranes, normal mucous production, and ostial patency. Disease processes which alter these factors can predispose a person to sinus disease. Processes that lead to abnormal ciliary function include cystic fibrosis and immotile cilia syndrome. The mucous membrane surface may be compromised by trauma or diseases such as Wegener's granulomatosis or presence of a neoplasm. Normal production of secretion can be impaired with the sicca syndrome (e.g., Sjögren's syndrome) or use of anti-cholinergic medications. When mucus is hyperviscous or a sinus mass (i.e., nasal polyps or neoplasm) is present, ostial obstruction may occur.

The clinical scenario described in this case is a classic presentation of acute sinusitis. Although acute sinusitis is one of the most common outpatient diagnoses, other diseases may present simi-

larly and, therefore, should be considered when evaluating a patient such as this. Nasopharyngeal tumors can obstruct ostial drainage (as mentioned above) as well as destroy the nasal mucosa, allowing the growth of bacteria or other pathogens likely to cause sinusitis.

Immunodeficient patients, such as those with X-linked agammaglobulinemia or common variable immune deficiency, commonly develop bacterial sinusitis (see Allergy/Immunology Case 3). Fortunately, the vast majority of patients with acute bacterial sinusitis are healthy immunocompetent individuals. However, the clinician should be aware of other possible underlying pathologic states.

The spectrum of disease mentioned above is reason to be suspicious of a patient with recurrent infection or atypical symptoms including bleeding, excessive pain, CNS symptoms, or visual presence of a mass. In this scenario a full examination is necessary (refer to Fig. 1-1-1).

QUESTION 2 The physical examination revealed a well-nourished, well-developed woman in no acute distress. Vital signs were T 101.4°F, P 84 bpm, RR 16/min, BP 110/60 mm Hg. Head and neck examination revealed no conjunctival infection, tympanic membranes translucent and normal canals, edematous and erythematous inferior nasal turbinates without obstruction of nasal passages. Purulent green nasal discharge was seen draining anteriorly. A 5 mm polyp was noted in the left nasal passage; tenderness to palpation in paranasal areas bilaterally but no tenderness in frontal area; no oral ulcers or exudates were seen. The remainder of the examination was normal. Which signs and symptoms are helpful in the diagnosis of acute sinusitis?

The most common clinical presentation includes persistent URI symptoms. Nasal congestion and clear rhinorrhea often progress to facial pain and purulent yellow-green nasal drainage. Positional headache, increased pain with the head dependent, may also be associated with acute sinusitis. Facial tenderness over affected sinuses may be seen; however, pain may be referred to other areas in the head. For example, pain due to maxillary sinusitis can radiate to the frontal head area or the upper teeth instead of typical pain under the affected maxilla. Disease of the ethmoid sinuses may lead to periorbital or temporal headaches. Some patients with frontal sinusitis will develop pain and tenderness in the frontal area. Sphenoid disease usually has a less defined pattern of pain.

Excessive nasal secretions may lead to postnasal drip altering the usual presentation and resulting in complaints of cough and chest congestion. Patients with asthma may experience an exacerbation of their respiratory symptoms during an episode of sinusitis. Fever and other constitutional symptoms such as fatigue may also be present.

A diagnosis of sinusitis is difficult on physical examination. Patients may have a paucity of findings compared to their symptomatology. Purulent secretions may not be obvious when examining the nose. Evidence of nasal polyposis could suggest a possible anatomic obstruction of the ostia as a cause of suspected sinusitis, but it is not specific for sinusitis.

QUESTION 3 You are able to obtain a swab of nasal secretions. The microscopic examination reveals a predominance of polymorphonuclear leukocytes with a few eosinophils. How do you interpret this finding? Which diagnostic tests may be performed in the office to support the diagnosis of acute bacterial sinusitis?

Nasal cytology is a quick and inexpensive procedure that may yield useful information in a patient thought to have sinusitis. Nasal secretions are swabbed from below the middle meatus and then examined microscopically. An abundance of neutrophils would be suggestive of a sinus infection. Eosinophils on the smear are commonly associated with either allergic causes of inflammation or nasal polyposis.

Transillumination of the sinuses has poor sensitivity and specificity for sinusitis, and it should not be used routinely as a diagnostic tool.

Fiberoptic rhinoscopy is an office procedure that may be performed by well-trained allergists, otolaryngologists, and primary care physicians. This technique allows one to better define the nasal anatomy and identify abnormalities that may predispose the patient to developing sinusitis (e.g., nasal polyps). Purulent secretions draining from the ostia can also be visualized in some patients with sinusitis. Direct sampling of purulent secretions can be carried out with less threat of contamination and certainty that purulent material was recovered.

QUESTION 4 What imaging techniques aid in the diagnosis of sinusitis?

Plain radiographs of the sinuses evaluate the maxillary and frontal sinuses in which air fluid levels and mucosal thickening supports a diagnosis of a sinus infection. Unfortunately, ethmoid sinus involvement is often difficult to evaluate with standard radiographic techniques. Computed tomography (CT) scans are much more sensitive as compared to plain films. The coronal views of sinus CT precisely defines the nasal sinus anatomy. The high resolution imaging afforded by CT also aids the surgeon if a patient requires surgical treatment. CT scans also offer the advantage of evaluating paranasal sinus bone in those severe cases of sinusitis where osteomyelitis is a concern.

Magnetic resonance imaging (MRI) of the sinuses does not provide additional useful information than CT does; therefore, at this time MRI is not recommended as a routine imaging procedure for patients with sinus disease.

QUESTION 5 What is the therapy for acute sinusitis?

Therapy is targeted primarily at eradicating the bacterial pathogens that are usually responsible

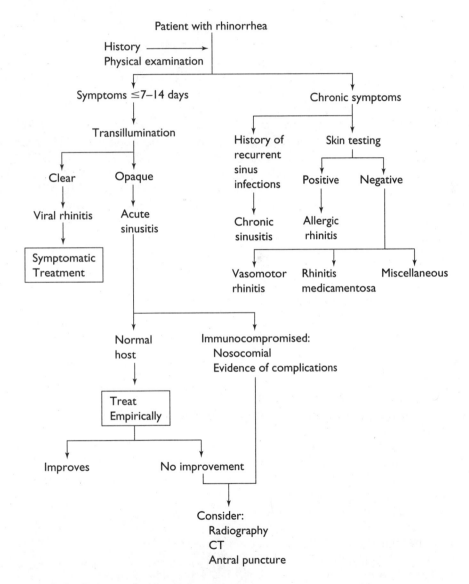

1-5-1 Patient with rhinorrhea.
(From Greene HL, Johnson WP, Maricic MJ: *Decision making in medicine,* St Louis, 1993, Mosby.)

for acute sinusitis. In adults, these organisms include *S. pneumoniae, M. catarrhalis,* and *H. influenzae.* Therefore, antibiotic therapy is the mainstay of treatment for acute sinusitis. A 10- to 14-day course of amoxicillin is the first choice. If β-lactamase producing organisms are of concern, a drug such as amoxicillin/clavulinate should be prescribed.

Trimethoprim/sulfamethoxazole is an alternative antibiotic for the penicillin-sensitive patient. Second generation cephalosporins, such as cefuroxime and cefaclor, and macrolides, particularly clarithromycin, are also effective in treating acute sinusitis. Longer courses of antibiotics, 3 to 4 weeks, are occasionally necessary for chronic or recurrent infections.

In addition to antimicrobial agents, patients require analgesics for the pain that commonly exists with sinus infections. Pain is a result of swelling and increasing intrasinus pressure because the bony sinus cannot expand. Decongestants, topical for short courses and oral for longer therapy, reduce mucosal edema that can be the exacerbating factor in sinusitis. Topical and oral corticosteroids are important antiinflammatory agents that are usually utilized more with chronic sinus disease. Antihistamines should not be prescribed routinely for patients with acute sinusitis. The drying effect of these medications may actually worsen the clinical condition. Some patients appear to attain benefit from other therapies such as mucolytics, steam, and saline sprays.

If improvement of symptoms is not seen within 7 days of initiating therapy, the patient should be switched to an alternative antibiotic. Symptoms persisting after a 21-day course of antibiotics should be further evaluated (i.e., rhinoscopy and/or CT scan). Other pathogens such as anaerobes, gram negative bacteria, and fungi should also be considered at this time.

QUESTION 6 What complications can arise from sinusitis?

Early diagnosis and treatment of acute sinusitis may avoid the development of more severe complications. Direct extension of the infection can lead to a periorbital cellulitis, dural sinus thrombosis, thrombophlebitis, and direct involvement of the globe. Patients presenting with chemosis, retinal engorgement, and oculomotor dysfunction should be evaluated for possible cavernous sinus thrombosis. In these situations, the patient may require surgical decompression and drainage in addition to antibiotic therapy. Special attention should be given to the preservation of visual acuity.

Invasion of the bony structure of the sinuses may lead to osteomyelitis. Sinusitis may also be a source for subdural or intraparenchymal brain abscess formation. In this case the sinus infection has eroded through bone and fascial planes, broken through the blood-brain barrier, and invaded the brain parenchyma. Treatment may require repair of the dural coverings to avoid presence of a chronic fistula.

CASE SUMMARY The patient was diagnosed with bacterial sinusitis and culture revealed growth of *Streptococcus pneumoniae.* The patient was treated with a 10-day course of amoxicillin and recovered without complications.

• •

BIBLIOGRAPHY

Bolger WE, Kennedy DW: Current perspectives on sinusitis in adults, *J Respir Dis* 13(3):421-448, 1992.
Calhoun K: Diagnosis and management of sinusitis in the allergic patient, *Otolaryngol Head Neck Surg* 107:850-854, 1992.
Druce HM: Diagnosis of sinusitis in adults: history, physical examination, nasal cytology, echo, and rhinoscope, *J Allergy Clin Immunol* 90:436-441, 1992.
Kaliner MA: Human nasal host defense and sinusitis, *J Allergy Clin Immunol* 90:424-430, 1992.
Polmar SH: The role of the immunologist in sinus disease, *J Allergy Clin Immunol* 90:511-515, 1992.
Slavin RG: Asthma and sinusitis, *J Allergy Clin Immunol* 90:534-537, 1992.
Slavin RG: Medical management of nasal polyps and sinusitis, *J Allergy Clin Immunol* 88:141-146, 1991.
Wagenmann M, Naclerio RM: Complications of sinusitis, *J Allergy Clin Immunol* 90:552-554, 1992.
Zinreich SJ: Paranasal sinus imaging, *Otolaryngol Head Neck Surg* 103:863-868, 1990.

CARDIOLOGY

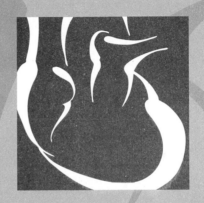

JOHN BARRON
SECTION EDITOR

Kevin Maquiling
John Barron

The patient is a 64-year-old male with a 15-year history of hypertension, noninsulin dependent diabetes mellitus (NIDDM), and an 8-year history of angina. This patient now presents to his private physician's office with a chief complaint of four episodes of anginal pain in the last month. The patient states that for the first three episodes, pain was relieved quickly with one sublingual nitroglycerin as is usual with his previous anginal episodes. The last episode, which occurred 4 days ago, required three sublingual nitroglycerin tablets before the pain was completely resolved. Prior to 1 month ago, the patient experienced three to four episodes of angina per year. The recent episodes occurred with moderate physical exertion; however, he denies any chest pain at rest. This level of exertion had not previously caused chest pain. Since the episode 4 days ago he has been "taking it easy" without any further episodes. He is currently pain free.

His coronary disease risk factors include NIDDM, hypertension, and 40 pack-year smoking history (quit 2 years ago). He denies any family history of premature cardiac disease and is uncertain of his cholesterol level.

QUESTION I What is the clinical syndrome with which this patient is presenting, and what historical factors support this diagnosis?

Though this patient does not currently complain of chest pain, the history of progressing symptoms is very worrisome. The clinical entity of "unstable angina" describes a dynamic constellation of symptoms intermediate between stable angina and acute myocardial infarction. Though

particular definitions have changed, three characteristic patterns have remained essential to the diagnosis of unstable angina: (1) new onset severe angina, (2) crescendo angina, and (3) angina at rest. The diagnosis of unstable angina therefore is made on the basis of a history of a progressive or changing anginal pattern in the absence of an acute myocardial infarction.

Inasmuch as the diagnosis of unstable angina demands accuracy and specific therapy, sharp clinical judgment is essential. The interviewer should bear in mind that not all patients with coronary artery disease manifest the same pain syndrome. These symptoms include left arm numbness, dyspnea, diaphoresis, nausea and vomiting, symptoms construed as indigestion, and back pain. Additionally, some patients, commonly diabetics, may not manifest any symptoms.

To support one's clinical suspicion of unstable angina, one should inquire about changing exercise tolerance, time until recovery from symptoms, frequency and number of sublingual nitroglycerin tablets used, and the changing nature and frequency of symptoms.

Additional history regarding cardiac risk factors was obtained that showed a history of NIDDM, hypertension, and tobacco use. The risk of death from coronary artery disease is 2 to 6 times higher in smokers than in nonsmokers. Smoking cessation helps to ameliorate the overall risk of developing coronary insufficiency; however, this benefit accrues only gradually. Individuals who have recently quit (SBP <5 years ago) should still be considered to be at increased risk as compared to nonsmokers. Though this patient does not have a positive family history, patients who have first-degree relatives manifesting vascular disease (myocardial infarction, cerebrovascular accident, transient ischemic attacks) before age 55 have up to a 5 times increased risk of developing coronary artery disease.

QUESTION 2 The patient is afebrile, P 88 bpm and regular; RR 12/min; BP 158/86 mm Hg. In general the patient is a slightly obese black male in no acute distress. He is lying in bed, head elevated at about 30 degrees. Xanthomas were not present on the skin, and the lungs were clear to auscultation bilaterally. Evaluation of the peripheral vasculature revealed no carotid, renal, or femoral bruits. The dorsalis pedis, posterior tibial, and radial pulses were 2+ bilaterally and symmetrically. There was no jugular venous distension on examination of the neck. The cardiac point of maximal intensity (PMI) was displaced 2 cm lateral to the midclavicular line and was diffuse. The cardiac examination did not demonstrate any heaves, thrills, or additional heart sounds. The abdomen was benign. His extremities revealed trace pretibial edema. The rectal examination was hemoccult negative. What are the important parts of the physical examination that underscore a suspicion of cardiac disease?

The physical examination contains abundant information to help the clinician assess the cardiovascular system. First, the patient's vital signs are essential. The patient who has ongoing cardiac ischemia may manifest tachycardia because of the autonomic sympathetic response to pain. Left ventricular failure with an elevated pulmonary capillary wedge pressure may lead to pulmonary edema and tachypnea. The blood pressure represents overall cardiac function or needed autonomic reflex compensation.

Examination of the skin and peripheral vasculature is also important. Examination should include palpation of the strength and symmetry of the distal pulses and auscultation for the presence of bruits. In this way, gross information regarding function of the left ventricle, degree of atherosclerotic disease, and the presence of aortic disease (i.e., dissecting hematomas, critical valvular ste-

nosis, etc.) can be attained in short order. In addition, the patient with impending cardiogenic shock will demonstrate acral cyanosis and vasoconstriction with cool, clammy skin.

As the left ventricle becomes increasingly ischemic, it first stiffens (producing the S_4), losing the ability to accept blood from the pulmonary circulation during diastole. This elevates the pulmonary capillary wedge pressure and leads to interstitial/alveolar edema that may compromise oxygenation. On examination one may auscultate rales (crackles) and detect basilar foci of decreased vesicular breath sounds as a result of the presence of a pleural effusion. The patient may be more dyspneic while supine (orthopnea), use accessory muscles of breathing, produce auto-positive end-expiratory pressure (pursed lip breathing) to recruit additional alveoli, and feel more comfortable with exogenous oxygen supplementation.

QUESTION 3 The ECG showed normal sinus rhythm, rate of 80 bpm, and left ventricular hypertrophy with a strain pattern. His medications included one enteric-coated aspirin per day, Isordil 20 mg po tid, Procardia XL 90 mg po q day. He had no known allergies. The patient was transferred to the coronary care unit for treatment and workup of unstable angina. What is known about the pathophysiology of unstable angina? How are these concepts translated into designing a plan for therapy?

Recent work has helped to elucidate the pathophysiologic processes leading to coronary insufficiency and, in particular, the mechanism behind acute progression of symptoms. Common to all concepts of unstable angina is the imbalance of myocardial oxygen supply and demand. Abnormal coronary stenoses have been shown in up to 90% of patients with unstable angina. Plaque rupture and fissuring exposes the circulation to subendothelial components (collagen) that are highly thrombogenic. This is the mechanism by which an acute clot can form in the vicinity of an asymmetric, narrowed atherosclerotic plaque.

Given these mechanisms for unstable angina, specific intervention can be applied on three fronts: antithrombotic treatment, antiischemic treatment, and direct intracoronary intervention.

QUESTION 4 The patient's admission labs were significant for creatinine of 1.4 mg/dl, cholesterol of 298 mg/dl, hemoglobin of 12.6 g/dl, white blood cell count of 10,500 mm^3. What is the hemodynamic pathophysiology in cases of myocardial ischemia? What is your initial approach to the treatment of this patient's anginal complaints?

Myocardial oxygen needs (MVO_2) are determined by the heart rate, contractility, and wall stress. The catecholamine response increases the heart rate and causes vasoconstriction, leading to increased wall stress (afterload).

First-line therapy is the use of supplemental oxygen. This overcomes hypoxia (goal Pao_2 < 60 mm Hg, Sao_2 < 90%) and makes the patient feel much more comfortable. In addition, there is bronchodilatation and vasodilatation, reduction in the pulmonary artery pressure and preload, leading to improved cardiac output. As renal perfusion improves, the stimulus for angiotensin and aldosterone secretion is gradually removed. A decline in secretion of angiotensin produces peripheral vasodilatation that reduces left ventricular afterload.

Usual practice dictates the use of sublingual nitroglycerin (SLNTG) tablets (0.4 mg) and topical nitrates. The former produces a constant serum level of nitrates through the transcutaneous route (Fig. 2-1-1). When the patient's symptoms remain refractory to this regimen, intravenous nitroglycerin (IV NTG) may be used. IV NTG has been shown to significantly reduce the number of anginal attacks experienced by patients with critical coronary lesions. IV administration is the route of choice and allows for rapid delivery and titration of NTG. IV NTG also has the advantage of a short half-life and may be stopped if serious hypotension occurs. NTG, primarily a venodilating agent, reduces pulmonary artery pressure and

decreases preload. The beneficial effects of continuous IV NTG, though, is diminished after the first 24 hours because of the development of nitrate tolerance.

IV NTG is dosed to clinical response: full alleviation of the patient's symptoms. When patients experience exacerbations of their symptoms, a sublingual tablet should be given along with an increase in the drip rate. SL NTG acts as a loading dose to elevate serum levels and allows time for the patient to receive the increased dose via the intravenous infusion. The managing physician should not be satisfied until the patient's symptoms are totally alleviated. Particular caution should be used in patients who are preload dependent such as those with hypovolemia, right ventricular infarction, pericardial constriction or effusion, pulmonary hypertension, and stenotic valvular lesions (aortic or mitral). Use of nitrates frequently leads to hypotension of a mild degree, which is easily counteracted with IV saline use.

Further antiischemic effects can be achieved by the use of beta-blocking agents. Beta-blockers reduce myocardial oxygen demand by preventing catecholamine-induced increases in heart rate, blood pressure, and myocardial contraction. Other beneficial features of beta-blockers in patients with unstable angina are the antiarrhythmic properties, the ability to reduce platelet aggregation, and alterations that shift metabolism from aerobic free fatty acids toward anaerobic glucose utilization. Beta-blockers, therefore, should be used in patients with unstable angina unless contraindications such as poor ventricular function, asthma/COPD, AV block, bradycardia, or prinzmetal syndrome exist. A regimen of metoprolol given in 5 mg IV boluses every 5 minutes for a total of 3 doses is an appropriate loading dose. If the initial 3 doses are tolerated, qid dosing of 25 to 50 mg can be instituted depending upon heart rate and blood pressure responses.

Another class of antiischemic agents, the calcium channel blockers, can be used in combination with or instead of the beta-blockers. The calcium entry blockers differ in their abilities to produce peripheral vasodilation (nifedipine), negative inotropy (diltiazem), and negative chronotropy (verapamil). The choice of calcium entry blocker, therefore, must be made with these features in mind. Nifedipine-induced tachycardia should be avoided in patients with coronary insufficiency. Concomitant use of a beta-blocker may offset this chronotropic effect. Diltiazem and verapamil have been shown to have equal efficacy when compared to nitrates in a treatment of coronary artery vasospasm. Diltiazem may be used to prevent subsequent ischemia events in patients with nontransmural MIs, provided the ejection fraction is greater than 35%.

Based on our understanding of the initiation of unstable angina, (plaque rupture and intracoronary thrombus formation) anticoagulation with aspirin and heparin have been shown to protect against myocardial infarction (MI) in men with this syndrome. Studies have shown a 51% lower incidence of death or infarction in patients with unstable angina treated with aspirin. The benefits of heparin used during the first week of therapy are evidenced by an 80% reduction in the number of transmural infarctions seen in a group treated with heparin. Further studies have shown a decrease in the incidence of myocardial infarction in patients treated with either aspirin or heparin with a trend toward greater benefit in those treated with heparin. No clear-cut benefits are noted in those treated with combination therapy. Care must be taken to consider the patient's risk before heparin is begun. Adequate anticoagulation requires prolongation of the activated partial thromboplastin time (aPTT) to 1.5 to 2 times control.

Despite the well-proven presence of the intracoronary thrombus, thrombolytic therapy has not proven beneficial in patients with unstable angina. Though there is angiographic improvement with thrombolytics, little clinical improvement has been noted.

QUESTION 5 The patient was initially started on IV NTG at a rate of 10 µg/minute but complained of a recurrence of anginal pain. The NTG was titrated

up to 50 µg/minute. He also received metoprolol 5 mg IV X 3 q 5 minutes. The patient was given 1 aspirin to chew and started on full-dose heparin anticoagulation.

The patient continued on his current therapy without chest pain or ECG changes until approximately 18 hours after admission when he complained of a recurrence of anginal pain. His symptoms continued despite three SL NTG tablets and increasing the IV NTG rate to 120 µg/minute. The patient's blood pressure was noted to be 170/95 mm Hg with a heart rate of 110 bpm. The ECG at that time showed new ST-segment depression in the V4, V5, and V6 of approximately 3 mm. An additional dose of metoprolol was given, but the pain continued to escalate over the next half hour without improvement. What is the next level of appropriate therapy for this patient?

This patient demonstrates the dynamic nature of the coronary lesion that defines unstable angina. At this point, the patient has pain refractory to medical treatment, and revascularization should be considered. Early studies confirmed that percutaneous transluminal coronary angioplasty (PTCA) was as efficacious as bypass surgery in those patients with unstable angina and single vessel disease. Later studies have also shown that emergency PTCA is as efficacious as coronary bypass in patients with single and multivessel disease in the immediate control of pain with a success rate of approximately 90% to 95%. However, long-term survival appears improved in patients with triple vessel disease who choose coronary artery bypass grafting rather than PTCA.

When a delay is encountered before revascularization is attempted, an intraaortic balloon pump may serve as a temporizing measure. The balloon pump is inserted via femoral arterial access and positioned just distal to the aortic arch. By its inflation during diastole and deflation during systole, the balloon pump reduces afterload, unloading the left ventricle, and reducing myocardial oxygen demand. Likewise a diastolic pressure gradient is achieved that may improve coronary flow by decreasing left ventricular end

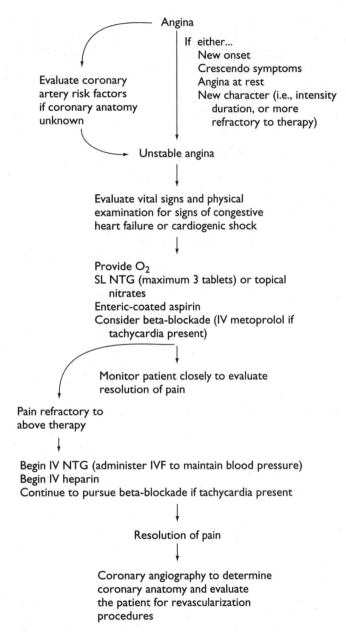

Angina

If either...
New onset
Crescendo symptoms
Angina at rest
New character (i.e., intensity
    duration, or more
    refractory to therapy)

Evaluate coronary
artery risk factors
if coronary anatomy
unknown

Unstable angina

Evaluate vital signs and physical
examination for signs of congestive
heart failure or cardiogenic shock

Provide O_2
SL NTG (maximum 3 tablets) or topical
    nitrates
Enteric-coated aspirin
Consider beta-blockade (IV metoprolol if
    tachycardia present)

Monitor patient closely to evaluate
resolution of pain

Pain refractory to
above therapy

Begin IV NTG (administer IVF to maintain blood pressure)
Begin IV heparin
Continue to pursue beta-blockade if tachycardia present

Resolution of pain

Coronary angiography to determine
coronary anatomy and evaluate
the patient for revascularization
procedures

2-1-1   Algorithm for treatment of myocardial ischemic syndromes.

diastolic pressure and increasing intraaortic diastolic pressure. It is necessary to monitor for
vascular complications including ischemia, hematoma, and mesenteric artery occlusions.

QUESTION 6   The patient was taken to the cardiac catheterization lab where a 90% mid left
anterior descending artery lesion was treated by
PTCA. The patient promptly reported relief of his

anginal symptoms. Ventriculography showed preservation of LV function. No other significant lesions were noted. The patient returned to the CCU and remained pain free. Cardiac enzyme analysis demonstrated a peak CK of 350 with MB fraction of 7%. Serial ECGs remained stable and showed resolution of the ST depression without any development of Q waves. What are the prognostic factors applicable to patients after a myocardial ischemic event?

Approximately 10% of patients admitted with unstable angina go on to develop myocardial infarction during that admission. This patient benefitted from quick revascularization in the catheterization lab and suffered only a small non-Q wave MI. In patients who have undergone acute MI, several clinical factors may forbode a poor long-term prognosis. Particular among these are poor left ventricular function, the presence of spontaneous ventricular ectopy or the presence of inducible ventricular tachyarrhythmias. An ejection fraction of less than 40% is an independent risk factor for sudden death as are spontaneous ventricular ectopy of greater than 10 PVCs per hour and nonsustained ventricular tachycardia. An abnormal signal averaged ECG independently predicts an eight-fold increase in risk of arrhythmic events postmyocardial infarction.

CASE FOLLOW-UP   The patient was discharged 2 days after PTCA. He participated in a cardiac rehabilitation program and has returned to an active lifestyle. He is maintained on antihypertensive therapy, lost 8 pounds, and continues to abstain from smoking.

• •

BIBLIOGRAPHY

Braunwald E: Unstable angina: a classification, *Circulation* 80:410-414, 1989.

Munger TM, Oh JK: Unstable angina, *Mayo Clin Proc* 65:384-406, 1990.

Schaer GL: Unstable angina pectoris, *Current Ther Crit Care Med* 26:112-115, 1991.

Theroux P: Aspirin, heparin, or both to treat unstable angina, *N Engl J Med* 319:1105-1111, 1988.

CASE

2

Kevin Maquiling
John Barron

. . . .

The patient is a 52-year-old female with a history of hypertension who presents with a 3-month history of "palpitations and skipped beats." They usually occur at rest with sudden onset, lasting a few seconds up to 1 to 2 minutes. The symptoms are usually relieved on their own. This morning the patient felt similar symptoms lasting approximately 1½ hours, leading to an emergency room visit. She complained of slight shortness of breath and dizziness with the episode. She denied chest pain and has no history of medications, though she recently cut back on caffeine. She has no history of tobacco use or of thyroid disease.

QUESTION 1 The patient's chief complaint is "palpitations." What does this term mean and how is the etiology of palpitations best documented?

Palpitations, or the conscious awareness of cardiac activity, is a common nonspecific complaint that may accompany a broad range of noncardiac and cardiac conditions with significance ranging from the sinus tachycardia of deconditioning to life-threatening ventricular tachycardia. Only one third of patients with complaint of palpitations actually have associated arrhythmias accompanying their symptoms during ambulatory ECG monitoring. While history and physical examination may occasionally give clues to the etiology of such episodes, they are unfortunately often normal. The key, therefore, to the diagnosis of palpitations is the ECG recorded during symptoms (Fig. 2-2-1 on p. 36).

Though physical examination may be unremarkable save for a tachycardia, one should look

for signs that, if present, may help to delineate the etiology of the palpitations. The examination of the neck veins may reveal the cannon A-waves of atrioventricular (AV) dissociation. Atrial flutter waves are occasionally seen in the JVP. Vagal maneuvers such as carotid sinus massage, Valsalva, gag, and facial cold water immersion, may decrease the rate or change the p to r relationship, a clue which will be discussed later. Attention to the first heart sound may reveal the variable intensity of S1 seen in ventricular tachycardias.

QUESTION 2 Physical examination revealed: T 98.4°F; RR 14/min; HR 160 to 180 bpm; BP 130/80 mm Hg. In general, this is a slightly anxious woman, HEENT examination normal; lungs clear to auscultation. Cardiovascular examination showed no JVD; venous pulsations normal; regular S_1, S_2, no S_3, S_4; no murmurs. Abdomen was benign. Laboratory examination showed normal SMA 18 magnesium and thyroid functions. Is the patient hemodynamically stable? What other studies should be undertaken?

At present the patient is hemodynamically stable as determined by blood pressure. If she had not been, the next step would be electrical cardioversion, regardless of whether the tachycardia is of ventricular or supraventricular origin.

As with the physical examination, laboratory tests are often normal. On occasion, electrolyte imbalance, in particular potassium and magnesium abnormalities, may be seen. Screening thyroid function tests should be performed. Screening for pheochromocytoma may also be warranted in the appropriate clinical setting.

QUESTION 3 Rhythm strips demonstrated a narrow complex tachycardia at a rate of 180 as in Fig. 2-2-2 on p. 37. How is the differentiation between a supraventricular and ventricular tachyarrhythmia ascertained? Describe the inciting mechanism for establishing a supraventricular tachycardia (SVT).

A determination of the particular rhythm is aided by examination of the 12-lead ECG during the tachycardia and if available, an ECG recorded prior to the arrhythmia. The vast majority of narrow QRS complex tachycardias are supraventricular in nature. Rhythms that possess wider complexes may be ventricular or supraventricular in origin. Criteria as established by Wellens, and recently modified by Brugada, are useful in delineating the locus of origin in most instances. The presence of a QRS duration greater than 0.14 sec, left axis deviation, A-V dissociation, or a mono or biphasic bundle branch block pattern suggests ventricular tachycardia.

Other general findings to look for on the ECG are as follows: (1) evidence of preexcitation such as a shortened PR interval and a delta wave as seen in Wolff-Parkinson-White (WPW) syndrome, (2) prolongation of the QT interval associated with congenital or drug-induced arrhythmias, or (3) evidence of previous infarction. The latter two findings favor a ventricular origin.

Determination of the mechanism of the supraventricular tachycardia is important both for the short-term management of SVT and in the long-term treatment of this condition. By understanding the mechanism of the SVT, one can direct intervention at either the AV node or an accessory pathway.

The two most common mechanisms of regular narrow complex tachycardia are AV nodal reentrant tachycardia (AVNRT) and orthodromic AV reentrant tachycardia (AVRT). AVNRT is dependent upon the presence of dual conduction pathways within the AV node. In the most common form (90% of cases), a slow-fast sequence is present. Impulses travel from the atrium to the ventricle via the slow pathway and return to the

atrium via the fast pathway. In AVRT, a concealed (Kent) accessory pathway is present. Impulses travel to the ventricle via the AV node, but return to the atrium via the accessory pathway. In this sequence a narrow complex tachycardia is the result. Patients with WPW may also be vulnerable to narrow complex tachycardias. In addition, these patients may also display wide complex tachycardias.

QUESTION 4 Vagal stimulation was performed with the Valsalva maneuver without change in either rate or rhythm. Adenosine was administered in a 6 mg IV bolus immediately followed by saline flush. This was repeated after one minute with a 12 mg bolus after which the patient converted to sinus rhythm. What is the treatment for SVT?

The treatment of narrow complex SVT is focused on the temporary interruption of AV nodal conduction by use of either vagal maneuvers or pharmacologic intervention. In the two most common types of SVT, the AV node accesses either one or both legs of a circuit allowing re-entrant circus type rhythms to be generated. Vagal stimulation includes carotid massage, Valsalva maneuver, gag reflex, or facial cold water immersion. Pharmacologic alternatives include calcium channel blockers, beta-blockers, cardiac glycosides, or more recently, adenosine. While these interventions are usually reserved for the hemodynamically stable patient, some of them may themselves be destabilizing. The calcium channel blocker verapamil is used commonly but is associated at times with hypotension, prolonged bradycardia, or AV block. This drug is contraindicated in patients with accessory pathways because of the risk of diverting impulses of atrial flutter/fibrillation directly to the ventricle via the bypass track. Similar side effects have been seen with beta-blockers and Digoxin.

Adenosine also causes depression of AV nodal activity but is free of the previously mentioned hazards because of its very short half-life. As opposed to the half-life of several hours seen with the other drugs, the half-life of adenosine is approximately 1 to 6 seconds, and it is totally cleared within 30 seconds. Other than transient feeling of flushing in up to one third of patients, there is little hazard in its use. Studies comparing adenosine and verapamil show them to be equally effective in terminating SVT, though the average time to termination was shorter with adenosine, approximately 30 seconds.

Because of its very rapid clearance, adenosine must be given as a rapid bolus immediately followed by a rapid saline flush. Likewise, the more centrally the injection is given, the higher the relative dose reaching the heart. Dosage adjustment may be necessary in patients receiving theophylline or other methylxanthines that competitively bind to adenosine receptors and in those receiving dipyridamole, which potentiates the effect of adenosine.

ECG following adenosine conversion showed normal sinus rhythm without evidence of acute ischemia or ventricular preexcitation.

As mentioned earlier, the ECG must be used to identify the mechanism of the SVT. The type of chronic prophylactic therapy will depend on the type of SVT.

QUESTION 5   What is an accessory pathway and what is the significance of this anatomic finding?

An accessory pathway is an alternate conduction circuit co-existing with the usual SAN → AVN → His-Purkinje system. An example is the Wolff-Parkinson-White (WPW) syndrome. This tachycardia is due to the presence of a pathway of conduction from the ventricle to the atrium, known as a Kent bundle. This allows an electrical impulse to be generated from the SAN to the AVN to the ventricle and back to the atrium, establishing a reciprocating circuit of conduction. This accessory bundle is not apparent on the scalar ECG and is therefore called "concealed." Because the reciprocating impulse activates the atrium before it would be expected from the normal specialized conduction system, this is known as a preexcitation syndrome.

The electrocardiogram may harbor clues to the presence of an accessory pathway. Normal sinus rhythm, a shortened PR interval, and a wide QRS complex with a delta wave suggest an accessory path. During tachycardia the presence of atrial activity 100 to 140 msec after the start of the QRS complex suggests an accessory pathway since impulses traveling via the accessory pathway are delayed by their root across the ventricle back to the atrium and are therefore not buried in QRS complex as is common in AVNRT. If vagal stimulation is performed, the A/V ratio may change, suggesting a mechanism other than reentry such as atrial tachycardia or atrial flutter. If an accessory pathway is present, further localization may be obtained from the ECG by closer scrutiny of the P-wave axis and its timing.

QUESTION 6   The patient was started on verapamil and tolerated it well without further episodes. What is the accepted mode of long-term therapy for patients with this type of tachycardia?

The chronic prophylaxis of AVNRT involves drugs aimed at slowing the conduction of both fast and slow pathways and decreasing precipitating events such as PVCs and PACs. Chronic prophylaxis of AVRT includes *Ia* or *Ic*, antiarrhythmics directed toward the accessory pathway.

While life-long use of such antiarrhythmics often has satisfactory results, the advances of electrophysiologic studies and radiofrequency ablation offer alternatives to those patients intolerant of medication or refractory to treatment. Intracardiac catheters can be used in either a palliative manner, to control the ventricular response, or in a curative manner, to ablate the source of the SVT or the myocardium necessary to maintain the reentrant tachycardia.

CASE FOLLOW-UP   The patient was discharged after being placed on a stable dose of verapamil. Two weeks after discharge, she has experienced good relief from her "palpitations" and is currently scheduled for her first follow-up visit to the cardiology clinic next week.

• •

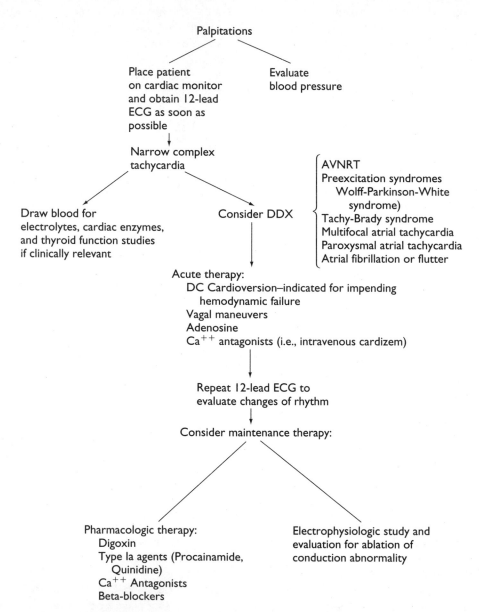

2-2-1 Algorithm for diagnosis and treatment of patients presenting with "palpitations."

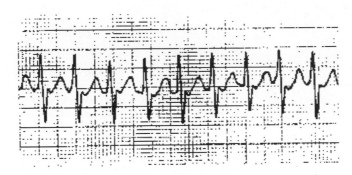

2-2-2

BIBLIOGRAPHY

Barrington WW, Greenfield RA, Bacon ME, et al: Treatment of supraventricular tachycardias with transcatheter delivery of radiofrequency current, *Am J Med* 93:549-557, 1992.

Brugada J, Atie J, Gursoy S, et al: Diagnosing regular tachycardias, *Intern Med* 13:23-28, 1992.

Brugada P, Brugada J, Mont L, et al: A new approach to the differential diagnosis of a regular tachycardia with a wide QRS complex, *Circulation* 83:1649-1659, 1991.

Caruso AC: Supraventricular tachycardia: changes in management, *Postgrad Med* 90:73-82, 1991.

Faitelson L, Ewey GA: Clinical algorithm: treatment of supraventricular tachycardia, *Hosp Med* 12:37-44, 1991.

Knopp DE, Wilber DJ: Palpitations and arrhythmias, *Postgrad Med* 91:241-254, 1992.

Rankin AC, Brooks R, McGovern BA: Adenosine and the treatment of supraventricular tachycardia, *Am J Med* 92: 655-664, 1992.

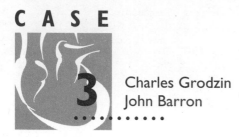

CASE

3

Charles Grodzin
John Barron

A 61-year-old male presents to the emergency room with the acute onset of lightheadedness, diaphoresis, nausea, and a fluttering sensation in his chest that began suddenly 2 hours prior to presentation. He denies alcohol abuse, but the odor of alcohol on his breath is strong. History includes a myocardial infarction 6 years previously without intercurrent angina, high blood pressure treated with a calcium channel blocker, and intermittent smoking. He denies chest pain or lower extremity pain. Physical examination finds him to have a blood pressure of 85/50 mm Hg and an irregularly irregular pulse. The cardiac monitor illustrates a narrow complex tachycardia.

QUESTION I What is your initial approach to a patient with the preceding presentation?

Initial consideration must be given to the patient's hemodynamic stability and to the assurance of end-organ perfusion. Signs and symptoms of hypotension include pallor, diaphoresis, and altered mental status. The patient may complain of nausea and vomiting, palpitations, and orthostasis when assuming an upright position. Organ systems that depend on a rich bed of capillaries may be compromised by systemic hypotension, especially in the bettering of diffuse atherosclerosis. This includes the renal, nervous, and cardiac systems. Specific screening examination should be carried out to assess each system's functional integrity.

When hypotension is suspected, a large bore IV line should be secured for the administration of saline; the patient should be placed supine to improve cerebral blood flow (Trendelenburg po-

sition if necessary); and vasopressors should be used if necessary to maintain a blood pressure greater than 70 mm Hg. Several etiologies of hypotension should be investigated immediately: acute blood loss, sepsis, third-spaced fluid, myocardial infarction, dysrhythmia, and clues for anaphylaxis. These diagnoses require immediate specific intervention.

In this clinical setting, the temporal relationship of both low blood pressure and the onset of the irregularly irregular cardiac rhythm suggest a causative relationship. Therefore, this can be taken as the presumptive etiology and warrants specific intervention.

QUESTION 2 The initial rhythm strip is shown below (Fig. 2-3-1). What is your interpretation of this rhythm, and how does this impact on your diagnosis and treatment?

The rhythm strip demonstrates a narrow complex tachycardia without obvious P wave activity with a ventricular response of 120 to 140 bpm that is irregularly irregular. In addition, there is a variable RR interval and an irregular baseline. Therefore, this rhythm qualifies as a supraventricular tachycardia (SVT). This term refers to any tachycardia of supraventricular origin. It is commonly taken to identify an AV nodal reentrant rhythm.

An expanded differential diagnosis of SVT includes Wolff-Parkinson-White (WPW) syndrome, multifocal atrial tachycardia, and sinus tachycardia. Electrocardiographic features of SVT are alterations in P wave morphology, a narrow QRS width, and a 1:1 association of P wave to QRS when P waves are present. Atrial fibrillation (AF)

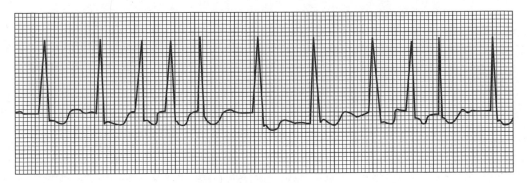

2-3-1 Initial rhythm strip.

and atrial flutter, however, present with an irregularly irregular rhythm and either an absent or variable P-QRS relationship, respectively. Only automatic atrial tachycardias and sinus tachycardias show a gradual increase in rate as the circuit warms up. Other SVTs are paroxysmal and begin abruptly.

The most common mechanism of SVT is AV nodal reentry (Fig. 2-3-2). Vagal maneuvers, including carotid massage, pressure on the orbits, immersion of the face in cold water, and Valsalva may provide enough parasympathetic tone so as to inhibit AV nodal conduction and convert the rhythm back to normal sinus or slow the rhythm, allowing identification of underlying P wave activity.

This end can also be reached pharmacologically with the use of adenosine. IV bolus adenosine has similar vagal properties as the above maneuvers. It is used most easily via the two-syringe method. Initially, one syringe is prepared with 6 mg of adenosine, and a second syringe is prepared with 10 ml of saline. Both needles are placed into the most proximal available port of the IV line and the distal portion pinched off to avoid backflow. In rapid succession the adenosine, over 2 seconds, followed by the saline, are injected to maintain bolus integrity. One needs to remember that the presence of methylxanthines inhibits adenosine, whereas dipyridamole and carbamazepine can augment the degree of heart block. Side effects include facial flushing, acute dyspnea, chest pressure, headache, lightheadedness, and nausea. If no response is attained, a second trial of 12 mg may be repeated twice before another agent is used.

QUESTION 3 You correctly diagnose the patient's problem to be hypotension secondary to the onset of atrial fibrillation with a rapid ventricular response. What is the pathophysiology of this dysrhythmia and what etiologies need be considered?

Atrial fibrillation is the product of multiple concurrent atrial foci of reentry with heterogeneous refractory periods producing multiple wave-fronts spreading over the atrial myocardium causing chaotic contraction. Impulses bombard the AV node and are translated, influenced by its refractory period, into ventricular contractions. Patients lose about 15% to 20% of their ventricular filling and cardiac output because of loss of coordinated atrial function and shortening of diastolic filling time. For those patients with borderline cardiac function, this decrement may be enough to lead to cardiac decompensation.

The most common predisposing condition is coronary artery disease (CAD). It is important to consider other diagnoses, especially in patients who do not have an underlying history of chronic cardiopulmonary disease (cardiomyopathy, CAD, aortic stenosis, rheumatic heart disease). Other etiologies include thyrotoxicosis, pulmonary embolism, myocardial infarction, ethanol abuse, poorly controlled hypertension, pericarditis, myocarditis, tachy-brady syndrome, or preexcitation syndromes. A screening battery including thyroid function tests, cardiac enzymes, ETOH level, blood pressure measurement, ESR, and cardiac monitoring can elucidate an underlying predisposition.

QUESTION 4 In the emergency room the patient's heart rate slowed but remained irregularly irregular with stabilization of the blood pressure. Echocardiogram reveals a 5.8 cm left atrium without other structural abnormality. What is the correct maintenance management of this patient?

In hemodynamically stable patients, optimal therapy includes rate control followed by elective cardioversion. Multiple pharmacologic agents exist that are useful in the management of AF. Digoxin acts by blocking atrioventricular conduction at the AV node. Digoxin is not a cardioversion agent. However, this drug will decrease the atrial refractory period and increase the rate at which the AV node is bombarded by impulses. Overload of the AV node leads to down-regulation of AV transmission and a slowed ventricular rate. An important caveat pertains to the use of adenosine as a therapy for AF. Use of this agent may lead to long pauses and further hemodynamic instability.

Other agents include the class Ia antiarrhythmics, which block the fast sodium channel. Quinidine enhances AV conduction via a vagolytic mechanism, abolishes atrial ectopy, and increases atrial refractory time. Levels should be followed closely to avoid toxicity: cinchonism (tinnitus, blurred or distorted color perception, diplopia, scotomata, and night blindness), nausea, vomiting, postural hypotension, and possible respiratory arrest. Electrocardiographic monitoring should raise alarm if the QRS complex widens by 25%. In cases of fast atrial rates, digitalization is necessary to avoid a rapid ventricular response. Procainamide decreases atrial excitability, slows conduction, and prolongs the atrial refractory period. Accurate levels are arrived at by cumula-

tive procainamide and NAPA (a metabolite of procainamide) levels.

Propafenone, a Na-channel blocking agent, has shown promise. It has been found useful in preventing recurrent AF, reducing symptoms related to the SVT and prolonging the refractory period of accessory pathways that may participate in development of SVT. Propafenone is not currently approved for the treatment of AF by the FDA.

Amiodarone also has played a role in the treatment of chronic AF. By slowing AV nodal conduction, this agent may be used with success in patients who do not respond to class Ia agents. Because of the large volume of distribution when loading with amiodarone, a clinical response may take up to 2 weeks. Side effects may include skin photosensitivity, pulmonary fibrosis, corneal micro-deposits, and hypothyroidism or hyperthyroidism. A panel of thyroid and pulmonary function tests and an evaluation of visual acuity as baseline values are necessary. Low dose therapy has fewer side effects.

In situations of more profound hemodynamic embarrassment, electrical cardioversion is the treatment of choice. Application of an electrical current to the heart results in a generalized depolarization with a resultant asystole that allows the sinus node to resume function as the pacemaker. Usually no more than 100 to 200 joules is necessary. The success of this procedure is related inversely to left atrial size (SBP <5 cm) and the length of time one has persisted in AF (SBP <1 yr). Patients with mitral/aortic stenosis or hypertrophic cardiomyopathy may require repeated attempts. Approximately half of the patients remain in sinus rhythm at 1 year.

If these modalities fail, electrophysiologic study with endocardial catheter fulguration of the AV node or HIS bundle may be necessary. Another alternative is surgical ablation of a concealed or manifest nodal bypass tract (i.e., Wolff-Parkinson-White syndrome).

QUESTION 5 What population of patients with AF require systemic anticoagulation?

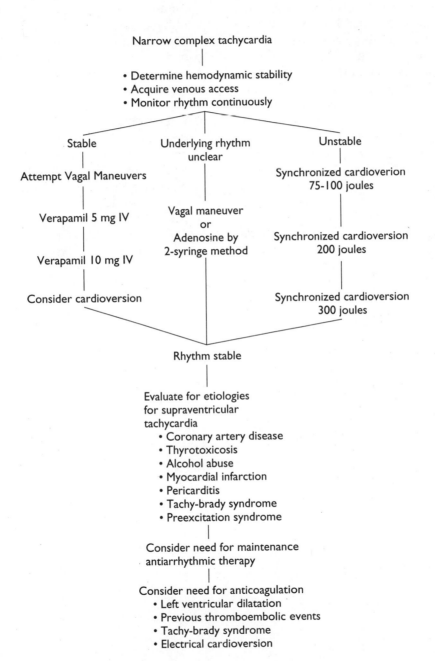

Narrow complex tachycardia

- Determine hemodynamic stability
- Acquire venous access
- Monitor rhythm continuously

Stable | Underlying rhythm unclear | Unstable

Attempt Vagal Maneuvers

Verapamil 5 mg IV

Verapamil 10 mg IV

Consider cardioversion

Vagal maneuver
or
Adenosine by
2-syringe method

Synchronized cardioverion
75-100 joules

Synchronized cardioversion
200 joules

Synchronized cardioversion
300 joules

Rhythm stable

Evaluate for etiologies
for supraventricular
tachycardia
- Coronary artery disease
- Thyrotoxicosis
- Alcohol abuse
- Myocardial infarction
- Pericarditis
- Tachy-brady syndrome
- Preexcitation syndrome

Consider need for maintenance
antiarrhythmic therapy

Consider need for anticoagulation
- Left ventricular dilatation
- Previous thromboembolic events
- Tachy-brady syndrome
- Electrical cardioversion

2-3-2 Diagnostic approach to the patient with atrial fibrillation.

AF is the most common cardiac abnormality leading to embolic disease. There is a 5.6-fold increase in stroke as compared to those without AF. There is a propensity for embolization with prosthetic valves and a 17-fold increase in embolic risk in those with associated rheumatic valvular disease.

Patients deemed to have a clear indication for systemic anticoagulation include those patients with a prior history of a thromboembolic event secondary to AF, rheumatic mitral valve disease, tachy-brady syndrome, and electrical cardioversion. In the thyrotoxic patient most emboli result as cerebral emboli.

The presence of a dilated left ventricle, especially of prolonged duration, adds to the risk of clot formation. This group is recommended to receive long-term anticoagulation also. There is a clustering of embolic phenomena around initiation of new onset AF, which may indicate the need for short-term anticoagulation until definitive therapy is applied or an underlying etiology is successfully treated.

It is important to anticoagulate for 1 to 4 weeks before DC-countershock as the risk for embolization is as high as 1% to 5%. New-onset AF, greater than 1 week's duration, requires short-term anticoagulation. After the procedure, anticoagulants can be stopped after an additional 4 weeks (target prothrombin time 1.3 to 1.5 times control). This is due to a temporal delay between electrical conversion and coordinated mechanical atrial contraction. In the thyrotoxic patient the best time to cardiovert is in week 16 after establishing the euthyroid state. Anticoagulation is not indicated in those with lone/transient AF and AF associated with hypertension.

Maintenance anticoagulation is indicated in patients with chronic AF in the presence of heart disease, prior embolism, or documented atrial clot.

CASE FOLLOW-UP The patient was loaded with digoxin and then procainamide and subsequently converted to normal sinus rhythm. Subsequent electrocardiograms did not reveal any further supraventricular ectopy. Thyroid function tests and cardiac enzyme assays were negative. He was not deemed a candidate for systemic anticoagulation. The onset of his AF was thought to be secondary to alcohol indiscretion. He was discharged in good spirits after 6 days of hospitalization.

● ●

BIBLIOGRAPHY

DiMarco JP, Miles W, Akhtar M: Adenosine for paroxysmal supraventricular tachycardia: dose ranging and comparison with verapamil, *Ann Intern Med* 113:104-110, 1990.

Dunn M, Alexander J: Antithrombotic therapy in atrial fibrillation, *Chest* 95(2):118S-127S, 1989.

Kastor JA: Multifocal atrial tachycardia, *N Engl J Med* 322(24): 1713-1717, 1990.

Pritchett ELC: Management of atrial fibrillation, *N Engl J Med* 1264-1270, 1992.

Repique LJ, Marais GE: Atrial fibrillation, *Chest* 101:4, 1992.

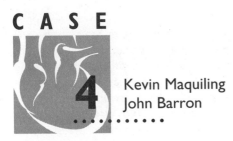

CASE

4
Kevin Maquiling
John Barron

The patient is a 28-year-old woman with a past medical history remarkable for hypertrophic cardiomyopathy who is referred to your cardiology clinic for examination and to arrange follow-up during her pregnancy. Specifically, she has not experienced any dyspnea, orthopnea, or PND. She has not developed any peripheral edema or suffered a decrease in her exercise tolerance. She is currently 4 weeks pregnant.

QUESTION I What are the important cardiovascular physiologic changes during pregnancy, labor, and delivery, and what is the impact on the cardiovascular system?

Prior to deciding on how to manage any cardiac abnormality in pregnancy, it is necessary to understand the normal physiologic changes associated with pregnancy. Because of substantial hemodynamic changes, women with certain types of heart disease are at risk for greater morbidity and mortality during their pregnancy and in the postpartum period. One major change is a substantial increase in blood volume that ranges from 20% to 100% of the usual intravascular volume in the nonpregnant state. This begins early in pregnancy and rises rapidly until midpregnancy, when the rate of volume expansion slows. Because the increase in blood volume occurs more rapidly than the increase in red cell mass, a phenomenon known as the "physiologic anemia of pregnancy" occurs. Hemoglobin levels generally drop to approximately 11 to 12 g/dl.

Cardiac output also increases during pregnancy to approximately 30% to 50% over the nonpregnant state. With the progressive increase in size of the gravid uterus, body position begins to

play an important role in determining cardiac output. Cardiac output declines significantly in the supine position because of decreased preload from inferior vena cava (IVC) compression by the enlarged uterus. Cardiac output is maximized when the patient assumes the lateral decubitus position.

A substantial increase in heart rate also occurs. This is most marked during the third trimester. The increased heart rate compensates for the decreased stroke volume seen secondary to IVC compression. On the average, heart rate increases 10 to 20 beats per minute during pregnancy. Systemic arterial pressure falls during pregnancy, reaching its nadir in midpregnancy. The decline in systemic vascular resistance is due to the vasodilatory effects of gestational hormones, prostaglandins, heat production by the developing fetus, and the low resistance circulation through the uterus.

Considerable hemodynamic changes occur during labor and delivery. Cardiac output increases by up to 50% during uterine contractions concurrent with a threefold increase in oxygen consumption. Postpartum hemodynamic changes are often significant. There is increased venous return after delivery of the fetus and relief of IVC compression. Likewise, a phenomenon known as auto-transfusion occurs as blood shifts back from the uterus to the systemic circulation leading to an increase in the preload and stroke volume. Approximately 24 hours postpartum, the stroke volume returns to normal.

With these physiologic changes, it is not surprising that women with heart disease may be at increased risk during pregnancy. In the past, as many as 22% of women with heart disease died during pregnancy, most frequently around the time of delivery. Mortality varies depending upon New York Heart Association functional classification. Class I and II have a mortality of approximately 0.4%, whereas classes III and IV have an associated mortality of 6% to 8%. Given that up to 4% of pregnant women have evidence of heart disease, it is incumbent upon physicians to recognize symptoms early and provide careful follow-up care, so as to make any necessary adjustments to reduce the risk of maternal mortality.

QUESTION 2   The patient reports doing well on verapamil 240 mg a day for the past 2 years. Her initial complaints had been shortness of breath and occasional dizziness, but since beginning with verapamil, she has been generally asymptomatic without any limitations except for the avoidance of very strenuous physical activity. The patient denies any other medical problems, denies tobacco or alcohol use, but reports a family history of two uncles with hypertrophic obstructive cardiomyopathy (HOCM), one of whom died at age 23. The patient denies any current symptoms associated with her pregnancy such as nausea, vomiting, or swelling. Given the family history, you are concerned about HOCM. What are the presenting symptoms of HOCM and what are the important genetic elements?

The symptoms described by the patient are common in those with hypertrophic cardiomyopathy. Though most patients are asymptomatic, initial symptoms usually occur in young adulthood. Dyspnea is the most common presenting symptom, often with associated chest pain, dizziness, palpitations, or syncope. Symptoms of congestive heart failure often progress over time. Unfortunately, sudden arrhythmic death may be the initial presentation without any previous suggestion of heart disease. This patient's family history of hypertrophic cardiomyopathy is consistent with recognized patterns in which HOCM occurs either sporadically or in familial clusters. The hereditary form of HOCM is autosomal dominant with varying penetrance. The risk of inheritance is as high as 50% in some families.

QUESTION 3   The patient is a well-developed woman in no acute distress. Her temperature and vital signs were normal; her lungs were clear. The cardiovascular examination did not demonstrate jugular venous distension; the carotid arteries had a good upstroke with a bifid carotid pulse. The PMI was forceful, sustained, and displaced laterally. There was crescendo-decrescendo systolic murmur along the left sternal border that decreased with hand grip. There was no S_3 or S_4 present. No peripheral edema was noted. What is the pathophysiology of HOCM and the associated findings on physical examination?

As with any cardiac problem, the key to understanding the physical examination is to understand the underlying pathophysiology. On the microscopic level, myocardial fiber disarray is the hallmark of hypertrophic cardiomyopathy. In addition, myocardial scarring and abnormal thickening of the intramural coronary arteries is seen in hypertrophic cardiomyopathy. It should be noted though that these changes may also be seen as sequelae of coronary artery disease or ventricular hypertrophy from chronic pressure overload. On a macroscopic level, characteristic changes in hypertrophic cardiomyopathy include a hyperdynamic left ventricle, dynamic obstruction to left ventricular outflow, and a diastolic compliance abnormality impairing left ventricular filling.

With these underlying hemodynamic abnormalities in mind, it is easy to understand the typical physical findings in hypertrophic cardiomyopathy. Physical examination may be entirely normal as some patients do not have a demonstrable outflow tract obstruction.

Typically, the jugular venous pulsation is normal unless there is right ventricular hypertrophy, in which case prominent A waves will be seen. The carotid upstroke is normally brisk but may, in patients with outflow obstruction, show a typical spike and dome or bifid carotid pulsation. A forceful PMI is consistent with the hyperdynamic left ventricle.

The characteristic murmur of HOCM is a

crescendo-decrescendo systolic murmur along the left sternal border. This reflects the dynamic outflow obstruction which may be increased with maneuvers that increase contractility, decrease ventricular volume, or reduce peripheral vascular resistance. The murmur therefore increases in intensity with exercise or tachycardia or upon straining with Valsalva's maneuver. Squatting or isometric hand grip decreases the intensity of this murmur. The third heart sound is occasionally heard. Impaired ventricular filling due to the diastolic compliance abnormality almost always yields a fourth heart sound. A murmur of mitral regurgitation is also often heard.

QUESTION 4 The electrocardiogram showed left ventricular hypertrophy, and the rhythm strip showed occasional premature ventricular contractions. An echocardiogram showed generalized left ventricular thickening with a septum:posterior wall ratio of 1.7. The presence of systolic anterior motion of the mitral valve was noted. An outflow gradient of approximately 30 mm was measured. How are these findings explained by HOCM?

This patient's electrocardiogram and echocardiogram are typical of patients with hypertrophic cardiomyopathy. Ventricular hypertrophy develops because of the chronic pressure overload from outflow tract obstruction. Ventricular ectopy is also a common finding. In addition to electrocardiography, Holter monitoring should be done if ectopy is discovered.

The echocardiogram is used to make a definitive diagnosis. A septum:posterior wall ratio of >1.5 supports the diagnosis of asymmetric septal hypertrophy. The term systolic anterior motion (SAM) describes the dynamic obstruction caused during midsystole by the abnormal movement of the septum and the leaflets of the mitral valve. Convergence of these structures during systole narrows the aortic outflow tract. Doppler flow studies can help to assess the severity of the outflow obstruction by estimating the peak velocity through this area.

QUESTION 5 What other elements of HOCM are important to discuss with this patient in terms of her pregnancy?

At this point, having made an initial evaluation, the physician should discuss certain points with his patient. First, the outcome of pregnancies in patients with hypertrophic cardiomyopathy is good. However, new onset or worsening of cardiac symptoms during the pregnancy is not uncommon. Second, fetal outcome also seems unaffected by the presence of hypertrophic cardiomyopathy. Medications that may be required to treat worsening cardiomyopathy during pregnancy pose potential risk to the fetus. This must be balanced with the risk of maternal sudden death related to hypertrophic cardiomyopathy independent of the pregnancy. Last, given the hereditary nature of hypertrophic cardiomyopathy, family screening and genetic counseling should be undertaken.

QUESTION 6 The patient did well continuing on her verapamil. At approximately the fourth month of gestation, the patient began to note shortness of breath and intermittent chest pain. What is your approach to the patient with these symptoms? What is your approach to pharmacologic therapy for this patient?

When evaluating a pregnant woman with cardiac disease, it is sometimes difficult to separate those signs and symptoms due to cardiac disease from those normally associated with pregnancy. Though shortness of breath is the most common symptom in hypertrophic cardiomyopathy, hyperventilation is also very common in pregnancy. Additionally, bibasilar rales may be caused by bibasilar compression of the lungs secondary to enlargement of the uterus and increased abdominal pressure and are not necessarily due to heart failure. Further confusion may arise as pressure on the diaphragm may also displace the heart causing the PMI to be displaced laterally. Other findings during pregnancy that mimic congestive heart failure include an elevation of the jugular venous pressure, which is normally seen about the 20th week of pregnancy, and leg and ankle edema, which is common late in pregnancy. These signs are secondary to the fall in colloid osmotic pressure and increased femoral venous pressure. A third heart sound has been reported in up to 90% of pregnant women, usually heard after the 20th week of gestation. Grade 1/3 systolic ejection murmurs are very common in pregnant women secondary to increased intravascular volume and flow state. Elevated intravascular volume may augment preload and support ventricular filling pressure. Increased heart rate, normally associated with pregnancy, may have deleterious effects by decreasing the diastolic filling time. At this point, a repeat echocardiogram may be useful to objectively assess ventricular systole and diastolic function.

Though verapamil is the most commonly used and investigated drug in patients with symptomatic HOCM, its safety in pregnancy has not been thoroughly investigated. So far, there are a few reports from European investigators that have failed to show any teratogenic effects with the use of verapamil. Traditional teaching recommends propranolol for symptomatic patients during pregnancy. Cardioselective beta-blockers are preferred during pregnancy because nonselective agents may cause premature uterine contractions. However, it is important to try to avoid beta-blocker use because of its propensity to cause abnormalities of the fetus.

Sudden death is the most common cause of death in young patients with hypertrophic cardiomyopathy. A Holter monitor should be placed in the initial evaluation to look for complex ventricular rhythms. If they are present, the preferred antiarrhythmics would be quinidine or procainamide because of their proven safety during pregnancy. Beta-blockers should be reserved for acute situations as their long-term use, particularly during the first trimester of pregnancy, has been associated with teratogenic effects. Amiodarone should be reserved for life-threatening arrhythmias because of potential maternal and fetal adverse effects including pulmonary toxicity.

QUESTION 7 Repeat echocardiogram did not show deterioration of cardiac function, and the patient's symptoms did not progress. She went into labor on schedule and underwent an uncomplicated vaginal delivery. What is the impact of labor and delivery on patients with HOCM?

Though in the past cesarean sections had been used routinely in patients with HOCM to reduce the stress of delivery, it is accepted that vaginal delivery does not pose increased risk to the mother or fetus. Forceps may be used to shorten the second stage of labor, but cesarean section need only be employed in those patients with obstetric indications. HOCM patients should be kept euvolemic or slightly hypervolemic to maximize their cardiac output. One should avoid the use of prostaglandins because of their strong vasodilatory effect. Likewise, if labor is to be induced, one would prefer ergonovine over oxytocin because of the latter's vasoconstrictive properties. If tocolytic agents are required, magnesium sulfate is recommended over the beta-agonists because of their potential to worsen outflow obstruction. One must also avoid spinal or epidural anesthetics because of their potential vasodilatory effects that can compromise preload. Instead, inhalation agents or paracervical and pudendal blocks are recommended. Because of the variety of potential hemodynamic complications, symptomatic patients with known outflow obstruction may benefit from pulmonary artery catheterization during their delivery.

HOCM is associated with an increased risk for bacterial endocarditis. Opinions differ on whether routine prophylaxis is necessary in all patients with hypertrophic cardiomyopathy prior to uncomplicated vaginal delivery. The standard antibiotic prophylaxis for gastrointestinal or genital urinary procedures is 2 grams of ampicillin, IM or IV, plus 1.5 mg/kg of gentamicin IM or IV one-half hour before the procedure with a second dose 8 hours later. A diagnostic algorithm for congestive heart failure is shown in Fig. 2-4-1.

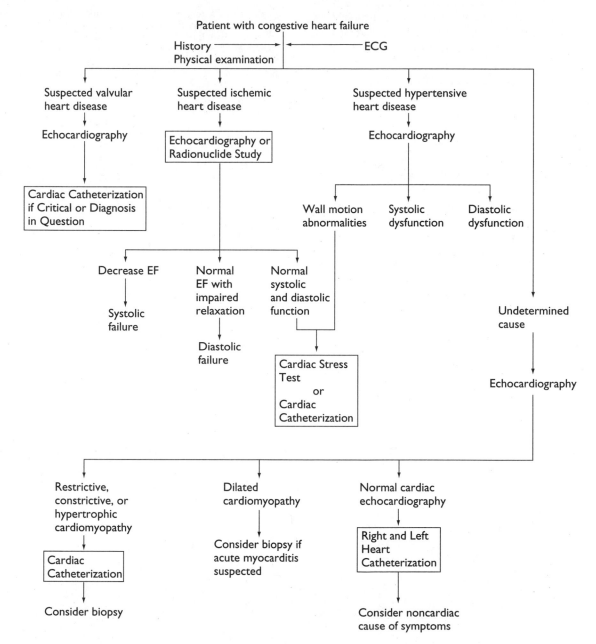

2-4-1 Diagnostic algorithm for congestive heart failure.
(From Greene HL, Johnson WP, Maricic MJ, editors: *Decision making in medicine,* St Louis, 1993, Mosby.)

CASE FOLLOW-UP   The patient was discharged from the hospital 2 days after delivery of her baby. At the time of discharge she was breathing easily and remained on her maintenance dose of verapamil. She is scheduled for a follow-up appointment at your office in 3 weeks.

• •

BIBLIOGRAPHY

Elkayam U: Pregnancy and cardiovascular Disease. In Braunwald E, ed: *Heart disease: a text book of cardiovascular medicine,* ed 4, Philadelphia, 1992, WB Saunders.

Elkayam U, Kumar A: Hypertrophic cardiomyopathy in pregnancy, *Cardiac Probl Pregn* 129-136, 1990.

Sullivan JM, Ramanathan KB: Cardiovascular disorders, *Med Surg Probl Obstet* 11-25, 1987.

Wynne J, Braunwald E: The cardiomyopathies and the myocarditides. In Brauwald E, ed: *Heart disease: a textbook of cardiovascular medicine,* ed 4, Philadelphia, 1992, WB Saunders.

CASE

5

Kevin Maquiling
John Barron
. . . .

The patient is a 64-year-old white male with a past medical history of rheumatic fever and peptic ulcer disease. While taking his wife to the doctor's office, he suddenly became short of breath. His dyspnea got worse over the next hour, and he was transported to the emergency room for evaluation and treatment. The patient reports that he was in his normal state of health without any specific complaints. However, his family members, who arrived several minutes later, noted that over the previous 1 week, he seemed easily fatigued. On one occasion, he was found gasping for breath and frantically loosening his collar after taking out the garbage. He now admits to smoking one pack of cigarettes a day for the last 25 years and that he has a history of mild hypertension that has been intermittently untreated. He adamantly denies any episodes of chest pain, orthopnea, PND, or lower extremity swelling. You are the senior resident in the ER and are initially called to see this patient.

QUESTION 1 Given this patient's history of smoking and hypertension, what differential diagnosis must be considered in your approach to this patient's complaints of dyspnea?

In a 64-year-old male the most common causes of shortness of breath are related to the cardio-pulmonary system. Symptoms that occur over 1 week require consideration of the causes of both acute and subacute dyspnea. The pulmonary causes of acute dyspnea include pulmonary embolism, pneumothorax, rapid accumulation of a large pleural effusion, chest trauma, and acute necrotizing pneumonia. Pulmonary diseases that may present subacutely with a 1-week prodrome include a decompensation of chronic obstructive

pulmonary disease and pneumonia. The former should be considered when a history of smoking, chronic bronchitis, or asthma is obtained. Both community-acquired typical and atypical (*Mycoplasma, Chlamydia,* Legionella and Q Fever) pneumonias should be included. The patient does not admit to any immunologic, occupational, or idiopathic lung diseases. These may be discarded from the differential diagnosis unless additional information becomes available.

Acute cardiac causes of dyspnea are restricted mostly to the events surrounding a myocardial infarction or acute arrhythmia unrelated to myocardial ischemia. These include severe pulmonary edema from massive left ventricular infarction, tachy- or brady-arrhythmias, free wall or septal rupture, acute pericardial effusion with tamponade, and acute valvular (aortic and mitral) insufficiency. Acute dysrythmias that produce profound hypotension usually lead to syncope/ presyncope. A 1-week history of fatiguability raises the possibility of decompensating ischemic congestive heart failure, especially in light of the patient's history of high blood pressure. Idiopathic cardiomyopathy (dilated, hypertrophic, or restrictive), myocarditis, congenital cardiac malformations, tachy- or brady- arrhythmias, constrictive and restrictive cardiomyopathies, or pericardial diseases may also present. Upon presentation to the ER, the patient was noted to be cyanotic, diaphoretic, and extremely dyspneic. On physical examination vital signs were: HR 118 bpm; RR 24/min; T 99.4°F; BP 138/99 mm Hg. Bilateral rales to the apices were present on lung examination. Pulse oximetry showed a saturation in the low 50s and the patient was immediately intubated. Cardiovascular examination showed a PMI displaced toward the anterior axillary line and a jugular venous pulsation of 7 cm at 30°. A Grade 3/6 systolic ejection murmur was heard at the base; no diastolic murmur was noted. Auscultation of the carotid arteries revealed bilaterally transmitted murmurs and palpation revealed diminished upstroke. The S2 was single and soft. The background coarse breath sounds complicated cardiac auscultation. There was no edema present peripherally, and distal pulses were 1 to 2+ bilateral and were symmetrical.

QUESTION 2 The initial physical examination is as above. What is your interpretation of the findings demonstrated by this examination?

The physical examination is classic for acute left-sided heart failure. This is supported by the findings of pulmonary congestion with attendant hypoxia and cyanosis. Although no S3 was auscultated, it may be difficult to hear over the background of coarse breath sounds and tachycardia. Tachycardia is a sign of activation of the sympathetic nervous system. This is activated in cases of heart failure because of activation of the carotid baroreceptors in instances of hypotension and the juxtaglomerular apparatus in the face of renal hypoperfusion. This triggers activation of the Renin-Angiotensin-Aldosterone axis leading to sodium retention and vasoconstriction. The skin becomes cool and clammy because of shunting of blood from skin capillaries to the central circulation.

The cardiac examination is consistent with aortic stenosis (Fig. 2-5-1). This is supported by the findings of a weak and delayed carotid upstroke (pulsus parvus-et-tardus), a systolic murmur transmitted from the base to the carotid arteries, and a displaced PMI. Aortic stenosis is evident particularly in light of the patient's reported history of rheumatic fever. The murmur of aortic stenosis can often be confused with that of aortic sclerosis, a common finding in the elderly population. One way to make this differentiation is that the murmur of aortic stenosis, which is best heard at the upper sternal margins, becomes more holosystolic as it radiates to the apex. This phenomenon is known as the *Gallavardin phenom-*

enon. The murmur of aortic sclerosis is shorter with an earlier peak and a normal A2, whereas the aortic stenosis murmur is prolonged, peaking later in systole, and is associated with a decreased A2 when secondary to calcific degeneration. These fine points of auscultation are often difficult to discern, and the quality of the carotid upstroke tends to be more important in the diagnosis of aortic stenosis and evaluation of the severity of the stenosis. This is particularly true in young patients. In older patients, the classic parvus-et-tardus pulse may not be appreciated because of stiffening of the carotid arteries. As the stenosis becomes more severe, the murmur becomes more high pitched and lasts longer, and the carotid pulsation becomes weaker and later. These elements often disappear when blood flow becomes severely restricted. The displaced PMI is consistent with left ventricular hypertrophy from a chronic high afterload situation.

In this patient the lack of an elevated jugular venous pulse or peripheral edema support the presumptive diagnosis of acute left-sided heart failure, aortic stenosis, and activation of the sympathetic nervous system with minimal right-sided cardiac decompensation at this point.

QUESTION 3 The electrocardiogram is completed very soon. This showed normal sinus rhythm, normal intervals, and a pattern consistent with left ventricular hypertrophy (LVH) with strain. The chest x-ray demonstrates an enlarged cardiac silhouette and pulmonary vascular redistribution with diffuse fluffy infiltrates. Laboratory evaluation was otherwise normal. What is your interpretation of this new information?

The ECG and chest x-ray are consistent with congestive heart failure. As cardiac decompensation occurs, the ventricular chambers dilate, left-sided filling pressure rises until this hydrostatic pressure overwhelms pulmonary capillary wall integrity leading to alveolar edema, diminished gas diffusion, stiffening of the pulmonary parenchyma, and hypoxia. In this patient it is likely, given our findings on physical examination, that this process is secondary to aortic stenosis. The diagnosis of aortic stenosis is supported on ECG by the findings of LVH with a strain pattern. The CXR also lends support to this diagnosis given the findings of alveolar infiltrates, cardiomegaly, kerleys lines (demonstrating lymphatic distension), and pleural effusions.

It is important to recognize the increased incidence of dysrhythmias in patients with aortic stenosis. This is of particular concern in a patient with aortic stenosis because systemic perfusion is very dependent on adequate filling pressures, and loss of the atrial kick, as seen in AF, may precipitate congestive heart failure. Ventricular tachyarrhythmias may also be associated with aortic stenosis. There was no evidence of atrial or ventricular dysrhythmias on the 12-lead ECg or the continuous cardiac monitor. Additionally, there was no evidence of acute ischemia, one of the other considerations in our initial differential. The lack of jugular distension, low voltage on ECG, a bottle-shaped cardiac silhouette, and the presence of rales on lung examination make the diagnosis of pericardial effusion unlikely.

QUESTION 4 The patient was admitted to the coronary care unit where he was diuresed approximately 4 liters and successfully weaned from the ventilator. Echocardiography showed global left ventricular hypokinesis and severe aortic stenosis with a valve area calculated at approximately 0.7 cm^2. What is your interpretation of the echocardiographic data? What are the concerns regarding volume management in this patient?

The findings of the echocardiogram are consistent with advanced aortic stenosis. The etiology of the aortic stenosis can often be told by the history and echocardiographic findings. The etiologies may be divided into four categories. Congenital noncalcific aortic stenosis usually presents in childhood. This entity requires intervention early in life. The second type of congenital abnormality is the bicuspid aortic valve. This is a fairly common abnormality occurring in 1.5% of the population, affecting males 3 to 4 times as often as females. This lesion is, however, asymptomatic until later life when the valve undergoes degeneration with

dystrophic calcification. Patients present between the ages of 45 and 75. A third category of aortic valvular abnormality is the postinflammatory type that includes rheumatic heart disease. This lesion involves fusion of the commissures and fibrocalcific thickening of the cusps and is twice as common in men as in women. Degenerative calcific stenosis of a normal tricuspid aortic valve is produced by deposition of calcium along the aortic aspect of each cusp impeding the normal excursion of the valve. In this type of aortic stenosis there is little involvement of the commissures, and men and women are affected equally. In recent decades the spectrum of aortic stenosis has changed with a decrease in the incidence of rheumatic fever and increase in life expectancy of the U.S. population. Whereas rheumatic heart disease had once been the most common cause of aortic stenosis, degenerative calcific aortic stenosis is now the most common cause in the U.S.

In a patient such as this, diuresis can be very complicated and is often performed with the aid of a pulmonary artery catheter. This allows for close monitoring of fluid status. Patients in whom the diagnosis of a fixed cardiac obstructive lesion is considered should be approached very carefully. Overly aggressive diuresis may reduce the preload to such an extent that ventricular filling pressure may be inadequate to maintain systemic perfusion. Accordingly, monitoring of central blood pressures by the use of a Swan-Ganz catheter is often warranted. This allows direct measurement of left ventricular pressures and cardiac output. Understanding of the patient's exact position on the Frank-Starling curve helps to match the optimal filling pressure to the best cardiac output. This physiology is present in patients with other fixed cardiac lesions including mitral stenosis, hypertrophic obstructive cardiomyopathy, restrictive or constrictive pericarditis, and proximal coarctation of the aorta. This patient's initial blood pressure was stable, and he tolerated diuresis well without a hypotensive episode.

QUESTION 5 Now that the diagnosis has been confirmed, what conclusions can you come to concerning the etiology of aortic stenosis in this patient, and what is the natural history of aortic stenosis?

Clues to the etiology of aortic stenosis can often be found by considering the patient's age at presentation. As stated earlier, congenital aortic stenosis presents in childhood, whereas rheumatic heart disease normally presents in the 50 to 70 age group. The chest x-ray may reveal the presence of valvular calcifications. Calcification of a congenital bicuspid aortic valve presents slightly later, and degenerative calcification of a normal tricuspid valve usually occurs after the eighth decade. In this patient it is likely that his history of rheumatic fever is the most likely etiology.

The natural history of aortic stenosis is a slow narrowing of the aortic outflow tract, with a progressive loss of valve area. Values decline in diameter at a rate of approximately 0.1 cm^2 per year. With slow narrowing and the development of a pressure gradient across the valve, the left ventricle slowly hypertrophies as a compensatory mechanism to preserve left ventricular systolic function. Eventually, the hypertrophied ventricle becomes inadequate in the face of a persistent outflow obstruction and systolic function diminishes. The finding of severe hypokinesis in this patient is quite worrisome. The transvalvular pressure gradient also drops as the ventricle fails. Attendant to the ventricular decompensation, pressure across the valve may be inadequate to open the calcified leaflets, and the stenosis becomes relatively worse despite a drop in the valve gradient. This rapid spiral can be particularly pronounced in patients with degenerative calcific aortic stenosis.

QUESTION 6 The patient and family have been apprised about the diagnosis. They are concerned about his prognosis. What is your response to their questions concerning the usual prognosis for aortic stenosis?

The most important factor in determining prognosis for patients with aortic stenosis is left ventricular function. Left ventricular function is generally preserved in asymptomatic patients and even in those patients whose symptoms include angina or syncope. Thornwald described the natural history of aortic stenosis as a spectrum of symptoms including angina, syncope, and heart failure. He noted that the mean survival after the onset of symptoms was 5 years for angina, 3 years for syncope, and 2 years for congestive heart failure. It is important to note that patients with aortic stenosis may have chest pain in the absence of significant coronary disease so that the diagnosis of angina should not be definitively made until the coronary anatomy is studied. Elderly patients with severe symptomatic degenerative calcific aortic stenosis have a mean survival time of only 15 months. A distinction must be made between those patients who are symptomatic and those who are asymptomatic. Asymptomatic patients, even with critically reduced valve area and an elevated transvalvular gradient, have survival times nearly identical to age-matched controls without aortic stenosis.

The incidence of sudden cardiac death is approximately 3% to 5% in patients with aortic stenosis. Asymptomatic patients rarely succumb to sudden death.

QUESTION 7 What is the next step in evaluating the patient's clinical status and to help stratify the severity of his disease?

The extent to which this patient's coronary artery disease contributed to this congestive heart failure is unclear, as no segmental wall motion abnormalities were noted. With the increasing sophistication of 2D and Doppler echocardiography, an accurate evaluation of the stenosis gradient and valve area can be made without need for cardiac catheterization. The primary role of cardiac catheterization in this setting is for the evaluation of the coronary arteries prior to valve replacement. Fifty percent of patients with significant aortic stenosis have concurrent coronary artery disease. Therefore, the next most important evaluation for this patient is coronary angiography. This procedure is employed to definitively define the coronary anatomy and determine whether symptoms of chest pain are related to the

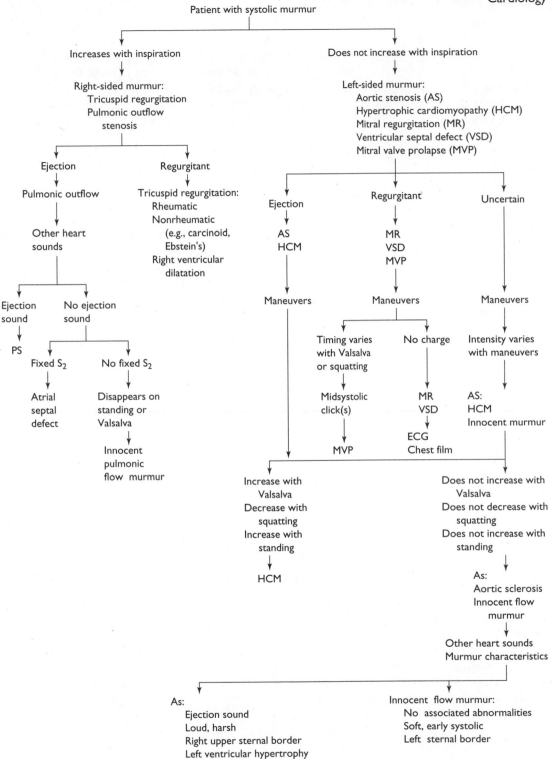

2-5-1 Diagnostic algorithm for aortic stenosis.
(From Greene HL, Johnson WP, Maricic MJ: *Decision making in medicine,* St Louis, 1993, Mosby.)

hypertrophied ventricle or to primary coronary insufficiency.

An additional consideration is the extent to which any ventricular dysfunction is due to an ischemic etiology. Even in the absence of significant coronary artery disease, patients can experience angina secondary to increased transmural pressures with decreased subendocardial blood flow and limited coronary filling at the source in the aorta. One must consider the possibility of hibernating myocardium that may regain function after restoration of adequate perfusion or stunned myocardium that may improve in the periinfarct period after revascularization. Either of these scenarios can yield some degree of improvement of ventricular function.

QUESTION 8 The patient underwent cardiac catheterization that confirmed the presence of severe aortic stenosis and global hypokinesis, but also revealed significant two vessel coronary disease involving the left anterior descending artery and the posterior descending artery. What is the impact of his findings on treatment?

As demonstrated by this case, medical therapy for heart failure, customized to the precise lesion present, is useful for the short-term treatment of congestive heart failure. However, medical therapy has no impact on long-term survival in patients with aortic stenosis. Aortic valve replacement is a curative measure that returns actuarial survival to that of age-matched and sex-matched controls. Surgical mortality in aortic valve replacement is approximately 5% to 8% and is slightly higher in those patients requiring bypass grafting as well as for patients over the age of 70. The decision to undergo valve replacement depends on the finding of "critical" aortic stenosis in a symptomatic patient. The definition of "critical" aortic stenosis is generally made when the aortic valve area is less than 0.75 mm^2. Patients are considered to have "moderate" aortic stenosis if the valve area is between 0.8 and 1.2 cm^2. These cutoffs are somewhat arbitrary and do not account for differences in body size.

As indexed valve area for body size may be more helpful. Values of less than 0.4 cm^2 per m^2 of body surface area may be more accurate in defining critical aortic stenosis. A grading scale of transvalvular pressure gradients is also used. A gradient of approximately 25 mm Hg would be considered mild stenosis, a gradient of 35 to 50 mm Hg is considered moderate, and a gradient above 60 to 70 mm Hg is considered severe. It is important to note that gradients depend upon left ventricular function and as the left ventricular function worsens, measurement of the valve gradient may underestimate the actual severity of the lesion.

Aortic balloon valvuloplasty has also been proposed for the treatment of aortic stenosis. This is accomplished by fracturing calcific bands on the aortic leaflets by insertion of a balloon-equipped catheter. This procedure has generally been reserved, though, for patients in whom perioperative risk is considered excessive. The mean valve area after valvuloplasty remains approximately 0.9 cm^2, and there is a 6-month re-stenosis rate of approximately 75%. Therefore, its uses are limited.

CASE SUMMARY The patient underwent successful aortic valve replacement and coronary artery bypass grafting. He was discharged home 6 days postoperatively and has done well for the last 6 months.

• •

BIBLIOGRAPHY

Bishop A, Wilkinson P: Problems in the diagnosis and investigation of aortic stenosis, *Postgrad Med J* 67:1039-1041, 1991.

Grayburn P: Hemodynamic assessment of aortic stenosis, *Am J Med Sci* 303:345-354, 1992.

O'Keefe TH, Nishimura RA, Lavie CJ, Edwards WD: Degenerative aortic stenosis, *Postgrad Med* 89:143-154, 1991.

Thibault GE: Too old for what? *N Engl J Med* 328:946-950, 1993.

Thibault GE, De Sanctis RW, Buckley MT: Aortic stenosis. In Eagle KA, Haber E, DeSanctis RW, Austen WG, eds: *The practice of cardiology*, ed 2, Boston, 1989, Little, Brown.

C A S E

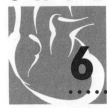

6

Paul Tamburro
John Barron

The patient is a 55-year-old white male with a past medical history remarkable for anterior wall myocardial infarction and coronary artery bypass graft surgery. A post-MI echocardiogram revealed an ejection fraction of 45%. He now presents complaining of progressive fatigue, 3 months in duration. He also notes a markedly diminished exercise capacity, becoming dyspneic upon walking one block. He had previously been walking 3 miles daily. In addition, he complains of vague abdominal symptoms including early satiety and dyspepsia.

Further questioning reveals only complaints of bilateral lower extremity edema that has increased in severity over the past 6 months. The patient denies any anginal symptoms, paroxysmal nocturnal dyspnea, orthopnea, or change in weight. He is compliant with his medical regimen. The remainder of his review of symptoms is unremarkable.

His medications included enteric coated aspirin 325 mg daily, Atenolol: 50 mg bid and Lovastatin: 20 mg bid. Additional past medical history included hyperlipidemia and Hodgkin disease 20 years before evaluation, treated with combined chemotherapy and irradiation. He had a cholecystectomy 20 years ago.

On physical examination the patient is a well-kept white male.

Height: 70 inches
Weight: 190 lbs
Vital signs: BP 144/90 mm Hg; HR 96 bpm; RR 20/min
HEENT: Normal
Neck: Jugular venous distension to the angle of the jaw, both x and y descents clearly visible

Respiratory: Dullness to percussion with diminished breath sounds in the right base
Cardiac: PMI is nondisplaced, S1 is normal, S2 is widely split, a third heart sound immediately following A2 is appreciated. A grade 2/6 systolic murmur is heard at the lower left sternal border and increases in intensity with respiration.
Abdomen: Normal bowel sounds are present. The liver is 14 cm in span, pulsatile, and mildly tender to palpation.
Extremities: 5 mm pitting edema is present in the lower extremities bilaterally extending to the mid thighs. A wellhealed scar is present on the left lower extremity.

QUESTION I What is the differential diagnosis at this point, and what additional features in the history and physical examination would be helpful in narrowing this list?

This patient with a history of myocardial infarction and cardiac surgery now presents with a constellation of findings suggesting systemic venous congestion. The differential diagnosis is expansive; however, the presentation contains several clues to help focus the clinician's further evaluation.

Right ventricular or biventricular dysfunction could account for the patient's symptoms. He had mildly impaired left ventricular function before surgery, with an ejection fraction of 45%. Cardiac function has not been evaluated postoperatively, and although anginal symptoms are denied, the possibility of silent ischemia or intraoperative myocardial damage cannot be excluded. The physical examination findings of peripheral edema and jugular venous distension are compatible with right ventricular failure. The third heart sound and possible pleural effusion noted on physical examination are also compatible with heart failure.

A tricuspid valvular lesion, either stenotic or regurgitant, must be considered in a patient with these systemic findings. The presence of a systolic murmur varying with respiration (Rivero-Carvello's sign) suggests the presence of tricuspid regurgitation. Signs of severe tricuspid regurgitation may include an S3 originating from the right ventricle and a hyperdynamic right ventricular impulse. Examination of the jugular veins typically reveals the absence of an x descent and the v wave and y descent are prominent. A venous systolic thrill or murmur may be auscultated over the jugular veins.

Cardiac tamponade can lead to a similar presentation as this patient's. Beck's triad of systemic hypotension, systemic venous distension, and a small quiet heart is typical of acute traumatic or hemorrhagic tamponade. In medical patients, however, tamponade is usually insidious in onset, and patients do not present in extremis, the most common complaint on presentation being progressive dyspnea. Jugular venous distension is the most common physical finding, and a characteristic waveform consisting of a prominent x descent and an attenuated or absent y descent may be noted. Tachypnea, tachycardia, and pulsus paradoxus are each noted in approximately 80% of cases. Constrictive pericarditis is caused by a thickened, fibrotic pericardium adhering to the myocardium and impairing diastolic filling. The disorder is associated with complaints of weakness, fatigue, and weight loss. Dyspnea is a common complaint as the disorder progresses and left heart filling pressures rise with associated pulmonary vascular congestion. Physical examination findings include jugular venous distension. The jugular venous waveform differs from that seen in pericardial tamponade in that a prominent y descent is present. An inspiratory decrease in venous pressure (Kussmaul's sign) is a classic finding of constrictive pericarditis, and a paradoxical pulse is observed in about one third of patients. The heart sounds may be distant, and a third heart sound, a pericardial knock, is often prominent, corresponding to a sudden deceleration in ventricular filling. Congestive hepatomegaly, splenomegaly, ascites, and peripheral edema are all common extracardiac findings associated with constrictive pericarditis.

Less common disorders that could account for the patient's symptomatology include restrictive cardiomyopathy, which is often difficult to distinguish from constrictive pericarditis. Vena caval obstruction is unlikely as venous congestion involving both the superior and inferior vena cavae is usually suggested by the physical examination. A right atrial myxoma could cause similar physical examination findings. Cor pulmonale can lead to this clinical syndrome; however, stigmata of advanced pulmonary parenchymal disease are not present in the history or physical examination of this patient.

QUESTION 2 The chest radiograph revealed a normal heart size, the presence of sternotomy wires, and a small right pleural effusion. The electrocardiogram is shown below. Do the findings on CXR and/or ECG aid in the diagnostic process (Fig. 2-6-1)?

The absence of cardiac chamber enlargement makes significant systolic dysfunction less likely. A large pericardial effusion may lead to an enlarged cardiac silhouette with a water bottle configuration, but the heart frequently appears normal in size. The cardiac silhouette may be normal, small, or enlarged with constrictive pericarditis. Calcification of the pericardium is seen in approximately half of patients with constrictive pericarditis, especially of tuberculous etiology.

The electrocardiogram is read as sinus rhythm, rate of 96, and normal axis. Nonspecific T wave abnormalities are present in the anterior precordial leads, and low QRS voltage is noted in the limb leads. No other abnormalities are noted. The differential diagnosis for low voltage includes

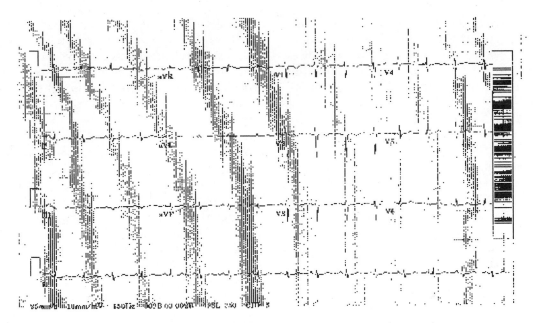

2-6-1 Initial electrocardiogram of patient with suspected pericarditis.

pericardial disease, both effusive and constrictive, infiltrative myocardial disease, pulmonary disease, hypothyroidism, and obesity. Of note, beat-to-beat variation in QRS voltage, termed electrical alternans, is absent. This finding is quite specific for cardiac tamponade in the presence of a concurrent pericardial effusion. Electrical alternans can also be seen with constrictive pericarditis, acute myocardial infarction, severe myocardial dysfunction, and tension pneumothorax.

This patient with a distant history of Hodgkin's disease, myocardial infarction, and coronary artery bypass surgery now presents with a constellation of findings consistent with systemic venous congestion. An extra heart sound and a small pleural effusion are also noted. The chest roentgenogram reveals a normal-size heart with pulmonary venous congestion and a small effusion, and the electrocardiogram is remarkable for low voltage. Likely diagnoses at this point include cardiac tamponade, constrictive pericarditis, and restrictive cardiomyopathy. Systolic ventricular dysfunction or significant tricuspid valvular disease are less likely based upon physical examina-

tion, roentgenographic and electrocardiographic findings.

QUESTION 3 What is the next logical step in evaluating this patient?

A transthoracic echocardiogram would be very useful in this situation. The absence of a significant pericardial effusion essentially rules out pericardial tamponade. If an effusion is present, echocardiography is useful in determining its hemodynamic significance. Echocardiographic evidence of right ventricular diastolic collapse and exaggerated respiratory variation in flow velocities seen with Doppler echocardiography suggest cardiac tamponade.

M-mode and two-dimensional echocardiography are also useful in the evaluation of constrictive pericarditis. The pericardium can appear thickened and dense, although echocardiography may overestimate pericardial thickness. Abrupt displacement of the interventricular septum (septal bounce), and dilatation of the inferior vena cava and hepatic veins have all been described in constrictive pericarditis. Doppler echocardiographic evaluation of hepatic venous and recently pulmonary venous respiratory flow variation have been found to be useful in discriminating constrictive pericardial disease from other disorders.

Finally, echocardiography provides invaluable information concerning ventricular and valvular function.

An echocardiogram is performed that reveals normal chamber sizes. The left ventricle has anterior wall hypokinesia, but normal global systolic function. Mild concentric left ventricular hypertrophy is present, and a prominent *a* wave is noted by Doppler interrogation of the left ventricular inflow tract, suggesting a diastolic filling abnormality. Mild tricuspid regurgitation is present. The pericardium appears thickened, but no significant pericardial effusion is noted.

The echocardiogram test effectively rules out pericardial tamponade as the etiology of this patient's symptoms. The examination confirms the presence of tricuspid regurgitation detected by auscultation, but mild regurgitation does not explain the patient's presentation. Left ventricular hypertrophy and a diastolic filling abnormality are consistent with restrictive cardiomyopathy; however, these are common findings in elderly patients. Pericardial thickening suggests the possibility of constrictive pericarditis but is also a nonspecific finding.

QUESTION 4 How can constrictive pericarditis be distinguished from restrictive cardiomyopathy?

Constrictive pericarditis is a disorder for which a surgical cure exists with pericardial resection; on the other hand, there is no definitive therapy available for restrictive cardiomyopathy. Therefore it is of paramount importance to distinguish between the two, and often a difficult clinical challenge.

Most authors recommend that left and right heart catheterization be performed in the evaluation of constrictive pericarditis (Fig. 2-6-2).

Typical findings of constrictive physiology include elevation and equalization of right- and left-sided end-diastolic pressures. A prominent early diastolic dip followed by a plateau (square root sign) is seen in the left and right ventricular hemodynamic tracings. The right atrial tracing typically demonstrates a preserved *x* and prominent *y* descent. The *a* and *v* waves are equal in size, giving the waveform an *M*- or *W*- shaped configuration.

A number of hemodynamic parameters have been proposed to discriminate constrictive from restrictive physiology. The three parameters commonly used suggesting constriction rather than restriction are: (1) Equalization of right ventricular and left ventricular end-diastolic pressure (<5 mm Hg), (2) ratio of right ventricular end-diastolic to systolic pressure of less than 1:3, and (3) right ventricular systolic pressure <50 mm Hg. The positive predictive value of all three criteria being positive is approximately 90%. If one or none of the criteria is positive, the negative predictive value is also approximately 90%. Unfortunately, the predictive value of two positive criteria is poor, and this includes one quarter of all patients.

Endomyocardial biopsy can also be performed at the time of cardiac catheterization. The procedure has a low associated morbidity and is useful in indeterminate cases.

Therefore, cardiac catheterization was performed with the following values obtained:
Right atrial pressure: 15 mm Hg
Right ventricular pressure: 42/18 mm Hg
Pulmonary artery pressure: 44/20 mm Hg
Pulmonary capillary wedge pressure: 20 mm Hg
Left ventricular pressure: 150/22 mm Hg
Cardiac output: 4.4 l/min

Based on echocardiographic evidence of pericardial thickening, with hemodynamic parameters suggesting constrictive physiology, the diagnosis of constrictive pericarditis was made.

QUESTION 5 What are the therapeutic options for constrictive pericarditis?

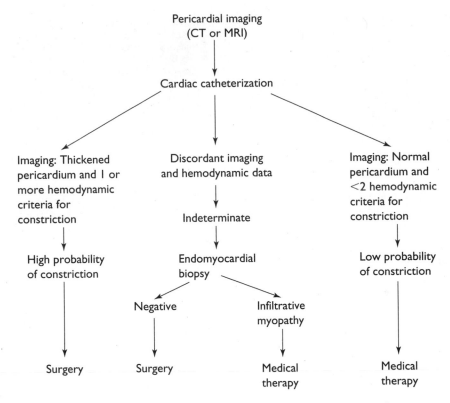

2-6-2 Diagnostic algorithm for evaluation of constriction or restriction.
(Reprinted from Vaitkus PT, Kussmaul WG: Constrictive pericarditis versus restrictive cardiomyopathy: a reappraisal and update of diagnostic criteria, *Am Heart J* 122:1431-1441, 1991.)

A minority of patients with constrictive pericarditis can be managed medically, diuretics and sodium restriction being the mainstay of therapy. However, most patients with clinically significant constriction require a surgical procedure; the definitive operation is a complete pericardial resection. The perioperative mortality is approximately 15%. Ninety percent of patients will experience improvement of symptoms, with complete resolution of symptoms occurring in half.

QUESTION 6 What were this patient's risk factors for developing constrictive pericarditis?

Constrictive pericarditis is most commonly idiopathic in nature, possibly developing after a clinically insignificant bout of viral pericarditis. Constrictive pericarditis following cardiac surgery is another common cause in developed nations, accounting for up to 39% of all cases in some series. Another common cause of constrictive pericarditis is mediastinal irradiation, with symptoms typically developing a decade or more after therapy. Tuberculous pericarditis, the most common cause of pericardial constriction a century ago, now accounts for approximately 15% of cases. Other less common etiologies include chronic renal failure and connective tissue disease. Neoplastic involvement of the pericardium by Hodgkin's disease, lung cancer, breast cancer, and other tumors can lead to constriction.

BIBLIOGRAPHY

Chandraratna PAN: Echocardiography and doppler ultrasound in the evaluation of pericardial disease, *Circulation* 84(suppl I):I-303-310, 1991.

Klein AL, Cohen GI, Pietrolungo JF, et al: Differentiation of constrictive pericarditis from restrictive cardiomyopathy by doppler transesophageal echocardiographic measurements of respiratory variations in pulmonary venous flow, *J Am Coll Cardiol* 22:1935-1943, 1993.

Lorell BH, Braunwald E: Pericardial disease. In Braunwald E, ed: *Heart disease*, Philadelphia, 1992, WB Saunders.

Vaitkus PT, Kussmaul WG: Constrictive pericarditis versus restrictive cardiomyopathy: a reappraisal and update of diagnostic criteria, *Am Heart J* 122:1431-1441, 1991.

Waller BF, Talierco CP, Howard J, et al: Morphologic aspects of pericardial heart disease: Part I, *Clin Cardiol* 15:203-209, 1992.

Waller BF, Talierco CP, Howard J, et al: Morphologic aspects of pericardial heart disease: Part II, *Clin Cardiol* 15:291-298, 1992.

Watkins MW, LeWinter MM: Physiologic role of the normal pericardium, *Annu Rev Med* 44:171-180, 1993.

C A S E

7

David Rabin
John Barron
· · · · · · · · · ·

A 55-year-old man presents to the emergency room with the chief complaint of approximately 8 hours of substernal chest pain that radiates to both of his arms. You are the emergency room physician on duty. The pain came on at rest and is associated with nausea, diaphoresis but not shortness of breath. He describes the pain as a burning, tight, occasionally scratchy sensation. The pain is not respirophasic, not positional in nature, and not reproducible by palpation. He denies any PND or orthopnea. He admits to a similar episode of discomfort occurring the previous night that resolved spontaneously. He denies any history of chest discomfort, exertional or otherwise before these two episodes.

Past medical history: Diet-controlled diabetes mellitus

Medications: None

Social history: Retired plumber, 45 pack-year cigarette smoker, occasional alcohol consumption

Family history: Negative for coronary disease

Cardiac risk factors: Male sex, age, cigarette smoking, diabetes

Physical exam: HR 80 bpm; BP 100/68 mm Hg; RR 20/min; T 99.5°F

Neck: No bruits, no evidence of increased JVP

Lungs: Clear

Heart: S1, S2 physiologically split, RRR, I-II/VI holosystolic apical murmur, no gallops or rubs, left ventricular impulse was 2+, non-displaced and non-sustained in the 5th intercostal space, mid-clavicular line.

Abdomen: Benign, no bruits

Extremities: Without cyanosis/clubbing/ edema, 2+ distal pulses, no bruits

ECG: As shown (Fig. 2-7-1)

Initial labs: CBC was normal, SMA: 20 was normal except for a glucose of 150

Initial CPK: 143 U/L with 28.8 ng/ml MB

QUESTION I   A 55-year-old man with several risk factors for CAD (male sex, age, cigarette smoking, diabetes) presents with a prolonged episode of fairly typical cardiac chest pain with the above ECG and initial laboratories. What is the differential diagnosis at this point?

First and foremost, on the differential, is an evolving Q wave anterolateral myocardial infarction (MI) with the ST segments elevated in leads V2-V6, I, and avL along with the loss of anterior forces (development of Q waves in the anterior leads). The ST segment depression in the inferior leads could either represent subendocardial ischemia in that myocardial distribution or "reciprocal changes." This diagnosis is further supported by the elevated MB of 28.8 ng/ml. The normal total CK should not mislead one as the elevated CKMB with a normal total CK can be found in approximately 15% of patients presenting with acute MI.

Another common cause of chest pain with elevated ST segments is pericarditis. However, the elevated ST segments in pericarditis tend to be more diffuse, concave in nature, and associated with PR depression. The clinical scenario and nature of the pain in this case is not consistent with pericarditis.

Unstable angina and subendocardial ischemia are also in the differential; however, they are

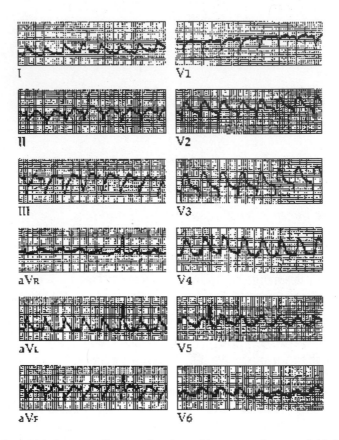

2-7-1 Initial electrocardiogram of patient with suspected myocardial infarction.

associated with ST segment depression and T wave inversion.

Other causes of chest pain such as pulmonary embolus, aortic dissection, peptic ulcer disease, esophageal spasm, musculoskeletal, etc., are not consistent with clinical presentation nor the laboratory data at this time.

QUESTION 2 What is the pathophysiology of AMI? (This topic has been covered to some extent in the Cardiology Case 1).

There are two major categories of MI: Q wave (also referred to as transmural) and non–Q wave (also referred to as subendocardial). The Q wave MI is usually an acute event, where a preexistent plaque ulcerates, ruptures, bleeds,

and a clot forms, with the subsequent occlusion of the coronary artery. This event frequently occurs in minimally to moderately diseased coronary arteries and usually involves a single artery's distribution. The non–Q wave MI usually occurs in the setting of moderate to severe preexisting single and multivessel CAD. If the period in which myocardial oxygen demand outstrips supply is prolonged greater than 30 minutes, the damage becomes irreversible and myocardial necrosis begins. Non–Q wave MI is also felt to occur in the setting of intermittent total coronary artery occlusion by thrombus that undergoes spontaneous lysis.

Many times patients suffering a non–Q wave MI have more severe underlying CAD than those suffering a Q wave MI. As the coronary arteries narrow, collateral circulation develops. This protects the myocardium supplied by the stenotic arteries if and when the latter become totally occluded. In the case of acute occlusion in the setting of the Q wave MI, there is no time for the development of adequate protective collateral circulation to support the area of myocardium supplied by the occluded artery. Therefore, a larger amount of myocardium is jeopardized.

Within 20 minutes of onset of ischemia, intracellular edema occurs. After 60 minutes, there is myocardial cell swelling and internal disruption of the myocytes. Over the subsequent hours the area of damaged myocardium becomes swollen and develops a neutrophilic infiltrate that ultimately extends through the entire infarct zone. Over the subsequent weeks to months the infarct zone thins as necrotic tissue is removed by monocytes. Eventually this region becomes an area of scar.

QUESTION 3 What would your initial management be at this point?

Initial management should be aimed at relief of pain while maintaining hemodynamic stability (Fig. 2-7-2). Ongoing pain reflects continued ischemia to viable myocardium; therefore, it is reasonable to assume that by relieving pain, one has reversed the ischemic process. Initial interventions short of reperfusion, with thrombolytics or mechanical revascularization (PTCA/CABG), include pharmacological maneuvers that decrease oxygen demand by decreasing preload/afterload, decreasing heart rate, lowering blood pressure, and decreasing sympathetic discharge (thus lowering the amount of circulating catecholamines).

The basics: oxygen, aspirin, nitroglycerin, analgesia and beta-blockers as discussed in Cardiology Case 1 should be routinely used. Nitroglycerin should be administered sublingually at first and then by IV if pain is not relieved. Topical and long-acting oral preparations should not be given in the unstable/acute setting as their time to onset of action is too long, and they are not titratable if hemodynamic instability ensues.

If, however, pain is not relieved and ST segments remain elevated in the setting of an evolving Q wave MI, then reperfusion therapy should be initiated either with thrombolysis or percutaneous transluminal coronary angioplasty (PTCA). If the patient is hemodynamically unstable and in cardiogenic shock (SBP <90, rales and an S3 on exam, cool and clammy), or contraindications to thrombolytic therapy exist, then the patient should be brought to the cardiac catheterization lab. The patient should be stabilized and angiography performed with the intent to do direct angioplasty. Thrombolytic therapy has not been shown to be of benefit in the setting of cardiogenic shock. If the patient is hemodynamically stable and has no contraindication for thrombolytic therapy, then the patient should be treated with thrombolytics.

QUESTION 4 Given the pathophysiology of the Q wave MI, why are thrombolytic agents effective? What are the contraindications/indications and proper time course for use of these agents?

As discussed previously, a Q wave MI is caused by the acute formation of an occlusive clot in a coronary artery. If the body's own fibrinolytic system could be activated and accelerated, by converting the proenzyme plasminogen to plasmin, the clot could be dissolved, reperfusion of the ischemic myocardium could be achieved, and the MI aborted. Agents currently in use include: *streptokinase* (SK), *anistreplase, anisoylated plasminogen streptokinase activator complex* (APSAC), *urokinase* and *tissue plasminogen activator* (TpA). The first three cause a general lytic state by extensively activating plasminogen to plasmin in the circulation. TpA has a binding site for fibrin and thus attaches preferentially to already formed thrombus and is therefore a "clot specific" thrombolytic.

There have been innumerable studies comparing the efficacies of all these agents. The question

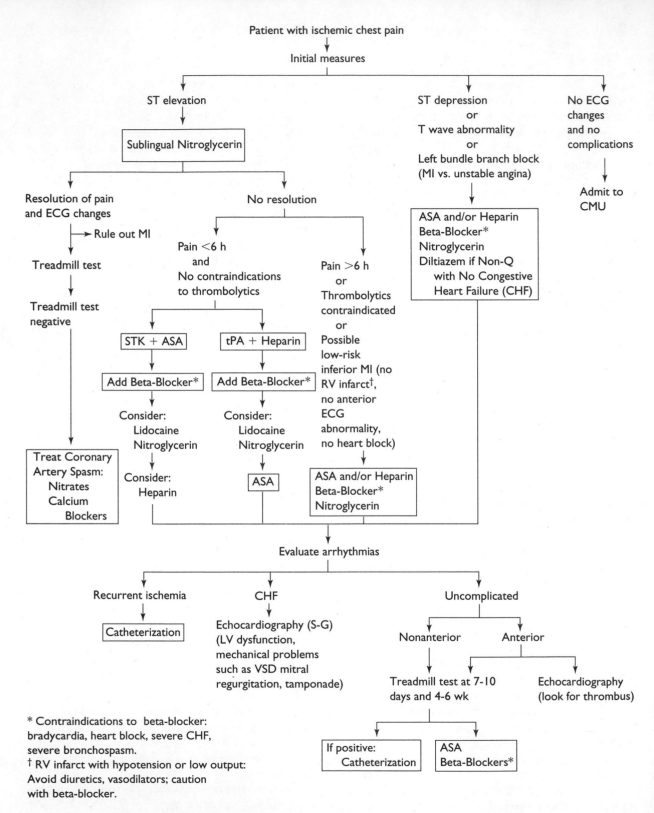

2-7-2 Diagnostic algorithm for ischemic chest pain.
(From Greene HL, Johnson WP, Maricic MJ: *Decision making in medicine*, St Louis, 1993, Mosby.)

of which agent to give is probably less important than the question of when and how to give it. These are the "guidelines" set out by the American Heart Association/American College of Cardiology regarding contraindications and indications for thrombolytic use:

Absolute contraindications
1. Active internal bleeding
2. Suspected aortic dissection
3. Prolonged or traumatic cardiopulmonary resuscitation
4. Recent head trauma or known intracranial neoplasm
5. Diabetic hemorrhagic retinopathy or other hemorrhagic ophthalmic condition
6. Pregnancy
7. Previous allergic reaction to the thrombolytic agent (SK, APSAC)
8. Recorded blood pressure >200/120 mm Hg
9. History of cerebrovascular accident known to be hemorrhagic

Relative contraindications
1. Recent trauma or surgery >2 weeks (trauma or surgery more recent than 2 weeks, which could be a source of rebleeding, is an absolute contraindication)
2. History of chronic severe hypertension with or without drug therapy
3. Active peptic ulcer disease
4. History of cerebrovascular accident
5. Known bleeding diathesis or current use of anticoagulants
6. Significant liver disease
7. Prior exposure to SK or APSAC (this contraindication is particularly important in the initial 6 to 9 month period after SK or APSAC use and applies to reuse of any SK containing agent but does not apply to TpA or urokinase)

Provided the patient does not have any of the above contraindications for the use of thrombolytics, the following are the Class I, II, and III indications for the use of thrombolytic agents. (Class I: usually indicated, always acceptable, considered usual and effective; Class II: acceptable, of uncertain efficacy, possibly controversial, IIa: weight of evidence in favor, IIb: not well established, can be helpful, probably not

harmful; Class III: not indicated, may be harmful.)

Class I
Patients <70 years old who present with chest pain consistent with the diagnosis of acute myocardial infarction and at least 0.1 mV (mm) of ST segment elevation in at least two contiguous ECG leads in whom treatment can be initiated within 6 hours of onset of pain.

Class IIa
1. Patients between 70 and 75 years of age who present with chest pain consistent with diagnosis of acute myocardial infarction and at least 0.1 mV (mm) of ST segment elevation in at least two contiguous ECG leads in whom treatment can be initiated within 6 hours of pain onset.
2. Patients with acute myocardial infarction >6 hours after symptom onset but with a "stuttering" pattern of pain.
3. Patients who suffer clinically apparent reinfarction in the days after the administration of thrombolytic therapy.

Class IIb
1. Patients who present with chest pain consistent with the diagnosis of acute myocardial infarction and at least 0.1 mV (mm) of ST segment elevation in at least two contiguous ECG leads in whom treatment can be initiated between 6 and 24 hours after pain onset.
2. Patients >75 years old who present with chest pain consistent with the diagnosis of acute myocardial infarction and at least 0.1 mV (mm) of ST segment elevation in at least two contiguous ECG leads in whom treatment can be initiated within 6 hours of pain onset where the impending infarct is extensive.
3. Patients who present with chest pain consistent with the diagnosis of acute myocardial infarction with ECG changes less profound than 0.1 mV of ST segment elevation in two contiguous leads who can be treated within 24 hours.

Class III
Patients who have chest pain when the following conditions are present:
1. Treatment cannot be initiated within 24 hours

of onset of chest pain, and pain has not recurred.
2. Chest pain is unknown and has receded.
3. The cause of the chest pain is unclear.

Our patient presents an interesting problem.
He presents with his pain approximately 8 hours
after its onset. The early *GISSI* trial showed a
nonsignificant reduction in mortality in patients
treated 6 to 9 hours after pain onset and actually
an increase in mortality in those who were treated
9 to 12 hours following onset of pain. *ISIS 2*,
however, showed a statistically significant benefit
in those treated 7 to 24 hours after pain onset, and
the recently completed *LATE* trial which looked
specifically at those treated >6 hours after onset of
pain found that there was a significant reduction
in 35-day mortality for those treated within 12
hours of onset of pain and for patients treated
even out to 24 hours after onset of pain.

QUESTION 5 If our patient had presented within
6 hours of pain onset, there would have been very
little debate about the benefit of thrombolytic
therapy. He is, however, 8 hours into his event.
How will lytic therapy benefit him?

Much attention has been paid to achieving a
patent infarct-related artery. Obviously, the earlier this is achieved, the better. The reduction in
mortality with early treatment (especially within
the first 1½ hours) is directly related to myocardial salvage. This makes sense when one considers
the pathophysiology of the evolving MI with
transmural necrosis becoming complete within
approximately 3 to 6 hours. Early reperfusion,
therefore, salvages myocardium that has not yet
become irreversibly damaged and thus limits infarct size and preserves left ventricular function.

In the case of those who present after 6 hours
from onset of pain, studies have not demonstrated
a significant improvement in left ventricular function with reperfusion therapy. The survival benefit in these patients is felt to be due to the effect
that a patent infarct-related artery has on the
other sequelae of transmural necrosis such as
reduced ventricular remodeling, infarct expan-

sion and aneurysm formation; improved healing;
reduced susceptibility to ventricular arrhythmias
and heart block; reduced incidence of thromboembolic complications, and finally that the patent
infarct-related artery serves as a source for collateral vessel formation.

QUESTION 6 What agents should be given as
"adjuvant" therapy with the thrombolytic?

There are a great many adjunctive agents to
thrombolytics, which can be divided into two
groups: those aimed at treating the infarct-related
artery (such as antiplatelet and antithrombin
agents as well as anticoagulants) and those directed at the myocardium (such as beta-blockers,
calcium channel blockers, angiotensin converting
enzyme inhibitors, etc.) The current recommendations for adjuvant therapy with thrombolytics,
based on the results of large-scale multicentered
trials, are as follows: Aspirin, chewable, at least
160 mg should be given immediately. ISIS-2
demonstrated the importance of aspirin in conjunction with streptokinase. Use of 160 mg of
aspirin accounted for a 23% reduction in the odds
of death; when used together, ASA/SK accounted
for a 42% odds reduction.

In addition, IV heparin should be used, especially with TpA to maintain vessel patency and
prevent reocclusion. Subcutaneous heparin
should not be used as the unreliable peaks and
troughs do not continuously affect the PTT. The
results from the *GUSTO* trial give some cogent
guidelines to the use of heparin. Heparin should
be given as a bolus (5000U IV were used in
GUSTO) followed by a constant infusion of
1000/hr with the dose adjusted to keep the PTT
between 60 and 80 seconds (or 1.5-2 times control). Adjunctive heparin was not associated with
any survival advantages with streptokinase, and
in fact there was a statistically significant excess in
hemorrhagic stroke in the heparin/SK groups
than in the heparin/TpA group. The lack of benefit
from heparin seen with SK may be due to the
more specific activity with TpA. Heparin, therefore, should not be used with streptokinase.

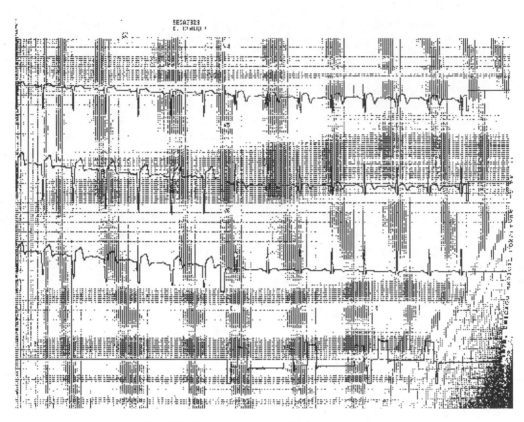

2-7-3 Electrocardiogram following treatment.

As far as acute therapy directed at the myocardium (reducing MVO2) in a Q wave MI, beta-blockers should be administered provided there are no contraindications such as bradycardia, hypotension, heart block, or bronchospastic disease. One can proceed with intravenous Lopressor at a dose of 5 mg × 3 doses 5 minutes apart until the desired heart rate or blood pressure effect. Calcium channel blockers have not been shown to be of benefit in Q wave MIs and therefore should not be used in the setting of a Q wave MI.

QUESTION 7 Our patient was given TpA along with aspirin, IV heparin, IV nitroglycerin, oxygen, and metoprolol. His pain resolved and his ST segments normalized. His serial CPKs (CpkMB) were as follows: 379 (483 ng/ml), 2350 (207 ng/ml), 1479 (253 ng/ml), 550 (143 ng/ml), and 260 (66 ng/ml). He has no arrhythmias (Fig. 2-7-3). Can we tell from this data that he has successfully reperfused with lytic therapy?

Thrombolytic therapy is highly effective for the treatment of Q wave MIs; however, reocclusion occurs approximately 25% of the time. The "gold standard" for assessing successful reperfusion is coronary angiography. However, given the inherent risks involved, along with the costs of the procedure, several "bedside" measures have been used to try to noninvasively assess reperfusion. These markers should optimally be available to the clinician within the first 90 minutes of reperfusion therapy. Arnold and Topol reviewed resolution of ST segment elevation; while highly predictive of angiographic reperfusion at 90 minutes, it actually only occurs in about 6% of patients.

Ventricular arrhythmias accompanying lytic therapy are frequently referred to as "reperfusion" arrhythmias. Although these arrhythmias seem to be linked to reperfusion in dogs, this finding has not been borne out in studies in humans. Many trials have looked at the question of reperfusion arrhythmias as a secondary question and therefore were not set up adequately to properly evaluate the question in a controlled setting. None of these studies found any consistent relationship between ventricular tachycardia or accelerated idioventricular rhythms and reperfusion. The TAMI trial is the largest trial to specifically address the utility of reperfusion arrhythmias and failed to find any significant resolution of ST segments to be highly predictive of reperfusion.

Early peaking of CK and CKMB known as "early washout" has not been shown to be predictive of the patency of the infarct-related artery. The rapid release of cardiac enzymes after reperfusion depends not only on reperfusion but the size of the area of necrosis, the time to reperfusion, and the degree of reperfusion. In addition, the delay in getting several sets of enzymes in order to establish the pattern of early washout is too long to be clinically useful in the decision regarding emergent catheterization.

In this patient's case, given the resolution of his pain and improvement of the ST segments, we can feel comfortable that he has reperfused. Alternatively, if the pain had continued with persistent ST segment elevation, then he would have needed cardiac catheterization with the intention to do rescue PTCA. Our patient continued to do well and was free of pain.

QUESTION 8 Our patient received a thrombolytic for treatment of his MI. What is the role of angioplasty (PTCA) for the acute MI?

Certainly, any patient with an evolving MI who has definite contraindications for throm-

bolytics should be considered for direct angioplasty. High-risk patients, those patients with associated higher mortality (>75 years old, persistent tachycardia) gain the most from direct PTCA. Those who present in cardiogenic shock have not been shown to benefit from thrombolytics and therefore should be considered for PTCA. What about those patients who would seem to benefit from either approach? Recently, three trials were published in the *New England Journal of Medicine* concerning this topic; two of them indicated that immediate PTCA had greater effectiveness in restoring vessel patency and preventing reocclusion. Patients treated with immediate PTCA were more likely to have a patent infarct-related artery and less likely to have a high grade residual stenosis several weeks after their infarct. In addition, those treated with immediate PTCA had lower incidence of recurrent ischemia, reinfarction, and death than those treated with thrombolytics.

It must be remembered, however, that these studies were done at centers that were well equipped to do emergent angioplasty. This involves having an interventional team experienced in emergent angioplasty as well as the ability to mobilize this team at a moment's notice. This involves not only the cardiologists but also nurses, technicians, and standby bypass surgery in case angioplasty is unsuccessful or associated with some complications. Approximately 18% of the hospitals in the U.S. are equipped to do angioplasty, even fewer can do it on an emergent basis. When a patient presents with an acute myocardial infarction, the most important goal is to achieve a patent infarct-related artery as soon as possible that will remain open. For the vast majority of patients, the therapy will remain intravenous thrombolytics.

This patient presented with an acute MI with a fairly typical story, clear ECG changes consistent with an evolving Q wave infarct, and with stable hemodynamics. Several other presentations of myocardial infarctions should be addressed as well.

QUESTION 9   Another patient presents to the ER with ongoing crushing substernal chest pain and profound shortness of breath. He has similar cardiac risk factors as the first patient. On physical examination his HR was 110 bpm, his BP was 85/60 mm Hg. His skin is cool and clammy; neck veins are not elevated, his lungs had crackles and wheezes throughout; there were dense crackles and dullness to percussion at the right base. The heart examination revealed a tachycardia S1 and S2, and an S3. He had no hepatosplenomegaly, hepatojugular reflux, ascites, or peripheral edema. His ECG showed marked anterior ST segment elevation. His chest x-ray shows pulmonary edema and a right-sided pleural effusion. How do you categorize this patient's clinical status?

This patient is in cardiogenic shock secondary to an acute Q wave myocardial infarction. He is tachycardic and hypotensive. His physical examination shows him to be in acute left heart failure. Pulmonary congestion is present as evidenced by a third heart sound indicating volume overload and the lung findings of crackles and right pleural effusion.

The major classifications of cardiogenic shock have been set out by Killip and Kimball. This classification system has four subsets, each with increasing mortality based on physical examination findings. Class I patients have no pulmonary congestion (as evidenced by auscultatory crackles) and no evidence of volume overload (as evidenced by lack of an S3); their mortality is 8%. Class II patients have either crackles or an S3 and a mortality of 30%. Class III patients have frank pulmonary edema with crackles >50% up the lung fields, and their mortality is 44%. Class IV patients are hypotensive with physical examination findings of "shock" (cool extremities, clammy skin, decreased urine production, mental status changes, etc.), and their mortality is 80% to 100%.

Autopsy studies have shown that cardiogenic shock occurs in the setting where there has been loss of function of approximately 40% of the left ventricular mass. This can occur in the setting of

one large myocardial infarction, a small infarct on a backdrop of previous ischemic cardiomyopathy, or an infarct in the setting of other metabolic derangements (DKA, sepsis, etc.). The goal in these patients is to relieve the ongoing ischemia, attain a patent infarct-related artery, and to reduce the work of the injured myocardium.

As stated earlier, thrombolytics have not been shown to be effective in the setting of cardiogenic shock. In the GISSI-1 trial, 25% of patients in Killip class II and 50% of Killip class III patients were dead at one year, despite thrombolytic therapy. The failure of thrombolytics to significantly affect mortality in the face of cardiogenic shock could be due to the more significant left ventricular dysfunction, lower perfusion rates, and other associated mechanical complications such as VSDs, acute mitral regurgitation or ventricular rupture.

The key is to quickly and accurately assess the patient's hemodynamic subset, and to tailor therapy appropriately. In order to do this, a right heart catheterization with a Swan-Ganz catheter should be done. This will help differentiate other causes of shock such as VSDs, tamponade, etc., as well as provide an accurate portrayal of the patient's hemodynamics and serve as a guide for subsequent therapies. The Swan-Ganz catheter provides hemodynamic verification of the Killip classifications. The hemodynamic subsets by Swan-Ganz measurements and their ultimate prognosis were set out by Forrester, et al. This was based primarily on pulmonary capillary wedge pressure (PCWP), by estimating the left ventricular end diastolic filling pressure, and cardiac index (CI), a measurement of pump function based on the cardiac output corrected for body surface area. Class I patients have normal hemodynamics (PCWP <18 mm Hg and CI >2.2) and have a mortality of 2%. Class II patients have evidence of pulmonary congestion but no evidence of peripheral hypoperfusion (PCWP >18 and CI >2.2). Their mortality is 10%. Class III patients do not have evidence of pulmonary congestion but do have peripheral hypoperfusion (PCWP <18 mm

Hg, CI <2.2). Their mortality is 22%. Class IV patients have both evidence for pulmonary congestion and peripheral hypoperfusion with PCWP >18 and CI <2.2, and their mortality is 56%.

Our patient is in Killip class IV by physical examination. A Swan-Ganz catheter is placed, and his PCWP is 22 mm Hg and the CI is 1.9, thereby making him a Forrester class IV as well. We are limited in our therapeutics as certain medications given to patients in congestive heart failure who are not in shock (i.e., lasix, morphine nitroglycerin), lower preload and dilate coronary arteries. These same medications are not tolerated in the setting of shock because of the limitations of hypotension. This requires improved forward blood flow in order to relieve pulmonary congestion and strain on the left ventricle. At the same time, patency in the distribution of the infarct-related artery is essential.

QUESTION 10 What pharmacological and mechanical interventions are useful in the treatment of patients in cardiogenic shock?

Medications are available to provide hemodynamic support such as dobutamine and dopamine. Dobutamine is predominantly a positive inotrope (beta-agonist) and exerts its beneficial effects primarily by increasing myocardial contractility as opposed to increasing heart rate. It also acts as a peripheral vasodilator and reduces total systemic vascular resistance (SVR) and, thus, afterload. The drawbacks here include potential exacerbation of existing hypotension by dropping the SVR and increasing the myocardial oxygen demand in the face of ongoing ischemia by increasing contractility.

Dopamine is an agent which, when used at low doses (1 to 5 µg/kg/min), acts as a dilator of mesenteric vasculature, improving renal blood flow and urine output. Because of this effect it acts as a sympatholytic agent. At higher doses (5 to 10 µg/kg/min) dopamine acts more as a chronotrope and increases heart rate (beta-agonist) and at still higher doses, (10 µg/kg/min) acts as a vasoconstrictor (alpha-agonist). In the face of ongoing ischemia, these higher doses have obvious deleterious effects on myocardial oxygen demand. A third commonly used medication is norepinephrine that acts mainly as a peripheral agent as well. All these medications have a role in the treatment of cardiogenic shock; however, in the setting of acute ischemia, all can easily exacerbate an already dire situation.

In this situation, an intraaortic balloon pump (IABP) may be indicated. This device is inserted percutaneously via the femoral artery in the aorta just distal to the arch. It is set to inflate during diastole and deflate during systole (timed off the patient's ECG). By inflating during diastole, the pump "augments" diastolic blood pressure, thus increasing the perfusion pressure to the coronary arteries, thereby increasing flow across stenotic coronary arteries and increasing perfusion to ischemic myocardium. By deflating during systole, the balloon pump has effectively lowered afterload and thus decreased the resistance the heart pumps against. This decreases myocardial oxygen consumption.

Newer devices are presently being employed called ventricular assist devices that totally take over the work of the ischemic left ventricle during the infarct period. These devices are merely bridges to definitive therapy and not a therapy in and of themselves. Studies have shown that patients who are treated with IABP alone without concomitant revascularized (either by PTCA or CABG) have a mortality as high as 80%, while those patients who are bypassed within a day or receive thrombolytics have mortality figures ranging from 25% to 55%.

Therefore, in this patient's case, quick assessment of the hemodynamic profile with a Swan-Ganz catheter, subsequent placement of an IABP, and appropriate pharmacologic agents as temporizing measures would be the initial management. While stabilizing this patient, arrangements should be made to bring the patient to the cardiac catheterization lab for catheterization and direct PTCA of the infarct-related artery or potential CABG if the coronary anatomy dictates such (i.e., left main or severe three vessel disease). Once successful reperfusion has been achieved, the patient should remain on IABP support to continue afterload reduction and augmentation of diastolic blood flow for several days or as his hemodynamics dictate.

QUESTION 11 A third patient now presents to the ER and initially tells you that he feels as if he is having a heart attack. He complains of waxing and waning chest pain of several hours duration, occurring at rest, relieved with sublingual nitroglycerin. The pain radiates to the neck, jaw, and down his arm, and is accompanied by diaphoresis. It is not associated with shortness of breath, nausea, or vomiting. He is currently complaining of pain as he arrives in the emergency room. His vitals are HR 100 bpm, BP 160/100 mm Hg, RR 20/min. His physical examination is remarkable only for an S4. His ECG shows a sinus tachycardia with 1 to 2 mm ST segment depression, with T wave inversion in V4-V6, I, and avL. His initial labs are normal except for a CK of 350 and an CKMB of 100. What is your diagnosis; what are your initial management strategies? Do thrombolytics play a role here?

The patient is in the midst of a non–Q wave MI. These used to be referred to as nontransmural MIs; however, it has been shown that the appearance of Q waves on the ECG is not a sensitive predictor of transmural cardiac ischemia. Studies have shown that although patients suffering non–Q wave MIs have lower in-hospital mortality, they have a much higher rate of reinfarction than patients with Q wave MIs. As discussed earlier in the pathophysiology of the acute MI, this has much to do with the underlying coronary anatomy of the patient. In the case of the non–Q wave MI, there is likely more extensive underlying coronary disease, with collateralization of the infarct-related artery. Instead of an acute thrombus formation on minimal underlying plaque, there is more than likely platelet rich thrombus forming on already severely narrowed coronary arteries, or clot forma-

tion with spontaneous lysis occurring on severe underlying lesions. It is evident then, that the non–Q wave MI represents a heterogeneous group of patients.

Initial management should be along the lines of unstable angina patients. Oxygen should be given and IV nitroglycerin administered to lower the double product (HR × BP). Calcium channel or beta blockade is indicated initially. In fact, the non–Q wave MI with preserved ventricular function is the only acute ischemic situation where calcium channel blockers are indicated. Diltiazem has been shown to be effective in preventing recurrent infarction in the setting of a non–Q wave MI. Antiplatelet therapy with aspirin is essential along with anticoagulation with heparin in the early stages or a non–Q wave MI has also been shown to be effective in reducing recurrent ischemia.

Given the heterogeneity of this population, thrombolytics have not been shown to be effective. There was no significant reduction in mortality in patients with ST depression in the GISSI trial and in the recent LATE trial; those patients who had their treatment with thrombolytics delayed were, in a large part, those with equivocal ECGs and non–Q wave MIs and in fact suffered a 15.3% increase in 35-day mortality.

Serious consideration should be given to bringing this patient to the cardiac catheterization lab for further assessment of his coronary anatomy with subsequent PTCA or CABG.

QUESTION 12 Another patient with a similar background as our first gentleman presents to the emergency room with complaints identical to the original case: prolonged substernal chest pain, radiating to his neck, jaw, and down his arms. He has associated nausea and vomiting with diaphoresis though no shortness of breath. The discomfort has been going on for about 2 hours. His physical examination is notable for a heart rate of 50 to 60 bpm and a blood pressure of 110/70 mm Hg. His neck shows JVP at 6 cm above the sternal angle at 45° indicating a CVP of 11 cm of H_2O. His lungs are clear and his heart examination reveals a regular S1,

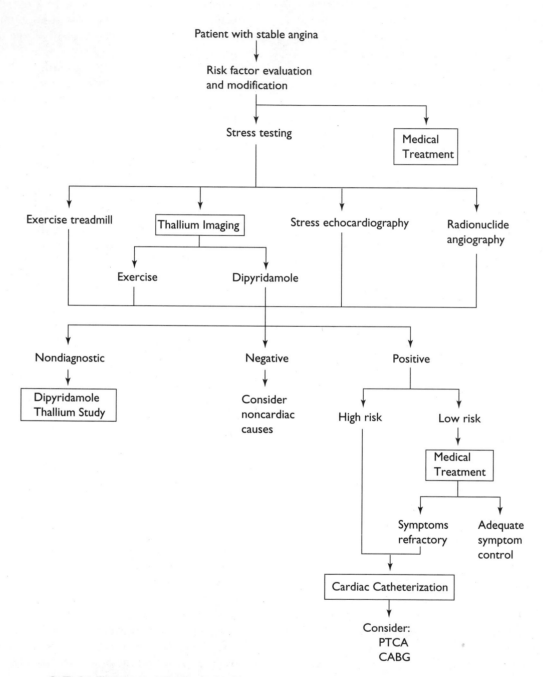

2-7-4 Diagnostic algorithm for stable angina.
(From Greene HL, Johnson WP, Maricic MJ: *Decision making in medicine,* St Louis, 1993, Mosby.)

physiological split S2, and absence of murmurs, gallops, or rubs. He has a large tender liver that is pulsatile and palpable several finger breadths below the costal angle. His extremities show trace pitting edema. His cardiac risk factors include cigarette smoking, male sex, and newly diagnosed diabetes. His initial ECG shows normal sinus rhythm with 2 to 3 mm of ST elevation in leads II, III, aVf along with an R wave in VI, and evidence of early R wave transition. There is ST segment depression V2-V6, I, and aVL. What is your diagnosis? What should your next diagnostic step be?

Our patient is suffering from an apparent acute inferior MI (IMI). The most important thing to determine at this point is the extent of the infarct (e.g., does it involve the right ventricle?). A second ECG with right-sided lead placement is essential when evaluating a patient with an IMI. A recent prospective study in 200 consecutive patients presenting with IMI found that ST segment elevation in V4R was present in over 50% of these patients and was highly predictive of right ventricular involvement. ST segment elevation in V4R indicates that the right coronary artery (RCA) is occluded proximally and that the right ventricle is involved. Lack of ST segment elevation in this distribution indicates that the occlusion is more distal or perhaps involves the circumflex artery. Those patients with ST segment elevation in V4R had a higher in-hospital mortality rate (31% vs 6%) and higher rates of in-hospital complications (64% vs 28%) than those patients without this electrocardiographic finding.

QUESTION 13 An ECG with right-sided leads was performed and demonstrated 2 to 3 mm of ST segment elevation in V4r-V6r. What are your management concerns and therapeutic options?

The strategy of treating the IMI with right ventricular infarct is different than treating an infarct involving the left ventricle. The ischemic right ventricle is particularly sensitive to changes in preload, such as administration of diuretics, and nitrates impair the filling of the noncompliant ischemic right ventricle and thus can precipitate profound hypotension and shock. In addition, since the AV nodal artery, a branch of the right coronary artery (RCA), is most often the major artery involved in IMIs and RV infarcts, high degree AV block is a common complication of these infarcts, and the administration of beta-blockers may exacerbate this problem.

Basic therapeutics, therefore, involve (1) maintenance of adequate right ventricular filling pressures through volume loading with normal saline and (2) the avoidance of agents which lower RV filling pressures such as nitrates, diuretics, and morphine. A Swan-Ganz catheter can be very helpful in guiding therapy. In the case of high-grade AV block, atrial or AV sequential pacing may be necessary if initial steps such as atropine are not successful. Inotropic support with dobutamine and afterload reduction with vasodilators (sodium nitroprusside) or IABP may be necessary. Reperfusion with thrombolytics or PTCA (if the patients are not candidates for thrombolytics) should be attempted given the high degree of in-hospital complications and high in-hospital mortality associated with IMIs with right ventricular involvement. A diagnostic algorithm for angina is shown in Fig. 2-7-4.

BIBLIOGRAPHY

Arnold AZ, Topol EJ: Assessment of reperfusion after thrombolytic therapy for acute myocardial infarction, *Am Heart J* 124:441-447, 1993.
Bosker HA, et al: Are enzymatic tests good indicators of coronary reperfusion? *Br Heart J* 67:150-154, 1992.
Cairns JA: Reperfusion therapy, *Chest* 11:142S-149S, 1991
Fuster V: Coronary thrombolysis: a perspective for the practicing physician *N Engl J Med* 329:23-725, 1993.
Gruppo Italiano per studio della streptochinasi nell' Ingarto Myocardico (GISSI): Effectiveness of intravenous thrombolytic treatment in acute myocardial infarction, *Lancet* i:39-401, 1986.
Guidelines for the Early Management of Patients with Acute Myocardial Infarction, August, 1990: A Report of the American College of Cardiology/American Heart Association Task Force on Assessment of Diagnostic and Therapeutic Cardiovascular Procedures (Subcommittee to Develop Guidelines for the Early Management of Patients

with Acute Myocardial Infarction), *Circulation* 663-707, 1990.

GUSTO Investigators. An International Randomized Trial comparing four thrombolytic strategies for acute myocardial infarction, *N Engl J Med* 329:673-682, 1993.

Hillis LD, et al: Risk stratification before thrombolytic therapy in patients with acute myocardial infarction, *J Am Coll Cardiol* 16:313-315, 1990.

ISIS-2 Collaborative Group: Randomized trial of intravenous streptokinase, oral aspirin, both or neither among 17,187 cases of suspected acute myocardial infarction: ISIS-2, *Lancet* i:397-402, 1986.

Kessler C: The pharmacology of aspirin, heparin coumarin, and thrombolytic agents: implications for therapeutic use in cardiopulmonary disease, *Chest* 99:97S-112S, 1991.

LATE Study Group: Late assessment of thrombolytic efficacy (LATE) with alteplase 6-24 hours after onset of acute myocardial infarction, *Lancet* 342:759-766, 1993.

Muller DW, Topol EJ: Selection of patients with acute myocardial infarction for thrombolytic therapy, *Ann Intern Med* 113:949-960, 1990.

Pasternak RC, et al: Acute myocardial infarction. In Brauwald E, ed: *Heart disease: a textbook of cardiovascular medicine*, ed 4, Philadelphia, 1992, WB Saunders.

Popma JJ, Topol EJ: Adjuncts to thrombolysis for myocardial reperfusion, *Ann Intern Med* 115:34-44, 1991.

Rapaport E: Thrombolytic therapy in acute myocardial infarction, *N Engl J Med* 320:861-864, 1989.

Rubinstein E, Federman D: *Scientific American Medicine*, p 144, New York, 1993, Scientific American, Inc.

Shah P: The role of thrombolytic therapy in patients with acute myocardial infarction presenting later than six hours after the onset of symptoms, *Am J Cardiol* 68:72C-77C, 1991.

Togoni G, et al: Thrombolysis in myocardial infarction, *Chest* 99:121S-127S, 1991.

CASE

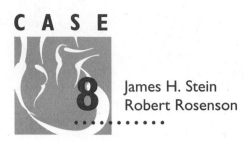

8

James H. Stein
Robert Rosenson
. . . .

A 46-year-old perimenopausal white female with hyperlipidemia presents to your cardiology clinic. Four years before presentation her total cholesterol (TC) was greater than 500 mg/dl, her serum triglycerides (TG) were approximately 300 mg/dl, and her HDL cholesterol was less than 35 mg/dl. She was treated with a National Cholesterol Education Program Step II diet and increasing doses of cholestyramine and lovastatin. After 2 years of unsuccessful lipid reduction, she was referred to a preventive cardiology clinic for further management.

At the time of referral, this patient's medications were lovastatin (40 mg bid), cholestyramine (4g bid), and levothyroxine (0.05 mg qd). She denied chest pain, shortness of breath, or symptoms of congestive heart failure. She denied claudication or transient ischemic attacks. She reported difficulty falling asleep with frequent early morning awakening. She denied myalgias, abdominal pain, constipation, or abdominal bloating.

Her past medical history did not include myocardial infarction, angina pectoris, cerebrovascular disease, peripheral vascular disease, diabetes mellitus, hypertension, liver disease, or gout. She was receiving treatment for hypothyroidism, which was discovered after a goiter was palpated 4 years previously. She denied symptoms of hypothyroidism. Her father had myocardial infarctions at ages 55 and 70 years old. Five of twelve paternal siblings had myocardial infarctions at early ages. She had a 24-year-old son with a TC level over 265 mg/dl and two first cousins with TC levels of approximately 350 mg/dl. Both first cousins had hypothyroidism. She smoked one pack of cigarettes daily and did not consume alcohol. She adhered to a low-fat, low-cholesterol diet; however, she did not exercise.

QUESTION 1 What are the important epidemiologic concepts concerning hyperlipidemia and vascular disease? What risk factors for ASVD are present in this patient?

Atherosclerotic vascular disease (ASVD) is a multifactoral process that begins in childhood and progresses throughout adulthood, when it manifests as coronary heart disease (CHD), cerebrovascular disease, and peripheral vascular disease. The lipid hypothesis of atherosclerosis maintains that hypercholesterolemia leads to endothelial "injury," which initiates a cellular cascade of events that eventually lead to atherosclerotic plaque. Epidemiologic studies consistently demonstrate a direct association between levels of serum cholesterol and the rate of CHD. In the Multiple Risk Factor Intervention Trial, the relationship between the age-adjusted CHD death rate and the serum cholesterol level was graded and continuous. A relative risk of 3.4 was demonstrated for patients with a serum cholesterol level ≥245 mg/dl. Of all CHD deaths, 46% were deaths attributable to serum cholesterol ≥180 mg/dl. Population studies have also demonstrated that lipoprotein abnormalities are present in up to 87.5% of patients with angiographic evidence of coronary artery disease prior to the age of 60 years.

This case illustrates the importance of understanding lipid metabolism and the value of the history and physical examination in determining the correct diagnosis and appropriate treatment for a patient with abnormal lipid levels. In addi-

- -

RISK FACTORS FOR CHD*

NONMODIFIABLE
AGE (MEN: ≥45 YEARS, WOMEN: ≥55
YEARS OR PREMATURE MENOPAUSE
WITHOUT ERT)
FAMILY HISTORY OF PREMATURE CHD
DEFINITE MYOCARDIAL INFARCTION OR
     SUDDEN DEATH BEFORE AGE 55 YEARS
     (MALE) OR AGE 65 YEARS (FEMALE) IN A
     FIRST-DEGREE RELATIVE
MODIFIABLE
CURRENT TOBACCO USE
HYPERTENSION (BP ≥140/90 MM HG OR
     USING ANTIHYPERTENSIVE
     MEDICATIONS)
DIABETES MELLITUS
HIGH LDL CHOLESTEROL (DISCUSSED
     WITHIN)
LOW HDL CHOLESTEROL (≤35 MG/DL)
IF THE HDL CHOLESTEROL LEVEL IS
     ≥60 MG/DL, SUBTRACT ONE RISK
     FACTOR

- -

(Adapted from National cholesterol education program second report of the expert panel on detection, evaluation, and treatment of high blood cholesterol in adults [adult treatment panel II], Circulation 89:1329-1445, 1994.)
*This patient's risk factors are in **bold**.

tion, this case demonstrates that all lipid-lowering drugs are not equal, even within the same pharmacologic class.

Clinically, the risk factors for ASVD are separated into those that are modifiable and nonmodifiable (see box). History, physical examination, and laboratory studies are used to characterize the CHD risk factors. The patient had four CHD risk factors—family history of premature CHD, current cigarette smoking, elevated LDL cholesterol, and low HDL cholesterol. Obesity, defined as a body mass index (weight in kg divided by height in meters squared) greater than 27 is not included as an independent risk factor because it operates through other accepted risk factors. Elevated triglycerides are also associated

with increased risk for CHD; however, the independent relationship between triglycerides and CHD remains unclear. Increased triglyceride levels were associated with low levels of HDL cholesterol and more atherogenic forms of VLDL and LDL.

QUESTION 2   Describe the key components of lipoprotein metabolism.

Effective diagnosis and treatment of patients with dyslipidemia require familiarity with the characteristics of the plasma lipoproteins and the pathways for cholesterol and triglyceride transport. Lipoproteins are heterogeneous particles composed of a lipid core of nonpolar cholesterol esters and triglycerides, surrounded by a polar shell of proteins, phospholipids, and unesterified cholesterol. The protein components of the lipoprotein particle are known as apoproteins. They serve as cofactors for enzymes and/or ligands for receptors. The lipoprotein particle transfers lipids to tissues where they can be used for steroid hormone production and bile acid formation or stored as energy sources.

Lipoprotein metabolism involves two major pathways (Fig. 2-8-1). In the exogenous pathway, dietary cholesterol and bile acids are absorbed by the intestine. In the intestinal cells, free cholesterol is esterified and free fatty acids are combined with glycerol to form triglycerides. These nonpolar lipids are then combined with apoproteins A-I, B-48, C-II, and E to form chylomicrons. Chylomicrons enter the bloodstream, where lipoprotein lipase hydrolizes the core triglycerides and free fatty acids are released. These free fatty acids can be used for energy, stored in adipose tissue, or converted to triglycerides. Chylomicron remnants are rapidly cleared by the liver through binding of their apo E components.

The endogenous pathway begins with hepatic synthesis and secretion of very-low-density lipoproteins (VLDLs), which are primarily composed of a triglyceride core and surface apoproteins B-100, C-II, and E. Apoproteins B-100 and E are ligands that interact with the LDL (or apo B/E)

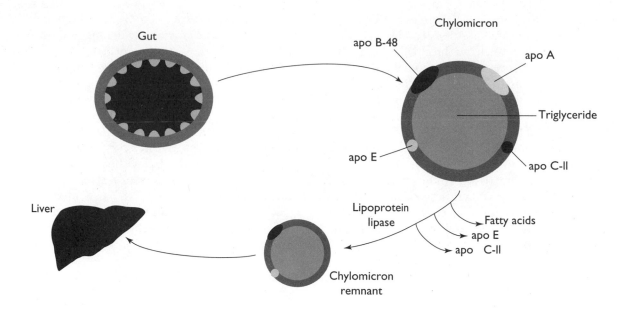

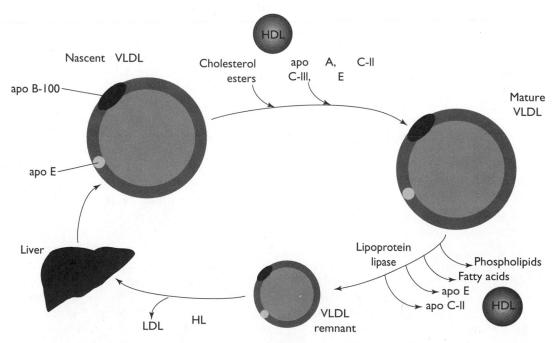

2-8-1 Lipoprotein metabolism. Upper panel: exogenous pathway, Lower panel: endogenous pathway

receptor. Circulating VLDL particles are hydrolyzed by lipoprotein lipase to release free fatty acids and intermediate-density lipoproteins (IDL). IDLs are cleared from the circulation by the liver via the LDL receptor or are converted by the liver into low-density lipoproteins (LDLs).

The LDL core is primarily cholesterol ester with a small amount of triglyceride. Apo B-100 is the only LDL apoprotein. Circulating LDL can be internalized by hepatocytes via the LDL receptor and converted into bile acids, or it can be internalized by peripheral tissues for hormone production, or cell membrane synthesis. LDL uptake is tightly regulated by cellular cholesterol requirements and negative feedback regulation of LDL receptor expression.

High-density lipoproteins (HDLs) are comprised of a lipid core that is predominantly phospholipid and cholesterol, and external apoproteins A-I, A-II, C-II, and E. HDLs are directly synthesized by the liver and intestines. They are also formed by procurement of surface components from the peripheral catabolism of chylomicrons and VLDL. When cell membranes turn over or cells die, unesterified cholesterol is released into the plasma where it is sequestered by HDL and is esterified with a fatty acid on the surface of the HDL particle. HDL particles maintain cholesterol balance and are the main effectors of cholesterol transport out of cells.

QUESTION 3   How are the dyslipidemias defined and classified? Based on the patient's pertinent medical history, what *primary* dyslipidemias should be included in the differential diagnosis of her disorder?

The laboratory diagnosis of dyslipidemia requires the demonstration of LDL cholesterol or triglyceride levels greater than the 90th percentile values, or HDL cholesterol levels lower than the 10th percentile values by age and sex The Fredrickson phenotypic classification of dyslipidemias is presented in Table 2-8-1.

Effective diagnosis and treatment of patients with dyslipidemias require familiarity with the

pathophysiology and classification of lipid disorders. Dyslipidemias can be primary (genetic) or secondary to other metabolic derangements.

Familial hypercholesterolemia (FH) is an autosomal dominant disorder caused by a mutation in the gene for the LDL receptor. Patients with FH typically have elevated total cholesterol (Fredrickson phenotype IIa), tendon xanthomata, and a family history of premature CHD. Homozygous FH has a phenotypic frequency of 1 in 1,000,000 and is associated with CHD within the first decade of life. Levels of total cholesterol typically exceed 500 mg/dl. Heterozygous FH has a phenotypic frequency of 1 in 500 and is frequently encountered in clinical practice. These patients have an increased risk of CHD beginning in their third decade of life. Heterozygous FH is found in 5% of males less than 60 years old with myocardial infarction.

Familial combined hyperlipidemia (FCH) is the most common dyslipidemia in the United States and is present in 1 in 100 patients. FCH is an autosomal dominant disorder caused by hepatic overproduction of apo B-100 containing particles. There is a preponderance of small, dense LDL subspecies that are highly atherogenic. FCH can be manifested as Fredrickson phenotypes IIa, IIb, or IV, because one-third of patients with FCH have an associated impairment in lipoprotein lipase.

Polygenic hypercholesterolemia is the most common cause of an isolated elevation in LDL cholesterol (phenotype IIa). The genetics are poorly understood but probably result from multiple abnormalities in LDL metabolism.

Familial hypertriglyceridemia is an autosomal dominant disorder manifested by moderate triglyceride elevation (less than 500 mg/dl). Patients manifest Fredrickson phenotype IV. This condition is often accompanied by obesity, hyperglycemia, insulin resistance, hypertension, and hyperuricemia. It is present in 5% of patients with CHD.

Familial multiple lipoprotein hyperlipidemia is an uncommon dyslipidemia that results from overproduction and reduced clearance of VLDL and

TABLE 2-8-1   **Classification Scheme for Common Lipid Disorders**

Lipoprotein	Fredrickson Phenotype	Dyslipidemia	Secondary Causes of Dyslipidemia
Chylomicrons	I	Lipoprotein lipase deficiency Apo CII deficiency	Diabetes mellitus
LDL	IIa	Familial hypercholesterolemia Polygenic hypercholesterolemia Familial combined hyperlipidemia	Nephrotic syndrome Hypothyroidism Cushing's syndrome Cholestatic liver Diseases
LDL and VLDL	IIb	Familial combined hyperlipidemia	Nephrotic syndrome Hypothyroidism Cushing's syndrome Glucocorticoid use
Remnants of VLDL and chylomicrons	III	Familial dysbetalipoproteinemia	Diabetes mellitus Hypothyroidism
VLDL	IV	Familial hypertriglyceridemia Familial combined hyperlipidemia	Diabetes mellitus Chronic renal failure Nephrotic syndrome Hypothyroidism Estrogen use Glucocorticoid use
Chylomicrons and VLDL	V	Familial hypertriglyceridemia Familial multiple lipoprotein hyperlipidemia	Diabetes mellitus Estrogen Nephrotic syndrome
HDL	Unclassified	Familial hypoalphalipoproteinemia	Cigarette smoking Obesity Physical inactivity Beta-blocker use Probucol use

chylomicrons. Multiple lipoprotein abnormalities, in conjunction with deficiencies or inhibitors of lipoprotein lipase (or its activator, apoprotein C-II), can lead to this disorder. Patients manifest Fredrickson phenotype V. The physical findings may include eruptive xanthomata, lipemia retinalis, and hepatosplenomegaly. Triglyceride levels commonly are greater than 1000 mg/dl, and patients may develop pancreatitis or the chylomicronemia syndrome.

Familial dysbetalipoproteinemia is an autosomal recessive disorder. Patients with this disorder manifest the type III phenotype and have two apo E2 alleles. Chylomicron and VLDL remnants are inefficiently cleared by the liver, and an atherogenic species of VLDL known as β-VLDL is formed. The expression of this dyslipidemia requires the coexistence of another metabolic abnormality such as diabetes mellitus, hypothyroidism, obesity, or gout. Physical findings include tuberoeruptive xanthomata and xanthomata of the palmar creases. This disorder is strongly associated with premature CHD and peripheral vascular disease.

Familial deficiency of lipoprotein lipase or apoprotein C-II leads to the extremely rare type I phenotype. There are also a variety of uncommon inherited disorders associated with low levels of HDL cholesterol. These result from inherited abnormalities in apoprotein A-I synthesis, increased apoprotein A-I catabolism, or enzymatic defects critical for the formation of HDL.

Familial hypoalphalipoproteinemia is associated with premature CHD and stroke. It is present in

31% of subjects with angiographically documented premature CHD.

A detailed family history can suggest a genetic etiology for a patient's dyslipidemia and improve CHD risk stratification. This patient's family members with elevated TG and coexisting hypothyroidism suggest a diagnosis of familial dysbetalipoproteinemia. Familial combined hyperlipidemia and familial multiple lipoprotein hyperlipidemia also were diagnostic considerations.

QUESTION 4 Based on this patient's medical history, what *secondary* dyslipidemias should be considered in the differential diagnosis of her disorder?

Secondary disorders of lipoprotein metabolism are common. In diabetes mellitus, insulin resistance and deficiency lead to elevated levels of triglycerides and low levels of HDL cholesterol. This results from impaired lipolysis of VLDL cholesterol and increased availability of glucose and fatty acids. Hypothyroidism is a common cause of hyperlipidemia. It is associated with elevated levels of LDL cholesterol and triglycerides and reductions in levels of HDL cholesterol. This patient had a history of hypothyroidism, but she was receiving adequate replacement therapy. Chronic renal failure is accompanied by hypertriglyceridemia in 30% to 50% of patients. The nephrotic syndrome is primarily associated with elevations of LDL cholesterol, although elevations in triglycerides can occur. Cholestatic liver diseases may be accompanied by severe hypercholesterolemia because of an accumulation of lipoprotein-X, a phospholipid micelle that forms around albumin. It can be accompanied by the hyperviscosity syndrome. Obesity and cigarette smoking are associated with reduced levels of HDL cholesterol.

The most common medications with adverse effects on lipid profiles include beta-blockers *without* intrinsic sympathomimetic activity (increase triglycerides, decrease HDL cholesterol), diuretics (increase LDL cholesterol and triglycerides), corticosteroids (increase LDL cholesterol and triglycerides), and high-dose estrogen (increase triglycerides). Cholestyramine, although effective at lowering LDL cholesterol, has a tendency to raise triglycerides, especially if impaired lipoprotein lipase activity is present. This phenomenon probably contributed to D.G.'s refractory hypertriglyceridemia.

QUESTION 5 What factors in this patient's social history contributed to her dyslipidemia?

The social history helps identify modifiable behaviors that contribute to an abnormal lipid profile. This patient smoked tobacco, lived a sedentary lifestyle, and had approximately 75% adherence to a Step II diet. Cigarette smoking is an independent risk factor for ASVD that also reduces HDL cholesterol. Alcohol (not used by this patient) elevates triglycerides. Although moderate alcohol consumption may raise levels of HDL cholesterol, alcohol consumption has many deleterious health effects. A detailed dietary history, with the assistance of a qualified nutritionist, should focus on the total daily intake of calories, carbohydrates, total cholesterol, saturated fat, and unsaturated fat. Because of the day-to-day variability in dietary fat intake, 21-day food records should be used. Levels of aerobic physical activity should also be ascertained.

QUESTION 6 Her blood pressure was 130/70 mm Hg and her heart rate was 70 bpm. The height was 63 inches and the weight was 155 pounds. Head and neck examination revealed bilateral xanthelasmas. Corneal arcus was not present and her fundoscopic examination was normal. The thyroid gland was not palpable. Neither eruptive, tendinous, nor palmar xanthomata were present. Cardiovascular examination revealed a nondisplaced cardiac impulse, a normal S_1, and a normal S_2 without murmurs. The abdomen was nontender; hepatosplenomegaly was not present. Peripheral pulses were normal and without bruits. Pedal edema was not present. What aspects of the physical examination assist in the diagnosis and management of her dyslipidemia?

The physical examination focused on signs of cardiac disease (e.g., no cardiomegaly, no murmurs), vascular disease (e.g., intact peripheral pulses without bruits), end-organ damage from other CHD risk factors (e.g., no diabetic or hypertensive eye disease), secondary causes of dyslipidemia (e.g., no goiter), and pathognomonic signs of specific dyslipidemias (e.g., no palmar or tendon xanthomas). Xanthelasmas were present on both of her upper eyelids; however, these are nonspecific signs of an elevated total cholesterol.

QUESTION 7 Fasting laboratory evaluation on her current medications revealed: (TC) 289 mg/dl, (TG) 287 mg/dl, (HDL) 43 mg/dl. LDL cholesterol (LDL) was 189 mg/dl, as calculated by the Freidewald formula (LDL = TC-HDL-TG/5, provided TG <400 mg/dl). Fasting glucose was 94 mg/dl; renal and liver function tests were normal. Uric acid and TSH levels were normal. Apoprotein E isoform analysis revealed the E3/E3 genotype. Discuss the laboratory evaluation and its role in classifying her disorder.

The pathophysiology and classification of this dyslipidemia were clarified by obtaining a fasting blood sample (Fig. 2-8-2). The marked elevation in total cholesterol and triglyceride levels noted 4 years previously, raised the suspicion of familial dysbetalipoproteinemia (phenotype III); however, the normal apo E isoform analysis effectively excluded this disease. Familial multiple lipoprotein hyperlipidemia (phenotype V) was unlikely because the triglyceride level was less than 1000 mg/dl and because there was no evidence of a creamy supernatant (chylomicrons) in a plasma sample refrigerated overnight. The lipid profile most closely fits Fredrickson phenotype IIb, so the most likely diagnosis was familial combined hyperlipidemia (FCH). Familial hypercholesterolemia or polygenic hypercholesterolemia with a co-existing lipoprotein lipase abnormality (to explain the increased TG) were less likely considerations.

Laboratory evaluation should always include liver function tests to detect cholestatic liver diseases as many lipid-lowering medications have hepatic side effects. Assessment of renal function and thyroid function to detect secondary dyslipidemias is essential. The fasting blood glucose and uric acid levels should also be determined because their elevations are associated with type III and type V dyslipidemias. Nicotinic acid therapy can worsen hyperglycemia and precipitate gout.

QUESTION 8 What is the rationale for lipid-lowering therapy in patients with dyslipidemias?

Clinical trials have demonstrated the utility of lipid-lowering therapy for both the primary and secondary prevention of CHD. *Primary prevention* refers to the treatment of patients without clinical evidence of ASVD in an effort to prevent its development. The Lipid Research Clinics Coronary Primary Prevention Trial included over 3800 men with elevated total and LDL cholesterol after dietary therapy. This landmark study showed that treatment with cholestyramine reduced the risk of cardiac death or nonfatal myocardial infarction by 10%. Overall, each 1% reduction in total cholesterol was associated with a 2% decrease in CHD risk. In the Helsinki Heart Study and the World Health Organization Trial, men with elevated cholesterol who were treated with a fibric acid derivative had significant reductions in CHD events as compared to men receiving placebo.

Secondary prevention refers to treatment strategies for patients with established ASVD to prevent recurrent cardiac events. In the Coronary Drug Project, patients treated with nicotinic acid had a significantly lower rate of recurrent myocardial infarction. A survey performed 10 years after termination of the study showed that the overall mortality rate in the group receiving nicotinic acid was reduced significantly.

The National Heart Lung and Blood Institute Type II Coronary Intervention Study demonstrated that treatment with a low-fat diet and cholestyramine resulted in less angiographic progression of coronary artery disease. Regression and diminished progression of established CAD have been demonstrated in many angiographic trials of lipid-lowering agents.

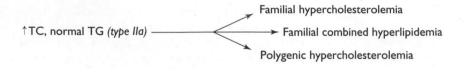

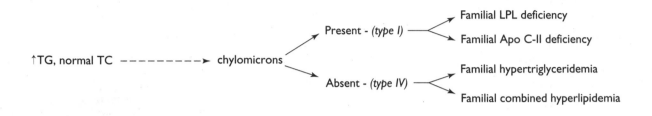

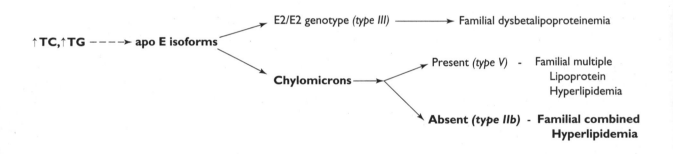

*This patient's risk factors are in **bold***

2-8-2 Differential diagnosis of primary dyslipidemias based on laboratory evaluation.

The Pravastatin Multinational Study Group for Cardiac Risk Patients demonstrated that treatment with pravastatin resulted in fewer cardiovascular events than placebo in 6 months. The rapidity by which lipid-lowering therapy reduced cardiovascular events suggests that aggressive treatment should begin early.

QUESTION 9 Discuss the initial approach to lipid-lowering therapy in this case.

In general, initial treatment decisions are based on screening for levels of total and HDL cholesterol. Levels of triglycerides and LDL cholesterol are determined if the screening HDL cholesterol is ≤35 mg/dl or if the screening total cholesterol is ≥240 mg/dl, or if the total cholesterol is ≥200 mg/dl and two or more CHD risk factors are present. Treatment decisions are based on LDL cholesterol level (Table 2-8-2). For primary prevention, a Step I diet (Table 2-8-3) is recom-

TABLE 2-8-2   Treatment Guidelines for Patients With and Without CHD

	LDL Cholesterol	
	Level to Initiate Treatment	Goal of Therapy
Without CHD and with fewer than 2 risk factors	≥190 mg/dl	<160 mg/dl
Without CHD and with 2 or more risk factors	≥160 mg/dl	<130 mg/dl
With CHD	≥130 mg/dl	≤100 mg/dl

Adapted from National cholesterol education program second report of the expert panel on detection, evaluation, and treatment of high blood cholesterol in adults (adult treatment panel II), *Circulation* 85:1329-1445, 1994.

TABLE 2-8-3   Dietary Therapy of Hyperlipidemia

Nutrient	Step I Diet	Recommended Intake	Step II Diet
Total fat	<30% of total daily calories		<7% of total daily calories
Saturated fatty acids	8% to 10% of total daily calories		
Polyunsaturated fatty acids		Up to 10% of total daily calories	
Monounsaturated fatty acids		Up to 15% of total daily calories	
Carbohydrates		≥55% of total daily calories	
Protein		Approximately 15% of total daily calories	
Cholesterol	<300 mg/dl		<200 mg/dl
Total calories	←	To achieve and maintain desirable weight	→

Adapted from national cholesterol education program second report of the expert panel on detection, evaluation, and treatment of high blood cholesterol in adults (adult treatment panel II), *Circulation* 85:1329-1445, 1994.

mended, and the lipid profile is reevaluated after 3 months. If the LDL cholesterol goal is not achieved, a Step II diet is initiated, and the lipid profile is reassessed at 6 months, before initiating drug therapy. More frequent visits with the nutritionist and/or other health care professionals may yield more effective lifestyle changes. The primary prevention treatment goals for this patient included an LDL cholesterol level less than 130 mg/dl, an HDL cholesterol level greater than 45 mg/dl, and a normal triglyceride level (less than 200 mg/dl). Although she was already on a Step II diet, she was referred to a nutritionist for ongoing assistance with weight reduction and to improve her compliance. Aerobic exercise, in addition to burning calories and assisting with weight loss, improves triglyceride utilization and

increases levels of HDL cholesterol. A supervised exercise program was recommended and adhered to by the patient. She also stopped smoking with the help of a smoking cessation support group and temporary use of a nicotine patch.

For secondary prevention, treatment should begin with a Step II diet. Although 6 months of dietary therapy are recommended before initiating drug therapy, drug therapy can be *added* to diet therapy earlier in patients with severe lipid abnormalities or ASVD.

Lovastatin and cholestyramine were discontinued, and treatment with pravastatin (40 mg qhs) and gemfibrozil (600 mg bid) was initiated. She entered a smoking cessation program and by repeat evaluation had decreased her tobacco use by 50%. She also entered a cardiovascular fitness

TABLE 2-8-4   **This Patient's Laboratory Values***

	TC	TG	HDL	LDL
Baseline	>500	>300	>35	Not calculated
Lovastatin/Cholestyramine	289	287	43	189
Pravastatin/Gemfibrozil	266	131	47	193
Pravastatin/Gemfibrozil/Estrogen	212	70	46	152
Pravastatin/Gemfibrozil/Estrogen/Cholestyramine	196	112	47	127

*All values in mg/dl.

program. After 8 weeks of treatment her lipid profile was: TC 266 mg/dl, TG 131 mg/dl, HDL 47 mg/dl, LDL 193 mg/dl. Her xanthelasmas and her sleep disturbances resolved. She denied myalgias and liver function tests remained normal.

She was prescribed ethinyl estradiol (0.625 mg qd) and medroxyprogesterone (2.5 mg qd), she quit smoking, and performed 30 minutes of aerobic exercise three times each week. After 8 more weeks of treatment, her weight had decreased by 6 pounds and her lipid profile was dramatically improved: TC 212 mg/dl, TG 70 mg/dl, HDL 46 mg/dl, LDL 152 mg/dl.

Cholestyramine (4 mg bid) was prescribed and her TC decreased to 196 mg/dl, TG 112 mg/dl, HDL 47 mg/dl, and LDL 127 mg/dl (Table 2-8-4).

QUESTION 10 What are the options for lipid-lowering pharmacotherapy and how were they selected for the patient?

Drug therapy was initiated early because of the magnitude of the patient's lipid abnormality and her strong family history of premature CHD. The dosing regimens and common side effects of lipid-lowering agents can be found in Table 2-8-5. Their efficacy is described in Table 2-8-6.

HMG-CoA reductase inhibitors include lovastatin, pravastatin, simvastatin, and fluvastatin. These agents competitively inhibit hydroxy-methylglutaryl-CoA reductase, the rate-limiting enzyme in cholesterol biosynthesis. Lowering of the intrahepatic cholesterol pool stimulates the synthesis of new LDL receptors, which facilitates

removal of LDL cholesterol from the plasma. This class of agents has highly potent LDL-lowering properties. Adverse reactions are less common than with other agents. Significant drug interactions with gemfibrozil, nicotinic acid, erythromycin, and cyclosporine have been reported for lovastatin and simvastatin, but these do not appear to occur with pravastatin. The data on fluvastatin are incomplete. Pravastatin is associated with less frequent sleep disturbance and is the only reductase inhibitor with FDA approval for combination therapy with gemfibrozil. The combination of pravastatin and gemfibrozil causes less hepatotoxicity and myositis than the combination of lovastatin and gemfibrozil. The patient tolerated combination therapy without evidence of hepatocellular or muscle injury. She experienced severe sleep disturbance with lovastatin that did not reoccur when she received pravastatin.

Gemfibrozil is a fibric acid derivative that inhibits hepatic synthesis of VLDL and improves VLDL catabolism, resulting in substantial reductions in triglycerides and increases in HDL cholesterol levels through stimulation of apoprotein A-I synthesis. It is effective for treating hypertriglyceridemia and is generally well tolerated. In combined dyslipidemias, reduction in triglyceride levels will facilitate reduction in LDL cholesterol levels and elevation of HDL cholesterol levels. Triglyceride reduction should be attempted first, especially if triglyceride levels are greater than 500 mg/dl. For the patient, gemfibrozil reduced triglyceride levels into the normal range, which facilitated LDL cholesterol reduction with pravas-

TABLE 2-8-5   Use of Lipid-Lowering Agents

Drugs	Dosage	Dosing	Side Effects	Drug Interactions

Bile acid sequestrants
  Cholestyramine
  Colestipol
	4-24 g/day
	5-30 g/day
		Within 30 minutes of a meal
		A double dose with dinner produces equivalent LDL lowering as bid dosing
			Nausea, bloating, cramping, and constipation
			Elevations in liver function tests
				Impaired absorption of fat soluble vitamins, digoxin, warfarin, thiazide diuretics, beta-blockers, thyroxine, phenobarbital

Nicotinic acid	1-12 g/day	Given with meals Begin with 100 mg tid and titrate to effect Closely monitor liver function studies, glucose and uric acid	Prostaglandin-mediated cutaneous flushing, hot flashes and pruritus Hyperpigmentation, acanthosis nigricans, and dry skin Nausea, vomiting, and diarrhea Myositis	

HMG-CoA reductase inhibitors
  Lovastatin
  Pravastatin
  Simvastatin
  Fluvastatin
	
	20-80 mg/day
	10-40 mg/day
	20-40 mg/day
	10-40 mg/day
		Given with evening meal, twice daily dosing for doses >20 mg
		Taken at bedtime
			Headache, nausea, sleep disturbance, myositis
			Elevations in liver function tests
				Lovastatin and simvastatin potentiate effect of warfarin and elevate digoxin levels:
				  pravastatin—none
				  fluvastatin—none

Gemfibrozil	600 mg bid	30-60 min before meals	Abdominal cramping and bloating	Potentiates effect of warfarin absorption Decreased by bile acid sequestrants
Probucol	500 mg bid		Loose stools, eosinophilia, QT interval prolongation, angioneurotic edema Lowers HDL	

tatin. The normalization of triglyceride levels with gemfibrozil allowed reinitiation of cholestyramine therapy and increased the HDL cholesterol level into the acceptable range.

Bile-acid sequestrants include cholestyramine and colestipol. These agents bind with bile acids in the intestinal lumen and interrupt enterohepatic cycling. The reduction in intrahepatic cholesterol levels stimulates synthesis of LDL receptors that clear LDL from the plasma. The intestinal synthesis of apo A-I is stimulated. Bile-acid sequestrants are indicated for mild or moderate elevations in LDL cholesterol. They are effective as monotherapy and are synergistic with

TABLE 2-8-6   Effects of Lipid Lowering Medication

Drug	LDL	HDL	TG
HMG-CoA reductase inhibitors	↓ 20-40%	↑ 5-10%	↓ 10-20%
Gemfibrozil	↓ 10-15%	↑ 15-25%	↓ 35-50%
Bile acid sequestrants	↓ 15-30%	↔ ↑	↔ ↑
Nicotinic acid	↓ 10-25%	↑ 15-30%	↓ 25-30%
Probucol	↓ 10-15%	↓ 20-25%	↔
Estrogen replacement therapy	↓ 15-25%	↑ 15-20%	↑ 10-70%

nicotinic acid and HMG-CoA reductase inhibitors for the treatment of severe elevations of LDL cholesterol. The tolerability of bile-acid sequestrants can be improved by using "light" preparations, combining them with small doses of psyllium hydrophilic mucilloid (Metamucil), and taking doses with meals. Use of bile-acid sequestrants is limited by significant intralumenal binding of other medications. Because the patient had FCH and probably had an associated lipoprotein lipase abnormality, cholestyramine probably contributed to her hypertriglyceridemia. After this agent was withdrawn and her triglycerides were reduced with gemfibrozil, cholestyramine was added back to her regimen to help achieve an LDL cholesterol level ≤ 130 mg/dl.

Nicotinic acid inhibits production of VLDL cholesterol by the liver, and LDL cholesterol levels are reduced as a consequence. HDL cholesterol levels also increase because of delayed catabolism. The HDL cholesterol-raising properties are seen at low doses (1 g daily); however, the VLDL cholesterol reductions typically require higher doses (3 g daily). Nicotinic-acid therapy is appropriate for most dyslipidemias and is inexpensive; however, it is poorly tolerated by most patients. Its adverse metabolic effects are elucidated in Table 2-8-5. Therapy must be started at low doses (100 mg tid) and gradually increased to prevent cutaneous and gastrointestinal side effects. Pretreatment with aspirin (325 mg) can be helpful. Nicotinic acid could also have been considered for primary therapy.

Probucol is a weak LDL cholesterol-lowering agent that has antioxidant properties. Its role in the management of hypercholesterolemia is controversial because it is associated with marked reductions in HDL cholesterol.

Estrogen replacement therapy (ERT) is associated with decreased CHD risk. In postmenopausal women, ERT lowers LDL cholesterol levels by approximately 20% and elevates HDL cholesterol levels by approximately 21%; however, triglyceride levels may increase by as much as 70%. In addition, ERT inhibits LDL oxidation, reduces fasting glucose levels, prevents osteoporosis, and may improve vascular endothelial function. For the patient, ERT caused a marked reduction in the level of LDL cholesterol. Triglyceride elevation was not seen because of concomitant use of gemfibrozil. Although the use of progestins partially attenuates the lipid-lowering effects of estrogen, they decrease the incidence of endometrial cancer, which may be more frequent in women receiving ERT. The use of ERT can be recommended for perimenopausal or postmenopausal women after consultation with the patient and carefully considering the relative risks of breast cancer, endometrial cancer, and ASVD.

CASE SUMMARY Aggressive therapy, including a Step II diet, cessation of cigarette smoking, increased physical activity, weight loss, and combination drug therapy allowed this patient to optimize her lipid profile and significantly reduce her risk of ASVD. In addition, her quality of life improved. This case demonstrates the importance of understanding lipoprotein metabolism when treating patients with dyslipidemias. This case also demonstrates the differences between and within the different classes of lipid-lowering agents.

Although all dyslipidemia cases are not as complicated as the one presented, the management principles are generally applicable. Despite its financial cost to the individual, lipid-lowering therapy is an investment that is returned as decreased morbidity and mortality from ASVD. As stated in the final section of the summary of the National Cholesterol Education Program Adult Treatment Panel II report, "The aggregate cost of CHD in the United States is enormous, costing the nation between $50 billion to $100 billion per year...the least expensive way to reduce CHD is through the public health approach.[1]"

• •

BIBLIOGRAPHY

Anderson KM, Castelli WP, Levy D: Cholesterol and mortality: 30 years of follow-up from the Framingham study, *JAMA* 257:2176-2180, 1987.
Applebaum-Bowden D, McLean P, Steinmetz A, et al: Lipoprotein, apolipoprotein, and lipolytic enzyme changes

following estrogen administration in postmenopausal women, *J Lipid Res* 30:1895-1906, 1989.

Assman G, Schulte H. Triglycerides and atherosclerosis: results from the prospective cardiovascular Munster study. In Gotto, AM, Jr, Paoletti R, eds: *Atherosclerosis reviews,* vol 22, New York, 1991, Raven Press.

Atmeh RF, Shepherd J, Packard CJ: Subpopulations of apolipoprotein AI in human high density lipoproteins: their metabolic properties and response to drug therapy, *Biochem Biophys Acta* 751:175-188, 1983.

Attman P-O, Alanpovic P: Lipid and apolipoprotein profiles of uremic dyslipoproteinemia-relation to renal function and dialysis, *Nephron* 57:401-410, 1991.

Austin MA: Plasma triglycerides and coronary heart disease, *Arterioscler Thromb* 11:2-14, 1991.

Babirak SP, Brown BG, Brunzell JD: Familial combined hyperlipidemia and abnormal lipoprotein lipase, *Arterioscler Thromb* 12:1176-1183, 1992.

The Bezafibrate Infarction Prevention Study Group: Lipids and lipoproteins in symptomatic coronary heart disease: distribution, intercorrelation and significance for risk classification in 6700 men and 1500 women, *Circulation* 86:839-848, 1992.

Blankenhorn DH, Azen SP, Kramsch DM, et al: Coronary angiographic changes with lovastatin therapy: the monitored atherosclerosis regression study (MARS), *Ann Intern Med* 119:969-976, 1993.

Blankenhorn DH, Nessim SA, Johnson RL, et al: Beneficial effects of combined colestipol-niacin therapy on coronary atherosclerosis and coronary venous bypass grafts, *JAMA* 257:3233-3240, 1987.

Brensike JF, Levy RI, Kelsey SF, et al: Effects of therapy with cholestyramine on progression of coronary arteriosclerosis: results of the NHLBI type II coronary intervention study, *Circulation* 69:313-324, 1984.

Brown G, Albers JJ, Fisher LD, et al: Regression of coronary artery disease as a result of intensive lipid-lowering therapy in men with high levels of apolipoprotein B, *N Engl J Med* 323:1289-1298, 1990.

Canner PL, Berge KG, Wenger NK, et al: Fifteen-year mortality in coronary drug project patients: long-term benefit with niacin, *J Am Coll Cardiol* 8:1245-1255, 1986.

Castelli WP, Doyle JT, Gordon T, et al: Alcohol and blood lipids: the cooperative lipoprotein phenotyping study, *Lancet* ii:153-155, 1977.

Castelli WP, Garrison RJ, Wilson PWF, et al: Incidence of coronary heart disease and lipoprotein cholesterol levels: the Framingham study, *JAMA* 256:2835-2838, 1986.

Committee of Principle Investigators: WHO cooperative trial on primary prevention of ischemic heart disease with clofibrate to lower serum cholesterol: final mortality follow-up, *Lancet* ii:600, 1984.

Coronary Drug Project Research Group: Clofibrate and niacin in coronary heart disease, *JAMA* 231:360-381, 1975.

Dannenberg AL, Keller JB, Wilson PWF, et al: Leisure time physical activity in the Framingham offspring study: description, seasonal variation, and risk factor correlates, *Am J Epidemiol* 129:76-87, 1989.

Davignon J, Nestruck AC, Alaupovic P, et al: Severe hypoalphalipoproteinemia induced by a combination of probucol and clofibrate, *Adv Exp Med Biol* 201:111-125, 1986.

DeJager S, Bruckert E, Chapman MJ: Dense low density lipoprotein subspecies with diminished oxidative resistance predominate in combined hyperlipidemia, *J Lipid Res* 34:295-308, 1993.

Domas A, Schuh D, Murtaugh M, et al: Determination of the minimum number of food records required to accurately estimate usual intakes of energy, fat, saturated fat, and cholesterol in preventive cardiology outpatients, *J Am Coll Nutr* 12:607a, 1993.

Gaziano JM, Busing JE, Breslow JL, et al: Moderate alcohol intake, increased levels of high density lipoprotein and its subfraction, and decreased risk of myocardial infarction, *N Engl J Med* 329:1829-1837, 1993.

Genest JJ Jr, Martin-Munley SS, McNamara JR, et al: Familial lipoprotein disorders in patients with premature coronary artery disease, *Circulation* 85:2025-2033, 1992.

Genest JJ Jr, McNamara JR, Ordovas JM, et al: Lipoprotein cholesterol, apolipoproteins A-I and B, and lipoprotein(a) abnormalities in men with premature coronary artery disease, *J Am Coll Cardiol* 19:792-802, 1992.

Gilligan DM, Quyyumi AA, Cannan RD III: Effects of physiological levels of estrogen on coronary vasomotion in post-menopausal women, *Circulation* 891:2545-2551, 1994.

Glueck CJ, Daniels SR, Bates S, et al: Pediatric victims of unexplained stroke and their families. Familial lipid and lipoprotein abnormalities, *Pediatrics* 69:308-316, 1982.

Glueck CJ, Oakes N, Speirs J, et al: Gemfibrozil-lovastatin therapy for primary hyperlipoproteinemias, *Am J Cardiol* 70:1-9, 1992.

Goldstein JL, Schrott HG, Hazzard WR, et al: Hyperlipidemia in coronary heart disease, *J Clin Invest* 52:1544-1568, 1973.

Grundy SM: Multifactorial etiology of hypercholesterolemia: implications for prevention of coronary heart disease, *Arterioscler Thromb* 11:1619-1635, 1991.

Grundy SM, Mok HYI, Zech L, Berman M: Influence of nicotinic acid on metabolism of cholesterol and triglycerides in man, *J Lipid Res* 22:24-36, 1981.

Grundy SM, Vega GL: Two different views of the relationship of hypertriglyceridemia to coronary heart disease, *Arch Intern Med* 152:28-34, 1992.

Hubert HB, Feinleib M, McNamara PM, et al: Obesity as an independent risk factor for cardiovascular disease: a 26-year follow-up of participants in the Framingham heart study, *Circulation* 67:968-977, 1983.

Keane WF, Kasiske BL: Hyperlipidemia in the nephrotic syndrome, *N Engl J Med* 323:603-604, 1990.

Kuhn FE, Rackley CE: Coronary artery disease in women: risk factors, evaluation, treatment, and prevention, *Arch Intern Med* 153:2626-2636, 1993.

Kwiterovich PO, Coresh J, Bachorik PS: Prevalence of hyperapobetalipo-proteinemia and other lipoprotein phenotypes in men (aged ≤50 years) and women (≤60 years) with coronary artery disease, *Am J Cardiol* 72:631-639, 1993.

Lavie CJ, Mailander L, Milani RV: Marked benefit with sustained-release niacin therapy in patients with "isolated" very low levels of high-density lipoprotein cholesterol and coronary artery disease, *Am J Cardiol* 69:1083-1085, 1992.

Lipid Research Clinics Program: The Lipid Research Clinic Coronary Primary Prevention Trial results, I. reduction in incidence of coronary heart disease, II. the relationship of reductions in incidence of coronary heart disease to cholesterol lowering, *JAMA* 251:351, 1984.

Luria MH: Effect of low-dose niacin on high-density lipoprotein cholesterol and total cholesterol/high-density lipoprotein cholesterol ratio, *Arch Intern Med* 148:2493-2495, 1988.

Manninen V, Elo MO, Frick MH, et al: Lipid alterations and decline in the incidence of coronary heart disease in the Helsinki Heart Study, *JAMA* 206:641-651, 1988.

Manson JE, Colditz GA, Stampfer MJ, et al: A prospective study of obesity and risk of coronary heart disease in women, *N Engl J Med* 332:882-889, 1990.

Nabulsi AA, Folsom AR, White A, et al: Association of hormone-replacement therapy with various cardiovascular risk factors in postmenopausal women, *N Engl J Med* 328:1069-1075, 1993.

National cholesterol education program second report of the expert panel on detection, evaluation, and treatment of high blood cholesterol in adults (adult treatment panel II). *Circulation* 89:1329-1445, 1994.

O'Brien T, Dinneen SF, O'Brien PC, et al: Hyperlipidemia in patients with primary and secondary hypothyroidism, *Mayo Clin Proc* 68:860-866, 1993.

Pravastatin Multinational Study Group for Cardiac Risk Patients: Effects of pravastatin in patients with serum total cholesterol levels from 5.2 to 7.8 mmol/liter (200 to 300 mg/dl) plus two additional atherosclerotic risk factors, *Am J Cardiol* 72:1031-1037, 1993.

Rosenson RS: Gemfibrozil-lovastatin associated myalgia, *Am J Cardiol* 71:497, 1993.

Rosenson RS, Baker AL, Chow M, et al: Hyperviscosity syndrome in a hypercholesterolemic patient with primary biliary cirrhosis, *Gastroenterology* 98:1351-1357, 1990.

Rosenson RS, Frauenheim WA: Safety of combined pravastatin-gemfibrozil therapy, *Am J Cardiol* 1994 (in press).

Rosenson RS, Goranson NL: Lovastatin-associated sleep and mood disturbances, *Am J Med* 95:548-549, 1993.

Sack MN, Rader DL, Cannon RD III: Oestrogen and inhibition of oxidation of low-density lipoproteins in postmenopausal women, *Lancet* 343:269-270, 1994.

Shepherd J, Packard CJ, Morgan HG, et al: The effects of cholestyramine on high density lipoprotein metabolism, *Atherosclerosis* 33:433-444, 1979.

Stalder M, Pometta D, Suenram A: Relationship between plasma insulin levels and high density lipoprotein cholesterol levels in healthy men, *Diabetologia* 21:544-548, 1981.

Stamler J, Wentworth D, Neaton JD: Is the relationship between serum cholesterol and risk of premature death from coronary heart disease continuous and graded? Findings in 356,222 primary screenees of the Multiple Risk Factor Intervention Trial (MRFIT), *JAMA* 256:2823-2828, 1986.

Stampfer MJ, Colditz GA, Willett WC, et al: Postmenopausal estrogen therapy and cardiovascular disease, *N Engl J Med* 325:756-762, 1991.

Stone NJ, Levy RI, Fredrickson DS, et al: Coronary artery disease in 116 kindreds with familial type II hyperlipoproteinemia, *Circulation* 49:476-488, 1974.

Wanner C, Frommherz WH: Hyperlipoproteinemia in chronic renal failure: pathophysiology and therapeutic aspects, *Cardiology* 78:202-217, 1991.

Wiklund O, Bergman M, Bondjers G, et al: Pravastatin and gemfibrozil alone and in combination for the treatment of hypercholesterolemia, *Am J Med* 94:13-20, 1993.

Wilson PWF, Anderson KM, Castelli WP: The impact of triglycerides on coronary heart disease: the Framingham study. In Gotto, AM, Jr, Paoletti, R, eds: *Atherosclerosis Reviews,* vol 22, New York, 1991, Raven Press.

Wood PD, Stefanick ML, Williams PT, et al: The effects on plasma lipoproteins of a prudent weight-reducing diet, with or without exercise, in overweight men and women, *N Engl J Med* 325:461-466, 1991.

Zavaroni I, Dall'Aglia E, Alpi O, et al: Evidence for an independent relationship between plasma insulin and concentration of high density lipoprotein cholesterol and triglyceride, *Atherosclerosis* 55:259-266, 1985.

CASE

9 Peter Kures

A previously well 65-year-old man presented to his physician with increasing breathlessness during routine daily activities and a 4 to 6 week history of weakness and fatigue. His symptoms have progressed to the point where he feels exhausted after climbing two flights of stairs and needs to rest to catch his breath. He also developed a chronic nonproductive cough and frequent nocturia.

QUESTION I What is the differential diagnosis for the above patient?

The major components of the differential diagnosis for such a presentation includes bronchitis, pneumonia, congestive heart failure, renal failure, and diabetes mellitus. Dyspnea and fatigue may be due to multiple etiologies. The first step in this patient's evaluation involves a careful history to verify the symptoms that are suggestive of congestive heart failure while excluding noncardiac possibilities. The most important noncardiac causes of exertional dyspnea are pulmonary diseases such as COPD and asthma (especially exercise-induced asthma), acute and chronic pneumonia, malignancy, and interstitial lung diseases. Renal disease and chronic liver disease often cause fluid retention that may lead to peripheral edema and fatigue. Less frequent noncardiac etiologies include neuromuscular and chest wall disorders and endocrine imbalances (thyroid and adrenal). The noncardiac etiologies require specific interventions and frequently respond to appropriate therapy. In addition, there are also multiple causes of acute deterioration in stable patients with previously

well-compensated heart failure. Myocardial ischemia and acute infarction, in particular, require immediate treatment and should be considered in all patients with chest pain or associated anginal symptoms.

The symptoms that are most suggestive of congestive heart failure are exertional dyspnea, orthopnea, and paroxysmal nocturnal dyspnea (PND). Unexplained fatigue, confusion, lethargy, and anorexia are frequent atypical symptoms in the elderly. Patients with these complaints should undergo a thorough evaluation for heart failure if a non-cardiac cause is not readily identifiable.

Since heart failure represents the final common pathway for most serious forms of heart disease, there are multiple etiologies and precipitating factors. The most common cause of heart failure is left ventricular systolic dysfunction. The major risk factors for the development of heart failure are advanced age, hypertension, coronary artery disease, diabetes mellitus, and tobacco use. The prevalence of heart failure has continued to rise over the last 20 years even though the death rates for myocardial infarction and stroke have been declining. More than 400,000 new cases of heart failure are diagnosed each year. The initial heart failure evaluation should also seek to define the severity of the clinical syndrome, and the New York Heart Association functional classification (Table 2-9-1) is commonly used for this purpose. Hospitalization is usually required if hypotension, hypoxemia (O_2 saturation less than 90%), pulmonary edema, acute coronary ischemia, or severe complicating medical illnesses such as pneumonia or gastrointestinal bleeding are present.

TABLE 2-9-1 New York Heart Association (NYHA) Classification

Class I	No limitation of routine physical activity
Class II	Slight limitation of activity; patients have fatigue, palpitations and dyspnea with ordinary physical activity, but are comfortable at rest.
Class III	Marked limitation of activity; less than ordinary physical activity results in symptoms, but patients are comfortable at rest.
Class IV	Symptoms are present at rest and they are exacerbated by any physical exertion.

(From Agency for Health Care Policy & Research Publication No. 94-0612, *Heart failure: evaluation and care of patients with left ventricular systolic dysfunction,* June 1994.)

QUESTION 2 The patient reported needing to sleep on 3 to 4 pillows to breathe comfortably at night over the last 1 to 2 weeks. He denied chest pain, palpitations, ankle swelling, or fever. He has no history of rheumatic fever in childhood or other heart trouble. There is no family history of myocardial infarction or heart failure, but his father died of a stroke at age 66. A younger sibling has hypertension. The patient smoked one pack of cigarettes a day for 20 years but none in the last 5 years. He drinks 2 to 4 cans of beer per day. His cholesterol and blood pressure were reportedly "borderline" elevated on a previous evaluation, and he was instructed to decrease dietary fat, salt, and alcohol intake. Are the clinical symptoms most compatible with NYHA Class III right ventricular (RV) failure, left ventricular (LV) failure, or biventricular failure?

The patient's clinical symptoms are most compatible with NYHA class III LV heart failure. The history and physical examination will usually determine whether the major clinical symptoms are due to left heart failure or isolated right heart failure. The major clinical symptoms of left heart failure are due to increased pulmonary venous congestion and result in orthopnea, paroxysmal nocturnal dyspnea, and exertional and rest dyspnea. Inadequate LV cardiac output is responsible for exercise intolerance, weakness, fatigue, and mental confusion. In contrast, the major symp-

toms of right heart failure are due to systemic venous congestion and result in dependent edema, right upper quadrant pain (due to stretching of the hepatic capsule), nausea, bloating, and anorexia. The most common causes of right heart failure are chronic left heart failure, pulmonary disease, cardiac valvular disease (tricuspid, pulmonic, or mitral stenosis), and congenital heart disease. Unless severe chronic obstructive pulmonary disease or ascites is present, orthopnea is not a prominent feature of right heart failure. The prognosis of patients with isolated right heart failure is dependent on the etiology. Extensive pulmonary parenchymal and vascular disease and advanced cyanotic congenital heart diseases are associated with increased mortality, and symptomatic therapy with oxygen and diuretics is only modestly efficacious. Right heart failure symptoms from tricuspid stenosis or constrictive pericarditis are often completely alleviated following appropriate surgery. Mitral stenosis is an important etiology of right heart failure that may be "silent" (the murmur may be difficult to diagnose) during examination. Often the only clue to excluding edema caused by primary liver disease is the presence of elevated jugular venous pressure (JVP) in the cardiac patients. Systemic venous congestion from right heart failure may lead to elevated liver enzymes and bilirubin, hypoalbuminemia, and coagulopathy. Since successful treatment of right heart failure often leads to complete recovery of liver function, passive liver congestion should be considered when the JVP is elevated.

QUESTION 3 Physical examination revealed a well-developed male who was slightly overweight but appeared comfortable at rest. Vital signs were BP 160/100 mm Hg (both arms), HR 96 bpm (no orthostatic changes), RR 14/min, and T 98.8°F. HEENT revealed fundi with grade 2+ arteriovenous (AV) nicking. The neck showed no jugular venous distension, and the carotid upstroke was normal without bruits or murmurs. The breath sounds were decreased in the basilar lung fields with scattered expiratory wheezing. The cardiac examination revealed a diffuse apical impulse in the 5th intercostal space displaced 2 cm lateral to the midclavicular line. The S_1 was decreased in intensity, and the S_2 was normal. A prominent S_4 and a soft S_3 were present at the apex. A grade 2/6 systolic ejection murmur was best heard at the base, and a grade 2/6 holosystolic apical murmur radiated to the axilla. The abdomen was nontender, and no organomegaly was present. Abdominal jugular reflux was not present. The peripheral pulses were normal and symmetrical, and the extremity examination revealed no edema. What are the possible etiologies of left ventricular failure in this patient?

The potential etiologies for LV failure in this patient include hypertension, coronary artery disease, mitral regurgitation, hypertrophic cardiomyopathy, and alcoholic cardiomyopathy. The clinician's goal is to define the reversible etiologies as early as possible in the heart failure evaluation. This examination reveals signs of long-standing HTN (AV nicking on funduscopy), LV enlargement (LV impulse displacement), LV volume overload (S_3), and mitral regurgitation (holosystolic murmur to the axilla). Even though an S_4 may be present in some normal persons, the clinician should also consider HTN, left ventricular hypertrophy, aortic stenosis, and CAD as possible causes. Hypertrophic cardiomyopathy with LV outflow tract obstruction may produce a marked accentuation of the systolic murmur following maneuvers that decrease LV cavity size (standing from a squatting position). The soft S_1 represents weak ventricular contraction but may also occur due to obesity, pericardial effusion, or first degree heart block. Alcohol history is notoriously inaccurate in heavy users, and the "holiday heart" syndrome often presents with atrial arrhythmias and heart failure after binge drinking.

The wide spectrum of clinical presentations of heart failure range from asymptomatic patients to pulmonary edema following extensive myocardial infarction (MI). Symptomatic patients with evidence of volume overload (dyspnea or edema) should have oral diuretic therapy initiated. Pulmonary edema requires oxygen supplementation, intravenous diuretic therapy, preload and afterload reduction with nitrates and morphine sulfate, and may require assisted ventilation, endotracheal intubation, intravenous inotropic agents, and intraaortic balloon counterpulsation in severe situations, until the underlying cause is identified and treated successfully.

This patient exhibits signs of mild volume overload with decreased basilar breath sounds, and expiratory wheezing (bronchial edema). However, there is no clear, acute, precipitating cause for his symptoms that requires hospitalization. Initially, the blood pressure must be controlled, and myocardial toxins (ethanol) completely eliminated. A focused evaluation should be performed to further define possible etiologies or precipitants of heart failure.

The Agency for Health Care Policy and Research has published guidelines that are helpful for the clinical evaluation and therapy of patients with left ventricular systolic dysfunction (Table 2-9-2).

QUESTION 4   The patient's laboratory evaluation revealed a normal CBC, urinalysis, electrolytes, serum creatinine and TSH. The serum glucose was elevated. The ECG revealed normal sinus rhythm with a premature atrial contraction (PAC) and voltage criteria for left ventricular hypertrophy (LVH). ST segment depression was present in leads I, AVL, V_5, and V_6 consistent with an LVH strain pattern. The chest radiograph (CXR) revealed an enlarged cardiac silhouette (60% cardiothoracic ratio) with prominent upper lobe vasculature and blunting of the right costophrenic angle. What are the predictors of mortality in heart failure?

A. NYHA functional class
B. Serum sodium concentration
C. Extent of coronary artery disease (CAD)
D. Left ventricular ejection fraction (LVEF)
E. Cardiothoracic ratio (CTR) on CXR
F. All of the above

The accepted predictors of mortality in heart failure include NYHA functional class, the serum sodium concentration, the extent of CAD, LVEF,

TABLE 2-9-2   AHCPR Recommended Tests for Patients with Suspected Heart Failure

Test Recommendation	Findings	Suspected Diagnosis
Electrocardiogram	Acute ST-T wave changes	Myocardial ischemia
	Atrial fibrillation, other tachyarrhythmia	Thyroid disease or heart failure due to
	Bradyarrhythmias	rapid ventricular rate
	Previous MI (e.g., Q waves)	Heart failure due to low heart rate
	Low voltage	Heart failure due to reduced left-ventricular
	LV hypertrophy	performance
		Pericardial effusion
		Diastolic dysfunction
Complete blood count	Anemia	Heart failure due to or aggravated by decreased oxygen-carrying capacity
Urinalysis	Proteinuria	Nephrotic syndrome
	Red blood cells or cellular casts	Glomerulonephritis
Serum creatinine	Elevated	Volume overload due to renal failure
Serum albumin	Decreased	Increased extravascular volume due to hypoalbuminemia
T4 and TSH (obtain only if atrial fibrillation, evidence of thyroid disease, or patient age >65)	Abnormal T4 or TSH	Heart failure due to or aggravated by hypo/hyperthyroidism

Note: TSH = Thyroid-stimulating hormone, MI = Myocardial infarction

(From Agency for Health Care Policy & Research Publication No. 94-0612, *Heart failure: evaluation and care of patients with left ventricular systolic dysfunction*, June 1994.)

and the CTR on CXR. The best predictor is the LVEF. The combined use of the history, physical examination, laboratory data, CXR, and ECG cannot be relied upon to consistently and accurately distinguish the pathogenesis of LV failure: i.e., systolic dysfunction with LVEF less than 35% to 40%, or diastolic dysfunction with LVEF greater than 40%. The LVEF predicts future mortality in heart failure, and NYHA Class III and IV patients have the worst prognosis. However, a large proportion of patients (20% to 40%) with signs and symptoms of heart failure will have an LVEF greater than 40%. These symptoms are then attributed to derangements in ventricular filling indices such as diastolic dysfunction or valvular disease, and the treatment is focused on the specific etiology. Some therapies used for systolic dysfunction (such as digoxin) may actually worsen heart failure symptoms that are due to diastolic dysfunction! The CXR is particularly valuable in predicting mortality from heart failure in myocardial infarction survivors who subsequently increase their cardiothoracic ratio. The presence of perivascular cuffing, pleural effusions, Kerley B lines, and pulmonary vascular redistribution to the apical vessels indicates elevated pulmonary venous pressures (more than 18 to 22 mm Hg) but does not accurately predict LVEF. The ECG is most useful in excluding acute ischemia, myocardial infarction, and arrhythmias as etiologies of heart failure but is a poor predictor of systolic function.

The use of echocardiography or radionuclide ventriculography can substantially improve diagnostic accuracy in defining the LVEF, and assessment of LV function is recommended in all patients who present with heart failure (Table 2-9-3).

Either of these two tests will identify patients with congestive heart failure symptoms and normal LV function. At the initial evaluation, echocardiography may be preferred because it not only estimates right and left ventricular systolic function, but also provides structural information such as LV wall thickness, valvular function, regional myocardial wall motion, and a physiologic assess-

TABLE 2-9-3   **AHCPR Comparisons of Echocardiography and Radionuclide Ventriculography**

Test	Advantages	Disadvantages
Echocardiogram	Permits concomitant assessment of valvular disease, left-ventricular hypertrophy, and left-atrial size Less expensive than radionuclide ventriculography in most areas Able to detect pericardial effusion and ventricular thrombus More generally available	Difficult to perform in patients with lung disease Usually only semi-quantitative estimate of ejection fraction provided Technically inadequate in up to 18% of patients under optimal circumstances
Radionuclide Ventriculogram	More precise and reliable measurement of ejection fraction Better assessment of right-ventricular function	Requires venipuncture and radiation exposure Limited assessment of valvular heart disease and left-ventricular hypertrophy

(From Agency for Health Care Policy & Research Publication No. 94-0612, *Heart failure: evaluation and care of patients with left ventricular systolic dysfunction*, June 1994.)

ment of diastolic function based on Doppler-derived velocity inflow patterns. This information may further define potentially reversible causes. The most frequent reversible etiologies of LV systolic dysfunction include coronary artery disease, valvular heart disease, and alcohol abuse. There is also a spectrum of cardiomyopathies (dilated, restrictive and infiltrative, and hypertrophic heart muscle diseases), metabolic diseases, infectious diseases, and myocardial toxins that have variable responses to specific therapy (see box). Patients with heart failure symptoms and normal LV systolic function are presumed to have diastolic dysfunction and have a better long-term prognosis. Symptomatic therapy for diastolic dysfunction should include heart rate lowering calcium channel blockers and beta-blockers to increase diastolic filling time and diuretics and nitrates to reduce pulmonary venous congestion. Antihypertensive agents that regress LVH are optimal long-term therapies if no other correctable etiology of abnormal diastolic filling is present (CAD, valvular disease, or pericardial disease).

In contrast, left ventricular systolic dysfunction with ejection fractions less than 35% to 40% are associated with significantly increased morbidity and mortality. Strong evidence from multiple large randomized trials demonstrates survival benefits with angiotensin converting enzyme (ACE) inhibitors, and all patients with CHF symptoms and depressed LVEF should be treated with these agents if no contraindications exist. Newer data have demonstrated benefit even in asymptomatic patients with depressed LV function in the prevention of overt CHF and the need for future hospitalizations. These agents act to normalize markers of neurohumoral activation (plasma norepinephrine, plasma renin activity, plasma arginine vasopressin, atrial natriuretic peptide, and low serum sodium) found in CHF by inhibiting the formation of angiotensin II, a potent endogenous vasoconstrictor shown to have a major role in the pathogenesis of peripheral vasoconstriction. This peripheral response to depressed cardiac output leads to increased left ventricular afterload, which in turn leads to more cardiac failure and further neurohumoral activation. This cycle is interrupted by the vasodilating ACE inhibitors and by combination hydralazine–nitrate therapy. The ACE inhibitors have demonstrated greater survival benefit than hydralazine–nitrates when compared directly in a large study.

In the Western societies where CAD prevalence is high, LV dysfunction due to ischemia offers a potential target for therapy. This patient has CAD risk factors including HTN, hypercholesterolemia, tobacco abuse, and possibly adult onset diabetes mellitus. Diabetic patients, in particular, may be more prone to "silent" coronary ischemia and

CAUSES OF SYSTOLIC DYSFUNCTION

ISCHEMIC HEART DISEASE AND MECHANICAL DEFECTS
- Acute myocardial infarction
- Chronic ischemic myocardium
- Papillary muscle dysfunction
- Papillary muscle rupture
- Ventricular septal defect
- Aortic insufficiency
- Aortic stenosis
- Papillary muscle dysfunction or rupture causing mitral regurgitation

PRIMARY MYOCARDIAL DISORDERS "IDIOPATHIC" DILATED CARDIOMYOPATHY INFECTIOUS
- Viral, rickettsial, Trichinella, bacterial, toxoplasmosis, trypanosomal

IMMUNOLOGIC/INFLAMMATORY
- Rheumatic fever, rheumatoid arthritis, systemic lupus erythematosus, sarcoidosis

ENDOCRINE
- Thyroid, pheochromocytoma, Cushing's disease, acromegaly, diabetes

TOXINS
- Ethanol
- Cobalt-beer
- Lead
- Cobalt radiation
- Adriamycin, daunorubicin
- Cocaine

NUTRITIONAL
- Thiamine deficiency
- Pellagra
- Kwashiorkor
- Keshan's disease

INFILTRATIVE
- Hemochromatosis
- Neoplastic
- Amyloid (late)

NEUROMUSCULAR
- Duchenne muscular dystrophy
- Myotonia dystrophia
- Freidreich's ataxia

FAMILIAL
- Familial cardiomyopathy

MISCELLANEOUS
- Obesity
- Peripartum
- Arteriovenous fistula
- Persistent supraventricular tachyarrhythmia

(From Kakavis PW, Barron JT, Parrillo JE: Severe heart failure, In Critical Care Medicine, St Louis, 1995, Mosby.)

therefore require careful evaluation. Elderly patients also tend to have atypical symptoms from coronary ischemia such as confusion, lethargy, and syncope. The left ventricle responds to acutely decreased coronary flow with diastolic dysfunction (decreased compliance) that precedes the systolic regional dysfunction (hypokinesis). In addition to these acute changes, ischemia may also result in chronic depression of myocardial function through stunning and hibernation mechanisms. Stunned myocardium refers to an acute ischemic injury and subsequent myocardial salvage. Temporary contractile dysfunction improves after a variable recovery period. Hibernating myocardium refers to chronically hypoperfused and ischemic myocardium that regains contractile function after adequate restoration of coronary blood flow, usually revascularization with coronary artery bypass graft (CABG) surgery, or percutaneous transluminal coronary angioplasty (PTCA).

QUESTION 5 The echocardiogram revealed moderate LV dilatation and concentric hypertrophy with severely depressed LV systolic function. LVEF was estimated at 30%. The anterior and septal LV regional wall motion was hypokinetic. The aortic valve was thickened but opened normally. The mitral valve was thickened, and moderate mitral regurgitation was present. The left atrium was moderately dilated. The right ventricle and right atrium were normal in structure and function. Which cardiac conditions can present with systolic dysfunction, diastolic dysfunction, or both?

Both systolic and diastolic dysfunction can be seen in cases of ischemic, hypertensive, and hypertrophic cardiomyopathy as well as aortic valvular stenosis. Many conditions that cause this clinical syndrome progress through stages. Acute ischemia, LV hypertrophy, and infiltrative processes often decrease LV filling parameters (diastolic dysfunction) before LV contractile failure (systolic dysfunction) is evident. The utility of objective measurement of LV function in selection of appropriate therapy, therefore, cannot be underestimated even when the clinical diagnosis is known!

This patient's echocardiogram revealed LV systolic dysfunction with dilation and LVH, anterior regional wall motion abnormality, and moderate mitral valvular regurgitation. The regional wall motion abnormality may indicate coronary ischemia or infarction, but regional variation may be present in dilated cardiomyopathy with patent coronary arteries. Acute and chronic mitral valvular regurgitation (MR) may be primary causes of LV systolic dysfunction; however, MR is often present when LV dilatation occurs and the mitral valve annulus is distorted. After treatment of heart failure the mitral regurgitation may decrease significantly. The question of primary MR leading to CHF versus secondary MR from ventricular dilation is often difficult to answer retrospectively. In acute situations the echocardiogram may reveal an acquired mitral valve structural defect (such as a torn chordae tendineae or a ruptured papillary muscle) which can be corrected with surgery. The presence of concentric LVH implies chronic pressure or volume overload and helps exclude hypertrophic cardiomyopathy.

Although multiple etiologies of LV dysfunction are still possible, the echo has excluded critical diagnostic possibilities of structural heart disease that would require specific therapy and in which ACE inhibitors would be contraindicated.

Aortic stenosis (AS) may present with chest pain, CHF, or syncope, and examination reveals a delayed carotid upstroke with a soft or absent aortic component of the second heart sound. Bicuspid aortic valvular stenosis can present in young and middle-aged adults. The use of ACE inhibitors for CHF in patients with AS may result in profound hypotension and possibly death. The therapy is based on surgical aortic valve replacement, and echocardiographic diagnosis based on Doppler data is very accurate when compared to invasive hemodynamics. In advanced AS, as the cardiac output falls, the valvular gradient decreases, and the murmur may be subtle.

Hypertrophic cardiomyopathy (HCM) presents with asymmetric septal hypertrophy leading to subvalvular LV outflow tract obstruction and mitral regurgitation. The LV outflow tract gradient may increase with exercise resulting in hypotension and possibly syncope. An increased risk of sudden death is present, especially in the familial forms. Beta-blockers and calcium channel blockers are used to depress the hypercontractile LV to allow for improved filling and to reduce the outflow tract gradient. AV sequential pacing has also been demonstrated to decrease the LV outflow tract gradient and improve exercise capacity. ACE inhibitors, in contrast, could increase the outflow tract obstruction and lead to hypotension. However, late in the clinical spectrum of this disease, some patients develop LV dilatation and systolic failure and would *then* be appropriate candidates for ACE inhibition.

High output heart failure presents with hypercontractile LV function in the setting of anemia, thyrotoxicosis, pregnancy, arterial-venous shunts (congenital, traumatic, Paget's disease of bone, or AV fistula for hemodialysis) and thiamine deficiency (beriberi). Malnutrition and alcohol abuse is a common cause of severe thiamine deficiency. Increased cardiac output causes heart failure in pregnant women with previously well-tolerated valvular or congenital heart disease. Therapy is based on correction of the underlying cause while decreasing pulmonary congestion with diuretics and nitrates.

Pericardial effusion that presents with predominant right heart failure, elevated JVP, and a pulsus paradoxus (systolic BP drop >10 mm Hg during inspiration) may indicate tamponade physiology. Diuresis and ACE inhibition can lead to profound hypotension. Patients with heart failure and echocardiographic evidence of a pericardial effusion with right heart chamber diastolic collapse should have urgent hemodynamic assessment and may require pericardiocentesis. Although severe chronic CHF may lead to significant pericardial and pleural effusions, an alternative etiology (malignancy or infection) should be excluded. Right pleural effusions are more common in heart failure due to the differential venous and lymphatic drainage capacity.

Heart failure due to inflammatory, infectious, or toxic etiologies usually demonstrates biventricular involvement on echocardiography. Endomyocardial biopsy may be necessary to confirm the diagnosis and select appropriate therapy.

QUESTION 6 The patient received counseling about his diagnosis and the prognosis of heart failure. Daily weight monitoring was started at home. The symptoms and medications (ACE inhibitor and diuretic) were explained. The patient was instructed what to do for worsening symptoms. Information was provided about dietary restrictions (less than 2 grams sodium per day) and the benefits of regular exercise such as walking or cycling. He was immunized for influenza and pneumococcal disease. Stress testing was considered in light of his risk factors for CAD. Which stress test predicts recovery of normal LV function following revascularization?

A. Exercise stress test (EST) with ECG
B. EST with myocardial perfusion scintigraphy (thallium)
C. Dobutamine stress test with echocardiographic imaging
D. Position–emission tomography (PET)
E. None of the above

None of these tests can predict the recovery of global LV function, but demonstrated viability increases the probability that revascularization will improve the regional myocardial wall function.

The benefits of revascularization are greatest in the setting of heart failure, angina pectoris, three vessel CAD or left main coronary stenosis greater than 50%, where CABG revascularization has demonstrated improved survival compared to patients treated medically. Many patients with a history of myocardial infarction have clinically important myocardial ischemia in areas supplied by the other coronary vessels. There are no data demonstrating survival benefits of revascularization in the absence of angina; however, patients with extensive areas of ischemia may benefit from revascularization and should undergo a physiologic test to evaluate for the presence of inducible ischemia.

The likelihood of CAD in patients without MI and without angina varies depending on individual risk factors, and the decision to proceed to physiologic testing should reflect the balance between the likelihood of CAD versus alternative etiologies such as alcoholic cardiomyopathy.

The physiologic stress test using thallium myocardial perfusion imaging is based on poststress, redistribution, and rest reinjection images that demonstrate regional viability by delayed redistribution of tracer to myocardial regions that demonstrated low tracer uptake in the poststress images. Transmural infarction (scar) does not concentrate thallium and appears as a persistent perfusion defect. Echocardiographic stress imaging uses wall motion response to exercise or dobutamine to differentiate infarcted myocardium from viable but ischemic myocardium than can be stimulated to contract with dobutamine infusion. Unfortunately, patients with dilated cardiomyopathy may have thallium perfusion defects and variable echocardiographic regional wall motion even in the presence of widely patent epicardial coronary arteries. Therefore, the noninvasive evaluation used to select patients for angiographic study has less predictive accuracy in

TABLE 2-9-4   Medications for Patient with LV Systolic Dysfunction

Medications	Initial Dose	Target Dose	Study
Captopril	6.25-12.5 mg tid	50 mg tid	SAVE
Enalapril	2.5-5.0 mg bid	10 mg bid	SOLVD
Ramipril	2.5 mg bid	5 mg bid	AIRE
Isosorbide dinitrate	10-20 mg qid	40 mg qid	VHeFT I
Hydralazine (Combination)	12.5-25 mg qid	75 mg qid	VHeFT I

(From Agency for Health Care Policy & Research Publication No. 94-0612, *Heart failure: evaluation and care of patients with left ventricular systolic dysfunction,* June 1994.)

heart failure patients than in patients who present with anginal symptoms.

Cardiac positron-emission tomography (PET) imaging can provide independent assessment of tissue perfusion via flow tracers and myocardial viability via metabolism of ^{18}Fluorodeoxyglucose (FDG). Since glucose utilization is increased in hypoperfused ischemic regions that remain viable, PET is useful in detection of myocardium that may regain contractile function after revascularization.

QUESTION 7 The patient with LV systolic dysfunction should expect symptomatic improvement following the initiation of which therapeutic agents?

A. ACE inhibitors
B. Diuretics
C. Digoxin
D. Hydralazine/nitrates
E. All of the above

Each of these agents will improve symptoms of CHF due to LV systolic dysfunction. Even asymptomatic patients with an LVEF less than 35% started on ACE inhibition benefit from this therapy. This can usually be safely accomplished by low dose ACE inhibitor initiation, (especially in volume depleted patients on diuretic therapy) followed by subsequent titration to target doses (Table 2-9-4). The target dosages were most often used in the clinical trials demonstrating a survival benefit. At present no trials that targeted lower dosages have demonstrated improved survival; therefore, when these agents are used for CHF, the

drug should be increased to target dose unless the patient has significant side effects. These include hypotension, azotemia, intractable cough, and hyperkalemia. Hypotension and azotemia can usually be corrected with diuretic and ACE inhibitor dose adjustments, and the ACE agent should be restarted when blood pressure and renal function are more stable. In renal artery stenosis the efferent glomerular vessels are maximally vasoconstricted by angiotensin II and ACE inhibition in patients with bilateral renal artery stenosis and can result in acute renal failure with anuria.

Diuretics are very effective for treatment of symptoms due to volume overload, and most patients will require a loop diuretic. In highly resistant patients metolazone (a diuretic that inhibits sodium resorption in the distal convoluted tubule) can be given 1 hour before the loop diuretic to improve the diuresis. Although potassium and magnesium supplementation may be necessary, diuretic-induced hypokalemia will be partially alleviated by the potassium-sparing effects of ACE inhibitors.

Digoxin has been used as symptomatic CHF therapy for 200 years without clear documented evidence of survival benefits in randomized clinical trials. Several studies have documented improvements in symptoms and exercise test time by the addition of digoxin, as well as the worsening of heart failure symptoms after digoxin withdrawal. For patients with persistent symptoms despite ACE therapy and diuretics, digoxin may be useful. In the setting of depressed LVEF and atrial fibrillation with a rapid ventricular response, digoxin is especially beneficial. Strong efforts should be directed at restoration and maintenance of normal sinus rhythm. Since the atrial contribution accounts for a large percentage of the LV stroke volume, new onset of atrial fibrillation and loss of the atrial "kick" can be associated with marked clinical deterioration.

Patients who remain symptomatic despite ACE inhibitors, diuretics, and digoxin, may benefit from the addition of nitrates for pulmonary congestive symptoms and hydralazine for symptoms of inadequate forward flow. The ACE inhibitor dose should be maximized before the addition of hydralazine, since greater survival benefits were demonstrated with the ACE inhibitors. Since the currently available direct vasodilators increase the neurohumoral activation and may decrease survival, newer vasodilating agents are now being evaluated in clinical trials.

Patients unresponsive to these agents may require inotropic therapy that can be optimally titrated with invasive hemodynamic monitoring. Two frequently used intravenous inotropic agents, dobutamine (beta receptor agonist) and amrinone (phosphodiesterase inhibitor), stimulate myocardial contractile reserve, decrease systemic vascular resistance, and decrease pulmonary venous congestion. In clinical practice dobutamine is associated with a greater frequency of atrial and ventricular tachyarrhythmias. Amrinone is associated with a greater frequency of hypotension because of its significant vasodilating properties. Although both agents are beneficial in the short-term therapy of severe CHF, they may increase mortality by arrhythmogenic mechanisms.

Cardiac transplantation is currently associated with a greater than 85% 2-year survival in selected patients and holds promise for patients with end-stage heart failure as a result of left ventricular systolic dysfunction.

QUESTION 8   The patient had an exercise thallium stress test that revealed anterior wall hypoperfusion immediately poststress and partial redistribution on delayed rest images. A cardiac catheterization was performed and revealed patent epicardial coronary arteries. ACE inhibitors, diuretics, digoxin, nitrates, and hydralazine at maximum tolerated doses were administered with moderate symptomatic improvement. The patient was considered for cardiac transplantation evaluation. What are the indications and medical contraindications for cardiac transplantation?

The indications for cardiac transplantation include severe angina not amenable to medical or revascularization therapy and symptomatic recurrent ventricular arrhythmias refractory to medical, surgical, and device-based (automatic implantable cardiac defibrillator) therapy. The CHF indications are based on maximal oxygen consumption (VO_2) during exercise rather than the NYHA functional class or the specific LVEF. Patients with maximal VO_2 less than 10 to 15 ml/kg/min with major limitation of daily activities or achievement of anaerobic threshold on stress testing are acceptable candidates for cardiac transplant evaluation. Exclusion criteria include coexistent systemic neoplasms and other illnesses with poor prognosis, active infection or bleeding, psychosocial instability, and alcohol or drug dependency. Pulmonary hypertension with elevated pulmonary vascular resistance (greater than 5 Wood units or 3 Wood units after treatment with vasodilators) requires evaluation before transplant. Chronically elevated pulmonary pressures from left heart failure lead to abnormal pulmonary vasculature and may progress to structural arterial changes. Chronically elevated pulmonary artery pressures may become irreversible and lead to right ventricular hypertrophy.

A donor heart that was not exposed to such high chronically elevated pulmonary artery pressures would develop right ventricular failure forced to contract against an abnormal afterload (without time to develop adequate hypertrophy) in the pulmonary arterial system. In cases of severe pulmonary arterial hypertension and end-stage heart failure, consideration should be given to a combined heart-lung transplant procedure.

BIBLIOGRAPHY

Agency for Health Care Policy and Research Publication No. 94-0612, *Heart failure: evaluation and care of patients with left ventricular systolic dysfunction,* June 1994.

AIRE Investigators: Effect of ramipril on mortality and morbidity of survivors of acute myocardial infarction with clinical evidence of heart failure, *Lancet* 342:821-828, 1993.

Cohn JN, Archibald G, Ziesche S, et al: Effect of vasodilator therapy on mortality in chronic congestive heart failure: results of a veteran's administration cooperative study, *N Engl J Med* 314:1547-1552, 1986.

Cohn JN, Johnson G, Ziesche S, et al: A comparison of enalapril with hydralazine—isosorbide dinitrate in the treatment of chronic congestive heart failure, *N Engl J Med* 325:303-310, 1991.

Kakavis PW, Barron JT, Parrillo JE: Severe heart failure. In Parrillo JE, Bone RC, editors: *Critical Care Medicine,* St Louis, 1995, Mosby.

Pfeffer MA, Braunwald E, Maye LA, et al: Effect of captopril on mortality and morbidity in patients with left ventricular dysfunction after myocardial infarction: results of the SAVE trial, *N Engl J Med* 327:669-677, 1992.

SOLVD Investigators: Effect of enalapril on mortality and development of heart failure in asymptomatic patients with reduced left ventricular ejection fractions, *N Engl J Med* 327:685-691, 1992.

SOLVD Investigators: Effect of enalapril on survival in patients with reduced left ventricular ejection fractions and congestive heart failure, *N Engl J Med* 325:293-302, 1991.

CRITICAL CARE

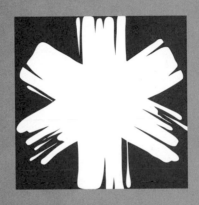

CHARLES J. GRODZIN
SECTION EDITOR

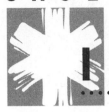
The patient is a 47-year-old African-American man who came to the emergency room with complaints of blurred vision, nausea, headache, and increasing shortness of breath for the past 2 days. The patient has a 10-year history of hypertension and gives the ER physician a history of noncompliance with his medications. The patient denies any history of chest, abdominal, or back pain. He reports a history of crack cocaine use in the past but states that he has "been clean" for the past 6 months. He also denies use of prescription drugs or over-the-counter medications.

Physical examination reveals a mildly confused man with the following vital signs: BP 270/130 mm Hg in both arms, HR 95 bpm, T 100°F, RR 20/min. The pupils are equal and reactive to light. The conjunctiva are injected. Funduscopic examination reveals bilateral flame hemorrhages with papilledema. There are no carotid bruits and there is no jugular venous distension. Cardiovascular examination reveals a normal S_1 and S_2. An S_3 is present, and the PMI is displaced laterally to the anterior axillary line. Pulses are brisk and palpable in all extremities. Pulmonary examination reveals bibasilar crackles. The patient's abdomen has normal active bowel sounds, is soft, and has no evidence of abdominal bruits. The chest x-ray reveals bilateral pulmonary vascular redistribution.

QUESTION 1 What is the difference between hypertensive emergency, hypertensive urgency, accelerated hypertension, and malignant hypertension?

Hypertensive emergencies and urgencies are defined on the basis of clinical data rather than absolute blood pressure measurements. The title *malignant hypertension* is synonymous with *hypertensive emergency* and has largely been replaced. This distinction is important due to the different consequences of an elevated blood pressure in a person with chronic compensated hypertension as opposed to a person who is previously normotensive and in the determination of treatment. Hypertensive emergency is defined as a severe elevation in blood pressure, usually with a diastolic pressure greater than 130 to 140 mm Hg and evidence of end-organ damage. This situation calls for a reduction in the mean arterial pressure by 25% or a reduction of diastolic pressure, 100 to 110 mm Hg.

End-organ damage as a result of severe hypertension may consist of the following: hypertensive encephalopathy with papilledema, acute left ventricular failure with pulmonary edema, aortic dissection, unstable angina, acute subarachnoid hemorrhage, intracerebral bleed, and azotemia.

Hypertensive urgency involves severe hypertension but without evidence of end-organ damage. This syndrome presents a less threatening prognosis. Oral medications are usually effective and control of blood pressure should be achieved within 24 to 48 hours.

The definition of *accelerated malignant hypertension* must also be addressed. This involves retinal hemorrhages and exudates with or without papilledema and is considered an emergency only if evidence of target organ damage is present.

The patient in the case presented is considered a hypertensive emergency as defined by severe hypertension with encephalopathy and left ventricular failure. Patients tend to be male rather than female and African-American with a peak between the ages of 40 and 50 years. The patient also has preexisting hypertension with non-compliance to treatment. Secondary causes of malignant hypertension should be suspected in patients with no prior hypertensive history and in those less than 30 or greater than 60 years of age.

QUESTION 2   What are the important historical points that should be elicited while interviewing this patient?

The patient's history should be geared toward determining the cause of the hypertensive crisis, as well as the presence of end-organ damage. The causes of a hypertensive crisis are many. However, it is most commonly seen in patients with preexisting essential hypertension that is poorly controlled. A thorough history of preexisting hypertension and compliance with medications, especially those with a potential for rebound (alpha antagonists and beta-blockers), is essential.

Use of medications that may precipitate hypertensive crisis must also be elicited. Illicit drugs are well-known causes of accelerated hypertension. A thorough history of cocaine, amphetamines, and other sympathomimetic drugs, including over-the-counter preparations, is essential. A history of prior use of prescription drugs such as oral contraceptives, corticosteroids, monoamine oxidase (MAO) inhibitors, and tricyclic antidepressants may be a cause of accelerated hypertension. A history of prior renal disease or vasculitis may also be helpful. With the history of noncompliance, a list of the specific agents the patient used is necessary to rule out malignant hypertension caused by abrupt antihypertensive withdrawal. It may be necessary to call the patient's family or home so that all the pharmocologic agents a patient has been taking can be found.

Other causes of hypertensive crisis include renovascular hypertension, acute or chronic renal failure, vasculitis, eclampsia, head injury, and burns.

QUESTION 3   What elements of the physical examination and laboratory evaluation are important in the evaluation of this patient?

Laboratory findings are as follows:
- Na 140 meq/dl K 3.4 meq/dl Cl 110 meq/dl
- CO_2 32 meq/l
- BUN 82 mg/dl Cr 2.3 mg/dl
- Urine - 2+ proteinuria
- 10 RBC/per high power field
- CBC hemoglobin of 13.2 g/dl with a moderate amount of schistocytes on the peripheral smear

- -

PHYSICAL EXAMINATION MANIFESTATIONS OF HYPERTENSIVE EMERGENCY

- Diastolic blood pressure >140 mm Hg
- Funduscopic examination: hemorrhage, exudate, papilledema
- Neurologic examination: headache, confusion, somnolence, stupor, visual loss, focal neurologic deficits, seizure, coma
- Cardiac examination: prominent apical impulse, cardiac enlargement, congestive heart failure
- Renal: oliguria, azotemia
- Nausea/vomiting

- -

(Adapted from Kaplan NM: Clinical hypertension, ed 5, Baltimore, 1990, Williams and Wilkins.)

The physical examination should target the determination of end-organ damage. The major foci of organ evaluation should concentrate on the optic fundi, central nervous system, heart, lung, and peripheral vasculature (see box).

A thorough ophthalmologic examination is vital in hypertensive crisis. Papilledema results from increased pressure surrounding the optic nerve inhibiting venous outflow. This causes decreased delivery of blood and subsequent injury to the cells of the optic disc. Intracellular swelling of nerve fibers results in papilledema. Flame hemorrhages are a result of arteriolar constriction damaging the capillary endothelium, resulting in hemorrhage into the area surrounding the optic disc. Cotton wool patches or exudates are due to an infarction of the nerve fiber layer in the retina as a result of arteriolar occlusion.

Siegrist's streaks are "chains of pigment spots along a sclerosed choroidal artery." Elschnig's spots, white areas in the retina, or black pigment over a yellow or red halo representing fibrinoid occlusion of choriocapillaries with overlying retinal detachment, may also be seen in malignant hypertension.

Physical examination should include blood pressure measurement in both arms to evaluate a pressure difference that might suggest aortic dissection or coarctation of the aorta. Orthostatic blood pressure measurements are important as patients with malignant hypertension tend to be volume depleted from a pressure associated diuresis. Some patients with pheochromocytoma may demonstrate lability of blood pressure upon standing.

The cardiovascular examination should revolve around cardiac manifestations of hypertension, chiefly signs of chamber enlargement and congestive heart failure.

The patient presents in mild to moderate left ventricular failure based on a history of increasing shortness of breath, presence of an S_3, bibasilar crackles, and findings on chest radiograph. Absence of chest, abdominal, or back pain decreases the likelihood of myocardial ischemia and dissecting aneurysm.

In patients with renal dysfunction one may observe Lindsay's "half and half" nails, identified by proximal pink or white discoloration and distal brown or dark red pigmentation with loss of the lunula. Livedo reticularis may be an accompanying finding in cases of vasculits or collagen vascular disease.

Signs of neurologic events should also be sought including stroke and transient ischemic attacks. The Cushing's reflex is seen in cases of significant brain injury and consists of hypertension and bradycardia.

A mild hemolytic anemia may result as a consequence of systemic vasoconstriction secondary to high levels of catecholamines, vessel wall injury, and deposition of fibrin. Schistocytes are produced when red blood cells are sheared by fibrin molecules leading to hemolysis.

The patient gives no history of renal problems and has no physical evidence of parenchymal renal disease. Laboratory values consistent with mild azotemia and proteinuria may indicate parenchymal renal disease as a cause or result of malignant hypertension. Hypokalemia may be a sign of hyperaldosteronism.

QUESTION 4 The patient is disoriented to time and place but answers questions slowly and appropriately. Reflexes are brisk but symmetric. The remainder of the neurologic examination is nonfocal. During the patient's stay in the emergency room he begins to refer to his daughter as his wife and states that you are his long-lost brother. He also complains of a pressure-like headache. What is accountable for this patient's altered mental status?

The patient's symptoms of disorientation and headache are consistent with hypertensive encephalopathy. The syndrome exists when patients have malignant hypertension with symptoms of headache, depressed alertness, impaired intellectual ability, delirium, generalized seizures, or cortical blindness without focal neurologic abnormalities. This syndrome is due to acute dilatation of cerebral arterioles leading to increased intracranial pressure and vessel wall damage with resultant increased vascular permeability and edema.

Cerebrovascular autoregulation is the reflex that maintains perfusion to capillary beds despite changes in perfusion pressure. This mechanism is intact up to a mean arterial pressure of 180 mm Hg. Above this level, known as the breakthrough barrier, vessels acutely dilate leading to cerebral edema and altered mental status. Patients who are usually normotensive develop encephalopathy more easily than those who are chronically hypertensive. The mental status changes are reversible with reduction of blood pressure if not explained by any other metabolic or neurologic abnormalities.

One may encounter mental status changes during the onset of therapy. In such a case, it is important to decide whether the alterations are due to hypertensive encephalopathy or a decrease in cerebral perfusion as the blood pressure is lowered. This may be differentiated by prompt improvement in mental status as the blood pressure is lowered. In this situation, the diagnosis is hypertensive encephalopathy. If the mental status deteriorates as the blood pressure is lowered, the blood pressure should be maintained to avoid cerebral hypoperfusion. One should then also consider the diagnosis of subarachnoid hemorrhage, intracranial hemorrhage, blunt head injury, or intracranial tumor as a source of hypertension and headache.

QUESTION 5 The electrocardiogram shows left ventricular hypertrophy with a strain pattern. What is the major risk of decreasing the blood pressure acutely in this patient? What is the differential diagnosis of a hypertensive crisis?

The mechanism of autoregulation (as described above) also harbors the responsibility of protecting distal capillary beds from systemic pressures via vasoconstriction. This response persists even after the blood pressure has been lowered. Therefore, if perfusion pressure falls before vasoconstriction resolves, the result may be severe end-organ hypoperfusion leading to end-organ ischemia (e.g., myocardial infarction, renal infarction, CVA, seizure, spinal infarction, or mesenteric ischemia).

Chronic elevation of the blood pressure leads to hypertrophy of the vascular intima leading to persistent vasoconstriction with inability to vasodilate, requiring an elevated blood pressure to maintain end-organ perfusion. This is the origin of the term "essential" hypertension. Necrotizing arteriolitis may follow and is appreciated in the optic fundus and juxtaglomerular apparatus (JGA). This can lead to irreversible retinal damage and stimulation of renin and angiotensin, further exacerbating hypertension. In such cases, an angiotensin-converting enzyme inhibitor may be useful therapy.

The differential diagnosis is broad, and there

DISEASE PROCESSES THAT MUST BE DIFFERENTIATED FROM HYPERTENSIVE CRISIS

- Left ventricular failure
- Uremia
- Cerebrovascular accident
- Subarachnoid hemorrhage
- Brain tumor
- Head injury
- Epilepsy - Postictal state
- Collagen vascular diseases (SLE, vasculitis)
- Encephalitis
- Overdose or withdrawal of narcotics or amphetamines
- Hypercalcemia
- Acute anxiety and hyperventilation syndrome

(Adapted from Braunwald E: Heart disease: a textbook of cardiovascular medicine, ed 4, Philadelphia, WB Saunders, 1992.)

are many syndromes that mimic hypertensive crisis (see box). The most common secondary cause of a hypertensive crisis is renovascular disease. This may be seen as the fibromuscular type in young women and as a manifestation of atherosclerosis in older men. Both Conn's syndrome (primary hyperaldosteronism) and pheochromocytoma are less common. Nonetheless, one should include questions about headache, hyperhidrosis, palpitations, and weight loss as part of the complete history. The physical examination should pay particular attention to such signs as tachycardia, lability of blood pressure on standing and a relative lack of retinopathy, glomerulopathy, and cardiac decompensation.

Additional causes include rebound after withdrawal of medications such as alpha-agonists, beta-blockers and, less commonly, calcium antagonists and minoxidil. Ingestion of tyramine found in aged cheese and Chianti wine may cause hypertension in individuals on MAO inhibitors. Use of oral contraceptives in young women should also be considered. Use of phencyclidine and cocaine may also cause hypertension.

Acute intermittent porphyria presenting with hypertension, abdominal pain and discolored urine may be confused with malignant hypertension with hematuria. In the obstetric population preeclampsia and eclampsia should be considered. IgA nephropathy, acute glomerulonephritis, systemic vasculitis, and 17-alpha hydroxylase deficiency should also be considered in the correct clinical settings.

QUESTION 6 What is the appropriate therapeutic management of patients with hypertensive crisis?

The most important aspect of the treatment of a hypertensive crisis is rapid control of the blood pressure with the ability to make minute-to-minute changes. Therefore, a short-acting IV preparation is the ideal therapeutic agent. The initial goal of therapy is to lower the mean arterial pressure by 15% or the diastolic blood pressure to 100 to 110 mm Hg or by 25% of the initial value, whichever is higher.

Successful treatment of hypertensive emergency requires IV infusion of antihypertensive drugs coupled with intra-arterial monitoring of blood pressure. This is best done in an intensive care unit. To some extent, the agent of choice varies based on the underlying disease process.

The treatment of choice in most settings is nitroprusside, which works as a potent balanced arterodilator and venodilator leading to reduction of afterload and preload. This drug has a very short half-life that allows easy titration and is very effective in decreasing blood pressure to desired level. The initial dose is 0.05 µg/kg/min and is increased by 0.05 to 0.1 µg/kg/min every 3 to 5 minutes until the desired blood pressure reduction. An alternate approach is to begin the infusion at 5 µg/min and titrate the dose upwards as dictated by the blood pressure response. When infusion is prolonged (greater than 48 to 72 hours) or there is underlying renal or hepatic insufficiency, one must be aware of thiocyanate toxicity. Thiocyanate is the metabolic end-prod-

uct of nitroprusside and leads to nausea, fatigue, and muscle spasms.

The next agent of choice is IV nitroglycerin (NTG). This agent is especially useful for patients with coronary artery disease, congestive heart failure, or angina. Delivery of this agent may be variable due to interaction with IV tubing compared to nitroprusside. This may make titration of the dose and smooth blood pressure control more difficult. Additionally, there is development of tachyphylaxis to nitrates that may lead to inadequate blood pressure control. One may need to empirically increase the dose to maintain tight blood pressure control.

Labetolol, a beta-blocker, may be administered by IV minibolus (25 mg → 50 mg → 100 mg) until the desired blood pressure effect is obtained or via continuous IV infusion. When this agent is used intravenously, the relative beta:alpha blockade shifts from 3:1 to 7:1. Therefore, one must be careful of exacerbating hyperglycemia or bronchospasm in some patients.

Certain clinical scenarios may be treated with specific agents (e.g., the use of the combination of alpha-blockade with phenoxybenzamine and subsequent beta-blockade in the management of pheochromocytoma). Beta-blockers are used in the treatment of a dissecting aortic aneurysm to decrease shear forces (dP/dT). Alternatively, trimethaphan may be used as an individual agent in this case. Left ventricular failure and volume overload are indications for the use of diuretics.

The transition to oral medications is the next step after satisfactory blood pressure control has been achieved. These should be initiated within the first 24 hours of hospital admission provided the blood pressure has come under adequate control. While there is no set guideline regarding which agent to use, the clinical history may provide clues. For patients who retain salt and water (renal insufficiency/failure), the combination of a vasodilator and diuretic is recommended. In cases of high sympathetic tone and hyperreninemia, an ACE inhibitor or beta-blocker may be useful. Cases of congestive heart failure leading to elevated blood pressure may be approached

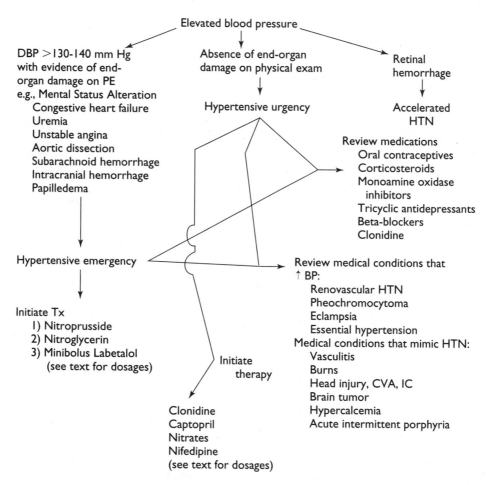

Elevated blood pressure

DBP >130-140 mm Hg
with evidence of end-
organ damage on PE
e.g., Mental Status Alteration
    Congestive heart failure
    Uremia
    Unstable angina
    Aortic dissection
    Subarachnoid hemorrhage
    Intracranial hemorrhage
    Papilledema

Absence of end-organ
damage on physical exam

Hypertensive urgency

Retinal
hemorrhage

Accelerated
HTN

Review medications
    Oral contraceptives
    Corticosteroids
    Monoamine oxidase
        inhibitors
    Tricyclic antidepressants
    Beta-blockers
    Clonidine

Hypertensive emergency

Initiate Tx
  1) Nitroprusside
  2) Nitroglycerin
  3) Minibolus Labetalol
      (see text for dosages)

Review medical conditions that
↑ BP:
    Renovascular HTN
    Pheochromocytoma
    Eclampsia
    Essential hypertension
Medical conditions that mimic HTN:
    Vasculitis
    Burns
    Head injury, CVA, IC
    Brain tumor
    Hypercalcemia
    Acute intermittent porphyria

Initiate
therapy

Clonidine
Captopril
Nitrates
Nifedipine
(see text for dosages)

3-1-1   Diagnostic algorithm for malignant hypertension.

with afterload reduction with nitrates or ACE inhibitors.

Hypertensive urgencies may be managed with oral medications. One method is to administer clonidine 0.2 mg followed by 0.1 mg/hr until control of blood pressure or until a total of 0.6 mg has been given. Oral captopril may be started with an initial dose of 6.25 to 25 mg with response seen in 15 to 30 minutes. Another method includes the use of calcium channel blockers (especially nifedipine) by the bite-and-swallow method. This provides a smooth onset of action as opposed to the sublingual administration that may abruptly decrease the blood pressure to unacceptably low levels. Other agents that may be used include nitrates and minoxidil. A diagnostic algorithm for malignant hypertension is shown in Fig. 3-1-1.

CASE FOLLOW-UP   The patient was admitted to the medical intensive care unit, and his blood pressure was controlled with IV nitroprusside. His mental status returned to normal. He underwent renal arteriography and collection of urine for metanephrines. However, both tests were normal. On the second hospital day, he was placed on enalapril and furosemide. He was discharged without complication on the fifth hospital day to follow-up in the general medical clinic daily for the next 3 days for blood pressure checks with a return appointment to see the physician in 1 week.

• •

BIBLIOGRAPHY

Braunwald E: *Heart disease: a textbook of cardiovascular medicine,* ed 4, Philadelphia, WB Saunders, 1992, p 843-847, 852-871.

Hall JB, Schmidt GA, Wood LH: *Principles of Critical Care,* New York, McGraw-Hill, 1992, p 1563-1571.

Wilkins EW: *Emergency medicine: scientific foundations and current practices,* Baltimore, Williams & Wilkins, 1989, p 133-142.

C A S E

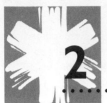

2

Catherine Dimou
Charles J. Grodzin
Robert Balk
• • • • • • • •

The patient is a 26-year-old white woman with a history of depression who was found by her parents in an unconscious state. She has been treated with 150 mg of amytriptiline daily for depression and was found with an empty prescription bottle next to her. Her parents state that when they left the house 1½ hours before finding their daughter, she appeared to be moderately depressed. The parents provided a history that the patient used marijuana while in college but, to their knowledge, has not used any other prescription, over-the-counter, or recreational drugs in the recent past.

QUESTION 1 What is the important epidemiologic data about toxic ingestions?

The evaluation of a patient having overdosed on illicit drugs or medications is commonplace. Seventy percent of such ingestions occur in children less than 5 years of age. In most circumstances, ingestions by children are accidental while ingestions in adults are usually deliberate and purposeful. Suicide is the third most common cause of death in adolescents, and poisonings are the most common cause of death in this age group. In addition to medical evaluation, it is important to also pursue psychiatric evaluation.

QUESTION 2 The patient's vital signs are as follows: T 102°F, HR 120 bpm, BP 110/70 mm Hg, RR 12/min. The patient breathes spontaneously and appears flushed. Her pupils are equal but dilated to 6 mm bilaterally and react weakly to light. Cardiovascular examination reveals tachycardia with a normal S_1 and S_2. Extra heart sounds and murmurs

are absent. The lungs are clear. Abdominal examination is remarkable for hypoactive bowel sounds with mild distension. Her belly is soft with no point tenderness. Neurologic examination reveals an obtunded patient who responds to pain, moves all four extremities, and has no focal abnormalities except for diffusely hyperactive reflexes. What are the important tenets in the treatment of a patient who is suspected of having a toxic ingestion?

The first priority is general support of the patient with emphasis on the airway and ventilation, maintenance of the blood pressure, the cardiac rhythm, and a rapid evaluation of the level of consciousness. Initially, specific management of the agent ingested is of secondary importance. The patient should be monitored continuously for signs of improvement or deterioration of mental status.

The next priority is to determine the specific agent(s) ingested, the number and strength of the pills, and the time frame of the ingestion. To determine this, one must not only take a history from the patient, but from objective observers (e.g., family, friends, paramedics, police, or pharmacists). It is important to obtain the pill bottles with special attention to the number of pills remaining and the date the prescription was last filled. It is common that patients are dropped off at the hospital once the patient is under medical care when illicit drugs are involved.

It is essential to send specimens of blood and/or urine for toxicologic screening as well as any pills possessed by the patient. Because this information usually takes several hours to return, treatment must begin before identification of the specific agent. Suspicion must remain high as to the concurrent use of alcohol as combined ingestion is common.

QUESTION 3   Anesthesia is called to intubate the patient to ensure an adequate airway. A large bore IV is placed and 100 mg thiamine, 1 ampule of D_{50}, 1 ampule of naloxone, and 1 ampule of flumazenil are given without an appreciable change in the patient's condition.

An ECG shows sinus tachycardia with right axis deviation, QRS interval of 0.12 msec, and QT interval of 0.42 msec. After the ECG, the patient suffered a generalized tonic-clonic seizure treated with 2 mg of Lorazepam intravenously with resolution of the seizure activity. The cardiac monitor showed a wide-complex tachycardia at a rate of 150 bpm. Her blood pressure dropped to 80 mm Hg systolic. The patient is hyperventilated, and 70 mg of lidocaine is given IV push and followed by an infusion at 2 mg/minute. The patient returns to a sinus tachycardia with a blood pressure of 110/70 mm Hg. What is the differential diagnosis and initial approach to evaluation of a patient suspected of a toxic ingestion? What criteria should be used to determine whether hospital admission is required?

Many clinical syndromes presenting with alteration of mental status may mimic or be a consequence of a toxic ingestion. Patients should be evaluated by laboratory examination to find a possible etiology to explain the alteration of mental status. Metabolic abnormalities such as hypoglycemia or hyperglycemia, electrolyte imbalances, thyroid dysfunction, rhabdomyolysis uremia, and hepatic failure may be suspected from the serum chemistries. Central nervous system disease, including a postictal state, blunt head injury, intracranial hemorrhage, and meningoencephalitis can account for similar changes. Evaluation of the patient's body temperature will detect hypothermia. Therefore, the initial laboratory evaluation should include serum electrolytes including calcium and glucose, and an arterial blood gas for determination of ventilation, oxygenation and pH, a creatine phosphokinase level (may support diagnosis of rhabdomyolysis), urinalysis

GUIDELINES FOR HOSPITAL ADMISSION

* Severe alteration of blood pressure
* Severe alteration of body temperature
* Anticholinergic crisis
* Cardiac arrhythmias
* Alterations of mental status
* Decreased urine output or uremia
* Alteration of gas exchange (hypoxia or hypercapnea)
* Suspected pulmonary edema or capillary syndrome
* Aspiration pneumonia
* Relapsing symptoms of the toxic ingestion

(Adapted from Wilkins EW: Emergency medicine, Baltimore, 1989, Williams & Wilkins.)

(pink discoloration also consistent with rhabdomyolysis), and urine and serum drug screening.

After consideration of the above differential diagnosis, patients should receive 50 to 100 ml of a 50% dextrose solution preceded by 50 to 100 mg of thiamine to avoid an acute exacerbation of the Wernicke-Korsakoff syndrome. Naloxone administration will rapidly reverse the respiratory depression and hemodynamic instability seen in narcotic overdose. Narcotic use may be suspected when needle tracks are present or when the pupils are pinpoint bilaterally. Administration of 1 to 2 ampules initially is followed by monitoring of a response. Because some agents are long lasting, the patient may require intermittent dosing of naloxone as determined by relapsing obtundation. Flumazenil is an analogous agent used for the reversal of the effects of benzodiazepines.

The decision concerning hospital admission is based on several tenets (see box). Largely, the level of consciousness is the determining factor. In addition, the patient's intent in ingesting the agent must also be considered. If suspicion remains that the patient is at high risk for harming himself or others, hospital admission is necessary.

TABLE 3-2-1 **Specific Antidotes for Some Toxic Substances**

Poison	Antidote
Acetaminophen	N-Acetylcysteine
Anticholinergic agents	Physostigmine
Carbon monoxide	Oxygen
Cyanide	Amyl or Sodium nitrate
Ethylene glycol	Ethanol
Iron	Desferoxamine mesylate
Narcotics	Naloxone
Nitrites or nitrates	Methylene blue
Organophosphates	Pralidoxime

(Adapted from Wilkins W: *Emergency medicine*, Baltimore, 1989, Williams & Wilkins.)

Depending on the degree of medical instability, patients may be admitted to the medical intensive care unit or the general medical floor as long as the patient can be continuously observed. When the ingestion is minor, direct admission to a psychiatric unit may be considered.

QUESTION 4 When the patient is stabilized, a nasogastric tube is placed. Gastric lavage is performed, and 30 to 50 grams of activated charcoal with sorbitol is administered. Dilantin 300 mg is also given by slow intravenous infusion. ECG at this time shows sinus tachycardia with a rate of 100 bpm, right axis deviation, and a QRS interval of 0.10 msec. What are the basic aspects of management of toxic ingestions?

Treatment of toxic ingestions focuses on removal of the drug from the patient's system. In some cases, specific antidotes exist and should be used when the ingested agent is known and the risk-benefit ratio is favorable (see Table 3-2-1). When patients present within 4 to 6 hours of ingestion, induction of emesis or gastric lavage is useful. Emesis may be induced by syrup of ipecac. Ingestion of 30 to 50 ml of ipecac with 8 to 12 ounces of water will induce emesis within 30 minutes. Contraindications include depression of

mental status that may predispose to aspiration. Gastric lavage also requires the patient to be awake and alert. An Ewald tube, or nasogastric tube with an internal diameter of at least 28 French, is used to remove pill fragments. The tube is inserted into the stomach with the patient in the left lateral decubitus position to facilitate mixing of stomach contents with 5 to 10 liters of physiologic saline. Contraindications to both of these procedures include ingestion of strong alkali or corrosives including lye, ammonia, and strong acids.

When the ingestion is greater than 6 hours before presentation or the patient ingests strong alkali or acidic material, use of activated charcoal may be effective. Thirty grams of activated charcoal is administered with sorbitol orally or via a nasogastric tube. Repetitive doses may be given every 2 to 6 hours as some toxins undergo enterohepatic circulation. Activated charcoal is most useful for nonprotein-bound water soluble agents (e.g., phenobarbital, theophylline, and carbamazepine).

Elimination of agents may be hastened by diuresis or manipulation of urinary pH. Water soluble nonprotein-bound agents (e.g., phenobarbital, meprobamate, amphetamines, and lithium) may be eliminated by administration of 200 to 400 ml of saline per hour followed by a loop diuretic. Alkalinization of the urine (pH greater than 8) may hasten the elimination of barbiturates, salicylates, and isoniazid. Acidification of the urine (pH less than 5) with the use of ascorbic acid or ammonium chloride may hasten the elimination of phencylcidine and amphetamines.

Hemodialysis is not believed to be better than forced diuresis as outlined above. However, hemodialysis rapidly removes methanol, ethylene glycol, and heavy metals in conjunction with chelating agents. Charcoal hemoperfusion, using a charcoal column, is useful in the removal of lipid-soluble or protein-bound drugs. However, this requires systemic anticoagulation and leads to consumption of clotting factors and should be saved for specific ingestions. In patients with renal failure, dialysis may be necessary for the general

INDICATIONS FOR INSTITUTION OF DIALYSIS AND TOXINS REMOVED BY DIALYSIS

INDICATIONS

* Ingestion of water-soluble poorly–protein-bound agents
* Extreme toxicity with renal failure and other organ failure
* Potential ingestion of lethal dose of agent

TOXINS WITH HIGH CLEARANCE WITH DIALYSIS

* Acetaminophen
* Amphetamines
* Ethanol, methanol, or ethylene glycol
* Lithium
* Phenobarbital
* Salicylates

(Adapted from Wilkins EW: Emergency medicine, Baltimore, 1989, Williams & Wilkins.)

support of the patient and the removal of toxins. (For more information see the box above.)

QUESTION 5 The patient is transferred to the intensive care unit for further monitoring. Hyperventilation is continued, and she is given bicarbonate to maintain pH at 7.5. The patient is given repeated doses of activated charcoal with sorbitol every 4 hours. The serum tricyclic antidepressant level is 115 ng/ml. The urine toxicology screen is otherwise negative. What are the medical complications associated with toxic ingestions and what is the specific treatment?

Hemodynamic instability may occur. Hypotension is usually due to dilatation of the venous capacitance vessels and should be treated with fluid resuscitation and use of vasopressor agents. Hypertension is commonly seen in overdose of tricyclic antidepressants and MAO inhibitors or secondary to brain injury (Cushing's reflex). It is best to use rapidly acting intravenous agents (e.g.,

nitroprusside) so that control of the blood pressure is rapid and flexible.

Respiratory failure may be due to central nervous system depression manifesting as hypoventilation with hypercapnea. Pulmonary edema may be a result of parenteral narcotic use because of the presence of adulterants or to high dose salicylate ingestion. Alveolar edema is due to alveolocapillary leak. When mental status is depressed, one must also consider aspiration pneumonia.

Hypothermia is most commonly a result of exposure of the comatose patient to the ambient environment below body temperature, phenothiazines, use of cold fluids for gastric lavage, or acute peritoneal dialysis. Hypothermia may lead to cardiopulmonary depression. Resolution may be achieved by use of warmed cardiopulmonary bypass, peritoneal dialysis, warmed IV fluid, and heated conditioned gas. It is important to avoid vigorous external rewarming as cutaneous vasodilatation may lead to hypotension. Hyperthermia may be a consequence of salicylates, tricyclic antidepressants, anticholinergic agents, ingestion-related seizures, or infection.

The patient's mental status may manifest agitation, hyperactivity, seizure, dystonia, and extrapyramidal syndromes. The treatment of choice for seizures is phenytoin as opposed to diazepam or barbiturates. One must be wary of using agents that may further cloud the patient's mental status. Seizure may be related to primary effects of the toxin, CNS hypoxia, head trauma, severe electrolyte imbalances, or exacerbation of preexisting seizure disorder. Prolonged seizures may lead to rhabdomyolysis and pigment-induced renal failure. Treatment of extrapyramidal syndromes is IV or IM antihistamine (e.g., dyphenhydramine). Restraints should be used for patients at risk for self-injury. As described previously, restraint is preferred as opposed to use of centrally acting depressants.

Renal failure is most commonly due to hypovolemia or pigment-induced nephrotoxicity. Anticholinergic agents may promote urinary retention. Bladder distension should be evaluated, and a Foley catheter placed if necessary.

Relapse of the toxic syndrome may be due to slow gastric emptying as seen with ingestion of anticholinergic agents. Relapse may be secondary to long half-lives, slowed metabolism due to liver disease, polyingestion, enterohepatic circulation of the agent, and high lipid solubility.

QUESTION 6 What are the important characteristics of tricyclic antidepressant overdose and what are the features of the anticholinergic syndrome?

Tricyclic antidepressant overdose occurs approximately 500,000 times per year with a mortality rate as high as 15%. The most common cause of death is related to cardiac toxicity. Tricyclic overdose is the leading cause of death by overdose. Life-threatening complications usually occur within 6 hours of presentation to the hospital but can still be seen up to 24 hours later. Close monitoring is needed during this time.

Cardiovascular toxicity presents with both anticholinergic and quinidine-like effects. The anticholinergic effect manifests itself as tachycardia. Quinidine-like effects may appear in the ECG including (in order of appearance) ST-T wave abnormalities; (including flattening T waves), QRS, QT, and PR prolongation; right bundle branch block; and atrioventricular block. Rhythm disturbances may include supraventricular tachycardias, ventricular tachycardia including *torsades de pointes*, and ventricular fibrillation. Heart block, junctional and idioventricular rhythms, and asystole have also been reported.

Central nervous system (CNS) toxicity is also a major consequence of tricyclic overdose and may take a variety of forms. Confusion, agitation, and visual hallucinations are thought to be related to a central anticholinergic effect. Increased muscle tone, hyperreflexia, clonus, the presence of a Babinski reflex, and extrapyramidal signs including choreoathetoid movement, nystagmus, coma, and seizures may also be observed. CNS toxicity usually resolves when not complicated by an accompanying ischemic encephalopathy.

Most seizures, even when recurrent, usually resolve without consequence. However, seizures can precipitate acidosis that increases the unbound concentration of tricyclics and may result in further cardiac toxicity and hypotension. Changes in mental status are not useful in predicting the occurrence of seizures. The majority of seizures occur early after admission, are not prolonged, and usually dissipate without the initiation of therapy. Treatment of seizures should involve small doses of intravenous benzodiazepines (e.g., diazepam or lorazepam) to initially extinguish the seizure activity if not self-limited. IV phenytoin should be administered next to prevent recurrent seizures. Phenytoin may give the added benefit of narrowing the QRS complex and as seizure prophylaxis. Physostigmine has also been used in the setting of status epilepticus.

Respiratory depression is the most common pulmonary complication seen. Hypoxemia without hypercapnea is usually seen in this situation. Patients, especially those with higher drug levels, are at risk for aspiration and the adult respiratory distress syndrome.

Other clues to tricyclic poisoning include presence of anticholinergic symptoms such as mydriasis with weak reactivity to light and decreased or absent bowel sounds secondary to delayed gastric motility. It is important to note that decreased gastric motility may decrease absorption of the ingested drug. Patients have also been known to exhibit hypothermia or hyperthermia.

Attempts have been made to predict the outcome of these cases. A recent study at the University of Louisville looked at the value of initial ECG findings. Despite the large number of changes that occur with overdose, ECG changes cannot predict the presence nor the degree of tricyclic interaction.

Management of tricyclic antidepressant overdose involves gastric lavage with a large-bore nasogastric/orogastric tube if the patient presents within the first 6 hours of ingestion. Gastric lavage may be performed if the patient presents later than 6 hours and pill fragments are suspected to be in the stomach. Since tricyclic antidepressant

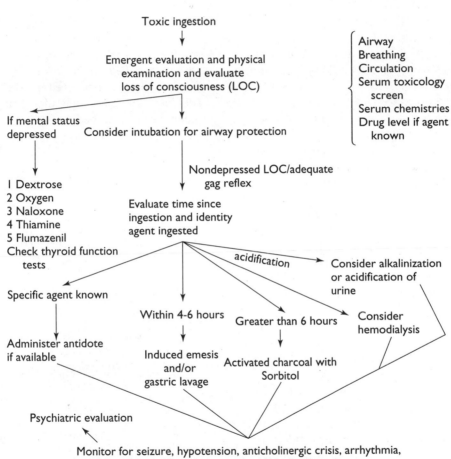

Toxic ingestion

Emergent evaluation and physical
examination and evaluate
loss of consciousness (LOC)

Airway
Breathing
Circulation
Serum toxicology
    screen
Serum chemistries
Drug level if agent
    known

If mental status
depressed

Consider intubation for airway protection

1 Dextrose
2 Oxygen
3 Naloxone
4 Thiamine
5 Flumazenil
Check thyroid function
tests

Nondepressed LOC/adequate
gag reflex

Evaluate time since
ingestion and identity
agent ingested

acidification

Consider alkalinization
or acidification of
urine

Specific agent known

Within 4-6 hours

Greater than 6 hours

Consider
hemodialysis

Administer antidote
if available

Induced emesis
and/or
gastric lavage

Activated charcoal with
Sorbitol

Psychiatric evaluation

Monitor for seizure, hypotension, anticholinergic crisis, arrhythmia,
respiratory depression, and consider ICU administration

3-2-1   Diagnostic algorithm for toxic ingestion.

drugs can lead to decreased gastric motility and the tricyclic antidepressant drugs undergo entero-hepatic circulation, patients should then be given serial doses of activated charcoal with sorbitol. It is estimated that 100 grams of charcoal binds 4 grams of the tricyclic agent.

The mainstay of treatment for cardiovascular toxicity is alkalinization of the serum. Alkalinization may be accomplished either by hyperventilation (goal pH = 7.50 with Pco_2 25-30 mm Hg) or by administration of intravenous sodium bicarbonate. Tricyclics are lipophilic and highly protein bound. Increasing the serum pH results in a decrease in the amount of free tricyclics.

When arrhythmias are present, alkalinization of serum is the first order of treatment. Lidocaine (class IB) is the antiarrhythmic drug of choice. Class IA and IC agents are contraindicated because they may have adverse effects additive to tricyclics. In addition, phenytoin has been shown to narrow the QRS complex; however, its use as an antiarrhythmic has yet to be proven.

QUESTION 7 What adjunct to the medical assessment is necessary in the treatment of a patient with a toxic ingestion?

In addition to the medical evaluation and treatment as described, it is equally important to evaluate the psychiatric stability of the patient. While interviewing the patient, one should inquire as to the purpose of the ingestion. It is also important to determine the social support of the individual. One must recall that even small ingestions may reflect a serious attempt at suicide. One should delay this evaluation until the patient's mental status has cleared. The patient should be separated from any potential hazardous device and placed in a soothing environment. Although ingestions by children are most commonly accidental, thorough questioning is necessary to rule out child abuse by parents, siblings, or peers. A diagnostic algorithm for toxic ingestion is shown in Fig. 3-2-1.

CASE FOLLOW-UP The patient's level of consciousness returns to normal, and the ECG changes resolve. The patient defervesced without a clear source identified for her fever. She is extubated after 18 hours, monitored in the ICU for an additional 24 hours, and then transferred to a monitored medical bed.

• •

BIBLIOGRAPHY

Braithwaite RA, Crome P, Dawlings CG: The invitro and invivo evaluation of activated charcoal as an absorbent of tricyclic antidepressants, *Brit J Clin Pharmacol* 5:389, 1978.

Dziukas L, Vohra J: Tricyclic antidepressant poisoning, *Med J Australia* 154:344-350, 1991.

Ellison DW, Pentel PR: Clinical features and consequences of seizures due to cyclic anti-depressant overdose, *Am J Emerg Med* 7:5-10, 1989.

Lavoie FW, Gausert GG, Weiss RE: Value of initial ECG findings and plasma drug levels in cyclic antidepressant overdose, *Ann Emerg Med* 19:696-700, 1990.

Lituritz T, Normann SA, Veltri JC: 1955 annual report of the American Assn. of Poison Control Center National Data Collection System, *Am J Emerg Med* 6:427-458, 1986.

Roy TM, Ossorio MA, Anderson WH, et al: Pulmonary complications after tricyclic antidepressant overdose, *Chest* 96:852-856, 1989.

Sutherland GR, Park J, Proudfoot AT: Ventilation and acid-base changes in deep coma due to barbiturate or tricyclic anti-depressant poisoning, *Clin Toxicol* 11:403-412, 1977.

Wilkins EW: *Emergency medicine,* Philadelphia, 1989, Williams & Wilkins.

CASE

3

Catherine Dimou
Charles J. Grodzin
Robert Balk

The patient is a 45-year-old woman with a history of lung cancer who came to the emergency room with increasing dyspnea on exertion. The patient was diagnosed with lung cancer 2 months before admission. An outpatient evaluation revealed a 4-cm tumor mass 3.5 cm from the carina, abutting the left mainstem bronchus. CT scanning with intravenous contrast also revealed ipsilateral bronchial lymphadenopathy. Bronchoscopic transbronchial biopsy revealed squamous cell carcinoma ($T_2 N_1 M_0$ or stage II cancer). The patient had a left pneumonectomy and was scheduled for hospital admission for chemotherapy; however, she came today, 3 days early. The patient noted shortness of breath while at home on climbing one flight of stairs. Her shortness of breath progressed until the patient had symptoms with only minimal movement. Her chest x-ray revealed opacification of the left hemithorax, shift of the cardiac silhouette to the left, and a clear but enlarged right hemithorax.

QUESTION I What is the differential diagnosis of shortness of breath in this patient?

Dyspnea is defined as the patient's perception of increasing shortness of breath. This patient is a young woman with recently diagnosed lung cancer. One must differentiate between cardiac and pulmonary causes of dyspnea.

The patient has an underlying malignancy and therefore is at increased risk of pulmonary thromboembolic disease. Pulmonary embolism is usually heralded by acute onset of shortness of breath, chest pain, and increased respiratory rate. This patient describes a progressive increase in

shortness of breath with exertion that would make the diagnosis less likely; however, it must still be considered.

The next process that must be considered is the patient's recent surgery. The patient had a significant smoking history and has had a pneumonectomy. The patient may have had increased shortness of breath while recovering from major surgery. However, the patient has progressive symptoms that make the diagnosis of pulmonary insufficiency secondary to pneumonectomy less likely. Other surgical complications include dehiscence of the tracheal stump or postoperative empyema. In addition, one must keep in mind that there may be progression of previously unknown tumor on the contralateral side.

Cardiovascular causes of dyspnea include ischemia, congestive heart failure, pericardial effusion, and constrictive pericarditis (for more information on pericardial disease see Cardiology Case 6). Pulmonary edema must also be considered in light of the chest x-ray that showed pulmonary vascular redistribution and interstitial edema. However, the patient gives no history of prior cardiac disease. Furthermore, she has recently survived major surgery without incident. Electrocardiograms have not shown evidence of ischemic cardiac disease. It is important to realize that blood flow through the nonsurgical lung is doubled. This may make interpretation of pulmonary vascular redistribution difficult.

A recent autopsy series showed that 15.4% of autopsies involving cancer patients had evidence of metastatic disease to the heart. Fifteen percent of those patients were found to have evidence of cardiac tamponade. Cardiac tamponade results from an accumulation of fluid within the pericardial sac. As the fluid accumulates, intrapericardial pressure is increased, leading to a decreased cardiac output secondary to impaired diastolic filling. This leads to pulmonary congestion, reduced lung compliance, and dyspnea. If this process has been gradually occurring, dyspnea may be of subacute onset.

QUESTION 2   In the emergency room the patient was found to have the following vital signs: T 98.4°F, HR 100 bpm, BP 120/80 mm Hg, and a RR of 32/min. Physical examination was remarkable for jugular venous distension to 5 cm above the sternal notch. Cardiac examination revealed a distant S_1 and S_2 with no S_3 or S_4. Pulmonary examination revealed decreased breath sounds at the left base with a "tubular" component and normal breath sounds throughout the right lung. Abdominal examination was normal. There was no lower extremity edema. Neurologic exam was grossly intact. The patient had a ventilation perfusion lung scan that was negative. Her shortness of breath gradually worsened. The patient was discovered to have a pulsus paradoxus of 20 mm Hg. Upon evaluation by the senior resident, her systolic blood pressure had dropped to 100 mm Hg. Physical examination was significant at that time for soft heart tones. The patient became progressively more dyspneic and obtunded and required elective intubation. How does the physical examination and hospital course to this point impact on your thoughts about the patient's complaint?

This patient manifests a collection of clinical findings highly suggestive of cardiac tamponade. This patient demonstrates the clinical triad of a small quiet heart, elevation of central venous pressure, and a decrease in systemic arterial pressure as described by Dr. Beck in 1935 (Beck's triad). Findings on physical examination vary both by the amount of fluid present in the pericardial space and the rapidity of fluid accumulation. The pericardium normally accommodates from 15 to 50 ml of fluid. Because of the steep pressure-volume relationship of the pericardium, small amounts of fluid may lead to high elevations of intrapericardial pressure. Chronic accumulation of pericardial fluid may be better tolerated as the pericardium stretches to accommodate larger amounts without symptoms.

In patients with a large pericardial effusion, symptoms may result from compression of adjacent organs by the fluid-filled pericardium. These symptoms may include dysphagia from esophageal compression, dyspnea and atelectasis from compression of adjacent lung tissue, cough from bronchial compression, hiccups from involvement of the phrenic nerve, and hoarseness secondary to recurrent laryngeal nerve involvement.

In patients with tamponade the physical examination is very important. In a series of 56 patients, tachypnea was seen in 80%, tachycardia 77%, pulsus paradoxus 77%, pericardial rub 29%, hepatomegaly 55%, and decreased heart sounds in 34%. Other symptoms include restlessness and cold or clammy skin. In addition, jugular venous distension and Kussmaul's sign may be seen. Kussmaul's sign is defined as a paradoxical rise in the jugular venous pressure detected by a rise in the jugular venous filling pressure during inspiration. Ewart's signs describe compression of the left lung base by pericardial fluid with alteration of breath sounds in the left basal area.

A pulsus paradoxus may be present. This is an exaggerated decrease in arterial pressure with inspiration. The maneuver to measure the pulsus paradoxus is as follows: the blood pressure cuff is inflated to the level just above the systolic blood pressure. The cuff is then deflated slowly until the point when the Korotkoff sounds are heard during inspiration. As the cuff is further deflated, one identifies the pressure at which the Korotkoff sounds are heard with the same intensity during both inspiration and expiration. The difference in mm Hg is the pulsus paradoxus. A positive pulsus is present when the pressure difference is greater than 10 mm Hg.

QUESTION 3   Laboratory evaluation revealed a normal electrolyte panel and complete blood count. An arterial blood gas revealed a pH of 7.45, a Pa_{CO_2} of 30 mm Hg, and a Pa_{O_2} of 90 mm Hg. The patient was admitted to the Intensive Care Unit for further evaluation. The patient had a Swan-Ganz pulmonary artery catheter placed that revealed the following:

Right atrial pressure 20 mm Hg
Pulmonary artery systolic/diastolic 40/20 mm Hg
Pulmonary capillary wedge pressure 20 mm Hg

What is a pulmonary artery catheter and what is your interpretation of the above hemodynamic information?

The Swan-Ganz or pulmonary artery catheter is a balloon-tipped, flow-directed, soft-tipped catheter with an associated pressure transducer system that is used to measure the hemodynamic parameters that describe the functional status of the cardiopulmonary system. The catheter is placed into the central circulation and cardiac chambers via the central venous route. The monitoring ports reside in the right atrium, right ventricle, and pulmonary artery. "Wedging" of the catheter is accomplished with inflation of the balloon at the tip of the catheter and occlusion of the pulmonary artery within which it is located. This provides that the distal tip of the catheter is in contact with the left atrium and ventricle via a continuous column of blood. This process allows for the measurement of the left ventricular end diastolic filling pressures and is known as the pulmonary capillary wedge pressure (PCWP) or pulmonary artery occlusion pressure. The normal range is between 8 and 12 mm Hg.

The hemodynamic parameters previously mentioned demonstrate equalization of diastolic pressure and is supportive of a diagnosis of cardiac tamponade. As fluid accumulates in the pericardial space, the pressure in the pericardial space rises. As long as the intrapericardial pressures are above the PCWP, this becomes the chamber's diastolic pressure. Since the right atrium and ventricle are thinner structures, they collapse more easily and cardiac output declines. Because right-sided filling is inhibited as a result of chamber collapse, central venous congestion follows. Early tachycardia may maintain cardiac output,

but as the intrapericardial pressure rises further, cardiac output falls precipitously.

Therefore, the hemodynamic profile of increased right atrial pressure and low cardiac output with equalization of diastolic pressures supports the diagnosis of cardiac tamponade. (See Table 3-3-1 for other hypotensive syndromes and their associated hemodynamic profiles.)

Right heart catheterization is an important diagnostic tool. In this case, the hemodynamic profile indicated the diagnosis directly. Additionally, it allows for the determination of the exact hemodynamic values, can guide pericardiocentesis, and may permit discovery of other cardiovascular alterations.

QUESTION 4 What are the major etiologies of cardiac tamponade? What other syndromes must be differentiated from cardiac tamponade?

The etiologies of cardiac tamponade are varied. The most common causative syndromes are malignancy, idiopathic pericarditis (usually viral), uremia, acute myocardial infarction in a patient on anticoagulants, and bacterial or tuberculous infections. In patients with a prior malignancy treated with radiation to the mantle area, pericardial inflammation may occur. Other causes include myxedema, leaking of a proximal aortic aneurysm, postpericardiotomy syndrome (Dressler's syndrome), serositis seen in systemic lupus erythematosus, and cardiomyopathy.

There are several syndromes that may demonstrate pulsus paradoxus, systemic venous distension, and clear lung fields that must be differentiated from cardiac tamponade. These syndromes include chronic obstructive pulmonary disease, constrictive pericarditis, restrictive cardiomyopathy, severe hypovolemia, and massive pulmonary embolism. This patient did not manifest signs or symptoms of these diagnoses.

QUESTION 5 The patient underwent an echocardiogram that showed a large pericardial effusion with diastolic collapse of the right ventricle during

TABLE 3-3-1   Hypotensive Syndromes and Their Hemodynamic Characteristics

Syndrome	Right Atrial Pressure	Pulmonary Artery Pressure	Pulmonary Capillary Wedge Pressure	Cardiac Index
Hypovolemia	Decreased	Decreased	Decreased	Decreased
Left ventricular failure	Elevated	Elevated	Elevated	Decreased
Right ventricular infarction	Elevated	Normal	Normal	Decreased
Cardiac tamponade	Elevated	Elevated	Elevated	Decreased
Sepsis	Decreased	Decreased, normal or increased	Decreased	Increased or normal

Normal hemodynamic values:

Right atrium 0-8 mm Hg

Pulmonary artery 15-30/3-12 mm Hg

Pulmonary capillary wedge pressure 1-10 mm Hg

Cardiac index 2.6-4.2 L/min/m^2

systole. The patient underwent a pericardial window and had an improvement in her blood pressure. The patient's diastolic cardiac pressures remain equalized. What are the roentgenographic, electrocardiographic, and echocardiographic manifestations of cardiac tamponade?

Roentgenographic findings in cardiac tamponade are variable. The pericardial sac can accumulate up to 250 ml of fluid without a change in the cardiac silhouette. Therefore, a normal cardiac silhouette on chest x-ray may not rule out a pericardial effusion. Classically, the heart may take the shape of a "water bottle." It is important to remember that the chest x-ray only provides a picture of the heart and does not give any functional information.

Electrocardiographic signs of tamponade may include generalized low voltage and electrical alternans. This phenomenon is described as electrical change in the polarity of the QRS complex and/or the T wave. This is a manifestation of the heart swinging in a pendular motion in the fluid-filled pericardium. While not solely due to tamponade (also seen in constrictive pericarditis, tension pneumothorax, and myocardial infarc-

tion), in the presence of a known pericardial effusion, this finding is very specific.

Echocardiogram is one of the mainstays of the diagnosis of cardiac tamponade. The role of echocardiography is to ascertain the presence and size of an effusion, ascertain the presence of pericardial constriction, wall motion abnormalities, right ventricular dysfunction, and visualize extracardiac processes. Another important finding is leftward movement of the interventricular septum reducing left ventricular size during inspiration. This finding correlates with the presence of a pulsus paradoxus. In addition to looking for the effusion, the echo can assist in ascertaining the importance of the amount of hemodynamic compromise. Right ventricular diastolic collapse is the most frequent sign of cardiac tamponade.

QUESTION 6 What is the correct management for the patient found to have cardiac tamponade and what is the physiologic reason for this?

As described previously, forward cardiac flow is obstructed as a result of compression of the cardiac chambers by the pressure in the pericardial space. To improve flow, one must either decrease

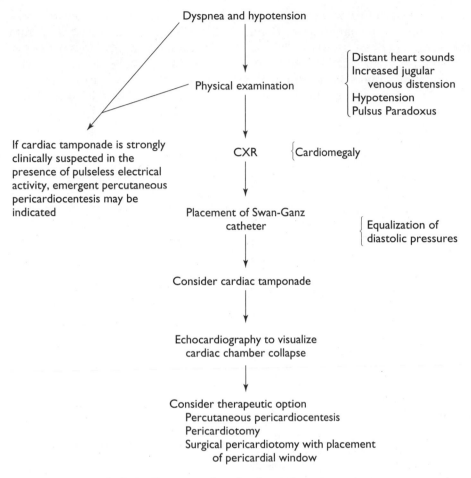

Dyspnea and hypotension

Physical examination

Distant heart sounds
Increased jugular
  venous distension
Hypotension
Pulsus Paradoxus

If cardiac tamponade is strongly
clinically suspected in the
presence of pulseless electrical
activity, emergent percutaneous
pericardiocentesis may be
indicated

CXR { Cardiomegaly

Placement of Swan-Ganz
catheter

Equalization of
diastolic pressures

Consider cardiac tamponade

Echocardiography to visualize
cardiac chamber collapse

Consider therapeutic option
    Percutaneous pericardiocentesis
    Pericardiotomy
    Surgical pericardiotomy with placement
        of pericardial window

3-3-1 Diagnostic algorithm for cardiac tamponade.

the intrapericardial pressure or increase cardiac chamber filling pressures. The latter can be accomplished by increasing the intravascular volume. The fluid of choice must have a high oncotic pressure (0.9 normal saline or albumin) so that it remains in the intravascular space. Another alternative may be to increase cardiac output by using pressor agents norepinephrine or isoproterenol. These agents can augment the available contractility. Hydralazine or nitroprusside can be used to achieve afterload reduction. However, this approach should be used cautiously, since afterload reduction could further reduce the blood pressure significantly.

QUESTION 7 What are the invasive treatment choices and how is a pericardiocentesis done?

In some cases, there is an indication for immediate evacuation of a pericardial effusion. The options include percutaneous pericardiocentesis, pericardiotomy, and surgical pericardiectomy. Percutaneous pericardiocentesis is the easiest and quickest treatment for stable or emergent cardiac tamponade. Potential complications include myocardial, coronary artery, or pulmonary laceration with development of hemothorax or hemopericardium. This procedure is less effective for the treatment of traumatic hemopericardium when there is less than 200 ml of effusion, absence of an anterior collection of fluid, loculated effusion, and clot or fibrin in the pericardial space. In the situation of a leaking ventricular laceration of aneurysm, wherein the fluid will reaccumulate rapidly, this should only be looked on as a temporizing measure.

The procedure should be done in a specialized procedure lab unless emergent. In elective cases, right-heart cardiac catheterization should be carried out first to document baseline pressures. The subxiphoid approach is best as it will avoid the internal mammary artery. An ECG V-lead or precordial lead should be attached to the needle so that recognition of contact with the myocardium can be noted. The skin should be prepared in a sterile fashion, and a small nick should be made with a No. 11 blade. A three-way stopcock should be placed on the end of the syringe with connections to a syringe and a pressure transducer. Once the needle is inserted past the bony xiphoid, the needle is moved to a 15° angle with the skin and advanced toward the head or shoulder. The needle is advanced slowly and smoothly, continually aspirating the syringe until the give of the pericardium is felt and fluid returns. When contact is made with the myocardium, the attached ECG will manifest ST-segment elevation and ventricular premature beats. If no fluid has been withdrawn at that point, the needle is slowly retracted with continual aspiration.

Once the needle is in the pericardial space, it is best to carry out aspiration with a soft plastic catheter 6 to 7 French in size. A guide wire may be inserted through the needle over which a catheter can be placed into the pericardial space. A glass vacuum bottle should not be used, as this may facilitate rapid movement of the heart against the catheter, leading to myocardial trauma. One can identify the fluid aspirated as coming from the pericardial space if it does not clot upon standing.

Fluid should be sent for biochemical analysis including protein, amylase, glucose, cholesterol, and hemoglobin and hematocrit. Microbiologically, gram stain and bacterial, fungal, and tuberculous culture should be sent. The patient should be followed in a critical care unit after the procedure. A diagnostic algorithm for cardiac tamponade is shown in Fig. 3-3-1.

CASE FOLLOW-UP Before these resuscitation efforts, the patient had stated that she did not want prolonged intubation. The patient's condition did not improve, and she was not able to be weaned from the ventilator. After discussion with the patient's family, the patient was made DNR (do not resuscitate). Three days later, the patient went into electromechanical dissociation and expired.

BIBLIOGRAPHY

Braunwald E: *Heart disease: a textbook of cardiovascular medicine*, Philadelphia, 1988, WB Saunders.
Chu H: Ketal left ventricular diastolic collapse, *Circulation* 83:1999-2006, 1991.
Guberman BA, Fowler NO, Engel PJ, et al: Cardiac tamponade in medical patients, *Circulation* 64:633, 1981.
Mukai K, Shinka T, Tominga K, Shimosato Y: The incidence of secondary tumors of the heart and pericardium: a 10 year study, *Japan J Clin Oncol* 18:195-201, 1988.
Okamoto H, Tetsu S, Yamakido M, Saijo N: Cardiac tamponade caused by primary lung cancer and the management of pericardial effusion, *Cancer* 71:938, 1993.
Smith T: *Pathophysiology: the biological principles of disease*, Philadelphia, 1985, WB Saunders.
Unverferth DV, Williams TE, Fulkerson DK: Electrocardiographic voltage in pericardial effusion, *Chest* 75:157, 1979.

CASE

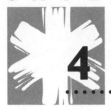

4

Catherine Dimou
Charles J. Grodzin
Robert Balk

•••••••••••

The patient is a 59-year-old man who came to the emergency room with fever of 102°F and urinary frequency. His medical history is significant for hypertension and benign prostatic hypertrophy. He underwent a biopsy of a prostatic nodule on the day before admission to the hospital. The patient is found to be diaphoretic with a respiratory rate of 30/min. His systolic blood pressure is 90 mm Hg. An electrocardiogram revealed sinus tachycardia.

QUESTION 1 What is the differential diagnosis of hypotension?

Shock can be classified into four basic types: cardiogenic, extracardiac obstructive, oligemic, and distributive. Cardiogenic shock may result from reduced systolic function secondary to myocardial ischemia or myocardial dysfunction in sepsis. It can also be caused by mechanical processes such as mitral regurgitation, ventricular septal defect, and left ventricular outflow obstruction.

Extracardiac causes include pericardial tamponade, constrictive pericarditis, severe pulmonary hypertension, and massive pulmonary embolism.

Oligemic shock may result from acute blood loss, massive urinary losses (e.g., postobstructive diuresis), massive GI losses, or from dehydration.

Distributive shock can be caused by sepsis, anaphylaxis, hypoadrenalism, and as a result of neurologic reflexes.

QUESTION 2 The patient received doses of both ceftazidime and vancomycin in the emergency room. The chest x-ray was clear, and the urinalysis

showed 50 WBC/hpf. The CBC was significant for a WBC count of 12,000/mm^3 with 66% segs, 24% bands, and 7% lymphs. What is meant by the SIRS syndrome? What is the definition of bacterial sepsis and what is the relation of sepsis to shock? What are the most common causative agents?

The SIRS syndrome stands for the Systemic Inflammatory Response Syndrome. SIRS may be caused by a variety of infectious and noninfectious causes. This syndrome refers to systemic inflammation related to such etiologies as infection, pancreatitis, visceral ischemia, trauma, hemorrhage, or immunologically mediated injury.

Bacterial sepsis is a systemic inflammatory response to a documented infection characterized by two or more of the following: temperature greater than 100.4°F or less than 96.8°F, heart rate greater than 90 bpm, respiratory rate greater than 20/min or a Paco$_2$ < 32 mm Hg, leukocyte count >12,000 mm^3 or <4000 mm^3 or greater than 10% bands. The term "bacterial" should only be used in situations where a bacterial isolate is cultured and felt to be the source of the SIRS response. The term *sepsis* is used to describe SIRS that is secondary to a documented infection.

Sepsis requires a source of infection which may include an abscess, pneumonia, urinary tract infection, etc. Some of the most frequent pathogens encountered in the intensive care unit include *E. coli, K. pneumoniae, P. aeruginosa* and *S. aureus* (associated with the highest mortality rate). Past studies have shown that greater than 50% of sepsis was caused by gram-negative organisms. More recent investigation has shown an equal distribution between gram-negative and gram-positive organisms. Approximately 49% to 56% of cases of sepsis are secondary to the enterobacteriaceae group and *P. aeruginosa*. Other microbes may also lead to sepsis including gram-positive organisms, fungi, parasites, and viruses. There may be various stages of SIRS or sepsis regarded as a continuum of severity of the inflammatory response. Adverse sequelae include septic shock and multiple organ dysfunction or failure. Sepsis may result in septic shock, which occurs in approximately 40% of patients. The mortality rate of patients with shock is between 40% and 90% and is the leading cause of death in the noncoronary intensive care unit.

QUESTION 3   Because of hemodynamic instability, the patient was transferred to the ICU. An arterial line was placed to monitor blood pressure. The patient had minimal urine output, and a 1000 cc fluid bolus of normal saline failed to improve systolic blood pressure.

A Swan-Ganz pulmonary artery catheter was placed with the following initial readings: pulmonary capillary wedge pressure was 8 mm Hg; systemic vascular resistance was 500 dyne-sec/cm^2. At that time lab results from the urine culture done at the time of the prostatic biopsy were received. The culture was positive for *Proteus mirabilis* sensitive to ceftazidime. What is the pathophysiology of septic shock?

While an infectious or inflammatory cause of sepsis and shock is necessary, it is the release of substances or mediators into the blood stream that leads to the SIRS response. These mediators include both portions of microorganisms and toxins. Endotoxin is a unique component of the gram-negative bacillus cell wall known as lipopolysaccharide (LPS). Regardless of the bacterial source, LPS maintains a common structural make-up, the lipid A and a polysaccharide component being the most conserved portion of the molecule. The lipid A portion is identical from organism to organism.

Endotoxin and other potential mediators and particles stimulate plasma monocytes, endothelial cells, neutrophils, and macrophages to produce the inflammatory cascade and other endogenous mediators of sepsis. Included in the group of potential mediators are interleukins 1, 2, 6, and 8; tumor necrosis factor; oxygen free radicals; hydrogen peroxide; nitric oxide and arachidonic acid metabolites (thromboxane A$_2$, leukotrienes, and prostacyclines); and platelet activating factor. This results in specific and nonspecific immune responses. Tumor necrosis factor (TNF) mediates tumor cell killing, fever, shock, and endothelial cell death. Interleukins 1, 6, and 8 produce similar inflammatory effects as TNF. Additional manifestations of this inflammatory cascade include microbial killing, hypotension, disseminated intravascular coagulation, and progression of the inflammatory cascade that may result in septic shock.

Michie demonstrated that healthy human volunteers, when given a 4 ng/kg IV bolus of endotoxin, released TNF between 60 and 90 minutes later. The amount of TNF released peaked at a level approximately 7 times normal. Furthermore, in some clinical conditions, there appears to be a relationship between the amount of TNF released and survival of the septic patient. In Waage's study of meningococcal meningitis, all patients with a TNF level greater than 440 units/ml died.

IL-1 stimulates pituitary hormone release, increases collagenase secretion, and stimulates prostaglandin production. Immunologically, T and B lymphocyte and marrow stem cells proliferate. IL-6 secretion is stimulated by TNF and mediates acute phase protein responses during inflammation. In some studies high levels of IL-6 have been found to be predictive of high mortality rates in critically ill patients.

These factors also result in arterial and venous dilatation, endothelial cell dysfunction, direct myocardial depression, and multiorgan dysfunction.

In addition to myocardial depression, multiple organs may be involved, resulting in renal failure, acute respiratory distress syndrome (ARDS, noncardiogenic pulmonary edema), and hepatic failure. Organ failure may be a result of the direct effect of the endogenous mediators on the organ or as a secondary result of profound hypotension or altered perfusion of the organ.

QUESTION 4 Results of the prostatic ultrasound showed a parenchymal abscess. What are the clinical and physiologic changes that result in sepsis?

Presenting symptoms in patients with sepsis almost always include fever and chills or hypothermia, lowered blood pressure, tachycardia, and tachypnea. One of the first signs may be a mild respiratory alkalosis that results from tachypnea and increased minute ventilation, probably secondary to mediator effects on the central nervous system respiratory centers. Specific organ system dysfunction appears to be a product of decreased visceral blood flow, with shunting of blood away from the viscera toward the central circulation, leading to ischemia and hypoxemia.

The usual hemodynamic profile accompanying septic shock is a low systemic vascular resistance (SVR) and elevated cardiac output. There is evidence that a direct myocardial depressant substance exists and circulates during sepsis. Thus, one may see a depressed ejection fraction with an increased cardiac output. Tumor necrosis factor has been shown to cause direct myocardial depression in vitro as well. Patients who develop ventricular dilatation early, but whose cardiac index returns to normal, have a faster resolution of hypotension and may have an improved outcome. The decrease in SVR is likely a direct result of the endogenous mediator cascade in sepsis. End products such as kinins and complement cause increased capillary permeability and vasodilatation. Nitric oxide can be synthesized from the amino acid L-arginine by the endothelial cells and leads to direct vasodilatation.

Changes in mentation occur in approximately half of patients with sepsis and may manifest as obtundation, stupor, irritability, confusion, or agitation.

The gastrointestinal systems may also be affected by a decrease in motility. This may be seen clinically as nausea, vomiting, or the development of an ileus. These changes are likely secondary to decreased blood flow with disordered perfusion. This same mechanism may cause renal insufficiency or failure and an increase in hepatic enzymes.

Hematologic consequences include increase in polymorphonuclear neutrophils with a left shift, thrombocytopenia and disseminated intravascular coagulation (DIC) as evidenced by a decrease in factors V, VIII, XII, fibrinogen, an increase in fibrin degradation products, and prolongation of the prothrombin time (PT) and activated partial thromboplastin time (aPTT). Assay of factor VIII is an important test in differentiating DIC from the coagulopathy of hepatic dysfunction as it is produced in endothelial cells and not in the liver. When factor VIII is normal, DIC is practically excluded, and coagulopathy may be due to liver failure. When decreased, a systemic consumptive process (e.g., DIC) is supported.

QUESTION 5 When the blood pressure fell to 70 mm Hg, norepinephrine and renal dose dopamine were started to maintain blood pressure and preserve renal perfusion. His vasopressor treatment was titrated to maintain a mean arterial pressure (MAP) of 65 mm Hg. Broad spectrum antibiotics were started consisting of vancomycin and ceftazidime. What is the classic treatment of sepsis and what are potential therapies that may specifically impact on the systemic inflammatory response?

In the setting of hypotension, one must use clinical judgment in the formation of a presumptive diagnosis to guide acute therapy. In such a scenario, when hypotension is severe, empiric therapy should be started rapidly. Objective testing should begin early and be guided by the presumptive diagnosis. It is most likely that this patient is manifesting distributive shock from gram-negative sepsis as a sequela of the development of a prostatic abscess after the biopsy.

Early clinical suspicion is an important component of the therapeutic regimen and leads to early initiation of antimicrobial therapy aimed at the most common causes of sepsis. In addition, supportive care for the hemodynamic consequences of septic shock is necessary.

Treating the underlying infection mandates the early institution of appropriate antibiotic coverage. Appropriate therapy is based on culture and sensitivity results. Gram-negative organisms have the most serious outcomes; however, sepsis can be caused by gram-positive organisms, fungi, myobacteria, and rarely viruses. The patient's clinical background may help to dictate therapy. For example, patients with surgically placed central access catheters should be covered for gram-positive organisms. Patients with T cell deficiency and a bilateral perihilar infiltrate should be covered for *Pneumocystis carinii* pneumonia. Local debridement and proper attention to the infective focus is also important.

Fluid resuscitation and maintenance of hemodynamic function are important aspects of the initial regimen. Cardiovascular support includes intensive monitoring with a Swan-Ganz catheter and intraarterial blood pressure monitoring. Fluid resuscitation with saline and/or colloids guided by the clinical examination or pulmonary artery catheter parameters is also important. If fluid resuscitation fails to improve hemodynamic function, vasopressors and/or inotropic agents should be used to support blood pressure and cardiovascular function.

It is important to maintain adequate oxygen delivery to the tissue. Administration of supplemental oxygen and, if necessary, mechanical ventilation when abnormalities of oxygenation or ventilation occur or when mental status deteriorates may be necessary. Controversy exists over the practice of maximizing oxygen delivery to tissues to "supramaximal" levels in an attempt to increase oxygen use or delivery to effect an improvement in survival.

QUESTION 6 What are the conclusions of the studies concerning use of newer agents including antiendotoxin and other agents?

The continued high mortality rate of patients with septic shock has stimulated the investigation of additional therapeutic agents. Monoclonal antibodies against endotoxin have been developed to add to conventional therapy. These agents do not have primary activity against bacteria, but attempt to offset the effects of lipopolysaccharide. The adjunctive use of nonsteroidal antiinflammatory agents and pentoxyfylline remains under investigation. Immunoglobulin has also been investigated. However, this modality neither prolonged survival or decreased the rate of complications.

Studies have shown that the monoclonal antiendotoxin antibody E5 decreased the 30-day mortality of patients with gram-negative sepsis who did not have refractory shock by 13%. HA-1A, another antiendotoxin monoclonal antibody, also improved the 28-day mortality of patients with gram-negative bacteremia by 39%. However, neither agent decreased the death rate among all patients given the drug. Both agents appeared to be useful in certain subgroups of patients, but it is often not possible to determine which patients will have refractory shock or whether bacteremia is present early. The conclusion regarding these modalities is such that they may be useful as an adjunctive agent but require further study.

Another option is the use of monoclonal antibodies directed against TNF (anti-TNF antibodies). This therapy has not become standard because of the difficulty in timing doses and the fact that definitive studies demonstrating a survival benefit have not been done. TNF may not be the only agent responsible for development of shock and may not be useful for all causes of shock. Because TNF stimulates release of IL-1 from monocytes, a major agent implicated in the sepsis cascade, an agent that blocks the receptor for IL-1 would theoretically be useful. In animal studies, when anti-TNF was given just before or after infusion of endotoxin, survival increased to 90%. Currently the safety of this agent is being evaluated for use in human subjects.

The current consensus pertaining to the use of these agents centers on the opportunity to interrupt the sepsis cascade at multiple levels. Investigation into the proper dosing, timing, titration of doses, and means of identifying impending sepsis

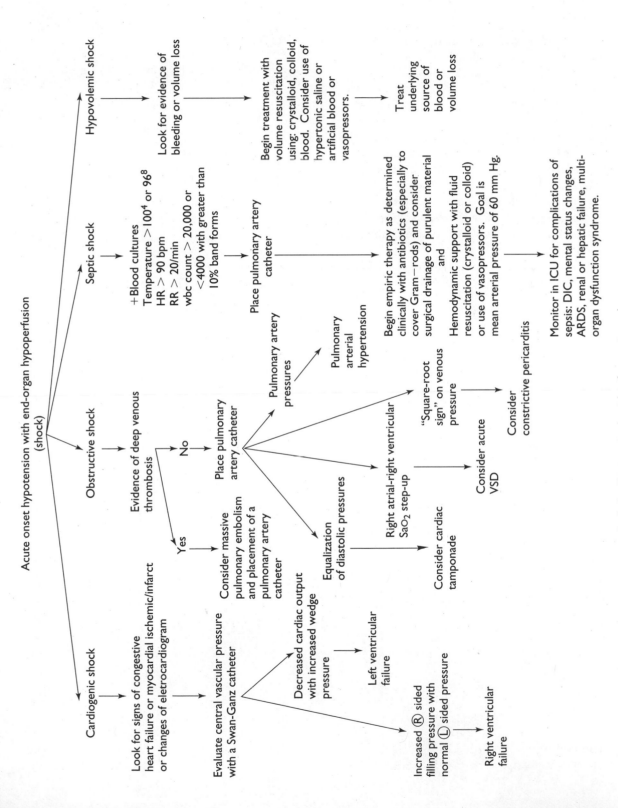

3-4-1 Diagnostic algorithm for sepsis syndrome.

Acute onset hypotension with end-organ hypoperfusion (shock)

Cardiogenic shock

Look for signs of congestive heart failure or myocardial ischemic/infarct or changes of eletrocardiogram

Evaluate central vascular pressure with a Swan-Ganz catheter

Decreased cardiac output with increased wedge pressure

Left ventricular failure

Increased ®️ sided filling pressure with normal Ⓛ sided pressure

Right ventricular failure

Obstructive shock

Evidence of deep venous thrombosis

Yes

No

Consider massive pulmonary embolism and placement of a pulmonary artery catheter

Place pulmonary artery catheter

Pulmonary artery pressures

Pulmonary arterial hypertension

Equalization of diastolic pressures

Consider cardiac tamponade

Right atrial-right ventricular SaO$_2$ step-up

Consider acute VSD

"Square-root sign" on venous pressure

Consider constrictive pericarditis

Septic shock

+Blood cultures
Temperature > 100[4] or 96[8]
HR > 90 bpm
RR > 20/min
wbc count > 20,000 or < 4000 with greater than 10% band forms

Place pulmonary artery catheter

Begin empiric therapy as determined clinically with antibiotics (especially to cover Gram—rods) and consider surgical drainage of purulent material and

Hemodynamic support with fluid resuscitation (crystalloid or colloid) or use of vasopressors. Goal is mean arterial pressure of 60 mm Hg.

Monitor in ICU for complications of sepsis: DIC, mental status changes, ARDS, renal or hepatic failure, multi-organ dysfunction syndrome.

Hypovolemic shock

Look for evidence of bleeding or volume loss

Begin treatment with volume resuscitation using: crystalloid, colloid, blood. Consider use of hypertonic saline or artificial blood or vasopressors.

Treat underlying source of blood or volume loss

earlier is underway. One must remember that normal physiologic mechanisms exist and that use of such agents may interfere with endogenous immunologic mechanisms. A diagnostic algorithm for sepsis syndrome is shown in Fig. 3-4-1.

CASE SUMMARY   The patients' blood pressure and cardiac output normalized on the second hospital day, and vancomycin was discontinued. The pulmonary artery catheter and intraarterial line were removed. He was transferred to the general medical floor when stable for 24 hours. The patient was discharged after a 10-day course of antibiotic therapy.

• •

BIBLIOGRAPHY

Bone RC, Balk RA, Cerra FB: Definitions for sepsis and organ failure and guidelines for the use of innovative therapies in sepsis, *Chest* 101:1644-1655, 1992.

Brody SL: State of the art in septic shock, *Emerg Med* 183-196, 1992.

Casey LC, Balk RA: Plasma cytokine and endotoxin levels correlate with survival in patients with the sepsis syndrome, *Ann Intern Med* 119:771-778, 1993.

Kuver A, Dimon C, Hollenberg SM, et al: Tumor necrosis factor produces a concentration—dependent depression of myocardial cell contraction in vitro, *Clin Res* 39:321A, 1991 (abstract).

Parrillo JE: Pathogenetic mechanism of septic shock, *N Engl J Med* 328:1471-1477, 1993.

Parrillo JE, Parker MM, Natanson C, et al: Septic shock in humans–advances in the understanding of pathogenesis, cardiovascular dysfunction, and therapy, *Ann Intern Med* 113:227-242, 1990.

Smith and Their *Pathophysiology: The Biological Principles of Disease*, Philadelphia, 1985, WB Saunders.

C A S E

5

M. Jeffrey Barkoviak
Robert Balk

A 45-year-old man came to the emergency room complaining of chest pressure and dizziness. The patient has a history of hypertension for which medication has been prescribed but that he takes sporadically. He has a 25-pack per year smoking history and was told that his cholesterol was elevated. He denies any family history of cardiac disease.

Further history reveals that the symptoms of chest pressure and dizziness became continuous approximately 3 hours before coming to the emergency department. They have also been occurring intermittently for 1 week prior to arrival but typically resolved after a few minutes. He describes his symptoms as a heaviness in the middle of his chest associated with an achy sensation in his left shoulder. He notes that he has episodic difficulty breathing and that he has experienced a fluttering feeling in his chest that, at times, is associated with dizziness.

The patient is immediately brought to the treatment area of the emergency room and a rapid physical examination is performed.

Vital signs: T 99.4°F; BP 100/74 mm Hg in both arms; HR 110 bpm, irregular; RR 24/min

General appearance: An anxious, diaphoretic slightly obese middle-aged man

HEENT: Normal; Neck: no JVD; Lungs: clear

Cardiac: Irregular rate, an S_4 gallop is heard, no murmur, PMI nondisplaced

Abdomen: Normal; extremities: pulses equal throughout, no edema

Neurologic: Normal

The patient is placed on a cardiac monitor; the rhythm is shown in Fig. 3-5-1.

QUESTION 1 Given this patient's history and physical examination findings, what is the differential diagnosis of this patient's symptoms? How would you proceed with confirming the diagnosis?

The differential diagnosis includes acute myocardial infarction (MI), unstable angina, pericarditis, pulmonary embolism (PE), and aortic dissection. A 12-lead ECG should be the initial test following acquisition of the history and physical examination. Other tests include cardiac enzymes, chest x-ray, and arterial blood gases.

In acute MI and unstable angina, symptoms include classic central chest heaviness or pressure associated with dyspnea, diaphoresis, and occasionally nausea. The pain may radiate to the neck, jaw, or arm. Studies have shown that pain with a pressure, ache or burning component, and substernal location in the correct clinical situation is strong evidence supporting myocardial ischemia. There may be a clinical response to sublingual (SL) or intravenous (IV) nitroglycerin. The ECG may reveal ST-segment elevation, depression, or may be normal. In a study of 114 patients with normal ECGs, only one patient proved to have a myocardial infarction. In another study, of 167 patients deemed to have a positive electrocardiogram, 57% had an infarction and 14% had acute complications. Diagnosis is made by using a combination of ECG findings in a patient with the appropriate history, risk factors, and cardiac enzymes that reveal an elevated MB fraction. In selected cases, echocardiography, technetium nuclear medicine scanning, and cardiac catheterization can confirm the diagnosis. In the case of cardiac catheterization, this provides a therapeutic opportunity.

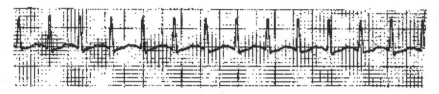

3-5-1 Rhythm strip.

Pericarditis often presents with central chest pain but is usually pleuritic (i.e., sharp and aggravated by position). Most patients characteristically find relief of their symptoms by sitting up and leaning forward. Some patients will have, however, presenting symptoms very similar to acute MI. The ECG classically shows diffuse ST-segment elevation without the reciprocal depression of ST segments seen in acute MI. Also, PR-segment depression characteristically accompanies the ST-segment elevation. Sequential ECGs may be useful in distinguishing pericarditis from acute myocardial infarction.

Patients with pulmonary embolism typically present with pleuritic chest pain and dyspnea. Many patients also have signs of a lower extremity deep venous thrombosis, that is, painful swelling of the leg. However, some patients have very nondescript symptoms that may be confused with myocardial ischemia. Most patients will have an increased alveolar-arterial oxygen gradient calculated from the arterial blood gas. ECG findings in pulmonary embolism are usually nonspecific. The classic finding is the presence of an S wave in lead 1 and Q wave in lead III (S_1Q_3 pattern). Diagnosis is made in patients with a high index of suspicion for PE by nuclear medicine ventilation/perfusion (VQ) scanning that would show multiple segmental or larger mismatches in ventilation and perfusion. If the V/Q scan is nondiagnostic, lower extremity Doppler studies or pulmonary angiography may be useful in making the diagnosis.

The symptoms of aortic dissection may mimic myocardial ischemia; however, a more classic description is of a "ripping" or "tearing" sensation radiating to the back in the interscapular area or abdomen. Often there is asymmetry of pulses or blood pressure in the extremities. Aortic dissection has no specific ECG findings. Diagnosis is

made by transesophageal echocardiography, CT scanning, or aortography.

QUESTION 2 A 12-lead ECG is performed and reveals sinus tachycardia with frequent premature ventricular contractions (PVCs), couplets, and 3 mm ST-segment elevation in lead V_1-V_4, with ST-segment depression and T wave inversion in leads II, III, and aVF. In light of this patient's symptom complex, history, and ECG findings, what is the most likely diagnosis?

The symptoms of myocardial ischemia and findings of ST-segment elevation in the anterior chest wall leads support the diagnosis of acute anterior wall MI. The symptom of central chest heaviness is a classic description of anginal pain. The finding of left shoulder or arm pain is seen in approximately 30% of patients with acute MI. The history is also remarkable for several cardiac risk factors: male gender, hypertension, hypercholesterolemia, and tobacco use. The ECG findings of ST-segment elevation in the anterior precordial leads are strongly suggestive of myocardial injury. Associated ST-segment depression and T wave inversion are likely to represent reciprocal changes. While no single modality is pathognomonic, the ECG findings in this clinical setting are highly suggestive, if not diagnostic, of acute myocardial infarction.

QUESTION 3 The patient is given supplemental oxygen at 4 LPM via nasal cannula. An IV is started, and the patient is given SL NTG. What other therapies need to be considered at this time?

Pain relief, a marker of resolved cellular ischemia, is of highest priority. It is important to interrupt the vicious cycle of myocardial ischemia

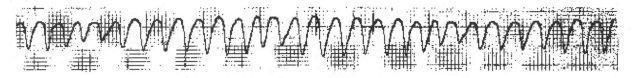

3-5-2 Rhythm strip.

→ ventricular stiffening and dysfunction → baro-receptor and juxtaglomerular apparatus activation → elaboration of renin and angiotensin → sympathetic nervous system (SANS) activation → tachycardia, arterial vasoconstriction → increased myocardial oxygen needs → further myocardial ischemia. NTG, by dilating coronary arteries, decreasing preload via venous pooling decreases myocardial oxygen requirements. One can turn off the SANS with the use of angiotensin converting enzyme inhibitors and beta-blockers. Diuretics used to treat pulmonary edema reduce dyspnea, increase patient comfort, and enhance arterial oxygen carriage. Exogenous oxygen also increases oxygen delivery to the myocardium.

Thrombolytic therapy needs to be considered as it has been shown to reduce morbidity and mortality in patients with acute transmural myocardial infarction, especially when given within 6 hours after onset of symptoms. Aspirin of 150 to 325 mg should also be given as soon as possible, as it has been demonstrated to reduce mortality and the rate of reinfarction.

Prophylactic lidocaine given in the presence of acute MI has been shown to reduce the incidence of primary ventricular fibrillation, but has not altered mortality rates. This, in addition to the delicate therapeutic index of lidocaine, has made the routine use of prophylactic lidocaine questionable. However, this patient has frequent (SBP >6 per minute) PVCs in the face of an acute MI. In this circumstance, the use of lidocaine is acceptable.

QUESTION 4 The patient has been in the emergency room for 15 minutes, and the decision is made to give thrombolytic therapy because he has had his symptoms for 3 hours and has no contraindications.

What are the indications and contraindications for thrombolytic administration?

The open artery hypothesis dictates that the sooner an occluded artery is opened, less myocardium is damaged. Ventricular function is preserved, less scarring occurs, and there is a decreased chance of an ectopic source of arrhythmia. Indications for the use of thrombolytic therapy include massive acute anterior wall MI with ST segment greater than 1 mm elevation in two contiguous leads and inferior infarction involving the right ventricle. At Rush-Presbyterian St. Luke's Medical Center thrombolytic therapy is considered up to 12 hours after symptom onset when the delay to primary coronary angioplasty is greater than 90 minutes and there are no contraindications to thrombolysis.

Absolute contraindications for thrombolytic therapy include active bleeding, known presence of intracranial lesions with potential for hemorrhage (such as a tumor, recent cerebrovascular accident, arteriovenous malformations, or aneurysm), and severe uncontrolled hypertension. Relative contraindications include major surgery within 10 days, postpartum state, liver disease, recent CPR, and recent needle biopsy.

QUESTION 5 His vital signs remain stable: BP 118/80 mm Hg, HR 116 bpm, RR 24/min. He still feels heaviness in the center of his chest, but the pain is not as severe after receiving 2 sublingual NTG tablets. As the lidocaine and thrombolytic medication are being prepared for administration, the rhythm in Fig. 3-5-2 is seen on the cardiac monitor.

The patient's vital signs remain stable: BP 112/80 mm Hg, HR 150 bpm, RR 24/min. The patient denies any new or worsening symptoms and is wondering why everyone is getting so excited. What rhythm is

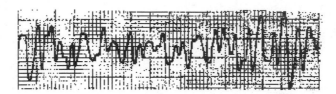

3-5-3   Rhythm strip.

now showing on the monitor and how would you treat it?

The rhythm strip shows a wide-complex (QRS >0.12 msec) tachycardia that is regular and lacks P waves. The possible etiologies include an atrial tachyarrhythmia with abberancy such as atrial flutter, atrial fibrillation, AV nodal reentrant tachycardia, or ventricular tachycardia (VT).

The differentiation of VT from supraventricular tachycardias (SVT) with aberrancy can be confusing and time consuming. The difference is important because the wrong therapy (e.g., a trial of verapamil to treat SVT) can be lethal to a patient with VT. On a 12-lead ECG, VT is supported by finding more than three consecutive ventricular beats, rate greater than 170 bpm, presence of fusion or capture beats, AV dissociation, a QRS complex greater than 140 to 150 msec, concordance, northwest axis, a monophasic or biphasic QRS in V1, and R/S ratio of <1. Lidocaine is recommended as the first agent to use for VT and all wide-complex tachycardias not known with certainty to be supraventricular in origin. Lidocaine is especially effective when VT is related to an ischemic etiology. Lidocaine is administered as an IV bolus of 1 to 1.5 mg/kg, followed as needed by reboluses of 0.5 to 0.75 mg/kg IV push every 5 to 10 minutes to a maximum total of 3 mg/kg. Once the arrhythmia has been terminated, a continuous infusion is begun.

QUESTION 6   The patient is given lidocaine 100 mg IV push. His vital signs remain stable, and the wide-complex tachycardia persists. An additional 50 mg of lidocaine is given IV push, then the patient reports feeling "funny," and suddenly becomes

unconscious. No pulse is detectable, and the rhythm shown on Fig. 3-5-3 is seen on the cardiac monitor.

What rhythm is present and how would you treat it?

The rhythm this patient now exhibits is ventricular fibrillation (VF). This rhythm is characterized by a coarse and chaotic pattern without organized conduction. VF and pulseless VT should be treated with immediate defibrillation at 200 joules (J). If the abnormal rhythm persists, electrical cardioversion should be repeated immediately with increasing energy at 200 to 300 J, and 360 J. Successive shocks are more important than drug therapy in this situation. Delays taken to administer medications or perform CPR decrease efficacy of further cardioversion.

QUESTION 7   The patient is defibrillated three times in a rapid, sequential manner with an escalating energy level up to 360 J. He remains pulseless, and his rhythm remains VF. CPR is begun, and the patient is endotracheally intubated. How do you further manage this patient?

The value of CPR should not be overlooked. The arrest situation is often chaotic. There should be one designated leader who gives specific orders and several colleagues who assume specific jobs as directed. CPR is a means of maintaining circulation via chest compressions, breathing by bag insufflation, and maintenance of the airway by correct jaw-thrust methods. These maneuvers allow time to assess the patient's status, organize the arrest team, establish IV access, and bring the appropriate equipment to the bedside.

When electrical cardioversion is ineffective,

the administration of epinephrine 1.0 mg IV push is indicated. The use of epinephrine at this standard dose is a high priority for patients in cardiac arrest. Epinephrine's beneficial effects are attributed primarily to its alpha-adrenergic receptor stimulating properties which increases myocardial and cerebral blood flow during CPR. The effects of epinephrine's beta-adrenergic receptor stimulating activity remains controversial as it may increase myocardial work and reduce subendocardial perfusion. Nevertheless, epinephrine hydrochloride 1.0 mg (10 ml or a 1:10,000 solution) IV is recommended every 3 to 5 minutes during cardiac arrest.

This standard dose of epinephrine has been questioned recently. A number of clinical trials have been performed looking at using higher dosages of epinephrine during cardiac arrest. These studies looked at prehospital settings and in-hospital cardiac arrests and found a higher rate of return of spontaneous circulation with higher dosages of epinephrine but no statistically significant improvement in survival rates when compared with standard dose epinephrine.

Based on these studies, it is recommended that epinephrine 1.0 mg be the first-line agent in cardiac arrest. Use of higher dose epinephrine (5.0 mg or 0.1 mg/kg) may be considered if 1.0 mg fails, but it can be neither recommended nor discouraged.

QUESTION 8 Epinephrine 1.0 mg is ordered IV push. However the peripheral IV line started when the patient was admitted to the emergency room has infiltrated. The staff is having difficulty restarting a peripheral IV line. What other options do you have for medication administration?

During cardiac arrest, cannulation of a peripheral vein (antecubital or external jugular) is the preferred choice because CPR would have to be interrupted to start a central line (subclavian or internal jugular). Central access would otherwise be preferred because drugs given via a peripheral line take 1 to 2 minutes to reach the central circulation. Other advantages of central venous access include a more rapid delivery of drugs and secure placement even when peripheral circulation is poor. Medications delivered via peripheral venous access should be given with a rapid bolus injection and followed by a 20 ml bolus of IV fluid and elevation of the extremity.

A consideration in this patient is the potential for increased risk of complication associated with central line placement if he were to receive a thrombolytic agent following his recovery from cardiac arrest. An unsuccessful central line attempt is a strong relative contraindication to thrombolytic therapy.

Another route of drug administration if venous access is delayed is via the endotracheal tube. Epinephrine, lidocaine, and atropine can be given safely via this route. Medications need to be administered at 2 to 2.5 times the recommended IV dose and should be diluted in 10 ml of normal saline or sterile water. A catheter should be passed beyond the tip of the endotracheal tube, and chest compressions should be stopped while the medication is injected. Several quick bag insufflations should be given to aerosolize the medication, and then chest compressions should be resumed. Intraosseous administration of medications is another alternative, especially in pediatric patients.

QUESTION 9 The patient is given epinephrine 2.0 mg diluted in 10 ml normal saline via the endotracheal tube. CPR is resumed after instillation of the medication and insufflation of the medication into the lungs. The patient remains pulseless and in VF. How would you proceed in managing this patient?

The patient should again be defibrillated at 360 J within 30 to 60 seconds of giving epinephrine if VF or pulseless VT persists.

At this point an antifibrillatory drug should be administered, followed by repeat defibrillation at 360 J. Lidocaine and bretylium have been studied the most as first-line antifibrillatory agents. Clinical trials have failed to demonstrate that one drug is superior to the other. Lidocaine is generally favored as the first agent as it is more familiar to most personnel and generally considered safer.

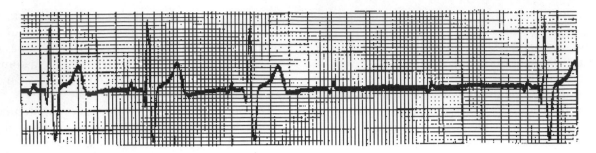

3-5-4   Rhythm strip.

In refractory VF, lidocaine is administered as a bolus of 1.5 mg/kg and may be repeated in 3 to 5 minutes as necessary to a total of 3 mg/kg. Additional boluses of 0.5 mg/kg may be given but not more often than every 8 to 10 minutes; however, it may lead to lidocaine toxicity.

If lidocaine and repeat defibrillation fail to convert VF, bretylium tosylate 5 mg/kg is administered as a bolus. After 1 to 2 minutes of CPR, repeat defibrillation is attempted. A second dose of 10 mg/kg can be administered in 5 minutes if the patient remains in VF. This can be repeated every 5 minutes to a maximum total dose of 30 to 35 mg/kg.

QUESTION 10   An IV has been successfully inserted into the patient's external jugular vein, and lidocaine 150 mg is given IV push (he received 150 mg before cardiac arrest) for a total loading dose of 3 mg/kg. He is then quickly defibrillated at 360 J but remains in VF. An arterial blood gas that was drawn at the onset of the cardiac arrest is completed and shows spH=7.10, Pco_2 = 60 mm Hg, Po_2 = 70 mm Hg. Given this arterial blood gas value, would you give sodium bicarbonate?

Acidosis that occurs during cardiac arrest is usually due to alveolar hypoventilation as well as lactic acidosis from inadequate tissue perfusion. As shown by the lower pH and elevated Pco_2, a respiratory acidosis is present along with a metabolic acidosis as the pH is lower than expected to accompany a Pco_2 of 60 mm Hg. Improvement of alveolar ventilation is the mainstay of the control of acid-base balance during cardiac arrest. There is

little data indicating that therapy with buffers improves survival. In fact, many studies have shown that bicarbonate therapy during cardiac arrest may be harmful. Bicarbonate can paradoxically produce a worsening of acidosis by increasing the production of CO_2 which can easily diffuse into myocardial and cerebral cells and depress function.

The tissue acidosis that occurs during cardiac arrest results from low blood flow and inadequate ventilation. The goals of therapy should be geared toward restoring adequate circulation and improving ventilation. Studies have failed to show that low blood pH adversely affects the ability to defibrillate, ability to restore spontaneous circulation, or short-term survival.

In this patient, correction of the acidosis should be geared toward correcting the respiratory component of the acidosis by endotracheal intubation and hyperventilation.

QUESTION 11   The patient remains endotracheally intubated and is being hyperventilated because of the presence of acidosis. The rhythm remains VF. Epinephrine 1.0 mg is given IV push (it has been 3 minutes since his last dose), and bretylium 500 mg is given IV push. After 2 minutes of CPR to circulate the medications, repeat defibrillation at 360 J is performed. Fig. 3-5-4 shows the rhythm that appears on the cardiac monitor. The patient remains unconscious, but a faint pulse is felt with a rate of approximately 40 bpm. The systolic blood pressure is faintly heard at 70 mm Hg. What rhythm is present? How would you manage this patient at this time?

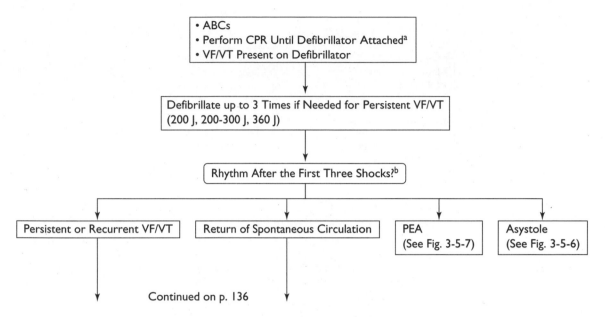

- ABCs
- Perform CPR Until Defibrillator Attached[a]
- VF/VT Present on Defibrillator

Defibrillate up to 3 Times if Needed for Persistent VF/VT (200 J, 200-300 J, 360 J)

Rhythm After the First Three Shocks?[b]

| Persistent or Recurrent VF/VT | Return of Spontaneous Circulation | PEA (See Fig. 3-5-7) | Asystole (See Fig. 3-5-6) |

Continued on p. 136

3-5-5 Ventricular fibrillation/pulseless ventricular tachycardia (VF/VT) algorithm. Class I, Definitely helpful. Class IIa, Acceptable, probably helpful. Class IIb, Acceptable, possibly helpful. Class III, Not indicated, may be harmful.

[a]Precordial thump is a Class IIb action in witnessed arrest, no pulse, and no defibrillator immediately available.

[b]Hypothermic cardiac arrest is treated differently after this point.

[c]The recommended dose of epinephrine is 1 mg IV push every 3-5 min. If this approach fails, several Class IIb dosing regimens can be considered:
- Intermediate: epinephrine 2-5 mg IV push, every 3-5 min.
- Escalating: epinephrine 1 mg-3 mg-5mg IV push, 3 min apart.
- High: epinephrine 0.1 mg/kg IV push, every 3-5 min.

[d]Sodium bicarbonate 1 mEq/kg is Class I if patient has known preexisting hyperkalemia.

[e]Multiple sequenced shocks are acceptable here (Class I), especially when medications are delayed.

[f]Medication sequence:
- Lidocaine 1.0-1.5 mg/kg IV push. Consider repeat in 3-5 min to maximum dose of 3 mg/kg. A single dose of 1.5 mg/kg in cardiac arrest is acceptable.
- Bretylium 5 mg/kg IV push. Repeat in 5 min at 10 mg/kg.
- Magnesium sulfate 1-2 g IV in torsades de pointes or suspected hypomagnesemic state or refractory VF.
- Procainamide 30 mg/min in refractory VF (maximum total 17 mg/kg).

[g]Sodium bicarbonate 1 mEq/kg IV:
Class IIa:
- If known preexisting bicarbonate-responsive acidosis.
- If overdose with tricyclic antidepressants.
- To alkalinize the urine in drug overdoses.
Class IIb:
- If intubated and continued long arrest interval.
- Upon return of spontaneous circulation after long arrest interval.
Class III:
- Hypoxic lactic acidosis.

(From *Textbook of Advanced Cardiac Life Support,* ed 3, The American Heart Association.)

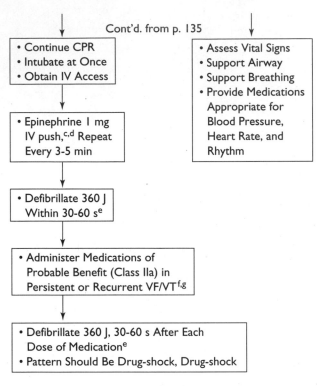

Cont'd. from p. 135

- Continue CPR
- Intubate at Once
- Obtain IV Access

- Assess Vital Signs
- Support Airway
- Support Breathing
- Provide Medications
  Appropriate for
  Blood Pressure,
  Heart Rate, and
  Rhythm

- Epinephrine 1 mg
  IV push,[c,d] Repeat
  Every 3-5 min

- Defibrillate 360 J
  Within 30-60 s[e]

- Administer Medications of
  Probable Benefit (Class IIa) in
  Persistent or Recurrent VF/VT[f,g]

- Defibrillate 360 J, 30-60 s After Each
  Dose of Medication[e]
- Pattern Should Be Drug-shock, Drug-shock

3-5-5 Cont'd.

The rhythm is second-degree heart block Mobitz type II. It is recognized by the absence of a ventricular beat unexpectedly without a preceding change in the PR interval. It is a serious rhythm most often associated with anteroseptal MI and is due to damage to the His-Purkinje system. The recognition of this rhythm is important because of the tendency for this block to rapidly progress to complete third-degree AV block.

Alternatively, Mobitz type I second-degree heart block (Wenkebach phenomenon) also is defined as an intermittent failure to conduct impulses to the ventricles. However, this type of block is characterized by progressive PR-interval prolongation prior to block of an atrial impulse. This block originates in the AV node and is commonly due to inferior wall MI or drug effect (digitalis or beta-blockers). This type of block is

generally well tolerated by the patient and rarely progresses to complete heart block.

Treatment of bradycardia should be geared toward treating complicating signs or symptoms and not the absolute heart rate. Bradycardia requires immediate treatment if associated with symptoms of chest pain, shortness of breath, mental status changes, or signs of hypotension, shock, pulmonary edema, or myocardial ischemia.

Symptomatic sinus bradycardia or type I second-degree AV block is initially treated with atropine, which reverses cholinergic mediated bradycardia and hypotension. The recommended dose is 0.5 to 1.0 mg IV every 3 to 5 minutes up to a total dose of 0.04 mg/kg (approximately 3 mg) that results in complete vagal blockade. Doses of atropine less than 0.5 mg are not recommended as they can be parasympathomimetic and result in

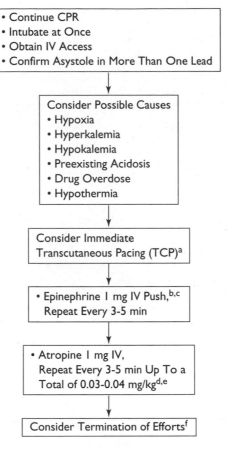

- Continue CPR
- Intubate at Once
- Obtain IV Access
- Confirm Asystole in More Than One Lead

↓

Consider Possible Causes
- Hypoxia
- Hyperkalemia
- Hypokalemia
- Preexisting Acidosis
- Drug Overdose
- Hypothermia

↓

Consider Immediate
Transcutaneous Pacing (TCP)[a]

↓

- Epinephrine 1 mg IV Push,[b,c]
  Repeat Every 3-5 min

↓

- Atropine 1 mg IV,
  Repeat Every 3-5 min Up To a
  Total of 0.03-0.04 mg/kg[d,e]

↓

Consider Termination of Efforts[f]

3-5-6 Asystole treatment algorithm. Class I, Definitely helpful. Class IIa, Acceptable, probably helpful. Class IIb, Acceptable, possibly helpful. Class III, Not indicated, may be harmful.

[a]TCP is a Class IIb intervention. Lack of success may be due to delays in pacing. To be effective TCP must be performed early, simultaneously with drugs. Evidence does not support routine use of TCP for asystole.

[b]The recommended dose of epinephrine is 1 mg IV push every 3-5 min. If this approach fails, several Class IIb dosing regimens can be considered:
- Intermediate: epinephrine 2-5 mg IV push, every 3-5 min
- Escalating: epinephrine 1 mg-3 mg-5 mg IV push, 3 min apart
- High: epinephrine 0.1 mg/kg IV push, every 3-5 min

[c]Sodium bicarbonate 1 mEq/kg is Class I if patient has known preexisting hyperkalemia.

[d]The shorter atropine dosing interval (3 min) is Class IIb in asystolic arrest.

[e]Sodium bicarbonate 1 mEq/kg:

Class IIa:
- If known preexisting bicarbonate-responsive acidosis
- If overdose with tricyclic antidepressants
- To alkalinize the urine in drug overdoses

Class IIb:
- If intubated and continued long arrest interval
- Upon return of spontaneous circulation after long arrest interval

Class III:
- Hypoxic lactic acidosis

[f]If patient remains in asystole or other agonal rhythm after successful intubation and initial medications and no reversible causes are identified, consider termination of resuscitative efforts by a physician. Consider interval since arrest.

(From *Textbook of Advanced Cardiac Life Support*, ed 3, The American Heart Association.)

Includes • Electromechanical dissociation (EMD)
• Pseudo-EMD
• Idioventricular rhythms
• Ventricular escape rhythms
• Bradyasystolic rhythms
• Postdefibrillation idioventricular rhythms

• Continue CPR	• Assess Blood Flow Using Doppler Ultrasound,
• Intubate at Once	End-tidal CO_2, Echocardiography, or
• Obtain IV Access	Arterial Line

↓

Consider Possible Causes
(Parentheses = Possible Therapies and Treatments)

• Hypovolemia (Volume infusion)
• Hypoxia (Ventilation)
• Cardiac Tamponade (Pericardiocentesis)
• Tension Pneumothorax (Needle decompression)
• Hypothermia (See Hypothermia algorithm)
• Massive Pulmonary Embolism (Surgery, Thrombolytics)

• Drug Overdoses such as Tricyclics, Digitalis, β-blockers, Calcium Channel Blockers
• Hyperkalemia[a]
• Acidosis[b]
• Massive Acute Myocardial Infarction

↓

• Epinephrine I mg IV
Push,[a,c] Repeat Every 3-5 min

↓

• If Absolute Bradycardia (<60 BPM) or
Relative Bradycardia, Give Atropine I mg IV
• Repeat every 3-5 min to a Total of 0.03-0.04 mg/kg[d]

3-5-7 Pulseless electrical activity (PEA) algorithm (electromechanical dissociation [EMD]). Class I, Definitely helpful. Class IIa, Acceptable, probably helpful. Class IIb, Acceptable, possibly helpful. Class III, Not indicated, may be harmful.
[a]Sodium bicarbonate I mEq/kg is Class I if patient has known preexisting hyperkalemia.
[b]Sodium bicarbonate I mEq/kg:
Class IIa:
• If known preexisting bicarbonate-responsive acidosis
• If overdose with tricyclic antidepressants
• To alkalinize the urine in drug overdoses
Class IIb:
• If intubated and continued long arrest interval
• Upon return of spontaneous circulation after long arrest interval
Class III:
• Hypoxic lactic acidosis
[c]The recommended dose of epinephrine is I mg IV push every 3-5 min. If this approach fails, several Class IIb dosing regimens can be considered:
• Intermediate: epinephrine 2-5 mg IV push, every 3-5 min
• Escalating: epinephrine I mg-3 mg-5 mg IV push, 3 min apart
• High: epinephrine 0.1 mg/kg IV push, every 3-5 min
[d]The shorter atropine dosing interval (3 min) is possibly helpful in cardiac arrest (Class IIb).
(From *Textbook of Advanced Cardiac Life Support,* ed 3, The American Heart Association.)

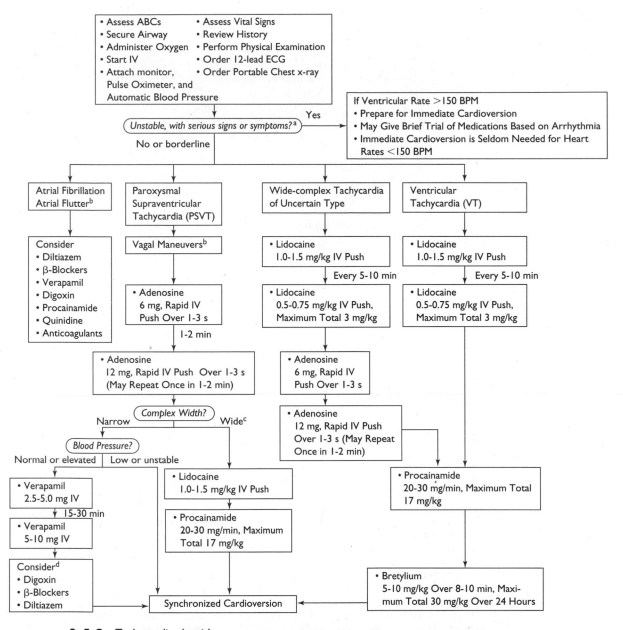

3-5-8 Tachycardia algorithm.

[a]Unstable condition must be related to the tachycardia. Signs and symptoms may include chest pain, shortness of breath, decreased level of consciousness, low blood pressure (BP), shock, pulmonary congestion, congestive heart failure, acute myocardial infarction.

[b]Carotid sinus pressure is contraindicated in patients with carotid bruits; avoid ice water immersion in patients with ischemic heart disease.

[c]If the wide-complex tachycardia is known with certainty to be PSVT and BP is normal/elevated, sequence can include verapamil.

[d]Use extreme caution with β-blockers after verapamil.

(From *Textbook of Advanced Cardiac Life Support*, ed 3, The American Heart Association.)

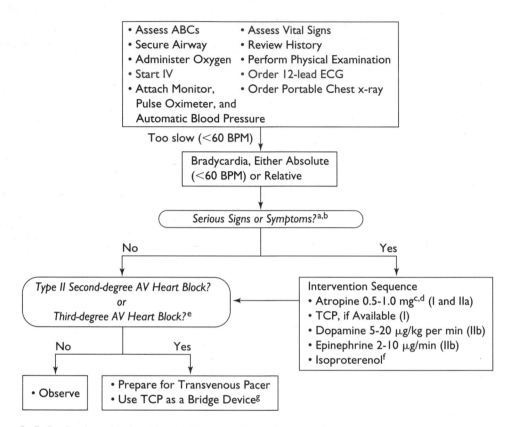

3-5-9 Bradycardia algorithm (patient is not in cardiac arrest).

[a]Serious signs or symptoms must be related to the slow rate. Clinical manifestations include

- Symptoms (chest pain, shortness of breath, decreased level of consciousness)
- Signs (low BP, shock, pulmonary congestion, CHF, acute MI)

[b]Do not delay TCP while awaiting IV access or for atropine to take effect if patient is symptomatic.

[c]Denervated transplanted hearts will not respond to atropine. Go at once to pacing, catecholamine infusion, or both.

[d]Atropine should be given in repeat doses every 3-5 min up to total of 0.03-0.04 mg/kg. Use the shorter dosing interval (3 min) in severe clinical conditions. It has been suggested that atropine should be used with caution in atrioventricular (AV) block at the His-Purkinje level (type II AV block and new third-degree block with wide QRS complexes) (Class IIb).

[e]Never treat third-degree heart block plus ventricular escape beats with lidocaine.

[f]Isoproterenol should be used, if at all, with extreme caution. At low doses it is Class IIb (possibly helpful); at higher doses it is Class III (harmful).

[g]Verify patient tolerance and mechanical capture. Use analgesia and sedation as needed.

(From *Textbook of Advanced Cardiac Life Support,* ed 3, The American Heart Association.)

further slowing of the heart rate. If atropine is not effective, transcutaneous pacing or catecholamine infusions (dopamine or epinephrine) are recommended.

In this patient with type II second-degree heart block and in those patients with complete heart block, the use of atropine may actually be detrimental. Atropine may act to increase the atrial rate and produce increased AV block that may be accompanied by a further decrease in heart rate. In addition, the use of atropine in these patients may exacerbate ischemia or induce VT or VF.

The treatment of choice in this patient is transcutaneous pacing used as a bridge until a transvenous pacer can be inserted. This technique is the method of choice for treating symptomatic bradycardias because of the noninvasive nature of the device and the ease of application. Many newer defibrillators are combined with transcutaneous pacing capabilities that increase the speed with which pacing can be performed. Diagnostic algorithms for ventricular fibrillation, asystole, electromechanical dissociation, sustained ventricular tachycardia (VT), and bradycardia are shown in Figs. 3-5-5 to 3-5-9.

CASE FOLLOW-UP A transcutaneous pacemaker is available and is placed on the patient. Adequate capture is achieved, and the patient is paced at a rate of 80. His blood pressure increases to 96/60 mm Hg, and he begins to regain consciousness. The patient is taken to the coronary care unit. The transcutaneous pacemaker is placed in a standby mode 30 minutes later when the patient regains a normal sinus rhythm with an adequate blood pressure. He is given thrombolytic therapy to treat his acute anteroseptal myocardial infarction and is eventually discharged home from the hospital.

BIBLIOGRAPHY

Aitkenhead AR: Drug administration during cardiopulmonary resuscitation: what route? *Resuscitation* 22:191-195, 1991.

Berenyi KJ, Wolk M, Killip T: Cerebrospinal fluid acidosis complicating therapy of experimental cardiopulmonary arrest, *Circulation* 52:319-32, 1975.

Bishop RL, Weisfeldt ML: Sodium bicarbonate administration during cardiac arrest, *JAMA* 235:506-509, 1976.

Callaham M, Madsen CD, Barton CW, et al: A randomized controlled trial of high dose epinephrine and norepinephrine versus standard-dose epinephrine in prehospital cardiac arrest, *Ann Emerg Med* 21:606-607, 1992.

Congolan HE et al: Depression of human myocardial contractility with "respiratory" and "metabolic" acidosis, *Surgery* 77:427-432, 1975.

Dauchot P, Gravenstein S: Bradycardia after myocardial ischemia and its treatment with atropine, *Anesthesiology* 44:501-518, 1976.

Ditchey RV, Lindenfeld J: Failure of epinephrine to improve the balance between myocardial oxygen supply and demand during closed chest resuscitation in dogs, *Circulation* 78:382-389, 1988.

Fisher, C: *Electrocardiography and vectorcardiography*. In Braunwald, E, ed: *Heart disease*, Philadelphia, 1992, W.B. Saunders.

Frederiuk CS, Sanders AB, Kern KB, et al: The effect of bicarbonate on resuscitation from cardiac arrest, *Ann Emerg Med* 20:1172-1177, 1991.

Gunnar R et al: Guidelines for the early management of patients with acute myocardial infarction, *J Am Coll Cardiol* 16:249-292, 1990.

Hayes RE, Chinn TL, et al: Comparison of bretylium tosylate and lidocaine in management of out of hospital ventricular fibrillation: a randomized clinical trial, *Am J Cardiol* 48:353-356, 1981.

Ketter F, Weil MH: Buffer agents do not reverse intramyocardial acidosis during cardiac resuscitation, *Circulation* 81:1660-1666, 1990.

Lindner KH, Ahnefeld FW, Prengel AW: Comparison of standard and high dose adrenaline in the resuscitation of asystole and electromechanical dissociation, *Acta Anaesthesiol Scand* 35:253-256, 1991.

Lorell B, Braunwald E: Pericardial disease. In Brauwald E, editor: *Heart Disease*, Philadelphia, 1992, W.B. Saunders.

Martin TS, Hawkins NS, Weigel JA, Rider DE: Initial treatment of ventricular fibrillation: defibrillation or drug therapy, *Am J Emerg Med* 6:113-119, 1988.

McMahon S, Collins R, Peto R: Effects of prophylactic lidocaine in suspected acute myocardial infarction, *JAMA* 260:1910-1916, 1988.

Michael JR, Geurci AD, et al: Mechanisms by which epinephrine augments cerebral and myocardial perfusion during cardiopulmonary resuscitation in dogs, *Circulation* 69:822-835, 1984.

Rankin AC, Rae AP, Cobbe SM: Misuse of intravenous verapamil in patients with ventricular tachycardia, *Lancet* 2:472-474, 1987.

Stiell IG, Weitzman BN, Wells GA, et al: A study of high dose epinephrine in human CPR, *Ann Emerg Med* 21:606, 1992.

The ASSET Study Group. Trial of tissue plasminogen activator for mortality reduction in acute myocardial infarction: The Anglo-Scandinavian study of early thrombolysis (ASSET), *Lancet* 2:525-530, 1988.

The ISIS-2 Collaborative Group. Randomized trial of intravenous streptokinase, oral aspirin, both, or neither among 17187 cases of suspected myocardial infarction: ISIS-2, *Lancet* 2:349-360, 1988.

CASE

6

Maureen Block
Robert Balk

A *63-year-old man is brought to the emergency room by his daughters because he is lethargic and appears to have labored breathing. The daughters explain that the patient has a history of alcohol abuse, but has never been hospitalized. He was in his usual state of health when they last visited 3 days ago. On arriving at his home on the evening of admission, they found him in bed, coughing, and breathing rapidly. He felt warm, and they suspected a fever. The patient was unable to tell them what had happened over the previous 3 days. In the emergency room, he admits that he is short of breath. He denies chest pain, abdominal pain, nausea, and vomiting. There is no history of cardiac disease, diabetes, or previous respiratory illness. There is no smoking history or occupational exposure.*

QUESTION 1 What is the differential diagnosis of this patient's acute illness?

In spite of the limited history, a number of explanations for the patient's fever, cough, and shortness of breath need to be considered. An infectious process is an important possibility. Acute infectious diseases of the respiratory system include bronchitis and pneumonia. The latter seems more likely here, since shortness of breath is such a significant component. Many etiologies of pneumonia, including viruses, community acquired bacterial organisms, and fungi can present acutely. There are additional causes that are especially important in the alcoholic patient, including gram-negative bacteria such as *Klebsiella pneumoniae* and *Mycobacterium tuberculosis*.

Other noninfectious etiologies include pulmonary embolism (PE), myocardial infarction (MI),

and congestive heart failure (CHF). All of these can present acutely with respiratory impairment as the prominent feature. Some temperature elevation is often associated with both MI and PE. The fever makes CHF less likely. Less common pulmonary diseases are also in the differential of fever, cough, and shortness of breath including pulmonary vasculitis, alveolar proteinosis, and hypersensitivity pneumonitis.

Another important feature of the patient's presentation is an apparent change in mental status. A number of possibilities exist here as well. If the lethargy and confusion are a result of the acute illness rather than the ingestion of alcohol or another drug, significant hypoxemia and/or hypercapnia may be present; therefore, the patient needs to be evaluated quickly.

QUESTION 2 The physical examination reveals a gentleman appearing older than his stated age, who is in moderate respiratory distress. The use of accessory muscles of respiration is noted. The following vital signs are obtained: T 101.6°F, HR 120 bpm, RR 28/min, and BP 110/76 mm Hg. A pulsus paradoxus of 14 mm Hg is measured. The HEENT examination is without signs of trauma. There is poor dentition. The neck is supple. The cardiac examination reveals a regular rate and rhythm without murmurs, rubs, or gallops. Percussion of the chest is unrevealing for areas of dullness or tympany. Coarse rales are heard at the right base. The abdomen is nontender, without organomegaly. There is no clubbing, cyanosis, or edema of the extremities. Neurologic examination reveals lethargy, but there are no focal findings. Does the physical examination narrow the differential diagnosis?

The examination confirms the presence of a febrile illness with focal findings on auscultation of the lungs. The presence of egophony, whispered pectoriloquy, or increased tactile fremitus would be helpful since they would confirm the presence of consolidation in the right lower lobe, where the rales were heard. Pneumonia, aspiration, and pulmonary embolism could all be associated with rales in a single lobe, and signs of consolidation would be most consistent with pneumonia if they were present. MI and CHF certainly cause the degree of illness observed in this patient, but the right lower lobe findings would be unusual. Diseases such as alveolar proteinosis and hypersensitivity pneumonitis are characterized by diffuse lung involvement.

There are multiple signs of respiratory impairment present that should focus further evaluation and therapy on the patient's ventilation and oxygenation. Accessory muscles are in use, possibly indicating fatigue of the intercostal muscles and diaphragm. A pulsus paradoxus is measured and determined to be greater than 10 mm Hg. This determination of the inspiratory fall in blood pressure can be a valuable addition to the examination of patients who are generating large amounts of negative intrathoracic pressure on inspiration. In patients with other corroborative findings, it may indicate pericardial tamponade as the cause of heart failure.

Once again, the patient's mental status is a significant finding that may be secondary to fever, hypoxemia, hypercapnia, or an ingestion. The physical examination does not point to a particular etiology.

QUESTION 3 What tests are required immediately in the evaluation of this patient?

The chest x-ray and arterial blood gas would add valuable information in terms of the diagnosis and direction of therapy. Each can be quickly obtained without moving a seriously ill patient from the emergency room. A toxicology screen from either serum or urine and a blood alcohol level could also be easily obtained. Sputum gram stain and a complete blood count are indicated because pneumonia seems likely. Serum electrolytes including glucose should be ordered since the patient is lethargic, has a history of alcohol abuse, and his recent intake of fluids and nutrition are in question. An ECG may also be helpful in a patient of this age with so little past history available.

QUESTION 4 The patient receives oxygen by face mask and intravenous fluids, and antibiotics are begun. Initially he appears improved and somewhat more responsive. The following morning, cyanosis is noted around the lips and the nail beds, and the patient's respiratory rate is increased to 32 bpm. A repeat arterial blood gas is obtained with a pH of 7.52, $Paco_2$ 30 mm Hg, and Pao_2 45 mm Hg. Oxygenation does not improve with 100% oxygen by face mask. The patient requires intubation and mechanical ventilation. His follow-up chest x-ray reveals diffuse bilateral infiltrates. Cultures of blood and sputum remain negative. A repeat ECG is unchanged. Initial results are as follows: arterial pH 7.51, $Paco_2$ 32 mm Hg, Pao_2 52 mm Hg; the chest x-ray reveals an infiltrate involving the right middle and lower lobes. The heart size is normal, and there are no pleural effusions. The white blood cell count is 15,0000/mm³. The blood alcohol level is zero. Serum glucose and electrolytes are within normal limits. The 12-lead ECG is without acute ST or T wave changes. Other results are pending. What are the possible causes of the deterioration in the patient's condition?

It is important to note that the patient has refractory hypoxemia; in other words, it does not improve with increases in the amount of inspired oxygen. Shunt is the likely physiologic explanation for this observation and is the result of the continued perfusion of lung units that are not being ventilated. Alveolar filling processes and circulatory abnormalities are causes of shunt. In view of the acuity of the illness and the chest x-ray findings, an alveolar filling process is likely. Pneumonia and pulmonary edema are alveolar filling processes that can progress rapidly. The possibility of a bacterial pneumonia has been appropriately investigated, and cultures are thus far negative. However, acid-fast organisms, viruses, and atypical bacteria have not been excluded. The patient's course could also be explained by either cardiogenic or noncardiogenic pulmonary edema. The former is the result of increased left-sided pressures (left ventricular end diastolic pressure and pulmonary capillary wedge pressure), which are transmitted to the pulmonary circulation, causing an increased flow of fluid from the intravascular space to the interstitium of the lung. The normal mechanisms of fluid removal are eventually overwhelmed, and the alveoli begin to fill with fluid. Noncardiogenic edema forms secondary to endothelial damage rather than increases in hydrostatic pressure. Normally, the vascular endothelium does not allow the passage of significant amounts of protein between the intravascular and interstitial spaces. However, in a number of diseases, this endothelial barrier is disrupted, and fluid and protein enter the interstitium and alveoli along a concentration gradient. The result is a type of pulmonary edema in which alveolar fluid has a high protein. When this type of permeability edema is due to acute lung injury causing respiratory failure, it is referred to as the adult or acute respiratory distress syndrome (ARDS). The typical features of this syndrome are (1) refractory hypoxemia, (2) diffuse bilateral infiltrates, (3) falling lung compliance, and (4) a normal or low pulmonary capillary wedge pressure.

The patient may have developed cardiogenic pulmonary edema secondary to aggressive fluid and electrolyte replacement; however, there is no prior history of cardiac disease, no ECG changes, and there are no new findings on physical examination that suggest congestive heart failure. At least three of the features of ARDS mentioned previously are present, and this type of edema seems more likely to be present. See the box for criteria in the diagnosis of ARDS.

QUESTION 5 What is the likely underlying cause of ARDS in this patient, and how can the diagnosis be made?

CRITERIA IN THE DIAGNOSIS OF ARDS

- Presence of a predisposing condition
- 5-lobed pulmonary infiltrates
- Normal cardiac silhouette
- Normal or low pulmonary capillary wedge pressure
- Refractory hypoxemia despite high inspired oxygen concentrations
- Low lung compliance

There are a number of predisposing conditions associated with the development of ARDS. These account for 150,000 cases in the United States annually. Trauma, inhaled toxins, and metabolic disorders are some broad categories of pathology known to cause ARDS. Most commonly, the condition is attributed to sepsis, which is complicated by ARDS in 5% to 40% of patients. Aspiration of gastric contents, pneumonia, and drug ingestions are other important associated conditions—all of which are possible in this patient. An additional cause, especially important in the alcoholic patient, is pancreatitis, although the lack of abdominal complaints and findings makes the diagnosis unlikely in this case.

The patient's initial presentation was one of respiratory compromise with focal abnormalities on lung examination. An attempt should be made to diagnose this initial process, possibly by using fiberoptic bronchoscopy. If the patient's oxygenation can be improved with mechanical ventilatory support, specimens for culture (including viral, fungal, and acid fast) and cytopathologic examination could be obtained from the distal airways by bronchoscopy. A protected specimen brush or bronchoalveolar lavage with quantitative cultures, if available, could also be used to further investigate the possibility of a bacterial process. See the box for a thorough list of the conditions associated with ARDS.

In addition, it may be necessary to attempt to confirm the diagnosis of noncardiogenic pulmonary edema. This can be accomplished with the

Acute shortness of breath

Physical examination   { Vital signs, cough with
                                purulent sputum, accessory
                                muscle use, signs of
                                respiratory or cardiac
Immediate evaluation   dysfunction
    CXR
    Arterial blood gas
    Electrocardiogram
    Toxicology screen
    Sputum gram stain
    Electrolytes and complete blood count
    Bedside spirometry with $FEV_{1.0}$

Immediate therapy options
    Oxygen
    Antibiotics – if clinically indicated by evaluation
    Hemodynamic support
    Intubation and mechanical ventilation
    Bronchodilators

Further respiratory deterioration
and refractory hypoxemia –
Suspect shunt physiology

Place Swan-Ganz catheter
to measure pulmonary capillary
wedge pressure (PCWP)

Normal PCWP   Elevated PCWP

Noncardiogenic pulmonary
    edema (ARDS)   Cardiogenic pulmonary
                                                                edema

Consider differential diagnosis: Treat heart failure
    Trauma
    Toxic inhalation
    Metabolic disease
    Sepsis
    Gastric aspiration
    Pneumonia
    Drug ingestion
    Neurogenic pulmonary edema

    Treat underlying disease

Therapeutic goals:
    Support respiratory system with O_2 and mechanical ventilation (if needed)
    Ensure adequate tissue oxygen delivery
    Prevent organ dysfunction
    Prevent complications (DVT/PE, undernutrition, stress-related GI ulceration,
        nosocomial infection) of critical illness

3-6-1   Diagnostic algorithm for respiratory failure.

CONDITIONS ASSOCIATED WITH ARDS

- Sepsis
- Trauma
- Near drowning
- Aspiration of gastric contents
- Respiratory infections
- Drug overdose
- Pancreatitis
- Toxic inhalations
- Shock
- Prolonged hypotension
- Multiple emergent blood transfusion

insertion of a pulmonary artery (Swan-Ganz) catheter. The catheter is inserted into a central vein and advanced to the right heart and pulmonary artery. Pressures can be monitored at any of the structures through which the catheter passes including the right atrium, right ventricle, and pulmonary artery. Of particular interest in this case is the pulmonary capillary wedge pressure, obtained when the balloon at the end of the catheter is inflated at the point in the pulmonary artery where it occludes flow. Since there is no forward flow at this point of occlusion, the measured pressure is a reflection of downstream pressure at the left atrium and the left ventricular end diastolic pressure. Normally, the wedge pressure ranges from 8 to 12 mm Hg; pressures greater than 18 to 20 mm Hg indicate hydrostatic edema. A normal or low pulmonary capillary wedge pressure supports the diagnosis of ARDS. The Swan-Ganz catheter is also beneficial for evaluating cardiac function and cardiopulmonary interaction. Serial calculations of the cardiac output and other hemodynamic parameters are necessary to use the catheter optimally.

QUESTION 6   What is the appropriate therapy at this point? How can the patient's oxygenation be improved?

At the present time, there is no known therapy that can reverse the process of lung injury responsible for ARDS. Therapy should be directed at the underlying cause and should support the patient's ventilation and oxygenation. In cases of diffuse lung disease with hypoxemia secondary to shunt, oxygenation may remain a significant problem even after mechanical ventilation is begun. If the patient continues to require a high level of inspired oxygen (Fio_2 >0.50), further lung injury may occur. In these instances, positive endexpiratory pressure (PEEP) can improve oxygenation by preventing alveolar collapse at end expiration and recruiting a greater number of alveoli to participate in gas exchange. As PEEP is administered, the patient should be carefully monitored for adverse effects of PEEP, including a fall in blood pressure and barotrauma. The hemodynamic effects of PEEP are largely a result of continuous positive pressure in the thorax that impedes venous return. PEEP should be administered at a level that allows reduction of the Fio_2 to less than or equal to 0.50 without causing a significant decrease in blood pressure or a dangerous increase in airway pressure. An assist-control or controlled mandatory ventilation mode of ventilation should be used to minimize the patient's work of breathing and oxygen consumption. Sedation and paralysis are also helpful in some cases. In spite of these measures, the mortality of ARDS remains high (50% to 70%) and is often the result of injury to other organs or episodes of infection that are superimposed on the respiratory failure. A diagnostic algorithm for respiratory failure is shown in Fig. 3-6-1.

BIBLIOGRAPHY

Bone R: The adult respiratory distress syndrome (ARDS). In Bone R, Dantzker DR, George RB, et al, eds: *Pulmonary and critical care medicine*, St Louis, 1993, Mosby.

Hudson LD, Schwarz MI: Acute respiratory failure without previous lung disease. In Schwarz MI, ed: *Pulmonary grand rounds*, Philadelphia, 1990, BC Decker.

Matthay MA, Matthay RA: Pulmonary edema: cardiogenic and noncardiogenic. In George RB, Light RW, Matthay MA, Matthay RA, eds: *Chest medicine: essentials of pulmonary and critical care medicine*, ed 2, Baltimore, 1990, Williams & Wilkins.

CASE

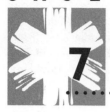

7

M. Jeffrey Barkoviak
Robert Balk

A 62-year-old man with a history of chronic obstructive pulmonary disease (COPD), diabetes mellitus, coronary artery disease, and CHF presents to the emergency room with a 1-week history of cough productive of green sputum, low grade fever, and worsening dyspnea. He was started on ampicillin orally 3 days ago by his internist. Since then, his cough has persisted and his dyspnea, which was initially associated with exertion, is now occurring at rest. He reports using his inhalers every 1 to 2 hours with only minimal relief of his dyspnea. He reports having intermittent chills, and his temperature yesterday was 100.9°F.

He reports smoking 2 packs of cigarettes a day for the last 40 years but quit 3 days ago. He has had a productive cough for "years" and was diagnosed with COPD 8 years ago when he began feeling short of breath at times. Since then he has used inhalers periodically for relief of his symptoms. He was hospitalized 1 year ago with an exacerbation of COPD and has required antibiotics every 2 to 3 months for bronchitis.

His medications include an albuterol metered dose inhaler (MDI), ipratroprium bromide MDI, furosemide 20 mg po q am, KCl 20 meq po q am, digoxin 0.125 mg po q am, NTG patch 0.4 mg q am, sustained-release theophylline 300 mg po bid, and ampicillin 500 mg po tid. He reports taking his albuterol regularly, but the others less frequently.

PHYSICAL EXAMINATION

Vital Signs: BP 184/98 mm Hg; HR 120 bpm; RR 32/min; T 100.2°F
General appearance: Elderly male in moderate respiratory distress
Skin: Pale, diaphoretic

HEENT: Remarkable for pursed lip breathing and circumoral cyanosis
Neck: Notable for use of the accessory muscles of respiration and the presence of JVD halfway to the angle of the mandible
Chest: Symmetric, increased anteroposterior diameter
Lungs: Distant breath sounds with prolonged expiratory phase, scattered rhonchi
Cardiac: Tachycardic, normal S_1, increased P2, II/VI systolic murmur at the left upper sternal border radiating to the carotid arteries, no gallops or rubs
Abdomen: Paradoxical breathing pattern noted; Hoover's sign present; abdomen flat, soft, and nontender
Extremities: 1+ pretibial edema; cyanosis of the nailbeds noted
Neurologic: Nonfocal

QUESTION 1 Considering this patient's history and physical examination findings, what would be the differential diagnosis of this patient's symptoms?

The differential diagnosis would include an exacerbation of COPD, pneumonia, congestive heart failure (CHF), pulmonary embolism, acute myocardial infarction (MI), and pneumothorax.

QUESTION 2 What is the most likely diagnosis given the history and physical examination findings?

The history of cough productive of purulent-appearing sputum in a smoker with known obstructive lung disease is strongly suggestive of an exacerbation of COPD triggered by a lower respiratory tract infection. Several signs on physical examination are suggestive of hyperinflation secondary to obstructive lung disease. Use of the accessory muscles of respiration, namely the scalene and sternocleidomastoid muscles, are commonly recruited into use to assist inspiration in these patients. Hyperinflation results in flattening of the diaphragm, which places it at a mechanical disadvantage, making its role in inspiration less efficient. Hoover's sign (the inward retraction of the lower rib cage during inspiration) can also be seen in severe hyperinflation and is due to the low, flattened position of the diaphragm that pulls the rib cage inward when it contracts. The presence of a paradoxical breathing pattern in which the abdomen is retracted inward during inspiration also supports this diagnosis. This pattern results when the accessory muscles of inspiration contract, generating a negative intrathoracic pressure, thereby pulling the diaphragm upward during inspiration rather than in the downward direction that normally occurs during inspiration. Pursed lip breathing, increased anteroposterior thoracic diameter and prolonged expiratory phase are other signs that are commonly seen in COPD and would support this diagnosis.

QUESTION 3 How would you proceed in diagnosing this patient?

A complete blood count is necessary to evaluate the white blood cell count that may be elevated in infection. An arterial blood gas is necessary to assess oxygenation and ventilation. A chest x-ray (CXR) is used to look for pneumonia, pulmonary edema, or pneumothorax. An ECG and cardiac enzymes will reveal a new ischemic event or recent MI leading to CHF.

QUESTION 4 The blood tests you ordered show an elevated WBC of 21,000 with a left shift. ECG shows sinus tachycardia with P pulmonale, RVH, RAD, inferior Q waves, and nonspecific ST-segment

changes; the ECG is unchanged from a previous tracing performed 1 year ago. The CXR shows flattened diaphragms and increased AP diameter; heart size is normal. A right middle lobe (RML) infiltrate is seen. A room air ABG shows pH 7.32, P_{CO_2} 65 mm Hg, P_{O_2} 40 mm Hg. How would you interpret the results of the ABG?

The arterial blood gas (ABG) shows hypoxemia and respiratory acidosis with a metabolic alkalosis. In acute respiratory acidosis, every increase in P_{CO_2} by 10 mm Hg should be accompanied by a decrease in pH by 0.08 units. Therefore, if this patient were experiencing an acute respiratory acidosis with a P_{CO_2} of 65 mm Hg, the pH should be 7.20. In this patient, the pH is not as low as one would expect with a pure acute respiratory acidosis; therefore, a concurrent metabolic alkalosis must also be present.

Given the scenario of this case, it is reasonable to speculate that this patient has had a chronic respiratory acidosis as a result of his COPD with metabolic compensation to keep the pH in the physiologic range. The increase in P_{CO_2} occurring as a result of this exacerbation of COPD is therefore associated with a decrease in pH that is not as extreme as it would otherwise be had there not been a metabolic alkalosis present.

QUESTION 5 The remainder of his blood tests are normal; his theophylline and digoxin levels are subtherapeutic. Blood cultures are also obtained. Given the above information, what is the most likely diagnosis? How would you treat this patient?

The most likely diagnosis is an exacerbation of COPD brought on by a lower respiratory tract infection. Treatment initially should be geared toward correcting hypoxemia and relieving airway obstruction. Special attention should be paid to the elevated P_{CO_2}, which may reflect the degree of airways obstruction or may be a sign of fatigue of the respiratory muscles.

Oxygen delivered in controlled amounts (i.e., with a face mask) is the initial treatment action.

Delivery of oxygen via a nasal cannula should be avoided in these patients during an acute episode as the amount of oxygen delivered depends upon the respiratory rate and the volume of gas inhaled, which can be variable in patients with respiratory distress.

Another goal of treatment would be relief of airways obstruction. Use of inhaled beta-2-bronchodilators would be the initial treatment of choice. Inhalation of these medications via an MDI can be difficult during an acute exacerbation, so the medication should be delivered via a nebulizer or with a MDI using a spacer device. The effectiveness of these medications in COPD patients depends largely upon the nature of their disease and the degree of reversibility of airways obstruction. Some patients with emphysema, for example, may have little reversibility. However, many patients have some overlap with reversible airways disease and do benefit from inhaled beta-2-agonist medications.

Repeat ABGs are essential in the early management of these patients to assess the progression of or recovery from the airway obstruction and respiratory muscle fatigue.

QUESTION 6 Since arrival in the emergency room, the patient has received two treatments with albuterol via med nebulizer. He has been placed on oxygen with an FiO_2 of 50% via Venti-mask. His dyspnea has progressed to the point that he is unable to speak in complete sentences. A repeat ABG shows pH 7.19, PcO_2 94 mm Hg, PO_2 85 mm Hg. How would you proceed in managing this patient at this time?

This patient's inability to speak in complete sentences is a strong indicator of progressive respiratory failure and should be an indicator of potential respiratory arrest. The arterial blood gas confirms this clinical suspicion and demonstrates progressive hypercapnic respiratory failure as indicated by the increase in PcO_2 and worsening respiratory acidosis.

At this point, the patient needs assisted venti-lation and should be intubated and placed on mechanical ventilation.

QUESTION 7 The patient is orally intubated but with difficulty due to his severe respiratory distress. A size 7.0 endotracheal tube is passed on the second attempt and is secured in place. The patient is placed on a mechanical ventilator. What parameters must be ordered to begin mechanical ventilation?

Four parameters must be considered when initiating mechanical ventilation: the mode of mechanical ventilation, the amount of oxygen to be delivered, the size of each breath, and the rate at which each breath is delivered.

The mode of mechanical ventilation can vary depending on the brand of ventilator in use. Most modern ventilators have several modes that can be used based upon the situation in which it is to be used and the level of support desired. Assist-control (A/C) is a form of ventilation in which every breath is fully assisted by the ventilator. If a patient chooses to breath at a rate that is faster than the rate programmed into the ventilator, he or she must trigger the ventilator with a small amount of effort (usually 1 to 2 cm H_2O pressure), and the ventilator will deliver a fully assisted tidal volume. This mode of ventilation is often used when patients are initially started on mechanical ventilation because it provides nearly full support. The patient is able to attain his or her desired minute ventilation with minimal effort.

Synchronized intermittent mandatory ventilation (SIMV) is another support form of mechanical ventilation. In this mode, the ventilator will deliver fully assisted tidal volume breaths at a set rate determined by the physician. If the patient chooses a rate faster than that set on the ventilator, he or she is able to take an additional breath, but without assistance of the ventilator. A patient can be fully supported in this mode of ventilation if the rate set on the ventilator meets or exceeds the respiratory rate of the patient. This mode can also be used to wean patients from mechanical ventilation. During weaning, the SIMV rate is gradually reduced, and the patient's own, spontaneous respirations replace the reduction in support by the ventilator.

Inspiratory pressure support ventilation (PSV) is a mode of mechanical ventilation that can provide partial or full support. In this mode each breath is patient triggered and supported by the ventilator. Inspiration begins when the ventilator senses that the patient is making an inspiratory effort, detected by a pressure drop or change in flow. The ventilator delivers a set level of pressure to the airways, and gas is delivered to the lungs. The volume of gas delivered to the patient depends on the pressure level set on the ventilator and the compliance (stiffness) of the patient's lungs. For a given level of pressure support, a decrease in compliance (increase in lung stiffness) will result in a reduction of delivered tidal volume. This form of ventilation can fully support a patient if enough pressure is set to minimize the inspiratory work the patient must perform. It can also be used as a weaning mode alone or in combination with SIMV. The amount of pressure support can be gradually reduced as is done with SIMV weaning until the patient is performing most of the ventilatory work. This mode is also used in small amounts (5 to 7 cm H_2O) in combination with SIMV to assist the patient's spontaneous ventilations by overcoming the resistance of the endotracheal tube and ventilator circuit. This mode of ventilation is limited in that it cannot be used in patients with altered mental status because each breath must be triggered by the patient.

The amount of oxygen to be delivered with each breath must also be ordered when beginning mechanical ventilation. This decision is based on the clinical situation, but in practice 100% oxygen is typically given at first to avoid unnecessary hypoxemia by underestimating the patient's requirements. The level of oxygen can be adjusted accordingly by following arterial blood gas measurements or oximetry.

The size of the delivered breath (tidal volume) must also be set on the ventilator. Traditionally, tidal volume size is based upon the size of the patient and has been in the range of 10 to 15 ml/kg. Recent studies suggest that tidal volumes in this range may promote lung injury by causing overdistention of the alveoli. Tidal volumes of 8 to 10 ml/kg are now considered a more appropriate size. Tidal volumes as low as 5 ml/kg, while tolerating the associated hypercapnea, are recommended in certain patients with acute lung injury to prevent further trauma to the lungs.

The desired respiratory rate must also be set on the ventilator if the patient is placed in the A/C or SIMV mode. This decision must be based on the clinical situation at hand, the degree of ventilatory failure, and is guided by ABG determinations. In general, rates in the range of 10 to 20 bpm are appropriate.

QUESTION 8   The patient is placed on the ventilator in the assist-control (A/C) mode, Fio_2 of 100%, RR of 16/min, tidal volume of 700 ml. Rapidly, the patient's RR becomes 32/min, he appears anxious, and his blood pressure drops to 80/50 mm Hg. On examination breath sounds are diminished bilaterally, and his expiratory phase remains prolonged. What are the possible etiologies of the hypotension and respiratory distress in this situation?

Hypotension and respiratory distress in a patient on mechanical ventilation must prompt an immediate search for a tension pneumothorax. Rupture of an alveolus or a bulla resulting from barotrauma can be life-threatening in patients who are receiving positive pressure mechanical ventilation. Air under pressure delivered by the ventilator can leak in this situation into the pleural space causing collapse of the lung. As further tidal volumes are delivered, more air leaks into the pleural space, resulting in further collapse of the lung and the development of increasing positive pressure in the pleural space. This can cause compression of the mediastinal structures, in particular, the superior and inferior vena cavae, resulting in decreased venous return to the heart and hypotension. A tension pneumothorax can be diagnosed clinically by the absence of breath sounds, hyperinflation of the chest, deviation of the trachea, and the presence of subcutaneous emphysema. If time allows, a chest x-ray can confirm the finding. The presence of a pneumothorax in a patient on mechanical ventilation mandates the placement of a chest tube to evacuate the air from the pleural space to prevent the development of a tension pneumothorax and hypotension.

The delivery of mechanical ventilator breaths under positive pressure can impair venous return even in the absence of a pneumothorax. Normally, individuals inspire by generating a negative intrathoracic pressure with the diaphragm and inspiratory muscles, which causes air to flow into the chest. During mechanical ventilation, inspiration is accomplished by forcing air into the chest using positive pressure. This positive pressure is transmitted to the entire thorax and can impede venous return. This scenario is typically seen in patients who are volume depleted and can usually be treated with IV fluids.

Dynamic hyperinflation or auto-PEEP (positive end-expiratory pressure) is another mechanism of hypotension and respiratory distress that can be seen in mechanically ventilated patients. This is usually found in patients with COPD or asthma who require mechanical ventilation. Auto-PEEP occurs because of the airway obstruction found in these patients and is due to their inability to completely exhale before the next breath is delivered by the ventilator. It is seen when the respiratory rate set by the patient or ventilator is too high or if the rate at which the gas is delivered during inspiration (inspiratory flow rate) is too low. When auto-PEEP is present, gas is trapped in the alveoli, which become overdistended. In order to trigger the next ventilator breath in the A/C mode, the patient has to overcome the pressure present in the alveoli as well as the triggering pressure on the ventilator. This can result in a significant work load for the patient and can lead to respiratory distress and eventually further ventilatory failure. The added positive pressure at end-expiration can impede venous return as previously described and result in hypotension. Auto-PEEP can be treated or

compensated for by treating the underlying obstruction with bronchodilators and antiinflammatory medications. Adjustments on the ventilator can also reduce the air-trapping induced by auto-PEEP. Increasing the inspiratory flow rate will allow a longer time for exhalation and will reduce air-trapping. Paradoxically, adding low levels of PEEP with the ventilator will ease the patient's work of breathing by decreasing the amount of pressure drop required to initiate the next breath.

Other diagnoses to consider in a critically ill patient such as this would be pulmonary embolism, myocardial infarction with or without CHF, and sepsis.

QUESTION 9 The patient is given an IV fluid bolus of 500 ml of 0.9% NaCl, and his blood pressure increases to 110/70 mm Hg and stabilizes. A CXR showed no evidence of pneumothorax. He is given albuterol via a medication nebulizer and becomes less tachypneic and appears more comfortable with an RR of 16/min.

An ABG is obtained 30 minutes after the patient is placed on mechanical ventilation and shows pH 7.54, P_{CO_2} 38 mm Hg, P_{O_2} 184 mm Hg. How would you interpret the ABG in this patient? Are any changes needed in the settings on the ventilator?

The ABG shows a metabolic alkalosis (elevated pH in the presence of a normal P_{CO_2}) and supranormal P_{O_2}. Considering this patient's history of COPD and probable chronic respiratory acidosis (chronically elevated P_{CO_2} compensated by elevation of serum bicarbonate levels), this blood gas suggests that this patient is being hyperventilated and in reality is a respiratory alkalosis in this particular case. If this level of ventilation is continued, the kidneys will respond by decreasing bicarbonate reabsorption, leading to a reduction of serum bicarbonate toward normal. At the time this patient would be ready to wean from the ventilator, he would become acidotic if he returns to his baseline elevated P_{CO_2} without the presence of his normally elevated bicarbonate levels to buffer. It would be prudent to decrease the level of ventilation in this patient by decreasing the respiratory rate and allow the P_{CO_2} to rise while aiming for a pH of 7.34 to 7.36. This strategy will maintain the chronic elevation of bicarbonate needed to compensate for this patient's chronic respiratory acidosis.

Reducing the F_{IO_2} is also needed with a goal of maintaining arterial saturation above 90% to 92% only. Supraphysiologic P_{O_2} levels have no clinical utility because they do not increase the oxygen content of the blood significantly. There are studies that show that use of high F_{IO_2} levels (SBP >60%) for prolonged periods of time can contribute to lung injury and may result in fibrosis.

QUESTION 10 The F_{IO_2} is decreased eventually to 40% while maintaining an oxygen saturation of 91% by oximetry. The respiratory rate is decreased to 10, and the patient's spontaneous rate is a total of 12 bpm. A repeat blood gas on these settings shows pH 7.34, P_{CO_2} 58 mm Hg, P_{O_2} 64 mm Hg. He is given albuterol via medication nebulizer every 4 hours and is started on IV Solu-Medrol for his exacerbation of COPD. Broad-spectrum IV antibiotics are started for treatment of his pneumonia.

Over the next 72 hours, the patient is maintained at the same level of ventilatory support and requires albuterol treatments less frequently. He has defervesced, and his sputum production is decreasing. What information is important in determining when a patient is ready to wean from mechanical ventilation?

An important initial determination is to decide if the reason mechanical ventilation was instituted has improved, resolved, or has been adequately compensated. Other factors that must be considered when deciding when to wean a patient from mechanical ventilation include level of consciousness, nutrition, amount of secretions, and degree of airway obstruction. It is important that patients be alert enough to comprehend what is occurring during the weaning process and that they be able to protect their airway if extubation is anticipated. Patients must be well-rested before a weaning trial and should have sedatives and paralytic agents discontinued at least 24 hours before a weaning trial. It is essential that proper nutritional support be initiated soon after a patient is started on mechanical ventilation. It may be necessary to perform metabolic analysis to assess the adequacy of nutrition. Patients must be able to handle the amount of secretions they produce with an adequate cough. Finally, if airway obstruction has complicated the patient's course, adequate treatment with bronchodilators and antiinflammatory medications is needed. It is also important that the patient's oxygen requirements have improved to the point that he or she requires no more than 50% oxygen while maintaining an adequate P_{O_2}. In this patient, the resolution of fever, the reduction of sputum production, and the decreasing frequency of bronchodilator requirements suggest that the underlying pneumonia and associated exacerbation of COPD is being adequately treated and the patient is improving.

QUESTION 11 The decision is made to wean the patient from the ventilation and weaning parameters are ordered. What weaning parameters are useful in determining when a patient is able to wean from mechanical ventilation?

"Traditional" weaning parameters include measurements of the patient's spontaneous tidal volume, vital capacity, peak negative inspiratory force, and minute ventilation (RR × tidal volume). It is generally believed that a patient is not ready to be weaned from the ventilator until he or she meets the following criteria:

Tidal volume of 4-5 ml/kg

Vital capacity of 10-15 ml/kg

Peak negative inspiratory force of −20 cm H_2O or more negative

Minute ventilation less than 10 l

Unfortunately, the predictive value of these indices is quite variable and are often not useful in patients who have been intubated and mechanically ventilated for more than a few days. As a result, other weaning parameters and indices have been investigated. These include complex indices that integrate a number of physiologic functions including measurements of compliance, maximal inspiratory pressure, and measures of gas exchange. Other variables assess the patient's work of breathing by using an esophageal manometer. Recently, an index was developed that assesses the respiratory pattern of spontaneously breathing patients who are weaning from mechanical ventilation. It relies on a measure of tachypnea and reduction in tidal volume that commonly occurs in patients who develop ventilatory failure. The rapid shallow breathing (RSB) index measures respiratory frequency (f) and spontaneous tidal volume (Vt) as the ratio f/Vt. It was found that an RSB index of 100 best differentiated patients who weaned or failed; a high RSB index indicates that a patient is likely to fail.

QUESTION 12 The patient's spontaneous tidal volume is 300 ml, he generates a vital capacity of 500 ml, his maximal negative inspiratory force is −18 cm H_2O, and the minute ventilation is 12 l. The RSB index (f/Vt) is 110. A weaning trial is planned. What methods of weaning are available?

There are numerous techniques and strategies available for weaning patients from mechanical ventilation. No one technique has been proven superior to another. The use of one strategy over another depends upon the clinician's familiarity and the clinical situation. T-piece trials involve removing the patient from the ventilator and connecting a high flow oxygen source to the endotracheal tube. The patient is placed on the T-piece for progressively longer duration until it is felt that he can sustain ventilation without the assistance of a mechanical ventilator. Patients can also be weaned by gradually decreasing the respiratory rate if the patient is in the SIMV mode or by gradually decreasing the set inspiratory pressure level if the patient is ventilated in the pressure-support mode. This method has the advantage that the patient remains connected to the ventilator and can be monitored with the equipment on the ventilator.

QUESTION 13 The patient's ventilator is switched from SIMV with a rate of 10 to a rate of 6. After 15 minutes the patient complains of dyspnea, develops tachycardia and an elevated blood pressure. His respiratory rate increases to 32 per min with spontaneous tidal volumes of 50 to 100 ml. The ventilator rate is increased to 10, and the patient becomes more comfortable. Over the next 4 days, further attempts at reducing respiratory rate are unsuccessful. What are some of the possible causes of this patient's inability to wean from mechanical ventilation?

In this patient, partial treatment of the pneumonia and COPD exacerbation could be the primary reason for failure to wean. Several more days of therapy with antibiotics, bronchodilators, and antiinflammatory agents may be necessary. It is important, however, to consider and evaluate for other occult reasons for failure to wean. Unsuspected respiratory muscle weakness is a common cause for inability to wean and can have many etiologies. Hypophosphatemia, hypomagnesemia, and hypokalemia occur commonly in ICU patients and cause respiratory muscle weakness. Serum chemistry profiles can identify this cause, which can be corrected with appropriate supplementation. Inadequate or inappropriate nutrition can contribute to failure to wean from mechanical ventilation. Inadequate caloric intake can cause respiratory muscle weakness, while excessive carbohydrate intake can lead to increased CO_2 production and may place a high ventilatory demand on the patient. This can be evaluated by performing a metabolic analysis and determining oxygen consumption and CO_2 production. Appropriate changes in nutritional supplementation can then be made. Unsuspected hypothyroidism, especially in elderly patients, can result in respiratory muscle weakness if not adequately treated. Excessive work of breathing because of airway obstruction as a result of bronchospasm, secretions, or an endotracheal tube

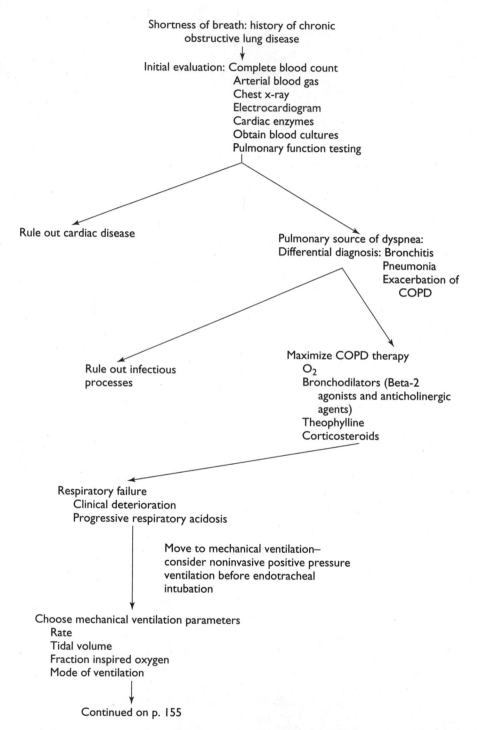

Shortness of breath: history of chronic
obstructive lung disease

Initial evaluation: Complete blood count
Arterial blood gas
Chest x-ray
Electrocardiogram
Cardiac enzymes
Obtain blood cultures
Pulmonary function testing

Rule out cardiac disease

Pulmonary source of dyspnea:
Differential diagnosis: Bronchitis
Pneumonia
Exacerbation of
COPD

Rule out infectious
processes

Maximize COPD therapy
O$_2$
Bronchodilators (Beta-2
agonists and anticholinergic
agents)
Theophylline
Corticosteroids

Respiratory failure
Clinical deterioration
Progressive respiratory acidosis

Move to mechanical ventilation—
consider noninvasive positive pressure
ventilation before endotracheal
intubation

Choose mechanical ventilation parameters
Rate
Tidal volume
Fraction inspired oxygen
Mode of ventilation

Continued on p. 155

3-7-1   Diagnostic algorithm for chronic obstructive pulmonary disease (COPD).

Cont'd. from p. 154

Monitor for adverse effects of mechanical
ventilation
Barotrauma
Hemodynamic compromise
Auto - PEEP
Determine necessary parameters needed
to provide respiratory support
FiO_2 Tidal volume
Respiratory rate

Treat source of respiratory failure
and avoid complications of critical illness:
Malnutrition
DVT/PE
Stop related GI bleeding
Nosocomial infection

Determine when weaning is appropriate
and evaluate weaning parameters
Tidal volume
Vital capacity
Negative inspiratory force
Minute ventilation
and
Ensure: Normal electrolytes (K^+, Mg^+, P^+, Ca^{++})
Adequate nutrition
Absence of sources of increased CO_2 production
Adequate rest for muscles of respiration
Unnecessary use of sedation or neuromuscular blocking
agents
Adequate removal of airway secretions
Avoidance of elevated airway pressures ($>40cm$ H_2O)
by manipulation of V_T; inspiratory flow rate
use of pressure support mode
Avoidance of undue hypercapnea with acidosis or
hypoxemia

3-7-1   Cont'd.

that is too small can cause a patient to fail. Finally, analgesics, sedatives, and tranquilizers are commonly given in the ICU setting and may cause central ventilatory drive suppression. Paralytic agents are also known to cause prolonged respiratory muscle weakness. Aminoglycoside antibiotics have been reported to cause neuromuscular paralysis, which is a potential cause for weaning failure, but is rarely seen today. A diagnostic algorithm for chronic obstructive pulmonary disease is shown in Fig. 3-7-1.

CASE FOLLOW-UP   The patient was continued on an aggressive regimen of bronchodilators, anti-inflammatory agents, and antibiotics. Serum chemistry profile revealed a phosphorus level of 1.0 mg/dl, which was corrected with supplementation. A metabolic cart study showed that the patient was receiving an adequate caloric intake and that he did not have excessive CO_2 production. His serum T_4 and TSH levels were normal. The size 7.0 endotracheal tube was noted to be kinked in the patient's posterior pharynx and was changed to a size 8.5 tube.

Attempts at weaning by reducing the SIMV respiratory rate were well tolerated by the patient with spontaneous rates of 10 to 16. The patient was eventually extubated 3 days later.

• •

BIBLIOGRAPHY

Benotti PN, Bistrain B: Metabolic and nutritional aspects of weaning from mechanical ventilation, *Crit Care Med* 17: 181-185, 1989.

Hickling KG, Henderson SJ: Low mortality associated with low volume pressure limited ventilation with permissive hypercapnia in severe adult respiratory distress syndrome, *Intensive Care Med* 16:372-377, 1990.

Jackson RM: Pulmonary oxygen toxicity, *Chest* 88:900-905, 1985.

Knochel JP: The clinical status of hypophosphatemia: an update, *N Engl J Med* 313:447-449, 1985.

Milic-Emili J: How to monitor intrinsic PEEP-and why, *J Crit Illness* 7:25-32, 1992.

Pinsky MR: The effects of mechanical ventilation on the cardiovascular system, *Crit Care Clin* 6:663-678, 1990.

Schmidt GA, Hall JB: Acute or chronic respiratory failure: assessment and management of patients with COPD in the emergency setting, *JAMA* 261:3444-3453, 1989.

Siafakas NM, Salesiotou V: Respiratory muscle strength in hypothyroidism, *Chest* 102:189-194, 1992.

Slutsky AS: Mechanical ventilation, *Chest* 104:1833-1859, 1993.

Sporn PH, Morganroth ML: Discontinuation of mechanical ventilation, *Clin Chest Med* 9:113-126, 1988.

Yang K, Tobin MJ: A prospective study of indexes predicting outcome of trials of weaning from mechanical ventilation, *N Engl J Med* 324:1445-1450, 1991.

C A S E

8

Charles J. Grodzin
Robert Balk

As the emergency room resident you are called to see a 66-year-old white man with a significant history of congestive heart failure, diabetes mellitus, and peripheral vascular disease. The patient came to the emergency room with complaints of progressive shortness of breath over the past week and recent inability to walk through his house.

In the emergency room vital signs are T 99.4°F, RR 36/min, BP 188/107 mm Hg, and P 122 bpm. Pulse oximetry reads 83% on room air but improves to 95% on a 100 Fio_2 nonrebreather mask. The patient is barely able to complete an entire sentence because of shortness of breath. He is diaphoretic, and is coughing up pink sputum. The physical examination reveals bilateral coarse crackles, 3+ lower extremity edema to the presacral area, a cardiac S3, and jugular venous distension to the angle of the mandible. Arterial blood gas taken on arrival returns: pH 7.20, Pco_2 60 mm Hg, and Po_2 49 mm Hg.

Soon thereafter, the patient demonstrates an escalating respiratory rate to 50 with perioral and acral cyanosis, increased tachycardia, and gradually increasing obtundation.

QUESTION I What is the appropriate treatment for the patient's deteriorating respiratory status? What are the physiologic responses to this treatment?

This patient requires immediate cardiopulmonary stabilization. In such a case, the definitive diagnosis is a secondary concern. The presentation of this patient is highly suggestive of congestive heart failure with the development of pulmonary edema leading to hypercapnea and hypoxemia. The development of progressive tachypnea, cyanosis, and obtundation along with the arterial blood gas analysis fulfills the criteria for acute respiratory failure. The most important immediate therapeutic intervention for the patient's deteriorating respiratory status is endotracheal intubation and mechanical ventilation.

There are two methods of augmenting ventilation: use of an external bag-mask apparatus or placement of an endotracheal tube (ETT). Use of a bag-mask system requires that the patient be stable and that the operator have significant skill and experience to assure airway patency and adequate ventilation. Maintenance of the airway is essential in providing adequate ventilation. Maneuvering the neck into extension and placing cephalad traction on the hyoid bone pulls the epiglottis and base of the tongue away from the posterior pharynx, opening the airway. An alternative maneuver is to place cephalad traction on the mandible to open the airway. Placement of an oral or nasal airway will help in maintaining airway patency. In placement of an airway, the nasal route is better tolerated. However, there is the attendant risk of nasal bleeding or fracture of a nasal turbinate. Iatrogenic injury can be minimized by making sure to push the nasal airway straight back rather than towards the top of the head. This facilitates entry into the nasopharynx as opposed to surrounding soft tissue structures.

In some situations wherein the patient has abnormal facial anatomy as a result of trauma or a congenital anomaly, it may be difficult to maintain an adequate mask seal. To help maintain mask seal, one can pull the cheeks over the sides of the mask. Leaving a patient's dentures in place or placing padding along the zygomatic process may also be useful to produce a tight seal. In some cases two people may need to participate: one to secure the mask in place with two hands and the other to ventilate the patient.

The other alternative to secure the airway is by placement of an ETT. There are five major indications for the placement of an ETT. First is maintenance of airway patency. In patients with compromised mental status, it is common for the soft tissue of the pharynx (tongue, epiglottis) to occlude the upper airway. The second indication is protection of the airway from passive regurgitation and aspiration of gastric contents. In situations of vomiting or bleeding, it is imperative to place an ETT to avoid aspiration if the patient is not able to close the glottis voluntarily. Massive aspiration is often unavoidable. An ETT is also necessary for the application of high levels of positive airway pressure or high levels of oxygen concentration. Finally, patients who require frequent suctioning to maintain pulmonary toilet may need an ETT for ease of care.

Placement of an ETT has attendant physiologic effects. Activation of either the parasympathetic or sympathetic nervous system can cause either bradycardia or hypertension and tachycardia. In addition, intubation may increase intracranial pressure because of decreased cranial venous return, transient elevation of CO_2 with cerebral vasodilatation, or increased cranial perfusion.

The pulmonary system may also be affected. The usual anatomic dead space in a healthy person is approximately 75 ml. Intubation can result in a decrease in the amount of dead space. A size 8 ETT that is 25 cm in length contains only 12.6 ml. However, attachment of the usual tubing may partially ameliorate this gain. Airway resistance is also affected. At low levels of airflow, airway resistance is small. However, as airflow increases and becomes more turbulent, ETT resistance can rise substantially. When the respiratory rate is very high, the resistance generated by the tube may be large enough to produce intrinsic PEEP. Coughing may be impaired because of an inability to close the glottis. Therefore, secretions

may accumulate in the airway, necessitating frequent suctioning to maintain pulmonary toilet and avoid ETT obstruction. Also, placement of an ETT may result in bronchospasm.

QUESTION 2   The chest x-ray taken before intubation reveals cardiomegaly, changes consistent with bilateral alveolar edema, and pleural effusions. Because of the clinical deterioration and hypoxemia, the decision is made to intubate the patient. Once the decision to endotracheally intubate a patient is settled upon, what are the indications for oral versus nasal intubation?

In general, it is preferrable to place an ETT orally. The oral route accommodates a larger size tube, allowing for a higher minute ventilation, easier access to secretions, and an easier route for the performance of bronchoscopy. Disadvantages of nasal tubes include a steeper dynamic resistance-to-air-flow curve, making high-flow breathing much more difficult for the patient. Occlusion of the ostia of the paranasal sinuses leads to more frequent paranasal sinusitis. In a comparison of the occurrence of sinus effusions, orally placed tubes were associated with effusions in 63% of patients as opposed to 95% in patients intubated via the nasal route.

The major indications for the placement of nasal tubes are cases in which oral hygiene is imperative, patients with prior laryngeal or cervical spine injury, and in patients who have demonstrated a propensity for self-extubation.

QUESTION 3   The respiratory therapist begins to ventilate the patient with an ambu-bag and opens the airway with mandibular traction. The Sao_2 monitor reads 87%. As you consider the intubation procedure, your attending asks you to recount the correct preparatory steps for intubation. What are the important aspects of patient preparation for intubation and what are the methods of tube placement?

Since the consequences of failed intubation may be catastrophic, adequate patient preparation is imperative. The patient should undergo bag-mask ventilation with care taken to ensure a patent airway to avoid hypoxia should tube placement be difficult. The patient should be positioned correctly, and the upper airway anesthetized well. Adjunctive pharmocologic agents are useful to blunt consciousness, provide an amnestic response for the procedure, minimize the muscular tone of the pharynx, and minimize activation of the sympathetic and parasympathetic nervous system in order to avoid cardiovascular and intracranial responses to intubation.

Correct position of the patient on the bed is essential to make the intubation process successful. The patient should be placed so that the head is at the end of the bed. Flexion of the cervicothoracic junction and extension of the atlantoaxial joint (the "sniffing position") allows the airway to assume a straight path. This facilitates visualization of the vocal cords upon direct laryngoscopy. In general, awake intubation can be done with ease as long as care is taken to anesthetize the upper airway and to diminish secretions by use of an antisialagogue (atropine). Use of lidocaine gel placed in the back of the mouth or coating the ETT will help anesthetize the mucosa in contact with the tube. Anesthesia of the trachea can be carried out readily by the use of nebulized lidocaine via nebulizer, bronchoscope, or the transtracheal route.

The agent of choice for muscle relaxation is succinylcholine. This depolarizing agent depletes the neuroendplate of neurotransmitters. This leaves the neurons refractory to further stimulation. This initial action is manifest as diffuse muscle fasciculations. This agent has an onset of action of 1 minute and duration of 3 minutes. Contraindications to use include paraplegia or other neurologic deficits and significant burn injuries that lead to hyperkalemia. Malignant hyperthermia may also occur. The usual dose is 1 mg/kg IV. The nondepolarizing agents and neuromuscular blocking agents have longer durations of action, making them less useful.

Use of sedation is also important. The agent of choice is midazolam as it provides short-term sedation with an amnestic element. In addition, it has little effect on the cardiovascular system. Doses of 1 mg IV may be given every 1 to 2 minutes successively until the desired level of consciousness is reached. Another alternative is a short-term barbiturate (thiopental). Because of high lipid solubility, this agent quickly enters the central nervous system, providing sedation with rapid redistribution and return of consciousness. In patients with depressed cardiac function, venous pooling may lead to significant hypotension in the hypovolemic patient. Other agents used less often include ketamine, which may be most useful in the patient with bronchospasm as it stimulates release of epinephrine. However, it may cause myocardial depression and ischemia. Etomidate is another short-acting agent that causes significant adrenocortical suppression. The toxic, adverse reactions to these agents makes them less useful.

The laryngoscope is held in the left hand, the blade is placed in the mouth and used to sweep the tongue to the left with traction applied at a 45° angle. This pulls the epiglottis away from the anterior pharynx to expose the glottis. In some cases, external cricoid cartilage pressure need be applied to move an anterior-placed glottis into clear view. The ETT is advanced into the airway only when the vocal cords can be seen clearly and during cord abduction.

Patient preparation for nasotracheal intubation differs in that it requires less sedation because it is a more comfortable procedure. A nasal vasoconstrictive agent should be used before tube placement to avoid nasal trauma. Warming the tube in warm water will increase the flexibility of the tube and allow easier passage and less mucosal injury. Once the tube has advanced into the oropharynx, it may be visualized through the mouth. At that time it may be helpful to advance the tube under direct vision with a Magill forceps.

There are several other less used methods of endotracheal intubation apart from the oral and nasal route. Blind nasal intubation can be carried out readily even in the presence of copious blood and secretions. The tube is guided into the glottis by listening through the tube for breath sounds and palpation of the neck to avoid lateral deviation. This technique requires little additional equipment.

Retrograde intubation is less commonly used. This procedure calls for introduction of a wire through a needle transtracheally until the end appears in the mouth or nose. Once established, this provides a guide for the antegrade placement of an ETT over the guide wire. Once the tip of the tube has reached the trachea, the wire is removed. This method may be particularly useful when facial anatomy is abnormal from either trauma, surgery, or a congenital anomaly.

Use of the fiberoptic bronchoscope allows for direct visualization of the airway and glottis in situations where direct laryngoscopic visualization was difficult. Special skill in the use of the fiberoptic bronchoscope is required.

Once the ETT has been placed, it is essential to ensure correct placement. Esophageal intubation is the major cause of morbidity resulting from failed endotracheal intubation. Consequences include severe hypoxia with cerebral and cardiac ischemia. Esophageal intubation may mimic tracheal intubation. Ventilation of the stomach may move the diaphragm and produce air movement via pressure on the diaphragm. Sounds from air moving into the stomach may be transmitted over the chest. Therefore, movement of the chest wall and the presence of breath sounds may be misleading. Clinically, one should make an effort to visualize passage of the tube through the glottis and note condensation on the walls of the tube. The gold standard of tracheal intubation is the detection of persistent carbon dioxide exhalation either by an in-line CO_2 monitor (capnographer) or by colorimetric means. During cardiac arrest, CO_2 may not return to the lungs and, therefore, may not be as valuable a marker in this situation.

The intubator must also take care not to advance the ETT too far. Once past the vocal cords, the tube should be advanced an additional 3 to 4 cm, approximately to a distance of 21 cm and 23 cm measured at the teeth in women and men, respectively. The chest x-ray can be helpful with the goal of noting the tip of the tube at the level of the aortic arch or projected over vertebral bodies C2-C4. Bronchoscopy may be used to definitively assess tube placement in the trachea.

QUESTION 4 The patient was stabilized in the emergency room and transferred to the medical intensive care unit. On the third hospital day, he develops a fever with a temperature of 102.6°F, and the chest x-ray remains clear. What are the major complications of intubation and extubation?

The complications of intubation can be separated into those occurring during the intubation procedure, the period wherein the tube is in place, and during or after extubation.

During endotracheal tube placement, complications usually arise secondary to trauma to upper airway structures. Often, mild injury can be made worse because of the stylet used to stiffen the ETT upon insertion. It is important to make sure that the tip of the stylet does not extend beyond the end of the tube and to remove the stylet as soon as the tip of the ETT has been seen to pass through the vocal cords. Injuries include nasal bleeding, dental trauma, pharyngeal laceration, bleeding, edema, and mucosal irritation. Perforation of the posterior pharyngeal wall is particularly significant. Important sequelae include bleeding, abscess formation, mediastinitis, subcutaneous emphysema, and potential cardiac arrest. The laryngeal structures (glottis, epiglottis, arytenoid cartilages, and vocal cords) can sustain abrasion, laceration, bleeding, and hematoma formation. The upper airways (trachea and mainstem bronchi) are also subject to perforation, laceration, abrasion, and rupture. Insertion of the ETT into the mainstem bronchi (right more commonly than left) can lead to pneumothorax, atelectasis, and significant hypoxia. Introduction of the ETT into the pharynx-larynx can stimulate central receptors and lead to vomiting.

Mistaken introduction of the ETT into the esophagus can have significant impact. Esophageal intubation is estimated to lead to one third of all deaths from anesthesia. Esophageal perforation may occur with development of mediastinitis and bleeding as well as hypoxia. Insufflation of the stomach can lead to vomiting and aspiration before adequate protection of the airway. This can lead to aspiration of gastric contents.

Neurologic complications also occur. Care for the cervical spine must be exercised in patients with bone disease, acute neck injuries, rheumatoid arthritis or primary disorders of the cervical spine. Dislocation or vertebral body crush fracture from neck hyperextension can cause acute spinal cord injury with catastrophic consequences. Acute elevation of intracranial pressure may exacerbate preexisting intracranial disease.

Sympathetic stimulation can produce hypertension, sinus tachycardia or bradycardia, supraventricular or ventricular tachycardia, and bronchoconstriction. In patients with underlying cardiopulmonary disease, these may be poorly tolerated.

Complications of intubation are greater when the patient is poorly prepared, in emergent situations, when intubation is performed by nonanesthesiologists, and when glottic structures are poorly visualized.

The most significant complications during the period during which the patient is intubated are development of sinus and middle ear infection, production of mucosal irritation, mainstem intubation, premature extubation, and aspiration pneumonia. Obstruction of sinus ostea leads to fluid accumulation and infection. Sinus infection may become a source of bacteremia and sepsis. The most commonly isolated organisms are gram-negative bacteria and *Staphylococcus aureus*. The rate of sinus infection development is greater with nasotracheal tubes than orotracheal tubes. Grindlinger found the rate of infectious sinusitis with nasal intubation was 51.6%, whereas it was 4.6% in patients intubated orally. Bach supported this finding by noting rates of 41.7% and 6.3%, respectively. Clinical signs include fever or purulent nasal drainage. CT scanning is believed to be the best way to determine the presence of sinus fluid as physical examination is insensitive.

Middle ear infection arises secondary to block-age of the eustachian tube drainage from the middle ear. Lucks found a rate of middle ear effusion in 29% of his patients. The most commonly isolated organisms are *Pseudomonas aeruginosa, Klebsiella oxytoca,* and *Enterobacter cloacae.*

Contact of the tube with oral, pharyngeal, laryngeal, supraglottic, glottic, and tracheal structures can lead to edema, inflammation, ulceration, hemorrhage, necrosis, and granuloma formation. Chronically, dilatation of the trachea, deterioration of cartilaginous structures, fistula formation, trachomalacia, abnormalities of ciliary clearance mechanisms, and colonization with bacteria occur. Potentially lethal complications include tracheo-arterial fistula formation and aspiration leading to acute lung injury and respiratory failure.

Pulmonary aspiration occurs clinically in 6.6% to 8% of cases. Low cuff pressure is the major determinant for allowing foreign materials into the lower respiratory tract. Actual aspiration probably occurs much more frequently than clinically appreciated. Elpern et al. demonstrated aspiration of blue dye placed in the GI tract in 77% of critically ill patients. While the criteria for the development of aspiration pneumonia are not well defined, pneumonia is thought to occur in 9% to 21% of cases with an estimated mortality rate of 55% to 71%. The most common organisms isolated are *Pseudomonas, Klebsiella,* and *Proteus* species.

After extubation, symptoms are most commonly a result of injury to pharyngeal and laryngeal structures. Symptoms include dysphonia, hoarseness, sore throat, cough, and occasional mild hemoptysis. The development of stridor, an inspiratory sound, represents an extrathoracic airway obstruction. Because of its uncommon frequency, routine prophylaxis is not required. Significant stridor was found by Mackenzie to occur in 0.1% to 0.6%. The most common causes were vocal cord edema or paresis or subglottic stenosis. Symptoms may occur between 5 minutes to 4 hours after extubation. For patients that have manifested postextubation stridor in the past, special consideration is warranted. Mackenzie found that this group required a mean of 2.9 reintubations due to recurrent stridor. Weymuller and colleagues developed a strategy for this population. They prescribed 50 to 100 mg prednisone and antibiotics for the preceding 1 to 2 days. There should be general anesthesia and an available operating room. Examination of the airway by direct laryngoscopy is necessary. Extubation was undertaken if the airway was deemed "safe." They also suggested consideration of tracheotomy should the airway display characteristics thought to preclude safe extubation. An additional predisposition to aspiration is a temporary loss of the gag reflex after aspiration.

QUESTION 5 Upon examination there is purulent drainage from the left nare. A diagnosis of acute sinusitis is made. Antibiotic therapy is started. The patient manifests a good response to intravenous diuretic agents. At 2 AM the nurse remarks that the tube has migrated from 23 cm to 20 cm at the lips and that the tidal volume has dropped to only 200 cc (initially set at 650 cc). What has happened to the ETT? How is the correct ETT chosen for a patient? What is the correct response to the patient's problem above?

The cuff of the ETT is an important part of equipment. It serves to anchor the tube in place and occlude the airway. However, there are also problems secondary to the ETT cuff.

One complication is laryngeal or tracheal cuff injury. This is a product of abrasive movement of the cuff across laryngeal mucosa or excessive cuff pressure on the tracheal mucosa leading to ischemic necrosis. In the larynx this may lead to abrasion, ulceration, or granuloma formation. Tracheal sequelae include dilatation, stenosis, cartilage necrosis, or tracheoesophageal fistula. Ischemic tracheal injury is also predisposed to by systemic hypotension. Ideal cuff pressure is less than 25 cm H_2O and should be monitored every shift. Injury to the trachea may also occur when the patient moves his or her head. Extension and flexion of the neck can move the tube from 1 to 2 cm upward and downward, respectively.

While the cuff should occlude the airway fully, aspiration still occurs (as previously described). Predispositions to aspiration include use of the wrong size tube because of folds in the cuff fabric, larger cuff diameters, stiffer cuff fabrics, and spontaneous extubations.

There are several important aspects of how to choose the correct ETT. The cuff should be high volume, low pressure. The materials should be pliable at body temperature to minimize pressure exerted on the mucosa. General guidelines include choosing a size 8.5 mm tube for men and 8.0 mm tube for women. The tube should be downsized by 0.5 to 1.0 mm for nasal insertion.

In this case it is apparent that the tube has slipped such that the cuff no longer occludes the airway. In such a situation, appropriate therapy includes noting the measurement of the tube at the teeth and full deflation of the cuff. The tube is replaced with attention to the measurement of the tube at the teeth, reinflation of the cuff with attention to cuff pressure, and reevaluation of tube function and adequacy of ventilation. A chest x-ray should be obtained after the tube is replaced.

Special care should be taken before advancing the tube to make sure that the cuff has not migrated proximal to the vocal cords as blind reintubation may impart undue trauma to the glottic structures. If this is the case, the patient should be fully extubated and undergo bag-mask ventilation with care to open the airway manually. The patient should then be reintubated as described previously.

QUESTION 6 The respiratory therapist tells you that the tube was initially at 23 cm. Now it is at 20 cm. You deflate the cuff and easily advance the tube to 23 cm. The cuff is reinflated, no air leak is heard, and the patient now returns 650 cc tidal volumes. A chest x-ray reveals the tip of the ETT at the aortic arch. What are the basic concepts concerning timing of tracheotomy? What are the most common methods of surgical airway maintenance?

The timing of a surgical procedure to maintain

the airway is determined by patient evaluation and clinical prognosis. It is accepted that there is a 5 to 7 day period of patient stabilization upon initial intensive care unit admission after intubation. Thereafter, if recovery is expected to occur within the next 7 to 14 days, patients are usually maintained on mechanical ventilation via an ETT. Surgical airways are usually only placed in these circumstances if there is intolerable patient discomfort or if there is extreme facial or upper airway swelling such that there is concern for adequate control of the airway should the patient fail extubation. If, on the other hand, recovery is expected to be a prolonged process (>3 weeks) or the point of extubation was not reached as expected, a surgical airway is suggested.

There are several surgical procedures that provide assurance of a patient airway. It is important to differentiate a few terms. A *tracheotomy* is a surgical procedure that provides temporary tracheal access. In this procedure the stoma closes upon decannulation. A *tracheostomy* is a surgical procedure that creates a permanent tracheal opening by suturing the surrounding skin to the tracheal wall.

The standard tracheotomy, partly described previously, is performed via horizontal incision between two tracheal rings with insertion of a tracheotomy tube. Specific indications include a mechanical upper airway obstruction, need for long-term tracheal access for pulmonary toilet, or long-term mechanical ventilation and prevention of recurrent clinically significant aspiration. The operative mortality is <1%.

A percutaneous tracheotomy is carried out via the Seldinger technique in which a wire is placed through a needle inserted into the trachea between two tracheal rings. Serially larger dilators are passed over the wire until an opening is large enough to accept a tracheotomy tube. Advantages include: it has a short procedure time, it may be done in the ICU at the bedside, limited personnel are required, it is less costly, it is more cosmetically pleasing, and it provides a more snug fit around the tracheotomy tube so that air leaks are prevented, bleeding is reduced, and the tube is better anchored. In comparison of the standard and percutaneous methods, Griggs found a 17.6% versus 3.9% morbidity rate, respectively, with one death in the standard group.

Cricothyroidotomy is the procedure of choice in emergent situations. A scalpel stab wound is made through the cricothyroid membrane. Space is created for the placement of a tracheotomy tube via cephalocaudal spreading. Brantigan and Grow found a 6.1% morbidity rate in 655 patients undergoing this procedure. Disadvantages include potential injury to the vocal cords with long-term hoarseness and scarring of the cricothyroid membrane. Contraindications include laryngeal pathology (infection, malignancy, or prior surgery), children, and endotracheal intubation for more than 7 days. However, in emergent circumstances, assurance of airway patency and ventilation overwhelm all other contraindications. After patient stabilization, the cricothyroidotomy should soon be converted to a more stable airway.

Minitracheotomy is a procedure that involves placement of a special 4 mm tube into the trachea percutaneously that has compatibility with a 10 French suction catheter. This procedure is specifically used for patients in whom secretion-related respiratory failure is feared. The patient should have a trial of chest physiotherapy or aggressive nasotracheal suction first. This access to the airway is not useful for ventilation. Adverse sequelae include abnormalities of the voice, stridor, pain, subcutaneous emphysema, and pneumothorax (rare).

QUESTION 7 Because of an intercurrent sinusitis and a myocardial infarction, the patient remained on mechanical ventilation for 20 days. He required 45% oxygen to maintain a P_{O_2} greater than 60 mm Hg. On day 22 he was converted to a fenestrated tracheotomy. What are the late complications of long-term endotracheal intubation or tracheotomy? What strategies may be used for tracheotomy weaning?

There are several important late sequelae of an artificial airway. Tracheal stenosis can occur at

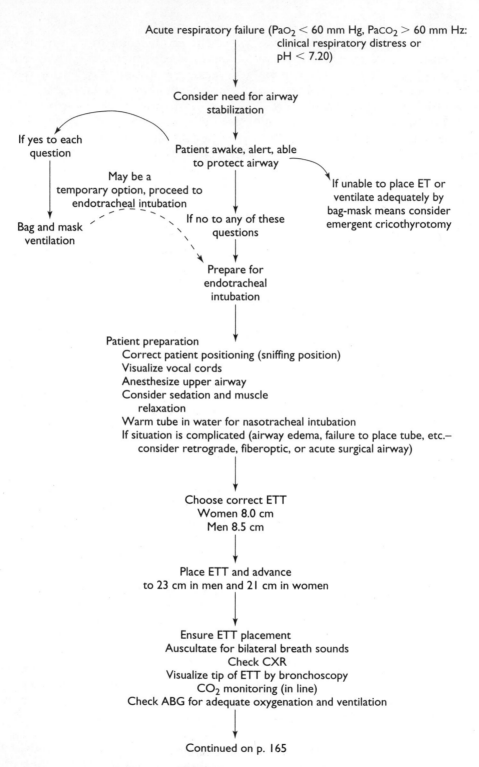

Acute respiratory failure ($PaO_2 < 60$ mm Hg, $PaCO_2 > 60$ mm Hz: clinical respiratory distress or pH < 7.20)

Consider need for airway stabilization

If yes to each question

Patient awake, alert, able to protect airway

May be a temporary option, proceed to endotracheal intubation

If unable to place ET or ventilate adequately by bag-mask means consider emergent cricothyrotomy

Bag and mask ventilation

If no to any of these questions

Prepare for endotracheal intubation

Patient preparation
 Correct patient positioning (sniffing position)
 Visualize vocal cords
 Anesthesize upper airway
 Consider sedation and muscle
  relaxation
 Warm tube in water for nasotracheal intubation
 If situation is complicated (airway edema, failure to place tube, etc.—
  consider retrograde, fiberoptic, or acute surgical airway)

Choose correct ETT
Women 8.0 cm
Men 8.5 cm

Place ETT and advance
to 23 cm in men and 21 cm in women

Ensure ETT placement
Auscultate for bilateral breath sounds
Check CXR
Visualize tip of ETT by bronchoscopy
CO_2 monitoring (in line)
Check ABG for adequate oxygenation and ventilation

Continued on p. 165

3-8-1 Diagnostic approach to airway management.

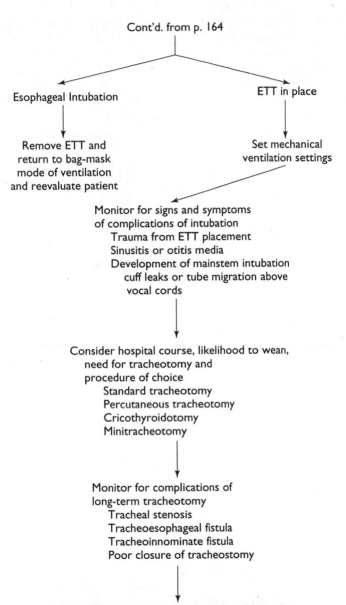

Cont'd. from p. 164

Esophageal Intubation

ETT in place

Remove ETT and
return to bag-mask
mode of ventilation
and reevaluate patient

Set mechanical
ventilation settings

Monitor for signs and symptoms
of complications of intubation
    Trauma from ETT placement
    Sinusitis or otitis media
    Development of mainstem intubation
        cuff leaks or tube migration above
        vocal cords

Consider hospital course, likelihood to wean,
    need for tracheotomy and
    procedure of choice
        Standard tracheotomy
        Percutaneous tracheotomy
        Cricothyroidotomy
        Minitracheotomy

Monitor for complications of
long-term tracheotomy
    Tracheal stenosis
    Tracheoesophageal fistula
    Tracheoinnominate fistula
    Poor closure of tracheostomy

Consider weaning - Rule out medical problems that
may prolong weaning: metabolic alkalosis, electrolyte
abnormalities, neuromuscular disease, endocrine
abnormalities, obstructive airways disease, malnutrition

3-8-1   Cont'd.

either the tracheotomy site (most common) or the area of the cuff. Predispositions include too large a cuff, too small a tube necessitating high cuff pressures, and excessive tube movement and abrasion of the mucosa. Clinically, signs may occur from at least 2 to 6 weeks after decannulation but may occur as late as 4 months (more rarely). Signs and symptoms include difficulty clearing secretions, exertion-related dyspnea, and cough and stridor. Radiographic means of evaluating tracheal diameter include use of a copper grid filter and computed tomography (CT). Pulmonary function testing may reveal a flow-volume loop consistent with an extrathoracic airway obstruction.

A tracheoesophageal fistula occurs in <1% of patients. This is a result of pressure necrosis of the trachea and esophagus as they are placed in opposition. Risk factors include high cuff or airway pressures, excessive tube movement, prolonged intubation, and diabetes mellitus. Clinical clues include increased cough, excessive abdominal distension, belching, and recurrent pneumonias. The x-ray may show a distended air-filled esophagus or persistent gastric distension. The presentation may simulate recurrent exacerbations of COPD. Diagnosis requires direct visualization via bronchoscopy. Alternatively, a communication may be demonstrated by placement of blue dye into the GI tract and recovery upon tracheal suction or via barium swallow radiography. Treatment is surgical.

A tracheoinnominate fistula is a particularly serious development. The innominate artery lies only about 9 to 12 tracheal rings below the cricoid cartilage. This is within reach of the ETT. Furthermore, unusual tube traction or patient positioning, a low tracheal window, sepsis, malnutrition, and steroid therapy may contribute to this condition. Clinical signs include seeing ETT pulsations or witnessing sentinel bleeding episodes. Endoscopy is necessary to visualize the source of bleeding. Acute therapy includes cuff hyperinflation to tamponade the vessel, translaryngeal tube placement, or use of digital compression via the tracheal stoma. Definitive therapy is sternotomy with arterial ligation.

A much less serious complication is poor closure of the tracheotomy known as a tracheocutaneous fistula. Unless heavily symptomatic, these are usually left alone.

Once a patient has been stabilized and has recovered respiratory function, weaning may be considered. The patient must manifest an ability to ventilate spontaneously for an extended period of time (24 to 48 hours). This should be done with the tracheotomy tube in place. If the tube size precludes breathing around the tube, one can replace it with a smaller size, cuffless, or fenestrated tube (a fenestrated tube has a hole in the greater curvature that allows air to move through the upper airway across the vocal cords). Control of patient's secretions provides a great advantage. Once this capacity is demonstrated, the patient may either be decannulated cold-turkey or be weaned to progressively smaller tracheotomy tubes. A diagnostic approach to airway management is shown in Fig. 3-8-1.

CASE FOLLOW-UP On day 29 after intubation the patient was taken off the ventilator and placed on a tracheotomy collar at 30% oxygen. Decannulation followed over the next 5 days. He was transferred to the rehabilitation center and was discharged to home 9 days later. He is currently completing a 2-week recuperative period. He plans to move to Florida to be closer to his son and daughter for the winter.

• •

BIBLIOGRAPHY

Bach A, Boehrer H, Schmidt H, Geiss HK: Nosocomial sinusitis in ventilated patients: nasotracheal versus orotracheal intubation, *Anesthesia* 47:355-359, 1992.

Brantigan CO, Grow JB: Cricothyroidotomy: elective use in respiratory problems requiring tracheotomy, *J Thoracic Cardiovasc Surg* 71:72-81, 1976.

Elpern E, Jacobs ER, Bone RC: Incidence of aspiration in tracheally intubated patients, *Heart Lung* 16:527-531, 1987.

Griggs WM, Myburgh JA, Worthley LIG: A prospective comparison of a percutaneous tracheostomy technique with standard surgical tracheostomy, *Intensive Care Med* 17:261-263, 1991.

Grindlinger GA, Niehoff J, Hughes SL, et al: Acute paranasal sinuis related to nasotracheal intubation of head injured patients, *Crit Care Med* 15:214-217, 1987.

Lucks D, Consiglio A, Stankiewicz J, O'Keefe P: Incidence and microbiologic etiology of middle ear effusion complicating endotracheal intubation and mechanical ventilation, *J Infect Dis* 157:368-369, 1988.

Mackenzie CF, Shin B, McAslan TC, et al: Severe stridor after prolonged endotracheal intubation using high-volume cuffs, *Anesthesiology* 50:235-239, 1979.

Rashkin MC, Davis T: Acute complications of endotracheal intubation: relationship to reintubation, *Arch Otolaryngol* 106:578-580, 1980.

Stauffer JL, Olson DE, Petty TL: Complications and consequences of endotracheal intubation and tracheotomy: a prospective study of 150 critically ill adults, *Am J Med* 70:65-76, 1981.

Tobin MJ, *Principles and practice of mechanical ventilation*, New York, 1994, McGraw-Hill.

ENDOCRINOLOGY

THEODORE MAZZONE
SECTION EDITOR

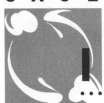
The patient is a 39-year-old woman who presents with complaints of depression, weakness, and weight gain. She has noted feeling depressed for the last several months and reports increased emotional lability. She has also felt tired and weak, and describes increased difficulty in climbing stairs. She feels that because of her depression she has been eating more and has gained 10 lbs. On closer questioning she notes easier bruising and development of "stretch marks" on her abdomen. There is no history of balding, menstrual irregularities, acne, skin pigmentation changes, headaches, visual field changes, polyuria, or known hypertension. She has never been treated with corticosteroids. She currently takes no medications.

On physical examination she is an emotionally labile woman, crying frequently.

BP 154/88 mm Hg, P 90.

Weight 185 lbs, obesity mainly central, with small buffalo hump and supraclavicular fat pads.

Skin: thin, many bruises, wide, deep red striae on lower abdomen. Full facies with plethora.

Chest: normal.

Heart: normal.

Abdomen: obese, no palpable masses.

Rectal: stool heme negative.

Extremities: thin arms and legs.

Neurological: visual fields fully intact, proximal muscle weakness noted in legs.

QUESTION 1 Based on this presentation, a diagnosis of hypercortisolism was suspected. What aspects of the history and physical examination are supportive of this diagnosis?

Features of this presentation that support a diagnosis of hypercortisolism include weight gain. Fat often accumulates in the abdomen, the dorsocervical areas, and the face. This leads to the classical "moon facies" and "buffalo hump." This patient also manifests fragile skin with easy bruisability. This also leads to the development of abdominal striae. Muscle wasting is evident leading to proximal muscle weakness and thin extremities. Furthermore, she complains of depression and emotional lability. Additional signs and symptoms of corticosteroid excess are summarized in the box on p. 172. These are often quite variable, and clinical presentation by itself is not adequate to diagnose Cushing's syndrome.

QUESTION 2 Initial laboratory evaluation of this patient included: Na 138 mEq/L, K 3.6 mEq/L, fasting glucose 118 mg/dl, calcium 9.4 mEq/L, albumin 3.2 g/dl, WBC 9,000 with 85% granulocytes and 10% lymphocytes. An 8 AM serum cortisol following an 11 PM dose of 1 mg of dexamethasone was 8 µg/dl (normal < 5), and a 24-hour urine collection contained 320 µg (normal 5 to 90) of free cortisol (creatinine 1.4 g/24 hr), confirming the diagnosis of hypercortisolism. A baseline 8 AM serum cortisol was 24 µg/dl (normal 5 to 25), with an adrenocorticotropic hormone (ACTH) level of 34 pg/ml (normal 9 to 52). The morning after the 11 PM administration of 8 mg of dexamethasone, the cortisol fell to 4 µg/dl. A pituitary MRI was obtained that did not show an obvious adenoma. Computed tomography (CT) scan of the chest and abdomen revealed only diffuse bilateral hyperplasia of the adrenal glands. Because of the initial concern regarding hypercortisolism, the above labs were drawn initially. How do you interpret the laboratory

MANIFESTATIONS OF CUSHING'S SYNDROME

INCREASED WEIGHT
- Obesity - not always present
- Central weight distribution
- Buffalo hump (dorsocervical fat pad)
- Supraclavicular fat pads
- Full (moon) facies

SKIN
- Thin
- Easy bruising
- Striae - abdominal, thigh
- Hyperpigmentation (with excessive ACTH secretion only)
- Facial plethora

MUSCLE WASTING
- Proximal muscle weakness
- Thin extremities

POOR WOUND HEALING

PSYCHIATRIC
- Emotional lability
- Depression
- Psychosis

INCREASED OPPORTUNISTIC INFECTIONS

GLUCOSE INTOLERANCE
OSTEOPOROSIS
CATARACTS
RENAL STONES
ABDOMINAL MASS - ADRENAL TUMOR ONLY
HEADACHE, VISUAL FIELD DEFECTS - PITUITARY MASS ONLY
LAB ABNORMALITIES
- Hyperglycemia
- Granulocytosis, lymphopenia,
- Eosinopenia
- Hypercalcemia
- Hypercalciuria
- Mineralocorticoid excess (if present)
- Hypertension
- Hypokalemia

ANDROGEN EXCESS (IF PRESENT)
- Acne
- Oligo/amenorrhea
- Male-pattern baldness
- Hirsutism
- Virilization

---

evaluation and radiographic data collected to this point?

There are two phases involved in the diagnosis of Cushing's syndrome (see the box on p. 173). The first is to demonstrate the presence of an excess of corticosteroids, and the second is to determine the etiology of the Cushing's syndrome in order to decide on therapy. Diagnosis is often complicated and may involve protracted testing.

For the diagnosis of hypercortisolism, random cortisol or ACTH levels are of little use in the diagnosis of hypercortisolism because of the pulsatile nature of their secretion. The simplest test to perform is the low-dose overnight dexamethasone suppression test, where 1 mg of dexameth-asone is taken orally at 11 PM, and the serum cortisol is checked at 8 AM the next morning. A value of less than 5 µg/dl suggests normal adrenal function with approximately 98% accuracy, but up to 15% of normals may not suppress adequately. Non-suppression suggests the presence of Cushing's syndrome. A 24-hour collection of urine for free cortisol is more specific, although undercollection of urine may critically affect the results. (A 24-hour urine creatinine should also be performed to help exclude this.) A normal value is 5 to 90 µg/dl for an adult, while most patients with Cushing's will be greater than 250. Patients with values between 90 and 250 can be further screened by looking for the loss of diurnal rhythm in cortisol secretion that occurs in Cush-

· ·

EVALUATION OF CUSHING'S SYNDROME

DEMONSTRATE HYPERCORTISOLISM
- 1 mg overnight dexamethasone suppression test
- 24-hour urine collection for free cortisol

DETERMINE ETIOLOGY
- Measure ACTH and perform 8 mg overnight dexamethasone suppression test

· ·

(Adapted from Kaye TB, Crapo L: The Cushing syndrome: an update on diagnostic tests, Ann Intern Med 112:434, 1990.)

ing's. Four blood samples are taken every half hour between 7 and 8:30 AM, and then again between 4 and 5:30 PM. The mean of the afternoon samples should be approximately half of the morning value.

Once hypercortisolism has been established, it is useful to draw a morning serum ACTH to divide the Cushing's into ACTH-independent (undetectable to low) or ACTH-dependent (normal to elevated). A normal value is from 9 to 52 pg/ml. A useful classification of Cushing's syndrome breaks down the causes into ACTH-dependent and ACTH-independent (Table 4-1-1). The classic dexamethasone suppression test is also a useful way of initially evaluating Cushing's syndrome; however, to be done correctly requires patient hospitalization for at least 3 days. Recent data indicate that the high-dose overnight suppression test provides equivalent information in a simpler manner. A baseline 8 AM serum cortisol is obtained, the patient takes 8 mg of dexamethasone at 11 PM, and another serum cortisol is obtained the following morning at 8 AM. Patients with pituitary adenomas should suppress to less than 50% of their baseline values, while those with adrenal tumors or ectopic ACTH secretion should not suppress.

We recommend performing both the high-dose overnight dexamethasone suppression test and obtaining an ACTH level once hypercortisolism is

demonstrated. Patients with adrenal tumors or nodular disease should have low to undetectable levels of ACTH and not suppress to high-dose dexamethasone. An abdominal CT scan should be obtained next in this group. Patients with Cushing's disease should have normal to elevated levels of ACTH and should suppress. A pituitary MRI scan should be performed to document an adenoma. Patients with ectopic ACTH secretion should have normal to very elevated levels of ACTH and should not suppress to the dexamethasone. A chest and abdominal CT scan should be done next to attempt to document the source of the ACTH.

QUESTION 3 Lack of suppression of cortisol production with the 1 mg dexamethasone test and suppression of cortisol production with the 8 mg dexamethasone test suggest Cushing's disease as the etiology of the hypercortisolism. What is the difference between Cushing's disease and Cushing's syndrome and what is the differential diagnosis of hypercortisolism?

This case illustrates a classic presentation of Cushing's disease and underlines the frequent complexity involved in determining the etiology of hypercortisolism. The syndrome of hypercortisolism is named after Harvey Cushing who first published a description of "the consequences of hyperadrenalism" in 1910. Cushing's *disease* refers specifically to those patients with ACTH-producing pituitary tumors, while Cushing's *syndrome* includes all patients showing the effects of elevated corticosteroids. Patients with Cushing's syndrome may also overexpress other adrenal steroids such as aldosterone or androgens. ACTH-secreting pituitary adenomas are the most common form of Cushing's syndrome (if the very common iatrogenic cause is excluded). These are typically microadenomas that occur predominantly (80% to 90%) in women. Macroadenomas may occur and cause mass effects (headache, optic nerve compression, pituitary stalk compression, and hypopituitarism). On the opposite end of the spectrum, there are cases in which excessive

TABLE 4-1-1 **Differential Diagnosis of Cushing's Syndrome and Frequency (Frequency Excludes Iatrogenic Patients)**

ACTH-dependent	Frequency	ACTH-independent	Frequency
Pituitary adenoma	60%	Adrenal carcinoma	15%
Ectopic secretion of ACTH	15%	Adrenal adenoma	10%
Ectopic secretion of CRH	Very rare	Micronodular adrenal disease	Very rare
		Macronodular adrenal disease	Very rare
		Iatrogenic	Common
		Factitious	Rare

ACTH can be shown to be coming from the pituitary gland. Pituitary surgery apparently cures the problem, yet no adenoma can be documented by pathology. These cases are postulated to be secondary to ectopic CRH secretion, primary corticotroph hyperplasia, or intermediate lobe tumors.

Excessive ACTH may be secreted from different types of tumors, causing ectopic ACTH-dependent Cushing's syndrome. These are most commonly small-cell lung carcinomas but also include thymic carcinomas, pancreatic carcinomas, pheochromocytomas, and bronchial carcinoids. The ACTH in these cases may be abnormally large ("big" ACTH) or small.

Adrenal carcinomas are malignant tumors that are frequently large enough at presentation to be externally palpable. They are also frequently associated with secretion of androgens. Adrenal adenomas are typically smaller than 3 cm at diagnosis and rarely secrete other hormones than corticosteroids. Adrenal incidentalomas (apparently nonfunctioning adrenal adenomas) may occasionally be associated with subtle glucocorticoid excess, which is defined as normal basal levels but failure to suppress after administration of low-dose dexamethasone.

Bilateral, apparently ACTH-independent adrenal hypertrophy may also rarely occur. Micronodular adrenal disease typically occurs in younger patients, with the glands often hyperpigmented from accumulation of lipofuscin. This condition may be familial and can occur as part of the Carney complex (with associated cardiac mxyomas, blue nevi, pigmented lentigines, Schwannomas, and testicular tumors). Bilateral macronodular disease also occurs. It is not clear if this condition is truly an ACTH-independent subtype, or whether prolonged ACTH stimulation causes adrenal hypertrophy, which then develops into an autonomous condition where the high levels of corticosteroids suppress further ACTH secretion.

Pseudo-Cushing's is a condition found in ethanol abusers, in which clinical manifestations suggestive of Cushing's syndrome are found in association with elevated cortisol levels and abnormal dexamethasone suppression of cortisol. The laboratory abnormalities will resolve, however, with withdrawal from alcohol. Other conditions that may be associated with increased serum cortisol levels are obesity, anorexia nervosa, anxiety, and acute stress. These elevations are transient or mild and without pathologic significance.

QUESTION 4 What is the underlying physiology of the hypothalamic-pituitary-adrenal axis?

In the normal state the hypothalamus and pituitary regulate the secretion of corticosteroids by the adrenals. Hypothalamic release of CRH (which is increased by stress) causes the anterior pituitary to release ACTH, which in turn stimulates the adrenals to synthesize and secrete corticosteroids of which cortisol is the most important. The effects of cortisol are diverse and complex, and are primarily catabolic and insulin-antagonistic. Cortisol functions through binding to nuclear receptors regulating gene expression. Excessive levels of corticosteroids will normally inhibit CRH and ACTH release by negative feedback. Normal release of ACTH and cortisol is both pulsatile and diurnal, with the highest cortisol levels occurring in the early morning. Pathologic hypersecretion of corticosteroids may be induced by excessive ACTH secretion with resultant bilateral adrenal hyperplasia, or autonomous adrenal secretion, in which case ACTH levels will be suppressed.

QUESTION 5 Unfortunately, imaging studies do not always confirm the results of the laboratory evaluation. When equivocal, what are additional tests used to provide further diagnostic information?

The patient was then sent for inferior petrosal sinus sampling, where simultaneous sinus and peripheral blood ACTH levels were obtained before and after administration of corticotropin releasing hormone (CRH). Generally, the most problematic cases will be in differentiating pituitary from ectopic ACTH sources, especially from bronchial carcinoids that may suppress to high-dose dexamethasone. Sampling of blood from the bilateral inferior petrosal sinuses should reveal an increased sinus:peripheral ratio of ACTH in Cushing's disease (greater than 1.7). This test is more accurate if CRH stimulation is performed simultaneously, although CRH is only available experimentally at this time. Inferior petrosal sinus sampling may also help to lateralize a pituitary adenoma.

QUESTION 6 What is the appropriate treatment for this patient?

Treatment of choice of Cushing's disease is a transsphenoidal adenectomy, leaving the remainder of the pituitary intact and functional postoperatively. Remission rates approach 90% if the adenoma can be localized. Complications include cerebrospinal fluid (CSF) leakage, men-

ingitis, damage to optic or extraocular nerves, diabetes insipidus, and hypopituitarism. Radiation therapy (either internal or external) may be used for macroadenomas or recurrent disease. Full effects of the radiation therapy may take up to 9 months to occur, and the patient will need to be managed medically initially. Hypopituitarism is common following radiation. Bilateral adrenalectomy will cure the hypercortisolism but results in symptomatic growth of the pituitary adenoma (Nelson's syndrome) in up to 40% of cases, and for that reason has been largely supplanted by pituitary surgery. Ectopic ACTH secretion should be treated by excision of the primary tumor. If the tumor is unresectable or cannot be localized, medical management will be required. Adrenal adenomas should be curable by unilateral adrenalectomy. Adrenal carcinomas are frequently impossible to completely resect, and mean survival is only 10 to 14 months following diagnosis. If residual disease is present, the adrenolytic agent O,P-DDD is usually given, although side effects are significant, and there is debate whether survival or quality of life is improved.

All forms of Cushing's syndrome will result in suppression of the hypothalamic-pituitary-adrenal axis. Even if this is left intact following curative surgical therapy, full recovery often will not occur for 9 to 15 months, and patients will require temporary corticosteroid replacement therapy. Recovery may be monitored by measuring an early morning cortisol level before the morning replacement dose is taken.

Medical management of Cushing's is often only partially successful, although there have been reports of spontaneous remission of Cushing's disease with only medical therapy. There are several agents that inhibit various enzymes in the adrenal synthetic pathway including ketoconazole, metyrapone, trilostane, and aminoglutethamide. The adrenolytic agent O,P-DDD has already been mentioned. Octreotide may be of benefit in Cushing's disease and ectopic ACTH secretion. Valproate and cyproheptadine may occasionally be useful in Cushing's disease.

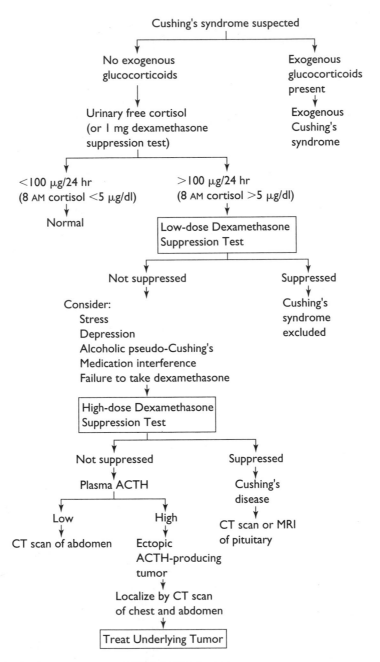

4-1-1   Diagnostic algorithm for Cushing's syndrome.
(From Greene HL, Johnson WP, Maricic MJ: *Decision making in medicine,* St Louis, 1993, Mosby.)

CASE SUMMARY An increased sinus:peripheral ACTH ratio supported the pituitary as the source of the ACTH. A transsphenoidal exploration of the pituitary was performed, where a 3-mm adenoma was found and removed. Following surgery, the patient's cortisol levels dropped quickly, and she was placed on replacement hydrocortisone that was gradually tapered off over 9 months. There was no recurrence of hypercortisolism, and pituitary function remained intact. A diagnostic algorithm for Cushing's syndrome is shown in Fig. 4-1-1.

• •

BIBLIOGRAPHY

Atkinson AB: The treatment of Cushing's syndrome, *Clin Endocrinol* 34:507, 1991.

Flack MR, Oldfield EH, Cutler GB, et al: Urine free cortisol in the high-dose dexamethasone suppression test for the differential diagnosis of the Cushing syndrome, *Ann Intern Med* 116:211, 1992.

Grua JR, Nelson DH: ACTH-producing pituitary tumors, *Endocrinol Metab Clin North Am* 20:319, 1991.

Kaye TB, Crapo L: The Cushing syndrome: an update on diagnostic tests, *Ann Intern Med* 112:434, 1990.

Limper AH, Carpenter PC, Scheithauer B, et al: The Cushing syndrome induced by bronchial carcinoid tumors, *Ann Intern Med* 117:209, 1992.

Loriaux DL: Cushing's syndrome. In Becker KL, ed: *Principles and practice of endocrinology and metabolism*, Philadelphia, 1990, JB Lippincott.

Stewart PM, Penn R, Gibson R, et al: Hypothalamic abnormalities in patients with pituitary-dependent Cushing's syndrome, *Clin Endocrinol* 36:453, 1992.

C A S E

2

Peter G. Curran
Theodore Mazzone

········

The patient is an 18-year-old man with type I (insulin dependent) diabetes mellitus who is brought to the emergency room by his family because of persistent vomiting and, most recently, progressive lethargy. The patient has been vomiting for 24 hours and unable to keep fluids down; he has also had a fever for several days, and throughout this period his blood sugars measured at home have been climbing. Because of his vomiting and decreased mental status, he has received no insulin for the past 12 hours. He has no known diabetic complications (specifically no renal, neurologic, or cardiac disease).

Medications included NPH insulin 30 units q AM, 7 units q PM and regular insulin 10 units q AM, 3 units q PM. Physical examination revealed a well-developed young man, pronounced odor of ketones on breath, responsive only to shouted commands. Vital signs were BP 88/40 mm Hg, P 136 bpm, T 96° F, RR 30/min and deep. Skin with decreased turgor, mucous membranes dry, neck supple, chest clear, heart exam reveals only tachycardia, abdomen is diffusely tender without bowel sounds or masses, neurologic examination reveals only lethargy.

A bedside glucometer reads greater than 400 mg/dl. A urethral catheter is placed, with immediate drainage of 300 ml of urine that is positive for glucose and ketones. An IV is placed and normal saline run in at 1 l/h.

QUESTION 1 As the emergency room physician, you have taken the above history and done the physical examination. The glucometer reading reveals an elevated glucose while other stat labs are still pending. Based on this information, what is your provisional diagnosis and main therapeutic and diagnostic concern about this patient?

This patient presents with mental status changes associated with hyperglycemia and a recent period without insulin administration. His vital signs reveal hypotension and tachypnea with deep respirations. The skin and mucous membranes are dry. Initially, one should be concerned about hemodynamic stability and airway maintenance. This patient has a low blood pressure so that fluid resuscitation with normal saline is the first priority. Once stable the next concern is diagnosis and treatment of the primary disease: the provisional diagnosis is diabetic ketoacidosis (DKA). At this time achieving control of the blood glucose is paramount.

Evaluation of presumed DKA concerns the patient's volume and acid-base status. Volume depletion is a product of the patient's persistent vomiting, decreased oral intake, and presumed osmolar diuresis leading to low blood pressure. A clue to the patient's acid-base status is the presence of Kussmaul's respirations: deep and rapid breathing. In addition, the odor of ketones on the patient's breath is due to the metabolic production of ketones produced in the insulinopenic state.

QUESTION 2 Soon the following laboratory values are available: glucose 685 mg/dl, Na 135 mEq/L, K 5.7 mEq/L, Cl 98 mEq/L, HCO_3 8 mEq/L, BUN 25 mg/dl, creatinine 1.4 mg/dl, calculated anion gap 29, calculated effective serum osmolarity 364 mOsm/L, serum ketones are large. Arterial blood gas reveals pH of 7.12, Po_2 of 110 mm, Pco_2 of 22 mm. WBC is 18,000 cells/mm^3, Hb 17 g/dl, Hct 48%. ECG shows sinus tachycardia, chest x-ray is without abnormalities, stool is heme negative. Describe the patient's acid-base status and provide a differential diagnosis for his current status. Does the measured, as compared to the calculated, serum osmolarity provide additional diagnostic value?

The patient has an anion gap of 29 (Na + K – Cl – HCO_3) and a HCO_3 of 8 mEq/dl. This is an anion gap metabolic acidosis. There are many conditions that can produce such an acid-base abnormality. They include ketoacidosis; uremia; salicylate toxicity; starvation; methanol, ethanol, paraldehyde, ethylene glycol; alcohol intoxication, and lactic acidosis. These etiologies can be further separated by calculation of the osmolal gap. The serum osmolality can be calculated by 2(Na) + glucose/18 + BUN/2.8. If the calculated osmolality differs from the measured value by more than 10 mosm/kg/H_2O, unmeasured particles are present that are osmotically active. In the setting of an anion gap acidosis a widened osmolal gap is due to the presence of ethanol, methanol, ethylene glycol, or other toxic alcohols.

Because of the metabolic acidosis serum, potassium is elevated although the total body potassium store is probably depleted. Nevertheless, concern about the effects of hyperkalemia is warranted. The main problem concerns the effect on the cardiac conduction system with the potential for heart block, bradycardia, and cardiac arrest. An ECG will first reveal peaked T waves followed by prolongation of the P-R and QRS intervals that, when severe, may develop into a sine-wave pattern. Rapid and temporary movement of potassium into the intracellular space can be stimulated by insulin use or use of beta-2 agonists (Med-Neb treatments). IV calcium gluconate can serve to stabilize the membranes of electrical cells to avoid disordered function.

QUESTION 3 Based on the preceding differential diagnosis, what is the primary diagnosis and what are the major clinical and laboratory manifestations?

DKA is a potentially lethal complication of uncontrolled diabetes, characterized by hypergly-cemia, dehydration, and overproduction of ketone bodies resulting in a metabolic acidosis. In the United States there are approximately 3 to 8 admissions per year for DKA for every 1000 diabetics. DKA is usually defined as a state in which the blood glucose is greater than 300 mg/dl in combination with a ketone body-induced acidosis with a pH of less than 7.2 and a bicarbonate of less than 15 mEq/L.

In about 80% of cases an event may be identified as causing or contributing to the development of DKA by increasing the level of insulin-opposing stress hormones or reducing the availability of insulin. As many of these precipitants are organic, it is important to identify and to treat them. An associated infection is found in up to 50% of cases of DKA, most commonly in the pulmonary and urinary systems. In the case above the DKA was apparently precipitated by a viral gastroenteritis. An elevated temperature in DKA usually indicates infection. Insulin deficiency in new-onset diabetics or noncompliant patients is another important precipitant and is involved in approximately 20% of cases of DKA. The case discussed underlines the importance of maintaining insulin therapy even if the patient is ill and not eating (although insulin dosage will need to be modified). Other important precipitants to consider include myocardial ischemia or infarction, cerebrovascular accident, gastrointestinal bleed, trauma, burns, dehydration, and use of such drugs as beta-blockers, glucocorticoids, ethanol, and anesthetic agents.

As noted, an osmotic diuresis typically occurs in DKA secondary to the marked hyperglycemia. If these fluid losses are not replaced, this will result in dehydration that may lead to orthostasis, frank hypotension, and shock. Prerenal azotemia often develops and may progress to acute tubular necrosis. Fluid losses in DKA are usually 5% to 10% of body weight, and fluid replacement is the critical initial step of therapy. Fluid and electrolyte losses are less significant in cases of oliguric renal failure.

The hyperglycemia and dehydration seen in DKA causes a syndrome of hyperosmolarity. Increased osmolarity may induce neurologic symptoms such as decreased alertness, obtundation, coma, and seizures. These symptoms generally occur when the plasma osmolarity exceeds 340 mOsm/L (the effective plasma osmolarity = 2 [Na + K] + glucose/18 + BUN/2.8, normal is 280 to 295 mOsm/L). It is important to consider other causes of neurologic impairment such as meningitis and stroke in the obtunded patient with DKA, especially if the serum osmolarity is less than 340 mOsm/L.

The osmotic diuresis also causes marked sodium and potassium losses. Sodium values on admission tend to be low despite the excessive free water losses. This is primarily due to a shift of free water out of cells because of the hyperglycemia and may be corrected for by increasing the sodium by 1.6 mEq/L for every 100 mg/dl increase in glucose. Despite significant potassium losses, serum potassium levels at presentation tend to be normal or elevated. However, cellular depletion of potassium is usually present, and hypokalemia typically develops with insulin therapy unless potassium replacement is instituted.

Acidosis in DKA is primarily due to accumulation of the ketone bodies acetoacetate and beta-hydroxybutyrate. These organic acids will be partially buffered by bicarbonate, causing a decreased serum bicarbonate value with an increased anion gap (anion gap = Na − [Cl + HCO$_3$], normal 8-16 mEq/L). Acetone, frequently detected on the breath of a patient in DKA, is neutral and does not contribute to the acidosis. The acid-base picture in these patients is usually complicated by other conditions. In response to the metabolic acidosis, deep rapid respirations (Kussmaul breathing) occur causing a respiratory alkalosis. A hyperchloremic metabolic acidosis may be present on admission and frequently develops during initial therapy. Other causes of metabolic acidosis should also be considered, including accumulation of lactate, uremic acidosis, or following ingestion of ethanol, methanol, ethylene glycol, or salicylates. Marked acidosis is associated with depressed myocardial contractility, increased cardiac irritability, reduced response to pressor agents, and decreased insulin sensitivity.

There are often gastrointestinal symptoms at presentation of DKA. Vomiting occurs in approximately 70% of patients before admission probably because of gastric stasis or an ileus. Diffuse abdominal pain is associated with severe ketoacidosis. If there is no underlying gastrointestinal pathology, this should resolve rapidly with therapy. Underlying problems are more likely to be present in older patients (>40 years old) and if the bicarbonate is greater than 10 mEq/L. Mild, self-limited gastrointestinal bleeding occurs in up to 25% of patients in DKA. Because of these problems, nasogastric suction is often indicated.

Other common laboratory abnormalities include a nonspecific leukocytosis of up to 20,000 cells/mm (this does not necessarily indicate an infection), a nonspecific increase in both amylase and lipase, and an increased CPK that may be associated with myoglobinemia and rhabdomyolysis. Serum phosphate levels are typically elevated at presentation, but decrease with therapy.

QUESTION 4 What is the normal physiologic mechanism of normal glucose control and what happens when this mechanism breaks down because of relative insulin deficiency?

Normal fuel metabolism is regulated mainly by the balance between the hormones insulin and glucagon and insulin-antagonist roles played by the catecholamines, growth hormone, and glucocorticoids. The effects of insulin predominate in the fed state, where it works to increase cellular glucose uptake and metabolism, and facilitates glycogen and triglyceride formation. Glucagon becomes more important in the fasting state, where it breaks down glycogen and fat stores to maintain fuel (glucose and ketone body) availability. Insulin will inhibit ketone body production, and in the normal state excess ketone body accumulation is prevented by the ketone bodies stimulating insulin secretion. Important signs and symptoms are summarized in Table 4-2-1, and an initial evaluation is summarized in Table 4-2-2.

In uncontrolled diabetes there is not only a relative insulin deficiency, but also a marked excess of the insulin-opposing hormones. This leads to both decreased glucose utilization and increased glucose production with resultant hyperglycemia. The increased plasma glucose causes an oncotic shift of free water out of cells, and induces an osmotic diuresis with resultant dehydration and electrolyte losses. The hyperglycemia and dehydration increase serum hyperosmolarity, which may lead to changes in mental status. Ketone body formation is stimulated, and without insulin, ketone bodies accumulate causing a metabolic acidosis. There are some patients with marked hyperglycemia who do not develop ketoacidosis (hyperosmolar nonacidotic diabetes). They are generally older, type II diabetics.

QUESTION 5 The patient was initially given a bolus of 20 units of regular insulin IV and was begun on a drip of 10 units per hour. He was transferred to the intensive care unit for further management. What is the definitive management plan for this patient?

As with any condition in which many factors are involved, therapy needs to be individualized. Use of the intensive care setting is frequently indicated, unless the DKA is mild and the nursing staff can provide vigilant observation. Meticulous record-keeping including labs, insulin doses, fluid intake and output, and vital signs will facilitate

TABLE 4-2-1   Important Signs and Symptoms of DKA

Dehydration: thirst, decreased skin turgor, orthostasis, possible hypotension	Frequent
Neurologic impairment	If hyperosmolarity or other CNS pathology present
Temperature	Often decreased
	Fever indicates infection
Vomiting	Frequent
Gastric stasis/ileus	Frequent
Abdominal pain	Frequent
Acetone odor on breath	Present
Kussmaul respirations	Present

TABLE 4-2-2   Initial Diagnosis and Evaluation of DKA

Search for precipitants	History and physical Obtain chest x-ray Urinalysis Electrocardiogram for cardiac ischemia and potassium status Stool sample for blood Consider blood/urine cultures
Fluid status	Estimate degree of dehydration Calculate serum osmolarity Estimate current urine output
Neurologic	Consider other causes of depressed mental status, especially if serum osmolarity <340 mOsm/L
Gastrointestinal	Consider surgical consult for tender abdomen, especially if patient >40 years old or HCO_3 >10 mEq/L
Pulmonary	Chest x-ray for pneumonia, edema, ARDS
Laboratory	Glucose, initially bedside monitor, confirm with laboratory sample Arterial blood gas Calculate anion gap Ketones, urine, and serum Electrolytes Renal profile Calcium, phosphate, magnesium Liver profile CPK CBC

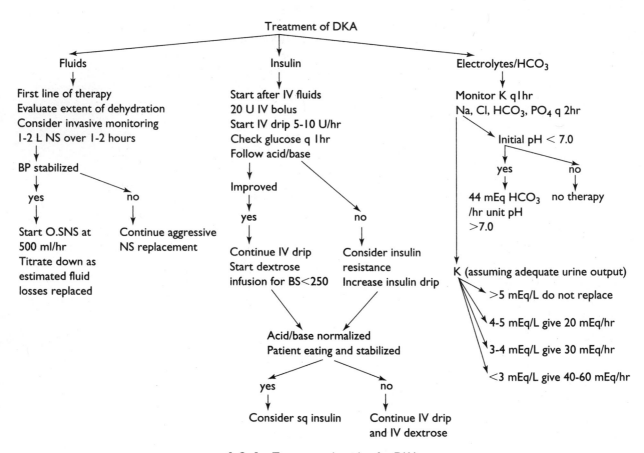

4-2-1   Treatment algorithm for DKA.

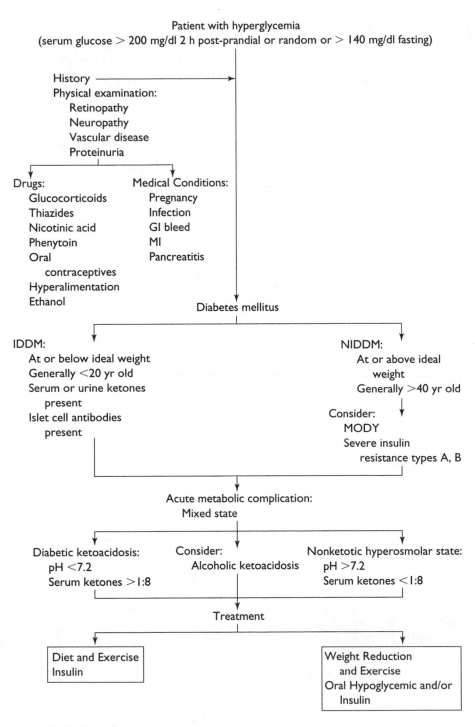

Patient with hyperglycemia
(serum glucose > 200 mg/dl 2 h post-prandial or random or > 140 mg/dl fasting)

History
Physical examination:
   Retinopathy
   Neuropathy
   Vascular disease
   Proteinuria

Drugs:
   Glucocorticoids
   Thiazides
   Nicotinic acid
   Phenytoin
   Oral
      contraceptives
   Hyperalimentation
   Ethanol

Medical Conditions:
   Pregnancy
   Infection
   GI bleed
   MI
   Pancreatitis

Diabetes mellitus

IDDM:
   At or below ideal weight
   Generally <20 yr old
   Serum or urine ketones
      present
   Islet cell antibodies
      present

NIDDM:
   At or above ideal
      weight
   Generally >40 yr old

Consider:
   MODY
   Severe insulin
      resistance types A, B

Acute metabolic complication:
   Mixed state

Diabetic ketoacidosis:
   pH <7.2
   Serum ketones >1:8

Consider:
   Alcoholic ketoacidosis

Nonketotic hyperosmolar state:
   pH >7.2
   Serum ketones <1:8

Treatment

Diet and Exercise
Insulin

Weight Reduction
   and Exercise
Oral Hypoglycemic and/or
   Insulin

4-2-2   Diagnostic algorithm for hyperglycemia.
(From Greene HL, Johnson WP, Maricic MJ: *Decision making in medicine,* St Louis, 1993, Mosby.)

management. An hourly flowchart of important parameters (pH, K, HCO$_3$, anion gap, insulin dose, fluid type) may be very helpful.

The major areas to focus on in treating DKA are aggressive fluid replacement, insulin therapy, electrolyte (mainly potassium) monitoring and replacement, and identifying and treating any possible precipitants (such as cardiac ischemia or gastrointestinal bleeding). The primary complications to avoid are therapy-induced hypokalemia and hypoglycemia. The development of cerebral edema should be suspected if there is an acute worsening of mental status during therapy (although this is uncommon in the adult population).

Fluid therapy should be started before insulin use in DKA (Fig. 4-2-1). The tonicity of the lost fluid is equivalent to half normal saline, but if hypotension is present, use normal saline until hemodynamic stability has been achieved. Urine output, serum sodium, and vital signs should be carefully followed; in cases of cardiopulmonary disease invasive monitoring is frequently indicated. Insulin therapy is best delivered as a constant intravenous infusion of short-acting insulin at an initial rate of .1 U/kg. An initial bolus of 10 to 20 units will shorten the time until steady state levels are obtained. If the acid-base status is not improved after 4 hours, significant insulin resistance is most likely present, and the insulin dose should be increased. As the serum glucose falls, the infusion should be gradually tapered. Intravenous insulin therapy needs to be continued until the acid-base status is normalized, and intravenous dextrose should be added when the blood sugar has decreased to about 250 mg/dl to prevent hypoglycemia. Potassium replacement is extremely important to anticipate and should be started when potassium levels reach the normal range. Routine bicarbonate therapy has not been shown to be of benefit and should be reserved for cases where the pH is less than 7.0 when significant hemodynamic effects may occur. Phosphate replacement should be considered when levels become subnormal.

Current mortality from DKA in the United States is from 2% to 4.5%. Increased mortality is associated with increased age and hyperosmolarity. Primary causes of death are bacterial pneumonia, myocardial infarction, adult respiratory distress syndrome, and thrombosis. A diagnostic algorithm for hyperglycemia is shown in Fig. 4-2-2.

BIBLIOGRAPHY

Androgue JH, Eknoyan G, Suki WK: Diabetic ketoacidosis: role of the kidney in the acid-base homeostasis re-evaluated, *Kidney Int* 25:591, 1984.

Campbell IW, Duncan LPJ, Innes JA, et al: Abdominal pain in diabetic metabolic decompensation, *JAMA* 233:166, 1975.

Curran PG, Mazzone T: Diabetic ketoacidosis, hyperosmolar nonacidotic diabetes, and hypoglycemia. In Parrillo JE, Bone RC, eds: *Critical care medicine: principles of diagnosis and management*, Philadelphia, 1994, Mosby.

Foster DW, McGarry JD: The metabolic derangements and treatment of diabetic ketoacidosis, *N Engl J Med* 309:159, 1983.

Kitabchi AE: Low-dose insulin therapy in diabetic ketoacidosis: fact or fiction? *Diabetes/Metab Rev* 5:337, 1989.

Matz R: Hyperosmolar nonacidotic diabetes (HNAD). In Rifkin H, Porte D, eds: *Diabetes mellitus, theory and practice*, New York, 1990, Elsevier.

Rosenbloom AL: Intracerebral crises during treatment of diabetic ketoacidosis, *Diabetes Care* 13:22, 1990.

Schade DS, Eaton RP, Alberti KGMM, Johnston DG: *Diabetic coma, ketoacidotic and hyperosmolar,* Albuquerque, 1981 University of New Mexico Press.

Siperstein MD: Diabetic ketoacidosis and hyperosmolar coma, *Endocrinol Metab Clin North Am* 21:415, 1992.

Wachtel TJ, Tetu-Mouradjian LM, Goldman DL, et al: Hyperosmolarity and acidosis in diabetes mellitus: a three-year experience in Rhode Island, *J Gen Intern Med* 6:495, 1991.

Wetterhall SF, Olson DR, DeStafano F, et al: Trends in diabetes and diabetic complications, 1980-1987, *Diabetes Care* 15:960, 1992.

CASE

3

Peter G. Curran
Theodore Mazzone

·········

The patient is a 32-year-old woman with a history suggestive of hypoglycemia who is referred for evaluation. About 8 months ago, her husband noted that one morning she was very lethargic and diaphoretic. After about 15 minutes this resolved, but it recurred several times over the next month. Six months ago, the morning after an evening of drinking alcohol, she was lethargic all morning, refusing to get out of bed. An ambulance was called, and she was admitted to a hospital where work-up included a normal head magnetic resonance imaging (MRI) and electroencephalography (EEG). Routine blood work was only significant for a glucose of 54 mg/dl. Despite the normal EEG, she was given a diagnosis of complex partial seizures and placed on tegretol. Her symptoms of early morning lethargy persisted, however, becoming more frequent. She was evaluated by a physician who administered a glucose tolerance test, significant only for a fasting glucose level of 42 mg/dl. She was placed on a diet of predominantly complex carbohydrates, with three meals and three snacks with improvement of her symptoms, and referred for further evaluation.

Her husband was asked to bring her to the clinic fasting in the early morning. She was alert, although somewhat irritable. Despite her job in finance, she was unable to do simple calculations. She was not taking any medicines, specifically denying use of insulin or oral hypoglycemic agents. She had no known renal, hepatic, or adrenal disease and had not had abdominal surgery. She drank about six beers per week. Her past history was otherwise unremarkable. There was no family history of hypoglycemia or endocrine tumors. Physical examination was com-

pletely normal with the exception of impaired mental status, with poor short-term memory, and diminished mental ability.

QUESTION 1 What is the normal regulatory response to hypoglycemia?

Hypoglycemia is variously defined as a blood sugar below 40 or 50 mg/dl. Once blood sugar falls below these levels, cerebral function begins to become impaired. With prolonged hypoglycemia this impairment may become more severe and irreversible and may eventually cause coma or death.

The response to hypoglycemia is stimulated by neuroglycopenia and is largely hormonal. In a normal person the liver stores enough glycogen to maintain the serum glucose for several hours. Fuel metabolism is closely regulated to maintain blood sugar levels within a narrow range. A lowered blood sugar will inhibit pancreatic insulin release and stimulate counterregulatory hormone release (catecholamines, cortisol, growth hormone). Catecholamines mobilize muscle glycogen and provide increased amounts of free fatty acids from lipolysis for the synthesis of glucose. Glucagon is derived from pancreatic A cells and secretion is stimulated by catecholamines and the sympathetic nervous system. This hormone increases hepatic glucose secretion and facilitates gluconeogenesis and glycogenolysis. States in which insulin levels are inappropriately elevated or when the counter regulation is impaired may lead to hypoglycemia.

A secondary response is elicited from the secretion of adrenocorticotropic hormone (ACTH) and growth hormone (GH). ACTH stimulates increased cortisol secretion leading to protein catabolism, release of amino acids, and glucose synthesis. Growth hormone antagonizes the activity of insulin on glucose.

QUESTION 2 Does this patient manifest Whipple's triad? What is the differential diagnosis of fasting symptomatic hypoglycemia? What is the appropriate laboratory evaluation?

Whipple's triad is a clinical constellation of findings that support hypoglycemia as a diagnosis (Fig. 4-3-1 on p. 189). This triad includes signs and symptoms of hypoglycemia, a serum glucose <45 mg/dl, and a clinical response to glucose infusion. Symptoms associated with hypoglycemia may be divided into two broad groups: those related to hypoglycemic-induced altered cerebral function (neuroglycopenic) and those related to adrenergic stimulus in response to the hypoglycemia. Neuroglycopenic symptoms include confusion, lethargy, somnolence, decreased vision, irritability, and amnesia. Profound hypoglycemia may induce seizures, focal neurologic disorders, coma, and death. Nocturnal hypoglycemia may induce nightmares. Neuroglycopenic symptoms may be subtle or misleading; in one series, 26% of patients with insulinomas were given a neurologic or psychiatric diagnosis at their first medical encounter for hypoglycemia. Adrenergic symptoms include anxiety, palpitations, headaches, weakness, and tremor.

Symptoms of organic hypoglycemia typically occur in the fasting state, and so are common in the early morning. They may also be brought on by exercise. As these symptoms resolve with eating, patients who have learned to control their symptoms by eating more frequently may gain weight. In retrospect, there typically is a slow progression of severity and frequency of hypoglycemia over time until diagnosis is made.

A number of different states may lead to hypoglycemia (see box), and the etiology is often multifactorial. Drugs are an especially common cause, especially insulin and oral sulfonylureas in the diabetic population. Liver disease and etha-

MAJOR CAUSES OF HYPOGLYCEMIA

STARVATION
- Hospitalized patients
- Pregnancy

DRUGS
- Insulin
- Oral hypoglycemics
- Ethanol
- Salicylates
- Adrenergic blockers
- Quinine
- Pentamidine
- Warfarin
- Acetaminophen
- Ritodrine
- Disopyramide

FACTITIOUS

ENDOCRINE
- Hypopituitary
- Hypoadrenal
- Hypothyroid
- Insulin/insulin receptor antibodies

HEPATIC FAILURE

SEPSIS

RENAL FAILURE

INSULIN HYPERSECRETION
- Insulinoma
- Nesidioblastosis

EXTRAPANCREATIC NEOPLASMS

POSTPRANDIAL
- Gastric surgery
- Idiopathic

DEFECTIVE COUNTERREGULATION

ENZYME DEFECTS (PRESENT IN INFANCY)

nol use may impair glycogenolysis and gluconeogenesis. Patients with renal disease are more prone to hypoglycemia, primarily as insulin and sulfonylurea metabolism are decreased. When evaluating a patient for a possible insulinoma (organic hypoglycemia), it is important to also

MULTIPLE ENDOCRINE NEOPLASIA TYPE I

PANCREATIC TUMORS
- Insulinoma
- Gastrinoma
- Glucagonoma
- Vipoma
- Somatostatinoma
- Serotoninoma

PARATHYROID ADENOMA OR HYPERPLASIA
PITUITARY ADENOMA

consider these other factors as primary or contributing causes.

Endogenous hypersecretion of insulin may also result in hypoglycemia. The majority of these cases are due to insulinomas, although from 8% to 22% of cases may be due to diffuse pancreatic involvement (nesidioblastosis, adenomatosis, and islet cell hyperplasia). Ninety percent of insulinomas are solitary benign lesions. They typically present in the 40 to 60 year age group with slowly progressive symptoms of hypoglycemia. Patients with insulinomas and the syndrome of multiple endocrine neoplasia type I usually present at a younger age, and frequently have multiple insulinomas along with one or more of the other tumors listed in the box above. Malignant insulinomas occur in about 5% of patients with organic hypoglycemia and metastasize to local lymph nodes and the liver. Nesidioblastosis is a rare condition in which the insulin-producing cells from the pancreatic ductules proliferate and hypersecrete insulin. It is typically found in infants, but has been reported in adults. Finally, antibodies to insulin or the insulin receptor have been reported to cause hypoglycemia.

Hypoglycemia may also be a component of chronic renal failure, hypercoritsolism, alcohol abuse, nonpancreatic tumors secreting insulin or an insulin-like factor, and inborn errors of carbohydrate metabolism.

The initial laboratory work-up should be done when the patient is hypoglycemic. One should draw an insulin level along with serum glucose, c-peptide and proinsulin assays. These results must be interpreted together in the presence of hypoglycemia (Fig. 4-3-2 on p. 190).

QUESTION 3 Initial capillary blood glucose on arrival was 34 mg/dl. Venous samples were drawn for glucose (32 mg/dl), insulin (45 µU/ml), C-peptide (0.66 mg/dl), proinsulin (130 pmol/L) (proinsulin 41% of total insulin). These were repeated three more times over the next 30 minutes with similar results. Insulin antibodies were not present, urine sulfonylurea screen was negative. What is the correct interpretation of this laboratory evaluation?

The diagnosis of hypoglycemia caused by excessive endogenous insulin secretion is made by obtaining simultaneous blood samples showing a low blood sugar with inappropriately elevated insulin. If symptoms are reliably induced by an overnight fast, as in the case above, this may be done as an outpatient. However many patients, especially older ones with other medical conditions, may need to be admitted. Greater than 95% of patients with insulinomas will develop hypoglycemic symptoms with a 72-hour fast, about 80% of them within the first 24 hours. If hypoglycemia has not been induced by 72 hours, the patient may be further challenged with exercise. Serum glucose levels should be obtained every 4 to 6 hours (both venous and capillary) during the fast, more frequently if the patient feels symptomatic or if the blood sugar is less than 50 mg/dl. When the blood sugar is below 40 to 45 mg/dl, simultaneous insulin, C-peptide, and proinsulin levels should also be collected. If possible, this collection should be repeated for a total of 3 to 4 sets of samples over 30 to 60 minutes. Following this, the patient should be fed and observed before discharge. An important caveat is that normal women may exhibit blood glucose as low as 40 mg/dl during an extended fast; however, they should not be symptomatic, and the insulin levels should be appropriately suppressed. If the fast is unsuccessful in inducing hypoglycemia, there are a number of provocative tests available, although they are often difficult to interpret and less reliable. An oral glucose tolerance test is not useful in the diagnosis of fasting hypoglycemia.

A normal insulin level with the blood glucose around 40 mg/dl is from 3 to 7 μU/ml. The insulin to glucose ratio may also be used and should be less than 0.3. Proinsulin levels aid in confirming the diagnosis of insulinoma. Normally the percentage of proinsulin compared to total insulin is from 10% to 15%; a percentage of greater than 22 is highly suggestive of an insulinoma. C-peptide, a longer-lived cometabolite of insulin, should also be elevated and is useful to exclude surreptitious insulin injection (where C-peptide levels will be low). Surreptitious use of sulfonylureas, however, will result in an elevated C-peptide, so a urine screen for these drugs should routinely be sent. Finally, it is useful to exclude the presence of insulin antibodies.

QUESTION 4   What is the appropriate therapy for hypoglycemia?

The primary treatment of organic hypoglycemia is surgical excision of the lesion. Proper excision of a single adenoma should be curative. Malignant disease will recur following initial surgery in about 63% of cases, but growth is indolent, and disease-free periods following surgery average 5 years (underlining the need for long-term follow-up). Resection of extensive malignant disease will also palliate hypoglycemia. Diffuse pancreatic disease (islet cell hyperplasia or nesidioblastosis) is usually treated with removal of 80% of the pancreas. Cures rarely result, however, and these patients typically require medical therapy postoperatively.

There is much controversy regarding the issue of how extensive a preoperative evaluation needs to be performed to attempt to localize the tumor, as well as which procedures are the most reliable. Since 85% to 95% of lesions may be detected

intraoperatively using palpation complemented by intraoperative ultrasound, some argue that preoperative testing is neither necessary nor cost effective. On the other hand, knowing the location of the tumor, or whether diffuse disease or multiple lesions exist, should help the surgeon operate more effectively. Localizing techniques include external or endoscopic ultrasound, isotope scanning, dynamic CT scanning, MRI, angiography, and transhepatic portal vein sampling (THPVS) for insulin. There is marked variation in reported reliability of these techniques, presumably dependent to a large extent on operator experience. External ultrasound, CT, and angiography appear to detect from 30% to 75% of lesions, with angiography being especially useful at detecting multiple lesions. Endoscopic ultrasound appears more sensitive, but is still in the experimental stage. The published experience with MRI is also limited, but it appears promising. THPVS appears very sensitive, and has the benefit of localizing the approximate area of the pancreas secreting the excess insulin, but this technique is perfected at only a few centers. In conclusion, it seems reasonable to perform an ultrasound or dynamic CT scan before surgery to attempt to localize a tumor. Angiography might best be used in possible cases of MEN I where multiple tumors are more likely. THPVS appears most useful before a reoperation, either in cases where a partial pancreatectomy was performed with recurrent disease postoperatively, or where no lesion could be found in the operating room and so no resection was attempted.

Medical therapy may be used in cases where surgery is not feasible or unsuccessful. Frequent meals (three small meals with three snacks per day) emphasizing complex carbohydrates are frequently helpful in alleviating symptoms. Diazoxide is a useful drug which both inhibits insulin release and enhances glycogenolysis. As it may cause sodium retention, it is often given with a thiazide diuretic. Octreotide given subcutaneously 2 to 3 times a day will suppress insulin release. Other agents with some reported success are phenytoin, propranolol, glucagon, verapamil,

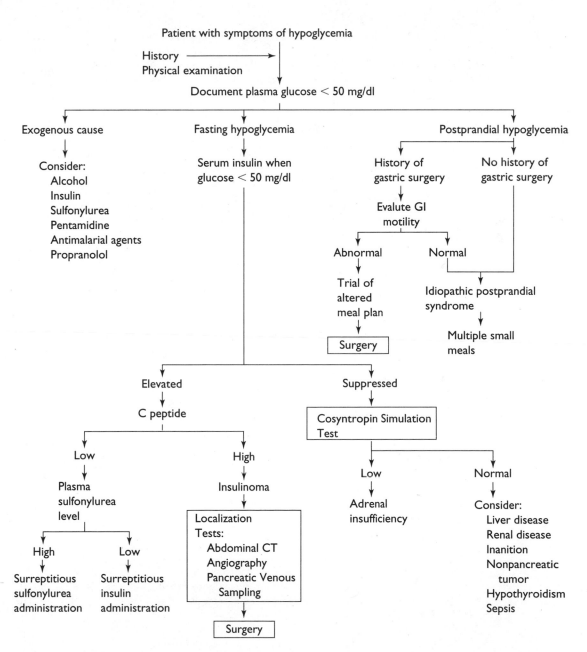

4-3-1 Diagnostic algorithm for hypoglycemia.
(From Greene HL, Johnson WP, Maricic MJ: *Decision making in medicine,* St Louis, 1993, Mosby.)

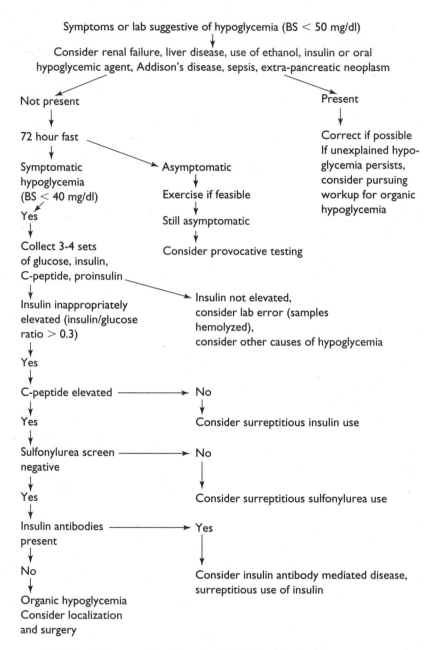

Symptoms or lab suggestive of hypoglycemia (BS < 50 mg/dl)

Consider renal failure, liver disease, use of ethanol, insulin or oral hypoglycemic agent, Addison's disease, sepsis, extra-pancreatic neoplasm

Not present

72 hour fast

Symptomatic hypoglycemia (BS < 40 mg/dl)

Asymptomatic

Exercise if feasible

Still asymptomatic

Consider provocative testing

Yes

Collect 3-4 sets of glucose, insulin, C-peptide, proinsulin

Insulin not elevated, consider lab error (samples hemolyzed), consider other causes of hypoglycemia

Insulin inappropriately elevated (insulin/glucose ratio > 0.3)

Yes

C-peptide elevated ⟶ No

Consider surreptitious insulin use

Yes

Sulfonylurea screen negative ⟶ No

Consider surreptitious sulfonylurea use

Yes

Insulin antibodies present ⟶ Yes

Consider insulin antibody mediated disease, surreptitious use of insulin

No

Organic hypoglycemia Consider localization and surgery

Present

Correct if possible If unexplained hypo-glycemia persists, consider pursuing workup for organic hypoglycemia

4-3-2   Diagnostic algorithm using lab results of a hypoglycemic patient.

and glucocorticoids. Chemotherapeutic agents for malignant disease include streptozocin and 5-FU.

CASE SUMMARY   An abdominal MRI was performed with evidence of a 1 cm mass in the tail of the pancreas. The patient went to surgery where this mass was resected. No other pancreatic masses were detected, lymph node sampling was negative for metastases, and pathology of the mass was consistent with an insulinoma. Postoperatively she required exogenous insulin for hyperglycemia for several weeks, but then became euglycemic, and since that time has no further episodes of hypoglycemia.

• •

BIBLIOGRAPHY

Archambeaud MF, Huc MC, Nadalon S, et al: Autoimmune insulin syndrome, *Biomed Pharmacother* 43:581, 1989.

Binder C, Bendtson I: Endocrine emergencies: hypoglycemia, *Baillieres Clin Endocrinol Metab* 6:23:1992.

Bittger TC, Weber W, Beyer J, Juninger T: Value of tumor localization in patients with insulinoma, *World J Surg* 14:107, 1990.

Comi RJ, Gordon P: Approach to hypoglycemia in adults, *Compr Ther* 13:38, 1987.

Fajans SS, Vinik AI: Insulin-producing islet cell tumors, *Endocrinol Metab Clin North Am* 18:45, 1989.

Field JB: Hypoglycemia, definition, clinical presentations, classification, and laboratory tests, *Endocrinol Metab Clin North Am* 18:27, 1989.

Fraker DL, Norton JA: The role of surgery in the management of islet cell tumors, *Gastroenterol Clin North Am* 18:805, 1989.

Fraker DL, Norton JA: Localization and resection of insulinomas and gastrinomas, *JAMA* 259:3601, 1988.

Grama D, Dkogseid B, Wilander E, et al: Pancreatic tumors in multiple endocrine neoplasia type 1: clinical presentation and surgical treatment. *World J Surg* 16:611, 1992.

Grungerger G, Weiner JL, Silverman R, et al: Factitious hypoglycemia due to surreptitious administration of insulin: diagnosis, treatment, and long-term follow-up, *Ann Intern Med* 108:252, 1988.

Harrison TS, Fajans SS, Floyd JC, et al: Prevalence of diffuse pancreatic beta islet cell disease with hyperinsulism: problems in recognition and management, *World J Surg* 8:583, 1984.

Liessi G, Pasquali C, D'Andrea AA, et al: MRI in insulinomas: preliminary findings, *Eur J Radiol* 14:46, 1992.

Pasieka JL, McLeod MK, Thompson NW, Burney RE: Surgical approach to insulinomas, assessing the need for preoperative localization, *Arch Surg* 127:442, 1992.

Samaan NA: Hypoglycemia secondary to endocrine deficiencies, *Endocrinol Metab Clin North Am* 18:145, 1989.

Seltzer HS: Drug-induced hypoglycemia, *Endocrinol Metab Clin North Am* 18:163, 1989.

Shakir KMM, Amin RM: Hypoglycemia, *Crit Care Clin* 7:75, 1991.

Rosch T, Lightdale CJ, Botet JF, et al: Localization of pancreatic endocrine tumors by endoscopic ultrasonography, *N Engl J Med* 326:1721, 1992.

Vinik AI, Moattari AR: Treatment of endocrine tumors of the pancreas, *Endocrinol Clin North Am* 18:483, 1989.

CASE

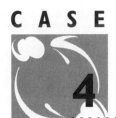

4

Peter G. Curran
Theodore Mazzone

....

A 48-year-old man presents to the emergency room with sudden onset of excruciating right flank pain and hematuria. He has no history of renal or urinary tract disease and no prior history of renal stones. He does recall being told several years ago that his calcium level was elevated, but this was not pursued further. He is otherwise well, with no history of bone fractures, muscle weakness, depression, recent dehydration, or gout. He was on no medications and specifically denied use of over-the-counter calcium supplements, vitamin D, glucocorticoids, lithium, or diuretics. The family history was negative for known cases of hypercalcemia, renal stones, hyperparathyroidism, pituitary disease, pancreatic tumors, medullary thyroid tumors, and pheochromocytomas.

Physical examination revealed a well-developed man in intense pain. BP 185/104 mm Hg, P 112 bpm. Eyes were normal, neck was without masses, significant right flank and lower abdominal pain was present, neurological exam was intact.

QUESTION 1 What features of the history and physical examination are most important?

The patient presents with an acute onset of symptoms, specifically right-flank pain and hematuria. Symptoms of acute onset usually include mechanisms such as infarct or ischemia, trauma, acute occlusion, or distension of a closed viscus or perforation. In addition, the site of symptoms helps to localize the area of abnormality: the right flank. However, one must also consider that this is the site of a referred pain syndrome. The presence of hematuria further localizes the lesion within

the genitourinary tract. One must closely inspect the perineum in both men and women to make certain there is not an anatomically closely related source of bleeding before settling firmly on the genitourinary tract. Additional questioning should try to elicit whether the pain radiates, what makes it better or worse, and if the patient has ever had similar symptoms.

The physical examination demonstrates pain in the same areas as the patient's complaints. It is most important to rule out the presence of an impending intraabdominal disaster. Signs of peritonitis include rebound tenderness, pain reproduced by shaking the bed, abdominal rigidity, and intense pain. A subtle sign is asking the patient whether riding in the car and going over bumps in the road was enough to cause similar pain. In some situations, the patient may not be able to tolerate even the weight of the stethoscope resting on the abdomen. Immediate surgical consultation is necessary.

QUESTION 2 What is the differential diagnosis at this point?

There are many causes of hypercalcemia (see the box on p. 193), and the possibility of other contributing causes needs to be considered, even if hyperparathyroidism (HPT) appears to be present. Initially, it is important to ensure that hypercalcemia does truly exist by repeating a serum calcium level (Fig. 4-4-1 on p. 197). Artifactually elevated calcium occurs with prolonged tourniquet administration, dehydration, and elevated serum binding proteins, in which case an ionized calcium is helpful.

HPT and hypercalcemia of malignancy are the

CAUSES OF HYPERCALCEMIA

- Hyperparathyroidism
- Hypercalcemia of malignancy
- Thyrotoxicosis
- Pheochromocytoma
- Addison's disease
- Vasoactive intestinal peptide secreting adenoma
- Vitamin D intoxication
- Vitamin A intoxication
- Lithium
- Thiazide diuretics
- Theophylline
- Granulomatous disease
- Immobilization
- Milk-alkali syndrome
- Parenteral nutrition
- Familial hypocalciuric hypercalcemia
- Acute renal failure
- Idiopathic hypercalcemia of infancy
- Artifactual

most common causes of hypercalcemia, accounting for over 90% of all cases. HPT is diagnosed with an elevated calcium accompanied by an elevated parathyroid hormone. Parathyroid hormone is generally quantified by immunoassay, with antibodies available against the N-terminus portion of the molecule (the bioactive part), the mid-portion or the C-terminus. Double antibody assays measure the intact molecule. All are relatively reliable, although the double antibody intact molecule assay is significantly more sensitive and specific and should be regarded as the assay of choice. In renal disease where inactive fragments from the C-terminus and mid-portion of PTH accumulate, the N-terminus or intact molecule should always be used. The only other causes of hypercalcemia where the parathyroid hormone level is elevated are lithium or thiazide use. In HPT the phosphate may be normal to decreased (a chloride/phosphate ratio of greater than 33 is associated with HPT), and markers of bone activity are often increased (alkaline phosphatase,

osteocalcin, urinary hydroxyproline). Creatinine clearance and an abdominal x-ray should be obtained to evaluate renal function and screen for nephrolithiasis. A high urine calcium excretion may be a risk factor for stone formation. Parathyroid hormone may also alter renal acid-base handling, and cause hyperchloremia with a metabolic acidosis. Urinary cyclic AMP and blood 1,25-dihydroxyvitamin D levels tend to be elevated, although these tests are usually unnecessary. Twenty-five percent of patients will have a normochromic normocytic anemia.

Hypercalcemia may occur with malignancies in three ways. The most common (50% to 70%) is secondary to osteolytic lesions, especially with metastatic breast carcinoma and multiple myeloma. Other neoplasms, primarily lymphomas, may synthesize excessive amounts of 1,25-dihydroxyvitamin D. In contrast to HPT, the phosphate levels with these two groups are often elevated. The third group, usually squamous, renal, bladder, or ovarian cancers, secrete peptides that have parathyroid hormone-like activity (parathyroid hormone related peptides). These peptides do not cross-react with parathyroid hormone assays, so parathyroid hormone levels should be depressed. As malignancy may coexist with primary HPT, it is recommended to at least obtain a serum protein electrophoresis and mammogram (in women) to exclude these common causes. If bone disease is suspected by history or symptoms, bone x-rays may prove helpful, although brown tumors may resemble lytic lesions and require a biopsy for final diagnosis.

Familial hypocalciuric hypercalcemia is an uncommon autosomal dominant condition that may be misdiagnosed as HPT. These patients tend to display a mildly elevated serum calcium with normal parathyroid hormone levels, normal phosphate and 1,25-dihydroxyvitamin D levels, normal to increased magnesium levels, and relative hypocalciuria. As this is benign and does not require therapy, it is important to distinguish it from HPT, especially in cases where the parathyroid hormone levels are not frankly elevated. This is best done by family screening and obtaining a

24-hour urine collection. The renal calcium clearance/creatinine clearance should be less than 0.01 in this disease.

QUESTION 3 The patient was given narcotic analgesia, and collection of his urine revealed several hard, black, mineralized fragments that were sent out for analysis. Abdominal x-ray showed two right renal pelvic densities compatible with renal stones. Initial blood work showed a calcium of 12.5 mg/dl (normal 8.5 to 10.5), phosphate 2.3 mg/dl (normal 2.5 to 4.5). Urine was grossly bloody, dip-stick and culture did not reveal an infection. Albumin, BUN, creatinine, and alkaline phosphatase were all normal. The CBC showed a mild normochromic, normocytic anemia. Stool was heme negative.

The patient passed the stone in the emergency room and became pain-free. The stone analysis returned as primarily calcium oxalate. He was seen several days later, at which time a repeat calcium was 12.9 mg/dl and a parathyroid hormone (PTH) immunoassay (double antibody, intact molecule) returned as 8.5 pmol/L (normal 1.6 to 6.8). IVP showed no residual urinary tract obstruction; 24-hour urine collection revealed a creatinine clearance of 65 ml/min (normal 70 to 140), with 440 mg of calcium/24 h (normal <250). Alkaline phosphatase, bone densitometry studies of the distal radius and spine, and x-rays of the skull and hands were all normal. Serum protein electrophoresis was normal. Based on this additional laboratory evaluation, what are the unifying diagnosis and the features of this disease? What is the normal calcium metabolism?

The most frequent cause of hypercalcemia in the outpatient setting is primary hyperparathyroidism (HPT). While HPT was originally considered a rare disorder, the advent of routine, multichannel screening of blood chemistries has led to the diagnosis of asymptomatic HPT much more frequently, with HPT being estimated to occur in 0.1% of the general population.

Calcium metabolism is closely regulated to maintain a constant level of serum calcium. Net gastrointestinal absorption of calcium averages about 200 mg/day, with a similar amount being excreted in the urine. In the blood about 50% of calcium is ionized or "free," 45% is protein-bound (predominantly to albumin), and 5% is complexed to anions such as phosphate and bicarbonate. The major reservoir of calcium is the skeletal system.

Parathyroid hormone is the primary regulator of serum calcium levels. It is secreted from four parathyroid glands that are usually located adjacent to the thyroid gland, although there may be variation both in their number and location with glands being found within the thyroid, in the esophageal groove, and in the mediastinum. Parathyroid hormone secretion is stimulated by slight decreases in the level of serum calcium, with maximal release occurring when calcium drops below 7.5 mg/dl. The hormone increases serum calcium concentration at several levels: (1) increases renal calcium absorption, (2) increases renal 1-alpha hydroxylation of 25-hydroxy-vitamin D to the active 1,25-dihydroxyvitamin D form, thus facilitating gastrointestinal calcium absorption, and (3) both directly and indirectly through increasing 1,25-dihydroxyvitamin D, increases bone resorption. Secretion of the hormone is decreased by negative feedback from increasing calcium levels. Parathyroid hormone also affects phosphate metabolism by increasing phosphate release from bone, increasing gastrointestinal phosphate absorption, and increasing renal phosphate excretion.

Primary HPT occurs when the parathyroid gland secretes excessive levels of parathyroid hormone, despite high levels of serum calcium. The most common etiology is a single parathyroid adenoma (80%), with multiple adenomas occurring in 5% of cases. Primary hyperparathyroid hyperplasia with diffuse enlargement of the glands occurs in about 15% of cases. Parathyroid carcinomas may also occur but are rare. Even less common is "normocalcemic hyperparathyroidism" in which there are signs suggestive of HPT and the parathyroid hormone level is elevated, but the serum calcium is normal. These cases are generally due to either calcium-binding abnormalities (where the ionized calcium would indeed be high) or associated with a nutritional or vitamin D deficiency inhibiting the characteristic increase in calcium.

The etiology of primary HPT remains unclear. It is postulated that in HPT the glands escape normal physiologic regulation in one of two ways: either by developing a higher set-point to shut off parathyroid hormone secretion in response to calcium, or by increasing the number of hormone-secreting cells without altering the set-point (or both). Other protein regulators of parathyroid hormone secretion may also be involved. HPT may occasionally be associated with several familial syndromes (multiple endocrine neoplasia [MEN] I and IIa, familial primary HPT, familial cystic parathyroid adenomatosis) and is seen following neck irradiation (secondary to mutations on chromosome 11). It is useful to consider the possibility of other endocrine tumors when evaluating patients with primary HPT; these include pituitary and pancreatic tumors in MEN I and medullary thyroid carcinomas and pheochromocytomas in MEN-IIa.

Secondary HPT occurs primarily in patients with renal failure, where phosphate retention, low levels of 1,25-dihydroxyvitamin D, and hypocalcemia stimulate parathyroid hormone secretion and may lead to bone disease (renal osteodystrophy). It may also be seen with abnormal gastrointestinal absorption of calcium or vitamin D. Occasionally, autonomous parathyroid hormone secretion may result, termed tertiary HPT.

QUESTION 4 What are the clinical features of primary hyperparathyroidism and what are the supportive features our patient demonstrates?

Primary HPT occurs with greatest frequency in women in the 50- to 60-year age group. Renal stones and bony changes are classically associated with the disease. Renal stones and nephrocalcinosis (diffuse renal calcifications) occur in 10% to 15% of patients with HPT. These are radiodense calcium-based stones that form secondary to the persistent hypercalciuria found in HPT. (Despite the increased renal calcium resorption in HPT, the hypercalcemia and increase in filtered calcium load leads to hypercalciuria.) There may be a decrease in renal function associated with renal involvement, and it is useful to check the creatinine clearance. Following therapy for HPT, residual renal stones usually dissolve and disappear.

Prolonged hyperparathyroidism will cause histologic bony changes in a majority of patients. The changes are primarily in cortical bone; in fact, HPT may even protect against cancellous bone loss in postmenopausal women. Severe bone involvement occurs in about 5% of patients and may be associated with pain or fractures. This is termed osteitis fibrosa cystica and is characterized by multifocal subperiosteal bone resorption with bone cysts and brown tumors (benign collections of osteoclasts with poorly mineralized colloid). Alkaline phosphatase will be elevated, and x-rays show characteristic resorption in the distal phalanges, tapering of the distal clavicles, and "salt and pepper" changes in the skull.

Complaints of proximal muscle weakness and fatigability may be associated with HPT, and there appears to be an element of depression in many of these patients, even those judged asymptomatic, which may resolve after therapy. Dementia may be brought on or worsened in the elderly. There may also be an increased incidence of peptic ulcer disease, acute pancreatitis, hypertension, gout, and pseudogout. Calcium elevation is usually mild; however, marked hypercalcemia (acute primary HPT) may occur with gastrointestinal symptoms (nausea, vomiting, constipation), polyuria, polydypsia, lethargy, obtundation, and the characteristic shortened QT interval on ECG.

The physical examination may reveal hypertension, band keratopathy, bony pain, proximal muscle weakness, decreased vibration sense, and hyperreflexia. A palpable neck mass suggests a parathyroid carcinoma.

QUESTION 5 What is the correct therapy for primary hyperparathyroidism?

Primary HPT is curable by surgery, and this is the treatment of choice for patients with symptomatic HPT (nephrolithiasis, symptomatic bone disease, marked hypercalcemia). Controversy exists as to whether patients with asymptomatic HPT should also undergo parathyroidectomy. Patients with mild untreated disease certainly may live many years, and while patients with HPT diagnosed when less than 70 years old may have a slightly decreased life expectancy, there is no evidence that surgery will prolong life expectancy. In addition, there is no good evidence that surgical treatment of asymptomatic HPT will reduce the future risk of fractures or renal failure. It has been reported that both nonspecific symptoms of depression and dementia may be relieved by surgery, even in mild cases. Although surgical cure rates may approach 95% with an experienced parathyroid surgeon, morbidity at 5 years has been reported at 19% (persistent hypercalcemia, negative exploration, recurrent laryngeal nerve damage, and hypoparathyroidism being the major problems). This problem was addressed by an NIH consensus group, who agreed that close observation rather than surgery could be recommended to patients who met the following criteria: (1) asymptomatic disease, (2) creatinine clearance greater than 70% predicted, (3) bone mass greater than 2 SD below the mean, (4) calcium not greater than 1 mg/dl above the normal range, (5) urine calcium of less than 400 mg/day, and (6) no previous life-threatening episode of hypercalcemia. In patients who meet all these criteria, surgery could be considered if the patient desired it, if they were less than 50 years old, or if it was judged that they would not return for requisite close follow-up.

Surgery should be performed by an experienced parathyroid surgeon, as all the glands need to be identified, and they may be ectopic and difficult to find. Enlarged glands should be removed (frozen section may be helpful to diagnose adenoma or hyperplasia in the operating room), while normal glands may be left in place. If all the glands are enlarged and hyperplastic, they should all be removed with one autotransplanted to the forearm to prevent hypoparathyroidism. Preoperative localization studies are not necessary, unless a reoperation is required for persistent HPT. Postoperatively, the patients generally require short-term calcium replacement. Persistent hypocalcemia may be secondary to hypoparathyroidism or "hungry-bone" syndrome, and a serum parathyroid hormone level should distinguish these. Hypomagnesemia may also be present following surgery for prolonged HPT, and if this is not corrected will interfere with the proper function of parathyroid hormone postoperatively.

If patients are not treated surgically, they should be advised to eat a moderate calcium diet. A low calcium diet may stimulate increased parathyroid hormone secretion, and a high calcium diet may exacerbate hypercalcemia. They should maintain adequate hydration, avoid thiazide diuretics and lithium, and avoid immobilization. Estrogen replacement in postmenopausal women will decrease serum and urine calcium levels, and will have beneficial effects on bone mineralization. Phosphate ingestion may stabilize bone and lower 1,25-hydroxyvitamin D levels, but may also increase PTH levels and cause soft tissue calcification, so is not usually recommended. A diagnostic algorithm for hyperparathyroidism is shown in Fig. 4-4-2.

CASE SUMMARY   Based on this evaluation, the patient was believed to have primary hyperparathyroidism. He was referred to an experienced parathyroid surgeon who on neck exploration found one of four parathyroid glands to be enlarged. This gland was resected, with pathology consistent with a parathyroid adenoma. Postoperatively, he required intravenous calcium supplementation for several days, at which time his calcium and phosphate levels remained stable without therapy. Follow-up over the next 5 years revealed normal calcium, phosphate and PTH levels, no change in his creatinine clearance, and apparent resolution of the renal stones previously noted on abdominal x-ray.

• •

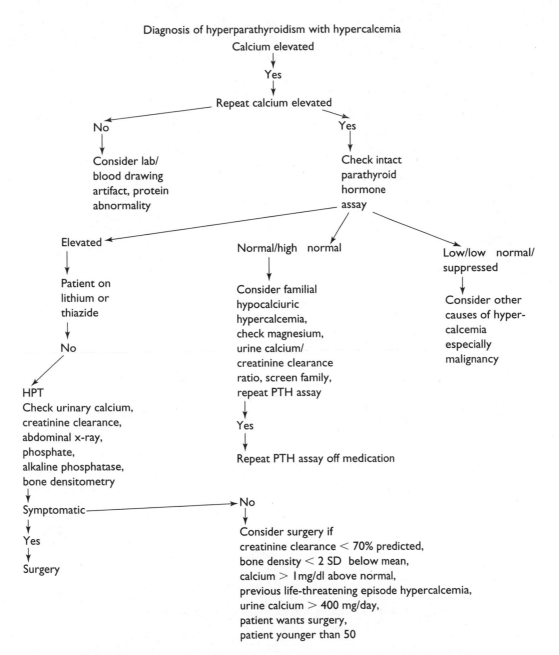

Diagnosis of hyperparathyroidism with hypercalcemia

Calcium elevated

↓

Yes

↓

Repeat calcium elevated

No ← → Yes

No → Consider lab/ blood drawing artifact, protein abnormality

Yes → Check intact parathyroid hormone assay

Elevated ←

Normal/high normal

Low/low normal/ suppressed

↓

Patient on lithium or thiazide

↓

No

↓

HPT
Check urinary calcium, creatinine clearance, abdominal x-ray, phosphate, alkaline phosphatase, bone densitometry

↓

Symptomatic ——————————→ No

↓

Yes

↓

Surgery

Consider familial hypocalciuric hypercalcemia, check magnesium, urine calcium/ creatinine clearance ratio, screen family, repeat PTH assay

↓

Yes

↓

Repeat PTH assay off medication

Consider other causes of hyper-calcemia especially malignancy

No

↓

Consider surgery if
creatinine clearance < 70% predicted,
bone density < 2 SD below mean,
calcium > 1 mg/dl above normal,
previous life-threatening episode hypercalcemia,
urine calcium > 400 mg/day,
patient wants surgery,
patient younger than 50

4-4-1   Diagnostic algorithm for hypercalcemia.
(From Greene HL, Johnson WP, Maricic MJ: *Decision making in medicine,* St Louis, 1993, Mosby.)

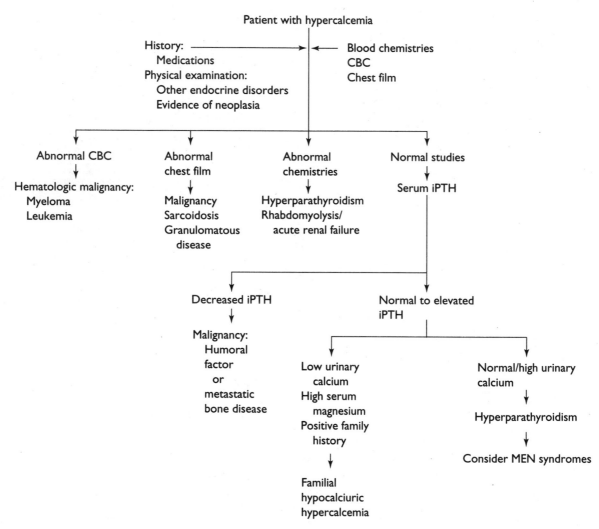

4-4-2 Diagnostic algorithm for hyperparathyroidism.

BIBLIOGRAPHY

Bilezikian JP: Hypercalcemic states, their differential diagnosis and acute management. In Coe FL, Favus MJ, eds: *Disorders of bone and mineral metabolism,* New York, 1992, Raven Press.

Davies M: Primary hyperparathyroidism: aggressive or conservative treatment? *Clin Endocrinol* 36:325, 1992.

Delmez JA, Slatopolsky E: Recent advances in the pathogenesis and therapy of uremic secondary hyperparathyroidism, *J Clin Endocrinol Metab* 72:735, 1991.

Erdman WA, Breslau NA, Weinreb JC, et al: Noninvasive localization of parathyroid adenomas: a comparison of x-ray, computerized tomography, ultrasound, scintigraphy and MRI, *Magn Reson Imaging* 7:187, 1989.

Kaplan EL, Yashiro T, Salti G: Primary hyperparathyroidisim in the 1990's: choice of surgical procedures for this disease, *Ann Surg* 215:300, 1992.

Klee G, Kao PC, Heath H: Hypercalcemia, *Endocrinol Metab Clin North Am* 17:573, 1988.

Lafferty FW, Hubay CA: Primary hyperparathyroidism, a review of the long-term surgical and nonsurgical morbidities as a basis for a rational approach to treatment, *Arch Intern Med* 149:789, 1989.

Marx SJ, Spiegel AM, Levine MA: Familial hypocalciuric hypercalcemia: the relation to primary parathyroid hyperplasia, *N Engl J Med* 307:416, 1982.

NIH Consensus Development Conference Panel: Diagnosis and management of asymptomatic primary hyperparathyroidism: consensus development conference statement, *Ann Intern Med* 114:593, 1991.

Potts JT: Management of asymptomatic hyperparathyroidism, *J Clin Endocrinol Metab* 70:1489, 1990.

Shane E: Medical management of asymptomatic primary hyperparathyroidism, *J Bone Miner Res* 6(Suppl 2):S131, 1991.

Silverberg SJ, Shane E, Jacobs TP, et al: Nephrolithiasis and bone involvement in primary hyperparathyroidism, *Am J Med* 89:327, 1990.

Stewart AF, Broadus AE: Parathyroid hormone-related proteins: coming of age in the 1990's, *J Clin Endocrinol Metab* 71:1410, 1990.

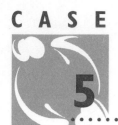

CASE

5

Peter G. Curran
Theodore Mazzone

The patient is a 74-year-old woman who was brought to the emergency room (ER) from a nursing home with a history of 2 weeks of a progressive decline in her mental status. She had become depressed since the death of her husband and subsequent placement in the nursing home 1 year ago. For the several weeks preceding this admission, she had stopped interacting with the other residents of the nursing home, and the staff had noted that she had increasing weakness and difficulty ambulating. After 2 days of being unable to rise from bed without assistance, she was found unresponsive in her room and sent to the ER for evaluation. The patient was taking only Xanax.

Past medical history included prolonged depressive adjustment reaction and hyperthyroidism in distant past, treated with thyroid surgery, and possible coronary disease.

PHYSICAL EXAMINATION:

In the ER she was unresponsive. BP 105/60 mm Hg, P 54 bpm, RR 12/min, T 35°C. Her skin was cool and dry. There was an anterior cervical scar without palpable goiter. Pulmonary examination revealed decreased breath sounds in the right lower lung field. The abdomen was distended without bowel sounds. Neurologic examination was significant for loss of the gag reflex and delayed relaxation of deep tendon reflexes.

LABS:

Na 122 mEq/L, glucose 56 mg/dl, BUN 18 mg/dl, CPK 412 IU/L, LDH 485 IU/L, cholesterol 314 mg/dl, WBC 5,600/ml with 56% segs, ABG pH 7.32, Pco$_2$ 48 mMol/L, Po$_2$ 54 mMol/L. The toxicology screen was negative. Thyroid function tests are pending.

QUESTION I Given the above presentation, how does the finding of hyponatremia and its attendant diagnosis help to define the primary diagnosis? Interpret the results of the arterial blood gas.

Often, evaluation of initial laboratory testing can shed light on the underlying primary diagnosis. In this case the patient presents with obtundation that had gradually progressed over the preceding 2 weeks, and she was then found acutely unresponsive in the nursing home. She is found to be markedly hyponatremic. Additionally, she appears on physical examination to be isovolemic. The calculated serum osmolarity equals 270 mOsm/kg. This falls into the category of isovolemic hypoosmolar hyponatremia. Underlying etiologies include water intoxication, renal insufficiency, SIADH, hypothyroidism, adrenal insufficiency, drugs, and emotional stress. Of these, only water intoxication has a urine Na <10 mEq/L.

The arterial blood gas reveals a respiratory acidosis with elevation of the Pco$_2$ and hypoxemia. Hypoventilation is present, and the accompanying pH suggests an acute onset for the level of hypercarbia. This differential diagnosis includes hypoperfusion of the lung, decreased ventilation, CNS depression, and neuromuscular weakness.

Both of the above signs could be caused by thyroid disease. This is made further suspicious by the patient's history of thyroid surgery without current replacement hormone therapy.

There are a number of other endocrine diseases that may also cause coma that are worthwhile to consider here. The most important of these is diabetes mellitus, where many metabolic abnormalities may contribute to altered mental status.

These include hypoglycemia, hyperosmolarity, ketoacidosis and lactic acidosis, uremia, hypophosphatemia, and hypotension. States of adrenal dysfunction, particularly hypoadrenalism, may also cause altered consciousness. Again, as with diabetes, there are most likely multiple factors involved, including hypotension, hyponatremia, as well as the direct effects of the loss of cortisol on the central nervous system. Finally, marked deviations in serum calcium concentrations as may occur in hyperparathyroidism or hypoparathyroidism may also alter mental status.

QUESTION 2 The ECG revealed a sinus bradycardia with decreased voltage without ischemic changes or evidence of prior infarct. The chest x-ray revealed a right lower lobe infiltrate with bilateral pleural effusions, and a head computed tomography (CT) revealed no significant findings. What factors are present in this patient's presentation that predispose her to acute thyroid insufficiency and myxedema coma, as an etiology of her acute mental status changes?

Many physiologic stresses necessitate normal thyroid function to maintain homeostatic function. Some of these include myocardial function, trauma, gastrointestinal bleeding, hypothermia, anesthesia, sedation and surgery, cerebrovascular accidents, and infection. This patient presented with hypoxemia, and the initial chest x-ray revealed a right lower lobe infiltrate with bilateral pleural effusions. Distinguishing this as a primary or secondary phenomena to acute thyroidal insufficiency is problematic. However, each entity should be approached as a potentially different problem because the treatments are different. In addition, it is very likely that pneumonia could trigger myxedema coma, and this entity should be treated specifically as well.

In a clinical situation where a disease process is present along with its sequela, if the sequela is benign, it may be observed. However, if the secondary phenomenon is potentially dangerous, it may require classification as an independent problem with a separate approach to therapy. An example would be a severely hypothyroid patient with a pericardial effusion. If the effusion is known to be minimal and not causing hemodynamic compromise, it may be observed. However, if tamponade is suspected or of any concern, a therapeutic maneuver, apart from rendering the patient euthyroid (i.e., pericardiocentesis or pericardial window placement) is warranted.

QUESTION 3 The thyroid function tests returned later that evening and revealed a T4 of 1.4 µg/dl (normal 4.5 to 10.7), FTI 1.1 (5.0 to 10.6), TSH 74 µU/ml (0.38 to 6.15) confirming the diagnosis of myxedema coma. What is the pathophysiology of myxedema coma?

Myxedema coma is a complicated metabolic emergency. Although rare, the condition should be considered in all patients with unexplained obtundation and coma, especially the elderly and those with a known risk of hypothyroidism (see the box on p. 202). While myxedema coma may occur from protracted hypothyroidism alone, in most cases there is some accompanying, precipitating event (box). Early thyroid hormone replacement and intensive supportive care are the cornerstones of therapy. With improved therapeutic techniques and advances in critical care, mortality rates have fallen from the 80% reported in 1963 by Forester; however, 30% to 50% of patients diagnosed with this condition still die.

Myxedema coma is associated with widespread organ dysfunction. Hypothermia is common, secondary to a decrease in basal metabolic rate as well as dysfunction of the thermoregulatory center. Hypoventilation occurs through a combination of upper airway edema, an impaired respiratory response to both hypercapnia and hypoxia, pleural effusions, and decreased efficiency of the respiratory musculature. Hypotension may occur from a combination of diminished cardiac contractility, bradycardia, and pericardial effusion resulting in a decreased cardiac output. Paralytic ileus or megacolon may develop. Hyponatremia is common, most likely from a combination of decreased glomerular filtration rate with subse-

RISK FACTORS FOR HYPOTHYROIDISM

- Thyroiditis: autoimmune, suppurative, subacute, postpartal
- Radioactive iodine
- Thyroid surgery
- Drugs: iodine, lithium, amiodarone, PTU
- Infiltrative disease: Tb, sarcoid, tumor
- Congenital thyroid disease
- Pituitary or hypothalamic disease

FACTORS PRECIPITATING MYXEDEMA COMA

- Infection
- Cerebrovascular accident
- Surgery
- Anesthesia, sedatives
- Hypothermia
- GI bleeding
- Trauma
- Myocardial infarction

quent impaired delivery of water to the distal tubule, as well as inappropriate secretion of ADH. Adrenal insufficiency from autoimmune adrenal disease may be associated with autoimmune hypothyroidism, and this may exacerbate the hypoglycemia often found in severe hypothyroidism. Infections are common in myxedema coma, possibly because of impaired leukocyte function.

The etiology of the central neurologic dysfunction-causing coma in this complicated disease is multifactorial. The well-recognized psychomotor retardation and lethargy of hypothyroidism can only be exacerbated by a combination of hypotension, hypercapnia, hypoxia, hypoglycemia, and hyponatremia.

QUESTION 4 What are the specific findings on physical examination and laboratory evaluation that support a diagnosis of myxedema coma?

As early therapy with thyroid hormone appears to improve survival in myxedema coma, it is important to attempt the diagnosis before thyroid function tests (TFTs) may be available. Any history that might suggest predisposition to hypothyroidism should be elicited (box). Important physical signs include: hypothermia; the thickened, doughy, yellowish skin changes characteristic of myxedema; thinning of the hair with loss of the lateral eyebrows; macroglossia; goiter or scars from prior neck surgery; evidence of pleural or pericardial effusions; decreased or absent bowel sounds; and delayed relaxation of deep tendon reflexes (best elicited at the ankle).

Lab abnormalities found in myxedema coma include: hyponatremia, hypercapnia, hypoglycemia, elevated CPK and LDH (isoenzymes may mimic the profile found in myocardial infarction), elevated SGOT, and elevated cholesterol. The WBC is usually normal even if infection is present. The ECG often reveals bradycardia, with decreased voltage and QT prolongation.

Thyroid function tests should reveal a low T4 and FTI, with an elevated TSH (>20 µU/ml). The main challenge in interpreting the TFTs is differentiating myxedema coma from the much more common euthyroid sick syndrome (ESS), where thyroid hormone replacement is generally not felt to be indicated. In the ESS the T4 and FTI are also decreased, but the TSH is not elevated, reflecting the general belief that these patients are not hypothyroid. In interpreting the TSH in the critical care setting it is important to note that both dopamine and glucocorticoids can cause TSH suppression. The TSH will also not be elevated in truly hypothyroid patients with pituitary or hypothalamic dysfunction. These cases are best differentiated from ESS by radiologic studies of the pituitary or by looking for other evidence of hypopituitarism.

QUESTION 5 What are the important elements of treatment of myxedema coma (Fig. 4-5-1)?

Effective treatment of myxedema coma requires an intensive care setting. The patients frequently need prolonged intubation and aggressive blood pressure support. Because of the frequent association of myxedema coma with infec-

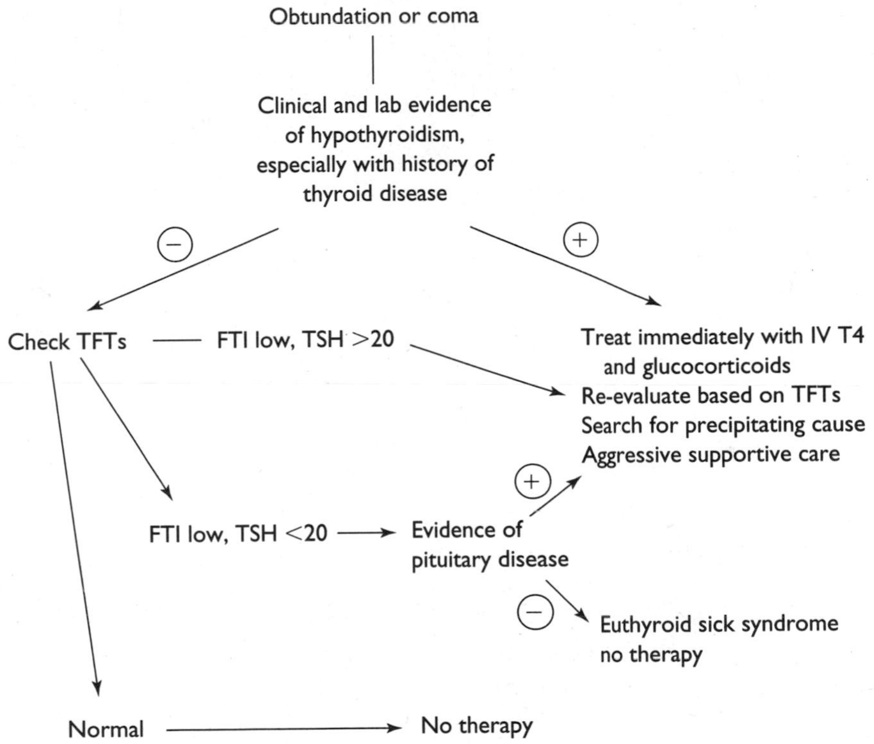

Obtundation or coma

Clinical and lab evidence
of hypothyroidism,
especially with history of
thyroid disease

$\ominus$ $\oplus$

Check TFTs —— FTI low, TSH >20

Treat immediately with IV T4
and glucocorticoids
Re-evaluate based on TFTs
Search for precipitating cause
Aggressive supportive care

$\oplus$

FTI low, TSH <20 ⟶ Evidence of
pituitary disease

$\ominus$

Euthyroid sick syndrome
no therapy

Normal ⟶ No therapy

4-5-1   Treatment/diagnostic algorithm for obtundation or coma.

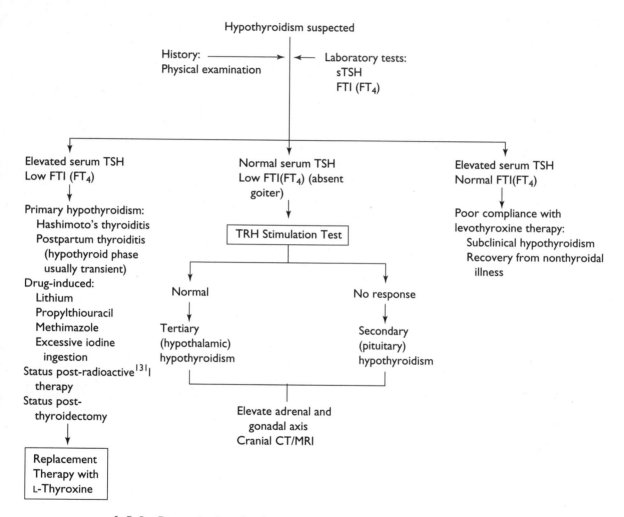

4-5-2 Diagnostic algorithm for hypothyroidism.
(From Greene HL, Johnson WP, Maricic MJ: *Decision making in medicine*, St Louis, 1993, Mosby.)

tion without leukocytosis or fever, antibiotics should be considered early. Medications are usually given intravenously because of potential ileus. The associated hypothermia is best treated with hormone replacement, as active warming may cause peripheral vasodilatation and shock.

Thyroid hormone replacement should be initiated in patients where strong clinical suspicion exists of myxedema coma, even before confirmation by TFTs. The reason for this is that early thyroid replacement may improve survival in this often lethal disease, while euthyroid people can tolerate temporarily elevated thyroid hormone levels. The most commonly used agent for replacement is IV-T4 (300-500 µg, then 50-100 µg/day). IV-T3 may also be used alone or in combination with T4. The T3 would theoretically have a quicker onset of action; however, there is no evidence that it improves survival, and it may be associated with an increased risk of cardiac arrhythmias. No matter what agent is picked, continuous ECG monitoring is important. Because of the association of hypoadrenalism with hypothyroidism, it is recommended that glucocorticoid replacement (100 mg hydrocortisone tid IV) be initially given with the thyroid hormone until the status of the hypothalamic-pituitary-adrenal axis is known.

Within 12 hours of initiating therapy the temperature and pulse should begin to respond. Mental status should begin to improve within 24 hours, and the TSH should begin to decrease in the first 1 to 2 days.

CASE SUMMARY The patient was admitted with the diagnosis of aspiration pneumonia, obtundation possibly secondary to hypoxia, and possible hypothyroidism. She was given oxygen and appropriate antibiotics. Because of concern about her possible cardiac disease, the decision was made to hold off on thyroid hormone replacement until the thyroid function tests were available. Several hours into her admission, her respiratory status was judged to have declined, and she was moved to the ICU and intubated. Her BP fell despite aggressive fluid management. The patient's condition continued to worsen over the next several hours, and she expired.

This case illustrates several important points. The first is the frequent occurrence of unrecognized hypothyroidism in the geriatric population, many of whom are misdiagnosed as depressed. Typically, the progression of symptoms is usually slow, although an event such as the aspiration pneumonia that occurred here may precipitate myxedema coma. The second is that thyroid hormone replacement should be given early. In this patient with history, physical examination, and lab results all supporting hypothyroidism, immediate hormone replacement might have changed the outcome. A diagnostic algorithm for hypothyroidism is shown in Fig. 4-5-2.

• •

BIBLIOGRAPHY

Forester CF: Coma in myxedema, *Arch Intern Med* 111:100-109, 1963.

Gavin LA: Thyroid crises, *Med Clin North Am* 75:179-193, 1991.

Hickman PE, Silvester W, Musk AA, et al: Cardiac enzyme changes in myxedema coma, *Clin Chem* 33:622-624, 1987.

Hylander B, Rosenqvist U: Treatment of myxedema coma—factors associated with fatal outcome, *Acta Endocrinol* 108:65-71, 1985.

Ladenson PW, Goldenheim PD, Ridgeway EC: Prediction and reversal of blunted ventilatory responsiveness in patients with hypothyroidism, *Am J Med* 84:877-883, 1988.

McCulloch W, Price P, Hinds CJ, Wass JAH: Effects of low dose oral triiodothyronine in myxoedema coma, *Intensive Care Med* 11:259-262, 1985.

Myers L, Hays J: Myxedema coma, *Crit Care Clin* 7:43-56, 1991.

Rapoport B: Myxedema coma. In Bardin CW, ed: *Current therapy in endocrinology and metabolism,* Philadelphia, 1991, BC Decker.

Smallridge RC: Metabolic and anatomic thyroid emergencies: a review, *Crit Care Med* 20:276-291, 1992.

Tachman ML, Guthrie GP Jr: Hypothyroidism, diversity of presentation, *Endocr Rev* 5:456-465, 1984.

C A S E

6

Peter G. Curran
Theodore Mazzone

A 52-year-old man complains to his physician of excessive flushing. He describes a deep red discoloration of his face and neck with associated tearing, lasting for about 5 minutes. This has been occurring with increasing frequency over the last several months and appears to be more frequent when he drinks red wine. In response to questioning, he also notes frequent watery bowel movements, especially in the afternoon. He has no cough, wheezing, dyspnea, abdominal distention or pain, bone pain, or neck mass.

Medications: aspirin prn, specifically no chlorpropamide.

Past history: noncontributory.

Family history: no endocrine neoplasia.

Physical examination: Well-appearing white male, with normal skin coloration. Vital signs normal. HEENT normal, thyroid normal, chest clear, normal physiologic flow murmur without gallop, abdomen without masses, no hepatomegaly.

QUESTION I   What is the differential diagnosis of facial flushing and what is the impact of the patient's history of watery diarrhea?

Facial flushing can be seen in a variety of conditions (Fig. 4-6-1 on p. 209). These include response to fever, alcohol ingestion, stress, and as an allergic reaction to some foods. The presence of abnormally high levels of carboxyhemoglobin produces facial flushing. Hormones, including catecholamines, pentagastrin, and serotonin can also produce flushing. One cause of hyperserotonemia is the carcinoid syndrome.

The patient's history of watery diarrhea lends

suspicion to the provisional diagnosis of the carcinoid syndrome.

QUESTION 2   What is the appropriate laboratory evaluation in the work-up to evaluate the presence of carcinoid syndrome?

To evaluate a patient for the presence of the carcinoid syndrome, it is necessary to evaluate both a serum serotonin level and a 24-hour collection of urine for 5-HIAA. The patient should be warned to abstain from consumption of chocolate, bananas, tomatoes, pineapple, walnuts, kiwi, pecans, and avocados as well as medications including acetaminophen, robitussin, and salicylates as these can elevate the level of serum serotonin. Certain pharmacologic agents including mephenesin, methocarbamol, reserpine, acetaminophen, glycerol, and guiacolate can have similar effects. Furthermore, diseases including Whipple's disease and nontropical sprue also can demonstrate elevated levels of serotonin.

QUESTION 3   Soon thereafter, the following laboratory results are available. The patient was asked to return with a 24-hour urine collection for 5-hydroxyindoleacetic acid (5-HIAA). The serum calcitonin is 24 ng/L (normal <100), the serotonin 8.4 micromol/L (normal <1.13), and the 5-HIAA 138 mg/day (normal 2 to 8). What is the correct interpretation of these laboratory tests?

Carcinoid tumors should be an important part of the differential diagnosis in patients with flushing, chronic diarrhea, or those with small tumors or nodules found in the lungs, intestines, or liver.

As an example, carcinoid tumors make up 13% to 34% of all small bowel tumors.

Diagnosis is based on finding elevated levels of serotonin in the blood, with increased amounts of the serotonin metabolite 5-HIAA in a 24-hour urine collection (Fig. 4-6-2 on p. 210). For this testing, patients should avoid the previously mentioned foods and medications to avoid false-positive tests. Approximately 87% of carcinoids will have elevated serum serotonin, and 75% will have an elevated 5-HIAA. These tests are an adequate screen; however, in cases where they are normal but carcinoid is still suspected, other peptides such as 5-hydroxytryptophan, neurotensin, or substance P may also be checked. In addition, provocative testing with calcium or pentagastrin may be performed. Finally, as medullary carcinoma with resultant high calcitonin levels frequently causes both flushing and diarrhea, it is useful to check a blood calcitonin level.

It should be noted that foregut carcinoid tumors (gastric and bronchial) are usually deficient in the L-amino-acid-decarboxylase enzyme that mediates degradation of 5-hydroxytryptophan (5-HT) to 5-hydroxytryptamine (serotonin) so that diagnosis rests on elevated 5-HT levels rather than an elevated 5-HIAA level.

QUESTION 4   What are the important features of the carcinoid syndrome?

Carcinoid tumors arise from enterochromaffin cells that are of neural crest origin and widely distributed throughout the body. They are classed with other hormone-secreting tumors of neural crest origin such as medullary thyroid carcinomas, islet cell tumors, and pheochromocytomas (amine precursor uptake and decarboxylation or APUDomas).

Although carcinoid tumors may secrete a variety of hormones, 80% to 90% hypersecrete serotonin. Others, apparently lacking the enzyme dopa decarboxylase, secrete instead the serotonin precursor 5-hydroxytryptophan. In addition, a wide variety of other hormones may be co-

HORMONES SECRETED FROM CARCINOID TUMORS

- Serotonin
- 5-hydroxytryptophan
- Dopamine
- Histamine
- Kallikrein
- Motilin
- Substance P
- Vasoactive intestinal peptide
- Adrenocorticotrophic hormone (ACTH)
- Growth hormone
- Growth hormone-releasing hormone
- Human chorionic gonadotropin
- Calcitonin
- Insulin
- Glucagon
- Somatostatin
- Parathyroid hormone

secreted (box above). Carcinoid tumors may also be associated with the multiple endocrine neoplasia type 1 syndrome. The incidence of clinically detected carcinoid tumors is only 1.5/100,000. However, in autopsy series it has been reported as high as 1%, suggesting that many small, clinically silent tumors are never detected. It is also probable that many carcinoids are misdiagnosed as small cell carcinomas or adenocarcinomas. Carcinoid tumors may be benign or malignant, metastasizing mainly to regional lymph nodes, liver and bone. The peak age of diagnosis is from 60 to 70 years old.

Because of the wide dispersion of enterochromaffin cells throughout the body, carcinoid tumors have been reported in almost every organ. The most frequently identified sites are the bronchus (22%) and the intestinal submucosa (47%). In almost one quarter of cases the primary site is never identified. In terms of predicting behavior and response to therapy, it is useful to divide the tumors into three groups based on their site of embryological origin: foregut (including bronchus, thymus, stomach, duodenum, and pancreas), midgut (ileum, jejunum, and right colon), and hindgut (transverse and left colon, and rectum).

The classic components of the carcinoid syndrome include flushing, diarrhea, right-sided cardiac valve abnormalities, and wheezing. Obvious carcinoid syndrome occurs in only 10% of patients with carcinoid tumors. Many patients present instead with vague abdominal pain or intestinal obstruction. In these cases, carcinoid is often a postoperative diagnosis, although in retrospect they may have had subtle symptoms.

Flushing occurs in about 85% of those with carcinoid syndrome. The type of flushing described in this case (short duration, localized to the face and neck) is typically associated with ileal carcinoids. The flushing may be more prolonged, darker in hue, or affect other areas such as the back. In addition, there may be significant lacrimation and facial edema that may become permanent ("leonine facies"). Bronchial carcinoids are often associated with this more severe flushing. Flushing may be spontaneous or induced by emotion, ethanol, or tyramine-containing foods such as chocolate, coffee, and blue cheese. Flushing is, of course, not specific to the carcinoid syndrome, and other causes should be considered. These include the postmenopausal state, panic attacks, medullary thyroid carcinoma, the combination of chlorpropamide and ethanol, autonomic instability, mastocytosis, and idiopathic flushing.

Diarrhea occurs in about 70% of patients with the carcinoid syndrome and is secondary to increased intestinal motility and secretion. Severe cases may be associated with steatorrhea. In addition, intraperitoneal fibrosis frequently occurs with gastrointestinal carcinoids that may cause diffuse abdominal pain, weight loss, and intestinal obstruction. Hepatomegaly may result if hepatic metastases are present.

Fibrosis may also occur in the heart, and cardiac valvular function may become compromised. This most commonly leads to tricuspid regurgitation or pulmonic stenosis. Wheezing occurs in about 17% of those with the carcinoid syndrome. Other less common findings include hyperpigmentation of the skin (pellagra dermatosis), myopathy, fibrosis of other organs (such as Peyronie's disease), hypercalcemia, and glucose intolerance or diabetes. Bone metastases may cause bony pain.

As these tumors may co-secrete other hormones, they are occasionally associated with other syndromes of excessive hormone secretion. The most important of these are Cushing's syndrome from ectopic ACTH secretion and acromegaly due to ectopic growth hormone secretion.

QUESTION 5 What imaging studies are useful in determining the location of the tumor?

Imaging studies are important in the evaluation of carcinoids to determine the location of the primary tumor as well as to evaluate for the presence of metastases. CT of the chest and abdomen is an effective way of locating pulmonary tumors, hepatic metastases, and lymph node involvement. If the primary tumor is in the small intestine, it may be difficult to localize the actual site, as local areas of fibrosis often obscure it. In these cases, superior mesenteric angiography is often useful. ^{131}I-metaiodobenzlyguanidine (MIBG) is concentrated by carcinoids (as well as other APUDomas) and is recommended along with CT for initial screening and localization. Once localized, ultrasound or CT-guided biopsy should be considered to provide cytologic confirmation of the diagnosis. ^{99}Tc-bone scanning is effective to evaluate for bony metastases. If right-sided heart disease is suspected clinically, an echocardiogram should be performed.

QUESTION 6 With a presumptive diagnosis of carcinoid syndrome, CT scans of the chest and abdomen are obtained that reveal a 2-cm fibrotic mass of the ileum with several enlarged adjacent lymph nodes without evidence of metastases to the liver. MIBG scanning demonstrates uptake only in

Facial flushing
↓
Patient history: fever
                alcohol ingestion
                stress
                allergic reactions
                catecholamine, pentagastrin, serotonin
                   excess
↓
Hyperserotonemia
↓
Consider carcinoid syndrome
↓
Check serotonin and urine 5-HIAA levels
(Instruct patients to avoid chocolate, bananas, tomatoes,
pineapple, walnuts, avocados, kiwi, pecans, and drugs
including acetaminophen, robitussin, and salicylates)
↓
If negative check additional enzymes
    i.e., 5-hydroxytryptamine
            Neurotensin
            Substance P
                OR
Carry out calcium or pentagastrin stimulation
    tests
↓
Carry out localizing procedures
    i.e., CT chest
        Mesenteric angiography
        I-131 metaiodobenzyguanidine (MIBG) scanning
        TC-99 bone scanning
↓
Obtain tissue for histologic diagnosis
↓
Begin treatment
↓
Surgical extirpation for localized disease or
    in metastatic disease when not extensive

Medical therapy with octreotide,
    methysergide, or cyproheptidine

Chemotherapy: streptozotocin, 5-FU, Alpha-
    interferon, cisplatinum, and etoposide

4-6-1   Diagnostic algorithm for facial flushing.

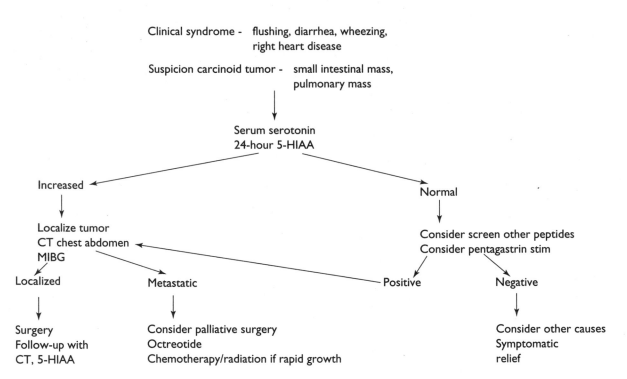

Evaluation of carcinoid tumors

Clinical syndrome -   flushing, diarrhea, wheezing,
right heart disease

Suspicion carcinoid tumor -   small intestinal mass,
pulmonary mass

Serum serotonin
24-hour 5-HIAA

Increased

Normal

Localize tumor
CT chest abdomen
MIBG

Consider screen other peptides
Consider pentagastrin stim

Localized

Metastatic

Positive

Negative

Surgery
Follow-up with
CT, 5-HIAA

Consider palliative surgery
Octreotide
Chemotherapy/radiation if rapid growth

Consider other causes
Symptomatic
relief

4-6-2   Diagnostic algorithm for carcinoid tumors.

the ileal region. ^{99}mTc bone scan did not reveal metastases. He is referred for surgery and undergoes a partial ileal resection with lymph node dissection. Pathology confirms the diagnosis of carcinoid tumor metastatic to local lymph nodes. What is the appropriate therapy for the patient's condition?

Although carcinoid tumors are regarded as fairly indolent neoplasms, they do frequently cause death, and therapy should be aggressive. Surgery should be considered as the primary modality for localized disease and is frequently curative. If metastatic disease is not extensive, surgery will often provide extended periods of symptomatic relief. In cases where surgery is unsuccessful or impossible, medical therapy includes the long-acting somatostatin analog octreotide (the most successful drug currently available), as well as the serotonin antagonists methysergide and cyproheptadine. Octreotide may also inhibit growth of the tumor.

. In cases of rapid growth of the tumor, chemotherapy may provide some benefit. Suggested regimens are streptozotocin and 5-FU for tumors of foregut origin, alpha-interferon for midgut, and cis-platinum and etoposide for poorly differentiated or unresponsive lesions. Radiation or arterial embolization has also been used if metastatic disease is unresponsive to chemotherapy.

Survival depends largely on how widespread the tumor is on diagnosis. Median 5-year survival ranges from 48% to 82%. If the tumor is localized, it is approximately 94%, with regional lymph node involvement 64%, and with metastatic disease 18%.

CASE FOLLOW-UP Following surgery, his symptoms disappeared. While his urinary 5-HIAA levels remain somewhat elevated, follow-up CT scans at 6 and 12 months show no signs of recurrence of gross disease. The patient is told no further therapy will be required unless symptoms recur or a mass is found on further follow-up.

• •

BIBLIOGRAPHY

Aldrich LB, Moattari R, Vinik AI: Distinguishing features of idiopathic flushing and carcinoid syndrome, *Arch Intern Med* 148:2614, 1988.

Feldman JM: Carcinoid tumors and the carcinoid syndrome, *Curr Probl Surg* 26:829, 1989.

Gordon P, Comi RJ, Maton PN, Go VLW: Somatostatin and somatostatin analog (SMS 201-995) in treatment of hormone-secreting tumors of the pituitary and gastrointestinal tract and non-neoplastic diseases of the gut, *Ann Intern Med* 110:35, 1989.

Hanson MW, Feldman JM, Blinder RA, et al: Carcinoid tumors: iodine-131 MIBG scintigraphy, *Radiology* 172:699, 1989.

Kvols LK, Moertel CG, O'Connell MJ, et al: Treatment of the malignant carcinoid syndrome, *N Engl J Med* 315:663, 1986.

Lamberts SWJ, Chayvialle JA, Krenning EP: The visualization of gastroenteropancreatic endocrine tumors, *Metabolism* 41:111, 1992.

Leinung MC, Young WF, Whitaker, Michale D: Diagnosis of corticotropin-producing bronchial carcinoid tumors causing Cushing's syndrome, *Mayo Clin Pro* 65:1314-1321, 1990.

Limper A, Carpenter PC, Scheithauer B, Staats BA: The Cushing syndrome induced by bronchial carcinoid tumors, *Ann Intern Med* 117:209, 1992.

Saini A, Waxman J: Management of the carcinoid syndrome, *Postgrad Med J* 67:506, 1991.

Vinik AI, McLeod MK, Fig L, et al: Clinical features, diagnosis, and localization of carcinoid tumors and their management, *Gastroenterology Clin North Am* 18:865, 1989.

C A S E

7

Peter G. Curran
Theodore Mazzone

A *22-year-old woman presents for evaluation of hirsutism. Since age 14 she has noted increasing facial hair growth and now needs to shave twice a week. She also notes heavy hair growth on her legs and for the last several years has developed hair on her back and chest. Her menarche was at age 13; however, her menses have typically been irregular, usually occurring about 4 times a year. She has never been pregnant, despite unprotected intercourse. There is no other history of virilization, specifically no temporal balding, acne, increased muscle mass, deepening of the voice, clitoromegaly, or breast atrophy. She has a history of obesity and was once told to lose weight as her "blood sugar was high." She has no hypertension, and there is no other history that is suggestive of Cushing's disease and nothing to suggest hyperthyroidism or hypothyroidism.*

Medications: none.

Family history: Mother with slight mustache. No known congenital adrenal hyperplasia (CAH).

Physical examination: Obese white woman with obvious facial hirsutism.

BP 128/84 mm Hg, P 88 bpm, weight 195 lbs, height, 5'4".

Skin: hypertrophic folds at neck and axillae consistent with acanthosis nigricans, no striae or acne, terminal hair growth on upper lip, chin, sideburns, back and chest, with male escutcheon.

HEENT: visual fields intact.

Neck: no hump, thyroid 20 g.

Breasts: normal.

Abdomen: no masses.

Pelvic: no clitoromegaly, normal vaginal mucosa, normal uterus, ovaries possibly enlarged.

Motor strength intact.

QUESTION 1 This patient presents with a combination syndrome of hirsutism and hyperandrogenism. What is the differential diagnosis of this syndrome?

Careful consideration needs to be given to the causes of hyperandrogenism and hirsutism (Fig. 4-7-1). Cushing's syndrome may be associated with hirsutism and increased levels of androgens, particularly DHEA-S. Thus a 1-mg overnight dexamethasone screen is often useful. Ovarian or adrenal virilizing tumors need to be considered, particularly if the levels of androgens are high (testosterone greater than 200 ng/dl suggests an ovarian tumor, and DHEA-S greater than 8000 μg/L suggests an adrenal tumor). Late-onset congenital adrenal hyperplasia may also present with elevated levels of DHEA-S. It is useful to screen for the most common form of this group, 21-hydroxylase deficiency, with a ACTH stimulation test for 17-hydroxyprogesterone. Use of androgen-containing drugs also needs to be considered. Other drugs not containing androgens may also cause hirsutism; these include diphenylhydantoin, minoxidil, corticosteroids, and diazoxide. Finally, hypothyroidism, porphyria, and anorexia nervosa may all be associated with mild hirsutism.

QUESTION 2 Laboratory testing revealed testosterone 130 ng/dl (normal 20 to 80), free testosterone 2.4 ng/dl (normal 0.1 to 2.0), DHEA-S 3110 μg/L (normal 820 to 3380), LH 74 mIU/ml (normal 0-30), FSH 20 mIU/ml (normal 5 to 25). Thyroid function tests and screening chemistries were normal, with a fasting blood glucose of 130 mg/dl. A 1-mg overnight dexamethasone suppression test (rule out Cushing's) and 17-hydroxyprogesterone pre- and post-ACTH (rule out late-onset 21-hydroxylase CAH) were all normal. What is the correct interpretation of this laboratory profile?

Women with polycystic ovarian syndrome (PCOS) often present for evaluation of infertility or hirsutism. While the diagnosis is often strongly suspected from the history, laboratory data will help both to confirm this as well as to exclude other causes. An androgen profile will usually reveal an increased androstenedione and free testosterone. Because of shifts in the concentration of sex hormone binding globulin, the total testosterone may frequently be only in the high normal range. DHEA-S will be elevated in about 50% of cases. The LH level is typically elevated, with the FSH level suppressed. An LH/FSH ratio often exceeds 3, although this is not necessary for diagnosis. Because of pulsatile secretion of the gonadotropins, repeated testing will give a more accurate estimation of the actual gonadotropin profile. Although it is rarely necessary to check estrone levels, these are typically elevated, with estradiol levels remaining in the normal mid-follicular range. Because of the variability in ovarian anatomy, it is rarely helpful to obtain an ovarian ultrasound.

QUESTION 3 What is the most likely diagnosis to explain the presentation of this young woman and what is the hormonal aberration demonstrated by this disease?

On the basis of her history and evaluation, the patient was felt to most likely have polycystic ovarian syndrome with probable insulin resistance. PCOS, described by Stein and Leventhal in 1935, is estimated to affect about 5% of women of reproductive age. It is a heterogeneous syndrome of ovarian hyperandrogenism associated with menstrual irregularities, infertility, hirsutism, and often with obesity and insulin resistance.

The underlying physiological defects in PCOS are difficult to define. To a large extent this is due to the marked heterogeneity of presentation found in this syndrome. Although many theories have been proposed as to its etiology, it is generally agreed to be a functional disorder of gonadotropin (luteinizing and follicle stimulating hormones) dependent ovarian hyperandrogenism.

Typically, the woman with PCOS has an elevated luteinizing hormone (LH) and a lowered follicle stimulating hormone (FSH) as compared to a normally menstruating woman in early follicular phase. This altered hormone profile is part of an abnormal cycle that results in chronic stimulation of the androgen producing cells (thecal cells) of the ovary. The increased androgens are partially converted to estrogens in the periphery, typically resulting in chronically high normal to high levels of both androgens and estrogens. The net effect of the increased levels of these sex steroids feeds back on the hypothalamus and pituitary, stimulating LH and inhibiting FSH secretion. The increased LH will further stimulate thecal cell production of androgens, and the decreased FSH will inhibit follicular maturation, resulting in follicular atresia, chronic anovulation, and infertility. While the primary defect appears to be in the regulation of the hypothalamic-pituitary-ovarian axis, adrenal androgen levels may also be somewhat elevated, contributing to the overall hyperandrogenism.

The ovaries are typically bilaterally enlarged, with multiple "cysts" that are actually the atretic follicles. Although these changes are characteristic of PCOS, they are not diagnostic. Similar ovaries may be found in nonhirsute women with normal menstrual cycles, and women with clinical PCOS may have normal appearing ovaries. Hyperthecosis of the ovary, where islets of luteinized cells are scattered throughout the ovarian

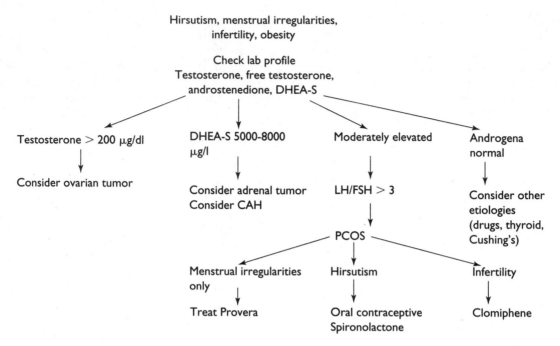

Hirsutism, menstrual irregularities,
infertility, obesity

Check lab profile
Testosterone, free testosterone,
androstenedione, DHEA-S

Testosterone > 200 μg/dl → Consider ovarian tumor

DHEA-S 5000-8000 μg/l → Consider adrenal tumor / Consider CAH

Moderately elevated → LH/FSH > 3 → PCOS

Androgena normal → Consider other etiologies (drugs, thyroid, Cushing's)

PCOS →
- Menstrual irregularities only → Treat Provera
- Hirsutism → Oral contraceptive Spironolactone
- Infertility → Clomiphene

4-7-1 Diagnostic algorithm for hirsutism.

stroma rather than collected around the follicles, is a subset of PCOS typically associated with more severe clinical disease.

QUESTION 4 Are the findings of insulin resistance and skin hyperpigmentation consistent with the presumptive diagnosis of PCOS or does this finding require further evaluation?

There is an interesting association with insulin resistance in about 50% of women with PCOS. Although much of this may be attributed to the obesity that frequently accompanies this syndrome, it is also found in nonobese women. It appears that the insulin resistance and increased levels of insulin contribute to the hyperandrogenism through a number of mechanisms. In addition, increased levels of insulin and androgens cause a characteristic hyperplastic response of the skin, acanthosis nigricans. This results in hyperpigmented and hypertrophic areas of the skin, particularly at the neck and axillary folds.

QUESTION 5 What are the maturational, hormonal, and body habitus characteristics of a woman with PCOS?

Women with PCOS typically have a normal menarche; however, their menses following this are usually irregular, and they may develop frank amenorrhea (in 50%). Only about 12% of these women will have cyclic menses, and the great majority (up to 95%) are infertile. Hirsutism occurs in about 70% of cases, but there are rarely any further signs of virilization (temporal balding, acne, clitoromegaly, increased muscular mass). In fact, if these other signs appear, an androgen-secreting tumor should be suspected. There are a number of formal ways to quantify hirsutism (such as the Ferriman-Gallwey scale); however, a written description of the areas involved usually suffices. Obesity occurs in 40% to 50% of these cases, and as mentioned previously, obese women with PCOS have an increased likelihood of insulin resistance (20% of obese PCOS patients will develop impaired glucose tolerance of diabetes mel-

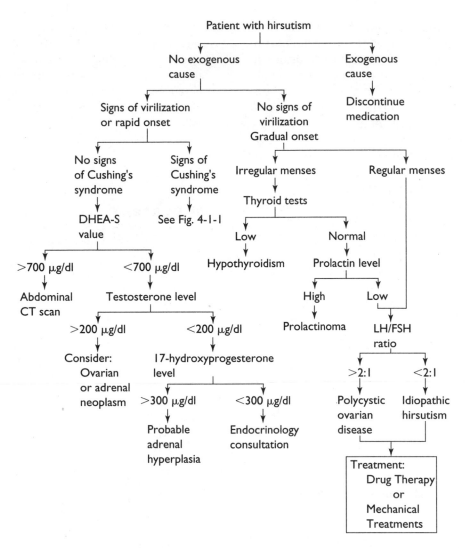

4-7-2 Diagnostic algorithm for hirsutism.
(From Greene HL, Johnson WP, Maricic MJ: *Decision making in medicine,* St Louis, 1993, Mosby.)

litus by the age of 40). As estrogen levels are not decreased by the menstrual irregularities, breast development and the vaginal mucosa are typically normal.

QUESTION 6 What is the correct method of therapy for women with polycystic ovary disease?

Treatment of patients with PCOS will vary because of the heterogeneity in the presentation of the disease. The important aspects to consider are weight reduction, prevention of endometrial hyperplasia in oligomenorrheic or amenorrheic women, and treatment of hirsutism and infertility.

Weight reduction is an important first line of therapy in any obese patient with PCOS. Not only will weight loss often ameliorate hirsutism and menstrual irregularities, but it may help to prevent diabetes. In a woman with PCOS who has menstrual irregularities but does not wish to become pregnant and does not have hirsutism, intermittent progesterone therapy is indicated to prevent endometrial hyperplasia and potentially endometrial tumors. This is best given as medroxyprogesterone acetate (Provera), 5 mg for 10 to 14 days each month. Therapy of hirsutism may be approached in several ways. Use of a low-estrogen oral contraceptive will suppress gonadotropin levels and thus ovarian androgen secretion, and will also normalize menstrual cycles. In addition, anti-androgens such as spironolactone and flutamide may act synergistically. As flutamide does not appear to have any advantages over spironolactone and is much more expensive, the combination of oral contraceptives and spironolactone is often used as the initial therapy for hirsutism in PCOS. Dexamethasone suppression of adrenal androgens is less likely to be successful in ovarian overproduction, although it may be considered as adjunctive therapy in cases where the DHEA-S is elevated. In infertile patients, clomiphene citrate is the drug of choice and is successful in 60% to 85% of cases. Refractory cases are usually managed with various combinations of gonadotropins or gonadotropin releasing hormone. While ovarian wedge resection was used extensively in the past, it has a high association with pelvic adhesions and is not now commonly considered. The same principle is currently being applied with newer techniques, such as laparoscopic cautery or laser vaporization of follicles, and appears to be promising.

CASE FOLLOW-UP   She was placed on oral contraceptives and spironolactone (200 mg/day), and was also strongly encouraged to lose weight. Over the next 12 months she was able to lose 20 lbs and noted gradual improvement of her hirsutism. A diagnostic algorithm for hirsutism is shown in Fig. 4-7-2.

• •

BIBLIOGRAPHY

Barbieri RL: Polycystic ovarian disease, *Annu Rev Med* 42:199, 1991.

Barnes R, Rosenfield RL: The polycystic ovary syndrome: pathogenesis and treatment, *Ann Intern Med* 110:386, 1989.

Dunaif A: Insulin resistance and ovarian hyperandrogenism, *Endocrinologist* 2:248, 1992.

Ehrmann DA, Rosenfield RL, Barnes RB, et al: Detection of function ovarian hyperandrogenism in women with androgen excess, *N Engl J Med* 327:157, 1992.

Gjonnaess H: A simple treatment for polycystic ovarian syndrome, *World Health Forum* 11:214, 1990.

Goldzieher JW, Young RL: Selected aspects of polycystic ovarian disease, *Endocrinol Metab Clin North Am* 21:141, 1992.

Longcope C: Adrenal and gonadal androgen secretion in normal females, *Clin Endocrinol Metab* 15:213, 1986.

Martin C, Santoro N, Hall J, et al: Management of ovulatory disorders with pulsatile gonadotropin-releasing hormone, *J Clin Endocrinol Metab* 71:1081A, 1990.

Nobels F, Dewailly D: Puberty and polycystic ovarian syndrome: the insulin/insulin-like growth factor 1 hypothesis, *Fertil Steril* 58:655, 1992.

Rittmaster RS: Treating hirsutism, *Endocrinologist* 3:211, 1993.

Scully RE, Mark EJ, McNeely WF, McNeely BU: A 56-year-old woman referred because of male-pattern baldness and hirsutism, *N Engl J Med* 328:1770, 1993.

CASE

8

Peter G. Curran
Theodore Mazzone

A 37-year-old woman visited her gynecologist because of infertility. She was G2P2, with her second child born when she was 23 years old. For the last year she had been trying to conceive without success. On further questioning she described irregular menses for the previous 2 years, and 6 months of bilateral galactorrhea. Her gynecologist checked her prolactin level, which was 305 mg/L (normal 2.2 to 19), and referred her to an endocrinologist. Here she gave no history of headaches or obvious visual field defects. She had noted increased emotional lability and a 7-lb weight gain over the last 3 to 4 months. Otherwise there were no symptoms to suggest either increased growth hormone secretion, or increased or decreased thyroid or corticosteroid secretion. She was on no medications.

Physical examination was normal with the exception of milk being easily expressed from both breasts. Visual fields were normal to confrontation.

QUESTION 1 Outline the normal physiology of prolactin production, and how is the diagnosis of hyperprolactinemia confirmed?

The pituitary gland extends inferiorly from the hypothalamus, connected by the pituitary stalk, and normally rests in the sella turcica. It is bounded inferiorly by the sphenoid sinus, laterally by the cavernous sinuses, and superiorly by a diaphragm of dura mater and the optic chiasm. The pituitary may be divided into two distinct regions: posterior (the neurohypophysis) and anterior (the adenohypophysis). The posterior pituitary secretes the hormone vasopressin (antidiuretic hormone). The anterior pituitary secretes prolactin, growth hormone (GH), adrenocorticotrophic hormone (ACTH), luteinizing hormone (LH), follicle stimulating hormone (FSH), and thyroid stimulating hormone (TSH).

Prolactin, otherwise known as somatomammotropin, is produced by the anterior pituitary. The major role of prolactin is to ready breast tissue for lactation. At the time of parturition the decrease of estrogen and progesterone remove inhibition and allow prolactin to effect lactation. In abnormal states of elevated prolactin production, one outcome is hypogonadism with an attendant decreased luteal phase, anovulation, oligomenorrhea, amenorrhea, and infertility. The normal secretory patterns of LH and FSH are also altered. Additionally, patients may develop glucose intolerance. Hypothalamic control on pituitary prolactin production is inhibitory as is circulation dopamine. Alternatively, thyroid releasing hormone provides positive feedback. Prolactin is cleared from the serum 75% via the liver and 25% via the kidney.

Prolactin is normally secreted episodically, with a normal level of 1.9 to 11.7 µg/L in men, and 2.2 to 19.2 µg/L in women (higher in pregnancy and during lactation, lower in the postmenopausal woman). Pituitary prolactin release is inhibited by hypothalamic dopamine secretion, and stimulated by thyrotropin releasing hormone (TRH), and vasoactive intestinal peptide. Hyperprolactinemia may occur from other causes than prolactinomas (box on left, p. 218), and it is important to exclude these in the initial evaluation. Hyperprolactinemia from other causes is usually mild and rarely exceeds 150 to 200 µg/L. With prolactinomas, generally the higher the level of prolactin, the larger the tumor. Because of

CAUSES OF HYPERPROLACTINEMIA

INCREASED ESTROGEN STATES
- Pregnancy
- Estrogen supplementation
- Suckling
- Hypothalamic disease or pituitary stalk compression causing decreased dopamine secretion
- Pituitary prolactinoma

DRUGS
- Neuroleptics
- Antidepressants
- Alpha-methyl dopa
- Reserpine
- Opiates
- Verapamil
- Cimetidine

PRIMARY OR SECONDARY HYPOTHYROIDISM

NEUROGENIC
- Chest wall disease
- Chronic nipple stimulation
- Chronic renal failure
- Cirrhosis
- Stress

EXTRINSIC CAUSES OF PITUITARY DYSFUNCTION

CIRCULATORY
- Hemorrhage
- Infarction
- Necrosis

INFLAMMATORY
- Chronic lymphocytic hypophysitis
- Granulomatous disease
- Histiocytosis-X

NEOPLASTIC

Benign
- Infundibuloma
- Chordoma
- Lipoma
- Meningioma

Malignant
- Metastatic (breast, lung)
- Craniopharyngioma
- Germ cell tumor
- Glioma

the episodic secretion of prolactin, if hyperprolactinemia is suspected but a blood test returns normal, it is best to repeat it. In addition, because of the occasional co-occurrence of growth hormone hypersecretion with prolactin, a somatomedin-C level should be checked.

QUESTION 2   A repeat prolactin level was 285 µg/L. Free thyroxine index, TSH, AM cortisol, and somatomedin C levels were all within the normal range. Normal overnight suppression occurred in response to 1 mg of dexamethasone. Estradiol was 160 ng/L (normal > 400), and a bone density was reduced (73% of mean for age). Goldman visual field studies were normal. What is the differential diagnosis of hyperprolactinemia and what clinical features are significant in the patient's history and physical examination?

Dysfunction of the pituitary gland may arise from intrinsic or extrinsic causes and may result in either overproduction or underproduction of pituitary hormones. Extrinsic causes of pituitary dysfunction (see box above) typically interfere with pituitary or hypothalamic function and result in partial or total hypopituitarism. An exception to this occurs when the pituitary stalk is compressed, interrupting the inhibitory flow of dopamine to the pituitary, which may cause mild hyperprolactinemia (generally blood levels of less than 150 to 200 µg/L).

Prolactin can be elevated in a number of normal physiologic circumstances. These include pregnancy, nursing, nipple stimulation, exercise, stress, and after sleep. When levels are being monitored, it is important to keep the above circumstances in mind. Furthermore, there are many abnormal settings that result in increased prolactin production: pituitary tumors, section of the hypothalamic-pituitary stalk (anatomical or functional), hypothyroidism, chest wall lesions, chronic renal failure, and severe liver disease. Pharmacologic induction of prolactin production includes estrogen, TRH, dopaminergic antagonists, opiates, and H antagonists. A diagnostic algorithm for hyperprolactinemia is shown in Fig. 4-8-1.

QUESTION 3 What is the correct radiologic approach to evaluate a patient with hyperprolactinemia?

Intrinsic lesions of the pituitary include adenomas and rarely carcinomas. These occur almost exclusively in the anterior pituitary, and further discussion here will be limited to the relatively common anterior pituitary adenoma. These lesions make up 10% to 15% of surgical intracranial neoplasms; however, the incidence of clinically unrecognized pituitary adenomas is much higher. Autopsy studies reveal an incidence as high as 27% in unselected adults. The incidence increases with age and is the same in men and women.

Adenomas may be classified in a number of ways: by size, growth pattern, biochemical activity, and staining characteristics. Size and growth pattern are important, as larger lesions may extend out of the sella causing local symptoms including headaches (from stretching of the diaphragm), optic chiasm compression (typically causing a bitemporal hemianopsia), and cranial nerve compression (causing gaze palsies). Excessive growth of the adenoma within the pituitary and sella may also cause partial or total hypopituitarism. A microadenoma is defined as one less than 10 mm in diameter and thus unlikely to cause compression symptoms; larger lesions are termed macroadenomas. The adenoma may be localized to within the pituitary, may fill the entire sella (expansive), or may invade locally (invasive adenoma). As these adenomas are derived from hormone-secreting cells, it is not surprising that there are often symptoms of hypersecretion associated with them. The most common types of pituitary adenomas are prolactin-secreting (25%), null cell or nonsecreting (18%), growth-hormone secreting (15%), and ACTH-secreting (9%, although another 6% are "silent" and do not result in Cushing's disease). In addition, some adenomas may secrete several hormones or only part of a hormone such as the alpha-subunit that is common to TSH, LH, and FSH. Immunohistochemistry is currently used to identify the hormone-secreting cell type on pathology. The previously used system of pathologic staining may still be referred to and classifies cells as acidophilic (growth hormone- and some prolactin-secreting), basophilic (ACTH-, gonadotropin-, and TSH-secreting), and chromophobic (some prolactin-secreting and nonsecreting).

When a prolactinoma is suspected clinically, radiologic confirmation should be obtained. Although both CT and MRI scans of the pituitary appear to be adequate, the current consensus is that MRI is preferred. The MRI gives better visualization of the suprasellar region and of pituitary anatomy, and avoids radiation exposure. CT is less expensive, however, and will give better visualization of bone and calcium deposits. Adenomas that are larger than 6 mm should be detected. Even if optic nerve compression is not suspected, it is recommended to obtain a baseline formal visual field examination. When a large pituitary or suprasellar mass is seen, especially if the prolactin levels are not markedly elevated, it is important to consider other possible diagnoses (box). In addition, it is important to evaluate pituitary function in this situation. In contrast, a very small adenoma may not be seen. Hyperprolactinemia without an obvious cause and without a pituitary adenoma visualized, termed *idiopathic hyperprolactinemia*, is usually presumed to be caused by a tiny microadenoma and treated as such.

An MRI was obtained of the pituitary which revealed a 7-mm anterior pituitary mass, without suprasellar extension. A diagnostic algorithm for a suspected pituitary tumor is shown in Fig. 4-8-2.

QUESTION 4 What is the appropriate treatment for a patient with this disorder?

Therapy for prolactinomas should be initiated when there is reproductive dysfunction, hypogonadism (to avoid osteoporosis), when decreased bone mass is already present, or when macroadenomas are causing mass effects. Simply giving a hyperprolactinemic woman estrogen therapy to maintain bone mass is unsatisfactory as estrogen supplements may increase the size of the tumor. Dopamine agonists such as bromocriptine (Parlodel) and pergolide (Permax) are the mainstay of therapy for both microprolactinomas and macroprolactinomas. Microadenomas typically respond very well to medical therapy, with normalization of prolactin levels in about 90% of cases, resolution of infertility in about 80%, and a decrease in size in 70%. Remission may occur in about 20% of these patients after 1 to 2 years of therapy, and it may be worth a trial of stopping the medication at that point. The dopamine agonists may be difficult to tolerate, with the main side effects being nausea, constipation, and orthostasis. It is best to start therapy with a low nightly dose, with food, and slowly titrate up to tid (bromocriptine) or bid (pergolide) as needed.

Transsphenoidal resection of microadenomas is reserved for those who cannot tolerate the dopaminergic agents. The initial cure rate may reach 80%, but up to 50% of these may recur. Morbidity from transsphenoidal surgery includes possible hypopituitarism, diabetes insipidus, sinusitis, meningitis, and CSF rhinorrhea. Radiation therapy for pituitary neoplasms is usually reserved as a secondary line of therapy as it may cause permanent hypopituitarism. Macroadenomas are frequently complicated by mass effects, the most ominous being optic chiasm compression with visual loss. Although surgery will provide rapid decompression, except for emergencies, dopaminergic agents are also the preferred treatment in macroadenomas. About 67%

of patients will have reduction of prolactin to normal, 48% will have a reduction in tumor size of greater than 50%, and up to 90% will have some decrease in size. The reduction in size is often rapid and may begin to occur within days to weeks, and it frequently continues for up to 6 months. Higher doses of the dopamine agonists are frequently needed in macroadenomas, and they should not be discontinued as the tumor may rapidly increase in size. Surgery is less successful in macroadenomas, with only 10% to 30% of patients returning to a normal prolactin postoperatively. There is also a high recurrence rate, and a 40% occurrence of residual hypopituitarism. Surgery should usually be reserved for cases of rapid visual loss or demonstrated lack of efficacy of dopaminergic agents. Repeat surgery for recurrent disease has a significantly higher risk of complications, and radiation therapy may be useful in these cases to control growth of the tumor.

QUESTION 5 Are there any important issues concerning pregnancy for a woman found to have a pituitary adenoma?

Many women have prolactinomas diagnosed during infertility evaluations, and restoration of fertility is often attempted with the use of dopamine agonists. The question therefore arises of the safety of a pregnancy in a woman with a prolactinoma. The pituitary of a normal woman will increase in size by about 70% during pregnancy, and the concern in the woman with a prolactinoma is that the increased levels of estrogen present in pregnancy will stimulate excessive growth of the tumor. It is estimated that, in a woman with a microadenoma, the risk of developing symptoms during pregnancy is less than 5%; this risk rises to 25% in a woman with a macroadenoma. While bromocriptine is not apparently teratogenic, it is recommended that therapy be discontinued at the first missed menses. Follow-up during pregnancy should be done by physical examination, including visual field examinations. Prolactin levels are not helpful as they will increase because of the pregnancy. If

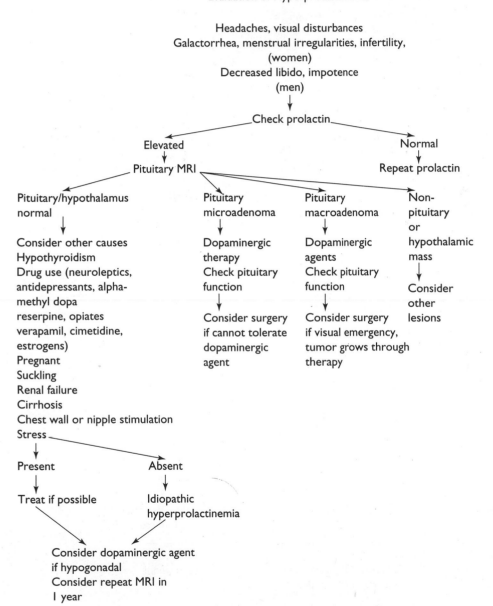

Evaluation of Hyperprolactinemia

Headaches, visual disturbances
Galactorrhea, menstrual irregularities, infertility,
(women)
Decreased libido, impotence
(men)
↓
Check prolactin

Elevated   Normal
↓   ↓
Pituitary MRI   Repeat prolactin

Pituitary/hypothalamus Pituitary Pituitary Non-
normal   microadenoma macroadenoma pituitary
                 or
↓   ↓   ↓   hypothalamic
Consider other causes Dopaminergic Dopaminergic mass
Hypothyroidism   therapy   agents
Drug use (neuroleptics, Check pituitary Check pituitary ↓
antidepressants, alpha- function   function Consider
methyl dopa   other
reserpine, opiates   ↓   ↓   lesions
verapamil, cimetidine, Consider surgery Consider surgery
estrogens)   if cannot tolerate if visual emergency,
Pregnant   dopaminergic tumor grows through
Suckling   agent   therapy
Renal failure
Cirrhosis
Chest wall or nipple stimulation
Stress

Present   Absent
↓   ↓
Treat if possible   Idiopathic
         hyperprolactinemia

Consider dopaminergic agent
if hypogonadal
Consider repeat MRI in
1 year

4-8-1 Diagnostic algorithm for hyperprolactinemia.

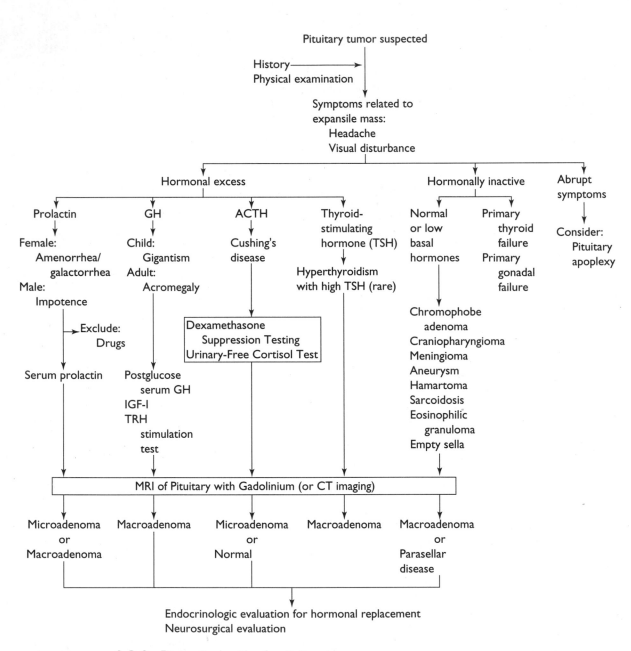

4-8-2   Diagnostic algorithm for pituitary tumors.
(From Greene HL, Johnson WP, Maricic MJ: *Decision making in medicine*, St Louis, 1993, Mosby.)

symptoms suggesting mass effect of the tumor are present, an MRI may be obtained, with treatment options being surgery or bromocriptine.

CASE SUMMARY She was placed on bromocriptine (Parlodel) therapy, and her dose was gradually titrated up to 2.5 mg tid, following which her prolactin level normalized, her menses became regular, and her galactorrhea resolved. She still wished to have another child, and the bromocriptine was discontinued with her first missed menstrual period. Beta-hCG levels were elevated, and she had an uneventful pregnancy without headaches or clinical evidence of optic nerve compression. Following delivery, a repeat MRI scan revealed an enlarged pituitary with a 9-mm adenoma; she was restarted on bromocriptine and continues to do well without further growth of the adenoma.

Clinical: Hyperprolactinemia associated with prolactin-secreting tumors classically presents in women with galactorrhea, amenorrhea, and infertility. Men may present with impotence, decreased libido, gynecomastia, and galactorrhea. There may also be associated weight gain and possibly increased emotional lability. Local extension of large prolactinomas may lead to headaches, visual loss, and cranial nerve palsies. Osteoporosis secondary to prolonged hypogonadism also occurs with hyperprolactinemia. Although clinically apparent, prolactinomas appear to be more common in women,

presumably because the manifestations are more apparent; in unselected autopsy series the incidence is equal in both sexes.

• •

BIBLIOGRAPHY

Klibanski A, Zervas NT: Diagnosis and management of hormone-secreting pituitary adenomas, *N Engl J Med* 324: 822, 1991.

Lamberts SWJ, Quik RFP: A comparison of the efficacy and safety of pergolide and bromocriptine in the treatment of hyperprolactinemia, *J Clin Endocrinol Metab* 72:635, 1991.

Melen O: Neuro-ophthalmologic features of pituitary tumors, *Endocrinol Metab Clin North Am* 16:585, 1987.

Melmed S: Pituitary tumors secreting growth hormone and prolactin, *Ann Intern Med* 105:238, 1986.

Molitch ME: Pregnancy and the hyperprolactinemic woman, *N Engl J Med* 312:1364, 1985.

Molitch ME, Elton RL, Blackwell RE, et al: Bromocriptine as primary therapy for prolactin-secreting macroadenomas: results of a prospective multicenter study, *J Clin Endocrinol Metab* 60:698, 1985.

Schwartzberg DG: Imaging of pituitary tumors, *Semin Ultrasound CT MRI* 13:207, 1992.

Serri O, Rasio E, Beauregard H, et al: Recurrence of hyperprolactinemia after selective transsphenoidal adenomectomy in women with prolactinemia, *N Engl J Med* 309:280, 1983.

Tran LM, Blount L, Horton D, et al: Radiation therapy of pituitary tumors: results in 95 cases, *Am J Clin Oncol* 14:25, 1991.

Vance ML, Thorner MO: Prolactin; hyperprolactinemic syndromes and management. In DeGroot LJ, ed: *Endocrinology*, Philadelphia, 1989, WB Saunders.

C A S E

9

Peter G. Curran
Theodore Mazzone

*T*he patient is a 24-year-old woman who presents to a general internist complaining of tiredness and weakness. For the past 2 months she has noticed increasing tiredness, malaise, and irritability. In addition, for about 2 weeks, she has been short of breath and felt weak in her legs when climbing the stairs to her apartment. Further questioning reveals a recent 18-lb weight loss, increased frequency of bowel movements, and irregular periods. The patient also wishes to discuss recent irritation and redness of her eyes, associated with persistent periorbital swelling.

She is on no medications and has no significant medical history.

Family history significant for two aunts with "thyroid problems."

Physical examination shows she is a thin, white woman, dressed inappropriately lightly for the cold day. She is anxious to please, jumping up to greet the interviewer, and discussing her problems without prompting.

BP 142/64 mm Hg, P 112 bpm. Skin is warm, fine, and diaphoretic. Eyes exhibit chemosis, conjunctivitis, a stare, and periorbital swelling, without exophthalmos, diplopia, or gaze palsy. Thyroid gland is 3 times normal size (45 g), without nodules. Extremities reveal well-demarcated plaques above the inferior tibia. She has a resting tremor, and deep tendon reflexes are brisk.

QUESTION I Because of the findings on the patient's neck examination, she was sent to see an endocrinologist. What are the important signs and symptoms in this presentation that support suspicion that the patient's symptoms are due to thyroid dysfunction?

Thyrotoxicosis is a state of excess free thyroid hormone, resulting in a recognizable syndrome of clinical and metabolic abnormalities. The spectrum of thyrotoxicosis is wide, ranging from thyroid storm, with the potential for multiple organ system failure, to states where mildly elevated levels of thyroid hormone cause no apparent clinical abnormalities.

The clinical diagnosis of thyrotoxicosis is rarely based on a specific finding but rather on a typical combination of many. As well as there being a wide spectrum of clinical severity, manifestations of thyrotoxicosis also vary with age, with the older patient typically having more subtle disease. When underlying cardiac disease is present, thyrotoxicosis often presents with cardiac symptoms.

The finding of an abnormally enlarged thyroid gland encourages the physician to explain the patient's problems based on abnormal function of the thyroid gland. Many of the patient's initial symptoms are reminiscent of hyperfunction of the thyroid gland. Specifically, she complains of being tired and weak, muscle weakness, weight loss, increased frequency of bowel movements, and irregular menses. In addition, she has noticed persistent swelling around her eyes.

In this case, the historical findings further heighten suspicion of a thyroid abnormality. When you first see this patient, it is apparent that she is dressed inappropriately lightly for the weather and you note that she is tachycardic. You are struck with her anxiety and impressed by her psychomotor agitation. Her skin is fine and moist.

SIGNS AND SYMPTOMS OF THYROTOXICOSIS

SIGNS
- Tachycardia or arrthymias
- Hyperactivity
- Tremor
- Weakness
- Brisk reflexes
- Warm, moist skin
- Stare

SYMPTOMS
- Anxiety or nervousness
- Weight loss
- Muscular weakness
- Menstrual irregularities
- Hyperdefecation
- Increased diaphoresis
- Palpitations
- Heat intolerance

The eye examination reveals conjunctivitis, and she appears to stare. She has plaque-like skin lesions on the anterior aspect of the lower extremity, and she has a tremor. Reflexes are brisk. A summary of the signs and symptoms is found in the box above.

QUESTION 2 Because of the preceding history and physical examination there was a high likelihood of hyperthyroidism. The following laboratory tests were received the next day: T4 16.4 µg/dl (normal 4.5 to 10.7), FTI 18.5 (5 to 10.6), T3 288 ng/dl (85 to 175), TSH 0.0 µg/ml (0.38 to 6.15). What is the correct interpretation of these lab tests?

Laboratory diagnosis is based on an elevated free thyroxine (FT4) or triiodothyronine (FT3), with a suppressed thyroid stimulating hormone (TSP). This illustrates a classic example of negative feedback: the end-product inhibiting the stimulatory hormone. Both the FT4 and FT3 should be checked, as T3 is often preferentially released by a damaged thyroid gland. In addition, cholesterol levels are frequently reduced, with an increased calcium (secondary to increased bone resorption) and elevated transaminases.

QUESTION 3 The laboratory evaluation assures a diagnosis of hyperthyroidism. In addition to the standard labs above, the antimicrosomal and anti-thyroglobulin antibodies are both strongly positive. What is the appropriate differential diagnosis?

There is a wide differential diagnosis for thyrotoxicosis (Fig. 4-9-1). This is important to consider, as diagnosis will affect treatment. Hyperthyroidism, or hyperfunctional thyroid gland that has escaped from pituitary-hypothalamic control, occurs with autoimmune thyroiditis, multinodular goiter, and toxic adenomas. In contrast, a damaged thyroid gland (silent thyroiditis, subacute thyroiditis, radiation thyroiditis, and lymphocytic thyroiditis) may release excess hormone through follicular cell damage. These disorders will have a reduced radioiodine uptake. Exposure to high levels of iodine or iodine-containing compounds (contrast dyes, amiodarone) may cause thyrotoxicosis, especially in an iodine-deficient state. Thyroid hormone may rarely be produced ectopically in struma ovarii or metastatic thyroid carcinoma. Finally, exogenous hormone use needs to be considered, either surreptitiously or iatrogenically.

There are also several rare conditions where the thyroid is supra-stimulated via an endocrine means resulting in thyrotoxicosis. These include TSP-producing pituitary adenomas and pituitary thyroid hormone resistance, in which cases the TSP is not suppressed, as well as stimulation by Beta-hCG secreted by trophoblastic tumors, which is a relatively weaker thyroid stimulator.

Multinodular goiter (Plummer's disease) results in thyrotoxicosis through autonomous follicular secretion. This occurs predominantly in older patients with large goiters and may be precipitated by an iodine load. As suggested by the name, the thyroid is enlarged with multiple nodules. A thyroid scan may reveal either increased, diffuse uptake or several hot nodules; however, these areas of increased uptake often do not correlate with palpable nodules.

Toxic adenoma (uninodular goiter). A hyperfunctional nodule may occasionally result in thyrotoxicosis. Thyroid scan will reveal a hot nodule, while the remainder of the gland is suppressed.

Silent thyroiditis usually presents as a mild thyrotoxicosis associated with a small, nontender goiter, low-level or no antithyroid antibodies, and with no uptake of radioactive iodine. The condition frequently occurs in the postpartum period and carries a strong predisposition to later hypothyroidism.

Subacute thyroiditis (de Quervain's) results in follicular damage and excess thyroid hormone release, probably secondary to a viral infection of the thyroid. It generally follows a 2- to 4-month course, and there is often a hypothyroid phase during recovery. Diagnosis is based on tenderness of the anterior neck, lack of radioactive iodine uptake by the thyroid, and an elevated ESR.

Although there are the above possible etiologies, by far the most common is *autoimmune hyperthyroidism,* illustrated in the case just discussed. Autoimmune hyperthyroidism (Graves' disease, Basedow's disease) accounts for anywhere from 60% to 90% of all cases of thyrotoxicosis. A defect in autoimmune regulation allows the production of TSP-receptor stimulating antibodies, which stimulate the thyroid gland, removing it from pituitary control. The patient frequently has a strong family history of thyroid disease, and the disease may be associated with other autoimmune conditions such as diabetes, adrenal failure, and pernicious anemia. Autoimmune hyperthyroidism occurs up to 10 times more frequently in women, and typically presents in the 20- to 50-year-old age group. The course of the disease is variable and often unpredictable.

A unique aspect of autoimmune thyroiditis is the frequent involvement of the eyes (in about 50% of cases). The affected patients exhibit varying amounts of swelling of retroorbital tissue and the extraocular muscles that may be due to antibodies against retroorbital constituents and extraocular muscles. This can cause impaired orbital venous drainage and extraocular muscle dysfunction. Clinically, this results in proptosis, chemosis, conjunctivitis, excess lacrimation, gaze palsies, and diplopia (especially on upward gaze). Therapy of this condition is complex, involving both local and systemic treatments. Localized myxedema may also occur in the skin of the lower leg (pretibial myxedema). The thyroid gland itself is typically hypertrophied, usually exhibiting diffuse enlargement.

Diagnosis of autoimmune hyperthyroidism is based on a combination of examination, including presence of eye disease or pretibial myxedema, family history, diffuse and increased uptake of radioactive iodine, and the presence of antithyroid antibodies. Beyond the standard thyroid function tests, assays for antimicrosomal and antithyroglobulin antibodies may both be found. However, these tests lack diagnostic sensitivity and specificity. Commercial assays specific for thyroid-stimulating antibodies are now becoming more readily available.

QUESTION 4 The young woman was judged to have autoimmune thyroiditis. What are the options available for treatment of this patient?

Decisions about therapy are based on the underlying cause of the thyrotoxicosis. The conditions that are self-limited, silent, and subacute thyroiditis are best treated symptomatically. Beta-blockade will reduce the severity of the adrenergic symptoms. In subacute thyroiditis, glucocorticoids may reduce the duration of the thyrotoxicosis. In contrast, to prevent the prolonged thyrotoxicosis associated with a hyperfunctional gland, patients with autoimmune thyroiditis, multinodular goiter, or toxic adenoma are best treated more definitively. This may be done by using drugs to reduce thyroid hormone production or release, thyroid gland surgery, through damaging the thyroid gland using radioactive iodine, or a combination of the above.

The most effective drugs available are the thionamides (propylthiouracil, methimazole),

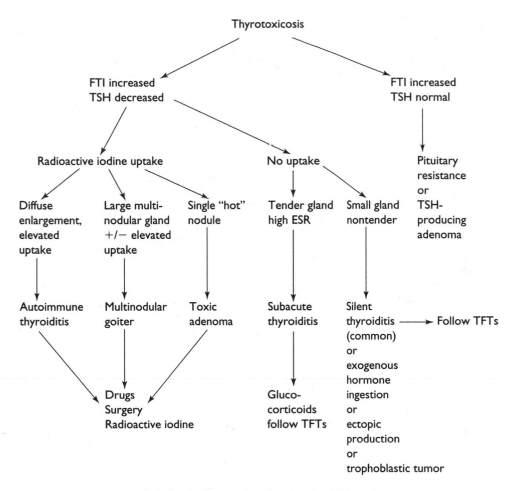

4-9-1 Diagnostic algorithm for thyrotoxicosis.

which act primarily by inhibiting thyroid hormone production. Major drawbacks to their use are a lack of permanent effect on the thyroid and the potential for severe side effects including agranulocytosis, hepatitis, rash, and arthritis. These agents are usually used in conjunction with surgery or radioactive iodine, although there are some cases where they may be used alone. These include mild thyrotoxicosis in an older and infirm patient, or a patient with autoimmune thyroid disease in whom remission is more likely to occur (small goiter, mild thyrotoxicosis). Other potential pharmaceutical agents include lithium, iopanoic acid, and iodine. The latter is particularly

effective in acutely lowering thyroid hormone release; however, as its effects are often short-lived, iodine is best used for short-term goals such as preparing a patient for surgery or in thyroid storm.

Surgery is an extremely effective means of quickly alleviating excess thyroid hormone production. Drawbacks include the expense, potential complications such as parathyroid gland or recurrent laryngeal nerve damage, and scarring. Because of the potential drawbacks and the availability of an attractive alternative in radioactive iodine, surgery is usually reserved for cases where there is a concern about malignancy in the thy-

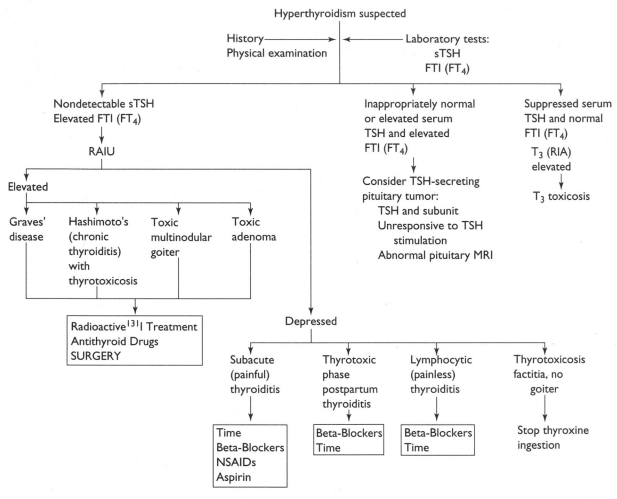

4-9-2 Diagnostic algorithm for hyperthyroidism.
(From Greene HL, Johnson WP, Maricic MJ: *Decision making in medicine*, St Louis, 1993, Mosby.)

roid, for glands that are excessively large resulting in cosmetic or obstructive concerns, and for those patients in whom medical compliance is judged poor.

The most commonly used therapy is [131]I. Uptake of this isotope by the thyroid gland will result in a radiation thyroiditis, with slowly progressive loss of function. This treatment is relatively inexpensive and is usually well tolerated. The major drawbacks are that most patients with autoimmune thyroiditis treated with radioactive iodine will eventually become hypothyroid, and that the effects are slow, thus requiring treatment with antithyroid drugs for at least several months following the radioactive iodine dose. There is no evidence that the radiation exposure causes any increase in cancer or infertility, although teratogenicity is a concern, and pregnant women should not be treated with radiation. There is much variability among physicians as to what dose of isotope should be used. Higher doses cause more hypothyroidism, while lower doses may require a second treatment and thus a more prolonged course of therapy.

CASE DISCUSSION   After a negative pregnancy test, radioactive iodine uptake was measured at 70%, and the patient was given a dose of [131]I. She was also placed on methimazole and propranolol. Within 4 weeks she was clinically much improved, and the propranolol was discontinued. Over the next 6 months the methimazole was gradually stopped. At this point she was judged euthyroid off all medications; however, because of the unpredictable course of the disease, she will need periodic thyroid function test follow-up. A diagnostic algorithm for hyperthyroidism is shown in Fig. 4-9-2.

• •

BIBLIOGRAPHY

Benker G, Esser J, Kahaly G, Reinwein D: New therapeutic approaches in thyroidal autoimmune diseases, *Klin Wochenschr* 68(Suppl XXI):44-54, 1990.

Carter JA, Utiger RD: The ophthalmopathy of Graves' disease, *Ann Rev Med* 43:487-95, 1992.

Cooper DS: Treatment of thyrotoxicosis. In Braverman LE, Utiger RD, eds: *The thyroid*, Philadelphia, 1991, JB Lippincott Co.

DeGroot LJ, Quintans J: The causes of autoimmune thyroid disease, *Endocrine Rev* 10:537-562, 1989.

Ferrar JJ, Toft AD: Iodine-131 treatment of hyperthyroidism: current issues, *Clin Endocrinol* 35:207-212, 1991.

Kuma K, Matsuzuka F, Kobayashi A, et al: Natural course of Graves' disease after subtotal thyroidectomy and management of patients with postoperative thyroid dysfunction, *Am J Med Sci* 302:8-12, 1991.

Nordyke RA, Gilbert FI Jr: Optimal iodine-131 dose for eliminating hyperthyroidism in Graves' disease, *J Nucl Med* 32:411-416, 1991.

Reiners C: Radioiodine treatment of Basedow's disease: interference and influence factors, risk estimation, *Exp Clin Endocrinol* 97:275-285, 1991.

Schicha H: Differential diagnosis of hyperthyroidism, *Exp Clin Endocrinol* 97:217-223, 1991.

Studer H, Gerber H, Peter HJ: Multinodular goiter. In DeGroot LJ, ed: *Endocrinology*, Philadelphia, 1989, WB Saunders.

Wolf PW: Thyroiditis, *Med Clin North Am* 69:1035-1048, 1985.

CASE

10

Peter G. Curran
Theodore Mazzone

The patient is a 37-year-old woman with systemic lupus erythematosus who is brought to the emergency room by her family because of recent weakness, nausea, and mental status changes. Approximately 3 months ago she was noted to have new proteinuria, with an active urinary sediment. Renal biopsy revealed diffuse proliferative glomerulonephritis, and she was treated with high-dose, IV, pulse methylprednisolone, and then placed on prednisone (60 mg/ day). When last seen by her internist, she complained bitterly about the side effects of the glucocorticoids: acne, increased facial hair, facial puffiness, and weight gain. She was told she needed to continue on the same dose of the prednisone to protect her kidneys.

In the emergency room, the patient's family notes that for the past week she has been increasingly tired, remaining in bed, and this morning she appeared confused. For the past several days she also experienced fevers, frequent coughing, bouts of nausea, and occasional vomiting. Upon initial examination, she is currently disoriented; BP 84/50 mm Hg, P 104 bpm, T 37.8° C, respiration 24/min. Skin is cool, with acne on the face and back. Her face is full, with increased facial hair growth. There is a buffalo hump; chest examination reveals decreased breath sounds in the left upper lobe, abdomen is diffusely tender. Stool is guaiac negative. Neurologic examination is nonfocal. Lab values include Na 135 mmol/L, BUN 31 mg/dl, creatinine 2.1 mg/dl, glucose 64 mg/dl, WBC 12.5 × 10⁹/L with a relative bandemia and eosinophilia.

QUESTION I What is your presumptive diagnosis based on the present history, physical examination and lab results?

The adrenal cortex secretes a variety of steroid hormones. They include the glucocorticoids, mineralocorticoids, and sex hormones. The sex hormones are mainly androgenic, and loss of their production is not critical. In contrast, loss of adrenal ability to secrete mineralocorticoids or glucocorticoids may be life-threatening. Mineralocorticoids regulate sodium and potassium balance, primarily by increasing active sodium resorption in the kidney, and thus protect against hypovolemia and hyperkalemia. Secretion of mineralocorticoids is primarily regulated through the renin-angiotensin system and the potassium concentration, and it is thus independent of pituitary control.

Glucocorticoids have multiple complex effects throughout the body via receptor-mediated regulation of gene expression. Major effects include increasing availability of glucose and immune-modulation. They also function to increase cardiac muscle contractility. Glucocorticoids are critical in the body's response to stress. Their secretion is regulated by negative feedback via the hypothalamic-pituitary-adrenal (HPA) axis. In this system, hypothalamic secretion of corticotropin-releasing hormone (CRH) stimulates the anterior pituitary gland to secrete adrenocorticotrophic hormone (ACTH), which in turn stimulates adrenal secretion of glucocorticoids. When circulation levels of glucocorticoids are high, CRH and thus ACTH release are inhibited.

Adrenal insufficiency may occur through failure of the adrenal gland itself (primary adrenal insufficiency, Addison's disease) or through failure of the hypothalamus or pituitary to stimulate the adrenal (secondary adrenal insufficiency).

Primary adrenal failure generally results in hyposecretion of all adrenal cortical hormones.

The most common etiologies of gland failure are destruction by autoimmune disease, tuberculous, or fungal infection, hemorrhage (often associated with meningococcal or Pseudomonal sepsis), metastatic neoplasia, and infiltrative processes such as amyloid or sarcoid. Several drugs can also interfere with corticosteroid synthesis (for instance, aminoglutethamide, mitotane, ketoconazolc). In the United States, 70% to 80% of primary adrenal disease results from autoimmune causes, and this condition is often associated with other autoimmune endocrinopathies (polyglandular autoimmune syndromes). If the HPA axis is intact, ACTH levels will be high in primary adrenal insufficiency.

Secondary adrenal failure may occur if hypothalamic or pituitary function are compromised. This can occur with mass lesions, vascular or infiltrative disease. Some of the most frequent causes of this condition are pituitary adenomas, brain tumors, pituitary apoplexy, and autoimmune hypophysitis. The most common form of secondary adrenal insufficiency, however, occurs when the HPA axis is suppressed iatrogenically by exogenous glucocorticoid use. Secondary adrenal insufficiency will primarily result in hyposecretion of glucocorticoids. As mineralocorticoid secretion is regulated through nonpituitary stimulation, it is usually unaffected. Because pituitary function is compromised in secondary adrenal insufficiency, ACTH levels will be low.

QUESTION 2 The patient is admitted to the critical care unit, where she is cultured (including a lumbar puncture) and placed on broad-spectrum antibiotics. Chest x-ray reveals a lobar infiltrate. A cortisol level is drawn, and she is placed on "stress" steroids (150 mg hydrocortisone IV q8h). Within 24 hours her condition has improved markedly, and she is transferred to the floor. What are the signs and symptoms that herald adrenal insufficiency?

Manifestations of glucocorticoid deficiency include weakness, malaise, weight loss, nausea, vomiting, diarrhea, abdominal pain, and emotional or mental status changes. On examination, the patient may be hypotensive and febrile. Typi-

cal lab abnormalities may include hypoglycemia, hyponatremia (secondary to decreased free water excretion), hypercalcemia, neutropenia, and eosinophilia. If mineralocorticoid deficiency is also present, hypotension is generally more severe, serum sodium will be more markedly decreased, and there will be an elevated potassium with an associated metabolic acidosis.

In primary adrenal disease, hyperpigmentation of the skin may occur from ACTH or beta-lipotropin stimulation of melanocytes (especially in sun-exposed areas, mucous membranes, and scars). In secondary adrenal insufficiency with hypopituitarism, the patient will often show signs of suggestive hypogonadism or hypothyroidism. Patients with hypothalamic-pituitary suppression from exogenous glucocorticoid use may show signs suggestive of glucocorticoid excess (full faces, buffalo hump, hirsutism, abdominal striae, centripetal obesity, muscle atrophy).

Adrenal insufficiency may present with slowly progressive development of the above symptoms, or a patient may present in acute adrenal crisis. This latter, potentially lethal condition is usually precipitated by an acute stress (surgery, trauma, infection) on top of adrenal insufficiency and is primarily manifested by hypotensive shock.

Adrenal insufficiency is an important differential in patients with weakness, fever, hypotension, and diffuse abdominal pain. It is especially important to consider in those who may have been on exogenous glucocorticoids and patients with other autoimmune endocrinopathies or neoplasia. The presence of a coagulopathy (including heparin administration) or thromboembolic disease increases the risk of adrenal failure from bilateral adrenal hemorrhage.

QUESTION 3 The cortisol level returns at 2.1 μg/dl. The patient admits to having rapidly reduced her prednisone doses over the last several weeks because of concern over the side effects. What are the means of assessing adrenal function?

Although there are several means of evaluating adrenal function, the best is the rapid ACTH stimulation test. Because of variability in secre-

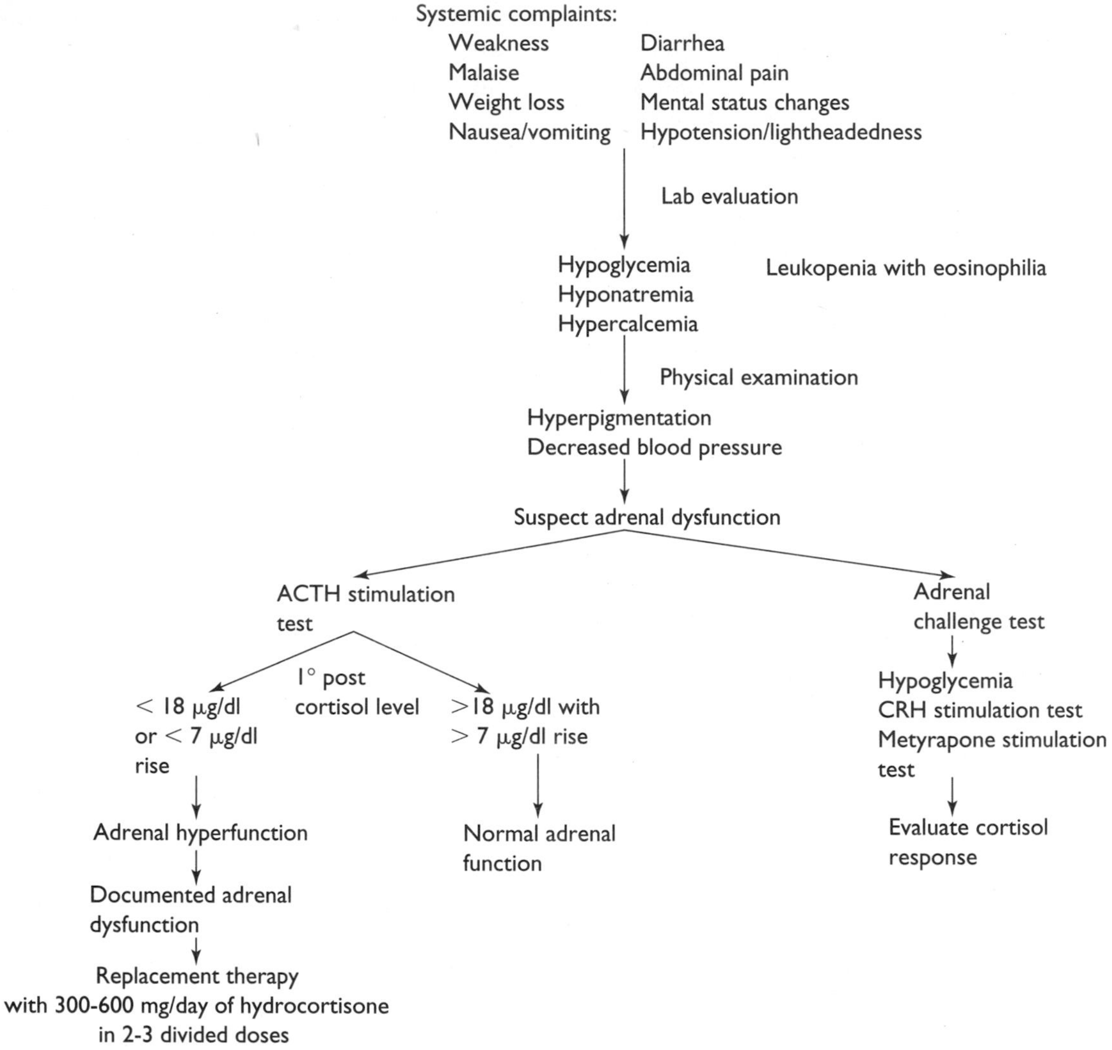

Systemic complaints:
>   Weakness   Diarrhea
>   Malaise   Abdominal pain
>   Weight loss   Mental status changes
>   Nausea/vomiting Hypotension/lightheadedness

Lab evaluation

Hypoglycemia   Leukopenia with eosinophilia
Hyponatremia
Hypercalcemia

Physical examination

Hyperpigmentation
Decreased blood pressure

Suspect adrenal dysfunction

ACTH stimulation   Adrenal
test   challenge test

1° post
cortisol level

< 18 μg/dl   > 18 μg/dl with   Hypoglycemia
or < 7 μg/dl   > 7 μg/dl rise   CRH stimulation test
rise   Metyrapone stimulation
                                         test

Adrenal hyperfunction   Normal adrenal   Evaluate cortisol
                        function   response

Documented adrenal
dysfunction

Replacement therapy
with 300-600 mg/day of hydrocortisone
in 2-3 divided doses

4-10-1   Diagnostic algorithm for adrenal insufficiency.

tion patterns, a random cortisol level is rarely helpful. A baseline and 30- or 60-minute serum cortisol sample are drawn around parenteral injection of 250 µg of synthetic ACTH (Cosyntropin). Adequate adrenal function is indicated by a 30- or 60-minute value of greater than 18 µg/dl, with an increase from baseline of greater than 7 µg/dl. Acutely ill patients with high baseline values may not show such an incremental increase. If pituitary disease is suspected, a baseline ACTH value may be helpful. Further evaluation of the HPA axis may be done using insulin-induced hypoglycemia, metyrapone, or CRH infusion. Pituitary or adrenal imaging may also be helpful. Dexamethasone will not cross-react in a cortisol assay, and so may be used before a diagnostic rapid ACTH test is performed.

QUESTION 4 After the patient awakes, she admits to having rapidly reduced her prednisone doses over the last several weeks because of concerns about side effects. What is the acute treatment for this patient?

Treatment of adrenal insufficiency is with glucocorticoid replacement and with fluid support and glucose replacement if necessary. Therapy should be initiated when clinical suspicion exists while awaiting test results. There is some debate about what dose of glucocorticoids should be used in adrenal crisis, but it appears that maximal possible adrenal output is equivalent to 150 to 300 mg of hydrocortisone per day (normal, unstressed output is approximately 30 mg/day). Based on this, most recommendations are to use in stress situations 300 to 600 mg/day in 2 to 3 divided doses (dexamethasone 12 to 24 mg/day) as adrenal replacement.

The patient described is a good example of how long-term glucocorticoid therapy may suppress intrinsic adrenal function and predispose to adrenal crisis. Suppression of the HPA axis begins within 5 days of initiating high-dose glucocorticoid therapy. Low-dose therapy (less than 4 mg/

day of prednisone or 16 mg hydrocortisone) does not appear to affect HPA integrity, although greater than 12.5 mg/day of prednisone will. After prolonged, high-dose glucocorticoid therapy, it may take greater than 12 months for the entire HPA axis to recover. Although a suppressed HPA axis may be able to function adequately under stress situations (breakthrough), it is best to treat even those off glucocorticoids for up to a year as potentially having adrenal insufficiency. In patients being treated with high-dose glucocorticoids it is also important to consider other possible side effects of these steroids. These include peptic ulceration, hyperglycemia, and the immunesuppression which makes it important to search aggressively for infection. A diagnostic algorithm for adrenal insufficiency is shown in Fig. 4-10-1.

BIBLIOGRAPHY

Chin R: Adrenal Crisis, *Crit Care Clin* 7:23-42, 1991.
Christy NP: Principles of systemic corticosteroid therapy in nonendocrine disease. In Bardin CW, ed: *Current therapy in endocrinology and metabolism*, Philadelphia, 1991, BC Decker.
Dixon RB, Christy NP: On the various forms of corticosteroid withdrawal syndrome, *Am J Med* 68:224-230, 1980.
Graber AL, Ney RL, Nicholson WE, et al: Natural history of pituitary-adrenal recovery following long-term suppression with corticosteroids, *J Clin Endocrinol* 25:11-16, 1965.
Hamaty D: Abrupt withdrawal of adrenal corticosteroids in patients with rheumatoid arthritis, *Southern Med J* 60:457-462, 1967.
Hartzband PI, Van Herle AJ, Sorger L, Cope D: Assessment of hypothalamic-pituitary-adrenal (HPA) axis dysfunction: comparison of ACTH stimulation, insulin-hypoglycemia and metyrapone, *J Endocrinol Invest* 11:769-776, 1988.
Helfer EL, Rose LI: Corticosteroids and adrenal suppression, *Drugs* 38:838-845, 1989.
Meikle AW: Secretion and metabolism of the corticosteroids and adrenal function and testing. In DeGroot LJ, ed: *Endocrinology*, Philadelphia, 1989, WB Saunders.
Muir A, Maclaren N: Adrenocortical insufficiency. In Bardin CW, ed: *Current therapy in endocrinology and metabolism*, Philadelphia, 1991, BC Decker.
Munck A, Guyre PM, Holbrook NJ: Physiological functions of glucocorticoids in stress and their relation to pharmacological actions, *Endocrine Rev* 5:25-44, 1984.

GASTROENTEROLOGY/ HEPATOLOGY

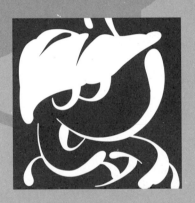

DONALD JENSEN (CASES 1 TO 4)

MICHAEL BROWN (CASES 5 TO 10)

SECTION EDITORS

CASE

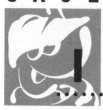

I

Panos Sechopoulos
Donald Jensen
. . . .

A 52-year-old woman is admitted to the hospital with complaints of fatigue and generalized itching. These symptoms have been present for several years with only occasional relief. On one occasion she sought the advice of a doctor who prescribed Benadryl for the itching, but this only had a temporary effect. She denied any history of jaundice, excessive alcohol consumption, blood transfusions, IV drug abuse, sexual promiscuity, weight loss, fever, cough, or recent travel. The patient believes she has arthritis but has never sought medical care for this problem as it has always been mild. Her initial physical examination was significant only for a liver span of 14 cm.

QUESTION I Because of the duration of her symptoms and her enlarged liver on physical examination, you are concerned about a presumptive diagnosis involving liver disease. What are the important historical features and physical findings associated with liver disease?

The liver is a central organ for many processes of metabolism and nutrition. There are many signs and symptoms that may suggest liver disease. For many individuals, chronic disease can lead to constitutional symptoms including fatigue, anorexia and weight loss, and fever, particularly those associated with chronic inflammatory or neoplastic processes. History may also be helpful in yielding clues to the etiology of liver disease. Excessive ingestion of alcohol can lead to steatosis, alcoholic hepatitis, or cirrhosis. Viral hepatitis may be suggested by a history of sexual promiscuity, blood transfusion, intravenous drug use, or close contact with infected individuals. Medications, recreational drugs, some herbs, and

industrial solvent exposures can cause liver injury and occasionally even fulminant hepatic failure. A family history of liver disease is important and may suggest Wilson's disease, hemochromatosis, or alpha-1-antitrypsin deficiency. Patients on chronic hemodialysis or hyperalimentation may develop liver dysfunction.

It is important to assess the duration and chronicity of elevated liver tests. One should try to find temporal relationships between the abnormal tests and the use of medications, travel, or toxin exposure. Liver disease may be suggested by a darkening of the urine or change of the stool to clay color. Pruritus in the absence of jaundice is not an uncommon presentation of chronic cholestatic disorders.

Physical examination can elucidate sequelae of liver disease. The skin examination may show jaundice, palmar erythema, spider telangiectasias, ecchymoses, and xanthelasma. Xanthomas may be observed in some cases of chronic cholestasis. Cirrhosis or excessive alcohol ingestion may lead to a loss of hair, gynecomastia, and testicular atrophy. Portal hypertension with the formation of gastroesophageal varices can lead to gastrointestinal bleeding. Elevated portal pressure may also produce ascites and splenomegaly. Excoriations may be a manifestation of pruritus. Patients can also develop anemia and leukopenia secondary to hypersplenism. Hepatic encephalopathy can lead to fetor hepaticus, asterixis, and changes of mental status.

QUESTION 2 The patient's admission labs were available soon after arrival. They revealed an elevated alkaline phosphatase and gamma glutamyl transferase (GGT) with normal SGOT, SGPT, and total bilirubin. How does one interpret this patient's liver enzyme tests and what is the significance of these findings?

The evaluation of liver function tests can be divided into several categories: synthetic function, clearance function, and cellular integrity. The liver is the chief organ for the production of clotting factors, cholesterol and protein, and for the production, and to a lesser extent, storage of glucose. In chronic disease these functions may become impaired. The patient may manifest a prolonged prothrombin time, vitamin K deficiency, and clotting-factor deficiency. The liver is also involved with the metabolism of ammonia and bile acids. In end-stage liver disease elevated levels of ammonia and other biogenic amines lead to hepatic encephalopathy. Additionally, poor hepatic function may lead to an elevated level of bilirubin.

Processes that lead to damage of the liver cell are characterized by an elevation of the serum aminotransferases (SGOT, SGPT) and lactate dehydrogenase (LDH). These enzymes, because of their intracellular location, are released into the bloodstream in cases of cellular necrosis.

Processes that lead to retention of bile or cholestasis are reflected by elevation of the alkaline phosphatase and bilirubin. Processes that impair bile drainage into the small intestine may lead to malabsorption of fat and the fat soluble vitamins (A, D, E, K). Hypovitaminosis K can cause a coagulopathy associated with clotting-factor deficiency; hypovitaminosis A can lead to night blindness; hypovitaminosis D can lead to metabolic bone disease. As circulating conjugate bilirubin increases as a result of the impairment in biliary excretion, this water soluble component may cause the urine color to darken. Conversely, absence of bile pigments in the stool may turn the stool clay colored.

The patient described above presents with signs and symptoms of liver disease and an elevated alkaline phosphatase (AP). This enzyme is also found in bone, intestine, placenta, and in some tumors (lung, ovary, colon, breast). Medications including phenytoin and dilantin are well known to increase AP levels. Elevations of the AP often accompany biliary obstruction and other cholestatic processes. In fact, a predominant rise in hepatic AP has become synonymous with cholestasis. Heat fractionation can separate the labile, bone type AP, from the stable, liver, and placenta types. Additionally, serum leucine aminopeptidase and 5'-nucleotidase are also increased in cholestatic processes and are more liver specific. Assay of gamma glutamyl transferase (GGT) is less specific and may be elevated in conjunction with the administration of certain drugs (anticonvulsants, tricyclic antidepressants, barbiturates) and heavy alcohol ingestion.

The initial approach to a patient with a predominantly cholestatic process involves determination of whether an obstruction is intrahepatic or extrahepatic. This can be easily answered by assessment of the size of the biliary ducts by ultrasonography. The presence of dilatation suggests an extrahepatic mechanical obstruction. This is most commonly due to gallstone disease or tumors of the bile ducts or pancreas. When the ducts are of normal size, the obstruction is more likely due to an intrahepatic process or to sclerosing cholangitis.

QUESTION 3 Further enzyme assays revealed an elevated GGT and 5'-nucleotidase. Ultrasound of the liver did not reveal ductular dilatation. Based on this additional information, what is the differential diagnosis of this enzyme elevation pattern?

Both the mild elevation of the AP and the absence of ductular dilatation suggest an intrahepatic process, although some cases of extrahepatic obstruction are missed by ultrasonography. Primary sclerosing cholangitis (PSC) is a nonneoplastic inflammatory narrowing of the intrahepatic and extrahepatic bile ducts. It is often associated with inflammatory bowel disease. The combination of jaundice and pruritus is a common form of presentation. Cholangiography reveals a "pruned tree" appearance that is characteristic of this disease. **Primary biliary**

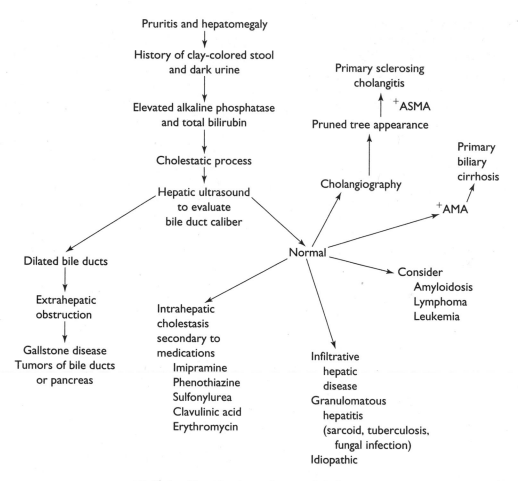

Pruritis and hepatomegaly

↓

History of clay-colored stool
and dark urine

↓

Elevated alkaline phosphatase
and total bilirubin

↓

Cholestatic process

↓

Hepatic ultrasound
to evaluate
bile duct caliber

Dilated bile ducts

↓

Extrahepatic
obstruction

↓

Gallstone disease
Tumors of bile ducts
or pancreas

Normal

Intrahepatic
cholestasis
secondary to
medications
    Imipramine
    Phenothiazine
    Sulfonylurea
    Clavulinic acid
    Erythromycin

Cholangiography

Pruned tree appearance

↑ +ASMA

Primary sclerosing
cholangitis

+AMA

Primary
biliary
cirrhosis

Consider
    Amyloidosis
    Lymphoma
    Leukemia

Infiltrative
hepatic
disease
Granulomatous
hepatitis
(sarcoid, tuberculosis,
    fungal infection)
Idiopathic

5-1-1   Algorithm for evaluation of cholestasis.

cirrhosis (PBC) is a disease that affects mostly women. The chronic obstruction leads to scarring and fibrosis of the portal areas, and ultimately to cirrhosis. Intrahepatic cholestasis can be seen as an adverse reaction to medications. Some of these include imipramine, phenothiazines, sulfonylureas, clavulanic acid, and erythromycin. Infiltrative hepatic processes including granulomatous diseases (sarcoidosis, tuberculosis, fungal infection, idiopathic), amyloidosis, lymphoma, leukemia, and abscess can produce a cholestatic biochemical pattern. This type of process may often be accompanied by an enlarged liver. Since these are systemic diseases, one should look for additional sites of involvement to support the

diagnosis. Chronic alcohol consumption may rarely produce isolated intrahepatic cholestasis as can sepsis and syphilis. One must keep in mind that no underlying liver disease is found in up to 30% of patients with an isolated elevation of the AP.

QUESTION 4   On the fourth hospital day the lab reports that the assay for antimitochondrial antibodies is positive. The results of the liver biopsy are reported as showing damaged interlobular and septal bile ducts surrounded by a dense infiltrate of lymphocytes and plasma cells. What is your diagnosis, and what are the important aspects of this disease?

The clinical constellation of pruritus, arthritis, elevated AP, GGT, and fatigue supports a diagnosis of primary biliary cirrhosis (PBC). PBC is a chronic cholestatic disorder affecting mostly women between the ages of 40 and 60. While the exact etiology is unknown, an autoimmune phenomenon is suspected. There is persistent destruction of interlobular ducts with eventual ductal fibrosis and cirrhosis. There is an association of PBC with Sjögren's syndrome, the presentation including xerostomia and dry eyes. CREST syndrome, thyroiditis, arthritis, pneumonitis, and renal tubular acidosis may also be seen in conjunction with this disorder.

The early stage of the disease includes fatigue, pruritus, hepatosplenomegaly, skin hyperpigmentation, and xanthomas. Ninety percent of patients are women. Late stigmata include jaundice, bone pain, osteoporosis, osteomalacia, ascites, variceal bleeding, malabsorption, and weight loss. These signs reflect gradually worsening liver function.

Serologic diagnosis rests on the demonstration of an elevated AP, usually 3 to 6 times greater than normal, with mild elevations of bilirubin later in the disease as the obstruction worsens. The serum cholesterol and ceruloplasmin can also be elevated. The presence of a circulating antimitochondrial antibody (AMA) is seen in >90% of patients.

The treatment of PBC is aimed largely at symptom control. Cholestyramine, used to bind bile salts in the GI tract and prevent their systemic absorption, can be used to treat pruritus. Both colchicine and ursodeoxycholic acid have an impact on liver tests but have not been shown to affect the progress of the disease. Ultimately, the best treatment for PBC is liver transplantation. In this group, the 1-year survival rates reach 80%.

CASE SUMMARY   The patient was placed on a regimen of cholestyramine and fat-soluble vitamins and discharged home. She expressed a wish to be placed on the list of patients eligible for liver transplantation. Two years later she received a liver transplant and is currently doing well 3 months postoperatively.

• •

BIBLIOGRAPHY

Braunwald E, et al: *Harrison's principles of internal medicine,* Section 2, Hepatobiliary disease, ed 12, New York, 1993, McGraw-Hill.

Clarke PJ, et al: Liver function tests in patients receiving parenteral nutrition, *J Parenteral Enteral Nutr* 15:54-59, 1991.

Cotran RS, Kumar V, Robbins SL: *Robbins pathologic basis of disease,* ed 4, Philadelphia, 1989, WB Saunders.

Herrera JL: Abnormal liver enzymes, the spectrum of causes, *Postgrad Med* 93(2):113-130, 1993.

Kaplan MM: Primary biliary cirrhosis, *Resident and Staff Physician,* 39(9):65-75, 1993.

Poupon RE, et al: A multicenter, controlled trial of ursodiol for the treatment of primary biliary cirrhosis, *N Engl J Med* 324:1548-1554, 1991.

Sherlock S, Dooley J: *Diseases of the liver and biliary system,* ed 6, Oxford, 1993, Blackwell Scientific.

Wyngaarden JB, Smith L, Bennett JC, eds: *Cecil, textbook of medicine,* Part XI: Diseases of the liver, gallbladder, and bile ducts, ed 19, Philadelphia, 1992, WB Saunders.

C A S E

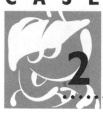

2

Panos Sechopoulos
Donald Jensen

A *21-year-old white man is brought to your office after experiencing a syncopal episode. The patient has otherwise been healthy. While in class today he felt weak, lightheaded, diaphoretic, cold, and "passed out." A classmate who observed the event states that the patient lost consciousness for a few seconds and that there was no head trauma or seizure activity. The patient's initial physical examination was negative except for icteric sclerae.*

QUESTION 1 Because of the short period of syncope, the patient is brought to the emergency room. You are the initial physician present. In your evaluation of jaundice, what is bilirubin and how is it metabolized?

Bilirubin, a bile pigment, is a product of the daily catabolism of hemoglobin, specifically the heme molecule. Every day about 4 mg/kg of bilirubin is produced, which is ultimately excreted in bile. The metabolism of bilirubin starts in the bone marrow and reticuloendothelial system with the destruction of red blood cells and liberation of hemoglobin. Hemoglobin is broken down to globin and heme moieties. The heme molecule is subsequently cleaved to biliverdin that is oxidized to bilirubin. Once bilirubin is formed, it is transported, complexed with albumin, to the liver.

Hepatic metabolism of this water-insoluble tetrapyrrhole molecule takes place in three stages. The first stage is uptake by hepatocytes. The bilirubin molecule dissociates from albumin as unconjugated bilirubin and is water-insoluble. In neonates this compound is particularly dangerous. Because it is able to cross the blood-brain

barrier, kernicterus may develop. This is a disease of the newborn with deposition of unconjugate bilirubin in the basal ganglia leading to lethargy, mental retardation, motor disturbances, and potentially death.

In the second stage of metabolism, conjugation, bilirubin combines with glucuronic acid (bilirubin monoglucuronide and diglucuronide) and becomes water soluble. The third stage of metabolism is excretion. The bilirubin reaches the intestine via the biliary tree where it is converted by intestinal flora to urobilinogen. This pigment is colorless and is excreted in the feces where, upon contact with air, it is oxidized to a characteristic brown pigment called urobilin, which gives stool its color. Part of urobilinogen is returned to the liver via enterohepatic circulation and excreted in the urine. In conditions of decreased excretion of conjugated bilirubin, blood levels increase, and some is filtered at the glomerulus. The conjugated bilirubin appears in the urine, imparting a characteristic dark-brown color. This becomes a very useful diagnostic clue.

QUESTION 2 While the patient is in the emergency room, further history is obtained. He reveals that he had a similar episode 2 years ago when, again, during a period of stress (final exams), he became jaundiced. He states that this year's final examinations are in 3 weeks and that he has been studying harder lately in preparation. He recalled that during routine physical examination, about 1 year ago, he was also found to have elevated bilirubin. Presently he has no complaints and denies any exposure to people with hepatitis, onset of dark urine or clay-colored stools, alcohol abuse, medication use, and states that there is no family history of liver disease.

The patient's physical examination remains unremarkable except for persistently icteric sclera. Laboratory tests are ordered. Repeat bilirubin remains at 3.5 mg/dl, while other standard liver chemistries (SGOT, SGPT, AP, and GGT) were normal. What are the causes of elevated bilirubin?

It is often helpful to divide the causes of hyperbilirubinemia into those disorders associated with predominantly conjugated hyperbilirubinemia and those associated with mostly unconjugated bilirubin. Unconjugated bilirubin will be elevated in three different situations. First, overproduction occurs during hemolysis or ineffective erythropoiesis, leading to an inability of the liver to keep conjugating the increased pigment load. There are multiple causes of hemolysis, but the most common ones include hereditary spherocytosis, sickle cell disease, pyruvate kinase deficiency, G-6PD deficiency, and transfusion-related, drug-induced, and mechanical (e.g., prosthetic valves) causes. Second, impaired hepatic uptake may lead to elevation of unconjugated bilirubin. This impairment is most commonly caused by medications (e.g., rifampin) that compete with bilirubin for the enzyme responsible for uptake. Third, decreased conjugation can occur during Gilbert's syndrome and Criggler-Najjar syndromes, types I and II. The latter is an inherited disorder characterized by the absence (type I) of hepatic UDP-glucuronyl transferase, the enzyme responsible for bilirubin conjugation. In type II disease the enzyme level is markedly decreased, and there are no clinical sequelae except elevated unconjugated bilirubin, which is easily treated with phenobarbital. Additional causes of decreased conjugation include drug inducement (chloramphenicol) and also hepatocellular disease (hepatitis, shock liver, alcoholic liver disease).

Bilirubin is conjugated in the hepatocyte and is excreted in the bile in the conjugated form. Serum levels of conjugated bilirubin are elevated during impaired hepatic excretion. Cholestasis refers to the impairment of bile formation or flow and is associated with elevated alkaline phosphatase activity and conjugated hyperbilirubinemia in advanced disease. Cholestasis may be subdivided into intrahepatic and extrahepatic causes.

The causes of intrahepatic cholestasis are multiple. Hepatocellular diseases including granulomatous hepatitis, primary biliary cirrhosis (discussed in Gastroenterology/Hepatology Case 1), sepsis, and drug-induced cholestasis are the most common and may be accompanied by elevation of transaminases. Impairment of secretory ability is also seen with drug ingestion via two separate mechanisms. Noninflammatory processes are due to ingestion of oral contraceptive pills and anabolic steroids. This defect is completely and rapidly reversible with discontinuation of the offending agent. Inflammatory lesions are associated with systemic signs of toxicity and may be related to phenothiazines, chlorpromazine, oral hypoglycemia agents, and macrolide antibiotics (erythromycin). Chlorpromazine is metabolized to several particularly toxic substances that can lead to a more aggressive necrosing cholestasis.

Other causes of intrahepatic cholestasis include Dubin-Johnson and Rotor syndromes, two uncommon benign autosomal recessive disorders. These syndromes are related to inability to excrete conjugated bilirubin with levels as high as 20 to 25 mg/dl, but more commonly are less than 7 mg/dl. There are no known detrimental sequelae.

In the correct clinical setting benign postoperative cholestasis also causes elevation of unconjugated bilirubin and typically follows major operations in severely ill patients who received multiple blood transfusions. It becomes evident on postoperative days 3 to 4 with jaundice and levels peak on days 10 to 14. This condition is aggravated by hyperalimentation and sepsis but is mostly a benign condition that resolves spontaneously. In evaluation of intrahepatic cholestasis, liver biopsy might be very helpful.

Extrahepatic biliary obstruction is caused most commonly by gallstones and less commonly by tumors of the head of the pancreas, bile duct, or ampulla of Vater. In evaluation of extrahepatic obstruction, imaging studies are essential in revealing ductal dilation indicative of obstruction. During complete obstruction bilirubin does not

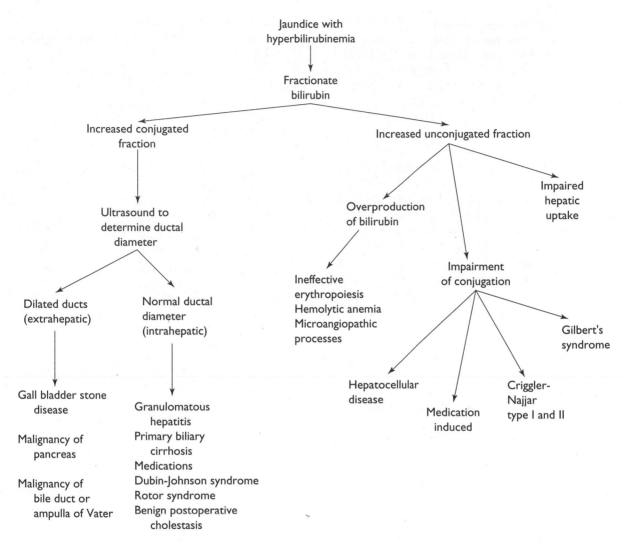

5-2-1 Decision tree for evaluation of jaundice.

reach the intestine, and as a result stool loses its characteristic brown color, becoming instead clay colored. Increased amounts of conjugated bilirubin reflux into the circulation and are filtered in the kidney, leading to darkening of the urine.

QUESTION 3 After hydration and glucose supplementation, the patient remained symptom free. Additional laboratory studies revealed that his bilirubin was predominantly unconjugated. The hemoglobin, MCV, and reticulocyte counts were nor-

mal. He was anxious and attributed the fainting episode to lack of food and long study hours. His physical examination did not change. What is your diagnosis?

Based on the information gleaned from his evaluation, his most likely diagnosis is Gilbert's syndrome. This is a common disorder affecting close to 7% of the population, with a male predominance. Enzymatically there is a decrease in the amount of UDP-glucuronyl transferase activity, slowed hepatic bilirubin uptake, and mild hemolysis. The condition is usually detected during the second to third decade. Clinically, patients are asymptomatic except during periods of stress or starvation (as with our patient). Bilirubin levels are typically less than 3 mg/dl. Diagnosis is suggested by several clinical clues. In Gilbert's syndrome, the tests of liver cell necrosis (SGOT, SGPT) and cholestasis (AP, GGT) remain normal. The bilirubin is elevated in response to fasting. At the end of a <400 kCal diet for 24 hours, repeat bilirubin should be obtained. This value should be about 2 times the baseline value to be consistent with Gilbert's syndrome. Liver biopsy proves to be normal and is unnecessary. Reduction of plasma bilirubin is seen with rest and adequate dietary calories. Prognosis is excellent without sequelae.

The patient's syncope was thought to be related to poor caloric intake because of his not eating for over 18 hours.

CASE FOLLOW-UP The patient returned home from the emergency room later that night and was advised to eat regularly. He was also informed that the key to studying is the quality of the effort rather than the quantity of time spent. He did very well on his examinations and is currently enjoying spring break.

• •

BIBLIOGRAPHY

Braunwald E, et al: *Harrison's principles of internal medicine,* Section 2: Hepatobiliary disease, ed 12, New York, 1993, McGraw-Hill.

Cotran RS, Kumar V, Robbins SL: *Robbins pathologic basis of disease,* ed 4, Philadelphia, 1989, WB Saunders.

Fevery J, et al: Unconjugate bilirubin and an increased proportion of bilirubin monoconjugates in the bile of patients with Gilbert's syndrome and Criggler-Najjar disease, *J Clin Invest* 60:970-979, 1977.

Ravel R: *Clinical laboratory medicine,* ed 4, Chicago, 1984, Year Book Medical Publishers, Inc.

Sinaasappel M, Jansen PLM: The differential diagnosis of Crigler-Najjar disease, types 1 and 2, by bile pigment analysis, *Gastroenterology* 100:783-789, 1991.

Sleisenger MH, Fordtran JS: *Gastrointestinal disease: pathophysiogy, diagnosis, and management,* ed 3, Philadelphia, 1983, WB Saunders.

Wyngaarden JB, Smith L, Bennett JC: *Cecil, textbook of medicine,* Part XI: Diseases of the liver, gallbladder, and bile ducts, ed 19, Philadelphia, 1992, WB Saunders.

C A S E

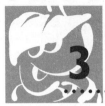

3

Panos Sechopoulos
Donald Jensen
. . . .

A 34-year-old man presents to the emergency room with a 1-month history of fatigue, malaise, fever, nausea, vomiting, and myalgias. The patient states that he has no other medical problems and takes no medications. He admits to IV heroin use for the last 5 years and states he often shares needles but insists that he sterilizes them thoroughly. He denies alcohol and tobacco use. On physical examination he is a thin, ill-appearing, jaundiced male who is alert and oriented. His examination is remarkable for icteric sclera; liver span measures 14 cm in the midclavicular line and is mildly tender to palpation. There are no other stigmata of chronic liver disease. He has multiple needle tracts on both arms. His initial laboratory values reveal SGOT 1250 mg/dl, SGPT 985 mg/dl, TB 2.2 mg/dl, and alkaline phosphatase 158 mg/dl. The electrolytes and complete blood count were normal.

QUESTION 1 What are serum aminotransfer-ases?

Aspartate (AST) and alanine (ALT) amino-transferases, SGOT and SGPT, respectively, are enzymes responsible for the transfer of the alpha-amino group from aspartate or alanine to the alpha-keto group of ketoglutarate. They are present in large quantities in the liver. AST is also found in cardiac muscle, skeletal muscle, kidney, pancreas, and red blood cells. ALT is found mainly in the liver and is therefore a more liver-specific enzyme. The aminotransaminases are released in the blood stream subsequent to hepatocyte membrane injury. These enzymes reflect active hepatocellular necrosis and are useful screening tests for liver disease.

QUESTION 2 Does that level of aminotransferase elevation have diagnostic significance? What is the differential diagnosis of elevated aminotransferase levels?

Clues to the etiology of liver disease may sometimes be inferred from the pattern and magnitude of aminotransferase elevation. For example, alcoholic liver injury frequently results in a modest increase in AST with a normal or only minimally increased ALT. Viral hepatitis on the other hand, typically gives rise to a more profound rise in both enzymes (5 to 20 times), with the ALT usually higher than the AST.

Very few conditions are associated with extreme (SBP >30 times) elevations of the aminotransferases. The most common is acute viral hepatitis, particularly types A and B. Hepatitis refers to inflammation of the liver and may be reproduced from a variety of agents including viral, toxins of pharmocologic agents, and immune-mediated processes. Viral hepatitis is caused by five hepatitis viruses A, B, C, D, and E and cytomegalovirus and Epstein-Barr virus. These organisms and hepatitis syndromes will be reviewed later in this case.

Drug hepatotoxicity may on occasion also lead to extreme hyperaminotransferasemia. Classically, acetaminophen is a medication causing such liver injury. Acetaminophen is metabolized in part by the cytochrome P-450 system. The initial metabolite is toxic but is quickly inactivated by glutathione. Concurrent use of alcohol or isonicotine acid hydrazide (INH) potentiates the cytochrome P-450 enzymes enhancing production of this toxic metabolite. Toxicity occurs when the amount of acetaminophen metabolite overwhelms the glutathione system, and this toxic metabolite causes hepatocellular necrosis. Treatment consists of gastric lavage to remove pill fragments and administration of N-acetylcysteine, which supports the activity of the glutathione system.

Other common substances causing liver damage leading to enzyme elevation include isoniazid, halothane anesthetic agents, carbon tetrachloride, aspirin, estrogens, allopurinol, alphamethyldopa, methotrexate, and many others.

The third condition leading to extreme aminotransferase elevation is hepatic ischemia or infarction. This situation can be encountered following a hypotensive episode (poor systolic function versus shock), or as result of congestive heart failure leading to passive congestion of the liver. During evaluation one must review the blood pressure trend and look closely for signs of heart failure, although in many cases the episode is transient. Typically, the extremely high levels of the serum aminotransferases return rapidly toward normal with restitution of the cardiac output, thus helping to differentiate this condition from viral or toxic liver injury. A quantitative evaluation of ventricular function may lead to a diagnosis.

The second pattern of aminotransferase elevation demonstrates mild, asymptomatic increases, usually less than 5 times normal. This may represent acute or chronic liver disease or neoplastic disease. Two common causes of acute liver disease in this category are drugs and alcohol. A persistent elevation of aminotransferases could reflect alcoholic fatty liver or alcoholic hepatitis. A careful history of alcohol consumption and physical manifestations of liver disease are important. It is important to remember that AST and ALT values greater than 8 to 10 times normal are very uncommon in alcoholic liver disease. During evaluation the ratio of SGOT/SGPT is helpful. A ratio greater than 2 is suggestive (but not diagnostic) of alcoholic liver disease. While not fully understood, this is believed to be due to damage to hepatocyte mitochondria specifically, the site of AST, and an absolute decrease in hepatic ALT synthesis.

Examples of chronic liver disease giving rise to modest ALT elevations include chronic viral hepatitis, Wilson's disease, and hemochromatosis. It is known that hepatitis B and C can ultimately lead to chronic hepatitis and mild, asymptomatic aminotransferase elevation. Serologic markers are helpful in establishing the diagnosis (to be discussed later).

Wilson's disease is an autosomal recessive disorder, seen in men and women less than 40 years of age, and characterized by impaired hepatic excretion of copper into bile. This abnormal copper metabolism leads to copper accumulation in the liver and deposition in the brain, cornea, and other sites. Clinically, patients may have neurologic signs, which include tremor, intellectual deterioration, dysarthria, muscle rigidity, and drooling. Other features of the disease include manifestations of liver disease, Kayser-Fleischer corneal rings, and renal tubular acidosis. Laboratory values reveal low (below 20 mg/dl) ceruloplasmin levels, urinary excretion of more than 100 μg/day of copper, and low uric acid and alkaline phosphatase levels. There may also be an associated hemolytic anemia. The liver biopsy reveals increased copper stores. Treatment consists of D-penicillamine, a chelating agent, that forms a ring complex with copper enhancing renal excretion. An alternate chelating agent called trientine can also be used. Prognosis is excellent if treatment is started before major neurologic manifestations.

A second chronic liver disorder that presents with moderate elevation of transaminases is hemochromatosis. Hemochromatosis is an autosomal recessive iron storage disorder usually presenting in the fifth or sixth decade in men. The cardinal presenting signs include hepatomegaly, skin hyperpigmentation, glucose intolerance, early onset impotence (hypopituitary hypogonadism), congestive heart failure, or arthritis. The etiology of the disease involves increased intestinal absorption of iron, leading to deposition in liver, pancreas, heart, pituitary, and other organs. Laboratory studies reveal an elevated transferrin saturation (TIBC/ferritin ratio), plasma iron greater than 200 µg/dl and high ferritin (usually >500 to 1000 ng/ml). Diagnosis is confirmed by liver biopsy that shows elevated iron stores. First-line therapy is phlebotomy that is used to maintain the hematocrit in the 30% to 35% range. If organ fibrosis has not occurred, organ dysfunction can be reversed. The second-line therapy is deferoxamine, a chelator that binds iron. The deferoxamine-iron compound is excreted in the urine, which turns dark red in color. In addition, restricting the dietary intake of iron is essential. Early detection and treatment prevent the life-threatening complications of the disease.

Neoplasm, primary or metastatic, involving the liver usually presents with elevated alkaline phosphatase. However, less commonly it may also present as mild aminotransferase elevation. Hepatic neoplasms can be benign or malignant. The benign neoplasms include adenomas (mostly affecting women and associated with use of oral contraceptive pills), hemangiomas (most common hepatic neoplasms), and focal nodular hyperplasia. Hepatocellular carcinoma is the most common primary malignant lesion affecting the liver and is associated with hepatitis B and C, cirrhosis, and aflatoxin ingestion. It is more common in men. Metastatic lesions are the most common hepatic malignancies and most often originate from stomach, pancreas, colon, lung, melanoma, and bladder. The clinical presentation of neoplastic disease is highly variable, and imaging studies with directed biopsy are essential in evaluation.

QUESTION 3 The patient remained stable in the emergency room. Additional laboratory tests were obtained, and the patient was started on intravenous fluids. He was subsequently admitted to the floor for further evaluation. Further history obtained was negative for any travel, blood transfusions, history of hepatitis, history of jaundice, homosexuality, or multiple sexual partners. The patient denied ingestion of toxins, medications, over-the-counter products, or herbal remedies. His physical examination remained unchanged. Laboratory tests revealed negative acetaminophen level; urine drug screen was positive for heroin; urinalysis was negative; and an alcohol level was absent. What is the preliminary diagnosis based on the above information?

The diagnosis in this case can be arrived at by first considering the patient's presenting symptom complex: an IV drug user with flu-like symptoms, jaundice, and very high transaminase levels. The most likely diagnosis is acute viral hepatitis.

The clinical features of acute hepatitis include fatigue, jaundice, darkening of the urine, anorexia, abdominal pain, nausea, vomiting, low-grade fever, and myalgias. On physical examination there is scleral icterus, hepatomegaly, right upper quadrant tenderness, and other signs of liver disease. Laboratory tests reveal elevated transaminases, elevated bilirubin, and normal or slightly elevated alkaline phosphatase. The complications include cholestatic hepatitis, fulminant hepatitis, and chronic hepatitis.

Viral hepatitis is caused by five viruses A, B, C, D, and E. Fecal-oral transmission is seen in hepatitis A and E viruses. The hepatitis A virus (HAV) is a small, nonenveloped, single-stranded RNA picornavirus that has a 2 to 6 week incubation period and causes benign, self-limited disease. Management is supportive. It is important to remember that infectivity lasts 2 to 3 weeks, starting late in the incubation period before clinical manifestations, underscoring the importance of proper blood and body fluid precautions in high-risk cases. Fulminant hepatic failure is an uncommon complication of hepatitis A. Chronic hepatitis does not occur.

The other hepatitis virus transmitted via the fecal-oral route is hepatitis E. This is a nonenveloped RNA virus that is epidemic to Burma, India, the countries of the former Soviet Union, North Africa, and Southeast Asia. This virus affects mostly young adults. The infection does not progress to chronic hepatitis; however, it can lead to fulminant hepatic necrosis in pregnant women.

Direct exchange of infected body fluid (blood, semen and saliva, vaginal fluid) is a common mode of transmission for hepatitis B and C. The hepatitis B virus (HBV) particle is a spherical, DNA virus (hepadnavirus), composed of an outer surface antigen (HBsAg) and an inner core consisting of circular DNA, DNA polymerase, and hepatitis B core antigen (HBcAg). The usual incubation period is 4 to 26 weeks. This virus is very versatile and can cause any of the following: asymptomatic carriage, acute hepatitis with complete resolution, persistence of HBV in 6% to 10% of patients and progression to chronic hepatitis in 30% of those, with possible progression to cirrhosis, fulminant hepatic failure, and hepatocellular carcinoma. Liver damage is due to the immune response to the virus and not direct viral cellular toxicity. Therefore, the extent of liver damage is proportional to the level of immunosurveillance. Clinically, the disease presents as typical acute hepatitis with a prolonged course and may also be associated with extrahepatic manifestation due to immune complex deposition including glomerulonephritis, arthritis, urticaria, and vasculitis (polyarteritis nodosa). Interferon therapy may be useful in cases of chronic hepatitis B with active viral replication (HBeAg-positive, HBV DNA-positive).

Hepatitis D is a small defective RNA virus that can cause disease only with concomitant HBV infection. This virus is found among intravenous drug users, transfusion recipients, and is endemic among HBV carriers in Africa, the Middle East, and other parts of the world. It can lead to massive hepatic necrosis or more active chronic hepatitis more often than hepatitis B alone. Management is supportive.

Hepatitis C (HCV) is a flavivirus-like RNA virus transmitted parenterally, though 40% of all cases have no known exposure history. This virus is the most common cause of posttransfusion hepatitis (90% of cases) and is also responsible for most cases of sporadic, community acquired hepatitis. The incubation period of this virus is 5 to 10

weeks. Infection may progress to chronic hepatitis or a carrier state and, uncommonly, leads to fulminant hepatic necrosis. Clinically the disease is similar to hepatitis B with a 50% rate of development of chronic hepatitis. Management of acute disease is supportive, and prevention is essential with close screening of the blood supply. Interferon therapy is useful in cases of chronic infection.

QUESTION 4 What is the definition of chronic hepatitis and what are the important pathophysiolgic processes?

Chronic hepatitis is a condition that causes hepatic inflammation for at least 6 months. The causes are multiple and include hepatitis B, C, and D; drugs (e.g., Aldomet and nitrofurantoin); Wilson's disease; autoimmune disease; or it may be idiopathic.

Chronic hepatitis is defined by elevation of aminotransferases for at least 6 months with characteristic histology. The severity of histologic lesions helps to differentiate the disease into mild, moderate, or severe chronic hepatitis. Clinically, stigmata of chronic liver disease might be present. Laboratory evaluation should include liver enzymes, ceruloplasmin, Fe/TIBC, ANA, ASMA, and hepatitis B and C. The diagnosis is confirmed by liver biopsy.

Treatment of autoimmune chronic hepatitis incorporates the use of corticosteroids with or without azathioprine. Stabilization or improvement of aminotransferase levels is seen in a majority of cases; however, the relapse rate at 2 years is roughly 50% to 90%. Steroids should not be used in hepatitis B or C because immunosuppression might enhance viral replication. Instead, interferon (as outlined above) might be beneficial in reducing viral replication.

QUESTION 5 The patient had an uneventful night, and the next day was feeling slightly better. His physical examination remained unchanged, and follow-up laboratory values revealed anti-HAV (IgM) negative, HBsAg positive, anti-HBc (IgM) positive, HBeAg positive, anti-HCV negative, and HIV negative. What is the significance of the above serologic markers and how is the diagnosis of viral hepatitis supported serologically for each type?

Serologic tests are essential in evaluation of viral hepatitis. In hepatitis A, antibodies in the serum are helpful markers. During acute infection, anti-HAV is of IgM type. Later, loss of IgM anti-HAV occurs with persistence of anti-HAV, indicating previous infection and immunity.

In the case of hepatitis B infection, HBsAg is positive in most cases of acute hepatitis or cases of chronic hepatitis. Anti-HBs is positive during recovery from acute hepatitis B and also after immunization with hepatitis B vaccine. Acute hepatitis B infection can be distinguished from chronic hepatitis B by the presence of IgM anti-HBc antibody at the onset of disease. HBeAg is positive during the period of high infectivity and reflects viral replication. In hepatitis D, acute or chronic, antibody to HDV antigen is positive along with HBsAg and anti-HBc antibody.

In hepatitis C, anti-HCV is positive about 2 to 15 weeks after clinical onset. The enzyme-linked immunoassay (EIA) test for antigen is only about 65% sensitive in acute hepatitis C and 90% to 95% in chronic cases. The EIA-II assay detects antibody to the c-200 and c-22 antigens produced from the HCV genome. Newer tests include RIBA II (recombinant immunoblot assay) and HCV RNA by PCR. RIBA II (recombinant immunoblot assay) and HCV RNA by PCR. RIBA II, a second generation test, utilizes four antigens, 5-1-1, c100-3, c33-C, c22-3 that detect and bind antibodies, indicating the presence of the virus. Matching four specific genomic sequences provides greater sensitivity. Polymerase chain reaction (PCR) uses primers as templates for the double polymerase chain reaction with hepatitis C RNA. The EIA-II is currently the best screening test for suspected cases because of its sensitivity and lower cost. RIBA-II is most often utilized as a confirmatory test for EIA-positive samples before initiating antiviral therapy. HCV RNA by PCR is sometimes used to follow the course of antiviral therapy, but is too expensive for routine application.

Correct interpretation of this patient's serology concludes that the patient has acute hepatitis B. Since the HBeAg is also positive, he is considered highly infectious.

QUESTION 6 What is the correct treatment for each of the hepatitis viruses?

Treatment of hepatitis A, B, C, D, and E is supportive.

Treatment of chronic hepatitis B includes use of alpha-interferon in cases that are HBeAg positive and HBsAg positive. Virus is cleared by inhibition of viral replication and enhancement of immune-mediated cellular destruction. Clearance of chronic hepatitis coincides with disappearance of HBV DNA and transition from presence of HBeAg to anti-HBe.

There is no good treatment for superinfection with the hepatitis D agent. Use of alpha-interferon provides only transient improvement in aminotransferase levels with relapse after discontinuation.

Treatment of hepatitis C includes interferon alpha. A 6-month course of interferon will normalize aminotransferase levels in approximately 40% to 50% of cases. However, about 50% of these patients will relapse within 6 months of discontinuation. Typically, milder disease responds better to interferon than does cirrhosis.

QUESTION 7 What are the indications for use of hepatitis B vaccine and/or immunoglobulin therapy?

As a result of the prevalence of hepatitis B, vaccination with recombinant HBsAg vaccines may be important for individuals at high risk. Preventive vaccination had been recommended only for high-risk groups (health professionals, dialysis patients, intravenous drug users, household contacts of infected patients, hemophiliacs, and sexually active homosexual males), but more recently, the recommendation has been extended to all newborns and adolescents in the United States.

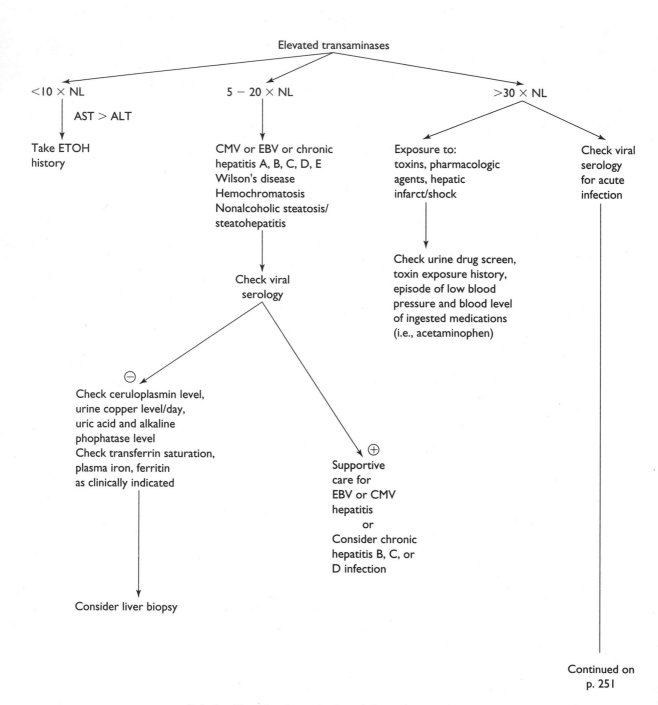

5-3-1 Algorithm for evaluation of elevated transaminases.

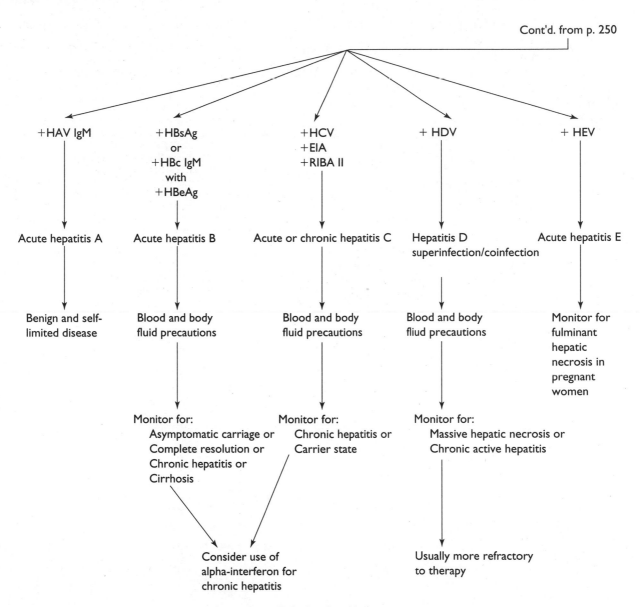

Cont'd. from p. 250

+HAV IgM	+HBsAg or +HBc IgM with +HBeAg	+HCV +EIA +RIBA II	+ HDV	+ HEV
Acute hepatitis A	Acute hepatitis B	Acute or chronic hepatitis C	Hepatitis D superinfection/coinfection	Acute hepatitis E
Benign and self-limited disease	Blood and body fluid precautions	Blood and body fluid precautions	Blood and body fliud precautions	Monitor for fulminant hepatic necrosis in pregnant women
	Monitor for: Asymptomatic carriage or Complete resolution or Chronic hepatitis or Cirrhosis	Monitor for: Chronic hepatitis or Carrier state	Monitor for: Massive hepatic necrosis or Chronic active hepatitis	
	Consider use of alpha-interferon for chronic hepatitis		Usually more refractory to therapy	

5-3-1   Cont'd.

In situations of exposure to a patient with acute hepatitis B, the spouse should receive HBIG, whereas other family members require only observation. Exposure of the spouse and other family members to patients with chronic hepatitis B should be treated with vaccination. Needle sticks are common in hospital accidents. If the recipient of a needle stick has already been vaccinated and the anti-HBs immune status is known, no further treatment is necessary. If the antibody status is unknown, HBIG should be administered. For those who have not been vaccinated, both vaccination and HBIG should be given.

CASE FOLLOW-UP The patient remains hospitalized for 7 days with resolution of abdominal tenderness and improvement in his liver enzyme tests. During his hospitalization he remained on strict body fluid isolation. He was unmarried, but was informed that any close household contacts should see their physicians to evaluate their need for testing and vaccination. His appetite gradually returned. He is scheduled to follow-up with you in the office in 2 weeks.

• •

BIBLIOGRAPHY

Adams PC, Kertesz AE, Valberg LS: Clinical presentation of hemochromatosis: a changing scene, *Am J Med* 90:445-449, 1991.

Bacon BR: Evaluation and management of iron storage diseases, *Pract Gastroenterol* 14(8):41-49, 1990.

Cotran RS, Kumar V, Robbins SL: *Robbins pathologic basis of disease,* ed 4, Philadelphia, 1989, WB Saunders.

DiBisceglie AM, et al: Recombinant interferon alfa therapy for chronic hepatitis C, *N Engl J Med* 321:1506-1510, 1989.

Herrera JL: Abnormal liver enzymes, the spectrum of causes, *Postgrad Med* 93(2):113-130, 1993.

Jensen DM, et al: Serum alanine aminotransferase levels and prevalence of hepatitis A, B, and delta in outpatients, *Arch Intern Med* 147:1734-1737, 1987.

Lambiase L, Davis GL: Treatment of chronic hepatitis, *Gastroenterol Clin North Am* 21(3):659-672, 1992.

Nakatsuji Y, et al: Detection of chronic hepatitis C virus infection by four diagnostic systems: first-generation and second-generation enzyme-linked immunoabsorbent assay, second-generation recombinant immunoblot assay and nested polymerase chain reaction analysis, *Hepatology* 16:300-305, 1992.

Scheuer PJ, et al: The pathology of hepatitis C, *Hepatology* 15:567-571, 1992.

Wyngaarden JB, Smith L, Bennett JC, editors: *Cecil, textbook of medicine,* part XI: Diseases of the liver, gallbladder, and bile ducts, ed 19, Philadelphia, 1992, WB Saunders.

CASE

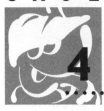

4

Panos Sechopoulos
Donald Jensen
. . . .

A 47-year-old woman is admitted to the hospital secondary to increasing shortness of breath. The patient has a history of alcoholic cirrhosis (diagnosed by liver biopsy 3 months ago) with ascites. She states that her abdomen has increased in size and that her breathing has become increasingly difficult. She has had mild abdominal discomfort for the last week but denies fever, nausea, vomiting, hematemesis, melena, or mental status changes. She denies excess fluid or salt intake and has been compliant with her medications, which include Lasix and Aldactone. Her social history is significant for heavy alcohol intake for 15 years. She denies current drug or tobacco use.

QUESTION 1 You are the resident on the floor admitting the patient. The patient carries a diagnosis of cirrhosis; however, you realize it is important to review the relationship between alcohol and liver function before examining the patient. How does ethanol damage the liver?

Alcohol abuse is the most common cause of liver disease in the Western world. Alcohol exerts its damaging effects by several different cellular pathways. Ethanol has a direct effect on membrane fluidity, leading to loss of membrane regulatory control and cell swelling. Another pathway involves the production of excess acetaldehyde from the metabolism of alcohol. Acetaldehyde exerts toxic effects on the hepatocyte and is responsible for a more severe lesion. During alcohol metabolism NADPH is formed, leading to an elevated redox potential favoring accumulation of hepatic triglycerides.

There are three patterns of alcoholic liver disease. Steatosis (fatty liver) involves the accumu-

lation of triglycerides in hepatocytes. This process begins within the first few days of alcohol intake and progresses with continued intake. This condition is completely reversible if alcohol intake is discontinued. Clinically it presents as moderate to massive hepatomegaly, right upper quadrant pain, and mild transaminase elevation (see Gastroenterology/Hepatology Case 3: differential diagnosis of mildly elevated aminotransferases). Diagnosis is confirmed by liver biopsy showing large droplet fat occupying most of the hepatocyte that resolves upon cessation of drinking.

Alcoholic hepatitis is a more serious pattern and implies acute liver cell necrosis with an inflammatory reaction. The histologic triad characteristic of this pattern includes (1) alcoholic hyaline (eosinophilic aggregates) also known as Mallory bodies, (2) infiltration by inflammatory cells, and (3) development of a network of intralobular connective tissue. The clinical presentation of this disease is highly variable, spanning the spectrum from asymptomatic to hepatic failure. Symptoms may include fever, jaundice, anorexia, nausea, vomiting, and weight loss. Physical examination reveals stigmata of liver disease. Laboratory evaluation reveals only mild elevation of transaminases SGOT:SGPT >2, leucocytosis, prolonged prothrombin time, and hypoalbuminemia. Diagnosis is confirmed by liver biopsy. The outcome is unpredictable but return to normal is possible with discontinuation of alcohol intake. Most commonly, alcoholic hepatitis leads to cirrhosis and may precipitate hepatic failure and death.

QUESTION 2 On physical examination her vital signs reveal a low-grade temperature and a respiratory rate of 28 breaths/minute. Her sclerae are icteric, and she has several spider nevi on the chest. She has bibasilar crackles and bilateral E-A changes. Her abdominal examination reveals tense distension and shifting dullness. Liver size is difficult to evaluate due to the ascites. There is mild right upper quadrant tenderness but no peritoneal signs. There is no peripheral edema, and rectal examination reveals brown stool, heme negative. What are the causes and clinical features of cirrhosis?

Cirrhosis is an alteration of the liver architecture and is characterized by the following: (1) interconnecting fibrous scars, (2) fibrous bands, (3) parenchymal nodules, and (4) formation of abnormal arteriovenous interconnections. Cirrhosis has been divided to micronodular and macronodular, but these are purely descriptive terms. The causes of cirrhosis in descending order of frequency follow.

Alcoholic cirrhosis (Laennec's cirrhosis) may be a sequela of alcoholic hepatitis. This type of cirrhosis is micronodular and accounts for close to 50% to 70% of cirrhosis in the Western world. **Chronic hepatitis** progresses to macronodular cirrhosis. The causes of chronic active hepatitis are multiple and include HBV, HCV, autoimmune injury, toxin exposure, and drug reactions (isoniazid, amiodarone). **Biliary cirrhosis** may be either primary (see Gastroenterology/Hepatology Case 1) or secondary. Secondary biliary cirrhosis develops after prolonged extrahepatic biliary tract obstruction that leads to bile retention, inflammation, fibrosis, and eventual cirrhosis. Inherited metabolic disorders can also lead to cirrhosis. These include Wilson's disease, alpha-1-antitrypsin deficiency and hereditary hemochromatosis (see Gastroenterology/Hepatology Case 3).

Alpha-1-antitrypsin deficiency (A1AT) is characterized by low levels of this protease inhibitor resulting in an imbalance favoring activity of destructive enzymes causing liver and lung injury. Hepatic congestion secondary to heart failure can cause cirrhosis known as *cardiac cirrhosis*. It is an uncommon complication of right heart failure and is mostly associated with constrictive peri-

carditis or rheumatic heart disease. Cryptogenic cirrhosis accounts for 10% of cases. In this circumstance, cirrhosis is found incidentally or presents as a complication of end-stage liver disease. The diagnosis is one of exclusion.

The clinical presentation of early cirrhosis is variable. Initially symptoms include anorexia, weight loss, weakness, and debilitation. Physical examination reveals a firm, large liver, jaundice, spider angiomas, gynecomastia, leukonychia, muscle wasting, and testicular atrophy. In the later stages of cirrhosis complications develop with additional clinical findings, which will be discussed later. Other physical abnormalities such as Dupuytren's contracture, xanthomas, Kayser-Fleischer rings, and a bronze discoloration of the skin are appreciated in specific forms of cirrhosis.

Laboratory evaluation of cirrhosis may reveal elevated bilirubin, mild transaminase elevation, hypoalbuminemia, and prolonged prothrombin time. Diagnosis is confirmed by percutaneous liver biopsy, which usually reveals distortion of hepatic architecture and the presence of nodules and scar tissue.

QUESTION 3 The laboratory data for your patient reveal a mild transaminase elevation, prothrombin time 16.2 sec, INR 1.9, albumin 1.8 g/dl, total protein 4.9 g/dl, WBC 13.3 K, plts 78 K, Hgb 10.8 g/dl, electrolytes are normal, viral hepatitis profile is negative, ammonia 32, total bilirubin 2.2 g/dl, and alkaline phosphatase 167. Arterial blood gas is consistent with respiratory alkalosis and a Pao_2 of 58. Chest x-ray shows small bilateral pleural effusions with compressive atelectasis but no infiltrates. Abdominal ultrasound shows a large amount of ascites, irregular liver surface, and splenomegaly. Upon receiving the above information, you place the patient on 2 L O_2 by nasal cannula and perform a therapeutic abdominal paracentesis. While waiting for the infusion you try to remember the complications of cirrhosis.

The manifestations of cirrhosis are divided into those related to hepatocellular injury (previously described) and to mechanical factors. The main complication of cirrhosis is portal hypertension. In the normal liver the resistance to portal venous flow is very low. However, when the liver architecture is altered (cirrhosis), resistance increases. This increase in resistance, along with the increase in portal venous inflow, is the mechanism for the development of portal hypertension. Cirrhosis is the main cause of this elevated resistance, but other causes include portal vein occlusion, hepatic vein occlusion (Budd-Chiari syndrome), veno-occlusive disease (seen after bone marrow transplant, or chemotherapeutic agents), schistosomiasis, alcoholic hepatitis, sarcoidosis, and other disorders that alter normal venous architecture. Varices form because venous blood flows to vasculature of lower resistance. These include the system connecting the portal vein to the azygos vein, gastric veins, and hemorrhoidal veins. The increase in flow to this system leads to varices in the submucosa of the lower esophagus and gastric fundus. These varices may bleed when the portal pressure is 12 mm Hg above the inferior vena cava pressure.

Variceal bleeding is the most lethal complication of portal hypertension. Clinically the varices are silent until rupture, which most commonly presents with hematemesis but can also present with melena or hematochezia. The bleeding may be massive with 40% fatality for each episode and 90% chance of recurrence within 1 year. Diagnosis is made by upper endoscopy. Endoscopy should focus on the lower esophagus, as well as the fundus of the stomach, since 10% of patients bleed from gastric varices. Diagnosis depends on high clinical suspicion in the right patient, presence of hematemesis or lower GI bleeding, and nasogastric tube recovery of heme-positive material. Management of variceal bleeding emphasizes restoration of circulating blood volume and control of the hemorrhage.

Pharmacologic agents used to control the bleeding include vasopressin and somatostatin. Vasopressin is a hormone derived from the posterior pituitary that causes vasoconstriction of the splanchnic circulation. NTG should be adminis-

tered concurrently to counteract its systemic vasoconstriction with end-organ ischemia. Other measures used to control bleeding include balloon tamponade (Sengstaken-Blakemore tube) and endoscopic-injection sclerotherapy. It is important to remember that balloon tamponade is only used as a temporary treatment. Emergency shunt surgery is reserved for variceal bleeding that is refractory to the above measures and is associated with 25% to 50% mortality.

Management of persistent or recurrent variceal bleeding may involve use of the transjugular intrahepatic portosystemic stent (TIPS), an experimental procedure. This stent, placed with the help of fluoroscopic guidance, shunts venous blood flow from the high resistance portal system to the right hepatic vein. This intervention reduces the portal venous pressure gradient (usually to less than 12 mm Hg), reducing intravariceal pressure and preventing rupture and further bleeding. The main complication of this procedure is encephalopathy because blood perfuses the central nervous system without having passed through the liver first. The incidence of encephalopathy depends on the shunt diameter (smaller shunts, 8 mm, result in decreased incidence of encephalopathy).

Variceal bleeding is associated with high morbidity and mortality; therefore prophylactic measures are essential. Prophylactic portosystemic shunts have been used and decrease the rate of rebleeding, but have not been shown to alter survival. Propranolol, a beta-adrenergic blocker, reduces mortality associated with bleeding. This drug has been shown to prevent the first episode of bleeding and to effect a decreased rate of rebleeding. Propranolol dosing needs to be sufficient to reduce the resting heart rate by 25%, which results in decreased variceal wall tension. Patient compliance is a major concern, since abrupt discontinuation can lead to rebound hypertension with acute rebleeding.

QUESTION 4 The initial physical examination revealed a protuberant abdomen with a fluid wave, shifting dullness, and prominent flanks. With what entity are these physical findings consistent and what are the associated complications?

Ascites refers to the accumulation of fluid in the peritoneal cavity. Ascites is appreciated on physical examination by detecting shifting dullness, bulging flanks, or a fluid wave. Cirrhosis is a common cause of ascites, but other causes include pancreatitis, a ruptured intraabdominal viscus, right heart failure, nephrotic syndrome, trauma, and Meigs' syndrome. In cirrhosis multiple factors lead to ascites, and these include: low albumin with loss of oncotic force within the vascular and interstitial spaces, renal retention of sodium and water, and portal hypertension with increased hepatic lymph production and transudation. Ascites resulting from cirrhosis is most commonly a transudate with protein content less than 1.1 g/dl. The diagnosis of ascites needs to be confirmed by ultrasound unless its presence is unquestionable by physical examination. Other imaging studies include CT scan and plain view of the abdomen (characteristic ground-glass appearance).

Management of uncomplicated ascites involves the following steps: (1) restriction of sodium and water (2 g Na/day and 2000 ml/day water) and (2) use of diuretics, specifically spironolactone. This is an aldosterone antagonist that has been proven to be more effective than loop diuretics because of its independence on blood flow for presentation to the nephron in patients with cirrhosis/ascites. Aldactone (spironolactone) is started at a dose of 50 to 100 mg bid and increased to 400 mg daily. If diuresis is not adequate with the 200 mg/day dose, then furosemide can be added (usual starting dose 40 mg/day). It is important to remember that spironolactone prevents the renal excretion of potassium and therefore should not be used in patients with renal insufficiency.

Ascites that is difficult to control by standard management is divided into two categories. In the first group, unresponsive ascites, diuretic use does not result in adequate natriuresis. In this group of patients the diuretic metolazone (Zaroxolyn) may be cautiously tried because it acts on the proximal tubule by inhibiting sodium reabsorption. In the second group, refractory ascites, natriuresis is achieved only in expense of a reduction in GFR. In this group a 4- to 8-week waiting period is necessary before labeling the patient refractory. During this waiting period reversible insults (alcoholic hepatitis, acute tubular necrosis, bacterial peritonitis) should be resolved before the diagnosis is accepted. Once ascites is confirmed to be refractory, peritoneovenous shunting should be considered. The LeVeen shunt is a subcutaneous stent that results in the transfer of fluid from the peritoneal cavity to the internal jugular vein via a one-way valve.

Large-volume paracentesis can also be used in the management of ascites. In many studies removal of large fluid volume, 4 to 6 L/day, resulted in shorter hospital stays and fewer complications than traditional diuretic therapy. In refractory ascites, large-volume paracentesis is equally as effective as the LeVeen shunt. One of the potential complications of this procedure is a decrease in the intravascular volume. It is, therefore, recommended that during large-volume paracentesis patients receive an intravenous infusion of albumin at the rate of 10 g/L of fluid removed. Finally, truly refractory ascites may be an indication for liver transplantation.

Spontaneous bacterial peritonitis (SBP) is an infection of the abdominal peritoneum and occurs in 10% to 25% of cirrhotic patients. The exact pathogenesis is unknown. The most likely mechanism involves the hematogenous seeding of the peritoneal cavity with enteric bacteria (translocation). These organisms enter the portal venous system via collaterals, avoiding the reticuloendothelial system of the liver. Another contributing factor is the low level of protein found in ascitic fluid. This reflects low complement levels (low opsonic activity), which in turn leads to decreased phagocytosis of bacteria. The incidence of SBP is higher in patients with ascitic fluid protein levels below 1.0 g/dl. The most common bacteria responsible are *Escherichia coli, Klebsiella pneumoniae, Streptococcus pneumoniae,* alpha-hemolytic streptococci and group D streptococci. Clinically, patients present with fever and/or abdominal pain; however, it is important to remember that one third of patients are completely asymptomatic. Laboratory data usually reveal a peripheral leukocytosis. Diagnosis is made by obtaining ascitic fluid for analysis. Direct inoculation of blood culture vials (broth) with 10 ml of fluid increased culture yield. Patients with suggestive clinical picture and fluid containing greater than 500 WBC/ml with 50% or higher granulocytes should be started on antibiotics before culture results confirm the presence of bacteria. Treatment of SBP involves intravenous administration of antibiotics astreonam + vancomycin or cefotaxime, with activity versus gram-negative bacilli. Follow-up examination of the fluid at 48 hours should be done to verify improvement. Prophylactic therapy for SBP is controversial. One antibiotic that has proven to decrease the incidence of recurrent SBP is norfloxacin (400 mg/day). This fluoroquinolone acts by selectively eliminating gram-negative bacilli from the intestinal flora, which is followed by a reduction in the rate of SBP.

QUESTION 5 The next day the medical student on the case comes to you concerned about the patient. She states that the patient thought that she was in Mexico and living on a tobacco farm and that the student was actually a mule used to haul the tobacco. What is the likely diagnosis leading to such a mental status change? What is another complication that may lead to renal failure?

One of the most difficult complications of cirrhosis is hepatic encephalopathy. This results from the portosystemic shunting of nitrogenous amines that can be neurotoxic. Precipitating factors include azotemia, use of sedatives/tranquilizers, gastrointestinal bleeding, infection, hypokalemic alkalosis, or excess protein intake. The symptoms and signs of this disease include (1) asterixis, a flapping motion seen when the patient is asked to hold his arms horizontally with the hands extended at the wrists, (2) fetor hepaticus, a feculent-fruity odor of the breath, and (3) mental status changes that vary from mood alter-

ations to lethargy, confusion, stupor, and finally coma. Ammonia levels may be elevated but do not correlate with the stage of disease. Hepatic encephalopathy can be classified in four categories: (1) agitation, (2) lethargy with asterixis, inappropriate behavior, and slurred speech, (3) stupor with hyperactive reflexes and nystagmus, and (4) deep coma with dilated pupils and opisthotonos.

Management of hepatic encephalopathy should emphasize correction of the precipitating factors. Other therapeutic measures should include temporary dietary protein restriction and use of lactulose or neomycin. Protein intake should be limited to 1 g/kg. Lactulose works by reducing intestine intraluminal pH and promoting diarrhea. The acidic environment created promotes protonation of ammonia to NH_4+, which is not well absorbed and is excreted in stool. Neomycin is an aminoglycoside antibiotic that decreases urease-producing bacteria and is as effective as lactulose. The use of neomycin is limited by attendant side effects of ototoxicity and nephrotoxicity.

The hepatorenal syndrome is another complication of cirrhosis. This is a potentially fatal complication and is defined by the presence of renal failure in combination with cirrhosis. This renal failure is characterized by decrease in GFR, azotemia, and oliguria. The exact pathogenesis is unknown, but precipitating factors include vigorous diuretic use, large-volume paracentesis without volume repletion and sepsis. These conditions all lead to decreased renal blood flow and GFR, both of which might precede overt renal failure. It is important to rule out prerenal azotemia before settling on the diagnosis of the hepatorenal syndrome.

Other complications of cirrhosis include gallstones, which form secondary to an increase in bilirubin from hemolytic anemia and hypersplenism. Peptic ulcer disease occurs with greater incidence in patients with cirrhosis. Hypoxia develops secondary to two possible mechanisms. Ascitic fluid may interfere with diaphragmatic movement, leading to the sensation of dyspnea, and retarding adequate ventilation. The second

TABLE 5-4-1 Child-Turcotte Classification

Child Classification	A	B	C
Serum bilirubin (mg/dl)	<2	2-3	>3
Serum albumin (g/dl)	>3.5	3-3.5	<3
Presence of ascites	Absent	Easily controlled	Refractory
Presence of encephalopathy	Absent	Minimal	Severe
Presence of malnutrition	Absent	Mild	Severe
Operative mortality rate (shunting procedure)	2%	10%	50%

(From Jarrell BE, Carabosi RA: *Surgery*, 1986, Harual Publishing Co., 156.)

mechanism is known as the hepatopulmonary syndrome. This is due to the formation of abnormal arteriovenous circuits in the lung, wherein perfusion is position dependent. Changes of position lead to alterations of ventilation and perfusion leading to hypoxemeia. Primary liver cell cancer is often seen in cirrhotic livers and is associated with hepatitis B and C and less commonly with cirrhosis due to alcohol.

Another manifestation of portal hypertension is splenomegaly, which results in thrombocytopenia and leukopenia. The decrease in platelets is clinically significant because of the usual concomitant coagulopathy of liver disease.

QUESTION 6 The large-volume paracentesis was completed without complications, and the patient tolerated the procedure well. You were able to remove 5 L of fluid that you sent for analysis. The cell count was normal, and the gram stain was negative. The patient is feeling and breathing much better and remains very stable for the next 24 hours. You are preparing to discharge the patient when the medical students ask you about liver transplantation for this patient. What are the indications and eligibility criteria for liver transplantation?

Orthotopic liver transplantation (OLT) has become routine therapy for advanced liver disease. This procedure has improved life expectancy, and most OLT recipients are able to return to work and have a relatively normal life. This success is due to

improvement in surgical technique, effective immunosuppressive therapy, and better guidelines regarding indications for transplantation. The most common indication for adult liver transplantation is end-stage cirrhosis. In evaluating a cirrhotic patient for liver transplantation, one should use the Child-Turcotte classification (Table 5-4-1). This classification uses albumin, bilirubin, control of ascites, degree of encephalopathy, and nutrition status to determine the patient's clinical condition. Worsening of the above parameters indicates clinical deterioration resulting in life-threatening events. Detection of such deterioration by the Child score is important in confirming candidacy for liver transplantation. Additional clinical events that may signal the need for transplantation include recurrent SBP, refractory variceal bleeding, hepatorenal syndrome, symptomatic coagulopathy, and the nonspecific but debilitating symptoms of fatigue and weakness. The above events are common to end-stage cirrhosis. Other more specific events that also signal the need for transplantation are progressive, severe bone disease, seen in primary biliary cirrhosis and primary sclerosing cholangitis, and recurrent bacterial cholangitis, often seen in patients with primary sclerosing cholangitis. The disease-specific indications for liver transplantation are acute liver failure, cirrhosis from previous alcohol abuse, cirrhosis from chronic hepatitis C, cryptogenic cirrhosis, primary biliary cirrhosis, cirrhosis from other viral hepatitis (B and D), primary sclerosing cholangitis, cirrhosis from autoim-

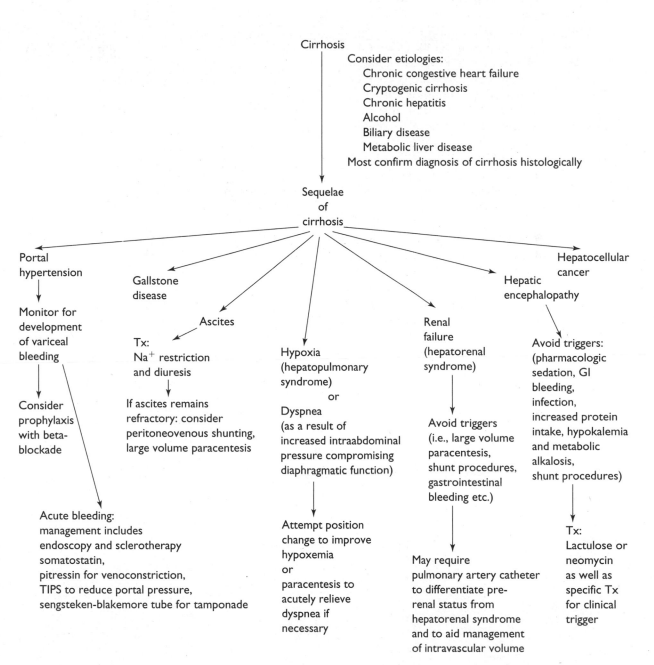

5-4-1 Complications of cirrhosis.

mune chronic active hepatitis, cirrhosis due to alpha-1-antitrypsin deficiency, Budd-Chiari syndrome, and hepatocellular carcinoma.

It is also important to consider other factors in determining candidacy for liver transplantation. The most common disease pre-OLT is alcoholic cirrhosis. Abstinence from alcohol is a requirement before consideration for liver transplantation. After transplant, patients need to be compliant with immunosuppressive medications. Patients must be emotionally capable to handle such a life-long commitment. Family support and adequate resources are also essential for successful liver transplantation.

CASE FOLLOW-UP   The patient was discharged 2 days after paracentesis with resolution of dyspnea. The patient was referred to a regional transplant center for evaluation and is currently on the waiting list for orthotopic liver transplantation.

• •

BIBLIOGRAPHY

Black M, Friedman AC: Ultrasound examination in the patient with ascites, *Ann Intern Med* 110(4):253-255, 1989(editorial).

Braunwald E, et al: *Harrison's principles of internal medicine*, ed 12, New York, 1993, McGraw-Hill.

Cotran RS, Kumar V, Robbins SL: *Robbins pathologic basis of disease*, ed 4, Philadelphia, 1989, WB Saunders.

Gines P, et al: Norfloxacin prevents spontaneous bacterial peritonitis recurrence in cirrhosis: results of a double-blind, placebo-controlled trial, *Hepatology* 12(4):717-723, 1990.

Gines P, et al: Paracentesis with intravenous infusion of albumin as compared with peritoneovenous shunting in cirrhosis with refractory ascites, *N Engl J Med* 325(12):830-842, 1991.

Gines P, et al: Randomized comparative study of therapeutic Paracentesis with and without intravenous albumin in cirrhosis, *Gastroenterology* 94:1493-1502, 1988.

Hoefs JC: Diagnostic paracentesis, a potent clinical tool, *Gastroenterology* 98:230-236, 1990.

Jensen DM: Portal-systemic encephalopathy and hepatic coma, *Med Clin North Am* 70(5):1081-1091, 1986.

Jensen DM, Payne JA: Patient selection for liver transplantation. In Williams JW, ed: *Hepatic transplantation*, Philadelphia, 1990, WB Saunders.

Kandel G, Diamant NE: A clinical view of recent advances in ascites, *J Clin Gastroenterol* 8(1):85-99, 1986.

Munoz SJ: Keeping current with the indications for liver transplantation, *Intern Med*, March 1994; 38.

Rikkers LF: Variceal hemorrhage, *Gastroenterol Clin North Am* 17(2):289-301, 1988.

Rossle M, et al: The transjugular intrahepatic portosystemic stent-shunt procedure for variceal bleeding, *N Engl J Med* 330(3): 165-171, 1994.

Runyon BA, Antillon MR, Montano AA: Effect of diuresis versus therapeutic paracentesis on ascitic fluid opsonic activity and serum complement, *Gastroenterology* 97:158-162, 1989.

Wilcox CM, Dismukes WE: Spontaneous bacterial peritonitis, a review of pathogenesis, diagnosis and treatment, *Medicine* 66(6):447-455, 1987.

Wyngaarden JB, Smith L, Bennett JC, eds: *Cecil, textbook of medicine*, ed 19, Philadelphia, 1992, WB Saunders.

CASE

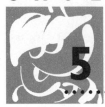

5

Panos Sechopoulos
Michael Brown
· · · · · · · · · · · ·

It is the first day of your gastroenterology rotation, and you are seeing patients in the outpatient clinic. There are four patients scheduled. The first patient is a 28-year-old white man diagnosed with AIDS 3 years ago. He was recently treated for pneumocystis pneumonia. He had been doing well until 1 week ago when he started to experience intermittent painful swallowing. His symptoms have progressively worsened, and he is now experiencing pain with every attempt to swallow solid food or liquids. He reports very poor oral intake with loss of 10 lbs. He denies fever and states that he has never had similar complaints in the past. His medications include Bactrim, AZT, and nystatin. His physical examination is unremarkable without oropharyngeal lesions.

QUESTION 1 What is your differential diagnosis for oral lesions that may present with dysphagia and/or odynophagia?

Dysphagia and odynophagia (Fig. 5-5-1 on p. 267) are common causes of poor oral intake in a patient with AIDS. A full physical examination should always start by examining the oral cavity. In AIDS patients, oral lesions may represent the initial manifestations of disease. The oral lesions are divided into fungal, bacterial, viral, neoplastic, and miscellaneous diseases including aphthous ulcers, idiopathic thrombocytopenic purpura, and xerostomia.

The term *thrush* describes white plaques on the oral mucosa. Fungal infection is most commonly due to Candida or, less often, *Torulopsis glabrata*. Diagnosis is made by visualizing hyphal elements after applying potassium hydroxide (KOH) to an oral smear. Treatment involves use of topical antifungal agents (nystatin, ketoconazole, or fluconazole).

Bacterial lesions usually manifest as gingivitis and/or periodontal disease. These lesions can be very troublesome since they may lead to complications including loose teeth and osteomyelitis. Treatment involves debridement and local antiseptic application.

Viral lesions are most commonly attributed to herpes simplex virus. This infection presents as small, painful vesicles that ulcerate. Diagnosis is made by culture or Tzanck smear. Treatment involves acyclovir. Resistant lesions may respond to Foscarnet. Another common viral oral lesion is oral hairy leukoplakia. This condition is asymptomatic and presents as white thickening on the tongue or oral mucosa. The etiology is Epstein-Barr virus. The treatment of this condition has been successful with high doses of oral acyclovir.

Aphthous ulcers are lesions of unknown etiology that are very bothersome and difficult to manage. These lesions present as recurrent crops of ulcers, approximately 1 cm in size. These lesions may affect the oral cavity as well as the esophagus, leading to odynophagia and poor oral intake. This is a diagnosis of exclusion. Management is aimed in providing symptom relief with topical steroids.

Neoplastic disorders that affect the oral cavity are rare but include Kaposi's sarcoma and lymphoma.

QUESTION 2 What lesions may be expected in the esophagus that present with similar complaints?

The patient previously described complained of dysphagia and odynophagia, two common complaints among AIDS patients (Fig. 5-5-2 on p.

268). Dysphagia refers to the difficulty swallowing solid or liquid foods, whereas odynophagia refers to painful swallowing. Both of these complaints are indicative of esophageal disease. The most common etiology of dysphagia in AIDS patients is Candida infection. The second most common fungal organism is *Torulopsis glabrata*. Esophageal candidiasis may be associated with oral thrush. Patients often do not experience odynophagia and cannot localize the level of the lesion in the esophagus. Diagnosis is made by barium contrast radiography that reveals an irregular mucosal texture corresponding to plaques with shallow ulcerations. Treatment is with ketoconazole 200 mg/day orally. The higher incidence of achlorhydria in AIDS patients may render ketoconazole less efficacious. Therefore, fluconazole is considered the first choice of therapy. Endoscopy is not necessary unless the patient fails oral antifungal treatment.

Odynophagia is more commonly seen with cytomeglovirus (CMV) and herpes esophagitis. CMV causes large ulcers (2 to 10 cm) with shallow ulceration. Diagnosis is made by endoscopy with biopsy revealing giant cells with viral inclusion bodies or via culture. Treatment with ganciclovir has been successful. However, there is a high relapse rate. Herpes simplex virus infection leads to esophageal ulcerations that are smaller but deeper. These lesions cause moderate dysphagia and severe odynophagia. The patient is often able to localize the affected level easily. These lesions may cause esophagospasm leading to substernal chest pain. Diagnosis is made by endoscopy and biopsy for viral cultures. Treatment with acyclovir 250 mg/m^2 IV q8h × 7 days is very successful, and recurrences are rare. Cryptosporidium is another infectious agent affecting the distal esophagus. Treatment with antiparasitic agents is recommended; however, responses are rare and the recurrence rate is high.

Other conditions affecting the esophagus leading to dysphagia and/or odynophagia and poor oral intake include dysmotility syndromes, achalasia, gastroesophageal reflux disease, malignancy, and strictures. AIDS patients have no increased predilection for these disorders; however, idiopathic ulcers often affect the esophagus, producing dysphagia and/or odynophagia. They are believed to be secondary to direct HIV injury. The management of these ulcers involves the use of steroids or thalidomide. These ulcerations should always be considered when evaluating the above symptoms in an AIDS patient.

Evaluation should consist of a thorough oropharyngeal examination and barium esophagram or upper endoscopy. The advantages of a radiologic study include lower cost, less risk to the patient and health worker; whereas endoscopy provides higher sensitivity, an opportunity to attain tissue for culture as well as better visualization of the upper gastrointestinal tract. Treatment is specific for each condition and should always be accompanied with nutritional supplementations as needed.

PATIENT SUMMARY   The patient described earlier had an upper endoscopy that revealed discrete large, shallow superficial ulcers in the midesophagus. Biopsies were obtained, and the rest of the exam was negative. The lesions observed were characteristic for CMV infection, and the patient was started on ganciclovir until tissue cultures confirmed the diagnosis.

• •

QUESTION 3   The next patient is a 34-year-old white man with AIDS diagnosed 10 years ago presenting with a 5-day history of jaundice, fever, and right upper quadrant pain. The patient has been unable to eat and has had one episode of vomiting. He denies coffee grounds emesis or hematemesis, diarrhea, melena, or previous similar symptoms. The physical examination reveals a thin male with icteric sclerae and right upper quadrant tenderness. Abdominal examination does not reveal rebound or guarding, and bowel sounds are hypoactive. The liver span is 10 cm without splenomegaly. Rectal examination revealed brown stool that was hemoccult negative. Laboratory evaluation revealed an alkaline phosphatase of 840 U, total bilirubin of 2.0 mg/dl, SGOT of 120 mg/dl and SGPT of 100 mg/dl.

What is your differential diagnosis, and how would you evaluate this patient?

The symptoms above fulfill Charcot's triad: right upper quadrant pain, fever, and jaundice (Fig. 5-5-3 on p. 270). Taken together with cholestatic lab values, this supports a suspicion of hepatobiliary disease. AIDS-related hepatobiliary disorders include acalculous cholecystitis, AIDS cholangiopathy, and neoplasia.

Acalculous cholecystitis is usually caused by infectious agents. The most common are *Cryptosporidium* and cytomegalovirus. AIDS cholangiopathy is a term used to include sclerosing cholangitis, papillary stenosis, or long extrahepatic bile duct strictures. While the underlying pathophysiology is not definitively known, there is suspicion of an infectious process producing ulceration with eventual scarring and obstruction. Neoplasms that most commonly affect the biliary tract include Kaposi's sarcoma and lymphoma. Both entities portend very poor prognosis. Non-AIDS-related processes should always be considered. These include gallstone disease, pancreatitis, hepatic abscess, viral or drug-induced hepatitis, and malignancy involving the biliary tract.

The evaluation of this patient includes a means of visualizing structures in the right upper quadrant. These include the gallbladder lumen, wall and pericholecystic region, the biliary ducts, pancreas, and liver. Both ultrasonography and CT scan are useful. If bile duct dilatation is found, the next step would be endoscopic retrograde cholangiopancreatography (ERCP). This allows direct visualization of tissue for culture and histologic examination and bile aspiration for culture and cytology. ERCP may also be used as a therapeutic tool to relieve obstruction by papillotomy or stent placement.

In cases of acalculous cholecystitis, ultrasound reveals thickening and edema of the gallbladder wall and dilatation of the common bile duct. If the diagnosis is delayed, potential complications include gallbladder perforation, abscess formation, fistulization, and peritonitis. Early surgical intervention is preferred treatment and carries excellent prognosis.

Pancreatic disease in the AIDS population should also be considered. In the AIDS population the most common etiology is an adverse drug effect. Dideoxyinosine (DDI) is the most common etiologic agent with a 25% incidence of pancreatitis. Other drugs include both Bactrim and pentamidine. The pancreas can be a recipient of infectious dissemination. Organisms most commonly seen include *Mycobacterium avium intracellulare,* CMV, and fungi. Neoplasm may also involve the pancreas, specifically Kaposi's sarcoma and lymphoma. The presentation of pancreatitis is similar to patients without AIDS. Iatrogenic causes of pancreatitis include long-term IV lipid infusion and ductal reflux after ERCP.

Hepatic parenchymal disease is common in HIV patients. Patients usually present with hepatomegaly, fever, abnormal liver function tests, and abdominal pain. Neoplasms involving the liver in AIDS patients include lymphoma and Kaposi's sarcoma. Skin lesions of Kaposi's sarcoma are usually present before GI involvement. Infection can also involve the liver parenchyma. *Mycobacterium avium intracellulare* leads to granulomatous hepatitis. Other agents include CMV, *Cryptococcus, Histoplasma, Entamoeba hystolytica, Pneumocystis carinii* and *Coccidioides.* Rickettsial infection of the liver results in peliosis hepatitis characterized by sinusoidal dilatation. Hepatitis B is usually mild or asymptomatic with persistent serological evidence for infection.

Drug-induced hepatitis is characterized by elevated aminotransferases and alkaline phosphatase. Common hepatotoxic drugs in the AIDS population include AZT, sulfonamides, antituberculous, antifungal, and antiprotozoal agents (including pentamidine).

Diagnosis of hepatic parenchymal disease is best made by liver biopsy. Special stains for organisms and evaluation for the presence of neoplastic cells should be sought before a diagnosis of drug-induced hepatotoxicity is accepted. Prognosis for intrahepatic disease is poor, and management is individualized to the specific disease.

PATIENT SUMMARY This patient had an abdominal ultrasound that revealed a thickened gallbladder wall with ductal dilatation. ERCP was performed and biopsy revealed cryptosporidium. The patient underwent laporoscopic cholecystectomy without complications and did well postoperatively.

• •

QUESTION 4 The next patient in your waiting room is a 28-year-old black man who has been HIV+ for 6 months without any AIDS-defining illness. He presents to the clinic feeling weak and unable to work. He has been on AZT and states he was doing very well until 2 days ago when he started feeling weak and experienced intermittent episodes of nausea. He denies abdominal pain and vomiting, but states he noticed black stools. There has been no blood per rectum and no diarrhea. His PMH is significant for HIV and also recurrent headache. The patient is evasive when asked about his alcohol intake but denies IV drug abuse or smoking. The physical examination was unremarkable except for slight nontender cervical lymphadenopathy. His rectal examination revealed melena without bright red blood. Laboratory evaluation was normal except for hemoglobin of 6 g/dl. What is the differential diagnosis of gastrointestinal bleeding in this patient?

Gastrointestinal bleeding is an unusual complaint in the HIV population. Non-AIDS-related diseases responsible for GI bleeding should always be considered and these include peptic ulcer disease, esophagitis, gastritis, Mallory-Weiss tears, varices, malignancy, diverticulosis, arteriovenous malformation, and hemorrhoids. Peptic ulcer disease however, is somewhat unusual in AIDS patients because of widespread hypochlorhydria in this population.

In AIDS patients the most common reason for upper gastrointestinal bleeding is gastric Kaposi's sarcoma followed by duodenal Kaposi's sarcoma and gastric lymphoma. Kaposi's sarcoma may involve stomach, colon, duodenum, and esophagus, in decreasing order of frequency. These lesions might become large and cause ulceration leading to bleeding, obstruction, or perforation. Cutaneous Kaposi's sarcoma lesions are present in 50% of patients with gastrointestinal Kaposi's sarcoma. Endoscopy confirms the diagnosis, and prognosis is poor. In immunocompetent hosts lymphomas are usually B-cell non-Hodgkin's type and involve the gastrum antrum. However, in HIV patients the lesions are more diffuse. Diagnosis is confirmed by endoscopy with biopsies.

Another cause of upper gastrointestinal tract bleeding in HIV patients is CMV esophagitis and gastritis. CMV is capable of producing deep ulceration that may result in massive hemorrhage. Additional infectious agents affecting the GI tract include Neisseria, Chlamydia, herpes simplex virus, and *Entamoeba histolytica*. Endoscopy, once again, is the best diagnostic test available. In addition, it is often therapeutic in acute gastrointestinal bleeding. Treatment is specific for each disease listed above.

PATIENT SUMMARY Because of the patient's anemia and severe weakness, you sent him directly to the emergency room (ER). In the emergency room, nasogastric tube lavage revealed large blood clots with no bright red blood present. Two IV lines were started and intravenous fluids were administered along with an H_2 blocker. After being typed and crossed the patient was transfused two units of packed red blood cells. The patient was kept NPO and had an endoscopic gastroduodenoscopy (EGD) that revealed erosive gastritis with stigmata of recent hemorrhage but no active bleeding. Biopsies were obtained, and the rest of the exam was unremarkable. After the procedure the patient was questioned again and admitted to recent intermittent headaches that he "treated" with ibuprofen and heavy alcohol intake. Biopsy results were negative and based on the additional history, diagnosis of erosive gastritis secondary to NSAIDS and/or alcohol was made. The patient was continued on H_2 blocker, and his hemoglobin remained stable. He was discharged after a couple of days feeling well on oral H_2 blocker. This case was selected to emphasize that non-HIV-related diseases should always be considered when evaluating an HIV-infected patient.

QUESTION 5 Your last patient of the day is a 20-year-old black man with a history of AIDS, pneumocystis pneumonia, CMV esophagitis, and retinitis who presents to your office complaining of diarrhea. The patient states he had been feeling well until the recent onset of fatigue and 8-lb weight loss. He has concurrently developed watery continuous diarrhea. He occasionally experiences periumbilical abdominal pain but denies fever, nausea, vomiting, blood per rectum, or melena. He describes his diarrhea as large volume, watery with no blood or blood clots and states that he has had over 10 bowel movements per day. He states he has not experienced similar episodes in the past and denies recent travel history or change in diet. Imodium provided no relief. His current medications include AZT, oral Bactrim, and ganciclovir. He is homosexual and denies alcohol or IV drug abuse. Physical examination reveals a thin ill-appearing male with temporal wasting. His examination is unremarkable and rectal examination is normal with brown stool, hemoccult negative. What is your differential diagnosis of noninfectious etiologies for diarrhea in this patient?

Early during the epidemic of AIDS the intestinal tract and rectum were known to be common sites of infection among the homosexual population. The "Gay Bowel syndrome" refers to intestinal or perirectal infections caused by sexually transmitted pathogens (e.g., Chlamydia, Neisseria, *Treponema pallidum,* herpes simplex virus) and also the common enteric pathogens (e.g., Campylobacter and Shigella). This syndrome was attributed to sexual practices among homosexual men before the AIDS epidemic.

The immunocompromised status in AIDS allows for a wide variety of opportunistic pathogens to infect the GI tract. Diarrhea has always been a common complaint among AIDS patients with an incidence of 30% to 60%. Small bowel infections/lesions are characterized by crampy, periumbilical abdominal pain with large volume diarrhea and weight loss. Colitic diarrhea, on the other hand, tends to be associated with frequent small volume stools, and pain is usually localized to the left lower quadrant and associated with rectal ur-

gency and sometimes painful defecation and bright red blood.

Noninfectious etiologies of diarrhea are unusual. The noninfectious causes are limited to neoplasms that include Kaposi's sarcoma, non-Hodgkin's lymphoma, cloacogenic carcinoma of the rectum, and squamous cell cancer of the anus/rectum. Each presentation may be variable, but diarrhea can be a presenting symptom. Other noninfectious causes of diarrhea in AIDS patients include medications, especially dideoxyinosine, and also AIDS enteropathy. AIDS enteropathy refers to a condition associated with morphologic alterations, blunted villi with low mitotic figures, in the small intestine without evidence of infection. Exact cause is unknown but believed to be secondary to direct invasion by the human immunodeficiency virus or increases in VIP or its receptor activity. Diagnosis is made by excluding infection and small bowel biopsy. Steatorrhea indicates malabsorption consistent with this condition. Treatment of AIDS enteropathy is mainly supportive.

QUESTION 6 What infectious agents should be considered as possible causes of diarrhea in this patient?

The infectious agents that affect the intestinal tract are divided into parasites, bacteria, viruses, and fungi. The most common organisms are *Cryptosporidium,* CMV, *Clostridium difficile,* MAC and *Isospora belli. Salmonella, Campylobacter,* fungi, *E. histolytica,* and *Giardia lamblia* are more unusual causes. The role of microsporidium as a pathogen is now controversial.

Cryptosporidium is a parasite transmitted via the fecal-oral route with ingestion of oocysts affecting the jejunum, colon, and biliary tract. Clinically, patients experience large volume, watery, profuse diarrhea, and malabsorption. Laboratory values are not helpful since peripheral and fecal white blood cells are usually not elevated. Stools may demonstrate oocysts, and ELISA (enzyme-linked immunoabsorbent assay), IFA (indirect fluorescent antibody), or acid-fast stains studies confirm the diagnosis. Treatment is supportive and emphasis should be placed on adequate nutrition and fluid repletion.

Isospora belli is another parasite transmitted via the fecal-oral route. This organism affects the small intestine and causes mucosal inflammation and villous atrophy. Clinically the disease presents as protracted diarrhea, colicky abdominal pain, flatulence, malabsorption, and fever. Diagnosis is made by multiple stool studies for parasites, and jejunal biopsy is confirmatory. Treatment with Bactrim yields good results; however, relapses are common.

E. histolytica only rarely affects AIDS patients. The mode of transmission is by direct ingestion of the cyst through oral or anal sexual practices. Clinically, patients present with bloody diarrhea, tenesmus (pain with defecation), and crampy abdominal pain. This organism is also responsible for extraintestinal manifestations, most commonly, liver abscess. Diagnosis is confirmed by stool studies revealing the parasite. Acute intestinal amebiasis is treated with metronidazole, while treatment of benign cyst carriers is with Iodoquinol.

Giardia lamblia is one of the major parasitic causes for diarrhea in the United States and a frequent cause of the "Gay Bowel syndrome" and traveler's diarrhea. This organism is transmitted via contaminated water as well as person to person. The clinical symptoms of this disease include abdominal pain, flatulence, non-bloody diarrhea, and weight loss. Diagnosis, once again, is made by identification of the parasite in the stool or in jejunal biopsy. Treatment with Quinacrine has proven to be slightly more effective than treatment with metronidazole.

The last protozoan organism affecting the intestinal tract leading to diarrhea is Microsporidium. This is an intracellular parasite with small unicellular spores which cannot be seen on stool examination by light microscopy but requires careful high power histologic examination or electron microscopy for visualization. In AIDS patients the specific microsporidial organism responsible is *Enterocytozoan bieneusi*. Clinically, patients present with malabsorption, wasting, and foul-smelling,

chronic diarrhea. Management is mostly supportive and includes the use of antimotility agents such as opiates. Lately, the exact role of Microsporidium as a pathogen has been questioned due to its high prevalence in AIDS patients without diarrhea.

Bacterial infections affect immunocompetent hosts and only recently have they been recognized as important pathogens in AIDS patients. The presence of achlorhydria is a risk factor for bacterial infection. The clinical presentation is very similar for all bacterial infections affecting the GI tract including abdominal pain, distension, fever and, ileocolitis. The common bacterial pathogens are *Salmonella, Shigella, Campylobacter* and *Clostridium difficile*. These agents are associated with severe diarrhea and colitis in AIDS patients. *Salmonella* bacteremia is common and represents an AIDS defining illness. Diagnosis is made by identifying the organism in stool studies. Therapy with Bactrim, third generation cephalosporins, and quinolones has been successful. *Shigella* may respond well to fluoroquinolone therapy.

Clostridium difficile is a common bacterial infection affecting AIDS patients and is associated with antibiotic use. Diagnosis is made by the presence of *C. difficile* toxin in the stool. Therapy includes the use of oral metronidazole or vancomycin.

Chlamydia trachomatis is a bacterium known to colonize the rectum and urethra of male homosexuals. HIV patients are more susceptible to chlamydia and other sexually transmitted diseases and may be responsible for causing diarrhea. Treatment with tetracycline or erythromycin needs to be initiated, and long-term therapy is required.

Mycobacterium avium complex (MAC) is the most common atypical mycobacterium in AIDS patients and can also lead to intestinal disease. The route of infection is via ingestion of contaminated water. These organisms are ingested by macrophages and cause a malabsorption syndrome, exudative enteropathy, and thickening of the bowel wall. Clinical manifestations of the infection include fever, progressive wasting, and diarrhea (foul-smelling). Diagnosis is made by cul-

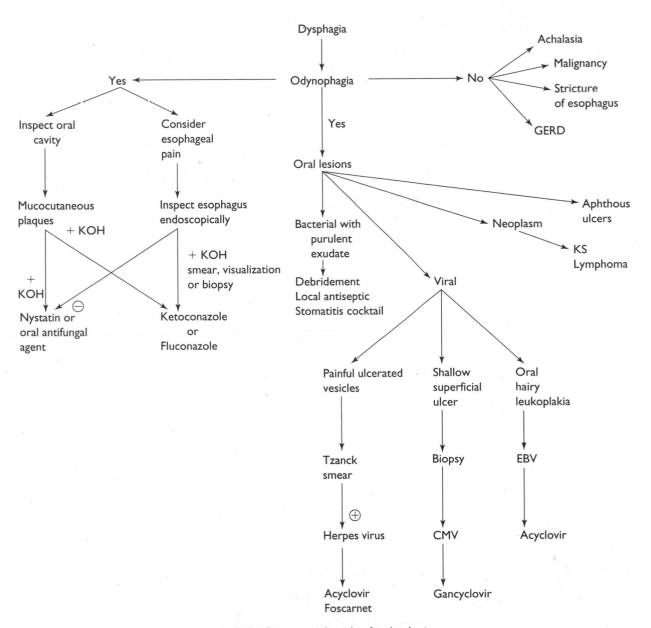

5-5-1   Diagnostic algorithm for dysphagia.

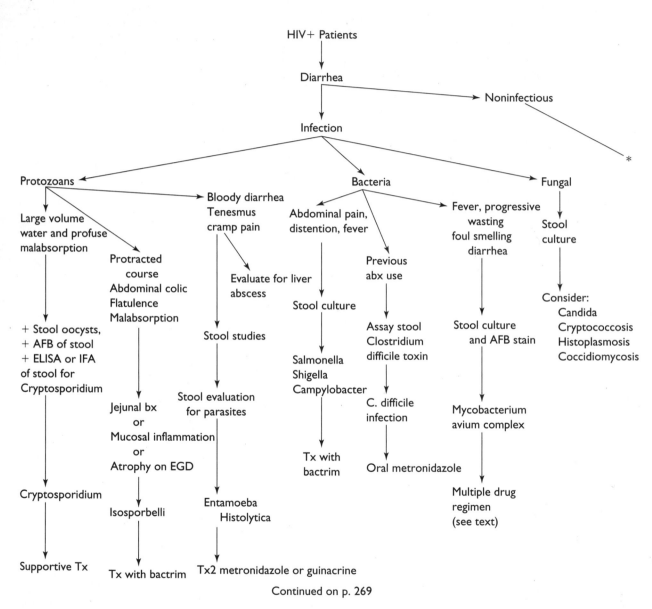

5-5-2 Diagnostic algorithm for AIDS patients.

Continued on p. 269

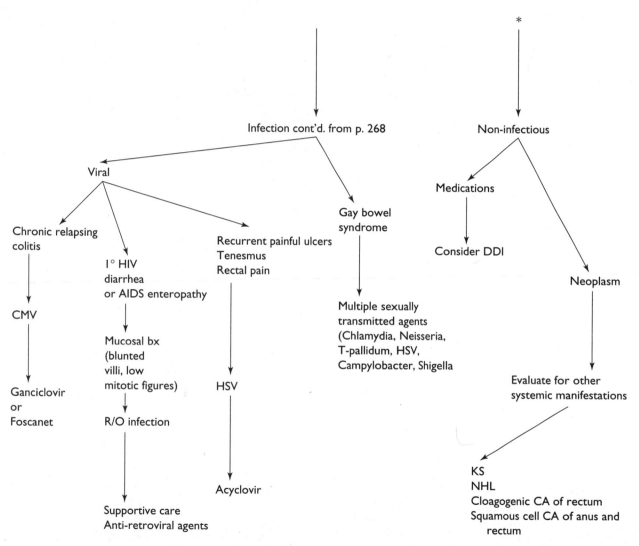

5-5-2 Cont'd.

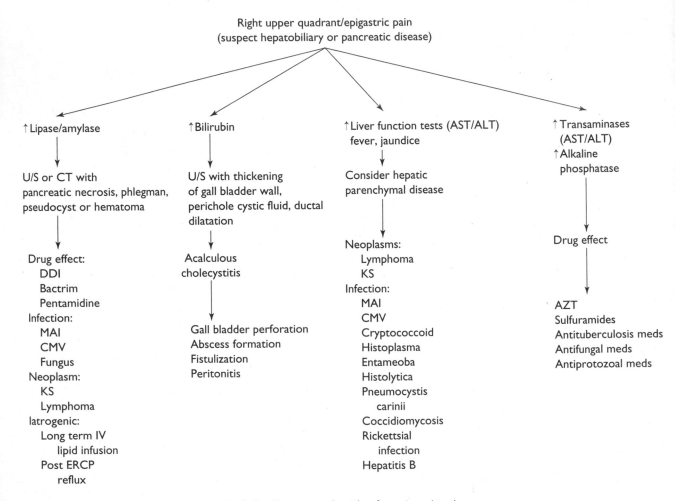

5-5-3   Diagnostic algorithm for epigastric pain.

tures and specific stains. Management is difficult and includes the use of multiple drugs such as rifampin, amikacin, ethambutol, ciprofloxacin, cycloserine, ethinonamide, streptomycin, and pyrazinamide. Treatment improves symptoms; however, long-term survival is not affected.

Viral causes of diarrhea in HIV patients are very important. CMV causes ulcerative lesions in the rectosigmoid area. The organism can be isolated in specimens obtained during endoscopy. CMV is responsible for chronic relapsing colitis leading to diarrhea. Treatment involves the use of ganciclovir or foscarnet. Herpes simplex virus commonly affects the anorectal area causing recurrent painful ulcers. HSV causes shallow ulceration, tenesmus, local pain, and rectal discharge. Treatment of the ulceration involves the use of oral or parenteral acyclovir since topical use of this agent has proven to be ineffective. HIV is also responsible for affecting the gastrointestinal tract and causing mucosal inflammation. The exact mechanism of action is unknown, and no effective treatment has been established.

Fungal infections are usually severe, necessitating rapid diagnosis and initiation of treatment. Candida infection is the most common, but others

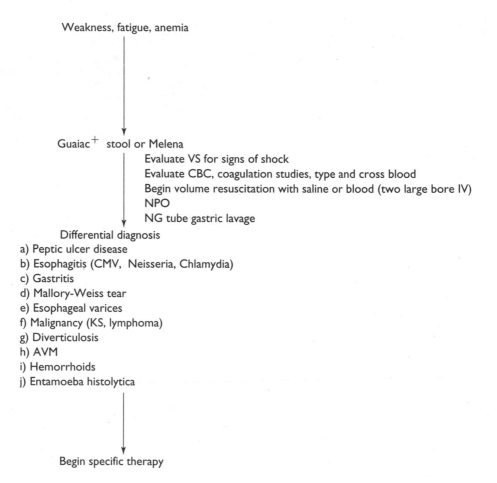

Weakness, fatigue, anemia

Guaiac$^+$ stool or Melena

    Evaluate VS for signs of shock
    Evaluate CBC, coagulation studies, type and cross blood
    Begin volume resuscitation with saline or blood (two large bore IV)
    NPO
    NG tube gastric lavage

Differential diagnosis
a) Peptic ulcer disease
b) Esophagitis (CMV, Neisseria, Chlamydia)
c) Gastritis
d) Mallory-Weiss tear
e) Esophageal varices
f) Malignancy (KS, lymphoma)
g) Diverticulosis
h) AVM
i) Hemorrhoids
j) Entamoeba histolytica

Begin specific therapy

5-5-4 Diagnostic algorithm for weakness, fatigue, and anemia.

include *Cryptococcus, Histoplasma,* and *Coccidioides.* Travel history to endemic areas is very important when considering fungal agents. Fungal infection manifests as a febrile illness with constitutional symptoms. Diagnosis is made by culture, and treatment involves the use of appropriate antifungal agents.

PATIENT SUMMARY The patient described had multiple stool studies looking for enteric pathogens, ova and parasites, and *C. difficile* toxin. He was admitted to the hospital for intravenous fluids and nutritional support. The patient continued to experience diarrhea but felt better once hydrated. Stool studies were positive for *Clostridium difficile* toxin.

He experienced immediate improvement on metronidazole therapy. The patient's diet was advanced as tolerated, and he was discharged in a stable condition to complete a 14-day course of oral metronidazole. A diagnostic algorithm for weakness, fatigue, and anemia is shown in Fig. 5-5-4.

• •

BIBLIOGRAPHY

Anthony MA, Brandt LJ, Klein RS, et al: Infectious diarrhea, *Dig Dis Sci* 33:1141-1146, 1988.
Cello JP: Acquired immunodeficiency syndrome cholangiopathy: spectrum of disease, *Am J Med* 86:539-546, 1989.

Edison SA, Kotler DP: How HIV infection and AIDS affect the gastrointestinal tract, *Critical Illness* 7(1):37-56, 1992.

Raufman JD: Odynophagia/dysphagia in AIDS, *Gastroenterol Clin North Am* 7(3):599-613, 1993.

Rodgers VD, Kasnoff MF: Gastrointestinal manifestations of the acquired immunodeficiency syndrome, *Western J Med* 146:52, 1987.

Sievert W, Merrell RC: Gastrointestinal emergencies in the acquired immunodeficiency syndrome, *Gastroenterol Clin North Am* 17:409-417, 1988.

Tanowitz HB, Simon D, Wittner M: Gastrointestinal manifestations: medical management of AIDS patients, *Med Clin North Am* 76(1):45-62, 1992.

Weber J: Gastrointestinal disease in AIDS, *Clin Immunol Allergy* 6:517-530, 1986.

C A S E

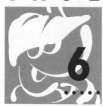

6 Karen S. Sable
Michael Brown
. . . .

A *42-year-old woman presents with a chief complaint of "food seems to stick when I swallow" and points to her upper sternum. Over the last several years she has progressively noticed a full sensation with eating and more recently appreciates a sticking sensation. She states that solids cause more symptoms than liquids. If she repeatedly swallows or straightens her back, the sensation is somewhat relieved. She has regurgitated food and noticed that cold liquids are more difficult to swallow. Because of the discomfort she has decreased her oral intake and lost 5 lbs over the last 3 months. She has been awakened at night with coughing spells. She denies nausea, vomiting, hematemesis, pyrosis, halitosis, food impaction, abdominal pain, or change in her bowel habits.*

Her past medical history is significant for two uneventful cesarean sections. She had an episode of pneumonia 6 months ago. She has no known allergies and no significant travel history. Her family history is remarkable for diabetes, CVA, and lung cancer. The patient has a 10-year history of cigarette smoking and consumes alcohol infrequently. She takes a multivitamin and ibuprofen periodically. Review of systems was significant for the absence of Raynaud's phenomenon, arthritis, skin lesions, neurologic diseases, caustic ingestion, diabetes, and lung disease.

QUESTION I What are the important unique anatomical features of the esophagus? Based on the patient's history and examination, create a differential diagnosis for the chief complaint.

The recognition of bolus arrest during swallowing, even if transient, indicates esophageal dys-

function. The patient may describe this sensation as food or liquid "sticking," "getting caught" or "hesitating" while they swallow. A special type of dysphagia that occurs when the bolus cannot be propelled from the mouth into the oropharynx, "transfer" or oropharyngeal dysphagia, is seen in neurologic disease or pharyngeal muscle weakness and must be differentiated from esophageal dysphagia. When one evaluates esophageal dysphagia, it is important to differentiate between symptoms related to solids or liquids, time course, progression of symptoms, chest pain, heartburn, and weight loss.

Esophageal dysphagia is produced by two different processes: mechanical narrowing or motor disorders.

STRUCTURAL/MECHANICAL OBSTRUCTIONS

- Esophageal carcinoma
- Gastric carcinoma
- Schatzki's ring
- Esophageal web
- Peptic stricture
- Diverticula
- Pseudoachalasia

MOTOR DISORDERS

- Nutcracker esophagus
- Diffuse esophageal spasm
- Esophagitis/GERD
- Collagen vascular disease/scleroderma
- Endocrine disorders
- Amyloidosis
- Chagas' disease
- Achalasia/pseudoachalasia

Mechanical narrowing may be due to tumors (esophageal carcinoma, gastric cardia tumors, infiltrating extraluminal tumors such as breast cancer), peptic or caustic strictures, esophageal rings or webs, Zenker's diverticula, or inflammatory disease. Mechanical dysphagia is caused by a structural obstruction and usually occurs with solids, unless the lumen is severely narrowed. The clinical course may be progressive or sudden. Patients with underlying malignancies may also experience weight loss. Other symptoms may include regurgitation, chest discomfort, or pulmonary complications (i.e., aspiration pneumonia).

Motor disorders which may produce dysphagia include Nutcracker esophagus, diffuse esophageal spasm, gastroesophageal reflux disease, collagen vascular disease (scleroderma, polymyositis), the consequences of endocrine disorders (hyperthyroidism, goiter, diabetes mellitus), amyloidosis, intestinal pseudoobstruction, Chagas' disease (*Trypanosoma cruzi* infection) and achalasia. Esophageal spasm and nonspecific esophageal motility dysfunction are usually associated with noncardiac chest pain although dysphagia may be a component of the presentation. Dysphagia associated with motor disorders is usually associated with liquids and solids. Cold liquids may trigger symptoms. Patients often are able to pass the retained bolus by repeated swallowing or changing their position. The clinical course is usually very gradual. There is some overlap in these categories. It is thought that a component of esophagitis is related to abnormal esophageal motility. Esophagitis can result in a peptic stricture and the patients' symptoms can then be associated to the mechanical obstruction. Similarly, esophageal diverticula have been associated with motor abnormalities of the esophagus.

QUESTION 2 For the mechanical disorders listed in the differential diagnosis, what are their pathophysiology, diagnosis, and treatment?

Gastroesophageal reflux disease (GERD) occurs when the balance between natural defenses in the esophagus (such as acid clearance, mucosal resistance) is overwhelmed by aggressive forces (such as acid flux, potency of refluxate, and local irritants). Esophagitis occurs when the epithelium becomes damaged by gastroesophageal reflux of predominantly acid and pepsin. This is thought to occur because of disruption of esophageal clearance by abnormal motility, alteration in the lower esophageal sphincter function, and abnormal cytoprotection at the epithelial level. Thus, GERD may begin as a motility disorder but may become a structural abnormality. In addition to experiencing heartburn (pyrosis), patients with GERD may experience extra-intestinal manifestations such as cough, asthma, pneumonitis, or laryngitis. Reflux disease may be detected on barium radiography, endoscopically if esophagitis is present, or confirmed by Bernstein acid perfusion test (exposure of the esophagus to acid to note recreation of symptoms). Ambulatory pH monitoring is generally accepted as the "gold standard" for identification of reflux. Therapy includes antireflux lifestyle modifications, high dose H_2 blockers, proton pump inhibitors, prokinetic agents, sucralfate, and antacids. Refractory patients may require antireflux surgery, the most common being the Nissen fundoplication which may be performed laprascopically.

Peptic stricture, pseudodiverticula, scar formation, and Barrett's esophagus result from the repair process following inflammation. Barrett's esophagus is a premalignant condition where specialized columnar epithelium replaces the stratified squamous mucosa that is normally present. Patients will need acid suppression therapy if inflammation is present and careful endoscopic follow-up as there is a 30- to 50-fold increase in the risk of esophageal adenocarcinoma occurring in this tissue. Peptic strictures may be found in a setting of peptic disease with or without Barrett's esophagus. The esophageal narrowing may be dramatically relieved by mechanical dilation; however, there is a high rate of restricturing requiring repeat dilatations.

Esophagitis may occur in patients taking oral medications, chemotherapy, or undergoing radiation treatments. Antibiotics, potassium, and quinidine account for 90% of reported cases. Tetracycline, aspirin, and iron salts cause damage because of their acidity. Others like quinidine have neutral pH but can cause severe injury. Caustic ingestions of strong alkaline (lye) or acidic agents may also result in intense esophageal inflammation with the potential for stricturing in approximately 15% to 25% of exposures.

Infectious processes may result in esophagitis and are most common in immunosuppressed individuals. Patients with AIDS, leukemia, lymphoma (especially after chemotherapy), congenital immunodeficiency syndromes, and endocrine disorders (diabetes, adrenal insufficiency) are predisposed to fungal infections of the esophagus. Patients on immunosuppressive medications or with conditions that predispose to stasis (achalasia, scleroderma) may also develop Candida esophagitis. Similarly, viral infections due to herpes simplex virus, CMV or varicella zoster may cause ulcerative esophagitis in immunosuppressed patients.

Esophageal carcinoma is one of the most lethal of all cancers. Epidemiologic studies suggest that squamous cell carcinoma of the esophagus may be related to the ingestion of tobacco, alcohol, nitrosamine, Candida infections, aflatoxin, deficiencies in riboflavin and vitamin A. There appears to be a definite relationship between esophageal carcinoma and other medical conditions like corrosive injury (such as lye) of the esophagus, iron deficiency in the Plummer-Vinson syndrome (Paterson-Kelly), Tylosis (hyperkeratosis of the palms and soles with autosomal dominant inheritance with 100% developing esophageal carcinoma), thyroid disease, and achalasia.

Squamous cell carcinoma of the esophagus most frequently develops in the midthoracic segment and tends to extensively invade before producing symptoms such as dysphagia. Lymph nodes are often involved at the time of diagnosis. Dysphagia is the classic symptom of the obstruction caused by esophageal carcinoma. The presence of dysphagia indicates extensive involvement, and the disease is incurable in most patients at presentation. Most patients have sustained weight loss because of decreased caloric intake and tumor cachexia. Hiccups may signal transmu-

ral invasion of the cancer with diaphragmatic or phrenic nerve involvement. Anemia and hemoccult positive stools may be present. Because the esophagus has no serosa, the tumor easily invades adjoining tissues, which may lead to an esophagopulmonary fistula with aspiration pneumonia or unexplained cough.

Diagnosis is often made endoscopically with biopsy and brushing. Double contrast barium radiography may be used to reveal nodularity, an abrupt luminal angulation, or shelving as well as to determine the length of the lesion. CT scan, endoscopic ultrasound, and laparoscopy are useful in staging the extent of invasion. The 5-year survival is 3% to 20%, regardless of the therapeutic course chosen. Surgery, radiation, and chemotherapy are often used to attempt a cure. Esophageal prostheses, laser, alcohol injection, and coagulation probes provide some palliation of symptoms.

Esophageal rings (thick structures composed of mucosa and muscle) and webs (thin structures composed of mucosa and submucosa) may manifest with intermittent, transient dysphagia. The classic Schatzki's ring may actually be classified as a web and usually presents with intermittent dysphagia. Patients have often consumed meat or bread just before the episode of dysphagia and may be able to regurgitate the offending bolus. Diagnosis may be made by barium radiography but usually requires the use of maneuvers such as valsalva or a barium marshmallow to visualize the ring. These rings are thin (several millimeters) and are located in the distal esophagus just above a hiatal hernia. Schatzki's rings are thought to occur because of reflux esophagitis. The ring may be disrupted endoscopically by bougienage with large dilators.

Esophageal webs may occur throughout the esophagus. When they are in the anterior cervical esophagus in patients with iron deficiency anemia, cheilosis and glossitis, a diagnosis of Plummer-Vinson syndrome (also called Paterson-Kelly) is made. This syndrome is associated with postcricoid carcinoma that may develop many years later. Barium radiography often with cineradiography is used to visualize these structures. The etiology of dysphagia may be related to a myopathy produced by iron deficiency, because iron therapy may relieve the dysphagia even when webs are still visible radiographically. Other upper esophageal webs occur that are not associated with iron deficiency. Some may be congenital, and others may arise in conditions such as graft versus host disease and dystrophic epidermolysis bullosa. Esophageal webs may occur elsewhere in the esophagus, and when located distally may be difficult to differentiate from the Schatzki's ring.

Esophageal diverticula may present with transient dysphagia and regurgitation. These may occur (1) immediately above the upper esophageal sphincter (Zenker's diverticulum), (2) near the midpoint of the esophagus (traction diverticulum), and (3) just above the lower esophageal sphincter (epiphrenic diverticulum). The midesophageal traction diverticulum is thought to result from extraluminal inflammation and scarring, which may produce motor abnormalities in this segment. Zenker's and epiphrenic diverticula are thought to be produced as a consequence of motor abnormalities, including incoordination of sphincter relaxation. Barium radiography will localize these outpouchings but may require rotating the patient so the column of barium does not obscure his visualization. The main method of treatment for Zenker's diverticulum is surgical with excision of the diverticulum and cricopharyngeal myotomy. More recently, endoscopic revisions have been reported with some success. Midesophageal and epiphrenic diverticulae are in a location where surgical intervention has significant morbidity and mortality. Simple myotomy may provide some relief.

QUESTION 3   For the motor disorders listed in the differential diagnosis, what are each disease's pathophysiology, diagnosis, and treatment?

Diffuse esophageal spasm, Nutcracker esophagus, hypertensive LES, and other nonspecific motility disorders comprise a group of esophageal motility disorders that are difficult to describe and characterize. Difficulty arises because of the overlap between these conditions as well as a lack of consensus in nomenclature.

Patients with abnormal esophageal motility because of these "spastic" disorders may present with dysphagia and noncardiac chest pain. Often these symptoms are intermittent. Most patients are approximately 40 years old and predominantly female. There is no known consistent pathologic change or anatomic abnormality. Barium esophogram may reveal dysmotility, "corkscrew esophagus," hiatal hernia, and reflux. Endoscopy reveals an essentially normal study. Esophageal manometry demonstrates various disturbances. During esophageal manometry patients with diffuse esophageal spasm may exhibit simultaneous contractions (nonperistaltic responses following >30% of swallows) and intermittent normal peristalsis. These simultaneous contractions occur at the distal esophagus and may be repetitive with increased amplitude or durations and may also exhibit incomplete LES relaxation. In Nutcracker esophagus there is normal peristalsis, but the waveform has an abnormally increased amplitude in the distal esophagus. Patients with hypertensive LES have normal peristalsis although the amplitude may be normal or increased.

Although symptoms may be difficult to control, patients with esophageal motility disorders do well, and their condition is not progressive. Therapy is aimed at normalizing the motility pattern. Nitrates and calcium channel blockers have potential benefits and may alter smooth muscle contraction. Antidepressants and psychotropic medications have also been employed. It is unclear if these medications alter esophageal function or the patient's perception of discomfort. Rare patients with incomplete relaxation of the LES may require dilation.

Esophageal involvement is seen in many (75% to 85%) patients with scleroderma. Patients describe heartburn and dysphagia. These patients have a significant motor disorder that may be due to fibrosis and muscle atrophy. Manometry often shows hypotension of the lower sphincter and aperistalsis of the distal (smooth muscle region) esophagus. Radiographic examination characteristically shows a dilated, aperistaltic segment of the distal esophagus with patulous gastroesophageal junction. Erosive esophagitis is seen in more than half of these patients, and thus therapy is directed to GERD in these patients. Other connective tissue diseases such as the CREST syndrome, dermatomyositis, polymyositis, and mixed connective tissue disease may present with similar findings. These patients will often experience Raynaud's phenomenon.

Achalasia was the first motility disorder clinically characterized. It is typified by aperistalsis of the esophagus and abnormal lower esophageal sphincter (LES) hypertension that creates resistance to the normal flow of solids and liquids. The majority of patients presenting with achalasia are between the ages of 25 and 60. Nearly all describe dysphagia to solids with the great majority also experiencing dysphagia to liquids. The onset of symptoms is gradual, and patients may describe vague symptoms of dysphagia, regurgitation, and chest pain for several years before diagnosis. Weight loss is common and usually increases with duration of the disease. Patients are often able to perform specific maneuvers to improve esophageal emptying, such as raising their arms and straightening their back, which increases intraesophageal pressure and improves emptying.

Abnormalities in both nerve and muscle can be detected in achalasia, although a neural lesion is thought to be the primary disorder. Neuroanatomic abnormalities have been found, including loss of ganglion cells within Auerbach's plexus, degeneration of the vagus nerve, and abnormalities on the dorsal motor nucleus of the vagus. Inflammatory cell infiltrates and decreased vasoactive intestinal peptide (VIP) have also been described. Decreased VIP may contribute to incomplete relaxation of LES characteristic in achalasia.

Diagnosis is suggested clinically. Radiographic studies done early in the disease may be essentially normal and only later reveal a dilated esophagus with tapering of the lumen at the level of the nonrelaxing LES. This smoothly tapered region is commonly called a "bird's beak." The more proximal striated muscle portion of the esophagus is often less dilated than the distal smooth muscle portions.

Endoscopy should always be performed even with classic x-ray and manometric findings to exclude diseases that mimic achalasia (pseudoachalasia) and to evaluate the esophageal mucosa before instituting therapy. The esophagogastric junction must be carefully examined to exclude the presence of a neoplasm. The most common malignancies producing pseudoachalasia are gastric adenocarcinoma (>65%), esophageal squamous cell, lymphoma, lung cancer, and pancreatic tumors. These may invade the esophageal wall without disturbing the luminal mucosa, making endoscopic detection difficult and necessitating other imaging studies. Other disorders that may produce pseudoachalasia include Chagas' disease (infection by the parasite *Trypanosoma cruzi* that damages the neural plexus of the esophagus and other organs and is endemic to South America, especially Brazil), chronic idiopathic intestinal pseudoobstruction, amyloidosis, sarcoidosis, postvagotomy syndromes, and multiple endocrine neoplasia (IIb).

Manometry is important in establishing the diagnosis of achalasia. Classically, there is aperistalsis in the distal esophagus. If waves are measured, they are simultaneous and low amplitude. The lower esophageal sphincter does not relax completely after swallowing. Although not required for the diagnosis, LES pressure may be elevated, and the esophageal baseline pressure may be greater than the gastric pressure.

The neural lesion in achalasia cannot be reversed medically. Treatment is directed towards palliation of symptoms and avoidance of complications. Pharmacotherapy aimed at smooth muscle relaxation includes nitrates, calcium channel blockers, anticholinergic agents, and hydralazine, with varying results. Pneumatic and hydrostatic dilators have been successfully employed and provide symptomatic relief in more than 60% of patients. Patients who fail to improve may undergo esophagomyotomy to disrupt the LES. Recent studies are exploring the use of Botulism toxin injections at the LES as therapy. The most common postoperative complication is esophageal reflux. There is an increased incidence of Candida esophagitis and esophageal carcinoma in patients with achalasia. This risk may be decreased by therapy, which relieves the obstruction and stasis.

QUESTION 4   On physical examination she was a well-developed female with normal vital signs. There was no temporal wasting. She had several white plaques in her posterior oropharynx, good dentition, no lymphadenopathy, or thyromegaly. Her lung, cardiac, and abdominal examination were unremarkable. Rectal examination was normal with guaiac-negative formed brown stool. Her extremities were without nail changes, telangiectasia, or skin lesions. Her neurologic examination was normal.

Laboratory findings included a normal CBC and general chemistries. Her internist ordered a chest x-ray that revealed normal lung fields and an air-fluid level in the midesophagus.

Given the preceding differential diagnosis and laboratory evaluation, analyze the patient's presentation and reevaluate the components of the differential as to their likelihood. What further diagnostic test would you order at this time?

A careful history is necessary in evaluating patients with dysphagia. Our patient presents with esophageal dysphagia for solids and liquids. Her dentition is good. Typically, cold liquids precipitate symptoms in patients with motility disorders, and patient maneuvers may relieve the sticking sensation. The patient's symptoms seem to be very slowly progressive with only recent slight weight loss. Each of these findings is suggestive of a motility disorder. The patient's symptoms are constant and progressive, which helps guide us toward achalasia as the diagnosis. Patients with diffuse esophageal spasm or Nutcracker esophagus have recurring episodes as opposed to constant, progressive symptoms. Pa-

tients with scleroderma typically describe heartburn because of the loss of lower sphincter competency, whereas patients with achalasia do not usually experience heartburn. In this group of patients endoscopy and radiography are important to rule out mucosal pathology, but esophageal manometry secures the diagnosis by revealing a typical motility pattern.

If our patients presented with dysphagia to solids alone or clearly preceding dysphagia to liquids, a mechanical stricture would have been higher on the differential. Dysphagia that is intermittent or sudden onset would have suggested an esophageal ring, web, or spastic motor disorder. A thorough review of medications, therapies, or prior ingestions is necessary to rule out caustic esophagitis with lumenal compromise. Our patient consumed a nonsteroidal anti-inflammatory agent that may predispose to gastrointestinal inflammation and ulceration. The patient's smoking history is a risk factor for esophageal carcinoma. Endoscopy and radiography usually provide the diagnosis in these structural lesions.

Physical examination and laboratory studies also aid in narrowing the differential diagnosis. Significant weight loss early in the presentation of dysphagia, anemia, or guaiac-positive stools presents more concern for a malignancy with a primary esophageal carcinoma or a lesion presenting as pseudoachalasia. Collagen vascular diseases may have esophageal motor abnormalities, and patients may present with telangiectasia, scleroderma or Raynaud's phenomenon. Nail changes (brittle nails and koilonychia) are seen in Plummer-Vinson syndrome. Our patient had none of these findings but did describe some pulmonary symptoms. Pulmonary complications may be seen in gastroesophageal reflux disease or achalasia, as regurgitated or refluxed material may cause laryngitis, nocturnal coughing, asthmatic episodes, and even aspiration with pneumonia. On the physical examination oral candidiasis was noted in our patient. Pharyngeal candidiasis may be seen when there is stasis in the esophagus as well as in immunocompromised patients.

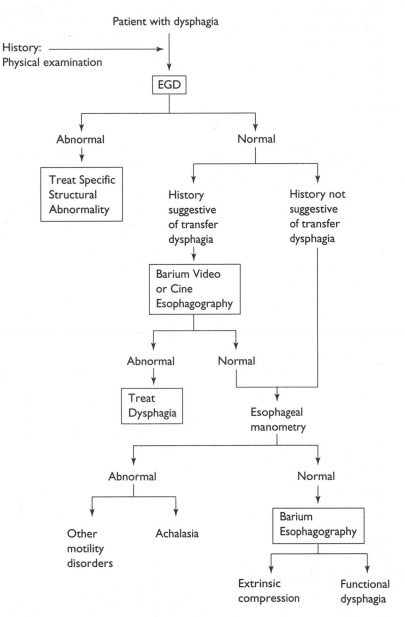

5-6-1 Diagnostic algorithm for dysphagia.
(From Greene HL, Johnson WP, Maricic MJ: *Decision making in medicine*, St Louis, 1993, Mosby.)

QUESTION 5 An upper GI series was ordered due to the suspicion of achalasia. What do you suspect that it revealed and what is your interpretation of the result? Are any other tests useful in the investigation of this diagnosis?

An upper GI barium x-ray was also performed and revealed a smoothly tapering narrowed distal esophagus with tubular dilatation of the body of the esophagus with some retained particulate matter. Barium slowly emptied into the stomach when the patient was upright. This is the classic radiographic finding seen in cases of achalasia.

An upper endoscopy was then performed. Endoscopy revealed retained secretions and fluid in the esophagus. The esophageal mucosa was normal, and the endoscope passed through the lower esophageal sphincter with gentle pressure. There were no esophageal lesions or gastric cardia lesions. The patient then underwent esophageal manometry. This revealed a loss of peristalsis in the distal esophagus and incomplete relaxation of the LES. These findings are all consistent with achalasia, and because pseudoachalasia had been ruled out, the patient underwent hydrostatic balloon dilation with significant improvement in her dysphagia, but requires an H_2 blocker for her new symptoms of esophageal reflux.

CASE SUMMARY: The patient returned home and experienced great improvement in her ability to swallow and gained 4 lbs in the first week. On follow-up in the clinic, she is smiling but complains of mild heartburn. She was placed on an oral H_2 blocker and called you to say that her symptoms are much relieved. A diagnostic algorithm for dysphagia is shown in Fig. 5-6-1.

• •

BIBLIOGRAPHY

Adelstein DJ, Forman WB, Beavers B: Esophageal carcinoma, *Cancer* 54:918-923, 1984.
Castello DO: Gastroesophageal reflux disease and its complication. In Fisher RS, ed: *Motor disorders of the gastrointestinal tract*, New York, 1993, Academy Professional Information Services.
Cluse RE: Motor disorders. In Sleisenger MH, Fordtran JS, eds: *Gastrointestinal disease: pathophysiology, diagnosis and management*, ed 5, Philadelphia, 1993, WB Saunders.
Earlam R: Pathophysiology and clinical presentation of achalasia, *Clin Gastroenterol* 5(1):73-88, 1976.
Feussner H, Kauer W, Siewert JR: The place of esophageal manometry in the diagnosis of dysphagia, *Dysphagia* 8(2):98-104, 1993.
Heitmiller F: Surgical solutions for esophageal dysphagia, *Dysphagia* 6:79-82, 1991.
Katz PO, Dalton CB, Richter JE, et al: Esophageal testing of patients with noncardiac chest pain or dysphagia, *Ann Intern Med* 106:593-597, 1987.
Levine MS, Rubesin SE: Radiologic investigation of dysphagia, *Am J Roentgenology* 154(6):1157-1163, 1990.
Marshall JB: Dysphagia, *Postgrad Med* 85(4)243-260, 1989.
Pope CE II: Rings, webs, diverticula. In Sleissenger MH, Fordtran JS, eds: *Gastrointestinal disease: pathophysiology, diagnosis, and management*, ed 5, Philadelphia, 1993, WB Saunders.
Reynolds JC, Parkman HP: Achalasia, *Gastroenterol Clin North Am* 18:223-255, 1989.
Richter JE, Castell DO: Gastroesophageal reflux, *Ann Intern Med* 97:93-103, 1982.
Richter JE: Motor disorders of the smooth muscle esophagus. In Fisher RS, ed: *Motor disorders of the gastrointestinal tract*, New York, 1993, Academy Professional Information Services.
Stuart RC, Hemmessy TPJ: Primary disorders of esophageal motility, *Brit J Surg* 76:1111-1120, 1989.
Vantrappen G, Hellemans J: Treatment of achalasia and related motor disorders, *Gastroenterol* 79:144-154, 1980.

CASE

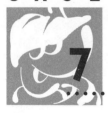

7 Kyoko Misawa
Michael Brown
• • • • • • • • • •

A *40-year-old man presents to the office with midepigastric pain for the past 2 weeks. He states that he had similar episodes in the past 2 years that were not as severe and would last for several weeks. Between episodes, he was essentially pain-free. He characterized the pain as an epigastric burning or "hunger pang" that usually occurred 1 to 3 hours after eating. The pain would awaken him from sleep approximately every other night. Food and antacids seemed to quell the discomfort. He noted occasional bloating, particularly with fatty foods. He admitted to mild, intermittent heartburn that would readily respond to antacids. He denied any nausea, vomiting, change in bowel habits, fever, rashes, arthritis, eye problems, or weight loss. He had no significant past medical history, and his only medication was occasional antacids.*

QUESTION I What is the differential diagnosis for abdominal pain as it applies to the patient presented thus far?

The differential diagnosis of midepigastric pain is broad. Of the gastrointestinal disorders, the discussion will be limited to: (1) gastric carcinoma, (2) gastroesophageal reflux disease, (3) biliary colic, (4) pancreatitis, and (5) peptic ulcer disease.

Gastric carcinoma has had a dramatic decrease in incidence over the past 50 years, although this has been less pronounced in the African-American population. There is marked variation in incidence worldwide with the United States having an incidence of approximately 7 per 100,000 persons. Incidence and mortality sharply increase as the patient's age rises over 50 years. Males are more likely to have gastric cancer than females, although this holds less true for the elderly. Immigrants from high incidence populations (e.g., Japan, Costa Rica, Chile, Hungary, Poland) appear to remain at increased risk for a couple of generations. Other etiologic factors include blood group A, familial clusterings, low socioeconomic status, and environmental factors. Of the latter, consumption of large amounts of starch, pickled vegetables, salted meats and fish, and smoked foods have been implicated. Controversy continues to surround whether the postgastrectomy state and pernicious anemia increase a person's risk of developing gastric cancer. Histologically, intestinal metaplasia and atrophic gastritis are believed to be precancerous lesions. Lately, *Helicobacter pylori* has been closely linked to both atrophic gastritis and gastric cancer. Gastric lymphoma may be even more closely tied to *H. pylori* infections.

Symptomatic gastroesophageal reflux disease (GERD) is the most common gastrointestinal complaint. As many as 33% of individuals suffer from symptoms in a month, and up to 7% of people experience heartburn on a daily basis. The etiologic factors for GERD have changed over the years. The reflux of acid into the esophagus is thought to be influenced by several factors. The amount and frequency of refluxed acid is affected, in part, by lower resting esophageal sphincter pressures and increased time of LES relaxation. Increased intraabdominal pressure, in this setting, can lead to more frequent episodes of reflux. The hiatus hernia is a possible contributor to the GERD equation. In addition, impaired esophageal motility decreases acid clearance resulting in GERD. Not all patients with reflux disease have esophagitis. Frequency and severity of symptoms do not correlate with endoscopic findings. There is more extensive erosive esophagitis in men. GERD complications occur with the highest incidence between the ages of 50 to 70.

Gallstone disease is another possibility. Sixty to eighty percent of all gallstones are thought to be asymptomatic at any time. There is a 2% per year incidence of stones becoming symptomatic in the first 5 years, a 15% incidence at 10 years, and 18% incidence at 15 to 20 years. When patients become symptomatic, 70% to 80% present with biliary colic. If the colic is due to acute cholecystitis, the typical patient is an overweight woman of childbearing age.

Pancreatitis can be due to a number of etiologies including biliary tract stone disease, ethanol abuse, infection, drugs, lipid abnormalities (hypertriglyceridemia), trauma, and pancreatic ductal obstruction. Ethanol abuse and biliary tract stones account for 60% to 80% of cases. An etiology is not identified in 10% to 15% of cases that are consequently labelled idiopathic pancreatitis. It is believed that acute pancreatitis is the result of injury caused by prematurely activated digestive enzymes. Recent data has demonstrated colocalization of digestive precursors with lysosomal hydrolases that could prematurely activate these zymogens within the acinar cells and when released into the cytoplasm would cause cell injury. The pain of chronic pancreatitis may be associated with acute inflammation, pancreatic ductal obstruction, perineural inflammation, mechanical compression due to a pseudocyst, and common bile duct stenosis.

There are 500,000 new cases of peptic ulcer disease (PUD) and 4 million recurrences every year. Genetic factors have been identified that put certain subsets of the population at increased risk. Concordance is higher in identical twins, as compared to nonidentical twins, then first degree relatives. Blood group O is associated with a mild increased risk, and a nonsecreting status of blood group antigens places a patient at even higher risk. There is an unexplained frequency of disease in the winter months. Nonsteroidal antiinflammatory drugs (NSAIDs) and tobacco use are primary offenders in ulcer genesis. More recently, *H. pylori* has been found to be the major etiologic factor for duodenal ulceration as well as its recurrence. Although infection with *H. pylori* is very common, it is not known why most infected persons never develop duodenal ulcers. Ninety-five percent of all duodenal ulcers not associated with NSAID use are positive for *H. pylori*. Equally impressive is the 78% to 83% decrease in the recurrence rate after treatment for the infection. Seventy to eighty percent of gastric ulcers are associated with *H. pylori*, and therapy for *H. pylori* reduces their recurrence as well.

QUESTION 2   On physical examination, he is a well-developed, well-nourished 40-year-old white man in apparent distress. His vital signs are stable, and he is afebrile. His cardiovascular and pulmonary examinations are normal. His abdomen is soft and nondistended with normoactive bowel sounds. He has mild epigastric tenderness with no rebound or guarding. He has no hepatosplenomegaly. Rectal examination reveals brown stool that is hemoccult negative. Laboratory examination demonstrates a Hgb 14.0/Hct 41.6, WBC of 6.5 with normal differential, and a platelet count of 207K. His electrolyte panel is normal with a BUN 12 and creatinine 0.8. The remainder of his chemical profile is normal. An amylase and lipase are unremarkable. For each of the diagnoses included in the differential diagnosis, what are their clinical signs and symptoms and what tests are used to distinguish each one?

Gastric cancer generally has a paucity of symptoms until the disease is advanced. With early gastric cancer, the symptoms range from none to only vague abdominal discomfort, epigastric fullness, and nausea. With advanced disease there is early satiety, sitophobia, weight loss, pain with eating, and sometimes obstructive symptoms. Physical findings and laboratory abnormalities are uncommon until late in the disease. As a result, most patients are diagnosed with advanced disease. Diagnosis can be suggested by UGI, but upper endoscopy is preferred since tissue can be obtained for histology. CT scan can be used to delineate disease extent. There is data to suggest that endoscopic ultrasound may also be of use in staging.

Classically, patients with gastroesophageal reflux disease complain of pyrosis that is generally retrosternal although it can also be epigastric. The symptoms are worse with eating and lying down. There may be nocturnal awakenings with acid regurgitation, water brash, or coughing. In a small subset of patients, there can be complaints of dysphagia or a globus sensation. On examination, there are usually no abnormal physical findings, and laboratory values are all normal.

The diagnosis of GERD can be made in a variety of ways. Clinical history is by far the most common method. If there is a doubt, radionuclide scintigraphy can help, although it has low sensitivity. UGI with esophagram is a poor test. The acid perfusion test has been used to elicit symptoms; however, it relies on the patient's ability to determine that the symptoms are being reproduced during blind acid infusion. Twenty-four hour pH monitoring is becoming the gold standard. This modality takes into account the intermittent nature of GERD, collects data in the patient's usual environment, and provides information on the correlation of symptoms with acid reflux. Upper endoscopy will not see reflux, but can identify some of its consequences and hiatus hernias. Patients with longstanding symptoms should undergo upper endoscopy to look for Barrett's esophagus. If this is identified, the patient will require long-term endoscopic surveillance since there is a 10% malignant transformation rate.

The pain of biliary colic results from intermittent obstruction and spasm of the cystic duct by a stone. Biliary colic is usually severe and episodic and most commonly located in the epigastrium. It can last for hours and is worsened by eating. It can radiate to other parts of the abdomen, interscapular region, or right shoulder. There is an occasional association with nausea, vomiting, and diaphoresis. The pain can occur at night as well. Biliary colic can be exacerbated by weight reduction and prolonged bed rest. Eighty percent of patients have associated dyspepsia. Physical examination may be unrevealing between episodes, but may demonstrate epigastric or right upper quadrant tenderness during a colic episode. If, however, the colic has progressed to obstruction, the patient may present with fever, chills, and localized tenderness.

In uncomplicated biliary colic, there are frequently no laboratory abnormalities. With progression to acute cholecystitis, there is generally leukocytosis and mild elevations (usually less than 2.5 times normal) of the transaminase, alkaline phosphatase, and GGTP. Elevation in serum bilirubin is usually not seen unless there is inflammation or obstruction of the common hepatic or bile duct.

Diagnosis can be aided by ultrasound, which may demonstrate gallstones, thickened gallbladder wall, pericholecystic fluid, common duct stones, biliary ductal dilation, or any combination of these findings. When gallstones are the only finding, HIDA scan is helpful. Hepatobiliary scintigraphy has a high sensitivity and specificity for acute cholecystitis. HIDA scans strongly suggest acute obstruction of the cystic duct when the gallbladder is not visualized by 90 minutes despite adequate visualization of the liver, common bile duct, and small bowel. False positives can occur in prolonged fasting states, chronic cholecystitis, and chronic alcoholism. Delayed scans at four hours can minimize the false positives and increase the sensitivity and specificity to 97% and 90%, respectively. When the diagnosis is not clear, endoscopic retrograde cholangiopancreatography (ERCP) can be helpful in identifying common bile duct obstructions due to stones or tumors that were not previously identified. If there is suspicion of a tumor causing the biliary colic, a CT scan is the test of choice.

Patients with pancreatitis typically present with epigastric pain that radiates through to the back. The pain is knifelike or boring in quality and can be somewhat alleviated by sitting forward or lying in a fetal position. There may be a pleuritic component. It is frequently associated with abdominal distension and nausea with vomiting. On physical examination, the patient is ill-appearing and may be jaundiced. Vital signs can range from mild fever to hypotension, tachycardia, and tachypnea. Auscultation of the lung can demonstrate basilar atelectasis. The abdominal examination is the most revealing with epigastric tenderness, guarding, distention, and hypoactive bowel sound. Laboratory tests can show hemoconcentration, leukocytosis, hyperglycemia, hypoalbuminemia, hypercalcemia, and hyperbilirubinemia. There may be evidence of prerenal azotemia as well as elevated transaminase and alkaline phosphatase. In severe cases, disseminated intravascular coagulation may develop. Elevated amylase and lipase are frequently seen in acute pancreatitis, although neither enzyme is diagnostic.

In patients with chronic pancreatitis, the only clue may be the abdominal tenderness. Severe chronic pancreatitis manifests with systemic symptoms when more than 90% of the gland is destroyed. Steatorrhea and subsequent weight loss occur when the lipase production is less than 10%. With compromise of endocrine function, brittle diabetes mellitus and its complications can result. Plain radiographs are helpful in alcoholic chronic pancreatitis, a simple upright KUB is crucial in the exclusion of other diagnostic possibilities such as perforated bowel and bowel obstruction. Ultrasound examination may detect gallstones, ductal dilation, pancreatic enlargement, and pseudocysts. Frequently, the pancreas is poorly visualized as a result of gaseous distension of bowel loops overlying it.

The severity of the attack and prognosis can be determined by Ranson's criteria, which assess the patient on admission and at 48 hours. At admission, these criteria include age >55 years, white blood cell count >16 K, glucose >200 mg/dl, SGOT >250 U and LDH >350 U. At 48 hours these criteria include a drop in the hematocrit by greater than 10%, an increase in the BUN by 5 mg/dl, serum Ca <8 mg/dl, Pao_2 <60 mm Hg, base deficit >4 mEq/L, and fluid sequestration >6 L. If fewer than 3 of these are present, mortality is less than 1%; however, if more than 4 are present, the mortality increases to 25% to 50%.

Severe episodes of pancreatitis can lead to multiple systemic consequences. These include hypotension and pericardial effusion, ARDS, pleural effusion, atelectasis, acute renal failure, gastritis, disseminated intravascular coagulation, hypocalcemia, hyperglycemia, fat necrosis, and alterations of consciousness. Local complications include pseudocysts, phlegmons, abscesses, severe hypocalcemia, and septic shock.

As opposed to pancreatitis, the patient with PUD has epigastric pain that is nonradiating, is relieved by food, and characterized as burning or gnawing. The pain awakens the patient at night. There can be mild heartburn, complaints of bloating, and fatty food intolerance. The patient may have discomfort for weeks and then be symptom-free for months. Some patients, in sharp contrast, are entirely asymptomatic, although this is more common with NSAID-induced PUD. These patients may present only when complications occur. Physical examination reveals only mild epigastric discomfort, and the laboratory values are usually unremarkable. Physical findings and laboratory values can be striking when patients present with hemorrhage, perforation, or obstruction.

In patients under the age of 40 with mild intermittent epigastric discomfort of short duration, a trial of H2-receptor antagonists is reasonable. In patients with symptoms of long duration or with any systemic symptoms, the diagnosis should be established. Diagnosis can be made either by upper GI x-ray or upper endoscopy. UGI can, however, miss smaller ulcers. Upper endoscopy has several advantages. In the case of duodenal ulcers, tissue can be taken for either Clotest or pathology. In the case of gastric ulcers, endoscopy permits the taking of requisite biopsies.

QUESTION 3 What would be the treatment of choice for each of these diagnoses?

Treatment of gastric cancer is dependent on stage. Surgery can provide the only possibility of cure in early gastric cancer and local disease. It also has a role for palliation of obstructive symptoms. In advanced disease, chemotherapy may be used as primary therapy or adjuvant to surgery. Results have been dismal. Radiation therapy has been used with limited success. Overall prognosis is exceedingly poor with a 5-year survival of <10%.

Treatment for patients with GERD is generally medical. First, patients are instructed to avoid those substances known to decrease LES pressure and inhibit acid clearance such as caffeine, chocolate, peppermint, tomatoes, and nicotine. Other preventive measures include raising the head of the bed, avoiding late meals and snacks, minimizing tight waistlines, and, if overweight, losing 10% of body weight. Not surprisingly, many people require more intervention. H_2-receptor antagonists are helpful to many patients. However, those with peptic strictures, severe erosive esophagitis, and smokers with severe mucosal damage frequently do not heal and experience persistent symptoms. Occasionally, these patients come under control with the addition of antacids, but this is rare.

Omeprazole, a proton pump inhibitor, inhibits 90% of acid production with a single daily dose. It is the most potent and effective medication for patients with severe symptoms and disease. Long-term use is becoming more commonplace as concerns regarding long-term hypergastrinemia fade. Data on long-term use should be forthcoming. In some patients, there is a role for prokinetic agents including metoclopramide, bethanecol, and cisapride. Surgery has a role in a select group of patients: those with poor healing despite adequate therapy, those who require long-term omeprazole therapy, and younger patients who will need lifelong, expensive therapy for a chronic disease. Laparoscopic approaches are making surgery more attractive.

Treatment of biliary colic is dependent on the cause. If the patient suffers from acute cholecystitis, surgery is the treatment of choice. Oral dissolution therapy may be used in highly selected patients, although stones almost always recur with termination of therapy. Extracorporeal shock wave lithotripsy (ESWL) has limited utility because of a significant complication rate and is not an FDA-approved device for this purpose in the United States. A recent study indicates that emergency ERCP can significantly reduce morbidity and mortality in acute gallstone pancreatitis. If the etiology of biliary colic is cholangiocarcinoma or pancreatic cancer, surgery provides the only possibility of cure although it more often provides only palliation.

Treatment of pancreatitis is largely supportive. Adequate fluid replacement, analgesia, and bowel rest are the mainstays. In the past, nasogastric suction was thought to hasten improvement, but has subsequently been found to provide only symptomatic relief of nausea and vomiting. Treatment ranges from supportive measures to antibiotics and surgery.

Treatment of peptic ulcer disease consists of stopping any offending agents (NSAIDs and tobacco) and prescribing H2-receptor antagonists, omeprazole, sucralfate, or antacids. In duodenal ulcers which are associated with *H. pylori*, treatment consists of colloidal bismuth subcitrate, amoxicillin, and metronidazole in addition to an H2-receptor antagonist or proton pump inhibitor. Colloidal bismuth subcitrate is given as two tablets qid, amoxicillin is given 500 mg tid, and metronidazole 250 mg qid; this regimen is given for 2 weeks. This results in eradication of the organism approximately 85% to 90% of the time. For those people who are penicillin allergic, amoxicillin is replaced by tetracycline 500 mg qid. Compliance rates with this regimen are less than 70%. Triple therapy with omeprazole (20 mg bid), metronidazole (500 mg bid), and clarithromycin (500 mg bid) for one week is an attractive alternative. In gastric ulcer patients, repeat endoscopy is required to document healing after 6 to 8 weeks of therapy.

QUESTION 4 The patient described in this case presents with midepigastric pain that is relieved by food and antacids. He is an otherwise healthy male. Physical examination revealed only mild epigastric tenderness, and his laboratory values were all normal. His symptoms, physical findings, and laboratory examination bring up the differential diagno-

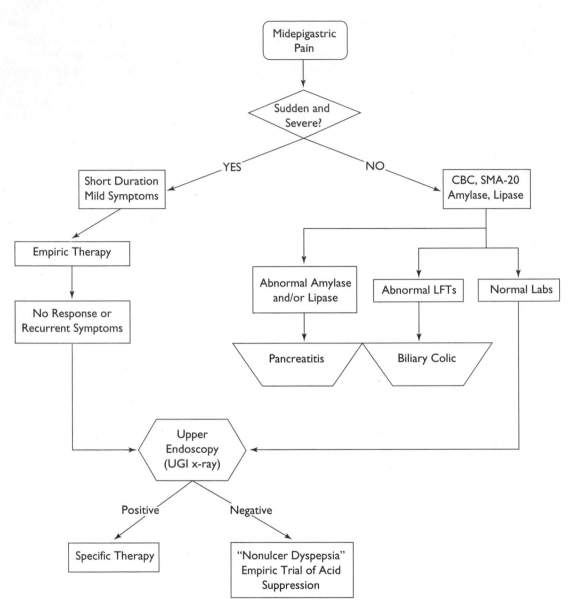

5-7-1 Diagnostic algorithm for midepigastric pain.

sis as outlined above. Based on the information obtained about this patient, how do you organize the differential diagnosis?

Gastroesophageal reflux disease and PUD are highest on the differential. These are difficult to distinguish at times and certainly may coexist.

GERD typically has worsening symptoms with eating. If pain is present, retrosternal location is more common. Symptoms, however, can cause nocturnal wakenings just as in PUD. In ulcer disease patients complain of a gnawing or burning pain that is improved with eating. The constant discomfort for weeks and months without symptoms is classical. Gastric cancer seems less likely given his age and lack of more generalized symptoms, although this could represent early gastric cancer. Biliary colic is another possibility, although his pain is not severe, does not radiate, and actually improves with eating. The lack of laboratory abnormalities can occur in uncomplicated biliary colic. Pancreatitis can also present with midepigastric pain. If this were acute pancreatitis, a more dramatic examination would be expected, and the amylase and lipase frequently elevated. In chronic pancreatitis, a prior history of pancreatitis or history of chronic heavy alcohol use should be sought. If this represents recurrent episodes, perhaps more systemic manifestations would have been elicited.

QUESTION 5   What is the CLO-test?

The CLO-test (Campylobacter-like organism test) is a rapid urease test done after gastric biopsy. The Helicobacter organism produces urease. Biopsy material is placed in a gel of urea, ammonium hydroxide, and a color indicator. If urease is present, the indicator turns red. An alternate means of diagnosing the presence of the organism is the carbon labeled CO_2 breath test. If the urease enzyme is present, labeled C^{13} or C^{14} is metabolized to $C^{13}O_2$ or $C^{14}O_2$, respectively. One caveat is that if the patient has been taking a bismuth subcitrate compound for symptomatic treatment, the urease enzyme can be inactivated. Serum measurements of IgG and IgA Helicobactor antibodies are also diagnostically useful.

QUESTION 6   What is the final diagnosis and the specific therapy for this disease?

Given the chronicity of the patient's symptoms, a definitive diagnosis should be sought. Upper endoscopy would be the test of choice. When an EGD was performed, a duodenal ulcer was found. Biopsies for Clo-test were positive for *H. pylori.*

Treatment consisted of an H_2 blocker for 2 months and triple therapy for 2 weeks. The patient was also advised to stop smoking. The patient's symptoms resolved during the course of therapy. He has been symptom-free except for mild intermittent pyrosis that responds promptly to antacids.

A diagnostic algorithm for midepigastric pain is shown in Fig. 5-7-1.

BIBLIOGRAPHY

Beaser MJ: Hypotheses in the pathogenesis and nature history of Helicobacter pylori-induced inflammation, *Gastroenterol* 102:720-727, 1992.

Calleja GA, Barkins JS: Acute pancreatitis, *Med Clin North Am* 77:1037-1056, 1993.

Gelfand MD: Gastroesophageal reflux disease, *Med Clin North Am* 75:923-940, 1991.

Graham DY, Lew GM, et al: Effect of triple therapy (antibiotics plus bismuth) on duodenal ulcer healing, *Ann Intern Med* 115:266-269, 1991.

Graham DY, Lew GM, et al: Effect of treatment of Helicobacter pylori infection on the long-term recurrence of gastric or duodenal ulcers, *Ann Intern Med* 116:705-708, 1992.

Hentschel E, Brandstatler G, et al: Effect of ranitidine and amoxicillin plus betronidazole on the eradicator of Helicobacter pylori and the recurrence of duodenal ulcers, *N Engl J Med* 328:308-312, 1993.

Holt S: Chronic pancreatitis, *So Med J* 86:201-207, 1993.

Kadakia SC: Biliary tract emergencies, *Med Clin North Am* 77:1015-1036, 1993.

Katz J: The course of peptic ulcer disease, *Med Clin North Am* 75:831-840, 1991.

Lai ECS, Mok FPT, et al: Endoscopic biliary drainage for severe acute cholangitis, *N Engl J Med* 326:1582-1586, 1992.

Peterson WL: Helicobacter pylori and peptic ulcer disease, *N Engl J Med* 324:1043-1048, 1991.

Rex DK: Gastroesophageal reflux disease in adults; pathophysiology, diagnosis and management, *J Fam Prac* 35:673-681, 1992.

Veldhuyzen van Zanten SJO, Sherman PM: Helicobacter pylori infection as a cause of gastritis, duodenal ulcer, gastric cancer, and non-ulcer dyspepsia: a systematic review, *Can Med Assoc J* 150:177-185, 1994.

CASE

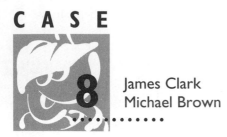

8 James Clark
Michael Brown
. . . .

A 78-year-old woman with a history of coronary artery disease, myocardial infarction 3 years ago, congestive heart failure, hypertension, and diabetes mellitus presents to the emergency room with abdominal pain. The patient felt fine until one day prior to admission when she developed left lower quadrant (LLQ) pain and several loose bloody bowel movements. She denies nausea, vomiting, upper abdominal pain, or melana. There was no recent shortness of breath, chest pain, palpitations, or dizziness. Her current medicines are digoxin, lasix, and glyburide.

QUESTION I   What is the differential diagnosis of abdominal pain presenting with bloody diarrhea?

Ischemic colitis is an important consideration in this patient. The colon is the most common site of ischemic injury in the GI tract. A wide spectrum of injury occurs and is related to both the duration and severity of the ischemia. The mildest changes include mucosal and submucosal hemorrhage and edema. This can be followed by ulceration of the overlying mucosa. Multiple ulcerations may lead to a transient segmental colitis that is completely reversible. With more severe or prolonged ischemia, the mucosa and submucosa are replaced by granulation tissue and may lead to a chronic segmental ulcerating colitis that can mimic inflammatory bowel disease. With a more severe ischemic insult, the muscularis propria is injured and healing with fibrosis may occur, leading to stricture formation. Finally, the most severe form of injury is transmural infarction with gangrene and perforation.

Over 90% of patients with ischemic colitis are over the age of 60. Most of these patients have underlying generalized atherosclerosis or impaired left ventricular function, which leads to a low flow state and poor tissue perfusion. However, in most cases, no dramatic precipitating event such as hypotension, volume depletion, acute myocardial infarction, or arrhythmia is found. Ischemic colitis affecting younger patients is usually due to unusual causes such as vasculitis, hypercoagulable states, and drug reactions (including estrogens, danazol, gold, psychotropic drugs, and vasopressin).

A special circumstance predisposing to ischemic colitis is a distal obstructing colonic lesion. It is estimated that 20% of patients with colonic ischemia have obstructing lesions such as colon cancer, diverticulitis, volvulus, or colonic stricture. The lesion is usually distal to the area of colitis. Finally, colonic ischemia may occur in 1% to 7% of elective abdominal aortic surgery as well as up to 60% of emergency surgeries done for ruptured aortic aneurysms.

Most patients present with sudden crampy LLQ pain and passage of bloody loose stools. Bleeding is usually not severe and rarely requires blood transfusion. On examination there is usually tenderness over the affected area of colon.

The most commonly affected areas are "watershed regions" between two adjacent arterial supplies. These areas of the colon are near the splenic flexure at the junction of the superior and inferior mesenteric arteries and the rectosigmoid region of the junction of the inferior mesenteric and hypogastric arteries. However, it is important to realize that any portion of the colon can be affected and that 10% to 15% of cases have involvement limited to areas proximal to the splenic flexure.

Even the highly vascular rectum can be involved in roughly 5% of cases.

Another important entity to include in the differential is infectious colitis. Infectious diarrhea is usually a mild self-limited disease, but even in the United States about 500 diarrheal deaths occur each year. Infectious diarrhea can be caused by either invasive or noninvasive pathogens. Invasive organisms penetrate the mucosa where an inflammatory exudate and ulcerations may occur. Clinically, these patients tend to present with tenesmus, lower abdominal pain, and frequent bloody diarrhea of low volume. Fecal leukocytes are usually present. These organisms include *Shigella, Campylobacter,* enteroinvasive *E. coli,* enterohemorrhagic *E. coli* (0157:H7), and *E. histolytica.*

Noninvasive organisms have toxic effects on the small bowel mucosa. Clinically, patients present with watery diarrhea and midabdominal pain. Bloody stool is absent, and they usually do not have significant numbers of fecal leukocytes. Cholera, for example, produces a toxin that activates adenylate cyclase to produce secretion of fluid and electrolytes into the intestinal lumen. Enterotoxigenic *E. coli,* rotavirus, Norwalk virus and *Giardia lamblia* are other noninvasive organisms. Finally, *Salmonella* and *Yersinia* do not fit these patterns well as they both tend to attack the ileum and colon. *Vibrio parahemolytica* causes an acute diarrhea associated with raw fish or shellfish. It usually produces an explosive watery diarrhea with nausea and vomiting but can also produce a bloody diarrhea associated with colonic ulcerations.

Inflammatory bowel disease (IBD) refers to the idiopathic chronic inflammatory disorders called ulcerative colitis and Crohn's disease. These diseases have a similar prevalence rate of 50 per 100,000 and are more common in Caucasians than non-Caucasians. Symptoms can begin at any age but have a peak incidence at the age of 15 to 30 years. There is a second smaller peak in the elderly.

The diseases are classified based on different pathologic characteristics. Ulcerative colitis always affects the rectum and extends proximally to varying degrees. The disease only affects the colon with the possible exception of patients with pancolitis who may have a mild ileitis (termed backwash ileitis). The disease is continuous without skip areas of normal mucosa. The epithelium is infiltrated with neutrophils leading to friability and superficial ulceration.

Crohn's disease, in contrast, can affect any portion of the GI tract from mouth to anus. About one third primarily involve the ileum, one third the colon, and one third both the ileum and colon. The rectum is involved in less than half of cases. The inflammation tends to be patchy with intervening "skip areas" of normal bowel between diseased segments. Pathologic findings included transmural inflammation with deep linear ulceration and an inflammatory infiltrate consisting of lymphocytes, macrophages, neutrophils, and, in up to 50% of cases, granulomas. Because of the transmural nature of the disease, adjacent bowel loops may adhere to each other leading to fistula and obstruction.

Many patients requiring radiation therapy will have exposure of the bowel to radiation as an innocent bystander. Radiation colitis is most commonly seen in patients with intraabdominal or pelvic malignancies who have received radiation therapy. Radiation can cause both an early colitis as well as a late chronic injury. Since radiation damage is greatest in rapidly dividing cells, the intestinal mucosal crypt cells are very sensitive to radiation. The acute changes can occur during or shortly after radiation therapy. This can lead to an extensive inflammatory infiltrate of the mucosa.

Endoscopically, these patients may have a dusky edematous and hyperemic mucosa with a poorly visible vascular pattern, and in more severe cases, they may have superficial ulceration. They present with tenesmus, diarrhea, and rectal bleeding. On occasion, extensive mucosal ulcerations occur, leading to severe bleeding and sepsis because of the loss of the epithelial barrier. Conservative measures such as antidiarrheal antispasmodics, topical analgesics, and warm sitz baths (for anal discomfort) are usually all that is required.

Chronic radiation toxicity occurs in at least 10% of patients and may present at any time from 2 months to 30 years after radiation therapy. This is thought to be due to damage of the intestinal endothelial and connective tissue cells. These changes may lead to an obliterative endarteritis and endophlebitis, which can cause chronic intestinal ischemia. Other conditions that impair the vasculature such as diabetes, hypertension, congestive heart failure, and atherosclerosis can exacerbate this radiation change. Other risk factors include the total dose of radiation (usually greater than 5000 rads), concomitant chemotherapy, and previous abdominal or pelvic surgery, which may produce adhesions that can immobilize bowel loops in the field of radiation. Endoscopically, these patients have a pale atrophic mucosa, friability, ulceration, and prominent submucosal telangiectatic vessels.

There are several other diseases that may present with bloody diarrhea. The presentation of colon cancer usually depends upon its location. Cancers in the cecum or ascending colon usually present with occult bleeding and iron deficiency, while rectal and low sigmoid tumors frequently present with red blood per rectum. This may be associated with diarrhea if the tumor produces a partial colonic obstruction. On occasion, colon cancer may perforate and present with abdominal pain and fever mimicking acute diverticulitis.

Diverticular disease of the colon is common in the United States. The sigmoid colon is involved in about 95% of cases with the proximal colon being involved less frequently. Colonic diverticulae are usually asymptomatic. Acute diverticulitis is usually related to retention of undigested food residues and bacteria in the diverticular sac, which may form a hard mass called a fecalith. This may lead to a small perforation (microabscess) and inflammation of the sac.

Angiodysplasia is a disease of the elderly characterized by dilated, distorted vessels lined by vascular endothelium that are usually 2 to 10 mm in size. These are usually multiple and found primarily in the cecum and ascending colon. While bleeding may occur, the presence of diarrhea is less common.

Toxin producing *Clostridium difficile* is the etiologic agent of pseudomembranous colitis and the cause of 15% to 25% of antibiotic associated diarrhea. Antibiotic use preceeds most cases of *C. difficile* disease although chemotherapy can cause the disease as well. In either case, there is disorganization of gut flora so that the *C. difficile* organism gains a selective advantage, and toxin A is produced in greater amount.

QUESTION 2 What are the clinical symptoms and signs on which a diagnosis is supported of each of the diseases considered in the differential diagnosis?

The diagnosis of ischemic colitis depends on early and serial radiographic and endoscopic findings. Plain abdominal x-ray may be unremarkable or show dilated loops of bowel with air-fluid levels. Thumbprinting is seen in 20% of cases and corresponds to submucosal edema and hemorrhage. It is important to realize that thumbprinting is not specific for ischemia and may be seen in other severe types of colitis. If the patient has no peritoneal signs and an unremarkable plain x-ray, then either colonoscopy or barium enema on the unprepped colon should be done. Colonoscopy is more sensitive in detecting erythema, exudate, and small ulcerations. Hemorrhagic nodules may also be seen. Biopsy of involved mucosa usually shows nonspecific inflammatory changes. Because insufflation of air to distend the colon may reduce colonic blood flow, neither barium enema nor colonoscopy should be done in patients with peritoneal signs. Alternately, in the correct clinical setting, demonstration of severe atherosclerotic disease of the superior or inferior mesenteric arteries can secure the diagnosis.

The etiologic cause of infectious diarrhea can only be established by microscopy and culture of the stool. A common approach is to check the stool for fecal leukocytes. The invasive organisms described above usually produce many polymorphonuclear neutrophil leukocytes (PMNs) while toxigenic organisms, virus, and *Giardia* produce few if any leukocytes in the stool. It should be understood that less than 10% of stool cultures submitted yield a pathogen. Even in hospitalized patients admitted with bloody diarrhea, only 40% to 60% will have a positive culture. This may reflect that either routine culture techniques lack sensitivity or that many cases of acute diarrhea are caused by unidentified pathogens.

Clinically, acute ulcerative colitis presents with fever, bloody diarrhea, tenesmus, and possibly lower abdominal pain. Severe disease may be associated with leukocytosis, electrolyte abnormalities, tachycardia, hypotension, and rarely perforation. Most patients have a remitting-relapsing course.

Crohn's disease usually has a more indolent presentation. With ileal disease, most present with low grade obstruction colicky pain, a right lower quadrant (RLQ) mass, and possibly watery diarrhea. With extensive colonic involvement, diarrhea is much more common, although bright red blood per rectum is not seen as frequently as with ulcerative colitis. Because of the transmural inflammation, patients may present with fistulae to the skin, urinary tract, and vagina.

Diverticulitis is characterized by fever, lower abdominal pain, and tenderness. While hemoccult positive stools occur in 25% of cases, red blood per rectum is unusual.

Diverticular bleeding, in contrast, is caused by erosion of a vessel by a fecalith within the diverticular sac. The bleeding is usually painless and not associated with signs and symptoms of inflammation as seen in diverticulitis. As in diverticular bleeding, there is no associated abdominal pain or inflammatory signs accompanying bleeding due to angiodysplasia.

Most patients with *C. difficile* diarrhea develop watery diarrhea 4 to 9 days after beginning antibiotics, but symptoms may occur up to 6 weeks after antibiotics are discontinued. Abdominal pain and fever occur in about 80% of cases while bloody diarrhea occurs in 5% to 10%. The best test for diagnosis is the detection of the *C. difficile* toxin in the stool although flexible sigmoidoscopy may suggest the diagnosis if the characteristic

pseudomembranes are present. Up to three stool examinations are necessary to reach a 90% sensitivity for *C. difficile* toxin.

QUESTION 3 As the senior resident you inform your intern that to include a disease process in the differential diagnosis one must understand the treatment of each process. What is the correct approach for treating the above-mentioned diseases?

The clinical course of ischemic colitis cannot be predicted by the initial presentation unless there are physical findings of peritonitis. Many cases will resolve within 24 to 48 hours. Up to 50% of cases, however, will have irreversible injury with development of either chronic segmental colitis, stricture, or gangrene. All patients should be monitored for worsening of symptoms by serial abdominal examinations. Findings of peritonitis should lead to exploratory laparotomy.

Conservative therapy consists mainly of bowel rest and IV fluids. In patients with a moderately severe attack, broad spectrum antibiotics may be indicated to reduce bowel damage. Cardiac performance should be optimized, anemia treated with transfusion if severe, and mesenteric vasoconstrictors such as dopamine and digoxin should be discontinued if possible. Patients with diarrhea or bleeding that persists for more than 10 to 14 days are at high risk for perforation and should undergo surgical resection. Ischemic strictures that cause obstructive symptoms should be resected.

The major goal of treatment for infectious diarrhea is to replace fluid and electrolytes. In patients with mild or moderate diarrhea, this may be accomplished with oral rehydration solutions. Various formulations have been produced, but all are based on the fact that glucose enhances sodium absorption in the small intestine. Nonspecific therapy includes avoiding lactose, caffeine, and methylxanthines. Antimotility drugs such as loperamide, diphenoxylate, and tincture of opium all decrease transit time, relieve cramping, and reduce fecal fluid losses. However, these drugs should never be used in patients with a severe colitis suggested either by endoscopic appearance or by the presence of bloody diarrhea. Antimotility drugs in these instances may precipitate a toxic megacolon with possibly fatal consequences.

Since the majority of patients with infectious diarrhea have a mild self-limited course, neither stool culture nor antibiotics are required in most cases. However, in immunocompromised patients or patients with severe colitis, especially those with bloody diarrhea, both stool cultures and antibiotics should be considered. Quinoline antibiotics are often used empirically as they have a broad spectrum of activity against all important bacterial pathogens except *C. difficile*. In general, symptomatic patients with Shigella, typhoid fever, traveler's diarrhea, amebiasis, Giardia, and cholera should be treated. Conflicting or inconclusive data exist concerning the treatment of *Campylobacter, Yersinia*, noncholera-Vibrio species and most forms of *E. coli*. Treatment of nontypical *Salmonella* usually does not alter the clinical course and, in fact, seems to increase the risk of developing a chronic carrier state. However, treatment should be considered in those with chronic debilitating diseases, malignancies, immunosuppression, prosthetic heart valves, or orthopedic devices and in those with findings suggestive of sepsis.

Medical management for IBD is similar in both diseases (ulcerative colitis and Crohn's disease). First-line therapy is generally sulfasalazine or related derivatives of pyridine-acetylsalicylic acid. For refractory or more severe disease, corticosteroid and even immunosuppressants such as azathioprine, 6-mercaptopurine, and cyclosporine may be necessary. Surgical treatment of ulcerative colitis is total colectomy with either an ileostomy or an ileoanal anastomosis to restore rectal continence. This is curative and is indicated in patients who fail medical management or who have severe dysplasia detected by biopsy to eliminate the risk of developing colon cancer. Surgical treatment of Crohn's disease is not curative and should be avoided whenever possible because the disease frequently recurs near the excision site. Surgery is

generally reserved for resection of fistulas, abscesses, and relief of obstruction. As little bowel as possible is removed because these patients may require multiple operations leading to a short bowel syndrome and malabsorption because of loss of ileal surface area.

Treatment of chronic radiation colitis is usually unsatisfactory. Steroid enemas, 5-ASA enemas, and sulfasalazine have all been tried with poor results. Rectal bleeding from telangiectasia may be treated endoscopically with the Nd:YAG laser or with formalin enemas that have shown promising results in controlling acute bleeding. Radiation strictures may respond to endoscopic balloon dilatation, but significant obstruction usually requires surgery. Surgery is also usually required for radiation-induced fistulous tracts as hyperalimentation and bowel rest usually do not lead to permanent closure of the fistula.

Many mild cases of pseudomembranous colitis will respond to discontinuing the precipitating antibiotic. The most commonly used drug therapy is metronidazole or vancomycin administered orally.

QUESTION 4   On examination, her temperature is 100° F, blood pressure is 130/70 mm Hg, pulse is 96 bpm, respiratory rate is 18/min. She has no JVD. The lungs are clear. Cardiac examination reveals a regular rhythm with an S4 gallop. There are no murmurs. The abdomen is mildly distended with hypoactive bowel sounds. Palpation revealed moderate LLQ tenderness without rebound or guarding. Rectal examination revealed red blood without any masses. Extremities were only remarkable for 1+ pitting edema. Laboratory examination showed a WBC = 11500 with 82% polys, 15% lymphs, 2% monos, and 1% eosinophil. Hb = 13.6 g/dl and plts = 256000. SMA 20, PT, PTT are normal. ECG reveals Q waves in V1-V3 with no acute changes from a previous ECG. How does the information from the physical examination and labs impact on the differential diagnosis? Are there any more tests you would like to carry out to investigate the cause of bleeding in this patient?

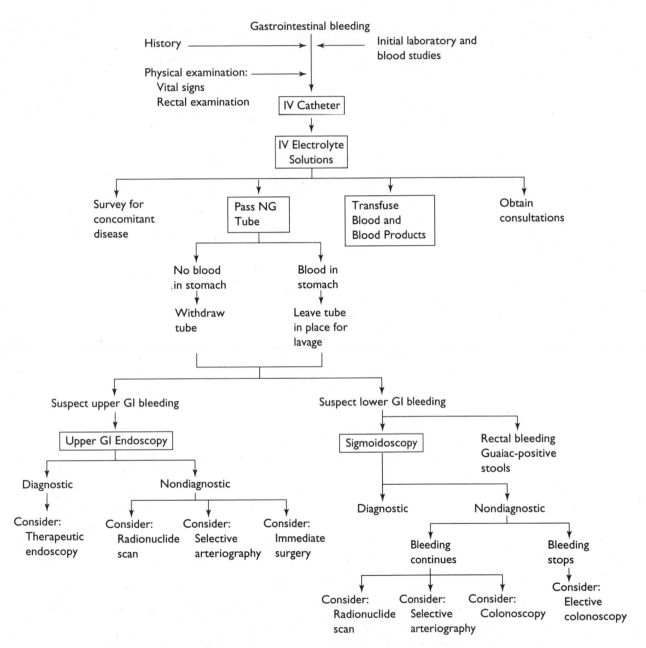

5-8-1   Diagnostic algorithm for gastrointestinal bleeding.
(From Greene HL, Johnson WP, Maricic MJ: *Decision making in medicine,* St Louis, 1993, Mosby.)

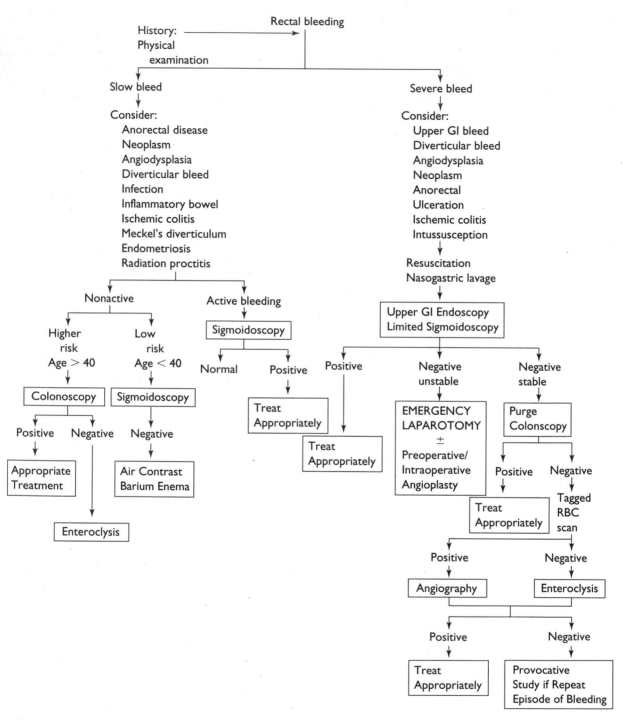

5-8-2   Diagnostic algorithm for rectal bleeding.

(From Greene HL, Johnson WP, Maricic MJ: *Decision making in medicine*, St Louis, 1993, Mosby.)

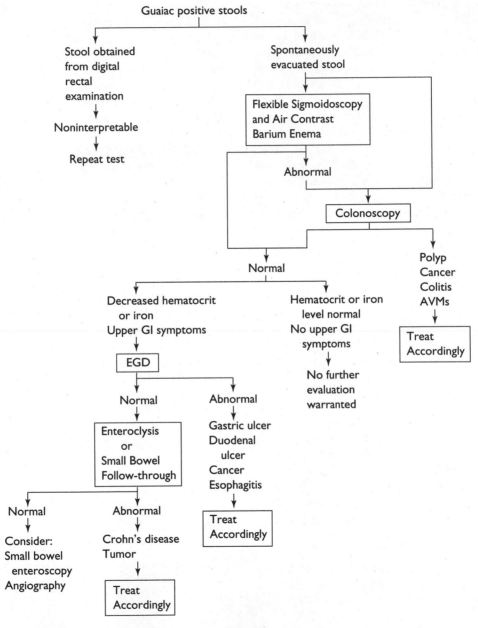

5-8-3   Diagnostic algorithm for guaiac-positive stools.
(From Greene HL, Johnson WP, Maricic MJ: *Decision making in medicine*, St Louis, 1993, Mosby.)

The major considerations are ischemic colitis, infectious colitis, and less likely inflammatory bowel disease. The lack of previous radiation obviously rules out radiation colitis as a cause in this patient. Given the clinical context of an elderly woman with atherosclerosis and CHF, the most likely diagnosis is ischemic colitis. However, stool should be sent for C + S and O + P as well to rule out an infectious source. An admission KUB should be done to evaluate for thumb-printing (negative in this case). The stool C + S and O + P came back negative the following day. Given the lack of thumbprinting on KUB and the absence of peritoneal signs on examination, the patient underwent an unprepped flexible sigmoidoscopy to determine the area and extent of involvement. The patient had erythema, exudate, and small ulcers from 20 to 35 cm at the rectosigmoid junction. The lack of rectal involvement rules out ulcerative colitis and makes infectious causes less likely, although infection is still possible based on these endoscopic findings. Crohn's disease can produce a similar segmental colitis, and there is a second peak in the incidence of IBD in the elderly. However, the acute presentation of bloody diarrhea would be somewhat unusual for Crohn's disease.

QUESTION 5 Because of persistent pain and bleeding, an angiogram of the mesenteric vessels was completed. The study revealed a 90% superior mesenteric obstruction and a near total occlusion of the inferior mesenteric artery just distal to its takeoff for the celiac plexus. A great deal of collateralization was noted at the time of angiography. What is the definitive diagnosis in this case?

This was an elderly patient with known cardiovascular disease who had a segmental colitis at the rectosigmoid junction with negative stool cultures. This most likely represents ischemic colitis. The angiographic findings further support this diagnosis. However, in the majority of patients with ischemic colitis, angiography is not necessary as most patients respond well to conservative therapy. The lack of any obvious hypotensive episode, volume depletion, or an acute exacerbation of CHF does not make ischemic colitis less likely as the majority of patients with this disease do not have an obvious precipitating event.

CASE SUMMARY The patient underwent angioplasty of the superior mesenteric artery with reduction of the stenosis from 90% to approximately 20%. The patient was followed with daily CBC and electrolytes as well as serial abdominal examinations. Her tenderness, pain, and diarrhea all resolved over the next 72 hours. Digoxin was discontinued in the hospital because of concern about its mesenteric vasoconstrictive properties. The patient was discharged and followed as an outpatient where she did well without any further diarrhea, pain, or obstructive symptoms to raise the question of a stricture or chronic segmental colitis. Diagnostic algorithms for gastrointestinal bleeding, rectal bleeding, and guaiac-positive stools are shown in Figs. 5-8-1, 5-8-2, and 5-8-3.

• •

BIBLIOGRAPHY

Barcewitz PA, Welch JP: Ischemic colitis in adult patients, *Dis Colon Rectum* 123:109, 1980.
Boley SJ, Schwartz S, Lash J, et al: Reversible vascular occlusion of the colon, *Surg Gynecol Obstet* 116:53, 1963.
Brandt LJ, Boley SJ: Colonic ischemia, *Surg Clin* 72:203, 1992.
Sakai L, Keltner R, Kaminski D: Spontaneous shock associated ischemic colitis, *Am J Surg* 123:109, 1980.

CASE

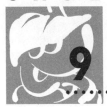

9

Scott Cotler
Michael Brown
• • • • • • • • • •

A 54-year-old businessman with a history of alcohol abuse, peptic ulcer disease, and gout presents with two episodes of vomiting blood followed by black tarry stools and severe dizziness upon arising. A duodenal ulcer was diagnosed by barium X-ray five years previously and treated with an H2 antagonist for one year. Previous ulcer symptoms have not recurred. There is no history of hematemesis or melana; however he does experience frequent nosebleeds.

The patient estimates that for the last 20 years he has had two double martinis at lunch and three glasses of cognac per evening. Over the last year he has attributed increasing abdominal girth to lack of exercise and middle age. Worsening heartburn has occurred, and his abdomen has become more distended. He recently completed a course of indomethacin for a flare-up of his gout.

The patient's wife states that he has become somewhat forgetful and that she has had to take over managing family finances. There is no history of blood transfusion.

QUESTION I What are the clues to an upper GI bleeding source? Generate a differential diagnosis for the patient's upper gastrointestinal bleeding.

It is important to make a presumptive diagnosis as to whether the source of bleeding is proximal (upper) or distal (lower) to the ligament of Treitz. It is more common, in a case of upper GI bleeding as opposed to lower GI bleeding, to encounter hematemesis (vomiting of bright red blood), melena due to digestion of blood components as it passes through the GI tract, and gastric lavage that returns bright red blood. These characteristics do not absolutely rule out the presence of a source of bleeding beyond the ligament of Treitz.

As in all patients it is best to analyze existing medical problems as a clue to the etiology of the current problem. In this case, with a history of alcohol abuse and progressive abdominal distension, one must consider the presence of cirrhosis and the development of esophageal or gastric varices. Furthermore, patients with liver failure often manifest a coagulopathy. This patient also has a history of a duodenal ulcer. Recent use of a nonsteroidal agent could exacerbate his ulcer disease. In addition, he has complaints of heartburn that may be a subtle clue to the presence of gastroesophageal reflux disease and distal esophagitis. Additional diagnoses to consider include Mallory-Weiss tear/Boerhaave's syndrome, and epistaxis. It is always essential to make certain that there is not a nasal or oropharyngeal source of bleeding.

QUESTION 2 The physical examination was as follows:

Appearance: Pale-appearing man with thin extremities and a protuberant abdomen

Vitals: Afebrile; supine P = 88 bpm, BP = 110/86 mm Hg; upright P = 110 bpm, BP = 96/62 mm Hg

Skin: Multiple spider angiomas over the upper chest and back, palmar erythema, and white nails

Eyes: Sclera anicteric

Nose: Dried blood present in the left nare

Chest: Gynecomastia

Respiratory: Clear to auscultation and percussion

Cardiac: Hyperdynamic precordium, 2/6 systolic murmur at left sternal border

Abdomen: Distended, hyperactive bowel sounds, nontender, dull flanks with shifting dullness, liver 8 cm to percussion, spleen palpated 2 cm below left costal margin

Extremities: No edema

Neuro: Mild asterixis

Rectal: Black, tarry stool

Labs: $\frac{Na^+\ 132/Cl\ 101/BUN\ 30}{K^+\ 4.4/HCO_3\ 25/Cr\ 1.2}\ \frac{Mgb\ 10.8}{Mct\ 31.6}$ WBC=5.1 Plt=68

PT=15.4   PTT=34   TP=7.7   TBili=1.2
SGOT=70   NH3=118   ALB=2.0   APhos=127
SGPT=30   Chol=120   GGT=96

What clinical or laboratory features of cirrhosis are present in this patient?

Skin changes seen in cirrhosis present on physical examination were spider angiomas (telangiectasiae), palmar erythema, and white nails (leuconychia). Vascular dilatation leads to the development of palmar erythema and cutaneous telangiectasias. Telangiectasias are most commonly seen on the face and anterior chest.

Gynecomastia is found most frequently in cirrhosis secondary to alcohol and is a sequela of impaired estrogen metabolism due to liver failure. This is also the etiology of hair loss and testicular atrophy. Although not present in this patient, fetor hepaticus, a sweet, musty smell to the breath is seen in cirrhosis and hepatic encephalopathy.

The patient's wife mentioned that he had been more forgetful as of late. Mental status changes are seen in hepatic encephalopathy. One means of assessing mental status is to check for the presence of asterixis. Asking the patient to extend his arms and hold his hands out as if to say *stop* will reveal tremor if asterixis is present.

The low albumin level and prolonged prothrombin time (evidence of compromised, hepatic synthetic function) and the elevated globulin level (total protein minus albumin) are suggestive of cirrhosis. Additional laboratories that may be seen in cirrhosis include a low cholesterol, metabolic acidosis, and hyperammonemia.

QUESTION 3   Do the history and physical examination provide evidence of portal hypertension?

Splenomegaly, documented in this patient, is the most important evidence of portal hypertension on physical examination. The associated thrombocytopenia is often present with secondary hypersplenism. Pancytopenia may also occur by the same mechanism.

The physical examination also revealed shifting dullness and splenomegaly. Shifting dullness is indicative of the presence of ascites. When the patient is placed in the left and right lateral decubitus position, ascites fluid flows dependently. Percussion over the dependent area is dull bilaterally in such a case. The presence of ascites suggests portal hypertension in conjunction with hepatocellular insufficiency.

Portal hypertension can also lead to the development of varices because of the marked increase in resistance of blood flow through the cirrhotic liver. Therefore, an assessment should be made for prominent veins on the abdominal wall known as a "Caput Medusae."

QUESTION 4   In the case of GI bleeding, what is the general management of this problem?

The acute management of GI bleeding is aimed at maintaining adequate circulation, intravascular volume, blood pressure, and determining whether or not the patient is actively bleeding. A nasogastric tube should be placed for gastric lavage with saline. Return of bright red blood implies that the source is in the upper GI (UGI) tract and that bleeding is active.

One means of determining the extent of intravascular volume is by assessing the patient for signs of orthostasis. If the blood pressure or pulse fall by 10 mm Hg or by greater than 20 beats/min, respectively, there has been approximately a 20% loss of intravascular volume.

Resuscitation is started immediately by the placement of at least two large bore intravenous catheters and administration of normal saline. When packed red blood cells are available, they should be used in cases of severe hypotension as opposed to saline. If the patient is known to have a coagulopathy (e.g., liver disease), fresh frozen plasma or cryoprecipitate would be optimal for replacement of clotting factors. Platelet transfusion should be done if the platelet count is below 20,000 if bleeding is persistent.

The medical intensive care unit is the optimal location for management of acute GI bleeding.

QUESTION 5 For each of these diseases in the differential diagnosis what is your approach to management and diagnosis, and what is the underlying pathology?

Variceal hemorrhage is the diagnosis with the highest risk of recurrence and mortality. Given that the patient has evidence for cirrhosis and portal hypertension, variceal bleeding should be considered first. However, one should keep in mind that up to one third of UGI bleeding in cirrhotics may be due to etiologies other than varices.

Intrahepatic resistance to portal blood flow in cirrhosis results in the development of collaterals that shunt blood to veins in the esophagus and proximal stomach. Dilated veins of varices arise because of increased flow with consequent increased pressure. Large variceal size (resulting in increased wall tension), portal pressure greater than 12 mm Hg, and degree of hepatocellular dysfunction are risk factors for variceal bleeding.

The patient's history of a duodenal ulcer puts him at risk for further ulcer disease. In fact, approximately 70% to 80% of duodenal ulcers recur in one year's time in the absence of maintenance therapy. Treatment of *Helicobacter pylori*, a bacterial pathogen implicated in the development of duodenal and gastric ulcers, markedly decreases recurrence rates. The use of nonsteroidal antiinflammatory drugs (NSAIDs) is a major risk factor for ulcer disease. The inhibition of vasodilatory prostaglandins leads to relative vasoconstriction leading to ischemia and hindering epithelial defense mechanisms. Cigarette smoking, present in this patient, is also a major risk factor for the ulcer occurrence. The role of corticosteroids in the pathogenesis of peptic ulcer disease remains controversial.

Hemorrhagic gastritis or gastric erosions accounted for nearly one quarter of cases of UGI bleeding in one large series. Superficial mucosal lesions are observed endoscopically, and massive bleeding can occur. Alcohol abuse and the use of NSAIDs, present in the patient under discussion, are predisposing factors. Physiologic stress is the other commonly encountered precipitant.

Prevention is the most important medical intervention with regard to hemorrhagic gastritis. The prostaglandin analogue *Misoprostol* has been shown to be effective in diminishing the risk of NSAID-related lesion, whereas H-2 blockers or proton pump inhibitors should be the agents of choice for treatment if an ulcer develops. Sucralfate and H-2 blockers reduce the incidence of bleeding in patients subjected to severe physiologic stress.

Esophagitis and esophageal ulcer are much less common causes of UGI bleeding, accounting for approximately 2% to 6% of cases. The patient under discussion had reflux symptoms, likely related to increased intraabdominal pressure secondary to ascites. Acid reflux into the esophagus is the most common etiology of mucosal damage leading to hemorrhage. NSAIDs are associated with esophageal ulceration and bleeding. Additional causes include pill esophagitis (seen with KCl, tetracycline, erythromycin, quinaglute, and NSAIDs) and infections such as Candida and herpes.

Mallory-Weiss tears account for 7% to 10% of cases of UGI bleeding. They occur near the gastroesophageal junction as the result of forces generated during retching. Of note, up to 50% of cases lack the classic antecedent history of retching. Use of alcohol and NSAIDs are commonly associated. The diagnosis is made endoscopically. A related syndrome is Boerhaave's syndrome. This syndrome is a through-and-through tear of the esophagus, usually above the GE junction on the left and presents as a sequela of vomiting, straining, or lifting heavy objects. Patients complain of chest pain and have a left pleural effusion and pneumomediastinum. This syndrome less commonly presents with bleeding.

Epistaxis is an uncommon cause of apparent UGI bleeding, accounting for less than 1% of cases of hematemesis and melana. However, given a history of epistaxis as in our patient, or the lack of another etiology after careful evaluation of the UGI tract, this diagnosis should be considered. Risk factors include coagulopathy and facial trauma.

QUESTION 6   What is the treatment for each of the entities mentioned in the differential diagnosis?

A number of modalities are used to treat acute variceal bleeding. Emergent sclerotherapy or banding is the preferred approach. Pharmacologic therapy is useful before or after endoscopic intervention or when an experienced endoscopist is not present. Vasopressin (used in conjunction with NTG) and somatostatin or the somatostatin analogue (octreotide) both have efficacy in reducing portal pressure and controlling bleeding. Somatostatin does not carry the risk of coronary vasoconstriction associated with vasopressin but is substantially more expensive.

Balloon tamponade with a Sengstaken-Blakemore tube can be useful in treating uncontrolled hemorrhage. Portal-systemic shunting provides effective therapy when endoscopic and pharmacologic intervention are unsuccessful. Transjugular intrahepatic portalsystemic shunt (TIPS) offers the advantage of lower morbidity than shunt surgery. The TIPS procedure entails creating a venous channel between the portal circulation and the inferior vena cava, thus decompressing portal pressure.

Endoscopic therapy for gastric varices is much less successful than for esophageal varices and is fraught with a higher complication rate. TIPS may be efficacious if medical and endoscopic approaches to bleeding gastric varices fail. Endoscopic therapy (sclerotherapy or banding) and shunt procedures are not indicated for primary prevention of variceal hemorrhage.

Nonselective beta-blocking agents (propranolol) have efficacy in preventing first variceal bleeds. Clinical endpoints for the use of beta-blockers include a decreased pulse rate by 20%. Both endoscopic intervention and beta-blocker therapy have proven beneficial in reducing the risk of recurrent variceal bleeding. Surgical shunts, and most recently TIPS, are typically reserved for patients with recurrent hemorrhage.

Therapy of peptic ulcer disease is somewhat different. Prompt endoscopy is desirable in the management of a bleeding ulcer disease. Endoscopy facilitates risk stratification. For instance, the presence of a visible vessel carries an approximate 60% to 70% chance of rebleeding. Furthermore, therapeutic measures performed through the endoscope, such as thermal coagulation and injection therapy, can be effective means of controlling active bleeding and preventing rebleeding.

Surgical backup is warranted in the management of bleeding peptic ulcers, and surgical intervention may become necessary if endoscopic therapy is unsuccessful. Radiographic embolization of a bleeding vessel is a further treatment option, though it carries a significant risk of complications.

The use of H-$_2$-blocker therapy is routine in the setting of acute bleeding. While of unproven benefit, such therapy is low in risk and is recommended. Once initial ulcer healing is achieved, patients with a history of life-threatening bleeding are candidates for prolonged maintenance therapy with an H$_2$-blocking agent or the H+K+ pump inhibitor omeprazole. *H. pylori* should be tested for and treated if present.

Therapy for hemorrhagic gastritis begins with cessation of alcohol or NSAID use or treatment of the process leading to physiologic stress. Pharmacologic agents (e.g., H$_2$ blockers) appear to promote healing and should be prescribed. However, as in the case of bleeding peptic ulcers, medications have not been shown to be of benefit in the acute setting. Therapeutic endoscopic techniques may be tried. Surgical intervention becomes necessary in cases of severe, refractory bleeding.

Endoscopic therapy for esophagitis, with or without the presence of an ulcer, has been shown to be effective in controlling active bleeding and diminishing the occurrence of recurrent bleeding

Approach to the cirrhotic patient with hematemesis

↓

History
(?Risk factors for UGI bleeding, including risk factors for liver disease)

↓

Physical exam
(Orthostatic measurements of pulse and blood pressure. A 10 mm Hg drop in BP
with postural change suggests an approximate 20% loss of blood volume)
(?Stigmata of liver disease, including evidence of portal hypertension)

↓

Resuscitation
(Large bore IV access. Intravenous fluid. Packed red blood cells if needed.
Fresh frozen plasma, platelet transfusion if needed)
(Laboratories should be drawn)

↓

Nasogastric lavage
(Assess for active bleeding and clear blood from stomach prior to endoscopy;
Orogastric lavage if needed)

↓

(Endotracheal intubation for airway protection prior to endoscopy in the
setting of massive bleeding or encephalopathy)

↓

Upper endoscopy
(Determine site of bleeding)

Varices
1. Sclerotherapy or banding
2. Vasopressin (and NTG) or somatostatin analog
   (while awaiting or after endoscopic intervention)
3. Balloon tamponade for controlled bleeding
4. TIPS or surgical portal-systemic shunt if above
   unsuccessful

Peptic ulcer disease
(active bleeding or visible vessel $^{+}/_{-}$ overlying clot)
1. Endoscopic therapy: thermal coagulation or injection
2. Intravenous H2 blocker by continuous infusion
3. Surgical or radiologic intervention if
   therapeutic endoscopy unsuccessful
4. Biopsy and treat for M. pylori if present

Hemorrhagic gastritis
1. Discontinue offending agents
2. Endoscopic therapy
3. Intravenous H2 blocker by continuous infusion
4. Surgical intervention if above unsuccessful

Esophagitis or esophageal ulcer
1. Discontinue offending agents
2. Therapeutic endoscopy
3. Continuous IV H2 blocker
4. Treat infectious etiology if present

Mallory-Weiss tear
1. Conservative management if
   hemodynamically stable
2. Therapeutic endoscopy for persistent bleeding

Epistaxis
1. Cauterization of bleeding
   vessels and nasal packing

5-9-1 Diagnostic algorithm for a cirrhotic patient with hematemesis.

of esophageal ulcerations. Initial medical therapy consists of IV H_2 antagonists. Of course, offending agents such as NSAIDs should be discontinued and infectious etiologies should be treated if present.

Conservative management of a Mallory-Weiss tear should be the initial approach in hemodynamically stable patients as the majority of these lesions stop bleeding spontaneously. Endoscopic therapy is indicated for persistent bleeding. Conversely, Boerhaave's syndrome necessitates immediate surgical repair of the tear.

CASE SUMMARY The patient underwent UGI endoscopy that revealed the presence of esophageal varices. There was no active bleeding at the time of the procedure. He was started on a regimen of Aldactone and Lactulose with reduction of the volume of ascites and improvement of the patient's mental status. He was discharged home on the 5th hospital day and is scheduled to follow up with you in the clinic in 10 days. A diagnostic algorithm for a cirrhotic patient with hematemesis is shown in Fig. 5-9-1.

· ·

BIBLIOGRAPHY

Conn HO: Transjugular intrahepatic portal-systemic shunts: the state of the art, *Hepatology* 17:148-158, 1993.

Friedman LS, ed: *Gastroenterology clinics of North America: gastrointestinal bleeding I,* Philadelphia, 1993, WB Saunders.

Graham DY, Schwartz JT: The spectrum of Mallory-Weiss tear, *Medicine* 57:307-318, 1978.

Hutchison SMW, Finlayson NDC: Epistaxis as a cause of hematemesis and melana, *J Clin Gastroenterol* 9:283-285, 1987.

Jensen DM, Cheng S, Kovacs TOG, et al: A controlled study of ranitidine for the prevention of recurrent hemorrhage from duodenal ulcer, *N Engl J Med* 330:382-386, 1994.

Saari A, Kivilaakso E, Inberg M, et al: Comparison of somatostatin and vasopressin in bleeding esophageal varices, *Am J Gastroenterol* 85:804-807, 1990.

Silverstein FE, Gilbert DA, Tedesco FJ, et al: The national ASGE survey on upper gastrointestinal bleeding, *Gastrointest Endosc* 27:73-79, 1981.

Sutton FM: Upper gastrointestinal bleeding in patients with esophageal varices: what is the most common source? *Am J Med* 83-273-275, 1987.

Wolfsen HC, Wang KK: Etiology and course of acute bleeding esophageal ulcers, *J Clin Gastroenterol* 14:342-346, 1992.

C A S E

10

Michael Brown

······

A 57-year-old man is in a reasonable state of health except for occasional arthritic complaints until 3 months before his visit to your office. He now complains of progressive diarrhea and weight loss. He has lost 21 lbs in that time period, and his appetite is poor. He has diarrhea characterized as a malodorous pale stool of semi-formed consistency. He has approximately 3 to 5 bowel movements per day. He has also noticed frequent abdominal cramping, but this improves with a bowel movement. He has not had diarrhea of this duration in the past. He notices no blood in the stool. He has not had fever or chills. The joint pains he experiences are intermittent and have been a problem for 2 years. The arthralgias affect several large joints and occasionally cause redness and swelling. He currently takes ibuprofen as needed. He smokes 1 pack of cigarettes per day and rarely drinks alcohol. He continues to work as an insurance salesman. His family history is noncontributory. In the review of systems he denied weakness, tinnitus, paresthesias, fatigue, nausea, vomiting, or cough.

The physical examination was remarkable for a temperature of 38° C, bilateral cervical lymphadenopathy, mild diffuse abdominal distension, and pain. The nodes are slightly tender, freely movable, and small. Clubbing is present. There was 2+ pitting edema in the lower extremities and a slight increase in skin pigmentation. The neurologic examination was normal.

QUESTION I What is the differential diagnosis in this patient presenting with signs and symptoms of malabsorption and arthralgia?

The differential diagnosis for malabsorption is broad but the preceding arthralgias help narrow the possibilities. Inflammatory bowel disease (IBD) is the most common disorder characterized by joint and malabsorptive findings. Acute arthropathy occurs in 10% to 15% of patients with IBD. The migratory peripheral monarthritis typically affects large joints and waxes and wanes with disease activity. Our patient has not noticed this association. However, joints in IBD become red and swollen as in this case. The central or axial arthritis manifested as ankylosing spondylitis or sacroiliitis tends to be progressive and is unaffected by the severity of bowel inflammation. In this case Crohn's disease would be the more likely diagnosis than ulcerative colitis because of the presence of malabsorption. Fevers are not uncommon in Crohn's disease, but peripheral lymphadenopathy is not seen.

Celiac sprue patients can develop osteopenic bone disease, which may present with bone pain that may be interpreted as arthralgias. Pain in the low back, ribs, and pelvis is common.

Patients with Whipple's disease often present with arthralgias starting from 2 to 5 years before the onset of malabsorption and characterized by red, swollen joints. Two thirds of Whipple's patient's will develop joint complaints during the course of their disease. An intermittent migratory arthritis is the most common presentation affecting large and small joints. As with IBD, sacroiliitis can occur. Low-grade fevers, hyperpigmentation, neurologic complaints, and lymphadenopathy are common in Whipple's disease.

Collagen vascular diseases can present with arthralgias or arthritis and malabsorption. The malabsorption may be secondary to an intestinal vasculitis, pancreatic insufficiency, amyloid, and/or bacterial overgrowth and lymphatic obstruction. This patient's constellation of symptoms including lymphadenopathy, low-grade fever, joint complaints, diarrhea, and abdominal pain certainly supports an autoimmune diagnosis. Clubbing is seen in most patients with advanced small bowel disease and malabsorption.

Pseudomembranous colitis and collagenous colitis have been associated with a polyarthritis similar to that seen in sprue. However, these disorders affect the colon and would therefore not be associated with significant steatorrhea and nutrient malabsorption. The iatrogenic malabsorption seen in patients with intestinal bypass operations for morbid obesity can also be associated with arthritis. The patient's history of the appropriate surgical procedure would lead to rapid identification of this gastrointestinal-rheumatic process.

Endocrinopathies are a consideration in this patient. Thyrotoxicosis may present with malabsorption, lymphadenopathy, neurologic abnormalities, edema, and fever. Clinical features of Addison's disease include hyperpigmentation, weakness, weight loss, malabsorption, abdominal pain, and anorexia. However, joint complaints are not seen in these disorders.

QUESTION 2   The patient undergoes a 24-hour stool collection that demonstrates a total volume of 567 ml and 14 g of fat. List the possible pathophysiologic mechanisms for the diarrhea and steatorrhea seen in this patient. What are examples of disease states that may produce these defects?

There are several pathophysiologic mechanisms that may lead to malabsorption. They are categorized with examples of each mechanism as follows.

Lumenal phase maldigestion

Pancreatic insufficiency: chronic pancreatitis (loss of enzymes)

Destruction of enzymes: Zollinger-Ellison syndrome (hyperacidity inactivates enzymes)

Rapid transit states: postgastrectomy syndromes (inadequate contact time), decreased bile salt synthesis and/or secretion, end stage liver disease, use of cholestyramine (inadequate fat

solubilization), increased bile salt deconjugation or absorption, bacterial overgrowth (inadequate fat solubilization), enhanced bile salt loss, terminal ileitis or ileal resection (inadequate fat solubilization)

Mucosal phase defects

Villous atrophy/destruction, celiac sprue, Crohn's disease, Whipple's disease (loss of brush border enzymes, loss of mucosal surface area), obstruction of epithelial transport, abetalipoproteinemia (inability to transport chylomicrons from brush border cells to lymphatics)

Transport phase defects

Lymphatic obstruction, tuberculosis, lymphoma (inability to transport chylomicrons through lymph drainage system), vascular damage, vasculitis, ischemia (impaired transport of nonfat nutrients)

QUESTION 3   Once steatorrhea has been defined in this patient, how should your work-up proceed? What initial blood work might be important?

Initial diagnostic blood work can shed light on the underlying diagnosis. Laboratories should include a complete blood count, serum Fe, ferritin, vitamin B_{12}, folic acid level, and electrolytes including magnesium, phosphorus, and calcium. Low levels of beta-carotene are supportive of significant steatorrhea in equivocal cases. Abnormalities of transaminases (SGOT/SGPT), alkaline phosphatase, and bilirubin may suggest bile salt inadequacy. Low protein and albumin levels suggest a protein-losing enteropathy. Furthermore, prolongation of the prothrombin time may be due to malabsorption of vitamin K.

Fig. 5-10-1 suggests a diagnostic algorithm for steatorrhea.

QUESTION 4   The patient undergoes small bowel biopsy when a D-xylose test suggests a small bowel absorptive defect. The pathologist's preliminary report suggests "flattened or atrophic villi." What disease processes might include this histologic abnormality and how would they be confirmed/refuted?

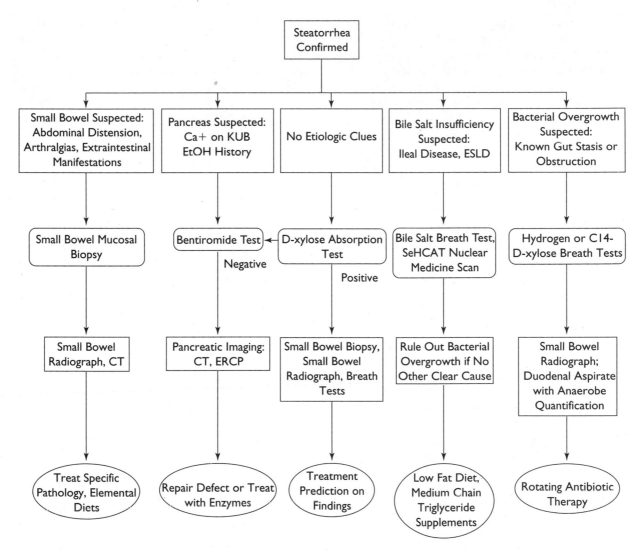

5-10-1 Diagnostic algorithm for steatorrhea.

Celiac sprue is characterized histologically by a loss of villous architecture. Crypts are elongated and hyperplastic. The mucosal surface is flat with remaining mucosal cells appearing cuboidal. Cellular cytoplasm is markedly basophilic with loss of typical basal nuclear polarity. There is an increase in the cellular infiltration of the lamina propria with lymphocytes and plasma cells. These abnormalities are usually diffuse. Diagnosis of this disorder now may rest on the finding of abnormal serum antibodies. IgA antigliadin antibodies are specific for sprue but are not as sensitive as their IgG counterparts. Smooth muscle endomysial antibody has been reported to be nearly 100% specific and sensitive for sprue. Improvement on a gluten-free diet would confirm the diagnosis and response may be seen in 3 to 4 weeks.

Tropical sprue is associated with a similar histologic picture of shortened villi and hyperplastic crypts. The inflammatory cell infiltrate is more diverse than in celiac sprue with lymphocytes, macrophages, plasma cells, and eosinophils. Flattening of the mucosa is usually not as severe. This patient lacks the usual travel history from a tropical to a temperate climate seen in tropical sprue. A response to empiric therapy with tetracycline and folic acid would be confirmatory.

Patients with Crohn's disease typically have a grossly abnormal endoscopic appearance with nodularity and ulceration. Villous atrophy and flattening are unusual with cryptitis being a more common histologic finding. The associated inflammatory infiltration is often intense with macrophages, lymphocytes, neutrophils, and plasma cells. Abnormalities may be segmental in Crohn's disease. Radiographic examination of the small bowel may be helpful in further eliminating Crohn's disease as a diagnosis.

The mucosal surface in Whipple's disease is typically flat with widened villi. The unique feature is an extensive infiltration of the lamina propria with large PAS-positive macrophages filled with glycoprotein granules. The increase in macrophages diminishes the presence of other inflammatory cells and is therefore pathognomic for Whipple's disease. Lymphatic dilatation and fat droplet accumulation is typical. The causative agent, *Tropheryma whippelii* can be seen just beneath the absorptive surface and lining the vessels. Response to antibiotic therapy can be dramatic and would be confirmatory. Current data suggest that trimethoprim-sulfamethoxazole is superior to tetracycline in the treatment of Whipple's disease. Treatment for 6 to 12 months is necessary to eradicate *T. whippelii* in the central nervous system.

Several other disorders may present with a similar small bowel histologic appearance including radiation injury, bacterial overgrowth, Zollinger-Ellison syndrome, AIDS enteropathy, viral gastroenteritis, ischemic bowel disease, and malnutrition. Of these, bacterial overgrowth may be the most difficult to diagnose. Quantitative anaerobic culture of the small bowel is difficult and is not widely available. Breath tests including the hydrogen and 14C or 13C-D-xylose breath test are used to assess bacterial metabolic activity in the proximal gut. The radiolabeled xylose tests are more accurate than hydrogen breath testing. Long-term treatment with rotating antibiotics may be necessary if no correctable cause for the overgrowth (stricture, isolated diverticula) is found.

CASE FOLLOW-UP Further details from the pathologist revealed the PAS-positive macrophages characteristic of Whipple's disease. He was begun on trimethoprim-sulfmethoxazole and responds with resolution of the steatorrhea and weight gain in 3 weeks.

• •

BIBLIOGRAPHY

Feurle GE, Marth T: An evaluation of antimicrobial treatment for Whipple's Disease. Tetracycline versus trimethoprim-sulfamethoxazole, *Dig Dis Sci* 39(8):1642-1648, 1994.

Fisher RL, ed: Malabsorption and nutritional status and support, *Gastrointest Clin North Am* 18(3):467-666, 1989.

Gaist D, Ladefoged K: Whipple's disease, *Scand J Gastroenterol* 29(2):97-101, 1994.

Gran JT, Husby G: Joint manifestations in gastrointestinal diseases, 2. Whipple's disease, enteric infections, intestinal bypass operations, gluten-sensitive enteropathy, pseudomembranous colitis and collagenous colitis, *Dig Dis* 10(5): 295-312, 1992.

Relman DA, Schmidt TM, MacDermott RP, Falkow S: Identification of the uncultured bacillus of Whipple's disease, *N Engl J Med* 327(5):293-301, 1992.

Riley SA, Turnberg LA: Maldigestion and malabsorption in gastrointestinal disease. In Sleisenger MH, Fordtran JS, eds: *Gastrointestinal disease: pathophysiology, diagnosis and management*, ed 5, Philadelphia, 1993, WB Saunders.

GENERAL INTERNAL MEDICINE

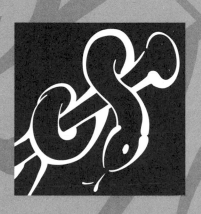

CHARLES J. GRODZIN (CASES 1 TO 7)
RICHARD ABRAMS (CASES 1 TO 7)
WILLIAM J. ELLIOT (CASE 8)
SECTION EDITORS

CASE

Charles J. Grodzin
Richard Abrams

A 61-year-old man presents with complaints of nausea, vomiting, and dizziness. He has a history of hypertension and diabetes. He relates a 2-week history of head congestion and rhinorrhea. He was able to stay at home and treat himself symptomatically, but became concerned when an episode of dizziness nearly led to him falling down a flight of stairs. For 3 days he had been taking generic aspirin and a decongestant he obtained from a local pharmacy.

QUESTION 1 At this point, what historical data would you like to gather to help understand the patient's complaints of dizziness?

Vision, vestibular sensation, joint position sense, touch-pressure sensation, and hearing are all involved in maintaining spatial orientation. Dizziness may result from distortion of any of these inputs. It is useful to classify the complaint of dizziness as presyncope (impending faint), vertigo, disequilibrium, and gait abnormalities. The difference may be more easily separated by asking the patient to describe his symptoms without using the word "dizzy."

Presyncope is a result of brain stem hypoperfusion associated with lightheadedness, diaphoresis, visual blurring or blindness, loss of lower extremity coordination, and difficulty maintaining posture. Consciousness is not impaired until syncope occurs.

Vertigo, produced by unequal bilateral vestibular input, is characterized by the illusion of spinning: the individual relative to the environment or vice-versa. However, patients may also complain of a "rocking" sensation, vague lightheadedness, or the illusion of a to-and-fro movement of the environment (oscillopsia). The patient may also develop tinnitus, fullness or stuffiness in the ears, or discharge from the external auditory canal. The review of symptoms should focus on additional psychiatric or neurologic symptoms, association with changes of head position, recent illness, medication use, or concomitant medical problems.

Disequilibrium is psychogenic in origin and is usually a feeling of dissociation between body movement and neural control without the illusion of movement. It is commonly present while walking, but disappears upon sitting down.

Gait disturbances manifest as ataxia. They are due to loss of coordination without the illusion of movement.

Vertigo may be either central or peripheral. *Central* causes present more insidiously. Episodes are of longer duration, demonstrate gait disturbance, headache, diplopia, unilateral loss of power or coordination, or other cranial nerve abnormalities. Nystagmus of central origin is not suppressed by visual fixation. *Peripheral* (labyrinthine) causes are characterized by unilateral tinnitus or decreased auditory acuity with normal periods of function between episodes. Symptoms are usually more severe and demonstrate adaptation of vertigo and nystagmus with time. Unilateral vestibulopathy may produce falling to one side (the side of the lesion). Bilateral vestibulopathy may present more so with abnormalities of tandem gait or Romberg testing. Importantly, vascular disorders present abruptly.

QUESTION 2 What findings on physical examination aid in characterizing the etiology of the patient's complaints? (box)

ETIOLOGIES OF VERTIGO AND ASSOCIATED PHYSICAL FINDINGS

ETIOLOGY	PATHOLOGY
Otogenic/acute vestibular	Meniere's syndrome, myringitis, otitis media, neuronitis, herpes zoster otitis, labyrinthitis, middle ear or labyrinthine tumors, petrositis, otosclerosis
Toxic	Alcohol, aminoglycosides, opiates
Psychogenic	Hysteria
Environmental	Motion sickness
Ocular	Diplopia
Circulatory	Vertebrobasilar insufficiency (VBI)
Neurologic	MS, skull fracture, temporal lobe seizures, encephalitis
Neoplasia (solid tumors)	Pontine tumors, CPA tumor, acoustic neuroma
Hematologic	Leukemic infiltration of the labyrinth

Physical examination should focus on the vestibular apparatus, which includes finger-to-nose, heel-to-shin, rapid alternating movements, Romberg and gait testing. Auscultation over the carotid artery, while both eyes are closed, the squamous portion of the temporal bone anterior to the ear and over the mastoid bones can reveal bruits suggesting vascular compromise. Otologic examination for the presence of tympanic membrane rupture, vesicles, or hemotympanum is essential. Neurological assessment with attention to visual dysfunction, cranial neuropathy, or a focal motor finding is necessary.

The Weber and Rinne tests are very useful. These tests investigate bone and air conduction. Air conduction (AC) depends on the integrity of the external and middle ear. Bone conduction (BC) depends on vibration of the skull to stimulate the inner ear directly. This bypasses the external and middle ear structures and makes use of CN VIII and central nervous system function. Therefore, if AC > BC, a deficit is present and resides in either the trochlear nerve or brainstem. If BC > AC, then the deficit is localized to the external or middle ear structures.

The Weber test is carried out by placing the stem of a vibrating tuning fork on the midpoint of the forehead and asking the patient on which side she or he hears the tone. In the presence of a conductive hearing loss, the tone is heard louder in the affected ear. In the presence of a sensorineural hearing loss, the tone is heard louder in the unaffected ear. The Rinne test comprises a comparison of air and bone conduction. The vibrating tuning fork is held with the tines near the ear, then the stem is placed in contact with the mastoid process when the vibrations are no longer audible. Normally, the vibration is heard louder and longer via air conduction than via bone conduction (AC > BC). In the presence of conductive hearing loss this is reversed (BC > AC). With a sensorineural lesion, air conduction is louder but both are reduced.

The *vestibuloocular reflex* may be assessed by rotating the patient's head at 1 cycle/second and asking him to read a standard eye chart. Loss of acuity of more than one line is evidence of dysfunction. The *Barany (Hallpike) maneuver,* done by changing patient position from upright to supine with the head hanging at 45° turned to the right, left, and in the central position, will reproduce vertiginous symptoms and induce nystagmus when the affected side is downward. When positive, this test demonstrates vestibulopathy. The *fistula test* involves placing a pneumatic otoscope into the external auditory canal. Inflation causes tympanic membrane fluctuation. If vestibulopathy is present, the result will be vertigo, nystagmus, and eye deviation. The effect of hyperventilation on decreasing cerebral perfusion is well-known. By asking a patient to hyperventilate, symptoms of presyncope can be produced for comparison to the patient's initial complaint.

QUESTION 3   After a complete history and physical, you are convinced that your patient is experiencing true vertigo. What is the differential diagnosis of vertigo? (box)

Meniere's disease is an abnormal accumulation of endolymphatic fluid leading to the classic triad of vertigo, tinnitus, and hearing loss. The tinnitus is usually low frequency and fluctuating. Attacks may recur every 2 to 3 days and may last from hours to days. Treatment may successfully reduce episodes of vertigo and associated symptoms, but hearing and vestibular function loss is inevitable. In some patients, recurrent symptoms may "burn out" over many years.

Benign positional vertigo (BPV) is the most common cause of vertigo. BPV is characterized by vertiginous episodes associated with sudden changes of head position (e.g., rolling over in bed). Episodes usually last less than 5 minutes, with symptom-free episodes between attacks and demonstrate adaptation and fatigue with recurrent challenge. The presence of symptom-free periods is an important diagnostic finding as vertiginous processes lead to persistent symptoms. The Barany maneuver duplicates symptoms and will produce nystagmus; physical findings will be fatigable.

Processes resulting in inflammation of labyrinthine structures (labyrinthitis) may produce vertigo. This may be the result of a viral infection (measles, herpes, mumps) or suppurative bacterial infection. Herpetic geniculate ganglionitis, the Ramsay-Hunt syndrome, produces long-lasting vertigo (days to weeks). Reactivation leads to vesicular involvement of the external auditory meatus and the geniculate ganglion. The syndrome includes loss of taste on the anterior two thirds of the tongue, ipsilateral facial palsy, and symptoms of vertigo. Inflammation may also be secondary to systemic illness, ototoxic medications/antibiotics (loop diuretics, quinine, caffeine, aspirin, aminoglycosides, phenytoin, cisplatinum), or alcohol ingestion. Hearing recovery occurs over 3 to 6 weeks.

Motion sickness, involving nausea and vertigo, is due to incongruous vestibular and optic neural input due to loss of fixation on the distant horizon. Symptoms are continuous throughout exposure and may last for a few hours after removal from the environment. *Traumatic etiologies* include labyrinthine concussion, fracture of vestibular or cochlear structures, development of a perilymphatic fistula (rupture of the perilymphatic sac) as middle ear ossicles are forced by trauma into the perilymphatic membrane. Deep sea diving can lead to decompression sickness, air embolism, or rupture of the oval window leading to symptoms of vertigo.

Processes that involve the *middle ear* include blockage of a eustachian tube creating negative pressure on the tympanic membrane, a situation approximated by the fistula test. Acute and chronic otitis media can also alter middle ear pressure producing vertigo. Otosclerosis, by virtue of stapedial immobilization, can produce vertigo associated with conductive hearing loss in a young person (second to third decade). A cholesteatoma is the result of growth of squamous epithelium into the middle ear from the external auditory canal.

Vascular insufficiency of labyrinthine structures will lead to vertigo. This etiology may be seen due to atherosclerosis, hypertensive, or diabetic vasculopathy, vasculitis, extrinsic compression, or arterial spasm. Symptoms may be temporally associated with transient ischemic attacks. The Wallenberg syndrome, infarction of lateral medullary structures in the distribution of the posterior inferior cerebellar artery, includes vertigo along with other deficits. The subclavian steal syndrome, unilateral subclavian artery occlusion with resultant ipsilateral retrograde vertebral ar-

VERTIGO: SUMMARY OF SYMPTOMS AND SIGNS

Physiologic vertigo (motion sickness, etc.)	Diaphoresis, nausea, vomiting, salivation, yawning, GI upset, hyperventilation, postural hypotension, and syncope. Need to match sensory input to cortex from different modes.
Benign positional vertigo	Brief, <1 min, with position change, fatigable paroxysmal nystagmus often rapid changes of body or head position. Can be fatigued, going through the same repetitive movements can eventually extinguish vertigo.
Acute peripheral vestibulopathy	Vertigo, nausea, vomiting, acute and lasts several days with neurological/auditory, symptoms Prodromal upper respiratory infection (URI)—question viral origin.
Meniere's syndrome	Fluctuating hearing loss and tinnitus, abrupt and severe vertigo, fullness/pressure in ear. Dilated endolymphatic duct and hair cell atrophy.
Posttraumatic vertigo	Labrynthine concussion following a blow to the head/occipital-mastoid area. Transverse fracture of temporal bone: passing through vestibular apparatus, hemotympanum; oval window fistula can follow acute changes in middle ear pressure— deep water diving, physical exertion, etc.
Postconcussive syndrome	Dizziness; less often vertigo associated with anxiety, decreased concentration, headache, and photophobia.
Chronic bacterial otomastoiditis	Invasion of middle ear by bacteria or erosion of a labyrinth by cholesteatoma otosclerosis.
Drugs	Aminoglycosides, alcohol.
Vascular insufficiency	VBI (abrupt, several minutes with nausea/vomiting) and may be associated with visual impairment due to ischemia of surrounding areas.
Brain stem and cerebellum	Infarcts. Positive cerebellar signs including extremity, gait ataxia and nystagmus.
Cerebellopontine angle tumors	Gradual vague disequilibrium or episodic vertigo, retrotrochlear hearing loss revealed by BSAEP. Find tumor with MRI.
MS	Involving brainstem, cerebellum, in vertebrobasilar (VB) vascular distribution - internuclear ophthalmoplegia (INO) on examination.
Parainfection, encephalomyelitis, cranial polyneuritis, Ramsay Hunt's syndrome	Geniculate ganglion herpes; vertigo, hearing loss and facial paralysis, and herpes lesions involving the external auditory canal.
Leptomeningeal metastasis	Involvement of cranial nerve VIII.
Miscellaneous	Vasculitis. Temporal lobe epilepsy. Granulomatous meningitis.

VBI, vertebrobasilar insufficiency; BSAEP, brainstem auditory evoked potentials; MRI, magnetic resonance imaging; INO, internuclear ophthalmoplegia.

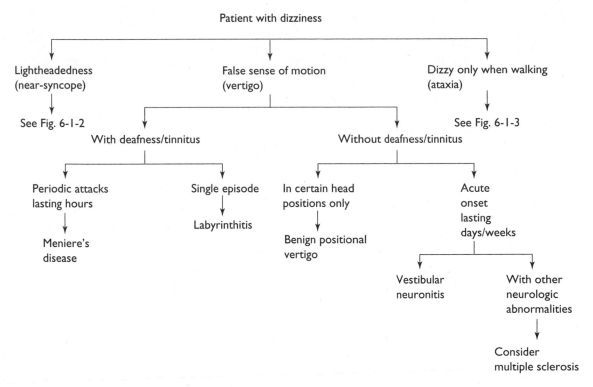

6-1-1 Diagnostic algorithm for dizziness.
(From Green HL, Johnson WP, Maricic MJ: *Decision making in medicine*, St Louis, 1993, Mosby.)

tery flow, will reduce labyrinthine perfusion and lead to vertigo. In this case, symptoms may occur with arm exercise. A subclavian bruit may be auscultated.

Intracranial tumors exert symptoms through structural compression. Cerebellopontine angle (CPA) tumors or acoustic neuromas (neurofibromatosis) impinging on cranial nerve VIII can lead to hearing loss and vertigo. Examination may discover facial or trigeminal nerve palsy, facial weakness, or numbness. An early sign of facial nerve involvement is loss of the corneal reflex.

QUESTION 4 What tests are useful in the evaluation of dizziness?

The first step is deciding, by history, whether the patient is complaining of vertigo, lightheadedness/presyncope, dissociation, or disequilibrium. One should also consider the diagnosis of hyperventilation syndrome with complaints of lightheadedness, especially when purposeful hyperventilation reproduces symptoms. Other psychiatric illnesses to consider include acute anxiety and panic attacks. Any focal findings on the neurologic examination demand neuroimaging with MRI. This imaging modality should be used unless acute hemorrhage (<24 hours) is highly suspected. If MRI is not available, CT with IV infusion is the next best study.

When the neurologic examination is nonfocal, audiometry should be the first test. An abnormal audiogram means that there is a problem either in the trochlear nerve (cranial nerve 8) or the retrotrochlear apparatus. The finding of sensorineural hearing loss can be investigated by doing brain stem auditory evoked responses (BAER). This examination tests the retrotrochlear apparatus.

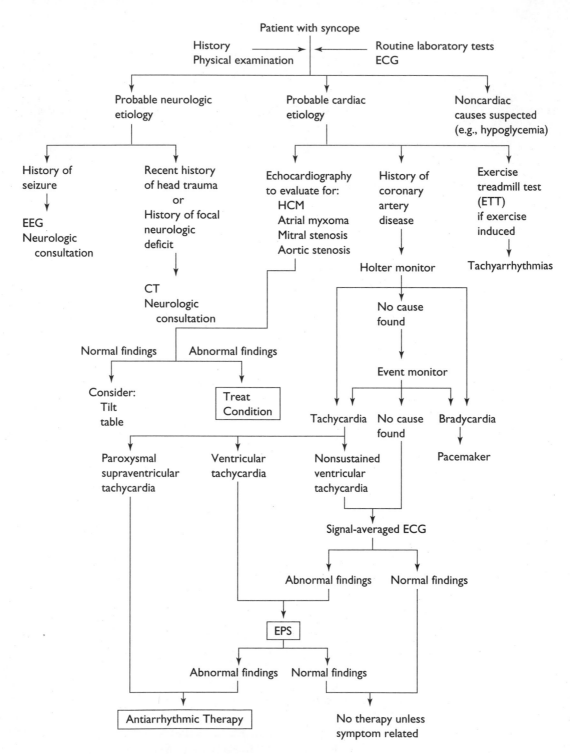

6-1-2 Diagnostic algorithm for syncope.
(From Greene HL, Johnson WP, Maricic MJ: *Decision making in medicine*, St Louis, 1993, Mosby.)

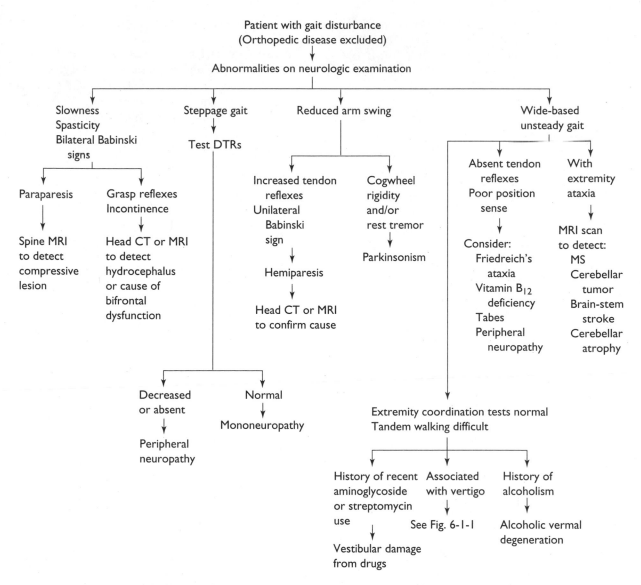

6-1-3   Diagnostic algorithm for gait disturbance.
(From Greene HL, Johnson WP, Maricic MJ: *Decision making in medicine*, St Louis, 1993, Mosby.)

Abnormality in this test suggests the presence of an acoustic neuroma or other C-P angle tumor.

When BAER are normal, this suggests the presence of labyrinthitis, Meniere's disease, endolymphatic fistula, or labyrinthine concussion. A normal audiogram should be followed by electronystagmography (ENG). Diseases including benign positional vertigo, peripheral vestibulopa-thy, physiologic vertigo, and ototoxicity are supported by an abnormal ENG.

If the patient's complaints are more suggestive of presyncope/lightheadedness, dissociation or disequilibrium, the test regimen is dictated closely by the neurologic examination or major complaint. If the examination discovers cardiac findings, testing should be aimed at arrhythmias, postural hypotension, and congestive heart failure. Complaints consistent with disequilibrium with a nonfocal neurologic examination require ENG testing to look for unusual presentations of ototoxicity or bilateral vestibulopathy.

QUESTION 5 Convinced of your diagnosis, acute peripheral vestibulopathy, how would you approach treatment?

Symptomatic therapy may be first-line treatment. Initially, acute symptoms of nausea and vertigo can be palliated by placing the patient in a dark quiet room, lying down, eyes closed. Many medications have anti-vertiginous qualities. Antiemetics are used to treat nausea and sedatives with antivertiginous properties (phenergan and diazepam) contribute to patient comfort and relief. Maintenance therapy may be necessary so that the patient may return to work and carry out daily activities. Both meclizine and scopolamine are much less sedating but have stronger antivertiginous properties. Disabling vertigo, unresponsive to pharmacologic therapy, may require surgical treatment to correct altered middle ear anatomy.

Treatment of secondary vestibulopathy is based on the underlying problem (e.g., infection requires antibiotics, sinus drainage). Vascular insufficiency may require anticoagulation or vascular surgery. Cerebellopontine angle tumors may require resection.

A diagnostic algorithm for dizziness is shown in Fig. 6-1-1.

BIBLIOGRAPHY

Baloh RW: Dizziness in older people, *J Am Geriatric Soc* 40:713-721, 1992.

Davis EA: Emergency department approach to vertigo, *Emerg Med Clin North Am* 5(2):211-225, 1987.

Slater R: How serious are recurrent and single attacks? *Postgrad Med* 84(5):58-67, 1988.

Warner E: Dizziness in primary care patients, *J Gen Intern Med* 7:454-463, 1992.

Wynngaarden JB, Smith LH: *Cecil's textbook of medicine*, ed 18, Volume 2, Philadelphia, 1988, WB Saunders.

C A S E

2

Charles J. Grodzin
Richard Abrams

A 47-year-old man comes to your clinic. He has become concerned about his health after the unexpected death of a friend. The initial evaluation, as well as several follow-up visits, reveal persistently elevated blood pressure.

QUESTION I In your initial history and physical examination what findings would you seek to identify the etiology and systemic effects of hypertension? What initial lab testing would you order to evaluate the patient's hypertension?

A blood pressure greater than 140/90 mm Hg on three occasions separated by at least 1 month confirms the diagnosis of hypertension. This approach is necessary to confirm the absence of false-positive findings on one evaluation. It is common to find that a patient's blood pressure is elevated because of anxiety provoked by seeing a physician (white coat hypertension), concern about the state of his or her health, or fear of illness.

Questions concerning factors that may be the source of, or complicate underlying hypertension, are important. These include family history of renal disease or cardiac disease, diabetes mellitus, Cushing's syndrome/disease, sickle cell disease, amyloidosis, and immune complex diseases (hepatitis B, systemic lupus erythematosus, endocarditis). In addition, use of nonsteroidal antiinflammatory agents, history of alcohol use (greater than 1 ounce per day), increasing obesity, use of salt indiscriminately, and smoking should be sought because of their propensity to elevate blood pressure.

Because high blood pressure contributes to end-organ failure, history and physical examination should seek signs of end-organ damage. Heart failure can be accompanied by complaints of orthopnea, paroxysmal nocturnal dyspnea, decreased exercise tolerance, dependent edema, and dyspnea on exertion. A patient who has required changing eyeglass prescriptions may in fact have advancing retinal microvascular disease. Macrovascular disease may stimulate complaints of lower extremity rest pain, distal coolness, muscle cramping or numbness, and tingling. Complaints of altered mental status, stroke or transient ischemic attack may be due to intracranial hypertension or cerebrovascular disease. Renal disease may manifest signs of volume overload with periorbital edema, more specifically related to renal failure opposed to other hypervolemic diseases, nausea, vomiting, or bleeding suggestive of platelet dysfunction (gingival or mucosal bleeding).

Macrovascular disease may involve coronary, carotid, renal, femoral, or cerebral vessels. Signs of heart failure should be sought (diminished arterial pulses, pulmonary congestion, cardiomegaly, valvular or anatomical murmurs, distended neck veins, a pulsatile liver, and peripheral edema). Signs of ventricular thickening are lateral displacement of the point of maximum impulse (PMI) and a fourth heart sound. Evaluation of symmetrical pulses as well as determination of a systolic pressure gradient between the arms and legs is important to help rule out the presence of aortic aneurysm or coarctation. Abdominal ausculatation can discover renal artery bruits. Neurologic examination may reveal focal deficits due to past cerbrovascular accidents. Microvascular disease may be reflected by funduscopic examination (copper-wire charges, A-V nicking, hypertensive retinopathy).

Initial laboratory testing includes electrolytes to measure the potassium concentration and creatinine, urinalysis, blood glucose, and a fasting lipid profile. Visual acuity should be determined, and an electrocardiogram should also be completed. This information is necessary to help ascertain the etiology and discover the extent of end-organ damage, and reveal other comorbid diseases. An elevated BUN and creatinine suggests renal insufficiency. Hypokalemia is found in some patients with primary hyperaldosteronism or hypercortisolism. Electrocardiography can provide information about ventricular hypertrophy as well as chamber size and conduction abnormalities caused by chronic hypertension. The blood glucose and glycosylated hemoglobin concentration yield information about the presence of diabetes.

Urinalysis can shed light on the presence of glomerular dysfunction (i.e., proteinuria) as a source of sequela of elevated blood pressure. The urinalysis sediment, when active, can suggest the presence of glomerulonephritis as a possible etiology of hypertension.

QUESTION 2 The history was significant for moderate alcohol use and diabetes he was told was due to obesity. The physical examination revealed a 2/6 systolic murmur loudest at the second left intercostal space, bilateral femoral bruits, and 1+ bilateral dorsalis pedis pulses. His electrolytes were normal, but his creatinine was 1.9 mg/dl. The ECG showed evidence of left ventricular hypertrophy. Because of the multiple physical findings, you decide to do a more extensive evaluation. What further testing would you carry out?

The goal of further testing is twofold. It is important to evaluate the degree of end-organ damage and the patient's risk factor profile for coronary, cerebral, and peripheral arterial disease.

Echocardiography is an excellent noninvasive means of evaluating left ventricular (LV) structure and function. In the face of heart failure, it is important to use this information to direct medi-

cal therapy. Segmental wall motion abnormalities require investigation with coronary angiography to evaluate the degree of coronary atherosclerosis. Systolic dysfunction is treated with afterload reduction, whereas diastolic dysfunction may be treated with calcium antagonists (e.g., verapamil) that aid ventricular relaxation.

Noninvasive arterial studies (pulse volume recording) assess lower extremity arterial sufficiency, vascular compliance, and degree of hypertrophy of arterial resistance vessels.

A 24-hour collection of urine for creatinine approximates the creatinine clearance and glomerular filtration rate. A collection of urinary albumin over a 24-hour period reflects glomerular integrity (>1 to 3 grams of protein is suggestive of a glomerular lesion as opposed to a tubular lesion).

Hypertension (HTN) is a significant independent risk factor for coronary artery disease (CAD). This finding should serve as the impetus to perform a health risk assessment aimed at quantitating the risk of CAD. Major risk factors also include a history of diabetes mellitus, smoking, hyperlipidemia, and male sex. Obesity and a sedentary lifestyle may add to an individual's risk but have not been isolated as independent risk factors. Risk factors act synergistically in the development of occlusive coronary disease. Patients with these risk factors require counseling about smoking cessation, weight loss, control of blood glucose, and the establishment of an open relationship with a primary physician.

QUESTION 3 What is the compelling evidence that treatment of HTN is useful?

A positive correlation exists between the severity of HTN and total cardiovascular mortality. An increased mean arterial pressure by 10% correlated with a 30% increase in risk of cardiovascular (CV) death. Framingham data revealed a threefold increase in sudden death in hypertensive patients without prior history of coronary heart disease (CHD). HTN is responsible for 15% to 20% of all cases of end-stage renal disease (ESRD).

Meta-analysis yields a significant reduction of overall mortality by 11%, and reduction of fatal and nonfatal stroke by 38% and 42%, respectively, when blood pressure is controlled. Fatal and nonfatal MI were decreased by 8% and 14%, respectively.

Normalization of blood pressure led to improvement of renal function or a slowed rate of progression to ESRD and coronary and cerebrovascular disease.

The Oslo study was done to answer the question of whether treatment of borderline/mild HTN would lead to a reduction in the incidence of CV disease. Treatment was initiated with hydrochlorothiazide. If blood pressure was not controlled, methyldopa and propranolol were added serially. Several conclusions were reached: There was a significant reduction in stroke, congestive heart failure, and electrocardiographic evidence of left ventricular hypertrophy. However, no protection from CHD was seen.

Isolated systolic hypertension is defined as a SBP >160 mm Hg with a DBP <90 mm Hg. The Build and Blood Pressure study in 1959 found a near-linear relationship between age and systolic HTN: 8% at 50 years old, 5% at 60 years old, 12% at 70 years old, 23.6% at 80 years old. Men were more affected than women, and blacks more than whites. Elevated systolic HTN is also associated with increased stroke and CAD than in normotensive individuals. The U.S. HTN Detection and Follow-up program supported a study that confirmed a 1% increase in mortality per mm HG increase in SBP. The Framingham study followed patients for 24 years and found an age-adjusted odds ratio for mortality at 2.1 for men and 3.1 for women with systolic hypertension. A European study found, paradoxically, that the very elderly (>78 years old) benefitted, in terms of survival, with elevated SBP.

The most recent study was conducted by the NHLBI: *Systolic Hypertension in the Elderly Program (SHEP)*. The study revealed a 26% decrease in stroke incidence and 27% reduction in incidence of nonfatal MI, with a 13% reduction of all cause mortality.

QUESTION 4 What are the significant side effects of antihypertensive therapy?

A constant concern about any medical intervention is the degree to which it carries other morbidity. Diuretics and beta-blockers have effects that exacerbate lipid abnormalities. Specifically, thiazide diuretics increase triglycerides (TG) and LDL, whereas beta-blockers increase TG and reduce HDL. Labetalol, a nonspecific beta-blocker with alpha-blocking qualities, has no significant lipid impact.

Glucose metabolism can also be affected. Thiazide diuretics lead to hyperglycemia because of diminished insulin secretion. Lasix has inhibitory effects on glucose transport. Beta-blockade (β-2), because of unopposed alpha-induced inhibition of insulin secretion, leads to hyperglycemia and can delay recovery time from hypoglycemia. The usual cardiac/autonomic responses to hypoglycemia may also be blunted because of antagonism to glucagon and catecholamine secretion, the main counter-regulatory hormones. Because of those effects, diabetics should only be given cardio-selective (β-1) agents (metoprolol and atenolol). An exception is pindolol (beta-blocker with intrinsic sympathomimetic effect) that does not lead to hypoglycemia. Paradoxically, acebutolol, a cardioselective agent, produces hypoglycemia.

Activation of the renin-angiotensin axis follows treatment with diuretics and vasodilators. The juxtaglomerular apparatus interprets decreased glomerular perfusion pressure as intravascular volume depletion and responds by activation of the renin-angiotensin-aldosterone (RAA) axis. Conversely, the RAA axis is antagonized by central alpha antagonists, beta-blockers, and ACE inhibitors. Because of salt and water retention associated with vasodilators, diuretics are useful adjuncts to therapy.

Diuretics can produce hypokalemic hypochloremic metabolic alkalosis or prerenal azotemia because of severe volume depletion. Replacement of intravascular volume in diuretic-treated, sodium-restricted patients with free water (mostly occurring at home) can lead to hyponatremia. In the bed-ridden patient, or one who has lost the thirst reflex, hypernatremia is a risk. For the volume-depleted patient treated with a loop or thiazide diuretic, volume replacement should include chloride in the form of potassium chloride or sodium chloride depending on the patient's serum electrolytes. Both ACE-inhibitor, due to inhibition of aldosterone secretion, and beta-blockers, can produce hyperkalemia. Potassium sparing diuretics (triamterene and spironolactone) can also elevate serum potassium by antagonism of aldosterone if left unchecked.

QUESTION 5 What are the endpoints for antihypertensive patients?

A study by Hartford in Sweden identified the goal-endpoints in antihypertensive therapy. In this small study, patients were begun on a cardioselective beta-blocker (metoprolol); if blood pressure was not controlled, hydrochlorothiazide (HCTZ) was added and then hydralazine if necessary. Thirteen patients were followed and compared with 37 controls over a 7-year follow-up period. Cardiovascular and renal parameters of the treated group compared to that of the untreated patient approached those of normotensive controls. In terms of hemodynamic improvement, there was a statistically significant improvement in mean arterial pressure, total peripheral resistance, systolic BP, diastolic BP, and heart rate. There was also significant vascular improvement as measured by compliance of large arteries and hypertrophy of arterial resistance vessels. Structurally, left ventricular (LV) wall thickness and mass improved. Improved diastolic blood pressure was chiefly due to normalization of LV relaxation time and LV filling distensibility. Systolic function improved as reflected by decreased peak and end systolic wall stress because of improved myocardial flexibility.

Evaluation of renal function discovered improved reno-vascular resistance and decreased microalbuminuria. However, the impact on clinical status is not known. The point at which development of end-stage renal disease is reached was found to be delayed.

QUESTION 6 What is the approach to the patient with refractory HTN? What are the causes of secondary HTN?

A patient is said to have refractory HTN when the blood pressure is above 140/90 mm Hg, there are no secondary causes suspected by routine testing, and the patient has been given full doses of two antihypertensives used for an appropriate period of time.

Of all patients with refractory HTN about 10% are found to have a treatable cause. Renovascular disease is often found in a stable patient who becomes suddenly uncontrolled. Atherosclerotic renal vascular disease usually occurs in white men over the age of 50 and in cigarette smokers. There is usually evidence of widespread vascular disease. Other causes of renovascular stenosis include fibromuscular dysplasia, more common in young women, vasculitis, neurofibromatosis, and tuberculosis.

Pheochromocytoma has variable presentations. Common signs and symptoms include palpitations, flushing, headache, cold and clammy skin, angina, and vomiting. Diagnosis depends on discovering the catecholamine metabolic products metanephrine and vanillymandelic acid in the urine over 24 hours. Secretion may be episodic and be secondarily elevated because of the use of rauwolfia alkaloids, methyldopa, catecholamines, or ingestion of large amounts of vanilla. Tumors greater than 2 cm in diameter can be localized by axial tomography. The radio-pharmaceutical agent, metaiodobenzylguanidine (MIBG), is picked up by pheochromocytoma tissue in 90% of cases. Treatment is necessary with both alpha and beta blockade simultaneously.

Primary hyperaldosteronism (Conn's syndrome) is due to an adrenal adenoma producing aldosterone independent of volume status or serum tonicity. The metabolic profile includes hypernatremia, hyperchlorhydria, and a hypokalemic metabolic alkalosis. The patient may complain of weakness, parethesias, muscle paralysis, or tetany. Persistent aldosterone secretion in the face of a high sodium diet supports the diagnosis. Renin levels are suppressed secondary to aldosterone feedback during situations where they would usually rise: after diuresis and assumption of the upright position. The best means of measuring aldosterone is bilateral renal vein sampling. Tomography may demonstrate an adrenal adenoma.

Secondary hyperaldosteronism is due to renin hypersecretion from an extrarenal stimulus. This is seen in edematous disorders including nephrotic syndrome, CHF, cirrhosis, and obstructive renovascular disorders. In the former group renin is stimulated due to the apparent intravascular volume depletion. The essential diagnostic difference between 1° and 2° hyperaldosteronism is depression, as opposed to elevation, of renin levels, respectively.

Coarctation of the aorta can lead to development of systemic HTN. Depending on the location of the stenosis, pulses may be asymmetrical in the upper extremity as opposed to the lower extremity. Auscultation of the posterior thorax may discover a continuous murmur. The chest radiograph may show rib notching and/or apical capping as a result of collateralization to the intercostal vessels. Echocardiography, digital subtraction angiography, and magnetic resonance angiography can visualize the stenosis. Treatment is necessary due to premature development of congestive heart failure, impending aortic rupture, intracranial hemorrhage, and the increased propensity for bacterial endocarditis. Surgical indications include a systolic pressure gradient between the arms and legs, visualization of a greater than 50% stenosis, and demonstration of adequate vascular collateralization. Without adequate collateralization, perfusion to the spinal cord during aortic cross-clamping can lead to spinal cord infarction. The absence of systemic hypertension or cardiomegaly should not discourage surgical correction.

Additionally, one should consider renal paren-chymal disease, thyroid hyperfunction, Cushing's syndrome, sleep apnea, acromegaly, carcinoid syndrome, porphyria, autonomic hyper-reflexia, central nervous system tumors, and hypercalcemia. Patients should be questioned concerning the use of over-the-counter medications including nasal sprays and decongestants that contain phenylpropanolamine, nonsteroidal antiinflammatory agents, and oral contraceptives. Psychotropic drugs and erythropoetin can also elevate blood pressure.

Additionally, one must rule out obesity, inadequate pharmacologic treatment, non-compliance to a medical regimen, and secondary drug resistance as the cause of refractory HTN. Secondary drug resistance is due to competitive interactions between antihypertensive agents. An example is activation of the RAA axis by diuretic-induced volume depletion. One approach to such a problem is to treat volume overload from vasodilators with diuretics; cardiovascular hyperkinesia can be treated with beta-blockade.

CASE SUMMARY The goal for this patient is long-term BP control, regular follow-up, and establishment of an open line of communication that allows the patient to communicate concerns to the doctor. These goals maximize compliance. Physical examination should monitor cardiac function, and periodic lab testing should monitor renal function and potential side effects of blood pressure lowering agents (potassium and sodium levels).

The patient subsequently lost 14 lbs over the next 6 months and brought his serum glucose into good control. He was initially started on Vasotec and hydrochlorothiazide but was able to tolerate decreasing doses concurrent with his weight loss. Over the next 3 months he had lost an additional 3 pounds and maintained a stable blood pressure off all medications. A follow-up ECG revealed diminishing findings of ventricular wall thickness. He no longer drinks excess alcohol.

A diagnostic algorithm for elevated blood pressure is shown in Fig. 6-2-1.

• •

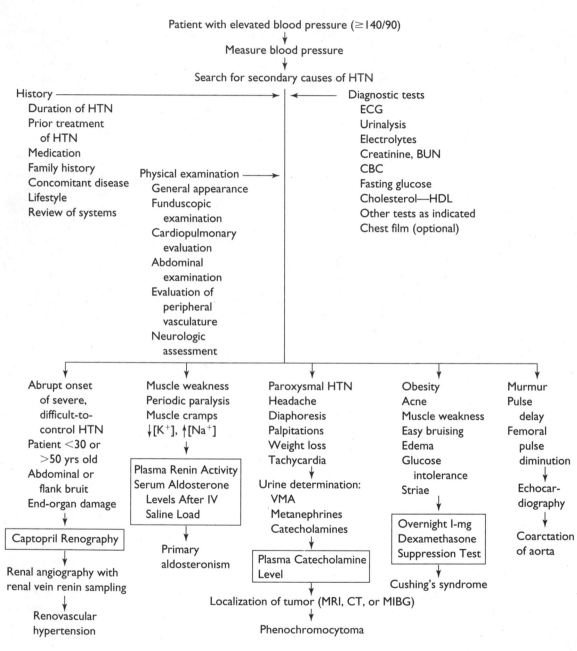

6-2-1 Diagnostic algorithm for elevated blood pressure.
(From Greene HL, Johnson WP, Maricic MJ: *Decision making in medicine*, St Louis, 1993, Mosby.)

BIBLIOGRAPHY

Asmar RG, Pdannier B, Sanntoni JP: Reversion of cardiac hypertrophy and reduced arterial compliance after converting enzyme inhibition in essential hypertension, *Circulation* 78(4):941-950, 1988.

Brazy PC, Fitzwilliam JF: Progressive renal disease: role of race and hypertensive medications, *Kidney Int* 37:1113-1119, 1990.

Feher MD: Hypertension in non-insulin dependent diabetes mellitus and its management, *Postgrad Med J* 67:938-946, 1991.

Fixler DE: Coarctation of the aorta, *Cardiol Clin* 6(4):561-571, 1988.

Flameanbaum W: Metabolic consequences of anithypertensive therapy, *Ann Intern Med* 98:875-880, 1983.

Fouad-Tarazi FM, Liebson P: Echocardiographic studies of regression of left ventricular hypertrophy in hypertension, Suppl II, *Hypertension,* 9(2 pt 2):II 65-68, 1987 Feb.

Hartford M, Wendelhag I, Berglund G: Cardiovascular and renal effects of long-term antihypertensive treatment, *JAMA* 259(17):2553-2557, 1988.

Helgeland A: Treatment of mild hypertension: a five year controlled drug trial, *Am J Med* 69:725-732, 1980.

Houston MC: Hypertension strategies for therapeutic intervention and prevention of end-organ damage, *Primary Care* 18(3):713-748, 1991.

Ryan C: Hypertension in the elderly, *Am Heart J* 122(4):1225-1227, 1991.

Setaro JF, Black HR: Refractory hypertension, *N Engl J Med* 327(8):543-547.

Silagy C, McNeill JJ: Epidemiologic aspects of isolated systolic hypertension and implications for future research, *Am J Cardiol* 69:213-218, 1992.

Viberti GC, Messent J: Introduction: hypertension and diabetes, *Diabetes Care* 14(11)(Suppl 4):4-7, 1991.

C A S E

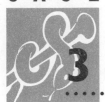

3

Charles J. Grodzin
Richard Abrams

On the general medical service you are asked to consult on the preoperative/postoperative management of a 72-year-old man hospitalized for a herniorrhaphy procedure. By history you find he has a 25 pack-year history of smoking, HTN, and diabetes.

QUESTION I On your initial examination no murmurs are detected, but you discover bilateral pretibial edema. He has been treated with hydrochlorothiazide for HTN. What are the important aspects that one must consider before surgery in this patient?

Patients with cardiac disease have a 25% to 50% greater risk of perioperative mortality. Risk is further heightened by procedures >2½ hours in length and for procedures done emergently. The most important predictive factor is left ventricular dysfunction. Careful attention should be given to signs of heart failure. Prudence warrants treatment of heart failure for 5 to 7 days before surgery. Be aware that treatment of congestive failure can lead to electrolyte imbalances and arrhythmia. Therefore it is important to evaluate ventricular function thoroughly.

Elective procedures should be put off at least 6 months after a myocardial infarction (MI). Patients who have had a recent MI (within the last 6 months) have a higher rate of reinfarction when surgery is carried out during that period.

When surgery is required sooner, risk can be assessed by submaximal thallium stress testing, ideally at 6 weeks post-MI. Patients without a history of MI, but who have cardiac symptoms, should be assessed with a treadmill stress test. The addition of thallium is indicated for women and those with either an abnormal ECG or known coronary artery disease. Patients unable to walk should undergo a dipyridamole thallium examination.

Several caveats exist depending on the patient's prior cardiac history or the discovery of significant coronary disease. Patients with stable angina and good exercise tolerance who would not otherwise undergo bypass grafting do not need preoperative coronary artery assessment. Patients having undergone uncomplicated coronary artery bypass grafting can undergo noncardiac surgery after 30 days. Patients with cardiac symptoms found to have significant coronary lesions (>70% occlusion) should be evaluated for revascularization.

Evaluation for valvular disease is important. Critical mitral or aortic stenosis predisposes to sudden death, especially in circumstances of increased cardiac demand such as surgery. The hemodynamic effects of valvular stenosis may be exacerbated by afterload reduction from anesthetic agents or venodilatation and decreased preload secondary to spinal/epidural anesthesia.

Conduction abnormalities may be significant. Isolated premature ventricular contractions (PVCs), well-controlled chronic atrial fibrillation, and chronic bifascicular block have little effect on risk. Supraventricular tachyarrhythmias are markers for perioperative complications. In elderly patients undergoing pulmonary surgery, or those with subaortic valvular stenosis or history of SVT, prophylactic digitalization may be beneficial. Patients with electrocardiographically identified 2° type II A-V block or transient 3° A-V block should be considered for temporary pacing. Pacemakers should be changed to the demand mode to avoid cautery induced intraoperative interference.

The most widely accepted criteria for cardiac risk assessment is the Goldman scale: a multifactorial assessment of perioperative risk. It is as follows:

I.	History:	Age >70	5
		MI within previous 6 months	10
II.	Physical	S_3 Gallop or JVD	11
	examination:	AS	3
III.	ECG:	Other than NSR/PAC	7
		>5 PVC/min	7
IV.	General:	$Po_2 < 60$ mm Hg or $Pco_2 > 45$ mm Hg	
		$K < 3.0/HCO_3 < 20$ mEq/l	3
		Bun >50 or Cr >3 mg/dl	
		Abn - SGOT, liver disease	
		Bedridden status	
V.	Procedure:	Intraperitoneal	
		Thoracic	3
		Aortic	
		Emergency	4
		Possible Total	53

The cumulative Goldman score is interpereted as such:

Class	Score	Major complication rate	Cardiac death
1	0-5	1%	.2%
2	6-12	4%	1%
3	13-25	14%	3%
4	>26	51%	39%

The Goldman scale is used for risk stratification. Allan Detsky modified the Goldman criteria to include a functional marker of coronary insufficiency. He found that the modified multifactorial index more accurately stratified perioperative cardiac risk. Both authors urge that these indices be used in combination with other information (i.e., potential for improvements in function after therapy and the urgency of the procedure before being applied uniformly).

Anticoagulation is often a component of treatment for cardiac disease. Patients who have been chronically anticoagulated must be treated to avoid thrombotic events while minimizing a hemorrhagic diathesis at the time of surgery. A practical approach is to discontinue coumadin 3 days before the procedure, then substitute intravenous heparin. The heparin should be withdrawn 6 hours before surgery and restarted 36 to 48 hours postoperatively and coumadin restarted 2 to 5 days later with the discontinuation of heparin when the prothrombin time is in the desired range. An orderly approach to the preoperative cardiac evaluation is found in Fig. 6-3-1 at the end of this chapter.

QUESTION 2 In your initial history the patient admitted to a 25-year history of smoking. He had quit for several months on several occasions but had been smoking consistently over the past 2 years. He would typically smoke 1 to 2 packs per day. How does this impact on his preoperative evaluation?

Patients with pulmonary disease invariably require aggressive preoperative therapy as this group has a morbidity rate of about 60%. The preoperative regimen should include discontinuation of smoking for 6 weeks, use of regularly scheduled inhaled bronchodilators, and antibiotics for patients with purulent sputum. Patients should not have been hospitalized for the preceding 3 weeks before an elective procedure. A course of systemic steroids should be considered in asthmatics to minimize airway inflammation. However, the length of the steroid course should be balanced with the risk of poor wound healing. Patients who have greater than a 20 pack-year history of smoking, $FEV_{1.0}/FVC <70\%$, $Pco_2 >45$ mm Hg, and PEFR <200 l/min benefit from preoperative/postoperative chest physiotherapy and bronchodilators. An initial determination of $FEV_{1.0}$ helps risk-stratify those patients with pulmonary disease. A severely decreased $FEV_{1.0}$ can identify patients for whom local anesthesia should be considered. Weight loss can decrease the risk of atelectasis postoperatively in the obese

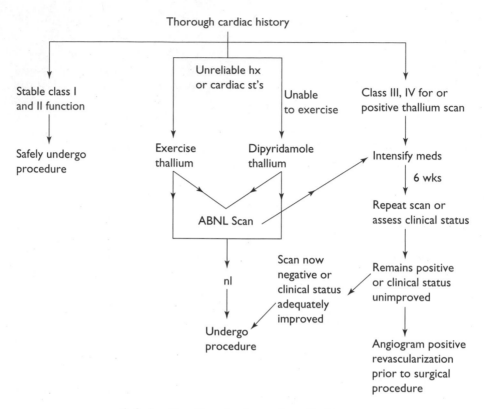

6-3-1 Algorithm of a thorough cardiac history.

patient; however, adequate nutrition is essential.

During surgery, periodic hyperinflation, prophylactic positive end-expiratory pressure (PEEP) or continuous positive airway pressure (CPAP), relatively large tidal volume (V_T), and epidural anesthesia may help decrease the likelihood of atelectasis. Upper abdominal incisions compromise respiratory mechanics the most. Incentive spirometry or CPAP, deep breathing, and chest physiotherapy improve postanesthesia respiratory function. Patients treated with CPAP develop atelectasis at one half the rate of patients using incentive spirometry. CPAP has been found to yield a better forced vital capacity (FVC) and Pa_{O_2} at 72 hours compared to incentive spirometry with only 23% of patients developing atelectasis, compared to 42% when not used.

Postoperatively, an early sign of atelectasis is a widened A-a gradient. For patients who require prolonged intubation, a preoperative arterial blood gas can help guide the manipulation of ventilator settings and provide goal gas tensions.

Prediction of residual function should be done for patients scheduled to undergo segment/lobe/pneumonectomy. Perfusion scanning is the best means of gathering data.

Pneumonectomy:
Postop $FEV_{1.0} =$

$$\text{Preop } FEV_1 \times \frac{\text{\% perfusion to remaining lung}}{100}$$

Lobectomy:
Loss of fcn =

$$\text{Preop } FEV_1 \times \frac{\text{\# total segments resected}}{\text{total segments of both lungs}}$$

A practical means of preoperative pulmonary evaluation is found in Fig. 6-3-2.

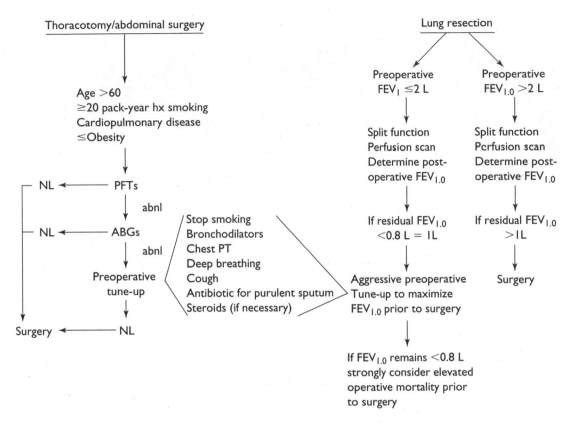

6-3-2 Preoperative algorithm for surgery.

QUESTION 3 On follow-up physical examination by a conscientious medical student, the patient is noted to have diminished arterial pulsations on the right lower extremity. Noninvasive arterial evaluation reveals a decreased ankle-brachial ratio on the right. Angiography shows a 5-cm stenosis of the middle one third of the right femoral artery. The vascular surgery consultant advises that a surgical revascularization is necessary. In a patient without known coronary disease, how does the presence of peripheral vascular disease change the preoperative evaluation and which procedure takes priority in this situation?

It is important to interpret peripheral vascular disease as a marker for systemic atherosclerosis. Limited exercise ability, due to intermittent claudication or previous amputation, can mask angi-

nal symptoms. McPhail found that only 30% of his patients undergoing treadmill stress testing could achieve 85% of their predicted maximum heart rate. The use of dipyridamole thallium testing adds significant information. Redistribution of thallium predicted perioperative events with 100% sensitivity and 73% specificity, while a normal scan or absence of reversible changes predicted an absence of perioperative events.

Therefore, it is practical to apply either the Goldman or Detsky multifactorial assessment followed by criteria that assign high, intermediate, or low cardiac risk. Both those assigned high risk via clinical criteria and patients from the intermediate group identified by the above qualities require angiographic evaluation. It is widely believed that significant coronary disease should be treated before the peripheral vascular lesion.

BIBLIOGRAPHY

Burke F, Francos C: Surgery in the patient with acute and chronic renal failure, *Med Clin North Am* 71(3): 1987.

Dajani S: Prevention of bacterial endocarditis: recommendations by the American Heart Association, *JAMA* 264:22, 1990.

Detsky A: Predicting cardiac complications in patients undergoing noncardiac surgery, *J Gen Intern Med* 1:211-219, 1986.

Fellen F: Hematologic problems in the preoperative patient, *Med Clin North Am* 71(3): 1987.

Friedman LS: Surgery in the patient with liver disease, *Med Clin North Am* 71(3):453-476, 1987.

Georgeson S: Prophylactic use of the intra-aortic balloon pump in high risk patients undergoing noncardiac surgery: a decision analytic view, *Am J Med* 92:665-678, 1992.

Jackson Maj CV: Preoperative pulmonary evaluation, *Arch Intern Med* 148:2120-2127, 1988.

Tisi G: Preoperative identification and evaluation of the patient with lung disease, *Med Clin North Am* 71(3):399-412, 1987.

Weits H: Noncardiac surgery in the patient with heart disease, *Med Clin North Am* 71(3): 1987.

C A S E

4

Charles J. Grodzin
Richard Abrams

. . . .

Several new patients are in your office waiting room as you arrive for your first day of work at a health department. The first patient is a 49-year-old woman who is concerned about her chances of developing breast cancer. She has never had a mammogram and only rarely performs breast self-examination. She is not sure if her technique is correct. Her grandmother had breast cancer, and she admits to smoking about 1 pack of cigarettes per day.

QUESTION 1 What is your approach to this patient?

Policy concerning cancer screening is evolving. For screening to be useful certain elements must be present. First, the disease must have a preclinical stage, during which time it may be identified and treatment be initiated before morbid events occur. Second, the disease must be prevalent enough in the society such that the predictive value of the test reaches an acceptably high level. Finally, testing must be simple, inexpensive, and accessible to the population at risk.

Among women, breast cancer is the most common malignancy. It is the second-leading cause of death in women in general. The cumulative lifetime probability of breast cancer is 9.3%. The risk doubles when family history is positive in the mother *or* sister and triples when positive in the mother *and* sister. The Breast Cancer Detection Demonstration Project (BCDDP) and the Health Insurance Plan (HIP) data suggest that for every 10,000 women screened annually for a period of 10 years, screening will make the difference between life and death for 25 women. Physical examination was estimated to add 10 to

30 days of life expectancy. Overall, when mammography was added, mortality was decreased by an additional 8% to 40%. In the Swedish trial screening mammography was identified to reduce mortality for women greater than 50 years old; additionally, the Malmo trial found a reduction in mortality by 20% in women greater than 55 years old. In a population of women 40 to 50 years old, about 60 new breast cancers will develop per million women, whereas 93,000 new cancers will be discovered during the same period.

The major controversy in breast cancer screening involves recommendations to women ages 40 to 50. A recent Canadian study demonstrated screening had no impact on mortality in this age group. Debate also concerns the role of breast self-examination (BSE) as a screening tool. Although it is simple, noninvasive, and inexpensive, no study has demonstrated its usefulness in decreasing cancer mortality.

The American College of Physicians recommends that Clinical breast examinations (CBE) begin at age 40 and be repeated annually. Mammography should begin at age 50 and also be carried out on an annual basis (Fig. 6-4-1).

QUESTION 2 The second patient is a 27-year-old woman who appears very apprehensive and complains of recurrent vaginal infections and occasional dyspareunia. She has only rarely seen a doctor and has never received a PAP smear. She relates a fear that her recurrent infections are related to cancer. What is your approach to this patient?

Cervical cancer is a disease of young women. Invasive cancer incidence peaks between ages 35 to 39 at 20/10,000 with a lifetime risk of 0.7%.

The general consensus is that if screening were not performed, the rates of invasive cancer would increase 2 to 3 times. The highest risk groups include those with an early age of first intercourse and multiple sexual partners. Smoking and the use of oral contraceptives have also been implicated.

Historical analysis of cervical cancer screening reveals that increased efforts to screen decreased rates of cervical cancer mortality. Case-controlled study underscores these results. Analysis of large screening programs suggests that screening programs, by identifying premalignant lesions, reduce a woman's chance of developing cancer by 90%. One potential problem is that laboratory consistency in cytological assessment has shown false-negative rates from 17% to 57% and false-positive rates were found to be between 0.24% and 1.3%. The Bethesda system for reporting cervical cytologic diagnosis has been endowed to promote uniformity among laboratories.

Screening for cervical cancer has been accepted as an effective means of reducing mortality and is cost effective. Evaluation should begin between the ages of 17 and 26. Screening at 3-year intervals retains 96% safety levels compared to continuing yearly PAP smears. Screening may terminate at age 65 as little benefit has been found in average risk females in this age group.

The American College of Physicians recommends PAP smears beginning at age 18 and 2 more annual exams, then, every 3 years until age 65 (Fig. 6-4-2).

QUESTION 3 The next patient is a 55-year-old man who has come to your office because he has not seen a doctor in many years. He has had no specific complaints. He asks your advice concerning his risk for colon cancer. How do you reply to this man's question?

For men, colon cancer is the second most common malignancy as well as the second leading cause of cancer death. Risk factors include family history of colon cancer, the family cancer syndrome, and familial polyposis coli. A personal history of endometrial, ovarian, or breast cancer, ulcerative colitis, adenomatous polyps, and previous colorectal malignancy increase risk.

Potential methods of colorectal screening are fecal occult blood testing (FOBT) and flexible sigmoidoscopy (FS). Use of FOBT has been reported to decrease cancer mortality by 30%. However, when done for cancer screening in asymptomatic people, the results are very nonspecific. In addition, false-negative results occur in the presence of antioxidants, lesions that bleed intermittently, or when blood is not evenly distributed in the stool.

Sigmoidoscopy comprises three separate examinations:

EXAMINATION	EFFICACY
• FS (35 cm)	• 50-70% of colon visible
• FS (60 cm)	• 80% of colon visible, 50%-60% of lesions found
• Rigid sigmoidoscopy	• 20%-35% of malignancies found

Data suggest that regular examination will identify lesions at an earlier stage and lead to better survival rates. Although present American College of Physicians recommendations include beginning FOBT at age 50 and every 3 years thereafter and flexible sigmoidoscopy every five years (Fig. 6-4-3), the value of screening for colorectal cancer remains controversial. Compliance to FS is diminished by cost, discomfort, and fear. The 60 cm FS examination is the investigation of choice, visualizing a greater proportion of the colon and finding more cancerous lesions and adenomatous polyps.

QUESTION 4 While you are making rounds in the hospital that afternoon, the housestaff engages you in a conversation about the efficacy of screening for lung cancer and its impact on morbidity and mortality. How do you respond to their question?

Lung cancer is the leading cause of cancer death in men and women. Screening procedures include chest x-ray, superior at identifying pe-

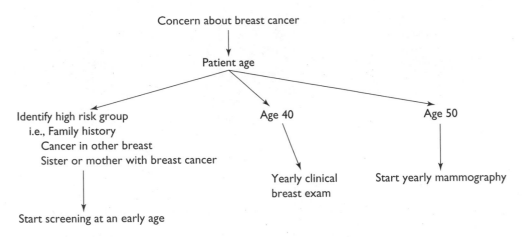

6-4-1   Algorithm of breast cancer screening recommendations.

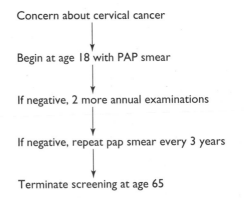

6-4-2   Algorithm of cervical cancer screening recommendations.

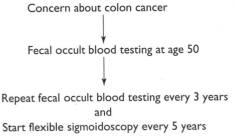

6-4-3   Algorithm of colon cancer screening recommendations.

ripheral lesions, and sputum cytology, best at identifying central lesions. An early study by the Mayo Clinic in 1970 found that malignancies identified by sputum cytology had a better 5-year survivability and resectability rate compared to those found by chest x-ray or presenting symptomatically. A European study designed to compare malignancy identification when chest x-ray was done every 6 months as compared to every 18 months, found that the biannual frequency also afforded a better resectability and 5-year survival rate. However, neither study was able to show decreased mortality rates from earlier identification.

Currently screening evaluation of asymptomatic individuals is not advocated by the American College of Physicians. The American Cancer Society suggests that screening resources should be aimed at high-risk age groups. This includes individuals greater than 45 years old with a greater than 20 pack-year history of smoking and/or exposure to carcinogenic substances, a chronic cough that gets worse, hemoptysis, and recurrent pneumonia. Therefore, recommendations for this group are to undergo yearly chest x-ray and sputum cytology (Fig. 6-4-4). The impact of screening on mortality is unknown.

QUESTION 5   You must evaluate a new admission to your service. He is a 67-year-old black man with low back pain. Prostate cancer is high in your

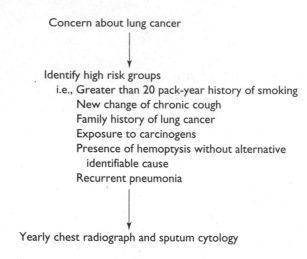

Concern about lung cancer

Identify high risk groups
  i.e., Greater than 20 pack-year history of smoking
      New change of chronic cough
      Family history of lung cancer
      Exposure to carcinogens
      Presence of hemoptysis without alternative
        identifiable cause
      Recurrent pneumonia

Yearly chest radiograph and sputum cytology

6-4-4   Algorithm of lung cancer screening recommendations.

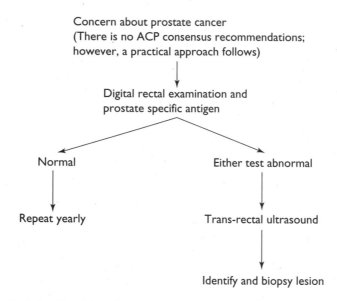

Concern about prostate cancer
(There is no ACP consensus recommendations;
however, a practical approach follows)

Digital rectal examination and
prostate specific antigen

Normal   Either test abnormal

Repeat yearly   Trans-rectal ultrasound

                          Identify and biopsy lesion

6-4-5   Algorithm of prostate cancer screening recommendations.

differential. How do you go about screening this man for prostate malignancy?

Prostate cancer is a common tumor in men and the most common cause of cancer death in men. Risk factors include increasing age, positive family history, and being of the black race. It is estimated that between the years 1980 and 2000, there will be a 90% increase in the total number of cases diagnosed and a 37% increase in prostate cancer-related deaths. The demand for better screening strategies is reflected by the fact that currently one third of lesions are confined to the prostate. When discovered, these lesions are felt to be curable.

Screening modalities include the digital rectal examination (DRE), prostate specific antigen

(PSA), and transrectal ultrasound (TRUS). DRE is simple and inexpensive. Its weakness is that, while able to detect palpable peripheral lesions, a significant number of lesions that were organ-confined and potentially curable were not detected.

PSA measurement has been able to find one third of cancers missed by DRE. PSA measurement is confounded because both benign and malignant processes may produce high levels of this antigen. One study has found a higher mean PSA in men with prostatic hyperplasia compared to men with organ-confined disease. Another study found 43% of men with prostate cancer to have normal values, and 25% with hyperplasia had elevated values. However, PSA values greater than 10 ng/ml increases specificity to 92% in support of malignancy. In one study, the PSA rate of change was found to be more useful with a 90% specificity when the rate of change was greater than 0.75 ng/ml/year. A small study, however, refutes the usefulness of this modality as it did not discriminate benign from malignant disease.

TRUS has been considered to have too low a sensitivity and specificity to be a lone screening test. Additionally, it is costly and operator dependent. But, unlike the DRE or PSA, it can detect intraprostatic lesions that were otherwise undetectable but that remain curable.

The American College of Physicians has no consensus recommendations for prostate cancer screening. A practical approach uses all three modalities together. Initially, the DRE and PSA are performed. When normal, these should be repeated on a yearly basis beginning at age 50. TRUS should be performed when either is abnormal for the purposes of identifying a lesion for biopsy (Fig. 6-4-5).

BIBLIOGRAPHY

Barnett K: Prostate cancer screening: what we know and what we need to know, *Ann Intern Med* 119:914-923, 1993.

Cupp MR: Prostate-specific antigen, digital rectal examination, and transrectal ultrasonography: their roles in diagnosing early prostate cancer, *Mayo Clin Proc* 68:297-306, 1993

Eddy DM: Screening for breast cancer, *Ann Intern Med* 111:389-399, 1989.

Eddy DM: Screening for cervical cancer, *Ann Intern Med* 113:214-226, 1990.

Epler G: Screening for lung cancer: is it worthwhile? *Postgrad Med* 87(6):181-186, 1990.

Fletcher A: Screening for cancer of the cervix in elderly women, *Lancet* 335:97-99, 1990.

Gupta T: Efficacy of screening flexible sigmoidoscopy for colorectal neoplasia in asymptomatic subjects, *Am J Med* 86:547-549, 1989.

Klein E: Prostate cancer: current concepts in diagnosis and treatment, *Cleveland Clin J Med* 56(4):383-389, July 1992.

McGee MC: Screening for lung cancer, *Semin Surg Oncol* 5:179-185, 1989.

Ochs M: Selected routine outpatient tests for older patients, *Geriatrics* 46(11):39-50, 1991.

O'Malley M: Screening for breast cancer with breast self examination, *JAMA* 257(16):2197-2207, 1987.

CASE

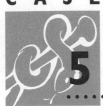

5

Charles J. Grodzin
Richard Abrams

• • • • • • • • • •

A 48-year-old man presents with lower back pain. He denies any past medical history and does not recall any episode of trauma. Over the past 2 weeks he has taken 500 mg Acetaminophen with only partial relief. Lately, the pain has gotten worse, and the patient is unable to sleep through the night.

QUESTION 1 What epidemiologic data apply to the patient with low back pain?

Low back pain is consistently one of the top 10 reasons people see primary care physicians. Eighty percent of people have back pain at some point in their life. It is the number one cause of activity restriction in people less than 45 years old. Because of the high prevalence, the medical cost of evaluation is enormous, approximately 5 billion dollars per year.

QUESTION 2 Upon further questioning he relates that the pain radiates down the posterolateral aspect of the thigh and knee and that he has occasional numbness in the same area. How is the history and physical examination useful and what are the important points to consider at this point in the evaluation?

The initial decision focuses on distinguishing pain as a result of mechanical versus systemic/visceral disease. Mechanical pain is usually exacerbated by movement and is relieved by rest while systemic/visceral pain is constant, aching, and difficult to relieve with standard analgesics. Disc herniation is a common example of a mechanical problem. Impingement on nerve structures can produce pain that is exacerbated with movement, is sharp, and radiates down the posterolateral aspect of the leg. Historical factors for disc herniation include repetitive mechanical movement of the lower spine, sedentary behavior, obesity, and cigarette smoking. History of fever or weight loss may signify an underlying infectious or neoplastic disease. Use of systemic steroids can lead to osteoporosis. Inflammatory spondyloarthropathies occur in younger individuals and are characterized by loss of spinal flexibility.

Physical examination should include a detailed breast, prostate, and urogenital examination as potential sources of metastatic neoplasia. Because 90% of disc herniations involve L4-L5 or L5-S1, absence of either the plantar reflexes or dorsiflexion of the foot suggests nerve root impingement. The straight-leg raise is a sensitive but nonspecific method of assessing disc herniation. A positive test is present when sciatic symptoms are recreated when the hip is flexed by the examiner to <60 degrees. The contralateral straight-leg raise is less sensitive but more specific.

The second important point to consider is the presence of neurologic compromise. The most important initial diagnosis to rule out is cauda equina syndrome. This manifests as incontinence of urine or stool, poor urethral or anal sphincter tone, and saddle anesthesia. This constitutes an emergency requiring immediate decompression of cord structures.

QUESTION 3 Upon further questioning the patient states that while playing football several weeks ago he noted a slight "twinge" in his back that became much more painful over the following 24 hours. What are the most appropriate next steps in the evaluation?

Complaints of low back pain

↓

Distinguish between mechanical and visceral pain
and identify risk factors for disc herniation, signs and symptoms
of infection, neoplasia, or osteoporosis

↓

Physical examination of the breast, prostate, and urogenital
tract, screening test for disc disease and neurologic
compromise in the lower extremities

↓

Laboratory tests specifically as indicated by patient history
(CBC, U/A, ESR, SPEP, Ca, Alkaline phosphatase, prostate specific
antigen)

↓

Spinal radiography in the subsets of age >50, fever, suspicion of
ankylosing spondylitis, weight loss or history of cancer, trauma,
neurologic deficits, steroid use, and failure of response to standard therapy

↓

Move to CT scanning to detect spinal stenosis, sacroiliitis,
facet degeneration, or anatomic guidance for surgery

↓

Conservative therapy with bedrest and analgesia

↓

Consider surgery for persistent symptoms, worsening
pain, persistent motor deficits

6-5-1 Diagnostic algorithm for low back pain.

In general, the yield of laboratory testing is low. It is more cost effective to reserve this testing for those with an initially abnormal examination.

Potential laboratory studies include a CBC, ESR, U/A, serum protein electrophoresis, calcium, alkaline phosphatase, and, in men, prostate specific antigen in the appropriate clinical setting. Liang found that the erythrocyte sedimentation rate was elevated more often than the white blood cell count in cases of osteomyelitis and was a more sensitive marker than radiography, except in cases of metastatic or primary bone disease. Park has suggested that the ESR may replace x-rays for initial screening evaluations. On urinalysis, the absence of protein by dipstick, but presence with use of sulfasalicylic acid (SSA), suggests the presence of multiple myeloma.

The appropriate use and timing of spinal x-rays is controversial. Disadvantages to routine x-rays include high gonadal doses of radiation, nonspecific findings that may not be related to the source of pain, and carrying a low yield since only 2% of patients have radiologically evident cancers or infectious/inflammatory arthropathy. In a study of 68,000 lumbar spine series, clinically unsuspected findings were present in approximately 1/2500 examinations. To increase specificity it has been suggested that x-rays should be obtained in the following sub-groups: age >50 years, fever, suspicion of ankylosing spondylitis, weight loss or history of cancer, trauma (especially in the elderly or those with risk factors for osteoporosis), neurologic deficits, steroid use, drug/alcohol use, and in patients with a clinical diagnosis who fail to respond to therapy in 3 to 4 weeks.

The CT scan carries a 92% sensitivity and 88% specificity in the diagnosis of a herniated disc. It is an excellent means of detecting spinal stenosis, sacroiliitis, and facet degeneration, and is better preoperatively for surgical guidance when neurologic deficits persist in the face of standard therapy. It appears that the combination of myelography and CT can demonstrate the level of neural entrapment and the cross-sectional geometry, respectively, of the spinal canal.

QUESTION 4 A CT scan revealed a bulging disc at the L4-L5 level. He is very concerned about his potential for long-term disability and asks if surgery is necessary. What do you advise him in this situation?

Conservative therapy begins with bed rest and analgesics. Studies have shown that 2 days of bed rest affords similar benefit as 7 days. The patient should ambulate for brief periods to avoid deconditioning. Sitting should be avoided as this maneuver increases intradiscal pressure. Analgesics should be given on a time-limited basis to promote a more active role in recovering function. Modalities including spinal traction and orthoses have not been found useful. Conservative therapy was equal to surgical intervention at 4-years follow-up.

To a large extent the effectiveness of any procedure designed to alleviate low back pain depends on patient selection. Those patients with pain of uncertain source, absence of sciatica, or psychologic dependence may have a less desirable outcome.

The use of epidural steroid injection is known to reduce pain and to improve function. However, in a study by Dilke, no difference was noted when compared to placebo at 24 hours. Chymopapain injection relieves sciatic pain in 85% to 90% of patients, but there is a risk of transverse myelitis, allergic reaction, muscle spasm, or infection such that this is no longer recommended. Debate exists about the effectiveness of diskectomy in terms of the duration of pain relief. The initial response is good in 90%, but falls to 70% over the next 10 years. Failure to note nerve canal stenosis or recurrent herniation will require reoperation in 5% to 15%. Spinal fusion has not been shown to afford better long-term relief.

Only 5% to 10% of people with a herniated disc and sciatic pain will require surgery for persistent symptoms. The major indications for surgery include persistent or worsening pain, persistent motor defects, and lack of response to conservative therapy. Surgically, patients receive complete pain relief in about 75% of cases and partial relief in 90% of cases. The primary advantage of surgical therapy is more rapid acquisition of pain relief.

A diagnostic algorithm for low back pain is shown in Fig. 6-5-1.

BIBLIOGRAPHY

Deyo RA: Early diagnostic evaluation of low back pain, *J Gen Intern Med* 1:328, 1986.

Deyo RA: Herniated lumbar intervertebral disk, *Ann Intern Med* 112:598-603, 1990.

Deyo RA, Diehl AK, Rosenthal M: How many days of bed rest for acute low back pain? *N Engl J Med* 315:1064, 1986.

Deyo RA: Lumbar spine films in primary care: current use and effects of selective ordering criteria, *J Gen Intern Med* 1: 20-25, 1986.

Frymoyer JW: Back pain and sciatica, *N Engl J Med* 318:291, 1988.

Liang M, Komaroff AL: Roentgenograms in primary care patients with acute low back pain: a cost-effectiveness analysis, *Arch Intern Med* 142:1108, 1982.

Scavone JG, Latshaw RF: Use of lumbar spine films, *JAMA* 246(10):1105-1108, 1981.

CASE

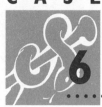

6

Charles J. Grodzin
Richard Abrams

· · · · · · · · · ·

A 56-year-old man presents with an elevated cholesterol level found on a recent insurance laboratory examination. His history also includes mild alcohol use and high blood pressure, for which he has been treated with Nifedipine. He denies any symptoms of angina, limitation to exertion, claudication, or symptoms of congestive heart failure. His physical examination reveals moderate obesity and a mildly displaced point of maximal impulse (PMI) on cardiac examination. There are no signs of heart failure.

QUESTION I What is the significance of an isolated elevation of the total serum cholesterol and what should be your next step?

Cholesterol measurement is an important component in the assessment of the risk factors that contribute to coronary heart disease (CHD). To accurately diagnose hypercholesterolemia, it is recommended to obtain two separate measurements. If the first two measurements differ by less than 30 mg/dl, an average should be taken as the accurate total cholesterol. A third assay should be carried out if the first two results differ by more than 30 mg/dl. Further risk stratification should be carried out by lipid fractionation. Care should be used to reproduce the circumstances of the test as closely as possible, including diet, time of day, measurement instrument, and specimen handling.

Coronary artery disease is a multifactorial condition such that risk is determined by the interplay of many factors. A formal risk factor analysis should be carried out to determine an overall level of risk. Major risk factors include a history of diabetes mellitus, hypertension, cigarette smok-

ing, and family history of coronary artery disease or cerebrovascular accident at an early age (<55 years). Other important factors to note are the presence of obesity, the daily level of exercise, and menopausal status. This patient carries two additional risk factors for coronary disease: hypertension and male sex.

An algorithm evaluation for coronary artery disease risk factors is shown in Fig. 6-6-1.

QUESTION 2 What is the evidence that reducing the serum cholesterol plays an important role in reducing cardiac morbidity and mortality?

Evidence to support the hypothesis that lowering one's cholesterol can reduce morbidity and mortality from CHD is controversial. Specifically, the World Health Organization (WHO) cooperative trial using drug therapy (clofibrate) achieved a 20% reduction in the overall rate of myocardial infarction. The Lipid Research Clinic Primary Prevention Trial found that reducing LDL-cholesterol with cholestyramine decreased the rate of CHD morbidity and mortality: a 25% reduction of total cholesterol or 35% reduction of LDL-cholesterol led to a 50% reduction of CHD. Finally, the Helsinki Heart Study found a 34% reduction in cardiac events in men whose cholesterol was lowered with gemfibrozil. These studies included men between the ages of 35 and 59 with cholesterol levels between 255 and 365.

It is evident from these studies that patients with different levels of risk respond differently to cholesterol reduction. What remains unclear is the risk/benefit received by treating individuals with moderate elevations of serum cholesterol.

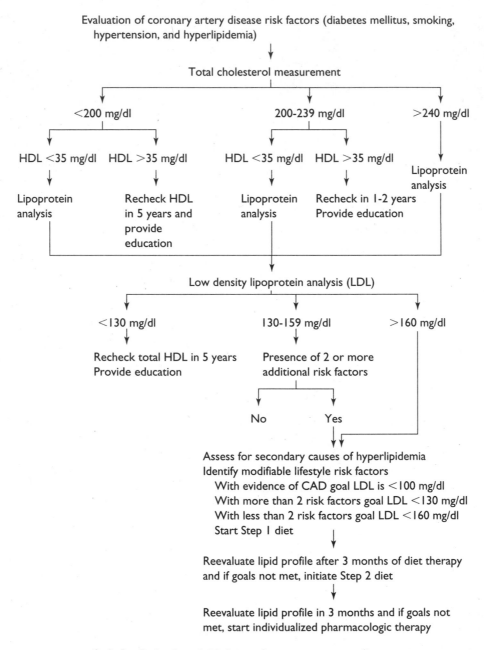

Evaluation of coronary artery disease risk factors (diabetes mellitus, smoking, hypertension, and hyperlipidemia)

Total cholesterol measurement

<200 mg/dl

HDL <35 mg/dl   HDL >35 mg/dl

Lipoprotein analysis

Recheck HDL in 5 years and provide education

200-239 mg/dl

HDL <35 mg/dl   HDL >35 mg/dl

Lipoprotein analysis

Recheck in 1-2 years Provide education

>240 mg/dl

Lipoprotein analysis

Low density lipoprotein analysis (LDL)

<130 mg/dl

Recheck total HDL in 5 years Provide education

130-159 mg/dl

Presence of 2 or more additional risk factors

No   Yes

>160 mg/dl

Assess for secondary causes of hyperlipidemia
Identify modifiable lifestyle risk factors
   With evidence of CAD goal LDL is <100 mg/dl
   With more than 2 risk factors goal LDL <130 mg/dl
   With less than 2 risk factors goal LDL <160 mg/dl
   Start Step 1 diet

Reevaluate lipid profile after 3 months of diet therapy and if goals not met, initiate Step 2 diet

Reevaluate lipid profile in 3 months and if goals not met, start individualized pharmacologic therapy

6-6-1   Evaluation of risk factors for coronary artery disease.

QUESTION 3 What factors should be considered when assessing an otherwise asymptomatic patient without other cardiac risk factors who is found to have an elevated total cholesterol and less than two additional risk factors?

While it is easy to determine a level of risk in patients with normal cholesterol and no other risk factors and those with elevated cholesterol and multiple risk factors, the approach to the group with a moderately elevated cholesterol and less than two risk factors is unclear. The question concerning efficacy of long-term use of lipid-lowering agents in these low-risk individuals is unanswered. No study has been done to elucidate the risk-benefit ratio of pharmacologic therapy versus a conservative approach. In patients found to have an elevated total cholesterol, risk can be stratified by evaluation of lipid fractionation. The Adult Treatment Panel of the National Cholesterol Education Program advises lipoprotein fractionation for this population using the LDL level as the determinant for treatment. When elevated >130 mg/dl or >160 mg/dl with or without two additional risk factors, respectively, they recommend a cholesterol-lowering treatment.

Another population comprises individuals excluded by these criteria. A practical approach begins with diet therapy. Instituting a low-cholesterol diet is safe, inexpensive, and if successful, may obviate the need for drug therapy. Physicians must educate patients that reduction of other risk factor behavior (e.g., smoking cessation, glucose and blood pressure control) may provide greater impact on longevity than modest reductions in cholesterol levels. Lower risk populations for which study has not been done include young men, women, elderly, and those with mild to moderate cholesterol elevation. Furthermore, long-term studies have not been done to evaluate the safety of lipid-lowering agents.

QUESTION 4 What are the recommendations for cholesterol measurements from the United States Preventive Services Task Force?

According to this task force, the primary intervention is counseling about dietary intake of fat and cholesterol. Secondly, periodic measurement of serum cholesterol may be targeted at middle-aged men and those with additional risk factors. The suggested frequency for a screening nonfasting total cholesterol is every 5 years; more often if a previously elevated cholesterol is found or treatment is underway. When a borderline or severe elevation is detected, information regarding the meaning of the results and dietary counseling as well as plans for follow-up measurement is necessary.

The recommended Step 1 diet prescribes that fat comprise no more than 30% of daily calories with no more than 10% being from saturated fat. Cholesterol should be minimized to less than 300 mg per day. Reevaluation after 3 months may warrant use of the Step 2 diet if lipid reduction is not achieved. This diet includes reducing saturated fat to less than 7% of daily caloric intake and keeping cholesterol to less than 200 mg/day. Patients may require close counseling by a dietitian to achieve these goals.

The task force also suggests that lipid-lowering agents be held until intense dietary therapy has failed a 6-month trial. The task force identified indications for drug therapy as cholesterol >240 with at least two risk factors and >265 without additional risk factors. Individuals with levels between 200 and 240 should be evaluated with regard to their lifestyle habits and risk factors and can be treated if their level of risk appears high despite diet modification. Medical follow-up is a key factor to support these behavior and lifestyle changes.

BIBLIOGRAPHY

The Expert Panel: Report of the National Cholesterol Education Program Expert Panel on detection, evaluation and treatment of high blood cholesterol in adults, *Arch Intern Med* 48: 1988.

Garber AM, Sox HC: Screening asymptomatic adults for cardiac risk factors: the serum cholesterol level, *Ann Intern Med* 110:622-639, 1989.

Guide to Clinical Preventive Services: An assessment of the effectiveness of 169 interventions report of the U.S. preventive services task force, *Screening for high blood cholesterol*, Baltimore, 1989, Williams and Wilkins, pp 11-21.

Lipid Research Clinics Program: The lipid research clinics coronary primary prevention trial results I and II, *JAMA* 251:351-364, 1984.

Multiple Risk Factor Intervention Trial Research Group: Multiple risk factor intervention trial: risk factor changes and mortality results, *JAMA* 248 (12):1465-1477, 1982.

Taylor WC, Pass TM: Cholesterol reduction and life expectancy, *Ann Intern Med* 106:605-614, 1987.

A 27-year-old female college student presents in your clinic with complaints of a sore throat. The patient states that her roommate has had a sore throat recently and was given antibiotics by her family doctor. She has no other medical problems and takes no medications.

QUESTION 1 What are the important clinical elements in the evaluation of pharyngitis?

Pharyngitis accounts for about 40 million visits to physicians each year by adults. Group A beta-hemolytic streptococci (GABHS) is the most important etiologic agent due to its suppurative and nonsuppurative complications.

The symptoms of pharyngitis are often nonspecific. Bacterial infection is associated with cervical lymph node swelling and tenderness, fever, odynophagia, and other systemic symptoms. Viral infections are often accompanied by cough, coryza, and throat irritation. A history of immunosuppression, current antibiotic use, diabetes mellitus, neck irradiation, HIV infection, or denture irritation predispose to candidal infection. Inability to handle secretions may signal acute epiglottis. A history of orogenital contact or a genital chancre can signal gonococcal or syphilitic pharyngitis. Angioneurotic edema is suggested by a family history of C-1 esterase deficiency, appropriate exposure, nonpitting edema, and pharyngitis.

Physical examination can suggest the etiology of sore throat. Unfortunately, the findings of tonsillar exudate, lymphadenopathy, and fever are not organism specific. GABHS infection typically presents with anterior cervical adenopathy, tonsillar exudate, fever, and in about 10% of cases, pharyngeal lesions with an erythematous rim and necrotic center (doughnut lesions). *Hemophilus influenza* can produce concomitant otitis media, laryngotracheitis, and epiglottitis.

A diagnostic algorithm for pharyngitis is shown in Fig. 6-7-1.

QUESTION 2 What is the differential diagnosis of pharyngitis that should be considered in this patient?

When patients present with severe throat pain and an inability to handle their secretions, epiglottitis (infection with *Haemophilus influenza* B) must be considered. The examiner must exercise care in the examination of such a patient because of potential airway obstruction. Acute airway closure is a realistic possibility and necessitates delay of examination until one is fully ready for immediate intubation. Epiglottitis can be suggested by pretracheal erythema. Diagnosis is by direct visualization of a "cherry-red" epiglottis or swelling of the epiglottis on lateral neck x-ray.

"Vincent's angina" is necrotizing ulcerative gingivitis with fusobacteria and a spirochete. It presents with gingiva-buccal ulceration, a membranous exudate on the interdental papillae and submandibular adenopathy. Diphtheria may present with a grey-green pseudomembrane that bleeds with manipulation and may extend into the upper respiratory tract with respiratory compromise and stridor. Additionally, toxin mediated sequelae include myocarditis, peripheral or cranial neuropathy, and hepatitis. Cervical adenopathy can produce the characteristic "bull-neck" deformity.

Infectious mononucleosis can present with hepatosplenomegaly, palatal petechiae, and uvular sparing. Laboratory analysis may show lymphocytosis with >10% atypical forms. *Mycoplasma pneumoniae* infection can present with laryngitis. Pharyngeal ulceration in the presence of pulmonary cavitation or miliary disease suggests tuberculosis. Candidal pharyngitis presents with characteristic white plaques with focal bleeding.

The distribution of lesions may be an especially important clue in viral infection. Herpangina, caused by Coxsackievirus, produces ulceration of the posterior oropharynx. Aphthous stomatitis produces round painful lesions in the middle oropharynx. Herpes virus typically only involves the anterior oropharynx. Coxsackievirus A-1b causes hand-foot-and-mouth disease dominated by a vascular eruption on the palms and soles.

Noninfectious etiologies should also be considered. Gastroesophageal reflux can produce irritation of the hypopharynx, arytenoids, and lead to posterior vocal cord edema. Thyroiditis may present as sore throat. Pemphigus can involve the mouth and throat with bullous lesions and a fibrous exudate. Erythema multiforme and Stevens-Johnson syndrome may present with oral vesicles and bullae that become necrotic with a white pseudomembrane. Cutaneous palmar and sole target lesions may also be present.

QUESTION 3   Since there has been an outbreak of GABHS infection in the community recently, your suspicion is high that the patient has streptococcal pharyngitis. How is this diagnosis of streptococcal pharyngitis made?

Diagnosis can be suggested by the clinical presentation. However, the development of rapid streptococcal antigen detection tests may also be useful. The sensitivity rate (the percent of patients with disease that test positive) is between 83% and 90%; the specificity (the percent of those without disease that test negative) is about 99%. If a microscope and gram stain materials are available, diagnosis can be made with about 73% sensitivity and 96% specificity. The gold standard remains bacterial culture with an accuracy rate of 90% to 95%. However, up to 56 hours may be required for a diagnosis with this method.

QUESTION 4   What considerations are necessary to begin therapy while awaiting results of the above tests?

The major reason to treat patients with GABHS is to prevent both suppurative (pharyngeal or peritonsillar abscess or infection of facial or cervical enclosed tissue spaces) and nonsuppurative sequelae including rheumatic fever. With penicillin therapy, suppurative sequelae have fallen from 8.6% to 1.1% compared to placebo. There are several strategies for deciding which patients to treat. First, patients can be assessed by symptom complex. Komaroff found that patients with fever, tender adenopathy, and tonsillar exudate had a 30% to 45% chance of having a positive culture for GABHS. The triad of pharyngitis, tender lymphadenopathy, and fever during an outbreak are highly suggestive of Group A beta-hemolytic strep infection. Experts concur that this method must be interpreted in light of the positive predictive value of the symptom complex as determined by disease prevalence, known exposure, seasonality, and past history of rheumatic fever.

The second strategy is the double swab technique. The first swab is for a rapid antigen detection test, and the patient is treated if positive. If the rapid test is negative, a second swab is sent for culture. Five to fifty percent of positive cultures may identify a chronic carrier state without symptoms or risk of sequelae. This method hopes to find and treat those individuals who have subclinical infection with minimal symptoms but who are at risk for sequelae. Non-GABHS do not lead to rheumatic fever. Data show that waiting for a culture to turn positive over 48 to 56 hours does not lead to further complication or spread.

The third method is to treat all sore throats with antibiotics. This may be an appropriate strategy in the emergency department or during an outbreak. However, there is a 1% to 2% rate of adverse reaction to penicillin with an estimated death rate of .001%.

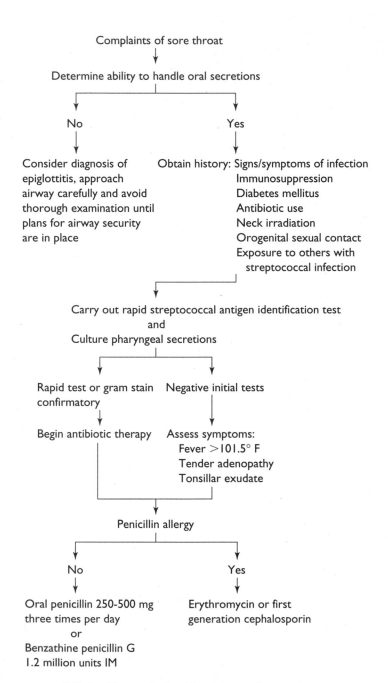

6-7-1   Diagnostic algorithm for sore throat pain.

QUESTION 5 What is the appropriate therapy once GABHS infection is confirmed?

Penicillin remains the drug of choice. A regimen of 250 to 500 mg 3 to 4 times/day for 10 days is suggested. A single intramuscular injection of 1.2 million units can be given if patient compliance is an issue. For penicillin allergic patients erythromycin is recommended. Because erythromycin can lead to abdominal discomfort, first generation cephalosporins are also useful as second-line therapy. An advantage of erythromycin use is the broadened spectrum of mycoplasma and chlamydial coverage.

Antibiotic therapy can fail if bacterial tolerance has developed, other beta-lactamase producing organisms are present, reinfection, and because of differences in antibiotic absorption. Persistent infection may require tonsillectomy. Local abscess formation also requires drainage procedures in addition to antibiotics.

BIBLIOGRAPHY

Berkow R, Fletcher AJ: *The Merck Manual,* ed 15, 1987 Merck, Sharpe and Dohme Research Laboratories.
Del Mar C: Managing sore throat: a literature review, *Med J Australia* 156:575, 1992.
Denny FW: Current management of streptococcal pharyngitis, *J Fam Prac* 35(6): 619-620, 1992.
Goldstein M: Office evaluation and management of the sore throat, *Otolaryng Clin North Am* 25(4):837-843, 1992.
Huovinen P: Pharyngitis in adults: the presence and co-existence of viruses and bacterial organisms, *Ann Intern Med* 110:612-616, 1989.
Huovinen P: Causes, diagnoses and treatment of pharyngitis, *Compr Ther* 16(10):59-65, 1990.
Kind A: Antibiotic treatment of pharyngitis, *Semin Respir Infect* 6(2):69-76, 1991.
Lang SDR: The sore throat, when to investigate and when to prescribe, *Drugs* 40(6):854-862, 1990.
Vukmir RB: Adult and pediatric pharyngitis: a review, *J Emerg Med* 10:607-616, 1992.
Walsh TB: Recognition of streptococcal pharyngitis in adults, *Arch Intern Med* 135:1493-1497, 1975.

CASE

8

Jong Y. Yi
William J. Elliott

A 57-year-old black man was referred from an ophthalmology clinic for management of "severe" hypertension. The patient gave a 1-week history of headache, and blurred vision intermittently for a year. His blood pressure was 200/110 mm Hg in the ophthalmologist's office. The patient stopped his methyldopa therapy for hypertension about 5 years ago "because it wasn't working." His wife indicated that he had stopped it because of sexual dysfunction. He denied nausea, vomiting, fever, chills, dizziness, palpitations, chest pain, shortness of breath, dyspnea on exertion, or transient ischemic attack symptoms.

His past medical history was otherwise unremarkable. His only medication was acetaminophen, which he took as needed for his headache. He claimed to have no known drug allergies. He works part time as a truck driver for a local short-haul transfer service. He has smoked 1.5 packs of cigarettes/day for the last 20 years and drinks only infrequent alcoholic beverages. The patient's health insurance comes from his wife and covers only inpatient costs; they have no pharmacy plan and pay for prescriptions out of pocket. The only pertinent family history was that his father had hypertension for 10 years before his death at age 82 of "old age." The review of systems is otherwise unremarkable.

Physical examination discloses a well-developed, well-nourished, slightly obese black gentleman, with BP 200/112 mm Hg (right arm, large adult-sized cuff) with pulse rate of 72 bpm in the supine position. It was 200/110 mm Hg (left arm, supine) and 196/100 mm Hg (right arm) with pulse rate of 78 bpm when standing. The respiratory rate was 20/min; the oral temperature was 98.5°F. He weighed 210 lb and was 70 inches tall.

HEENT examination was normal except for the fundi, which showed bilateral exudates and one hemorrhage in the right fundus 0.5 disc diameter wide, 2 disc diameters out at 3 o'clock. The neck was supple, without JVD; no carotid bruits were noted. The chest was clear to auscultation bilaterally. The heart had a regular rhythm and rate, no S_3, but an S_4 was noted. A 2/6 systolic ejection murmur was heard best in the aortic area; the PMI was slightly displaced laterally. The peripheral pulses were equal and strong. A femoral bruit was heard bilaterally with both systolic and diastolic components. The abdomen was normal, without bruits. The extremities were normal, without edema; the thigh BP was 220/118 mm Hg. The neurologic examination was nonfocal.

Laboratory studies included a hematocrit of 39%, platelet count of 353K, WBC 6.0. The chemistry panel disclosed Na 143, K 5.0, Cl 105, HCO_3 20, BUN 12, Cr 2.2, glucose 91, urate 9.4, Ca 9.3, and cholesterol 228. The urinalysis had a pH 7.0, specific gravity (S.G.) 1.010, ALB 2+, and no RBCs or WBCs. The ECG showed normal sinus rhythm with left axis deviation and LVH by voltage criteria. The posteroanterior (PA) and lateral chest x-ray showed a slightly increased cardiothoracic ratio but was otherwise normal.

QUESTION 1 Does this level of blood pressure need therapy? If so, what agent(s) should you recommend?

This patient presented with stage 3 hypertension (HTN) and target organ damage (TOD) with

TABLE 6-8-1   Classification of BP (age ≥18)

Category	Systolic, mm Hg	Diastolic, mm Hg
Normal	< 130	< 85
High normal	130-139	85-89
Hypertension		
Stage 1 (mild)	140-159	90-99
Stage 2 (moderate)	160-179	100-109
Stage 3 (severe)	180-209	110-119
Stage 4 (very severe)	≥ 210	≥ 120

Adapted from *Arch Intern Med* 153:161, 1993.

TABLE 6-8-2   Recommendations for Follow-up

Category	F/U
Normal	In 2 yrs
High normal	In 1 yr
Stage 1	In 2 mo
Stage 2	In 1 mo
Stage 3	In 1 wk
Stage 4	Care immediately

Adapted from *Arch Intern Med* 153:162, 1993.

renal, cardiac, and retinal involvement according to the new classification of BP for adults aged 18 years and older by the Fifth Report from The Joint National Committee on Detection, Evaluation, and Treatment of High Blood Pressure (JNC V). Previous reports have been published every 4 to 5 years over the last 20 years to guide physicians and other health care providers in the prevention and management of high blood pressure.

One of the biggest changes in this report was the new classification of hypertension (see Table 6-8-1). The "cutpoints" were based on levels of BP that correlated with future morbidity and mortality, especially as shown in the MRFIT screen follow-up. Previous descriptive classifications such as *mild* or *moderate* HTN had led some patients and even a few health care providers to underestimate the risk of consequences of the lower stages of hypertension, especially cardiovascular morbidity and mortality.

Diagnosis of hypertension should not routinely be based on a single measurement. Rather it needs serial (2 to 3 different days with an average of two or more readings each visit) measurements under nonstressful conditions to represent a patient's usual level of BP. Based on this initial set of BP measurements, the recent JNC V report gives recommendations regarding appropriate intervals for follow-up (Table 6-8-2).

Another change in the JNC V report is the emphasis on lifestyle modifications (previously referred to as "nonpharmacologic therapy") as definitive or adjunctive treatment for BP control. The recommended lifestyle modifications include weight reduction, exercise, limiting sodium and alcohol intake, and smoking cessation.

The ultimate goal of the management of hypertension is to decrease morbidity and mortality from elevated BP rather than just to decrease the numbers of millimeters of mercury. That is why optimal treatment of hypertension is not just random use of medications, like tossing bait before fishing with a net, but should be part of a comprehensive approach of all cardiovascular risk factors. Choice of drug therapy depends on coexisting conditions, unique features of each drug (Table 6-8-3), severity of BP, TOD, demographic characteristics, cost of medications, potential side effects, etc. The treatment algorithm recommended by JNC V is shown in Fig. 6-8-1 on p. 350.

In stage 1 and 2 hypertension, initial pharmacologic therapy is recommended only after aggressive lifestyle modification for 3 to 6 months and then only with a single drug. In JNC V, diuretics and beta-blockers are recommended as initial choices even among the first-line drugs because those are the only drugs shown to be effective in reducing morbidity and mortality in long-term trials. However, those studies included only patients with hypertension as their sole problem, so those may not represent the general hypertensive population, especially if they have

TABLE 6-8-3   **Various Effects of Major Antihypertensive Drugs**

Effect	Alpha-Blocker	ACE Inhibitor	Beta-Blocker	Calcium Antagonist	Diuretic
Hemodynamic[1]	+	+	+	+	+
Metabolic[2]	+	0	–	0	–
Antiproliferative[3]	+	+	0	+	0

1. Effects on BP

2. Effects on lipid and glucose metabolism

3. Effects on ability to inhibit adverse vascular wall proliferative changes

+ = beneficial, 0 = neutral, – = adverse. ACE = angiotensin converting enzyme

other clinical problems and concomitant diseases. The JNC V report relegates calcium antagonists, ACE inhibitors, and alpha-blockers to "alternative therapy" because these drugs have not yet been tested or shown to reduce cardiovascular morbidity and mortality; such studies (including ALL-HAT, the Antihypertensive and Lipid Lowering Heart Attack Trial) are being carried out now. The JNC V report also makes the obvious point that diuretics and beta-blockers are, in general, available in generic formulations, which generally cost less than "alternative therapy," although this will change in the near future.

For the patient discussed, a diuretic was prescribed initially because he had no other clinical conditions which might have been indications for another medication. The recent VA Comparative Trial showed no significant difference in efficacy regarding BP reduction between the calcium antagonist and the diuretic in older African-American men. There is concern regarding male sexual function and diuretics, but it is probably less of a problem with diuretics than with methyldopa. Especially because this patient expressed concern about the cost of medications, the diuretic was believed to be the appropriate first-choice drug.

The goal of BP control is generally <140/90 mm Hg, but some physicians may withhold drug therapy from patients within the range of 140-149/90-94 mm Hg.

In stage 3 and 4, as in this case, a shorter time interval may be appropriate before the addition of a second or even a third drug, and one may start with more than one agent. If significant, acute TOD is present, hospitalization or consultation may be needed. Overaggressive treatment increases the risk of adverse side effects such as stroke and MI, probably even with oral agents. Physicians should schedule frequent appointments with these patients and escalate therapy cautiously without panic.

A list of preferred initial therapy based on coexisting conditions is presented for quick reference in Table 6-8-4.

QUESTION 2   He was initially started on a loop diuretic (because of chronic renal impairment), which decreased his BP to about 168/100 mm Hg; a calcium channel blocker was added 4 weeks later. His blood pressure decreased to 140-150/80-90 mm Hg with two antihypertensive medications and lifestyle modification. He seemed to be doing well for a while. However, his BP became difficult to control (155-165/95-105 mm Hg) with the above regimen within a month. What do you do now?

Although the majority (about 90%) of all patients' BPs can be controlled with a combination of 2 to 3 appropriately-chosen drugs (preferably one of which is a diuretic), there is a substantial number (about 10%) of patients who repeatedly demonstrate lack of responsiveness to therapy. Causes of lack of responsiveness to therapy in-

TABLE 6-8-4   Suggested Initial Therapy for Hypertension Based on Coexisting Conditions

Condition	Diuretics	Beta-Blockers	CCBs	ACEIs	Alpha-Blockers
COPD/Asthma	–	– – – –	+	– (?)	±
CHF	+++	– – (or +?)	+ or – (?)	+++	+ or – –
IDDM	– –	–	±	++ (?)	+ (?)
Dysrhythmias	– (?)	+++	+++ or ±	±	+ (?)
Angina Pectoris	±	+++	+++	±	±
Post-MI	± (?)	+++	+	± or + (?)	?
"Silent Ischemia"	± or – (?)	++	++	±	?
DJD (NSAIDs)	– –	–	±	– – –	?
Renal Insufficiency	++	+	+	– – (?)	±
Benign Prostatic Hypertrophy	– –	–	±	±	+++

Key: – – – – = severely contraindicated; – – – = moderately contraindicated; – – = mildly contraindicated; – = possibly contraindicated; ± = no major effect; + = possibly beneficial; ++ = mildly beneficial; +++ = FDA-approved for this use; ? = uncertain effect depending on clinical circumstances.

clude nonadherence to therapy, drug-related problems, increased weight and alcohol intake, secondary hypertension, volume overload, or pseudohypertension. These conditions are considered as causes of resistant or refractory hypertension. In JNC V, resistant hypertension is defined "when the BP can not be reduced to <160/100 mm Hg by an adequate and appropriate triple drug regimen." Resistant hypertension is more common (up to 13%) in referral centers and less in community-based practice (<1%). According to one report from a tertiary referral clinic in 1992, the causes of refractory hypertension were identified in 90% of such patients; the most common cause was suboptimal medical treatment (diagnosed in 43%). Some other causes were drug intolerance (14%), secondary hypertension (11%), noncompliance (10%), psychiatric causes (8%), office hypertension (2%), alcohol abuse (2%), and drug interactions (1%). More than 60% of the patients presenting with resistant hypertension had their BPs controlled or improved simply by modifying or adding a diuretic (most frequently), ACE inhibitor, or calcium antagonist.

QUESTION 3   An angiotensin converting enzyme inhibitor was added, and his BP came down to 120-130/80-90 mm Hg range. His serum creatinine increased to 3.8 mg/dl and remained elevated after repeated testing 2 weeks later. Why did this happen? What do you do now?

The most common type of hypertension is the essential or primary form. As the name implies, the cause of this essential hypertension is uncertain. However more and more clinicians consider it as part of a syndrome with features of hyperinsulinemia with insulin resistance, dyslipidemia, truncal obesity, and reduced arterial compliance, often with microalbuminuria, and left ventricular hypertrophy with diastolic dysfunction as late features.

Only a small percentage (less than 5%) of patients have identifiable causes of their hypertension (i.e., secondary hypertension). However, this subset accounts for a significant proportion of resistant hypertension and is important to diagnose because their hypertension is potentially curable, with correction of the underlying cause. Certain findings in the history, demographic characteristics, physical examination, and laboratory values are suggestive of secondary hypertension in the patient discussed. Table 6-8-5 shows some of the features for the three most common causes of secondary hypertension: renovascular hypertension (RVHT), primary aldosteronism, and

TABLE 6-8-5   Some Features of the Three Most Common Causes of Secondary HTN

Features	RVHT	Pheochromocytoma	1° Aldosteronism
Etiology	Atherosclerosis vs. fibromuscular dysplasia	Adrenal medullary tumor vs extra adrenal origin	Adrenal cortical adenoma vs hyperplasia

History	Sudden onset of HTN
	Age <30, >50
	Resistant HTN in smoker or PVD[1] present (see below)
		Paroxysmal HTN
		Labile BP
		5H's
		  Hypertension
		  Headache
		  Hyperglycemia
		  Hypermetabolic state
		  Hyperhidrosis
			Similar to essential HTN, but seldom Stage IV

Physical examination	Abd. bruit (systolic and diastolic) PVD findings (peripheral bruits, decreased pulses)	Tachy/bradycardia, tremor, pallor, sweating, orthostatic hypotension	Similar to essential HTN, seldom with high-grade retinopathy
Routine Labs	Unexplained worsening of renal function Reversible renal insufficiency with ACE Inhibitor Unilateral small kidney (often incidentally found)		Spontaneous[2] hypokalemia <3.3
Diagnosis	Captopril renal scan (noninvasive) Angiogram Renal vein renin sampling bilaterally	Metanephrines in spot or 24 hr urine Urine and plasma catecholamines before and after clonidine CT/MRI/MIBG[3]	Plasma aldo/renin ratio Saline loading/suppression test CT Iodocholesterol scan
Treatment	PTRA[4] Revascularization Medical therapy	Phentolamine β-blocker only after α-blocker Surgery	Surgery for adenoma Hyperplasia: medical therapy

1. PVD: peripheral vascular disease

2. Administration of K-sparing diuretics, ACEI, or K+ supplements usually does not restore serum K$^+$ to normal

3. MIBG: metaiodobenzylguanidine scan; MRI: magnetic resonance imaging; CT: computed tomographic scan

4. PTRA: percutaneous transluminal renal angioplasty

pheochromocytoma. Other causes of secondary hypertension are shown in the box on p. 349.

In renal artery stenosis (RAS), the renin-angiotensin system is activated, which constricts the renal efferent arterioles. In bilateral RAS or a solitary functional kidney, pressure distal to the stenosis is lowered. This would be expected to cause an acute decrease in GFR. However in the subacute stage, angiotensin II acts on the efferent arteriole, resulting in potent vasoconstriction, which maintains adequate GFR. An ACE Inhibitor (ACEI) blocks the production of angiotensin II, causing dilatation of the efferent arteriole. This results in decreased renal perfusion pressure, a drop in GFR, and subsequently an increased serum creatinine. The increase in serum creatinine is, however, neither a specific nor sensitive indicator for renovascular hypertension, as it can be seen in essential hypertension as well.

QUESTION 4 Because of his history, clinical course, physical findings, and laboratory abnormalities, renovascular hypertension was considered and a captopril renal scan was obtained. The result of the scan showed near-total absence of uptake of radioactive tracer in the right kidney (representative panel [at 25 minutes after injection] from scan is shown in Fig. 6-8-2 on p. 351). The arrow indicates

CAUSES OF SECONDARY HYPERTENSION

COMMON

- Renal parenchymal disease
- Renal vascular disorders
- Thyroid disease
- Mineralocorticoid-excess states
- Glucocorticoid-excess states
- Pheochromocytoma
- Coarctation of the aorta
- Sleep apnea

RARE

- Hypercalcemia
- CNS tumors
- Porphyria
- Carcinoid syndrome
- Acromegaly
- Autoimmune hyperreflexia associated with spinal cord lesions

the left kidney, which fills and drains normally. Note the PA orientation. What do you do now?

RVHT is the most common cause of remediable hypertension. Because of recent improvements in technical procedures, it is often curable with either angioplasty or surgical procedures. After a technically successful procedure many patients (80%) require less medications or no (about 48%, overall) medications at all. Therefore, diagnosis of RVHT is very important. Clinical clues suggestive of the need for evaluation for RVHT include: (1) reversible impairment of renal function with ACEI, (2) incidental finding of unilateral small kidney, (3) accelerated or malignant hypertension (grade 3 or 4 retinopathy), (4) unexplained or sudden worsening of renal insufficiency (especially in a smoker or in the setting of peripheral vascular disease), (5) abdominal bruit (systolic/diastolic), (6) abrupt onset of stage 3 or 4 HTN before 30 or after 50 years old, and (7) BP refractory to an appropriate two or three-drug regimen. On detecting more than one of the above "clinical clues," some physicians proceed directly to a renal angiogram, but others prefer noninvasive "screening tests," especially if the suspicion of renal artery stenosis is not very high. It is worth remembering that anatomic renal artery stenosis does not necessarily cause RVHT; renovascular hypertension is, in fact, a diagnosis made by asymetric levels of renal vein renin associated with a stenotic vessel or retrospectively by measuring BP after a procedure to repair the stenotic artery. Prospective functional assessment of possible renal arteries has traditionally been done using renal vein renin (and several ratios), but recently several noninvasive functional "screening" tests for RVHT have been proposed. In a recent study of 150 patients with a high suspicion of renovascular disease, captopril renal scintigraphy (CRS) was more accurate than the "captopril challenge test." Other work also suggests that the captopril renal scintigram successfully predicts the outcome of therapeutic intervention: lack of postcaptopril changes showed a very high failure rate in controlling BP after revascularization or percutaneous transluminal renal angioplasty (PTRA).

In acute and subacute RAS, GFR is maintained largely by the renin-angiotensin system. An ACEI (captopril) inhibits formation of angiotensin II, which normally induces constriction of the efferent arteriole from the glomerulus, and causes a significant reduction in GFR with or without a delay in renal excretion. In CRS, the renograms are compared before and one hour after the administration of captopril (25 mg or 50 mg orally). If the renogram after captopril shows decreased renal uptake of radioactive tracer, it indicates deterioration in renal function and suggests the presence of renovascular disease; current data suggest it has about a 90% sensitivity and 91% specificity in selected patients.

The definite anatomic diagnosis of RAS can be done by renal arteriogram or digital subtraction angiography (DSA). The equipment for DSA is expensive and still does not avoid a substantial radiocontrast dye load, so many centers continue to perform direct aortography and selective renal

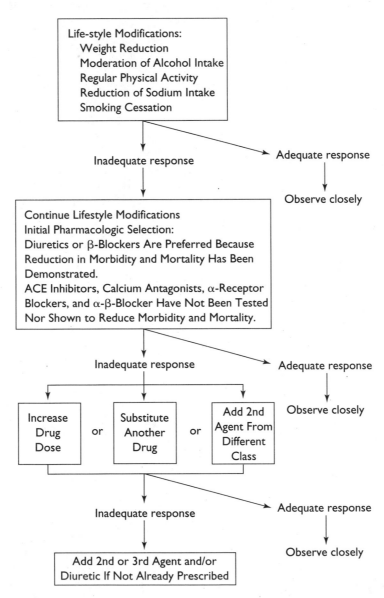

6-8-1 Joint National Committee on Detection, Evaluation, and Treatment of High Blood Pressure recommended treatment algorithm, *Arch Intern Med* 153:164, 1993.

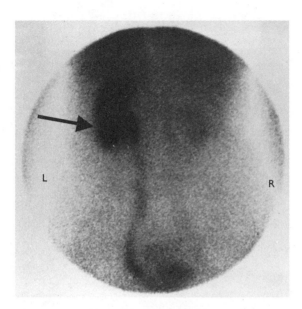

6-8-2   Illustrative panel (25 minutes after injection) from Renal Scintigram (using ^{99m}Tc-DTPA tracer) obtained an hour after oral captopril administration.

arteriography as their test of choice. Many angiographers prefer to attempt angioplasty during the same procedure as the diagnostic angiogram, arguing that it saves time, a second dye load, and a second arterial puncture. The counter argument is that renal vein renin ratios are not available so quickly, and some angiographers will proceed to angioplasty only when the ratios "lateralize." This may be of lesser importance if a captopril renal scan is obtained prior to angiography.

QUESTION 5   A renal angiogram was done ("aortic flush," Fig. 6-8-3). There was prompt and full filling of the left renal artery (*large arrow*), and the left kidney displayed a relatively normal nephrogram (limits of which are shown with the three *small arrows*), but the right renal artery was not visualized. The large artery on the right of the aorta is in fact the superior mesenteric (as shown on several other views). Extensive efforts to catheterize the right renal artery were made (taking about 40 minutes), and eventually were successful (as shown in negative, subtracted magnified spot film Fig. 6-8-4). The small arrow points out the near ostial stenosis; the

large arrow shows the area of poststenotic dilatation in the right renal artery: the diagnosis of renal artery stenosis was made. The angiographer was disappointed that he could not pass a wire through the stenosis despite a further 45 minutes of trying. What is your recommendation now?

The best management of RVHT is controversial. No one argues that revascularization (when successful) is excellent, but the less invasive PTRA is widely accepted as an alternative. Relative contraindications to PTRA include ostial lesions, multiple lesions in a single renal artery, and a lesion in one of several segmental renal arteries to the same kidney. PTRA in these settings has a high failure rate. Medical therapy is needed if the above procedures cannot be done, but renal failure may develop ultimately, even with adequate blood pressure control. If a patient must be managed medically, most physicians choose agents that block the renin-angiotensin system. ACEI and even beta-blockers are good choices, but ACEI may elevate serum creatinine if bilateral renal stenosis is present. Renal function should be

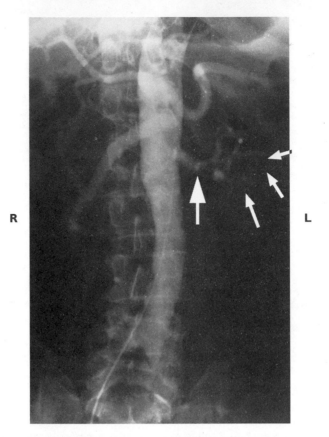

6-8-3 "Flush" aortogram obtained about 2 seconds after injection into aorta just superior to renal arteries. Note the absence of dye in the right renal artery, but filling on the left.

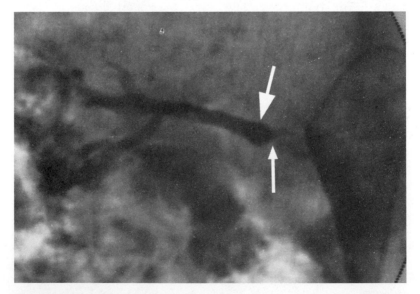

6-8-4 Selective digital subtraction angiogram of the right renal artery obtained about 3 seconds after injection. The slight arrow indicates the area of tight stenosis; the broad arrow points to the post-stenotic dilatation.

followed closely with any antihypertensive therapy, but especially with ACEI.

In this patient the diagnosis was made appropriately by angiogram, which was done after a highly suggestive captopril renal scan, and treated properly and successfully, given the normal blood pressures six weeks after surgery, and the need for no medications six months after the procedure. This case highlights some of the features of the JNC V guidelines.

CASE SUMMARY   He underwent surgical revascularization that resulted in a BP of 140/88 mm Hg immediately postoperative. The BP was 128/84 mm Hg 6 weeks later. Six months later, BP remained under control without any antihypertensive medications.

· ·

CASE COMMENT   In summary, treatment of HTN does not merely involve controlling BP, but more importantly requires surveillance of end organs. Many antihypertensive agents have been developed and control BP quite effectively. Since morbidity and mortality from HTN are also affected by coexisting conditions, overall assessment to obtain these aims are more critical than just choosing antihypertensive drugs. Before any form of therapy is initiated, several questions have to be raised, such as whether the patient has primary vs secondary HTN, whether there is TOD present, or whether there are other cardiovascular risk factors present. Cardiovascular disease-related morbidity and mortality attributed to HTN has markedly decreased in incidence since the beginning of the National High Blood Pressure Education Program

and the First Report of the Joint National Committee on Detection, Evaluation, and Treatment of High Blood Pressure. Secondary HTN can be diagnosed appropriately most of the time in a high-risk group (selected only on clinical grounds), and BP can be quite effectively controlled with drugs and/or invasive procedures, which only infrequently includes surgery.

A diagnostic algorithm for elevated blood pressure is shown in Fig. 6-2-1.

· ·

BIBLIOGRAPHY

Elliott WJ, Martin WB, Murphy MB: Comparison of two noninvasive screening tests for renovascular hypertension, *Arch Intern Med* 153:755-764, 1993.

Joint National Committee on Detection, Evaluation, and Treatment of High Blood Pressure: Fifth report of the Joint National Committee on Detection, Evaluation, and Treatment of High Blood Pressure (JNC V), *Arch Intern Med* 153:154-183, 1993.

Kaplan NM: Establishing control of refractory hypertension, *Hosp Pract* 29:115-120, 1994.

Navar LG: Renovascular hypertension: pathophysiology. In Izzo Jr JL, Black HR: *Hypertension primer*, Dallas, 1993 Council on High Blood Pressure Research American Heart Association, pp 99-101.

Prigent A, Froissart M: Current recommendations for diagnosis of renovascular hypertension, *Kidney: a Current Survey of World Literature* 3:138-144, 1994.

Ram CVS: Secondary hypertension: workup and correction, *Hosp Pract* 29:137-150, 1994.

Setaro JF, Black HR: Refractory hypertension, *N Eng J Med* 327:543-547, 1992.

Weber MA: Controversies in the diagnosis and treatment of hypertension: a personal review of JNC V, *Am J Cardiol* 72:3H-9H, 1993.

Yakovlevitch M, Black HR: Resistant hypertension in a tertiary care clinic, *Arch Intern Med* 151:1786-1792, 1991.

MEDICAL ONCOLOGY AND HEMATOLOGY

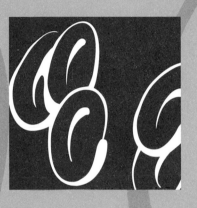

STEPHEN C. SCHWARTZ
SECTION EDITOR

CASE

Stephen C. Schwartz
Gary Schwartz

A 42-year-old woman came to her family physician with complaints of a burning sensation most prominently in her mid-chest and to a lesser degree, epigastrium, after meals and upon becoming recumbent. These symptoms began approximately 4 weeks ago and were accompanied by abdominal bloating and gas over the same time course. She believes that she has gained a substantial amount of weight without a commensurate increase in her appetite. She denies constitutional symptoms or shortness of breath. The patient's sensation of burning lasts greater than 30 minutes and is relieved promptly and temporarily by antacids. The pain does not radiate and is not associated with activity. The patient denies tobacco or ethanol abuse. She has no history of heart disease, diabetes, or hyperlipidemia.

QUESTION 1 Generate a differential diagnosis for patients with this character and distribution of pain.

Chest pain as a presenting complaint is commonly encountered in the practice of internal medicine. Because multiple diagnoses may manifest with this symptom, a thorough and methodical approach is always warranted. The patient profile (risk assessment) and presentation will initially direct the diagnostic strategy selected. Paramount in this regard is the necessity of ruling out coronary heart disease as an etiology. Because the consequences of a missed diagnosis in coronary heart disease may be profound, a low threshold should be maintained for initiating a cardiac workup.

Clinical history is often unreliable in differentiating cardiac and noncardiac chest pain. Noncardiac causes of chest pain include musculoskeletal disorders, gastroesophageal reflux, peptic ulcer disease, nonspecific esophageal motility disorders, diffuse esophageal spasm, esophageal mucosal disease, biliary tract disease, and pleuritic inflammation. Aortic dissection should always be considered in the differential diagnosis.

Chest pain may be described as burning, aching, sharp or stabbing, dull, heavy or pressure-like. Anginal pain is often described as pressure-like or crushing. Pleuritic pain may be characterized as sharp, often provoked by deep inspiration. Musculoskeletal pain may not infrequently be reproduced on physical examination. The proclivity to radiate, the specific location, or an association with exertional onset may not assist in the diagnostic process. None of these qualities are exclusive to a cardiac or noncardiac diagnosis.

The presence of risk factors may help to establish the diagnosis. Patients over 50 with a history of hypertension, diabetes, tobacco usage, or previously diagnosed coronary artery disease should be evaluated for coronary artery disease aggressively. Associated dysphagia or odynophagia may suggest esophageal disease, while symptoms provoked by recumbency or caffeine suggest gastroesophageal reflux. It is important to realize that esophageal chest pain may result from chemoreceptor stimulation by bile or acid, as well as smooth muscle spasm or dilatation.

The workup for chest pain should begin with a thorough history and physical examination. A significantly elevated blood pressure may signify hypertensive emergency with angina as a presenting symptom. Palpation of the musculature, ribs, and costochondral joints may aid in ruling out a musculoskeletal etiology. An initial ECG is helpful if abnormal but may, however, be unrevealing. Stress testing with thallium imaging may serve as a more sensitive technique for detecting coronary ischemia than conventional stress testing. Ultimately, in high-risk patients cardiac catherization will be required in selected cases with uninformative stress testing.

If a diagnosis is not established and cardiac disease deemed unlikely, a noncardiac source should be sought. Peptic ulcer disease can be ruled out by endoscopic evaluation. This procedure will also assess the esophageal mucosa. Ultrasound may help to exclude biliary tract disease as a source of noncardiac chest pain. Failure to achieve a diagnosis should lead the physician to institute a short course of anti-reflux therapy (elevate head of bed, avoid citrus and coffee, avoid bedtime eating, stop smoking, PRN antacids, and avoid drugs that decrease lower esophageal sphincter tone). If unsuccessful the patient may require 24-hour esophageal pH monitoring. This test allows the physician to correlate symptomatic episodes with changes in esophageal pH. If this test is negative, a CXR, if not already undertaken for a cardiac workup, should be obtained to assess for esophageal motility disorders. Esophageal manometry with edrophonium provocation may also be helpful. Approximately 60% of all noncardiac chest pain will have the esophagus as the primary etiology.

QUESTION 2 Physical examination revealed a well-nourished, well-developed woman in no distress appearing her stated age. The patient's vital signs were normal. Cardiac and pulmonary examination were within normal limits. No reproducible chest wall tenderness could be elicited. Examination of the abdomen revealed modest distension but was otherwise unremarkable. A genitourinary examination was deferred because the patient had a pelvic examination and PAP smear approximately 8 months ago. The rectal examination was negative for occult blood. A resting ECG was obtained and was unrevealing. The physician referred the patient for endoscopy given his low suspicion for the presence of coronary artery disease.

She was sent home with an H_2-antagonist and was given instructions for the prevention of reflux. Three weeks later the patient was seen by the gastroenterologist. She had gained moderate relief with the aid of the H_2-antagonist and her physician's instructions; however, she felt her abdominal girth to be increased in size over this 3-week period. Examination confirmed the presence of a distended abdomen with a probable fluid wave. The patient was sent for ultrasonography to assess for the presence of ascites and other pathology. What is in the differential diagnosis for a nonpainful or painful distended abdomen?

Distension of the abdomen is a common clinical entity. The internist must separate a patient's subjective sense of abdominal enlargement often described as bloating from an objective and sustained increase in abdominal girth. The former is usually a transient state produced by functional gastrointestinal disorders. In general, distension may be produced by the excess presence of (1) gas in the bowel or peritoneum, (2) ascitic fluid in the peritoneum, (3) blood in the peritoneal cavity, (4) bowel ileus, or (5) mass lesion(s) with or without disseminated carcinomatosis in the abdominal cavity.

Clinical presentations of abdominal swelling range from the acute to the insidious. In the acute setting hemoperitoneum may be encountered with traumatic abdominal injuries. In the latter scenario, the gradual accumulation of ascites may not be noticed by the patient for some time. Patients may present after the realization that clothes and belts no longer fit. Patients may develop a "pulling-like" sensation in the flank or groin region. New abdominal hernias or a newly everted umbilicus may be found. Common to abdominal distension are complaints of indigestion or retrosternal chest pain from gastroesophageal reflux as a result of increased intraabdominal pressure. Patients may also complain of tachypnea or dyspnea caused by limited diaphragmatic excursion with a raised diaphragm.

Nonpainful abdominal distension is common to patients with ascites secondary to cirrhosis, right-sided heart failure, and nephrotic syndrome. Bowel ileus is often painless and may be accompanied by emesis. Collections of gas in the bowel secondary to complete or partial obstruction may often be painful. Mass lesions invading or replacing a viscous may be painless or painful. Mass lesions may cause pain by bowel obstruction, distension, or rupture.

The diagnostic workup for abdominal distension should include a thorough history and physical examination. Issues to address in the history should include ethanol intake, a history of viral hepatitis, past surgeries, a history of heart failure or valvular disease, history of prior malignancy, and any current medications. Examination should be directed toward the confirmation and support of possible etiologies (i.e., the presence of peripheral stigmata of cirrhosis, the presence of an S_3 in heart failure, high-pitched tinkling bowel sounds in obstruction).

Radiographic assessment is often helpful in ascertaining the diagnosis. Abdominal films may demonstrate the presence of air-filled loops of bowel in obstruction or the absence of psoas muscle shadow in ascites. Ultrasonography is useful in assessing for ascites or mass as is computed tomography.

QUESTION 3 The patient underwent abdominal ultrasound that revealed the presence of ascites and probable omental masses. CT examination confirmed these findings delineating multiple omental masses that appeared to coalesce. The appearance of the ovaries, uterus, and bowel were within normal limits. The patient's internist performed a pelvic examination that was unrevealing. The physician recommended a diagnostic paracentesis as the next course of action. How can examination of ascitic fluid aid in establishing a diagnosis?

The analysis of ascitic fluid is mandatory in the workup of new onset ascites. Fluid should be assessed by paracentesis for overall appearance, protein concentration, specific gravity, and cell count with differential. Bacterial cultures, gram stain, and stains for acid fast bacilli are routine. Cytology should also be reviewed on a routine basis.

Ascites is characterized as being *transudative* or *exudative*. Transudative fluid has a protein concentration of less than 25 g/L and a specific gravity less than 1.016. Exudative fluid has greater than 25 g/L of protein with a specific gravity greater than 1.016. Transudative ascites is a feature of cirrhosis, nephrosis, and/or congestive heart failure. Exudative fluid is common in ascites related to neoplasm, pyogenic and tuberculous infections, and pancreatic pseudocysts. The presence of high cell counts with a predominance of PMNs suggests a bacterial infection. High counts with a large population of lymphocytes suggest TB. Cytology may be positive for malignancies that have a predilection for intraperitoneal spread such as ovarian, colorectal, and gastric cancers. Hepatoma may also produce ascites by producing portal hypertension.

Chylous ascites is milky white or cloudy. This fluid contains fat globules that stain with sudan black. High triglyceride levels are found in samples of chylous ascites. Chylous ascites is found in scenarios where lymphatic obstruction has occurred. This may result from tumor, trauma, tuberculosis, nephrosis, filariasis, and congenital abnormalities. *Pseudochylous* ascites is present when ascites appears turbid from tumor or high cell counts in infection. Alkalinization and ether extraction may help delineate the two entities.

QUESTION 4 The patient underwent paracentesis. The following results were obtained on routine analysis:
   Protein: 50 g/L
   Specific gravity: 1.020
   Cell count was positive for an abundance of lymphocytes
   Cytology: consistent with adenocarcinoma with papillary features
   Now that a malignancy has been identified, how should the search for a primary site be conducted?

The workup for a cancer of unknown primary site serves as a paradigm for the assessment of all newly diagnosed malignancies. Two tasks are incumbent upon the oncologist/internist in this setting. First, a diagnosis of malignancy must be established on pathologic grounds. Secondly, an origin or primary site must be sought that will permit classification of the malignancy. This will allow for prognostication and will eventually direct therapeutic intervention. Initial presentations of patients with unknown primary sites include lesions in the liver, lungs, lymph nodes, and bone. Other presentations may include pleural effusion and malignant ascites. Patients with cancers of unknown primary site often present with widespread metastatic disease. They may exhibit constitutional signs and symptoms including profound weight loss, cachexia, and fatigue. The initial workup should begin with a detailed history and physical examination. Pelvic and rectal examinations are mandatory. Routine laboratory analysis including CBC, electrolytes, and screening profile should be obtained as should chest radiograph and CT scan of the abdomen.

Biopsy of the most accessible site should be performed early. Open biopsies are considered superior to fine-needle aspiration as the former displays improved maintenance of histological features and provides more tissue for special analysis.

Pathologic assessment of a cancer of unknown primary site begins with an analysis by light microscopy. This technique will allow for the placement of the malignancy into one of five distinct categories. These will include *adenocarcinoma, squamous carcinoma, poorly differentiated malignant neoplasms, poorly differentiated carcinoma, and poorly differentiated adenocarcinoma*, each of unknown primary site. Approximately 60% of patients will be placed into the category of adenocarcinoma of unknown primary. Adenocarcinomas from various organs are not usually distinguishable by light microscopy and require other means to categorize them specifically. Five percent of all cancers of unknown primary site are recognizable as squamous cell carcinomas.

Light microscopy will not provide information regarding tumor lineage in the remaining 35% of patients assessed. Pathologic analysis will suggest poorly differentiated neoplasm, poorly differenti-

ated carcinoma, or poorly differentiated adenocarcinoma. Malignancies carrying these diagnoses should always undergo further pathologic assessment because identification of specific tumor types may allow curative therapy to be instituted. This is especially important in poorly differentiated neoplasms because 30% to 70% of these cases will ultimately be diagnosed as non-Hodgkin's lymphoma. These malignancies are chemosensitive tumors and are potentially curable. The tissue of origin for poorly differentiated carcinomas and poorly differentiated adenocarcinomas will not be identified by further analysis in a majority of cases. However, because approximately 20% of these cases will also be diagnosed as being non-Hodgkin's lymphoma, full analysis should be carried out. On occasion, patients demonstrate classic histologic features for specific tumors other than the five aforementioned distinct classifications. These cases should be assessed and treated in accordance with the particular tumor type involved (i.e., sarcomas or melanoma).

Those patients whose pathology suggests poorly differentiated malignancy, poorly differentiated carcinoma, or poorly differentiated adenocarcinoma should have their specimens assessed by immunohistochemistry (immunoperoxidase staining). This method, which relies on the detection of cell components or products by monoclonal and polyclonal antibodies, allows for the characterization and classification of cancers. Specimens staining positive for *cytokeratin* represent carcinomas or mesotheliomas. A distinction between mesothelioma, squamous cell carcinoma, and other carcinomas may be made on the basis of molecular weight. Squamous cell carcinomas and mesotheliomas have high molecular weight keratins, while adenocarcinomas, hepatocellular carcinoma, neuroendocrine tumors, thyroid, and renal cell carcinomas have low molecular weight keratins.

Antibodies to the *leukocyte common antigen (LCA)* possess a high degree of specificity for lymphomas. Patients whose specimens are positive for LCA should be treated for lymphoma accordingly.

Although some lymphomas stain positive for *vimentin*, this component is often associated with sarcomas.

Individual sarcomas may also be identified by immunoperoxidase staining. Rhabdomyosarcoma may stain positive for desmin, myoglobin, and SM actin. Angiosarcomas often express factor VIII antigen and ULEX. Melanomas may stain for vimentin and are often S-100 and HMB-45 positive. Spindle cell carcinomas, mesotheliomas, renal cell carcinomas, Wilms' tumor, synovial sarcoma, epithelioid sarcoma, and chordoma may stain for both keratin and vimentin. Although it is often not feasible to determine the primary site for most carcinomas, several specific stains exist that may lead to identification. These include stains for prostate-specific antigen in prostate carcinoma, thyroglobulin in follicular thyroid carcinoma, calcitonin in medullary thyroid carcinoma, neuron-specific enolase and chromogranin in neuroendocrine tumors, and HCG and AFP in germ cell tumors. While these stains may be specific in the appropriate clinical setting, only prostate-specific antigen carries enough specificity that the diagnosis may be made by the results of the stain alone.

Those specimens initially identified as adenocarcinoma or squamous carcinoma may also benefit from immunohistochemical analysis. However, the majority of these cancers will not be placed in a specific subgroup and will remain adenocarcinomas and squamous carcinomas of unknown primary site.

Electron microscopy (EM) may reveal specific ultrastructural features that may aid in the diagnosis of cancer of unknown primary site. EM may make the distinction of carcinoma from lymphoma. It may also distinguish neuroendocrine tumors by the presence of neurosecretory granules or melanoma by the presence of premelanosomes. Adenocarcinoma is identified by the presence of intracellular lumina or microvilli, while squamous cell carcinoma demonstrates tonofilaments.

Cytogenetics may define the malignancy when chromosomal abnormalities exist that are specific for a particular tumor type. Multiple cytogenetic abnormalities exist in lymphomas, which may present as a clue to the diagnosis. The 11, 22 translocation in Ewing's sarcoma and the isochromosome of chromosome 12 in germ cell tumors are two cytogenetic abnormalities specific for solid tumor malignancies. As more specific cytogenetic abnormalities and tumor-associated oncogenes are identified, techniques such as the polymerase chain reaction (PCR) and fluorescent in situ hybridization (FISH) will be used to identify various tumor types. When tumor type cannot be identified by immunohistochemistry, EM and cytogenetic analysis may be used in combination to establish tumor type. (See Fig. 7-1-1 on p. 364.)

QUESTION 5 What will the workup entail for identifying the primary site?

After pathologic assessment of the relevant biopsied tissue has been completed, the search for the primary site may be undertaken. The diagnostic strategy involved will rely heavily on the signs and symptoms, pathology, and the distribution of metastasis. As outlined in the aforementioned paragraphs, initial evaluation should include a thorough history and physical examination, routine labs, chest radiograph, and CT imaging of the abdomen.

If a primary site cannot be established by these means, further pursuit of the primary site may be unnecessary and nonproductive. The use of diagnostic imaging, invasive procedures, or random tumor marker determination is not prudent. However, in patients with relevant history or positive radiographic findings, further studies may be required. As an example, patients possessing CXRs with positive findings (parenchymal or mediastinal lesions) should be considered for CT scanning and possible bronchoscopy.

QUESTION 6 What is the approach to management of cancers of unknown primary site?

When the origin of a cancer of unknown primary site is subsequently identified, treatment is initiated based upon best therapy available for the particular stage of the primary cancer. The vast majority of patients with cancer of unknown primary site (the majority of which are adenocarcinomas) will not benefit from intervention except for good supportive care. There will be a small percentage of patients who will benefit from palliative measures and a small cohort for whom potentially curative therapy is available. In the approach to therapy for a truly unknown primary, patients are separated into four representative histologic groups: adenocarcinoma, squamous carcinoma, poorly differentiated carcinoma, and poorly differentiated adenocarcinoma. It is assumed that poorly differentiated malignancies will be grouped into one of these four histologies based upon light microscopy and immunohistochemistry obtained to date. Each of the aforementioned histologic groupings will have subgroups based upon the patient profile and the site of disease. Each subgroup in turn has a particular approach to therapy.

Patients with adenocarcinomas represent the largest of the unknown primary groups. Four subgroups are recognized: (1) women with axillary nodal metastases, (2) women with peritoneal carcinomatosis, (3) men with tumors staining for prostate-specific antigen or who have elevations in serum PSA levels, and (4) patients who possess a solitary peripheral nodal metastasis.

Women who possess *axillary nodal metastases* or who have them in combination with other metastatic sites are likely to have breast cancer. Those patients having only axillary nodal disease (stage II breast cancer) may be treated with intent to cure. There is data to support modified radical mastectomy in these patients even in the setting of a negative mammogram and physical examination. Between 40% and 60% of these patients will ultimately have an occult breast cancer identified. The use of adjuvant chemotherapy and/or hormonal therapy has been recommended in this subset of patients, although no data exists to establish efficacy. The prognosis for this subset of patients is similar to that of patients routinely diagnosed with stage II breast cancer. Those

patients who have axillary nodal metastasis, in conjunction with other sites, may benefit from treatment for metastatic breast cancer. This may include chemotherapy, hormonal therapy, or both.

Women with *peritoneal carcinomatosis* whose pathology is consistent with adenocarcinoma displaying papillary features often have ovarian cancer. There remains a segment of this subgroup in whom an ovarian lesion cannot be detected. These women have pathology identical to that of ovarian cancer. They possess a syndrome referred to as peritoneal papillary serous carcinoma or multifocal extraovarian serous carcinoma. This presentation is based upon the embryologic development of the ovarian epithelium which is derived from elements of the peritoneum. Women who present with peritoneal carcinomatosis identified as adenocarcinoma possessing papillary features with or without an identifiable ovarian source should undergo exploratory laparotomy and surgical cytoreduction. These same patients should also be treated with chemotherapeutic regimens active against ovarian cancer. Response rates ranging from 30% to 40% have been described for patients treated in such fashion.

Men who have metastatic lesions in the setting of an *elevated PSA or whose tumors are positive for PSA* by immunohistochemical means may have metastatic prostate cancer. These patients may benefit from a trial of hormonal therapy appropriate for prostate cancer. In the elderly age cohort, patients who develop osteoblastic metastasis whose tumors do not stain for or whose serum levels of PSA remain normal, may also be considered for a trial of hormonal therapy.

Patients presenting with an *isolated peripheral lymph node* in the cervical, axillary or inguinal region which reveals adenocarcinoma by pathology may benefit from an excisional procedure, radiation therapy, or a combination of both. These measures have produced long-term survival in a small proportion of these patients.

Those patients who present with adenocarcinomas not falling into one of these four subgroups may be considered for a trial of chemotherapy. It must be pointed out that response rates for these patients have been generally poor to date, with approximately 20% of patients achieving some kind of response. Chemotherapy should be reserved for those patients who possess an adequate performance status, which in the setting of unknown primary tumors, may be a small population of patients. Chemotherapeutic agents including cis-platinum, 5-FU, adriamycin, and mitomycin have been used alone or in various combinations. It has been suggested that two cycles of chemotherapy should be administered and adequacy of response assessed. If response is poor, best supportive care may be instituted. Those patients who are responders may continue therapy for up to 6 months if response is maintained.

The majority of patients who possess squamous cell carcinomas of unknown primary site have disease isolated to *cervical or inguinal lymph nodes*. It is important that these entities be recognized because they represent treatable and potentially curable malignancies. Although most often squamous cell carcinomas, adenocarcinomas may also arise in the supraclavicular region. Patients having right-sided supraclavicular involvement most often have disease in the lung or breast, while those with left-sided disease (Virchow's node) more commonly have gastrointestinal malignancies. Patients with *cervical lymph nodes* containing squamous cell carcinoma may have either head and neck or lung primaries. If a primary site cannot be established by panendoscopy, CT examination of the head, neck, and chest and thorough otolaryngeal evaluation, treatment will be based on the level of nodal involvement and will be directed toward the involved neck region. Patients with upper- or mid- cervical involvement should be treated by both radical neck dissection and radiation therapy (RT). Each modality has proven to be the others equal in terms of survival; however, high recurrence rates in the 30% range are observed in patients not receiving postoperative radiation. Therefore RT is added as standard therapy and should be given in the same field and dosage as that given to known primaries of head and neck cancer. Low cervical and supraclavicular nodes containing squamous cell carcinoma are more likely to represent lung primaries. The limited disease-free and overall survival seen in these patients is probably a reflection of their lung origin. These patients should be fully assessed for disease below the clavicle. If no site is found, treatment should follow guidelines established for patients with mid- and high-cervical disease.

Patients who have *inguinal lymph nodes* containing squamous cell carcinoma may have anal or perirectal tumors. If a thorough workup fails to disclose a primary, these patients should be treated by inguinal lymph node dissection and radiation therapy. Long-term survival has been reported in those patients so treated.

Patients whose initial pathology by light microscopy reveals poorly differentiated carcinoma or poorly differentiated adenocarcinoma may be given new diagnoses after immunohistologic analysis. The most often revealed new diagnosis is lymphoma; however the vast majority of patients will continue to have diagnoses of poorly differentiated carcinoma and poorly differentiated adenocarcinoma. A few young patients will have features of a germ cell tumor with disease in the mediastinum and retroperitoneum and elevations in serum B-HCG and/or AFP. Patients with lymphoma, suspected germ cell tumors, and other specifically identified malignancies initially diagnosed as poorly differentiated carcinomas and poorly differentiated adenocarcinoma should be given therapy appropriate for their tumors.

Treatment for those patients who remain poorly differentiated carcinomas and poorly differentiated adenocarcinomas has evolved significantly over the last 10 years. The introduction of platinum-based regimens in this group of patients has produced complete responses in the 50% range. Approximately 20% of these patients had long-term disease-free survival. It is felt that this group of responders represents a heterogeneous group of patients with malignancies that include atypical germ cell tumors, neuroendocrine tumors, and anaplastic carcinoids. The finding of an isochromosome 12 in germ cell tumors by cytogenetic analysis has helped to identify poorly

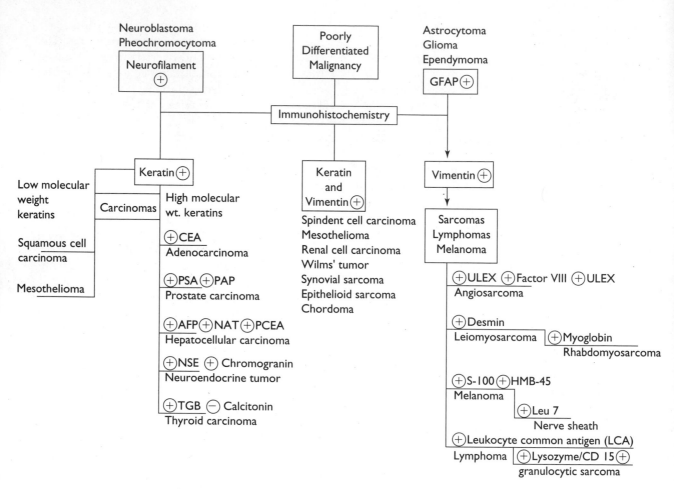

7-1-1   Diagnostic algorithm for cancer of an unknown primary site.

differentiated carcinomas and poorly differentiated adenocarcinoma of unknown primary origin. Those patients who were isochromosome 12 positive, responded well overall to platinum-based compounds. Neuroendocrine tumors can sometimes be identified by their neurosecretory granules on electron microscopy. The origin of these tumors is not well established. They are, however, chemo-sensitive tumors, especially to cis-platinum-based regimens.

Patients who are not placed in a specific category and remain poorly differentiated carcinomas and poorly differentiated adenocarcinomas

should receive a trial of platinum-based therapy. Two cycles are usually given initially to assess response. If a response is achieved, two additional cycles may be given. More than four cycles has never been shown to change outcome. Prognostic factors used to predict responders to platinum-based chemotherapy include location of tumor to the retroperitoneum or peripheral lymph nodes, less than two sites of metastasis, young age, and no history of tobacco exposure.

CASE FOLLOW-UP   This patient was taken to the operating room. At the time of surgery exploratory laparotomy, total abdominal hysterectomy, bilateral salpingo-ophorectomy, omentectomy, and surgical debulking were performed. The patient was considered optimally debulked (all disease remaining is less than 2 cm in diameter). The ovaries were without evidence of disease, placing the patient in the category of peritoneal papillary serous carcinoma. No individual mass had been greater than 5 cm in greatest diameter.

She began a chemotherapeutic regimen of cisplatinum and Taxol (standard therapy for advanced carcinoma) approximately 3 weeks after discharge. She received 6 cycles of this regimen followed by reassessment. Physical examination, chest x-ray, and CT examination of the abdomen were without evidence of disease after 6 cycles of chemotherapy.

The patient was taken back to the operating room where a second-look exploratory laparotomy was performed. At the time of surgery multiple 0.50 cm implants were noted on the surface of the small bowel. The patient was again cytoreduced. She then received intraperitoneal taxol on protocol. She is completing the 3rd cycle of a planned 6 cycles of this treatment.

BIBLIOGRAPHY

Allhoff EP, Proppe KH, et al: Evaluation of prostate specific acid phosphatase and prostate specific antigen in identification of prostate cancer, *J Urol* 129:315-318, 1983.

Dalrymple JC, Bannatyne P, et al: Extraovarian peritoneal serous papillary carcinoma: a clinicopathologic study of 31 cases, *Cancer* 64:110-115, 1989.

Hainsworth JD, Greco FA: Treatment of patients with cancer of unknown primary site, *N Engl J Med* 329:4, 257-263, 1993.

Hainsworth JD, Johnson DH, et al: Poorly differentiated neuroendocrine tumor of unknown primary site: a newly recognized clinicopathologic entity, *Ann Intern Med* 109: 364-371, 1988.

Hainsworth JD, Wright EP: Poorly differentiated carcinoma of unknown primary site: clinical usefulness of immunoperoxidase staining, *J Clin Oncol* 9:1931-1938, 1991.

Mohit-Tabatabai MA, Dasmahapatra KS, et al: Management of squamous cell carcinoma of unknown origin in cervical lymph nodes, *Am Surg* 52:152-154, 1986.

Nystrom JS, Weiner JM, et al: Metastaic and histologic presentations in unknown primary cancer, *Semin Oncol* 4:53-58, 1974.

Shildt RA, Kennedy PS, et al: Management of patients with metastatic adenocarcinoma of unknown origin: a southwest oncology group study, *Cancer Treat Rep* 67:77-79, 1983.

Strand CM, Grosh WW, et al: Peritoneal carcinomatosis of unknown primary site in women: a distinctive subset of adenocarcinoma, *Ann Intern Med* 111:213-217, 1989.

C A S E

Stephen C. Schwartz
Gary Schwartz

A 42-year-old woman with no significant medical history came to her private physician with a right breast mass discovered on self-examination. The patient performs this examination on a routine basis and states that the "lump" was not present last month. She describes a history of other masses in the past that were believed to be benign by her gynecologist. She states that she is mid-cycle in her menses and has experienced no other symptoms. The patient is a mother of three. Her last mammogram was performed 2 years ago and read as normal. No familial history of breast cancer in a first degree relative was elicited.

QUESTION 1 What is the initial evaluation of a solitary breast mass?

The detection and subsequent workup of a solitary breast mass must be approached methodically. Risk assessment must be ascertained from the clinical context of the patient. Ultimately, pathologic assessment must be undertaken by needle or surgical biopsy. A multitude of processes may produce discrete mass lesions in breast tissue. These include carcinoma, fibrocystic change, fibroadenomata, cysts, fat necrosis, and sclerosing papillary proliferations.

Fibrocystic change, the most common lesion at biopsy in the 30 to 65 age group consists of a constellation of pathologic findings including sclerosis, adenosis (increased glandular proliferation), hyperplasia, and cyst formation. Fibroadenomata are lesions most commonly seen in the younger population, their size often varying during the menstrual cycle.

A new breast lesion in a low-risk individual

may be observed over the course of 1 month. Changes occurring in lesions during the menstrual cycle are most prominent 7 days before menses and are least so just after menses. Dominant breast lesions are those that persist through the menstrual cycle. These types of lesions should always be further investigated. Breast masses are most prevalent in the perimenopausal age group. Lesions detected postmenopausally have a higher incidence of carcinoma.

A thorough physical examination should be performed. Inspection of both breasts including contour, presence of dimpling, nipple discharge, and skin changes should be routine. Measurements of the primary lesion must always be estimated. Careful palpation of both breasts is necessary to help rule out synchronous lesions. Inspection and palpation of the axillae and other nodal areas is necessary and may be helpful in documenting nodal disease. Metastatic disease, most commonly to the lung and bone, may also be discovered on examination. The finding of a supraclavicular node represents metastatic disease. Peau d'orange change in the skin represents T_4 unresectable disease by definition.

Mammography is often helpful in the evaluation of breast mass lesions. However given the false-negative rate of approximately 10% to 15%, this technique cannot be used to rule out breast cancer. This technique is most useful in delineating small and deep lesions in large fatty breasts where physical examination is often difficult. (See Fig. 7-2-1 on p. 372.)

QUESTION 2 Physical examination revealed a firm lesion in the 10 o'clock position of the right breast approximately 2.5 cm in greatest diameter.

The axillae and other nodal areas were free of ostensible disease. Nipple discharge was not present at that time. The remainder of the physical examination was within normal limits. The patient was followed through the end of her present cycle. At the time of follow-up 10 days after her menses, the lesion had not regressed in size. Bilateral mammography revealed a stellate lesion in the right breast. No other findings were present. What are the patterns on mammography that are suggestive of pathology?

The finding of a suspicious mass lesion on physical examination should prompt bilateral mammography before biopsy or needle aspiration. Mammography offers additional delineation of the lesion, helps to rule out synchronous lesions, and serves as a baseline before biopsy, ensuring adequate sampling. Patterns on mammography suggestive of breast cancer include stellate or crab-like densities and clusters of 5 or more calcifications measuring 1 mm or less individually in an area less than 1 cm. Distortion of normal breast architecture in proximity to scars or other anomalies should also be considered suspicious. Structures that are believed to be cystic should be confirmed by ultrasound. Subsequent aspiration with disappearance of the cyst suggests a benign process. Should frank blood be removed or should the cystic fluid reaccumulate rapidly, a high degree of suspicion for malignancy should be maintained.

QUESTION 3 The patient's physician recommends an expeditious biopsy procedure in order to establish the diagnosis. She was given the option of excisional biopsy for lumpectomy and nodal dissection if carcinoma is diagnosed or a fine-needle biopsy. The patient chose to have an initial needle biopsy in the surgical day hospital. What are the relative merits of needle aspirate versus an excisional biopsy?

Both needle aspiration and excisional biopsy are easily performed in the outpatient setting without the need for general anesthesia. By mak-

ing an initial diagnosis with fine-needle aspiration, the physician gives the patient an appropriate time interval in which to choose a course of therapy and adjust to the diagnosis. These issues are critical to the well being of the patient because she may be thrust into a definitive surgical procedure before being emotionally and intellectually equipped to undergo such a course. Patients must also understand that a negative result on a fine-needle aspirate in the setting of a suspicious lesion warrants a definitive biopsy procedure. A given center must also have the services of an experienced pathologist and cytologist in order to be confident in the diagnostic accuracy of the procedure. Both procedures deliver tissue that may be analyzed for the presence or absence of estrogen and progesterone receptors.

QUESTION 4 The patient underwent needle biopsy. A diagnosis of invasive ductal carcinoma was established. She was now given the option of undergoing a modified radical mastectomy with axillary nodal dissection versus a lumpectomy, axillary nodal dissection, and primary radiation as a breast-conserving procedure. What is her best option? Are there survival advantages?

The choice between a breast-conserving procedure consisting of lumpectomy, auxiliary nodal dissection and primary radiotherapy versus modified radical mastectomy and auxiliary nodal dissection will ultimately rest on the resectability of the tumor, the cosmetic result foreseen, the presence of ductal carcinoma in situ, and the patient's personal preference. No decision should be made until the patient is thoroughly informed of all risks and benefits. Breast cancer may be deemed resectable if all cancerous tissue may be extirpated from the primary site. The involvement of skin, underlying fascia, muscle, or distant site makes the situation inoperable. Primary sites less than 4 cm are usually amenable to lumpectomy. Tumors over 5 cm have not been studied in this setting. It is thought that their size may make for a less than adequate cosmesis. When compared with modified radical mastectomy the National Surgical Adjuvant Breast and Bowel Cancer Project (NSABP) found that lumpectomy with primary radiation paralleled the former in survival advantage. However, lumpectomy was not without its risks.

A significant proportion of local recurrence in the range of 5% to 15% was documented in those patients receiving lumpectomy and primary radiation. Higher recurrence rates in the 30% range were reported for those patients receiving lumpectomy, primary radiation, and whose biopsy specimens demonstrated *ductal carcinoma in situ (DCIS)*. The use of breast-conserving surgery with radiation remains controversial in those patients with DCIS in their biopsy specimens and has been deemed a relative contraindication.

Local relapse in patients undergoing breast-conserving procedures and radiation has not led to a decrease in survival as it has for those undergoing modified radical mastectomy. A salvage simple mastectomy for those with a local recurrence after a breast-conserving approach achieves a survival advantage equal to those who would initially receive a modified radical mastectomy.

QUESTION 5 The patient elected to have a lumpectomy, nodal dissection, and primary radiation therapy. Routine screens for advanced disease were negative including CBC, liver function studies, and CXR. A 2.5-cm mass was removed en bloc from the right breast. Four of twelve lymph nodes sampled were positive for malignancy. The specimens were confirmed pathologically as well-differentiated infiltrating ductal carcinoma exhibiting both estrogen and progesterone receptor positivity. What are the clinical and pathologic prognostic features available for risk stratification? Estimate a relative risk for recurrence given the clinical and pathologic data.

The most significant prognostic factor affecting overall survival and recurrence after resection is the number of involved axillary lymph nodes. Increasing numbers of involved nodes portends a worse outcome and increased likelihood of recurrence. Greater than three lymph nodes has been found to be a particularly poor prognostic factor.

Pathologic subtype may correlate with overall prognosis. Tumor types including mucinous, papillary, tubular, and combination tumors may have the best prognosis, while invasive lobular and medullary are intermediate when compared to invasive ductal carcinoma, which carries the worst prognosis. Some investigators believe that pathologic subtype does not correlate with overall prognosis, stating that differences seen in overall survival may represent earlier detection and thus lead time bias. Most agree that stage per stage the prognosis is equal with all pathologic types. In addition, large tumor bulk, perimenopausal status, absence of estrogen and progesterone receptors, high S-phase percentage, presence of various oncogenes (i.e., ERB-B2), and cell constituents (capthesin) represent poor prognostic variables. A high degree of aneuploidy, lymphatic and vascular invasion may also increase the probability of recurrence.

Lobular carcinoma in situ appears in a younger age population and is found in 0.8% to 8% of all breast biopsies. This entity has been likened to a field defect existing in the patient's mammary tissue, predisposing to bilateral invasive carcinoma. This marker for invasive disease has generated a significant degree of controversy in terms of its management. Therapeutic options have ranged from expectant observation to prophylactic bilateral mastectomy.

A useful, albeit simplistic approach to relative risk assessment uses primary size and absolute numbers of involved lymph nodes as a probability function for recurrence. For each 1 cm of primary size a recurrence rate of 10% is attached. Each lymph node involved represents a 6% relative risk for recurrence. For example, a patient with a primary of 2.5 cm and four involved nodes has a relative risk for recurrence of 49% $(2.5 \times 10\%) + (4 \times 6\%) = 49\%$. This, of course, provides only a rough estimate and does not take into account other pathologic variables nor the use of adjuvant therapy in minimizing recurrence risk.

QUESTION 6 How is breast cancer staged? What is this patient's appropriate stage?

Breast cancer is staged per the TNM classification of the International Union Against Cancer (IUAC) and the American Joint Committee on Cancer (AJCC). This system in based on the size of the primary tumor, the presence of nodal disease, and the existence of metastatic lesions. This formulation is invaluable in directing therapy and formulating a prognosis (see Table 7-2-1).

QUESTION 7 The patient's physician suggested a course of adjuvant chemotherapy. What are the indications for adjuvant therapy? What survival benefit can be bestowed?

Patients whose breast cancer is deemed operable who present with an increased risk for recurrence are candidates for adjuvant therapy. Up to 25% of patients with node negative disease will relapse and succumb to metastatic disease. Therefore it becomes paramount to identify patients with a high risk of recurrence. Those patients with nodal involvement, large primary tumors, and smaller tumors with aggressive characteristics (i.e., poorly differentiated, lymphatic and vascular invasion) often fall in to this cohort. Those patients with primary tumors of less than 1 cm have a recurrence risk of approximately 10% at 10 years. Patients falling into this group are usually not offered adjuvant therapy after assessing risk/benefit ratios. Adjuvant therapy often takes the form of a chemotherapeutic regimen intended to eradicate minimal residual disease. Alternatively, hormonal manipulation using a variety of estrogen blocking agents has also been a mainstay of therapy. The type of adjuvant therapy used will ultimately depend upon the probability of recurrence, the age and hormonal milieu of the patient (i.e., menopausal status), and the patient's personal preference.

Those patients with *node negative disease* with primary tumors greater than 1 cm in diameter may benefit from some form of adjuvant therapy. Multiple studies have demonstrated improved,

disease free, and overall survival in node negative breast cancer patients who undergo adjuvant therapy. Overall results reported by the Early Breast Cancer Trialists Collaborative Group (EBCTCG) suggest both a decrease in recurrence rate and improvement in overall survival. Of the pool of 12,910 patients from 133 randomized trials who received *tamoxifen* a 24+/−4% reduction in recurrence and a 17+/−5% reduction in mortality were established. A total of 2,710 patients were treated with combination chemotherapy showing a 26+/−7% reduction in recurrence and a 18%+/−8% decrease in mortality. Subgroup analysis from this and other studies suggest that postmenopausal patients with negative nodes and positive receptors benefit from a trial of tamoxifen. Receptor negative patients may benefit to a lesser degree. Although the EBCTCG results did not show a statistically significant decrease in mortality when looking at premenopausal node negative patients who received adjuvant therapy, the general trend suggests that this group of patients may benefit from 6 months of chemotherapy. In this instance multiple drug regimens have been found to be superior when compared to single agents. Combinations of tamoxifen and chemotherapy may be efficacious in postmenopausal patients with a more significant recurrence risk.

The use of adjuvant therapy in patients with *node positive disease* is well established. Current consensus would have premenopausal node-positive patients receiving systemic chemotherapy. The most impressive results were found in those patients having between 1 and 3 positive lymph nodes. Bonnadonna and colleagues reported a 12-year relapse-free survival of 28% for a control and 40% for a treatment arm in those patients receiving cytoxan, methotrexate, and 5-FU (CMF). Total survival in both arms was 38% and 50%, respectively. Postmenopausal estrogen receptor positive patients appear to derive most benefit from a 2-year course of tamoxifen. Because a small but definite risk of endometrial carcinoma has been found in patients on tamoxifen, current recommendations suggest tamox-

TABLE 7-2-1   TNM Staging for Breast Cancer

T	Primary tumor
T_X	Primary tumor cannot be assessed
T_0	No evidence of primary tumor
T_{is}	Carcinoma in situ: intraductal carcinoma, lobular carcinoma or Paget's disease with no tumor
T_1	Tumor 2 cm or less in greatest diameter a. 0.5 cm in greatest dimension b. Larger than 0.5 cm but not greater than 1.0 cm c. Larger than 1.0 cm but not greater than 2.0 cm
T_2	Tumor more than 2.0 cm but not greater than 5 cm in greatest dimension
T_3	Tumor more than 5.0 cm in greatest dimension
T_4	Tumor of any size with direct extension to the chest wall or skin. Chest wall includes ribs, intercostal muscles, and serratus anterior muscle but not pectoral muscle a. Extension to chest wall b. Edema (peau d'orange), ulceration of the skin of the breast, satellite skin nodules confined to the same breast c. Both of the above d. Inflammatory carcinoma
N	Regional lymph nodes
N_X	Regional lymph nodes cannot be assessed
N_0	No regional lymph node metastasis
N_1	Metastasis to movable ipsilateral axillary nodes
N_2	Metastasis to ipsilateral axillary lymph nodes fixed to one another or to other structures
N_3	Metastasis to ipsilateral internal mammary lymph nodes
M	Distant metastasis
M_0	No evidence of distant metastasis
M_1	Distant metastasis (including metastasis to ipsilateral supraclavicular lymph nodes)

Clinical staging per the AJCC

Stage		T	N	M
Stage 1		T_1	N_0	M_0
Stage 2				
	A	T_0	N_1	M_0
		T_1	N_1	M_0
		T_2	N_0	M_0
	B	T_2	N_1	M_0
		T_3	N_0	M_0
Stage 3				
	A	T_0	N_2	M_0
		T_1	N_2	M_0
		T_2	N_2	M_0
		T_3	N_1	M_0
		T_3	N_2	M_0
	B	T_4	Any N	M_0
		Any T	N_3	M_0
Stage 4				
		Any T	Any N	M_1

ifen courses limited to 2 years. Others suggest that the cardioprotective and osteoprotective qualities of tamoxifen outweigh the minimal risk of endometrial carcinoma imparted to the patient. The answer to this question will require further detailed analysis.

Some investigators have suggested the use of both chemotherapy and tamoxifen in high-risk postmenopausal patients. Theoretically, the combination of the cytostatic effects of tamoxifen and the use of chemotherapy may be antagonistic. Cytotoxic chemotherapy works best in cell populations that are rapidly dividing. Tamoxifen may limit this ability. Several studies using standard CMF regimens have suggested this relationship to be true. However, the use of doxirubicin or cytoxan together with tamoxifen may not be antagonistic. If both chemo and hormonal modalities are to be used, it is suggested that tamoxifen be started after chemotherapy is complete. Results from several trials have generated conflicting data on this question.

The proven efficacy of doxorubicin in metastatic breast cancer provided the rationale for its use in adjuvant therapy trials. A number of studies have demonstrated an increased disease-free survival when patients with greater than three positive lymph nodes received this drug incorporated into conventional CMF regimens. More importantly, this drug when delivered in a sequential fashion with CMF proved superior to an alternating strategy of CMF and adriamycin. This finding helped to modify the Goldie-Goldman model that espouses the superiority of regimens containing multiple non–cross-resistant drugs given in an alternating fashion. This hypothesis was based on the expansion of an absolute number of mutated clones in a tumor population providing resistance to a chemotherapeutic agent before the initiation of treatment. Although, the tenets of the Goldie-Goldman hypothesis were maintained, sequential delivery of chemotherapeutic regimen as suggested by Day have proven superior to alternating combinations when dose intensity is controlled.

Patients with 10 or more positive lymph nodes display exceedingly high rates of recurrence. Dose intensification has been used in an attempt to reduce this rate. Support has been lent to the concept that dose intensity correlates with improved response. Budman et al. described a disease-free and overall survival advantage for patients enrolled on a high dose arm of a 5FU, doxorubicin, and cyclophosphamide regimen. Peters et al. have investigated the use of high dose chemotherapy with autologous bone marrow support in the setting of 10 or more positive lymph nodes. This group achieved an increase in event-free survival when compared with historical controls. Randomized trials will be required to confirm trends in improved survival.

QUESTION 8 What surveillance procedures are appropriate for this patient?

Adequate follow-up remains essential in helping to assess for persistent or recurrent disease. Formal guidelines serve only as minimal recommendations. Patients who have undergone primary therapy should receive screening mammography on a regular basis. Many centers have suggested a yearly mammogram for patients with a low risk for recurrence. A mammogram should be obtained every 6 months for high-risk patients and those whose cancer was discovered on mammography initially. Other frequently used surveillance tools include the use of CXR and bone scan every 6 months for the first 3 years and subsequently at 1-year intervals. The use of tumor markers CEA and CA-15-3 has been advocated by some as a means to detect recurrent disease. Progressively rising values may signal persistent micrometastatic disease. However, persistently elevated and stable values after primary therapy often do not signal recurrent disease, and thus these values should be interpreted with caution.

CASE FOLLOW-UP The patient received sequential chemotherapy with adriamycin and CMF. She tolerated this regimen well, suffering only alopecia and mild nausea. MUGA studies performed initially and at completion of her therapy to assess for adriamycin-based cardiotoxicity remained

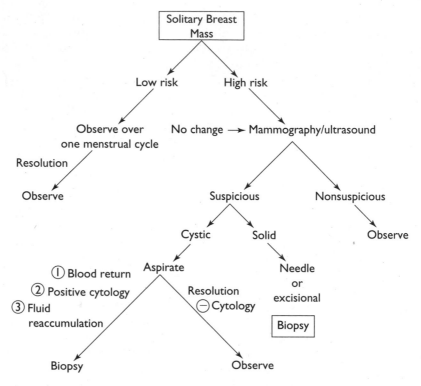

7-2-1 Diagnostic algorithm for a solitary breast mass.

within normal limits. She is currently free of disease 1 year from her initial diagnosis.

• •

BIBLIOGRAPHY

Bell D, Hajdu S, Urban J: The role of aspiration cytology in the diagnosis and management of mammary lesions in office practice, *Cancer* 51:1182-1189, 1983.

Bonadonna G, Valagussa P, Zambetti M: Sequential adriamycin-CMF in the adjuvant treatment of breast cancer with more than three positive axillary nodes, *Proc Am Soc Clin Oncol* 11:61, 1992.

Buzdar AU, Kau SW, Hortobagyi GN, et al: Clinical course of patients with ten or more positive nodes who were treated with doxorubicin-containing adjuvant therapy, *Cancer* 69 (2):448-452, 1992.

Carter Cl, Allen C, Henson DE: Relation of tumor size, lymph node status, and survival in 24,740 breast cancer cases, *Cancer* 63:181-187, 1989.

Chu K, Smart C, Tarone R: Analysis of breast cancer mortality and stage distribution by age for the Health Insurance Plan clinical trial JNCI 80:1125-1132, 1988.

Consensus Development Panel: Consensus statement: treatment of early stage breast cancer. In Early Stage Breast Cancer, pp 1-5. National Cancer Institute monograph number 11, Washington DC, 1992, U.S. Government Printing Office.

Early Breast Cancer Trialists Collaborative Group: Systemic treatment of early breast cancer, hormonal, cytotoxic, or immune therapy, *Lancet* 339:1-15, 71-85, 1992.

Fisher B, Bauer M, Margolese R, et al: Five year results of a randomized clinical trial comparing total mastectomy and segmental mastectomy with or without radiation, *N Engl J Med* 312:665-673, 1985.

Fisher B, Costatino J, Redmond C, et al: A randomized clinical trial evaluating tamoxifen in the treatment of patients with node negative breast cancer who have estrogen receptor positive tumors, *N Engl J Med* 320:479-484, 1989.

Fisher B, Slack N, Katrych D, Wolmar N: Ten year follow-up results in patients with carcinoma of the breast in a cooperative clinical trial evaluating surgical adjuvant chemotherapy, *Surg Gynecol Obstet* 140:528-534, 1975.

Harris JR, Morrow M, Bonnadonna G: Cancer of the breast. In De Vita VT, Hellman S, eds: *Cancer principles and practice of oncology,* Philadelphia, 1993, JB Lippincott.

Hughes P, Buzdar A: Early stage breast cancer and adjuvant therapy. In Paidur R, ed: *Medical oncology: a comprehensive review,* Huntington, NY, 1993, PPR.

Peters WP, Ross M, Vredenburgh J, et al: High dose alkylating agents and autologous bone marrow support for stage II/III breast cancer involving ten or more axillary lymph nodes, *Proc Am Soc Clin Oncol* 11:58, 1992.

Rosner D, Lane WW: Node negative minimal invasive breast cancer patients are not candidates for routine systemic adjuvant therapy, *Cancer* 66:199-205, 1990.

Schmitt SJ, Silen W, Sadowsky NL, et al: Ductal carcinoma in situ of the breast, *N Engl J Med* 318:898-903, 1988.

Trandon AD, Clark GM, Chamness GC: HER-2/Neu oncogene protein and prognosis in breast cancer, *J Clin Oncol* 7:1120-1128, 1989.

World Health Organization: Histologic typing of breast tumors, *Tumor* 68:181, 1982.

CASE

3

Stephen C. Schwartz
Gary Schwartz

A 57-year-old man with a long-standing history of chronic obstructive pulmonary disease came to his primary physician with complaints of incessant cough and profound weakness over a 5-week course. This patient was known to have a chronic cough but described his current cough as significantly changed in both the intensity and character. The patient stated that he had been fatigued as of late and was often unable to lift himself from a chair. He denied recent fever or chills and stated that he was producing scant amounts of green mucous, which he described as his usual amount. He denied any dyspnea or wheezing.

QUESTION 1 What elements of a cough should be focused on in the medical history? How will this help formulate a differential diagnosis?

The cough reflex functions as a mechanism of defense, clearing particulate matter and secretions from the airways. Afferent mucosal receptors that initiate the cough reflex extend from the nasopharynx to the level of the terminal bronchiole. These afferent networks may respond to multiple stimuli including mechanical, chemical, and inflammatory. The efferent loop of this reflex pathway serves to initiate the three phases of cough: (1) deep inspiration, (2) closure of the glottis with an increase in pleural pressure, and (3) forceful contraction of the diaphragm and other respiratory muscles leading to an explosive release of pressure.

A cough may be characterized by its acuity or chronicity, although a significant degree of overlap exists. Other defining features that may illuminate the underlying etiology of the cough include the presence of sputum production, pain or blood, time of occurrence, and any positional character.

The most common causes of acute cough include acute bronchitis, tracheitis, pneumonia, environmental irritants, and bronchospasm. Postnasal drip from a draining sinus is an exceedingly common cause of a new or chronic cough in the general population. A worsening cough superimposed on a chronic cough in a patient with chronic obstructive pulmonary disease (COPD) must also alert the physician to the possibility of acute bronchitis. The clinical picture with this entity is based on the presence of an antecedent upper respiratory tract infection with attendant purulent sputum, fever, myalgias, and malaise. Patients with COPD less commonly develop pneumothoraces. Cough as a presenting symptom for pneumothorax is much less common than is acute dyspnea.

The most common causes of a chronic cough include chronic bronchitis, cigarettes, environmental exposures, postnasal drip, heart failure, aspiration, bronchiectasis, and reactive airway disease.

A new or changing cough in a patient with an extensive tobacco history is an ominous finding. A physician must remain vigilant for the possibility of a malignant neoplasm. Other presentations commonly associated with a new pulmonary neoplasm include hemoptysis, wheezing, chest pain, stridor, hoarse voice from recurrent laryngeal nerve paralysis, phrenic nerve paralysis, esophageal compression with dysphagia, Horner's syndrome, and shoulder and arm pain in an ulnar distribution from a superior sulcus tumor. Other causes of chronic cough include chronic granulomatous disease, namely tuberculosis and fungal pathogens. A new lung abscess in a COPD patient with a concomitant alcohol history may superimpose an acute cough on a chronic one. Fever, recurrent pneumonias, and foul-smelling sputum are usually associated findings. Rarely, bronchial adenomas may present with cough; however, wheezing, recurrent pneumonias, and hemoptysis are the most common presenting symptoms.

A thorough physical examination and PA and lateral chest x-ray (CXR) are mandatory for proper initial evaluation. Other pertinent studies useful in arriving at a diagnosis include CBC, U/A, SMA-6, screening chemistry profile, sputum examination, ECG, PPD, and anergy panel. If these studies are not illuminating in the setting of a negative CXR, fiberoptic bronchoscopy can be safely employed. The goal here is to biopsy suspicious lesions and obtain cytology, brushings, and pertinent stains. Protected cultures should also be routinely obtained.

QUESTION 2 Physical examination revealed a normal head and neck examination with no pharyngeal pathology. Pulmonary examination was remarkable for bilateral wheezes and soft rhonchi. No adenopathy was present. The cardiac and GI examination were within normal limits. Neuromuscular examination was remarkable for proximal muscle weakness with diminished reflexes. Clubbing was not present. The CXR revealed a 3.0-cm irregular, solitary, noncalcified density in the right upper lobe. The right hemidiaphragm appeared elevated as did the minor fissure. Hyperinflation of the lungs was evident, consistent with COPD. What is to be considered in the differential diagnosis?

The appearance of a solitary pulmonary nodule is a common finding on CXR. These lesions are described as circumscribed lesions less than 6 cm in diameter. Approximately 35% of these lesions will be malignant. A multitude of processes may produce this roentgenographic appearance. Included in this list are neoplastic (benign and malignant), infectious, inflammatory, and vascu-

lar entities. The most common diagnoses for a solitary pulmonary nodule include healed granulomata, primary pulmonary malignancies, metastatic cancer, AV malformations, and hamartomatous lesions. Given the patient profile, the previously described findings are most suspicious for a newly diagnosed neoplasm in the right lung field. An obstructed bronchus is likely, given the indicators of right-sided volume loss. Malignancies to be considered include non-small cell and small cell lung cancer, a metastatic focus from a malignancy outside the lung, lymphomas, and rarely sarcomas arising from lung parenchyma. Benign lesions include both adenomas and pulmonary hamartomas. Approximately 80% of all pulmonary adenomas are carcinoids, which, although usually indolent, possess metastatic potential. Hamartomas are lesions appearing in the age 60 cohort. These lesions are composed of multiple elements including smooth muscle and connective tissue. They are clinically benign in most cases. Healed granulomata may give rise to a solitary pulmonary nodule. In endemic areas histoplasmosis and coccidiomycosis frequently give rise to this picture. Tuberculosis should also be considered in the appropriate clinical setting. Many malignancies metastasize to the lung. Breast, lung, colon, renal cell, bladder, germ cell tumors, and sarcomas are common offenders in this regard. Vasculitides may on rare occasion give rise to a solitary pulmonary nodules; however, multiple pulmonary nodules are more common (see Fig. 7-3-1 on p. 380).

QUESTION 3 What are the indications for biopsy? How should this be performed?

As a majority of solitary pulmonary nodules are benign, the resection of documented lesions may expose patients to unnecessary operative procedures with their concomitant morbidity. It is the charge of the physician to define those lesions that are unlikely to be malignant. Evaluation of the chest x-ray with regard to rate of change, size, and shape, and presence of calcification of the lesion is used in concert with the patient profile to help affirm the nature of the lesion. Whenever possible, old CXRs should be obtained for comparison. In general terms, lesions possessing doubling times of less than 500 days are suspicious for malignancy. Doubling times longer than 18 months are assumed to be benign. Calcifications are often telltale signs that a particular lesion is benign. Patterns of calcification denoting benign lesions include (1) a large central nidus, usually representing a granuloma, (2) small flecks of calcium in the center or periphery of a lesion, also suggesting granuloma, (3) concentric calcifications, and (4) popcorn calcifications commonly seen in hamartomas. Size and shape offer additional clues to the nature of the lesion, although their use is limited. Malignant lesions often have less well-defined boarders and may be lobulated or notched. Patients less than 30 years of age rarely have malignant, solitary, pulmonary nodules and can often be observed with serial CXR every 6 months. Patients over 50 have a higher incidence of malignancy, especially if they use tobacco. It is imperative that new lesions provoking some degree of suspicion be fully worked up in this group.

In light of the patient's age, the appearance of the lesion on CXR, and his smoking history, a significant amount of suspicion exists pointing toward the malignant nature of this lesion. Essential now is to obtain a pathologic diagnosis. This can best be achieved by any of several methods: (1) bronchoscopy and transbronchial biopsy, (2) CT-guided transthoracic needle biopsy, and (3) thoracotomy. The nature of the lesion and the clinical context will dictate the procedure selected. The proximal location of this lesion may make it accessible to transbronchial biopsy during bronchoscopy. Peripheral lesions may be more amenable to transthoracic needle biopsy. Inadequate sampling of tissue may require a mini-thoracotomy to establish the diagnosis. The sending of sputum for cytology can also help establish the diagnosis but remains much less sensitive than bronchoscopic biopsy. Referral to an experienced pulmonologist, interventional radiologist, or thoracic surgeon should be made depending on the procedure selected.

QUESTION 4 The patient ultimately underwent bronchoscopy. Exploration of the superior lingular bronchopulmonary segment revealed a mass lesion compromising that bronchus. Direct biopsy was obtained. Pathology confirmed a squamous cell carcinoma. The patient tolerated the procedure without complication. Discuss the various pathologic subtypes of lung cancer. Are there survival advantages when particular subtypes are compared stage per stage?

It is customary to distinguish nonsmall cell lung carcinoma (NSCLC) from the small cell (SCLC) variant. This distinction is clinically relevant as each possess vastly different biologies and require differing modalities of treatment. Pathologic subtypes including squamous cell, adenocarcinoma, and large cell carcinoma are classified as NSCLC. This group and its pathologic variants compromise approximately 80% of all lung primaries. Small cell (oat cell) lung cancer accounts for a majority of the remainder of lung primaries. *Adenocarcinoma* is the most frequently diagnosed lung primary in North America, accounting for 40% of all lung primaries. Improved histologic techniques may be responsible for the increased incidence of this entity. It is felt that many adenocarcinomas have been classified as poorly differentiated large cell cancers in the past. Adenocarcinomas often present as peripheral lesions. They have been found to arise from epithelial or glandular constituents and may also derive from scar. It is likely that adenocarcinomas have a worse prognosis when compared with other NSCLC primaries. *Bronchoalveolar* carcinoma is thought to represent a subtype of adenocarcinoma. This cancer may present as a pneumonic infiltrative pattern spreading intraparenchymally in addition to solitary nodules and multifocal disease.

Squamous cell carcinomas usually arise in proximal bronchi. They grow rather slowly and are often predated by in situ changes and metaplasia. This tumor's cells exfoliate, allowing for cytologic diagnosis to be made early in some cases. A period of 3 to 4 years is necessary for in situ lesions to progress to clinically detectable cancer. This histologic subtype represents approximately 30% of all lung primaries. *Large cell* lung cancers represent approximately 15% of all lung primaries. This number has decreased as immunohistochemical techniques have been refined. Previously described large cell cancers are now being placed into the adenocarcinoma and squamous categories.

Small cell lung cancers represent approximately 20% of all lung cancers. Pathologically, they are derived from neuroendocrine lineage. Their behavior is aggressive in nature with early metastasis being the rule. Small cell lesions are usually centrally located. Mediastinal involvement is common with many patients presenting with recurrent laryngeal and phrenic nerve entrapment. Superior vena cava syndrome is also a frequent presentation. These malignancies are exquisitely sensitive to chemotherapy and radiotherapy; however, they have an exceedingly high rate of recurrence and resistance to rechallenge with chemotherapy. Generally their prognosis is the poorest of all lung cancers. Because of their biology, SCLC is staged and treated in a different manner than NSCLC.

QUESTION 5 What are the staging procedures for NSCLC?

At this juncture an extent of disease and staging workup should be pursued. Determination of *resectability* becomes paramount. Staging should include CT imaging of the chest and upper abdomen to the level of the adrenals, CBC, SMA-18, and coagulation parameters. Bone scan or head CT should be undertaken if the appropriate clinical findings should suggest their utility. These tests, when performed in the correct clinical setting, should rule out all possible sites of metastatic disease including hilar and mediastinal lymph nodes, pleura, contralateral lung, liver, adrenals, bone, and CNS. If metastatic disease is not apparent, mediastinoscopy should be undertaken to rule out bilateral mediastinal nodal involvement, a finding that makes the patient unresectable. Other clinical settings that preclude resection include recurrent laryngeal or phrenic nerve paraly-

sis, scalene node involvement, SVC syndrome, primary involvement less than 2 cm from the carina, and contralateral lung involvement (M_1).

The assessment of *operability* must also be pursued. Complete pulmonary function studies are requisite in patients who may be compromised by pulmonary disease such as COPD. While no established criteria exist, a FEV_1 of less than 1 liter or a resting pCO_2 greater than 50 suggests a poor surgical candidate. The use of quantitative ventilation/perfusion scanning can help predict the postoperative functional capacity. A postoperative FEV_1 greater than 800 ml suggests adequate reserve allowing for resection.

QUESTION 6 This patient's staging workup demonstrated a 3.5-cm lesion greater than 2 cm from the carina. Right mediastinal adenopathy was present measuring 2 cm in greatest diameter. The left mediastinum and hilum were without evidence of disease. Both liver and adrenals were uninvolved by CT examination. PFTs revealed an obstructive pattern; however, forced expiratory volume in one second (FEV_1) was 2, and forced vital capacity (FVC) and maximal minute ventilation (MMV) were greater than 50% of predicted, suggesting that this patient is a viable operative candidate. Quantitative ventilation/perfusion scanning was performed giving a predicted postoperative FEV_1 greater than 1, suggesting this patient could tolerate pneumonectomy if required. All other staging parameters were unremarkable. How is lung cancer staged? What is this patient's pathologic stage?

Staging in lung cancer is per the American Joint Committee on Cancer (AJCC) and uses the standard TNM classification. This classification is based on the size of the primary tumor, the presence of nodal involvement, and the detection of metastatic disease (Table 7-3-1).

His workup now complete, this patient would be staged clinically as $T_2 N_2 M_O$ or stage IIIA according to the TNM classification and AJCC criterion. Increasing T, N, or M designation as well as increasing overall stage correlate with a poorer prognosis. Five-year survival rates for stages I and II are 55% and 35%, respectively. Survival for

TABLE 7-3-1   TNM Staging for Lung Cancer

Primary tumor

T_X	Primary tumor cannot be assessed or tumor proven by the presence of malignant cells in the sputum or bronchial washings not visualized by imaging or bronchoscopy
T_0	No evidence of primary tumor
T_1	Tumor 3 cm or less in greatest dimension, surrounded by lung or visceral pleura, without bronchoscopic evidence of invasion more proximal than the lobar bronchus
T_2	Any of the following: more than 3 cm in greatest dimension, involves main bronchus, 2 cm or more distal to the carina, invades the visceral pleura, associated with atelectasis or obstructive bronchitis that extends to the hilar region but does not involve the entire lung
T_3	Tumor of any size that invades the following: chest wall (including the superior sulcus), diaphragm, mediastinal pleura, parietal pericardium, tumor in the main bronchus less than 2 cm distal to the carina but without involvement of the carina, associated atelectasis, or obstructive pneumonitis of the entire lung
T_4	Tumor of any size that invades the following: mediastinum, heart, great vessels, trachea, esophagus, vertebral body, carina, or malignant pleural effusion

Regional lymph nodes

N_X	Regional lymph nodes cannot be assessed
N_0	No regional lymph node metastasis
N_1	Metastasis in the ipsilateral peribronchial and/or ipsilateral hilar nodes including direct extension
N_2	Metastasis in ipsilateral mediastinal and/or subcarinal nodes
N_3	Metastasis in the contralateral mediastinal, contralateral hilar, ipsilateral or contralateral scalene or supraclavicular lymph nodes

Distant metastasis

M_X	Presence of distant metastasis cannot be assessed
M_0	No distant metastasis
M_1	Distant metastasis

Stage groupings are as follows:

Stage 0	Tis	N_0	M_0
Stage I	T_1	N_0	M_0
	T_2	N_0	M_0
Stage II	T_1	N_1	M_0
	T_2	N_1	M_0
Stage IIIA	T_1	N_2	M_0
	T_2	N_2	M_0
	T_3	N_0, N_1, N_2	M_0
Stage IIIB	Any T	N_3	M_0
	T_4	Any N	M_0
Stage IV	Any T	Any N	M_1

stage III is 15% and less than 2% for metastatic disease.

QUESTION 7 The patient met with his surgeon and medical oncologist who offered the patient surgical intervention and postoperative adjuvant radiotherapy. He sought a second opinion at a major cancer center. There he was offered a protocol that would treat him with neoadjuvant (preoperative) chemotherapy to be followed by surgery and subsequent radiation therapy. He elected the investigational approach. He received 8 weeks of chemotherapy after mediastinoscopy revealed no evidence of left-sided mediastinal nodal disease. He tolerated it well while achieving a partial response. He was subsequently scheduled for surgery. Right middle and upper lobectomies were performed at the time of surgery. He tolerated the procedure well and after recuperation began a course of radiotherapy 4 weeks later. His performance status was excellent; however, his weakness persisted. What are the standard approaches to therapy for the various stages of NSCLC?

Patients with stages I and II of lung cancer are cured by surgical means. Often, clinical staging understages these patients. Only 65% of patients described clinically as stage I truly are at thoracotomy. Recurrences of stage I and II NSCLC are usually distant metastasis or new primaries. Few studies thus far have demonstrated any impact of adjuvant radiation or chemotherapy on recurrence rates or survival for stage I and II disease. Those patients deemed resectable who are medically inoperable (i.e., severe COPD) may occasionally achieve cure with radiation therapy. Twenty percent 5-year survivals have been reported in stage II NSCLC receiving radiation.

Intensive investigation into optimal therapeutic modalities for stage III disease is currently underway. The use of multimodality therapy in the neoadjuvant and adjuvant setting have been pursued. Cis-platinum-based adjuvant regimens with and without radiation have been explored by the Lung Cancer Study Group. Their findings suggest a benefit in disease-free survival in two studies with modest impact on overall survival in only one. The use of neoadjuvant or preoperative chemotherapy has shown promise. Disease-free survival has been shown to increase to 30% at 5 years, an increase from the 10% seen in historical controls. Preoperative radiotherapy appears to be of benefit only in patients with superior sulcus tumors. Concurrent and sequential chemoradiotherapy is another combination modality being actively pursued. Stage IIIb NSCLC by virtue of its unresectability is an optimal candidate for investigational studies. As in stage IV disease, cis-platinum-based regimens have activity; however, survival is only marginally improved. Radiotherapy in the patient with stage IIIb disease has seen some success in locally advanced disease with trends toward improved survival being demonstrated in work accomplished by the Radiation Oncology Study Group. At Memorial Sloan-Kettering Cancer Center (MSKCC) stage IV disease with adrenal metastasis and operable thoracic disease now are resected on an investigational basis with subsequent adjuvant chemotherapy. Preliminary results are encouraging.

QUESTION 8 What is the etiology for this patient's proximal muscle weakness?

Paraneoplastic syndromes are common findings in patients with lung cancer. Several syndromes have been described including ACTH secreting tumors, syndrome of inappropriate antidiuretic hormone, cerebellar and cortical degeneration, nephrotic and nephritic syndromes, and hypercalcemia. Proximal muscle weakness is a classic finding in patients with small cell carcinomas. This entity is referred to as the Eaton-Lambert (ELS) or myasthenic syndrome. These patients have proximal muscle weakness and overall fatigue. Muscles of the pelvic girdle and lower extremities are most affected. Dry mouth, muscle ache, and parasthesias are also encountered. Unlike cases of true myasthenia gravis, patients with ELS actually improve their muscle

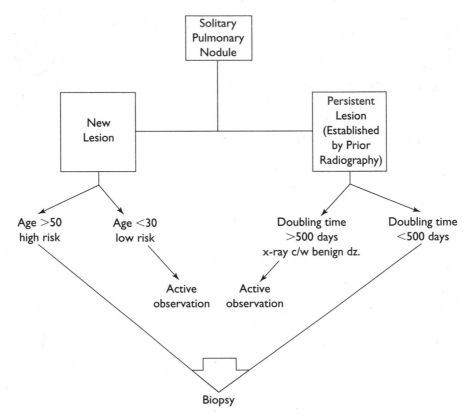

7-3-1 Diagnostic algorithm for a solitary pulmonary nodule.

strength with repeated exercise. ELS has been characterized as an autoimmune disorder. The use of plasmapheresis and guanidine HCL has been advocated in its management. Treatment of the underlying disease has also been shown to be effective in ameliorating the condition. In NSCLC, as well as a multitude of other tumor types, syndromes of polymyositis, dermatomyositis, and mixed sensor-motor neuropathies can lead to muscle weakness less disabling than Eaton-Lambert.

It is thought that between 7% and 34% of all cancer patients have one of these entities. Polymyositis is characterized by progressive weakness of the proximal musculature with diminished reflexes. Creatine phosphokinase, aldolase, and ESR are usually elevated with a concomitantly abnormal EMG. Steroids may have a role in the treatment of this syndrome, although no well-controlled studies have been accomplished.

It is highly likely that this patient had some component of polymyositis. Indeed, elevated CPK levels were found on laboratory investigation. Steroids were administered in small doses with a modest degree of improvement.

QUESTION 9 How should surveillance be performed in this patient?

Those patients with low risks for recurrence treated successfully for lung cancer may be seen at 3- to 4-month intervals for the first year and 4 to 6 months thereafter. Comprehensive physical examination with attention to pertinent nodal areas is mandatory. Routine CBC, screening profile, and PA and lateral CXRs should always be obtained.

Patients with a higher risk of recurrence should probably be seen on a monthly basis for the first year. It is uncertain whether CT examination of the chest bestows a survival benefit in this subset of patients. The physician must be vigilant not only for recurrence but for second primaries from the lung and aerodigestive tract in patients who are high risk.

CASE FOLLOW-UP This patient was free of disease at 1 year from his diagnosis, functioning with a performance status of 100%. He returned to work and is scheduled for a follow-up CXR in 3 months.

• •

BIBLIOGRAPHY

Coquhoun SD, Rosenthal DL, Morton DL: Role of percutaneous fine needle aspiration biopsy in suspected intrathoracic malignancy, *Ann Thorac Surg* 51:390-393, 1991.

Dillman RO, Seagren SL, Prppert KG, et al: A randomized trial of induction chemotherapy plus high dose radiation versus radiation alone in stage three non-small cell lung cancer, *N Engl J Med* 323:940-945, 1990.

Ginsberg RJ, Kris MJ, Armstrong JG: Cancer of the lung. In Devita VT, Hellman S, Rosenberg S, eds: *Cancer: principles and practice of oncology*, Philadelphia, 1993, JB Lippincott.

Green N, Kurohara SS, George FW, et al: Post resection radiation for primary lung cancer, *Radiology* 116:405-407, 1975.

Huber MH, Lippman SM: Non-small cell lung cancer. In *Medical oncology: A comprehensive review*, Huntington, NY, 1993, PRR.

Johnson DH: Chemotherapy for unresectable non-small cell lung cancer, *Semin Oncol* 17(supp 7): 20-29, 1990.

Lad T, Rubenstien L, Sadagh A, et al: The benefit of adjuvant treatment for resected locally advanced non-small cell lung cancer, *J Clin Oncol* 6:9-17, 1988.

Strauss GM, Langer MP, Elias AD, et al: Multimodality treatment of stage IIIa non-small cell lung carcinoma: a critical review of the literature and strategies for future research, *J Clin Oncol* 10:829-838, 1992.

Wang-Peng J, Knutsen T, Gazdar A, et al: Non-random structural and numerical chromosome changes in non-small cell lung cancer, *Genes Chrom Cancer* 3:168-188, 1991.

CASE

4

Stephen C. Schwartz
Gary Schwartz

. . . .

A 59-year-old man with a history of ulcerative colitis came to his private medical doctor with complaints of abdominal cramps over a 1-month course and, most recently, bright red blood in his stool. Upon questioning he reports no weight loss, hematemesis, change in stool caliber, fever, or other constitutional symptomatology. There are no complaints of dyspnea or chest pain. He describes his abdominal discomfort as crampy, nonfocal, and intermittent, bearing no relationship to the consumption of food. His last colonoscopy was conducted 3 years ago and was reported to be consistent with mild inflammatory bowel disease. He is presently taking no medications.

QUESTION I Generate an approach to lower gastrointestinal (GI) bleeding. What are the leading diagnoses to consider?

An accurate history and thorough physical examination may help to establish the site of GI bleeding. Hematochezia or the passage of bright red blood per rectum most often denotes a source of bleeding in a distal GI segment. Hematochezia is also reported with massive upper-GI sources. Under these circumstances blood acting as a mucosal irritant decreases bowel transit time. Melena or black tarry stool represents a source proximal to the mid-transverse colon.

Stool may appear red after the ingestion of beets or phenolphthalein. Black stools are also seen with ingestion of iron, charcoal, or bismuth-containing compounds. Emesis of bright red blood (hematemesis) or of coffee grounds localizes the source to the upper GI tract. A history of recent steroid or NSAID usage is important in the context

of upper GI bleed or hematochezia with rapid transit. The presence of fever and or diarrhea suggests an infectious source as an etiology for bloody stool. Resuscitative measures should begin immediately and include the placement of two large bore intravenous catheters and the administration of volume expanders (normal saline) and/or whole blood.

Full physical examination including a digital rectal examination and anoscopy should be undertaken. Initial laboratory studies should include a CBC, coagulation parameters, liver function tests, electrolytes, BUN, and creatinine. Stool culture for bacterial and parasitic pathogens should be obtained in the appropriate setting. Should an upper source be suspected, placement of a nasogastric tube is standard. Because hematochezia may appear in upper GI bleeding, all patients with GI bleeding in the acute situation should be considered for NG-tube. Return of fresh blood or a large volume of old blood should prompt gastric lavage. This technique will allow for better visualization with endoscopic techniques and may limit blood loss by causing contraction of the gastric musculature. If a lower source is suspected, a sigmoidoscopy may be performed initially. A colonoscopy may be held in reserve if a lesion is not detected by sigmoidoscopy. This procedure will require adequate preparation for feasibility, which will in turn increase its sensitivity. If a bleeding site is not identified by the above means, angiography or radionuclide scanning may be undertaken. The former will identify sites of bleeding with rates of 0.5 ml per minute or greater, while the latter is more sensitive, detecting bleeding at rates as low as 0.1 ml per minute. The use of selective angiography in GI bleeding allows for the infusion of vasopressin. This approach may be effective in controlling bleeding from an arterial site.

Entities to consider as a potential source of bleeding given this patient profile should include the following: (1) recrudescence of inflammatory bowel disease, (2) diverticular disease, (3) angiodysplasia, (4) hemorrhoids, and (5) colorectal carcinoma or adenomatous disease. A less likely cause is ischemic bowel disease.

Physical examination proved unrevealing in this patient except for a positive stool guaiac test. No masses were palpated in the rectum, and anoscopy demonstrated no internal hemorrhoids. Laboratory studies were significant for a HgB of 9 and a HCT of 29. The MCV was 78. After adequate preparation, a full colonoscopy was performed, revealing an erosive napkin-ring lesion at 30 cm from the anal verge. (See Fig. 7-4-1 on p. 387.)

QUESTION 2 How does this finding narrow the differential diagnosis?

At this juncture given this patient profile exclamated by the evident history of inflammatory bowel disease, colorectal carcinoma becomes the leading diagnosis to be ruled out. Other pathology, benign and malignant, must also be considered. Upon visual inspection diffuse large cell lymphomas arising from the large bowel can be mistaken for a typical adenocarcinoma. A nodular, thickened, and ulcerating bowel wall is a common finding in this lymphoma variant. Sarcomas may also arise from the wall of the large bowel. Carcinoid tumors have been reported in the rectum. Those lesions less than 2 cm rarely metastasize, and those that do, do not produce a classic carcinoid syndrome. Benign processes such as a diverticular inflammatory mass or inflammatory strictures related to the patient's ulcerative colitis must be ruled out. Entities such as adenomatous disease also may produce GI bleeding and indeed abdominal cramping.

Adenomas may be classified as (1) tubular, (2) villous, or (3) tubulovillous. Grossly, these tumors may be described as sessile with a broad base or pedunculated, with a fibrous thin pedicle containing blood and lymphatics.

The potential for tubular or tubulovillous polyps to undergo malignant transformation is as high as 30%. An increased risk exists for those polyps greater than 2 cm in greatest diameter. Data derived from the National Polyp Study suggest that removal of polyps greater than 0.3 cm has decreased the overall incidence of colon cancer.

A number of premalignant *familial polyposis* syndromes have been described and are now associated with a high incidence of colorectal carcinoma. These include familial adenomatosis polyposis coli (FAP), Gardner's and Turcot's syndromes. Recently, a gene has been identified that is thought to predispose to the development of colorectal cancer. The discovery of the APC gene, a tumor suppressor gene on the long arm of chromosome 5, may someday allow for early detection of this disease. Proctocolectomy and subtotal colectomy have been advocated in both FAP and Gardner's syndrome. With juvenile and hyperplastic polyps malignant transformation rarely occurs. Lipomas actually represent the second most common benign colonic neoplasm after adenomas. Leiomyomas are also described in the colon but with much less frequency than in the stomach or small intestine.

QUESTION 3 Subsequent pathology from biopsy and brushings revealed adenocarcinoma—poorly differentiated of probable colonic origin. Define the risk factors for colorectal carcinoma. What does the initial diagnostic workup for colorectal cancer entail?

Multiple risk factors have been found to be associated with colorectal cancer. These include genetic, dietary, lifestyle, and inflammatory bowel disease. As already mentioned several inherited familial polyposis syndromes increase risk to colorectal cancer including FAP and Turcot's syndromes. Other genetic predispositions exist that do not demonstrate polyposis. The hereditary non-polyposis colorectal cancers (HNPCC) types

1 and 2 (formerly Lynch syndromes 1 and 2) are also associated with genetic abnormalities. HNPCC type II is also associated with other malignancies including breast, ovarian, endometrial, and gastric cancers. The gene for HNPCC, also known as hMSH2, is the human analogue of the prokaryotic gene mutS, which assists in the repair of DNA mismatches.

Diets found to be high in fats and cholesterol have been associated with cancers of the colon and rectum. The role of increased fats in carcinogenesis is incompletely understood; however, it is thought that fat induces an increase in endogenous bile acid production, which may potentiate the process. Yellow and green vegetables are thought to serve a protective role in decreasing the incidence of colorectal cancer. Sedentary lifestyle and nulliparity have also been associated with increased rates of colorectal cancer.

At this juncture the patient should have an initial diagnostic workup including imaging of the abdomen and pelvis with computerized tomography, CXR, CBC, urinalysis, liver function studies, and carcinoembryonic antigen. Most recently, Satumomab Pendetide, a monoclonal antibody labeled with In111, has been approved for determining the presence of extrahepatic metastases in colorectal carcinoma. In a study by Collier et al. this method appeared more sensitive than CT scanning in detecting pelvic and extrahepatic disease. While its role in the routine diagnostic workup remains controversial, Satumomab may have utility in patients being considered for resection of solitary liver metastasis.

Most importantly consultation must be sought with a colorectal surgical oncologist for extirpation of the tumor. Pathological staging is critical because this remains the most important factor determining prognosis. Proper staging is also requisite for the correct choice of therapy. It must be pointed out that preoperative detection of metastatic disease does not obviate the need for surgical intervention because obstruction can often complicate a patient's course, making surgical removal of the primary often necessary as a palliative measure. Also new operative techniques are making it possible to resect liver metastases with a small but definable number of cures.

QUESTION 4 Preoperative CAT scan demonstrated only a solitary mass lesion in the left colon. Both CXR and LFTs were normal. A preoperative CEA was 120. The patient underwent a left-hemicolectomy with an end-to-end anastomosis. The pathologic specimen revealed tumor invading the pericolic fat. Two of five pericolic nodes were found to contain tumors. No other identifiable disease was present. Describe the staging schemes currently in use. Is overall pathologic stage correlated with survival?

Staging in colorectal carcinoma has traditionally followed the Astler-Coller-Dukes system, which relates depth of tumor invasion through bowel wall, number of involved nodes, and presence of distant metastasis to overall pathologic stage. Most recently the TNM staging classification as adopted by the AJCC/IUAC has been modified to correlate with the A-C-D classification. This patient's pathologic staging represents a $T_3N_1M_0$ or a Dukes C2 (Table 7-4-1).

In general terms pathologic stage is directly correlated with overall survival. Stages 1 and 2 have 5-year-survival rates of 90% and 80%, respectively. Five-year survival for stage 3 disease falls into the 40% range whereas metastatic disease has a 5% survival at 5 years. Conventional wisdom held that hemorrhage and rectal bleeding appeared to affect prognosis favorably. One explanation was that the erosion of a mucosal surface as an early manifestation may bring the presence of the malignancy to the attention of the physician with subsequent early intervention. Further analysis has proven this not to be the case. Overall prognosis is also improved in those cases where the carcinoma involves only colon. Five-year survival is lower for patients with rectal or rectal sigmoid carcinoma. Several studies have demonstrated an improved prognosis for right- versus

TABLE 7-4-1   Staging for Colorectal Cancer

Stage 0	T_{is}	N_0	M_0	
				Dukes A
Stage 1	T_1	N_0	M_0	
	T_2	N_0	M_0	
Stage 2	T_3	N_0	M_0	Dukes B
	T_4	N_0	M_0	
Stage 3	Any T	N_1	M_0	Dukes C
	Any T	N_2, N_3	M_0	
Stage 4	Any T	Any N	M_1	Dukes D

T_{is} = in situ, T_1 = invades submucosa, T_2 = invades muscularis propria, T_3 = through muscularis propria invading subserosa or invading into non-peritoneal pericolic or perirectal tissues, T_4 = perforates the visceral peritoneum or invasion of other organs

N_0 = no nodal involvement, N_1 = less than three nodes, N_2 = four or more nodes, N_3 = lymph nodes along the course of a named vascular trunk

M_0 = no distant metastasis, M_1 = distant metastasis

left-sided lesions; however, present data remain controversial. Obstruction and organ perforation are correlated with poorer prognosis.

QUESTION 5 Two weeks postoperatively the patient was seen by his surgeon. The patient has recovered well and now has a CEA that is unmeasurable. Clinically, the patient appeared to have no evaluable disease. What are the indications for adjuvant therapy? What modalities are employed?

Curative rates in stage I and most stage II colorectal carcinomas are without question exceedingly high. Approximately 75% of all patients present with a lesion that can be surgically cured. However, 50% of all patients with colorectal carcinoma die from metastatic disease. Micrometastatic disease must exist in a significant number of patients thought to be cured with surgery alone. No well-performed study to date would suggest that the addition of adjuvant chemotherapy for stage I and most stage II disease provides a survival advantage or decreases the recurrence rate. Stage III disease represents a subset of patients at high risk for ocult metastasis.

This seems likely given the advanced nature of their disease and perhaps an inherent biological difference predisposing to the metastatic phenotype.

Because the patterns of recurrence differ between colon and rectal carcinoma, differing strategies have evolved to optimize the eradication of minimal residual disease. Rectal carcinoma most often reoccurs in local-regional fashion. Efforts to eliminate occult metastasis have taken the form of bi-modality therapy. The Gastrointestinal Tumor Study Group (GITSG) found that postoperative fluorouracil chemotherapy and pelvic irradiation decreased local-regional recurrence and increased overall survival. This study enrolled stage III (C) and stage II (B2) rectal cancers. Present recommendations have all B2 and C rectal cancers receiving adjuvant fluorouracil-based chemotherapy (5FU in combination with mitomycin) and radiation. These measures remain a standard of care in patients so staged. Recent data support the superiority of infusional 5FU over bolus therapy.

Colon carcinomas most often recur at a distance. Metastatic sites include the liver, peritoneum, and bone. Control of occult disease requires a systemic approach. Standard therapy now consists of fluorouracil chemotherapy in conjunction with levamisole, an anti-helminthic agent described as a nonspecific immune modulator. A study performed by the North Central Cancer Treatment Group and the Mayo Clinic showed that Dukes B2 and C patients treated with 5FU/levamisole had decreased recurrence rates when compared to controls. A benefit in overall survival was enjoyed by those patients who were Dukes C treated in this fashion. Excellent evidence exists to validate the role of adjuvant therapy in Dukes C colon carcinoma. This same therapy has now been recommended for those patients with B2 disease at high risk for recurrence (perforation, obstruction, etc.). Trends in improved survival were seen in this high-risk cohort of patients although improvement in overall survival did not reach statistical significance. The recommendation for this patient would be a 1-year course of levamisole and 5FU.

QUESTION 6 This patient received 5FU/levamisol for a 1-year course tolerating his chemotherapy well. His CEA values remained unmeasurable during that period. How will surveillance be conducted for resected colorectal cancer?

Standard recommendations call for patients to undergo a full colonoscopy every year for 5 years and then 2 years thereafter to rule out recurrence or metachronus lesions. Serial determinations of CEA may help to detect an asymptomatic recurrence or new lesion; however, its routine use has yet to bestow a survival advantage. Serial CT scans may be of use in following those patients at high risk for recurrence. A CXR should be obtained yearly, and a mammogram, breast and pelvic examinations performed on female patients with no evidence of disease. It is unclear if any of these measures confer a survival benefit. Currently, several studies are accruing patients designed specifically to answer questions regarding the follow-up of completely resected patients treated with and without adjuvant therapy. A British study now underway randomized patients into two groups. The first group is being followed expectantly with periodic history and physical examinations. The second group is being followed with serial CEA and CAT scans. Overall survival will serve as a comparative endpoint. The results acquired from this study will help to better define future surveillance procedures.

QUESTION 7 What is the relationship of ulcerative colitis and colorectal carcinoma? How should this subset of patients be managed differently?

A well-established increase in relative risk for colorectal cancer has been documented in patients with ulcerative colitis. The relationship is thought to exist because of a tendency toward mucosal dysplasia, thus increasing the potential for malignant growth. The probability of a colorectal malignancy developing in these patients is directly related to the duration of disease, age of onset, and the extent and severity of disease. Patients with ulcerative colitis have a five times greater chance of developing colorectal carcinoma than the general population. Patients with the least risk are those with proctitis and left-side colitis. Those who manifest pancolitis are at greatest risk. Patients with pancolitis have a 35% chance of developing carcinoma 30 years into their disease. Moreover, approximately 40% of patients with pancolitis will succumb to colorectal cancer provided they survive their ulcerative colitis. Patients with ulcerative colitis should undergo full colonoscopy on a yearly basis. At that time all suspicious lesions should be biopsied, and biopsies should be taken randomly to assess for dysplasia. Total colectomy should be performed in patients who are felt to be high risk because of duration, onset, extent, or severity. Patients with Crohn's disease are also at risk for developing colorectal carcinoma, albeit to a lesser degree.

CASE FOLLOW-UP The patient has recently undergone surveillance colonoscopy at the 1-year

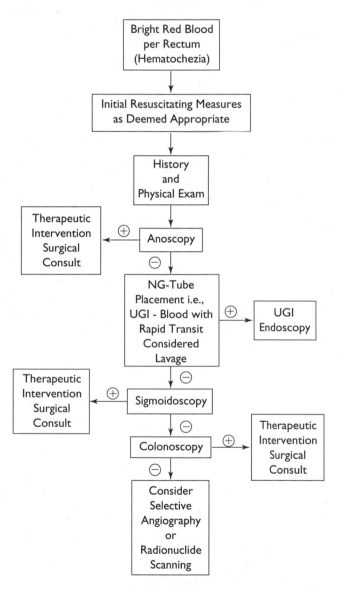

7-4-1   Diagnostic algorithm for lower gastrointestinal bleeding.

point. The results were negative. He now eats a healthy low-fat diet and has returned to work full time.

• •

BIBLIOGRAPHY

Cass AW, Million RR, Pfaff WW: Patterns of recurrence following surgery alone for adenocarcinoma of the colon and rectum, *Cancer* 37:2861-2865, 1976.

Cohen AM, Minsky BD, Schilsky RL: Colon cancer. In Devita VT, Hellman S, Rosenberg SA, eds: *Cancer: principles and practices,* ed 4, Philadelphia, 1993, JB Lippincott.

Coia LR, Hanks GE: The role of adjuvant radiation in the treatment of rectal cancer, *Semin Oncol* 18 (6):571-584, 1991.

Doerr RJ, Abdel-Nabi H, Krag D, et al: Radiolabeled antibody imaging in the management of colorectal cancer, *Ann Surg* 214:118-124, 1991.

Edwards FC, Truelove SC: The course and prognosis of ulcerative colitis, *Gut* 5:1-22, 1964.

Gastrointestinal Tumor Study Group: Adjuvant therapy of colon cancer: results of a prospectively randomized trial, *N Engl J Med* 310:737-743, 1984.

Jaiyesimi IA, Pazdur R: Colorectal cancer: diagnosis and managment. In Pazdur R, ed: *Medical oncology: a comprehensive review,* Huntington, NY, 1993, PRR.

Kane MJ: Adjuvant systemic treatment for carcinoma of the colon and rectum, *Semin Oncol* 18:421-442, 1991.

Kemeny N, Daly J, Reichman B, et al: Intrahepatic or systemic infusion of flurodeoxyuridine in patients with liver metastases from colorectal carcinoma: a randomized trial, *Ann Intern Med* 107:459-465, 1987.

McCormick PM, Burt ME, et al: Lung resection of colorectal metastses: ten year results, *Arch Surg* 127:1403-1406, 1992.

Nishisho I, Nakamura Y, Miyoshi Y, et al: Mutations of chromosome 5q21 genes in FAP and colorectal patients, *Science* 253:665-669, 1991.

Rao AR, Kagan AR, Chan PM, et al: Patterns of recurrence following curative resection alone for adenocarcinoma of the rectum and sigmoid colon, *Cancer* 48:1492-1495, 1981.

Rustgi AK: Hereditary gastrointestinal polyposis and nonpolyposis syndromes, *N Engl J Med* 331:1695-1702, 1993.

Skibber JM: New approaches to rectal cancer, *The Cancer Bulletin* 44:282-285, 1992.

Windle R, Bell P, Shaw D: Five year results of a randomized trial of adjuvant 5FU and levamisol in colorectal cancer, *Br J Surg* 74:569-572, 1984.

CASE

5

Stephen C. Schwartz
Gary Schwartz

A 28-year-old man presented to his primary physician with complaints of back pain over a 3-week course. The patient stated that the pain was left-sided, aching, and radiating across his back on occasion. He had treated himself with nonsteroidal agents with minimal improvement. He recalls no specific time at which his back was injured. He denies any weakness or parasthesias in his lower extremities and is continent of both bowel and bladder. The primary physician added a muscle relaxant to his existing pain regimen after a cursory physical examination was unrevealing. An appointment was made for a 2-week follow-up.

QUESTION 1 Generate a differential diagnosis. What is an approach to back pain in the ambulatory care patient?

Acute back pain in young and middle-aged patients often relates to traumas imparted to that region. Lumbosacral syndromes arising from trauma are accompanied by significant muscle spasm, tenderness, and limited range of motion. Complete bed rest for 48 hours along with muscle relaxants and NSAIDs may help to relieve the problem, although recent studies point to the beneficial effects of mobility and directed exercise.

Compromise of the spinal canal, the nerve roots, and intravertebral foramina may occur in many settings. Included here are herniated disks, degenerative changes, spondylarthropathies, and trauma. Herniated disks may arise from degenerative changes to the disk itself. Nerve impingement and symptoms including hyposthenia and weakness commonly involve the L4-L5 and L5-S1

disks. Compression fractures have mechanisms of injury that are unique to themselves. Significant falls, landing feet first, often give rise to this type of injury. Heritable diseases such as HLA-B27 related ankylosing spondylitis often present in the 20- to 30-year-old age group. Osteoarthritic changes seen in middle- and older-age groups may produce degenerative changes in disks, apophyseal joints, and vertebral bodies. Nerve root compression is seen when disks are compromised.

Connective tissue disorders such as juvenile rheumatoid arthritis, Reiter's syndrome, and inflammatory bowel disease may affect the lumbosacral spine-producing back pain. Infectious processes such as meningitis and osteomyelitis may also produce back pain. Lower back pain may arise from bone involvement with *M. tuberculosis* (Pott's disease). Patients with sickle cell anemia often experience back pain during a pain crisis and often require large amounts of narcotics. Avascular necrosis is seldom found in this setting.

Back pain that is unilateral may often have a urologic etiology. Pyelonephritis and obstructive nephropathy produce significant back pain in their usual clinical setting. Fibromyalgia refers to a constellation of clinical symptoms including aches, pain and stiffness in muscles, ligaments, tendons, and subcutaneous areas that may be exacerbated by manipulation of specific "trigger points." This entity accounts for a significant percentage of visits to rheumatologists and may present with back pain.

Back pain with associated neurologic findings is a medical emergency. Proper evaluation with MRI facilitates ruling out cord compression. Finally, back pain in the 20- to 30-age group should prompt the physician to evaluate the testis as this is a common presenting symptom in testicular carcinoma with retroperitoneal metastasis.

QUESTION 2 Approximately 1 week after the initial appointment, the patient called the physician's office stating that he had become short of breath over 2 days. Per the conversation the physician could appreciate his dyspnea and recommended that he come to the office immediately. Upon arrival the patient appeared dyspneic. Pulse oximetry demonstrated a saturation of 82%. Supplemental oxygen was added with improvement to 90%. Dry rales were appreciated on examination. The remainder of the cursory examination was normal. The patient was taken to the emergency room where a CXR was remarkable for bilateral, multiple, large-circumscribed nodular densities measuring from 3 to 6 cm. Discuss the differential of multiple pulmonary nodules in a young patient. What aspects of the examination will be central? What diagnostic tests will be informative?

Multiple pulmonary nodules in a 28-year-old man with back pain places a germ cell malignancy high in the differential. Classic for germ cell malignancies are bilateral pulmonary nodules with varying sizes. Other malignancies presenting in this fashion include metastatic melanoma, soft tissue sarcoma, rhabdomyosarcoma, and osteosarcoma. Lymphoma may also present with pulmonary symptoms. Most commonly, B-symptomatology and lymphadenopathy are present. In the proper clinical setting other entities should be considered: tuberculosis, histoplasmosis, blastomycoses, nocardia, and coccidiomycosis must always remain in the infectious disease differential. Septic emboli should be considered in young patients with intravenous drug habits, as the potential to seed right-sided cardiac valves always exists. Aspergillus in neutropenic patients can progress rapidly requiring the prompt initiation of systemic therapy with amphotericin. Collagen vascular disorders such as Wegner's granulomatosis may produce bilateral pulmonary nodules. Rheumatoid arthritis has also been known to

manifest in this manner. Pulmonary presentations as an initial finding in R.A. are uncommon. Both sarcoid and other granulomatous disease can present with pulmonary nodules. Along with a variety of roentgenographic findings that include hilar adenopathy and interstitial infiltrates, sarcoid may present with systemic symptoms, as well as arthralgias, arthritis, and erythema nodosum.

To establish a diagnosis in this patient, a repeat full history and physical examination should be undertaken. Genitourinary examination is indispensable here, as a testicular mass may be palpated. If no mass is palpated, bronchoscopy would be a high-yield procedure if biopsy and washings are obtained concurrently. A transthoracic needle biopsy is also an accepted procedure.

QUESTION 3 The patient was stabilized in the emergency room with supplemental oxygen. Testicular examination revealed a non-tender 2.5-cm mass arising from the left testicle. No other findings were remarkable. What is in the differential of a testicular mass? How will you confirm the diagnosis?

Testicular masses are seen commonly in clinical practice. Hydroceles, varicoceles, spermatoceles, epididymal cysts, and testicular tumors make up the bulk of testicular masses. Indirect hernias may also present as a mass in the scrotum. Epididymitis and orchitis may manifest as painful testicular swelling. Tuberculomata, metastatic disease, and lymphomas are rare findings. *Hydroceles* present as fluctuant masses that may be transilluminated distinguishing them from solid masses or indirect hernias. *Varicoceles* are enlarged venous plexi that extend caudally up the spermatic cord. These entities will decrease in size when the patient becomes supine and will not transilluminate. A new left-sided varicocele that does not diminish in the supine position should lead the clinician to suspect left spermatic vein obstruction relating to retroperitoneal malignancy. *Spermatoceles* are circumscribed lesions that do not transilluminate and will remain stable in size as the patient is placed in the supine position. *Epididymal cysts* arise from the epididymis, are smooth, and may transilluminate. *Epididymitis* and *orchitis* may be the result of a viral or bacterial infection. These entities are usually exquisitely painful. This pain may be relieved by elevation and support of the scrotum (Prehn's sign). Testicular masses that are firm and painless should be considered a testicular malignancy until proven otherwise.

Diagnosis can be established by obtaining a scrotal ultrasound followed by a transinguinal orchiectomy should the ultrasound suggest a mass lesion. A urologist with experience in dealing with germ cell tumors should be sought. A transscrotal surgical approach is contraindicated in these circumstances for two theoretical reasons. First, it remains mandatory to achieve control of the testicular blood supply before manipulating the testis lest the physician disseminate disease in this fashion. Secondly, transscrotal approach may subject the inguinal lymph nodes to contamination by tumor, which produces a high recurrence rate. Extirpation of the primary lesion should always be undertaken if identified by diagnostic means. This will allow for a diagnosis to be made and serves as a definitive therapeutic maneuver in certain stage I lesions. Even in the setting of metastatic disease, the primary lesion is removed for proper histologic identification. Serum markers for alpha-fetoprotein and beta-human chorionic gonadotrophin (HCG) should be drawn prior to surgery. (See Fig. 7-5-1 on p. 395.)

QUESTION 4 Scrotal ultrasound revealed a 2-cm left testicular mass. A left transabdominal orchiectomy was performed without complication. Pathology confirmed embryonal carcinoma. Preoperative AFP was 1200. β-HCG was 2000. The LDH was 980. Describe the pathologic subtypes and presentations of germ cell tumors. Are there risk factors for the development of germ cell tumors?

Germ cell malignancies are divided into *seminomatous* and *nonseminomatous* varieties. These account for 95% of all testicular malignancies, the remainder comprising stromal and sex cord tu-

mors. As a whole these tumors are the most common malignancies in the 15- to 35-year-old age group in males. Seminomas, thought to arise from primordial germ cells, represent approximately 45% of all germ cell tumors. Seminoma is divided into several variants including classic seminoma, spermatocytic, anaplastic, and giant cell with syncytiotrophoblasts. Classic seminoma possesses low metastatic potential. Most patients present with early stage disease. Patients with seminoma have a bimodal distribution with regard to age at presentation. Peak incidences are in the 30- and 50-year-old age groups. Pure seminomas may secrete beta-HCG, but do not secrete alpha-fetoprotein as do nonseminomatous germ cell tumors, which may secrete both.

Nonseminomatous germ cell tumors may be divided into several distinct categories. These include choriocarcinomas, embryonal carcinomas, teratoma, endodermal sinus tumors, and mixed germ cell tumors. There exists a high degree of varied biological behavior within these groups. In general, these malignancies have a proclivity to metastasize and secrete alpha-fetoprotein. Approximately 40% of all germ cell tumors are *mixed germ cell* tumors. The most commonly seen combinations include teratoma and embryonal carcinoma (25%), embryonal and seminoma (15%), and teratoma, embryonal, and seminoma (15%). *Embryonal cell* carcinoma represents between 15% to 30% of all nonseminomatous germ cell tumors. This variant presents as metastatic disease to paraaortic nodes, liver, or lung in up to one third of cases. *Teratomas* may be classified as mature or immature. Mature teratomas may be benign in prepubertal patients and aggressive in older age groups. Pathologically mature teratoma displays cystic structures with remnants of bone, cartilage, or nerve. Mucinous material is also a common finding. Immature teratomas do not demonstrate discernible tissue. This malignancy affects the prepubertal age group most often, but is commonly seen as a component of mixed germ cell tumors. *Choriocarcinomas* are uncommon malignancies in their pure form representing less than 1% of all germ cell tumors. Their peak incidence is in the

30- to 40-year-old age group. Pathologically, they are characterized by syncytiotrophoblasts and cytotrophoblasts and exhibit a high degree of necrosis. Endodermal sinus tumors (yolk sac tumors) are most commonly seen in childhood, representing 75% of all germ cell neoplasms in children. These tumors usually secrete high levels of alpha-fetoprotein.

Patients often present with a painless testicular mass. Gynecomastia is a presentation in up to 10% of all patients and results from the secretion of human chorionic gonadotrophins. Many mixed germ cell tumors (up to 25%) present with acute epididymitis. Germ cell malignancies may present with back pain because retroperitoneal nodes are a common site of metastasis. Patients who have evidence of undescended testis and abdominal pain should have an occult torsion of a mass ruled out. Because germinal epithelium traverses the midline during embryogenesis, areas of sequestered primordial germinal cells may be established. These areas may give rise to extragonadal germ cell tumors. This presentation has been described in such entities as Klinefelter's syndrome and acute megakaryoblastic leukemia (AML FAB M7).

Risk factors for the development of germ cell tumors include maldescent and abnormal development of the testis. Cryptorchidism increases the probability of developing a germ cell tumor by 10% to 40%. Individuals with testicular arrest in the abdomen have a 1:20 chance of developing this tumor, while those with arrest inguinally are approximately 1:80. Testicular feminization increases risk for germ cell tumors. Other putative risk factors include trauma, torsion, testicular atrophy from orchitis, radiation, exposure to diethylstilbestrol in early fetal life and diethylformimide.

Recently, Bosl et al. at Memorial Sloan-Kettering Cancer Center identified the isochromosome of chromosome 12 to be a cytogenetic marker for germ cell tumors. Interestingly, those hematological malignancies (AML FAB M7) associated with extragonadal germ cell tumors possess the same cytogenetic abnormality i(12)p.

QUESTION 5   Describe the extent of disease and staging workup for germ cell tumors? How are germ cell tumors staged? What is this patient's final staging?

After pathologic assessment has been made, an extent of disease workup should be undertaken. Routine studies include pretreatment measurement of beta-HCG, alpha-fetoprotein, and LDH. A chest x-ray to exclude pulmonary metastasis is obtained and followed by a CAT scan if the former is suspicious or positive. CAT scan of the abdomen is mandatory for assessment of the retroperitoneum. Blood work is obtained for CBC, electrolytes, BUN, and creatinine. A 24-hour urine collection for creatinine clearance is helpful in assessing renal function in the face of cisplatinum-based chemotherapy for advanced disease.

Staging of seminomatous germ cell tumors is relatively straightforward. Involvement limited to the testis represents stage A disease. Retroperitoneal spread denotes stage B disease, while metastasis above the diaphragm or to visceral organs represents stage C. As the size of retroperitoneal lymph nodes in seminoma has important treatment implications, stage B is often divided into three substages. Retroperitoneal lymphadenopathy of less than 5 cm denotes stage B_1, 5- to 10-cm stage B_2, and greater than 10 cm corresponding to stage B_3 (Table 7-5-1).

Nonseminomatous germ cell tumors are staged similarly. Stage A is confined to the testis. Stage B denotes spread to the retroperitoneum. Again, stage B is divided into several substages. Stage B1 has less than six positive nodes with no node greater than 2 cm, and with no extranodal extension. Stage B_2 includes disease with greater than six positive nodes, or any node greater than 2 cm or extranodal extension. Stage B_3 represents massive retroperitoneal lymphadenopathy. Stage C denotes metastatic disease.

This patient was found clinically to have metastatic disease in both lung and retroperitoneum. This denotes stage C disease by definition. The largest mass in the retroperitoneum measured

TABLE 7-5-1 Germc Cell Tumor Staging

Seminoma Staging (MSKCC)

Stage A	Tumor confined to the testis
Stage B	Spread to regional nodes
B_1	Nodes < 5 cm
B_2	Nodes > 5 cm, < 10 cm
B_3	Nodes >10 cm
Stage C	Spread beyond the retroperitoneal nodes

Non-Seminoma Staging (Skinner)

Stage A	Confined to the testis
Stage B	Spread to the retroperitoneum
B_1	< 6 nodes, no node > 2 cm, no extranodal extension
B_2	> 6 nodes, any node > 2 cm, extranodal extension
B_3	Massive retroperitoneal lymphadenopathy
Stage C	Metastatic disease

approximately 8 cm, while the largest mass in the lung was 6 cm by CT scan.

QUESTION 6 What are the treatment options for early stage germ cell tumors? For late stage? Are the approaches the same for both seminomatous and nonseminomatous germ cell tumors?

Because of their unique sensitivity to radiation, early stage seminoma is often managed differently than nonseminomatous germ cell tumors. Historically, *stage A seminoma* has been treated with orchiectomy followed by adjuvant radiation in the hope of eradicating occult retroperitoneal disease known to exist in 15% of all clinically staged patients. A total of 25 to 35 Gy is usually administered in 2 Gy fractions. Radiation ports are established depending upon the risk of spread to pelvic nodes (scrotal invasion) and extent of the stage A disease (i.e., spermatic cord involvement). Although this is generally a safe and effective strategy, adverse effects, although few, are observed. These include transient drops in sperm

count, nausea, and the possibility of second malignancies.

Recently several centers have developed cautious post-surgical surveillance of stage A seminoma in hopes of sparing patients the effects of radiation. This approach could only be undertaken because excellent salvage strategies exist, should observation fail. Results from the Royal Marsden Hospital suggest that this approach achieves similar success rates to that of orchiectomy and radiation.

Clinical *stage A nonseminomatous germ cell tumors* have been managed conventionally with orchiectomy and retroperitoneal lymph node dissection (RPLND). However, because RPLND is a major procedure with several untoward complications (retrograde ejaculation and infertility) with only 30% of patients harboring pathologic stage B disease, attempts have been made to define subsets of patients who may be spared this procedure. Patients with lymphatic or vascular invasion, large tumor bulk, and those with a component of embryonal carcinoma may represent a patient population at risk for harboring stage B disease. Therefore with these patients it would seem prudent to proceed with RPLND, which may prove curative in those with low-volume disease. Patients who are observed after orchiectomy should undergo exceedingly close surveillance.

In the era before cis-platinum–based chemotherapy, *stage B seminoma* was treated with orchiectomy and radiation. This approach was effective for patients with low-volume stage B_1 disease. Patients with stage B_3 disease suffered from recurrent disease in a substantial percentage of cases, stage B_2 less so. Currently, it is recommended that patients with stage B_1 receive orchiectomy with radiation only. Management of B_2 is more controversial. Some would advocate orchiectomy and initial radiation, with cis-platinum–based chemotherapy held in reserve for nonresponders and recurrent disease as a salvage measure. Others suggest up-front chemotherapy for stage B_2 in light of the 30% incidence of distant metastasis. Chemotherapy is the suggested up-front therapy for all stage B_3 and C patients and those with primary mediastinal seminoma patients who have superior vena caval syndrome and those with axillary or supraclavicular adenopathy should receive upfront chemotherapy.

Those patients with residual radiographic abnormalities after chemotherapy for bulky stage B disease may have residual seminoma. At MSKCC those patients with residual masses greater than 3 cm undergo an operative procedure with extirpation of the involved tissue. If seminoma is found, further chemotherapy or radiation is given. If patients are not taken to surgery, then abdominal RT is offered. Investigators at Indiana University offer no further therapy for residual masses unless radiographic or serologic evidence of residual tumor is present.

Clinical *stage B nonseminomatous germ cell* tumors may be treated with primary RPLND or up-front chemotherapy depending on extent of disease. Those patients clinically staged with low-volume B_1 and B_2 disease undergo RPLND. Patients found to have pathologic B_1 disease may receive close follow-up and are treated with four cycles of cis-platinum–based chemotherapy at relapse. Alternatively, those patients with pathologic stage B_2 may be treated with two cycles of adjuvant cis-platinum–based chemotherapy. Two drug combinations of platinum and etoposide appear to be as efficacious as multidrug regimens. Patients who have stage B nonseminomatous germ cell tumors with clinical B_3 disease are usually treated with primary chemotherapy. Those who obtain a complete response may be observed. Patients obtaining a partial response should undergo RPLND. If cancer is discovered on pathologic examination, two cycles of adjuvant therapy may be given. If teratoma or fibrosis is observed pathologically, the patient is observed. Patients progressing through therapy may be offered salvage therapy with VP-16, ifosfamide, and cis-platinum or go to autologous bone marrow transplant.

Patients with disease that is supradiaphragmatic, visceral, or greater than 10 cm possess stage C or advanced disease. The advent of cis-platinum–based chemotherapy revolutionized the treatment of advanced seminomatous and nonseminomatous germ cell tumors. Whereas 10% complete responses were obtainable with dactinomycin-based regimens, the addition of cis-platinum to vinblastine and bleomycin PVB resulted in 70% complete remissions. Cure rates remain in the 80% range with the addition of VP-16 to most regimens. All advanced seminomas are treated with cis-platinum–based chemotherapy.

For advanced nonseminomatous germ cell tumors, patients may be placed into good-risk and poor-risk prognostic groups based upon clinical information and mathematical models. These same models have not been found applicable to seminomatous disease. Seminomas are treated in the same fashion as good risk NSGCTs and respond similarly. At MSKCC, risk groups have been identified using a mathematical model incorporating the number of disease sites (N = 0,1,2), pretreatment beta-HCG, and pretreatment LDH. Treatment is formulated according to results obtained.

$$h = 8.514 - 1.973 \log (LDH + 1) - 0.530 \log (HCG + 1) - 1.111 \text{ TOTMET}$$
TOTMET = number of meastatic sites = 0,1, ≥ 2
probability of CR = exp h/(1 + exph)

Extragonadal germ cell tumors arise from remnant germinal epithelial cells deposited in a midline distribution during migration of these cells in embryogenesis. These tumors most commonly arise in the mediastinum and retroperitoneum and represent a poor-risk group of germ cell tumor.

Standard therapy for good risk patients at MSKCC relies on four cycles of VP-16 and cis-platinum. For good-risk patients at Indiana University three cycles of platinum, bleomycin, and vinblastine are offered as standard therapy. Cure rates are in the 90% range. Poor-risk groups have an overall cure rate of between 35% to 65%. Efforts have been made to improve upon these numbers by dose intensification of active existing agents and the use of newer active agents

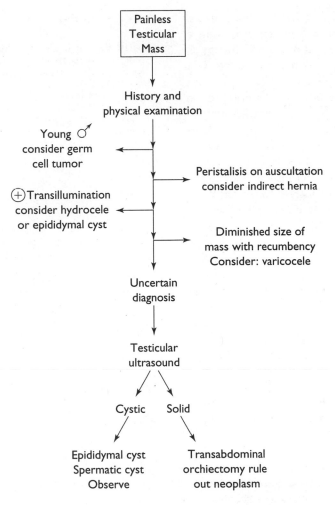

7-5-1   Diagnostic algorithm for a painless testicular mass.

shown to have activity in salvage regimens. Dose intensification of cis-platinum has not proven to be efficacious in poor-risk patients. The use of high-dose carboplatinum with autologous bone marrow transplant has met with some success as has the use of intensified ifosfamide regimens. Loeher et al. found a 33% complete response rate with VP-16, ifosfamide, and platinum.

At MSKCC the expected half-life decay of serological markers has been used to predict platinum-resistant disease. In an ongoing study, patients are treated up-front with two cycles of platinum and VP-16. If markers decay at expected rates, chemotherapy is continued. If markers do not decay appropriately, patients are given high-dose chemotherapy with autologous bone marrow rescue. Results of this study will be forthcoming.

As in stage B NSGCT, surgery remains a useful adjunct in rendering patients disease free with localized stage C disease after primary chemotherapy. Persistently elevated markers or radiographic changes of residual masses may prompt surgical and, in some cases, radiotherapeutic intervention. This will provide a significant group of patients with long-term survival.

QUESTION 7 This patient fits criterion for the good-risk subgroup. Probability for achieving a complete response with conventional therapy is greater than 70%. In light of this, the patient was offered four cycles of platinum and VP-16. The patient was also offered sperm banking prior to his chemotherapy, which he accepted. He tolerated the chemotherapy well with only mild hematologic toxicity. By the end of the patient's second cycle of therapy, his markers had normalized, diminishing appropriately by half-life. After his fourth cycle the patient's disease was not apparent by CT examination. How shall surveillance be conducted in this patient?

The use of serum markers, when initially positive, has served to make the early detection of recurrent or residual disease possible. Physical examination, CXRs, and tumor markers are performed every month for the first year, every 2 months for the second, and every 6 months thereafter. CAT scans of the retroperitoneum and all involved sites are obtained on an every 3-month basis for the first 24 months and every 6 months thereafter. Surveillance may be continued for as long as 10 years because late relapses have been reported.

CASE FOLLOW-UP The patient had no evaluable disease 2 years from his initial diagnosis. He maintained an excellent performance status subsequent to his chemotherapy. The patient's wife underwent artificial insemination resulting in a successful term pregnancy.

• •

BIBLIOGRAPHY

Babaian RJ, Zangers GK: Testicular seminoma: the M.D. Anderson experience. An analysis of pathological and patient characteristics and treatment recommendations, *J Urol* 139:311-314, 1988.

Bosl GJ, Dmitrovsky E, Renter VE, et al: Isochromosome 12: clinically useful marker for male germ cell tumors, *J Natl Cancer Inst* 81:1874-1878, 1989.

Bosl GJ, Gekker NJ, Bajorin D: Identification and management of poor risk patients with germ cell tumors: the MSKCC experience, *Semin Oncol* 15:339-344, 1988.

Bosl GJ, Lange PH, Fraley EE, et al: Human chorionic gonadotropin and alpha-fetoprotein in the staging of nonseminomatous testicular cancer, *Cancer* 47:328-332, 1981.

Einhorn LH: Treatment of testicular cancer: a new and improved model, *J Clin Oncol* 8:1777-1781, 1990.

Einhorn LH, Richie JP, Shipley WU: Cancer of the testis. In De Vita VT, Rosenberg SA, Hellman S, et al, eds: *Cancer: principles and practice of oncology*, Philadelphia, 1993, Lippincott.

Horwich A, Dearnaley DP: Treatment of seminoma, *Semin Oncol* 19:1711-180, 1992.

Mostofi FK: Testicular tumors: epidemiologic, etiologic and pathologic features, *Cancer* 23:1186-1201, 1973.

Pierce GB, Abell MR: Embryonal carcinoma of the testis, *Pathol Annu* 5:27-60, 1970.

Priti HA, Logothetis CJ: Testicular cancer in medical oncology: a comprehensive review. In Pazdur R, ed: Huntington, NY: PRR, 1993.

Strader CH, Weiss NS, Darling JR, et al: Cryptorchidism, orchioplexy, and the risk of testicular cancer, *Am J Epidemiol* 127:1013-1018, 1988.

Williams SD, Stablein DM, Einhorn LH, et al: Immediate adjuvant chemotherapy versus observation with treatment at relapse in pathological stage II testicular cancer, *N Engl J Med* 317:1433-1438, 1987.

CASE

6

Stephen C. Schwartz
Walter Fried

A previously healthy 52-year-old man came to his private physician with concerns regarding a painless lump under his right arm. The patient stated that the lump had been present for the preceding 8 to 12 months, although it had regressed in size on several occasions. Recently, a new lump appeared under the left arm. The right axillary lump appeared to increase in size. There were no complaints of fever, chills, or night sweats. He denied any significant weight loss. His appetite was good. No changes were noted in his bowel or bladder habits. He was questioned regarding intercurrent illness and denied any recent upper respiratory tract infections or exposure to infectious agents including tuberculosis or syphilis. He denied any risk factors for HIV infection. The patient had a 35-year tobacco history and drank alcohol on occasion. He took no medications.

QUESTION 1 The patient is presenting with a recent history of lymphadenopathy (LAN) in more than one anatomical region. What is your understanding of the physiology of lymphadenopathy?

The initial presentation of this patient would suggest a picture of generalized LAN. Lymph node enlargement is conveniently classified as being reactive or infiltrative and may be localized or generalized. Reactive processes are those in which the node demonstrates a proliferative response mainly to antigenic material. This response is most commonly seen with infection. Noninfectious sources of reactive nodal enlargement also exist. Examples of this process include connective tissue disorders, sarcoidosis, and pseudolymphoma caused by dilantin administration. An infiltrative

process enlarges lymph nodes by replacement of normal cells with other tissue. Lipid storage disorders and lymphoma are common offenders in this regard. Localized adenopathy denotes nodal enlargement confined to one node or nodal region. Generalized adenopathy describes involvement in more than one nodal region.

When stimulated, nodal blood flow may increase upwards of 20 fold. Total numbers of lymphocytes are increased by several mechanisms including (1) a sequestration of lymphocytes from the circulating blood, (2) a decreased nodal egress of lymphocytes, and (3) proliferation of stimulated lymphocytes. Together these mechanisms may increase lymph node size approximately 10 to 15 times their baseline.

QUESTION 2 Physical examination revealed a well-nourished, well-developed gentleman in no acute distress. Vital signs were T 98.9°F, BP 122/69 mm Hg, RR 14 bpm, and P 77 bpm. Examination of the head and neck was remarkable for cervical adenopathy with the largest node measuring 1.5 cm in diameter. Prominent LAN was present in both right and left axilla and in the inguinal area. The largest node, measuring approximately 2 cm, was in the right axilla. The nodes were firm, had a rubbery consistency, and were moderately tender to palpation. Cardiovascular and pulmonary examinations were within normal limits. The spleen tip was palpated 3 cm below the right costal margin. The liver was normal in size and consistency. What information can one glean from the physical examination that may provide insight into the diagnosis?

Physical examination may provide clues to the underlying diagnosis. It is extremely important to understand regional lymphatic drainage to localize sites of disease. An example is lymphangitic spread to epitrochlear and axillary lymph nodes from a distal source in the upper extremity. Such spread should always follow contiguous lymph node chains. Hard, matted nodes often accompany metastatic malignant disease. Tender nodes with surrounding dermal erythema usually indicate an infectious source. Firm, rubbery nodes may signify lymphomatous involvement. In lymphoma, nodes may also become matted and fixed to overlying skin. Processes involving the skin usually are not associated with directly underlying lymph node involvement. One must keep in mind, however, that advanced lymph node disease may progress to involve subcutaneous structures, ulcerate, and appear to primarily involve the skin.

Specific regional involvement may provide clues as to the site and type of disease process (i.e., posterior cervical chain involvement seen in rubella or Sister Mary Joseph's node at the umbilicus in GI malignancies). Virchow's node in the left supraclavicular fossa is also classic for GI malignancy.

Generalized LAN is a usual manifestation of systemic illness including infectious, autoimmune, and lymphoproliferative etiologies. A thorough diagnostic evaluation should be undertaken to exclude nonmalignant causes of generalized adenopathy. Even if subsequent etiologies are uncovered in a timely fashion, nodal biopsy may be warranted to rule out concurrent malignancy or to confirm diagnosis through culture and histology. (See Fig. 7-6-1 on p. 404.)

QUESTION 3 Routine laboratory analysis was remarkable for a WBC count of 20,000, hemoglobin 12 g/dl, and platelets 90,000. The chemistry panel included an LDH of 1210. A CXR was unrevealing. What is your differential diagnosis of generalized LAN?

Diagnostic studies should be undertaken to rule out infectious sources as a possible etiology to the patient's LAN. Various viruses may be implicated. Carriage of human immunodeficiency virus and/or frank AIDS presents with generalized LAN in a significant percentage of cases. Risk factors for HIV infection include exposure to blood or body fluids from infected patients, sexual promiscuity, and sharing needles used for intravenous drug abuse. When this etiology is suspected, individuals at risk must undergo HIV testing by ELISA with subsequent Western blot confirmation if the former is positive. Other viral diseases to consider include Epstein-Barr virus (EBV), cytomegalovirus (CMV), and infectious hepatitis. Both EBV and CMV produce a mononucleosis-like illness presenting in a young adult with fever, LAN, upper respiratory tract symptoms, and splenomegaly. A peripheral blood smear containing atypical lymphocytes helps to solidify the diagnosis of EBV. Both a monospot test and IgM for CMV should be obtained.

Multiple bacterial etiologies of generalized LAN exist. These include various staphylococcal and streptococcal infections, *Listeria monocytogenes*, Lyme disease, cat-scratch disease, and *Pasteurella multocida* infection. Appropriate blood cultures and serologies can help include or exclude these diagnoses. Typical as well as atypical *Mycobacterium* may present with generalized LAN. Other infectious agents classically presenting with LAN include secondary syphilis, toxoplasmosis, coccidioidomycosis, tularemia, brucellosis, and histoplasmosis. Connective tissue disorders such as rheumatoid arthritis often present with significant LAN, especially when the disorder presents with multisystem involvement. Sarcoidosis, although usually presenting with hilar LAN, can exhibit generalized LAN and is a diagnosis to consider.

Various drug exposures and serum sickness can present with LAN. Classically dilantin has been found to produce pseudolymphoma. This presents with generalized LAN known to regress upon discontinuation of the drug. However, several cases of lymphoma have been reported in the literature in association with this clinical picture. The immunogenic response to foreign protein gives rise to generalized LAN as seen in the Arthus reaction where an antigen-antibody complex is deposited in tissue.

Neoplasm, giving rise to LAN, usually represents metastatic phenomenon from a carcinoma, although a primary lymphoproliferative disorder such as malignant lymphoma or Hodgkin's disease must be ruled out. More generalized presentations are seen in lymphomatous processes.

This patient has a paucity of physical complaints and lacks fever and URI symptoms. Although the patient has a WBC count of 20,000 with a predominance of lymphocytes, no atypicals are present. This lack of findings lessens the chance of an infectious process. The patient described herein has no inherent HIV risk factors. There are no historical factors that suggest a drug or immunogen exposure. The absence of rheumatologic findings and lack of constitutional symptoms makes the diagnosis of a collagen vascular disease unlikely.

QUESTION 4 The patient was electively admitted to the hospital for evaluation. A general surgeon was consulted, and the patient underwent subsequent axillary nodal biopsy. A review of the pathology revealed a follicular small cleaved cell non-Hodgkin's lymphoma (NHL), and the patient was subsequently referred to an oncologist. What are the important epidemiological and pathophysiologic elements of lymphoma. What are the pathologic types of lymphoma?

In 1992 approximately 41,000 new cases of lymphoma were diagnosed. The ratio of men to women was approximately equal in these cases. It is also noteworthy that the incidence of lymphoma has increased by 50% between the years of 1973 to 1988, and it is thought that this is due, in large proportion, to the emergence of the acquired immunodeficiency syndrome (AIDS). The only well-documented etiology of NHL thus far has been viral etiologies. It has been shown that EBV is associated with a substantial percentage of high-grade lymphomas of the Burkitt's type. Other associations between HTLV-I and T cell leukemia-lymphoma have been demonstrated.

Lymphoma is also found very commonly in patients who have a high degree of immunosuppression such as AIDS, Wiskott-Aldrich syndrome, X-linked immunodeficiency, ataxia-telangiectasia, and other immunodeficiency disorders.

Multiple cytogenetic abnormalities have been identified in NHL. Most noteworthy is the 8,14 translocation in Burkitt's lymphoma. This involves the translocation of the C-myc oncogene to an area adjacent to the immunoglobulin heavy chain locus. Other translocations including an 8,2 and 8,22 have been described. These are associated with the translocation of the C-myc oncogene to light chain loci for kappa and lambda light chains. These translocations of the C-myc oncogene bring it into areas adjacent to the promoter region for these heavy and light chain loci and subsequently the expression of the C-myc oncogene is increased. The end result of the increased expression of C-myc is the increased production of a DNA binding protein that is thought to be important in the subsequent regulation of self-proliferation. The (14,18) translocation is seen in upwards of 80% of patients presenting with follicular small-cleaved cell lymphoma. This translocation brings the BCL-2 oncogene in proximity to the immunoglobulin heavy chain joining region. This BCL-2 gene product is upregulated and codes for an inner mitochondrial membrane protein that may inhibit programmed cell death.

The pathology of NHL rests on the determination of cell size and architecture of the lymph node. Generally speaking, cell types with smaller cells and a follicular or nodular pattern are related to better prognosis. Larger cell types and more undifferentiated cells are more aggressive and carry a worse prognosis.

Hodgkin's lymphoma (HL) is separated into four major groups that are differentiated by the amount of Reed-Sternberg (RS) cell infiltration. The lymphocyte predominant type has a paucity of RS cells and an increased percentage of lymphocytes. The mixed cellularity type has more equal amounts of RS cells and lymphocytes. Nodular sclerosing types are similar to the mixed cellularity type but with bands of fibrous tissue through the cellular infiltrate. Finally, the lymphocyte deplete type has numerous RS cells and few lymphocytes. The lymphocyte predominant and nodular sclerosing varieties generally carry the best prognosis.

QUESTION 5 What is the usual presentation of patients with lymphoma and what is the initial workup to determine the extent of disease?

The clinical presentation of most patients with NHL is usually similar: the presence of a painless nodal mass. Lymphomas often present with noncontiguous generalized lymphadenopathy that may regress and return over time. They may otherwise be asymptomatic; however, 15% to 20% may have other symptoms along with presenting lymphadenopathy. Known as B-symptoms, these include night sweats, fever, and loss of at least 10% of the baseline body weight. The presence of B-symptoms usually represents greater tumor mass and in many cases a poorer prognosis.

In NHL, nodes are usually rubbery and firm. Adenopathy may undergo a waxing and waning pattern over months to years before the diagnosis of lymphoma is made. On physical examination, one should not forget that tonsillar tissue is lymphatic and may be a subtle clue for other areas of GI involvement. Symptoms may be due to organ infiltration or compression from involved nodes. Other findings that may be seen in lymphoma include chylous ascites or pleural effusions from abdominal and mediastinal disease, respectively. Anemia and other cytopenias may be found when bone marrow involvement is present.

NHL patients usually have early involvement of oropharyngeal, cervical, skin, and gastrointestinal tissues. Low-grade lymphoma involves the bone marrow early on in a large percentage of patients who present with this subtype. The involvement of bone is most commonly seen in the high-grade lymphomas. Leukemic presentations occur in approximately 10% to 15% of patients with NHL. Patients may also develop Coomb's

positive hemolytic anemia, which is more commonly seen in NHL as compared to Hodgkin's disease.

Alternatively, HL commonly presents with lymphadenopathy involving contiguous lymph node chains. Characteristics of HL include the Pel-Ebstein fever pattern. This is a classic finding wherein high fever alternates with normal temperature every several days. Pruritus that is generalized and refractory to routine therapy can be seen and should raise suspicion for Hodgkin's disease. Additionally, pain localized to involved areas after consumption of alcohol is a classic sign associated with HL. Radiography may disclose the presence of "ivory" vertebrae resulting from vertebral osteoblastic changes. Other findings may include Horner's syndrome, paraplegia due to cord compression, intrahepatic or extrahepatic biliary obstruction, superior vena cava syndrome, ureteral and bronchial obstruction.

The initial workup for suspected NHL should always include tissue biopsy. This biopsy should be sent for appropriate marker studies to assess cellular identity. Bilateral bone marrow biopsy and aspirate are mandatory for a thorough evaluation of all lymphomas in order to rule out bone marrow infiltration. Cytogenetic studies may also be useful. The presence of an involved bone marrow in large cell lymphomas suggests the possibility of CNS involvement making lumbar puncture mandatory. In the setting of neurologic complaints, examination of the cerebrospinal fluid is always warranted. The patient should also have routine hematologic and chemistry parameters including a complete blood count, reticulocyte count, platelet count, ESR, and blood chemistries including liver function tests, BUN, and creatinine. Quantitative immunoglobulins should also be obtained because hypogammaglobulinemia is a frequent accompaniment of NHL.

Initial radiographic studies should include both PA and lateral chest radiography. If abnormalities are detected on this study, a CT scan of the chest is warranted. CT scans of the abdomen and pelvis are also considered essential in the routine work-up. These are helpful in delineating involvement of liver and spleen and in documenting the extent of regional lymph node involvement. Bone films are required if bone pain is obtained in the history; subsequent bone scan may also be helpful in detecting other sites of involvement.

The use of staging laparotomy in HL remains controversial. Its use is reserved for scenarios where findings from laparotomy will change treatment directions. It is thought that approximately 33% of patients with early stage HL have occult abdominal disease. The presence of B-symptoms and an increased number of upper torso nodal sites may portend a high likelihood of abdominal disease. Those patients not undergoing laparotomy in this setting should be considered as having abdominal disease and treated accordingly. The use of bipedal lymphangiography has found its place in the assessment of lymphadenopathy in HL that is poorly demonstrated by CT scan. This procedure may be necessary to detect abdominal disease or to separate patients with stage IIIA1 and IIIA2 disease and determine the need for chemotherapy. Abdominal nodes inundated with lymphangiography contrast material may be followed by conventional x-ray for response to chemotherapy. These films may also be used in generating fields for radiation therapy. Gallium scan has recently fallen out of favor with regard to its lack of specificity.

QUESTION 6 Further diagnostic evaluation by CT examination is remarkable for the presence of border-line mediastinal, mesenteric, periaortic, and inguinal lymphadenopathy. The presence of spleno-megaly was noted along with areas of low attenuation suggestive of splenic involvement with lymphoma. Histopathologic examination of the bone marrow biopsy reveals cells that were suspicious for lymphoma, morphologically identical to those seen on biopsy of the axillary lymph node. Describe the clinical staging for this patient. What are the important characteristics of the type of lymphoma seen in this patient?

Anatomic staging for patients with lymphoma is described per the Ann Arbor staging system. Stage I disease describes a lesion that involves a singular lymph node chain or extralymphatic site on one side of the diaphragm. Stage II disease includes the involvement of 2 lymph node chains or one extralymphatic site with one or more nodal regions located on the same side of the diaphragm. Stage III disease is found when lesions are present on both sides of the diaphragm involving lymph nodes or spleen. Stage IV disease represents systemic spread to extranodal organs including bone marrow. The presence of B-symptoms is denoted by fever, night sweats, and loss of more than 10% of the baseline weight (*b* after the numerical sign). Extralymphatic disease, contiguous from a lymph node, is denoted by *E* at the end of the numerical sign. For example, disease in cervical nodes and periaortic nodes with invasion into the left kidney in a patient with drenching night sweats is staged clinically as IIIEb.

Application to this patient places him as stage IV due to the patient's disseminated disease involving the bone marrow. From a histopathologic perspective, using the working formulation that divides lymphomas into low-, intermediate-, and high-grade types, this patient's follicular small cleaved cell lymphoma is placed into the low-grade category.

As are approximately 95% of all lymphomas, the follicular small cleaved cell lymphoma is of B-cell lineage. Both low-grade and several intermediate-grade lymphomas represent neoplasms that have a long natural history and good prognosis. The follicular small cleaved cell lymphoma represents approximately 40% of all NHL subtypes. It is the most common histologic subtype. Noteworthy is the fact that this subtype of lymphoma often presents in the advanced stage on initial presentation. Approximately 82% of patients with the follicular small cleaved cell type will present with stage III disease. In general, patients presenting with low-grade lymphomas often present in late stage III or IV disease. Patients who present with small lymphocytic lymphoma are felt to be indistinguishable from patients with chronic lymphocytic lymphoma. Those patients presenting with intermediate- and high-grade lymphomas, are just as likely to present with stage 1 and 2 as they are with stage 3 and 4. It should be noted that these patients often have less involvement in their bone marrow.

QUESTION 7 What is the current approach to treatment for nonHodgkin's and Hodgkin's lymphoma?

When considering therapy for NHL, one must understand the paradox of low-grade versus high-grade disease with regard to curability. Untreated, the prognosis of low-grade lymphomas is measured in years, high-grade tumors in months, and aggressive disease in weeks. While they exhibit a long natural history, low-grade lesions often recur and have little chance for cure with present chemotherapy. High-grade lesions, as well as the intermediate diffuse large cell lymphomas, are often responsive to present regimens and have a greater chance for complete cure, although left untreated prove rapidly fatal. Treatment for low-grade lesions may be held until disease is advanced or symptoms are present. Patients may live many years with a paucity of symptoms. Conversely, high-grade disease and most intermediate-grade lymphomas require immediate therapy.

Effective treatment of NHL calls for a multidisciplinary approach combining surgical, chemotherapeutic, and radiation modalities to produce an effective cure. Surgery in the treatment of lymphoma has been limited to anatomic staging via staging laparotomy in HL. There are, however, a number of special circumstances that are indications for surgical intervention. The resection of aggressive gastrointestinal NHL is widely recommended to significantly reduce the risk of possible perforation and/or bleeding complications. This is thought to be the standard of care, although no prospective randomized trials exist to confirm this strategy.

When radiotherapy is used in the treatment of

NHL, it is imperative that a complete and proper staging procedure is followed. The usefulness of curative radiotherapy is usually limited to the management of localized disease. This represents stages I, IE, and early stage II disease defined as a nonbulky or limited stage II involvement. Low-grade lymphomas have a lengthy natural history and are generally highly responsive to radiotherapy. Local control rates exceeding approximately 90% can be achieved with tolerable doses of radiation. Low-grade and intermediate-grade lymphomas rarely present with localized disease. Therefore, the use of radiotherapy may be limited. A review of the literature shows several groups demonstrating a 10-year survival of greater than 50% with extended field radiotherapy for localized stages I and II low-grade lymphomas. The Stanford experience demonstrates a 10-year survival for patients with follicular low-grade lymphomas to be approximately 68%. These same patients had a freedom from relapse at 10 years at approximately 54%. It must be pointed out that in this subset of patients, relapse is quite common. When stage I or II NHL is limited to the gastrointestinal tract, a majority of patients undergo surgical resection that is subsequently followed by low-dose radiotherapy with an additional dose to adjacent nodal sites. Radiation therapy is also an effective treatment in primary CNS NHL.

The role of palliative therapy with radiation in low-, intermediate-, and high-grade lymphomas cannot be underestimated. Scenarios in which palliative therapy becomes necessary include the relief of spinal cord compression, the treatment of superior vena cava obstruction, and the treatment of any painful tumor mass. Radiotherapy is also useful in primary lymphoma of the bone.

Chemotherapy in NHL is reserved for those patients who have disease not thought to be amenable to radiation therapy alone. As in the case under discussion, NHL of the low-grade type usually presents as a systemic disease. Stage III and IV disease, however, have a median survival approaching 7 to 10 years; hence in certain cases, chemotherapy has to be used judiciously. When presenting as asymptomatic disease, it is not uncommon to establish a "watch and wait" approach, withholding chemotherapy until the disease progresses or becomes symptomatic. The use of these chemotherapy regimens earlier in the course of low-grade lymphoma is also now being investigated. It is uncertain whether the early use of intensified or standard chemotherapy bestows a survival advantage in low-grade lymphoma.

The use of chemotherapeutic regimens including CVP, CHOP, M-BACOD and PROMACE-MOPP are considered standard therapy in advanced low-grade NHL. The use of the CHOP has become widespread. This particular regimen consists of cyclophosphamide, adriamycin, vincristine, and prednisone. Patients receive approximately six or more cycles of this regimen with each cycle being repeated every 4 weeks. With these particular chemotherapeutic regimens, clinical remissions can be realized in approximately 30% to 70% of all patients with low-grade disease. However, remissions in low-grade lymphomas are not durable, averaging approximately 2 to 3 years. The use of high intensity induction chemotherapy with adriamycin and vincristine is currently under investigation. Induction therapy is followed by consolidation with high-dose Cytoxan therapy.

Patients with intermediate (large cell lymphomas) and high-grade NHL without therapy have a poor clinical outcome. The use of combination chemotherapeutic regimens in early and late stages has altered the natural history of this aggressive disease. Although time to remission and duration may be extended, no survival advantage has been demonstrated when CHOP regimens are compared to more aggressive counterparts. A complete response of 40% to 80% have been reported in numerous series using CHOP-based combination chemotherapy. Large cell NHLs are exceedingly susceptible to this form of aggressive chemotherapy. Involved field radiation therapy has also been advocated in combination with chemotherapy in some cases of early-stage intermediate-grade lymphoma. Those who would subscribe to the finding of equal efficacy amongst various combinations when compared to CHOP must also consider the evidence that supports improved survival in dose intensified treatment of lymphoma. With the increase of aggressiveness of these chemotherapy regimens come concomitant potential toxicities. These include prolonged bone marrow suppression, infection, and bleeding diatheses. Specifically, neutropenia is seen due to myelosuppression. The use of Cytoxan can lead to severe hemorrhagic cystitis caused by the metabolite acrolein. The use of colony stimulating factors, such as GCSF, have helped to ameliorate neutropenia, while the use of MESNA has been found to limit bladder toxicity related to Cytoxan usage. The use of high-dose chemotherapy followed by either autologous or allogeneic bone marrow rescue is now being investigated in multiple centers. As such, bone marrow transplantation has been used in situations not amenable to salvage chemotherapy. Both lymphoblastic and Burkitt's lymphoma are treated with high dose regimens such as used in acute lymphoblastic leukemia.

In cases of HL, treatment plans may be based on pathologic stage of disease after laparotomy or on clinical staging. Radiation therapy may be curative in many patients. For pathologic disease stages I and IIA radiation therapy is the treatment of choice. Mantle radiation is used and includes all lymph node tissue above the diaphragm. Radiation technique in HL is based on the pathophysiologic tenet that HL spreads via contiguous node chains. The presence of bulky mediastinal disease ($> \frac{1}{3}$ the AP diameter of the chest) may be an indication for chemotherapy as are the presence of B-symptoms and hilar adenopathy. For clinically staged I and II disease most centers recommend a combination modality approach, although radiation or chemotherapy alone may accomplish the same task. The practice of prophylactic radiation to the abdomen for supradiaphragmatic presentations may be of limited usefulness in patients staged by laparotomy.

Stage III HL is separated into two categories: involvement of the celiac and portal nodes (III_1) and spread to the iliac, inguinal, and further periaortic disease (III_2). Stage $IIIA_1$ disease may be

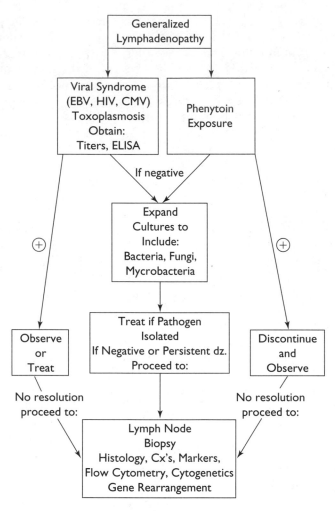

7-6-1 Diagnostic algorithm for generalized lymphadenopathy.

treated with radiation therapy with an extended field to include the ilioinguinal area. Disease-free survival approaches 65% to 75%. Stage IIIA$_2$ disease receiving radiotherapy had cure rates approaching 32%. Both groups of patients had a significant improvement in survival when treated with combined modality therapy (< radiation therapy and chemotherapy). Stage IIIB were also found to enjoy an improved survival when treated with combined modality therapy. Stages IVA and IVB are treated with combination chemotherapy. Standard chemotherapy regimens are

MOPP (mechlorethamine, vincristine, procarbazine, and prednisone) and ABVD (adriamycin, bleomycin, vinblastine, and dacarbazine) or altering combinations of the two. Complete remissions occur in about 70% to 80% of cases with a > 50% 5- to 10-year cure rate. Yahalom and colleagues at MSKCC have advocated the role of adjuvant radiation therapy in stage IV disease. Their recommendations are based on the finding that recurrence in advanced HL occurred often in previously unradiated sites.

Follicular small cleaved low-grade lymphomas

and other lymphomas of low-grade histology may indeed transform into the more aggressive histologies, most commonly diffuse large cell lymphomas. A study conducted by the NCI documented a progression to a more aggressive morphology more than 3 months from the original biopsy in approximately 41% of the cases of follicular small cleaved lymphomas. Data from Stanford suggest histologic conversion in approximately 50% of the cases at 8 years. Clonal evolution and effacement of nodal architecture by an increasing contingent of malignant cells is thought to be responsible for this transformation. When this transformation occurs in small lymphocytic lymphoma (CLL), a Richter's syndrome is said to have occurred.

CASE FOLLOW-UP   The decision to treat this patient was based upon the patient's degree of bone marrow involvement and concomitant anemia. The patient underwent six cycles of a CHOP regimen over the course of 6 months. No disease could be seen in his bone marrow, and his lymphadenopathy had fully regressed. He achieved complete remission for approximately 50 weeks thereafter. In the 51st week the patient developed significant lymphadenopathy in both axillae. Biopsy was performed at this time with pathology revealing a transformation to a diffuse large cell NHL.

This patient subsequently underwent further chemotherapy with a DHAP regimen that includes dexamethasone, high dose ara-c, and cis-platinum. He remains disease free at this juncture, approximately 24 months from his last chemotherapy.

• •

BIBLIOGRAPHY

Canellos GP, Nadler L, Takvorian T: Autologous bone marrow transplantation in the treatment of malignant lymphoma and Hodgkin's disease, *Semin Hematol* 25:58-65, 1988.

De Vita VT Jr, Hellman S, Rosenberg SA: Hodgkin's disease and non-Hodgkin's lymphoma. In Devita VT, Hellman S, Rosenberg SA, eds: *Cancer: principles and practices of oncology,* New York, 1993, JB Lippincott.

De Vita VT Jr, Longo DL, Hubbard SM, et al: The lymphomas: biological implications of therapy and therapeutic implications of the new biology. In *Malignant lymphoma,* Baltimore, 1987, Williams & Wilkins.

Glatstein E, Donaldson S, Rosenberg SA, et al: Combined modality therapy in malignant lymphomas, *Cancer Treatment Report* 61:1199-1207, 1977.

Goffinet DR, Warmke R, Dunnik NR, et al: Clinical and surgical evaluation of patients with non-Hodgkin's lymphoma, *Cancer Treatment* 61:981-992, 1977.

Miller TP, Dana BW, Weick JK, et al: The southwest oncology group clinical trials for intermediate and high grade non-Hodgkin's lymphoma, Third International Conference on Malignant Lymphoma (abstract).

Rosenberg SA, Berard CW, Brown BW, et al: The National Cancer Institute sponsored study of complications of non-Hodgkin's lymphomas. Summary and description of a working formulation for clinical usage, *Cancer* 49:2112-2135, 1982.

Rosenberg SA, Kaplan HS, eds: *Malignant lymphomas: etiology, immunology, pathology, treatment,* New York, 1982, Academic Press.

Stein RS: Clinical features and clinical evaluation of Hodgkin's disease and non-Hodgkin's lymphomas. In Bennett JM, ed: *Lymphomas I,* Boston, 1981, Marcus Nijhoff.

CASE

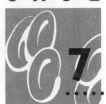

7

Stephen C. Schwartz
Walter Fried

A 46-year-old black man with an extensive tobacco history was evaluated by emergency services for a 2-day history of cough productive of yellow sputum with attendant wheezing. Three days before this evaluation he developed symptoms suggestive of an upper respiratory tract infection. There were no complaints of fever, chills, hemoptysis, nausea, vomiting, or diarrhea. On initial assessment the patient appeared in no apparent respiratory distress, was afebrile, and manifested stable vital signs. The pulmonary examination was remarkable for diffuse soft rhonchi with occasional wheezes. The remainder of the examination was unremarkable. A routine CBC was within normal limits: the WBC was 8.0, Hgb 15, and HCT 38. The mean corpuscular volume (MCV) was 90 Fl. A PA and lateral CXR was obtained demonstrating no consolidative changes. The patient was sent home on a 10-day course of Bactrim and ventolin inhaler for a presumed bronchitis with a component of reactive airway disease. Follow-up was arranged in the outpatient setting.

Approximately 18 hours after leaving, the patient was returned to the emergency room by family members who stated that the patient had complained of extreme weakness and lightheadedness and promptly collapsed while in his kitchen. On reevaluation the patient appeared stuporous with a blood pressure of 75/40 mm Hg which responded well to a 500 cc saline challenge. Physical examination was unchanged. ABGs drawn displayed excellent oxygenation and ventilation on 2 L O_2. ECG revealed sinus tach without acute changes. Repeat CBC was remarkable for a Hgb of 5 g/dl and a HCT of 17%. The MCV was 92 fl. A full chemistry panel was significant for a prominent increase in the unconjugated fraction of bilirubin and an elevated LDH. The urine was 4+ positive for blood although RBCs were not detected on microscopic examination.

QUESTION I What is the approach to patients with newly diagnosed anemia?

Anemia is the result of (1) effective blood loss, (2) inadequate bone marrow production of red cell mass, or (3) hemolysis. Anemia may result from the loss of red blood cells or from the loss of hemoglobin. A Hgb less than 14 mg/dl or HCT less than 42% in men, and a Hgb less than 12 mg/dl or HCT less than 37% in women is considered anemic. The evaluation of a patient with newly diagnosed anemia should begin with an extensive history and physical examination. Attention to race, sex, and ancestral origin should be routine. Individuals of color have a higher incidence of sickle cell anemia while patients of Mediterranean origins manifest glucose 6-phosphate dehydrogenase (G6PD) deficiency and thalassemias more frequently. Female patients will present with iron deficiency anemia in a high percentage of cases. Concomitant medical illnesses are also to be gleaned from the history as should present medications. Anemic patients may present asymptomatically or with signs or symptoms such as pallor, dyspnea, or chest pain.

Routine workup of anemia should always include a data base consisting of Hgb concentration, HCT value, mean corpuscular volume (MCV), mean corpuscular hemoglobin concentration (MCHC), and reticulocyte count. A peripheral blood smear is essential in providing morphology of red blood cells that may be diagnostic in particular cases. In approaching the patient with anemia, several key questions may help in identifying the underlying etiology of anemia. These include (1) what is the MCV, (2) what is the mechanism of anemia, and (3) what are the concomitant medical illnesses or pertinent historical facts?

The value of the MCV provides an index of the red cell size. This index represents an average over a large population of cells and may be misleading when two types of anemia with differing cell populations exist simultaneously. MCV values between 80 and 100 fl are considered within the normal range, and cells thus described are considered *normocytic*. Cells with an MCV less than 80 fl are described as *microcytic* and those greater than 100 fl *macrocytic*. The differential diagnosis of associated etiologies for each of these categories of cell size is relatively well-defined. Thus, the MCV is an excellent point from which to begin a diagnostic inquiry. Common entities causing anemia in patients with low MCVs include iron deficiency and thalassemia. High MCVs are seen in such entities as liver failure, megaloblastosis related to B_{12} or folate deficiency, myelodysplastic syndromes, alcoholism, myelophthisis, and a variety of drugs. Reticulocytosis may produce a MCV out of the normal range. The differential diagnosis of processes giving rise to normocytic anemia is extensive. The ability to divide this category into normocytic anemias with appropriate versus non-appropriate reticulocyte indices provides more manageability. The reticulocyte count assesses the marrow response to anemia. Reticulocytes make up 1% of new cells released from the bone marrow per day. High reticulocyte counts suggest a marrow response to anemia. The reticulocyte index provides a measure of appropriateness of that response for any given degree of anemia. Normocytic anemias with appropriate responses include hemolysis and bleeding. Inappropriate reticulocyte indices are observed in normocytic anemias such as those of chronic disease and renal failure.

The second question, that of defining the mechanism of anemia, can also be answered by using the reticulocyte count and index. In anemia of recent onset the bone marrow, under the stimulation of erythropoietin, may increase its production upwards of ten fold. This increase in production manifests in a high retic count. Anemia resulting from limited red cell production has reticulocyte indices of less than 3%. Patients suffering from hemorrhage or hemolysis demonstrate reticulocyte indices of greater than 3%.

The hematocrit is also useful in defining mechanisms of hemolysis. Patients whose marrow is completely unable to produce cells will, in the absence of hemorrhage or hemolysis, decrease their HCT approximately 4% per week. A greater rate of fall in the hematocrit suggests hemorrhage or hemolysis. The finding of an appropriate reticulocyte index in the setting of anemia in the absence of bleeding suggests hemolysis.

The association of anemias with particular diseases or medical problems is well-known. This fact allows the physician to focus on the history, culling out possible associations between symptoms and diseases while relating them to patterns of anemia. It is not uncommon for a newly discovered anemia to lead to an underlying diagnosis, while the corollary is also often true. Thus, the finding of a microcytic anemia in the setting of guaiac positive stool may lead one to consider colorectal cancer, while patients with hypertension on alpha-methyldopa should be followed for signs of hemolysis. (See Figs. 7-7-1, 7-7-2, and 7-7-3 on p. 411.)

QUESTION 2   The patient was transferred to the intensive care unit with a blood pressure of 100/60. A review of the peripheral smear demonstrated polychromasia, small numbers of spherocyte and bite cells. The reticulocyte count was estimated at 5.0. How is this patient's rapidly progressive anemia and cardiovascular compromise categorized?

The above profile is consistent with a hemolytic process. The elevated reticulocyte count, normal MCV, and rapidity of the event all suggest a hemolytic process. An elevated LDH is also in keeping with diagnosis. The determination of the haptoglobin may also aid in the diagnosis because a decrease in this parameter suggests a hemolytic process.

Red blood cells may undergo lysis in the intravascular space or more commonly they may be sequestered by the monocyte-macrophage system in both the liver and spleen where they undergo extravascular destruction and breakdown. Antierythrocyte-directed antibodies of the warm-agglutinin type are representative of this category. These antibodies may be associated with (1) autoimmune disorders of which SLE and RA are prominent, (2) neoplasms such as lymphoma and multiple myeloma, (3) infection most commonly from EBV and mycoplasma, and (4) idiopathic sources based on exclusion of other diagnosis and a number of drug reactions.

Erythrocytes may be cleared from the circulation in one of two ways. Bound immunoglobulin directed at red cell membrane antigen determinants may be present to which macrophages in the spleen or liver may specifically bind. In this case the bound antibody is usually an IgG molecule. Complement is not activated by IgG in this scenario, and the cell moves to the RE system where Fc receptors are present that attach to the Fc portion of the IgG and facilitate removal from the circulation. The peripheral smear may show microspherocytes. This is known as *warm antibody autoimmune hemolytic anemia* and is due to the presence of bound antibody on the cell surface. The direct Coombs' test is positive in these cases.

Cold antibody autoimmune hemolytic anemia occurs when IgM binds to the red cell surface and activates complement leading to intravascular hemolysis. Anemia is usually more moderate and cyanosis may occur in the tips of the fingers, earlobes, toes, and tip of the nose. This process may be secondary to infection with *Mycoplasma pneumoniae,* Epstein-Barr virus, cytomegalovirus, and immunoproliferative disease. If the IgM is found to be monoclonal, one must strongly consider the presence of an underlying immunoproliferative disease.

Abnormal physical properties of RBC membranes that limit their unimpeded traverse of splenic and hepatic capillary beds may produce a hemolytic picture. These defects usually reflect genetically determined abnormalities in RBC structure or function that manifest throughout the RBC lifespan. These defects may represent membrane abnormalities typified by the disorders paroxysmal nocturnal hemoglobinuria (PNH) and hereditary spherocytosis (HS). PNH is an erythrocyte abnormality that is manifest by absence of the complement activation inhibitors, C8 binding protein, decay accelerating factor, and factors H and I on the cell surface. The defect is brought out by the Ham's test or sugar water test wherein changes in pH or osmotic forces, respectively, activate complement and cause hemolysis to a greater extent than in normal cells. Both leukocytes and platelets may be similarly affected, and neutropenia or thrombocytopenia may be the presenting finding. This disease may be a preneoplastic process as a harbinger of future myelofibrosis, myelodysplasia, aplastic anemia, or acute leukemia. An interesting feature is marked abdominal pain due to hemolysis. This presentation may mimic an acute surgical abdomen. Alternately this must be distinguished from the propensity to develop large vessel thrombosis with resultant intestinal, cerebral, splenic, or hepatic thrombosis. Iron deficiency is common; however, replacement can stimulate the release of PNH cells and lead to massive acute hemolysis. Hereditary spherocytosis is an abnormality of the red cell cytoskeleton (deficiency of spectrin) that leads to membrane instability. This is similar to hereditary eliptocytosis.

Disorders of the erythrocyte interior represent intracorpuscular defects leading to hemolytic anemia. Included are the hemoglobinopathies, thalassemias, enzyme defects, and disorders of the hexosmonophosphate shunt such as G6PD deficiency. The presence of an intracorpuscular defect is suggested by (1) the presence of a similar hemolytic disorder in a relative, (2) a history of anemia since childhood, (3) a negative Coombs' test, (4) recurring jaundice or evidence of gallstones before the age of 30, and (5) individuals of Jewish, African, Asian, or Mediterranean extraction who, as a group, manifest a greater frequency of inherited RBC disorders.

Mechanical damage to the RBC membrane from a microangiopathic process occurs in disseminated intravascular coagulation, intravascular prostheses, idiopathic thrombotic thrombocytopenic purpura, as well as the hemolytic uremic syndrome. Red cell destruction may also result from trauma imparted by prosthetic heart valves. The peripheral smear will be useful in arriving at an eventual diagnosis. Confirmatory testing directed at the underlying disorder should be undertaken if any of the above diagnoses are entertained.

QUESTION 3 What are the mechanisms by which drug exposure causes antibody mediated hemolysis?

The use of medications can mediate immune hemolytic anemia. The first mechanism is the *hapten type.* In this situation, the combination of penicillin (as an example) and the red blood cell membrane contribute to the structure of the antigen to which the IgG antibody attaches, facilitating hemolysis. The direct Coombs' test will be positive. The second mechanism is the *quinidine type (innocent-bystander).* In this type, the quinidine-plasma protein complex acts as an immune complex and lands on the surface of the erythrocyte. Activation of complement destroys the erythrocyte as well as the immune complex. The third type is the *alpha-methyldopa variant.* In this case antibodies to erythrocytes are produced de novo leading to hemolysis.

QUESTION 4 How does the peripheral blood smear help the physician arrive at a diagnosis?

Attention to the peripheral blood smear may suggest a particular diagnosis. In general, the presence of schistocytes, burr cells, spherocytes, or microspherocytes may suggest the presence of hemolysis. The presence of spherocytes or eliptocytes may indicate antibody coating RBC membrane or the presence of hereditary spherocytosis or eliptocytosis. Basophilic stippling is common in thalassemia, and if found, warrants a subsequent hemoglobin electrophoresis to discern elevated levels of Hgb A2 and F. Sickling or the presence of Howell-Jolly bodies call for a sickle prep and hemoglobin electrophoresis to be undertaken in the appropriate clinical setting. If neutropenia is a feature, PNH must be strongly considered. A sugar water test and an examination of the urine for hemoglobin and hemosiderin helps confirm the diagnosis of PNH. If the marrow were to reveal ringed sideroblasts, one must consider the presence of a myelodysplastic syndrome.

Enzyme defects rarely manifest in morphologic changes in the peripheral blood smear. These disorders are discernible by their clinical association with provocative agents such as infection and drug exposure as seen with G6PD deficiency. Bite cells, characterized by asymmetric hemoglobin placement inside the cell, are seen in states of oxidative hemolysis such as G6PD deficiency.

QUESTION 5 What is the significance of finding positive blood without the presence of red blood cells on urinalysis?

The determination of blood by dipstick urinalysis depends on the lysis of red cells on the surface of the dipstick and reaction with free hemoglobin. Therefore, free hemoglobin also triggers a positive response without the presence of red blood cells. Furthermore, myoglobin will produce a positive test for blood on dipstick urinalysis. When the binding capacity of haptoglobin for hemoglobin is exceeded, free hemoglobin enters the glomeruli. Most hemoglobin is reabsorbed by the renal tubular cells; however, when hemolysis is severe and intravascular, the reabsorbtive capacity of the tubular cell is exceeded and free hemoglobin spills into urine. The result is urine positive for blood without the presence of RBCs. Urine free hemoglobin is responsible for the change in urine color. The key to clarifying this dilemma is the microscopic analysis. If red blood cells are not seen, the differential is limited to the presence of free hemoglobin as in hemolytic anemia or myoglobin in rhabdomyolysis. The clinical presentation must then dictate further workup.

QUESTION 6 What is the most probable diagnosis and what factors promoted the development of this process?

The patient under discussion presents with a rapidly progressive hemolytic anemia probably related to an underlying enzymatic G6PD deficiency. G6PD deficiency is the most common enzymopathy that leads to hemolysis (the second is pyruvate kinase deficiency). This is an X-linked disorder prominent in black and eastern Mediterranean populations. Because males will manifest the gene as hemizygotes, they will be afflicted more severely than females. There exist over 300 variant loci coding for this enzyme. The wild type is termed G6PD-B. Black populations exhibit two major variants: G6PD-A and G6PD-A–. G6PD-A is associated with normal levels of enzyme while the G6PD-A– variant loses stability over time and predisposes to hemolytic crises. The Mediterranean type is associated with more severe hemolysis and can lead to renal insufficiency. Those who manifest the deficiency have a dysfunctional cytosolic hexosmonophosphate shunt pathway in their RBCs. This pathway subserves the primary function of regenerating reduced glutathione. The maintenance of glutathione in the reduced state protects sulfhydryl groups on hemoglobin and erythrocyte membranes from oxidation. When these moieties are oxidized, Hgb precipitates in the cell (Heinz bodies) and membrane injury ensues, resulting in hemolysis. As G6PD activity is diminished over the course of the normal RBC life span, only older populations of cells are usually susceptible to hemolysis. Those patients with a normal narrow response may have episodic anemia without clinical sequelae.

A hemolytic crisis may be precipitated by environmental stressors such as viral or bacterial infections. It may also be induced by challenge with certain medications that act as oxidants,

COMMON MEDICATIONS ASSOCIATED WITH HEMOLYSIS IN PATIENTS WITH G6PD

- Nalidixic acid
- Nitrofurantoin
- Sulfanilamide
- Methylene blue
- Pamaquine
- Sulfacetamide
- Sulfapyridine
- Trinitrotoluene
- Primaquine
- Niridazole
- Sulfamethoxazole

especially in patients with hepatic and renal disease. In this case the hemolysis was related to the sulfa moiety on the trimethoprim-sulfamethoxazole used as a treatment for bronchitis. Agents that may trigger a crisis include antimalarial and other drugs, ingestion of raw fava beans, or recurrent infection. The clinical spectrum ranges from chronic intermittent anemia to acute episodes of shock, severe hemolytic anemia, and renal failure (see box).

QUESTION 7 What are the significant clues to the diagnosis in this case?

Clues to the diagnosis here include the rapid onset of the anemia and profound drop in hematocrit in the absence of hemorrhage and in temporal relation to exposure to provocating factors: the administration of a sulfa agent coincident with probable viral infection. This patient was also found to have an exceedingly low level of haptoglobin, a plasma protein and acute phase reactant taken up by the monocyte-macrophage system that functions to scavenge free hemoglobin. Exceedingly low or absent levels of haptoglobin suggests intravascular or extravascular hemolysis.

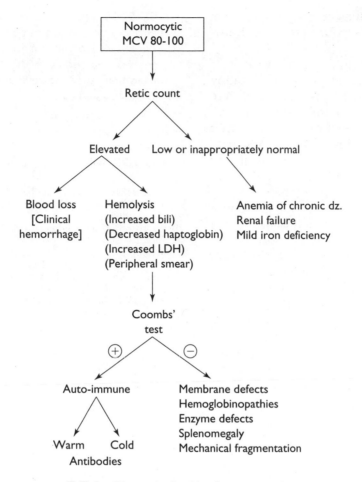

7-7-1   Diagnostic algorithm for normocytic anemia.

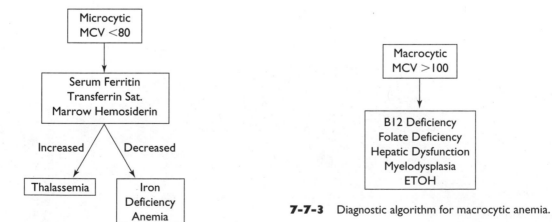

7-7-2   Diagnostic algorithm for microcytic anemia.

7-7-3   Diagnostic algorithm for macrocytic anemia.

QUESTION 8 What is the correct management of this patient once the hemolytic process is discovered?

Effective therapy was directed at eliminating the provocating agent, in this case Bactrim. Severe effective intravascular volume depletion can highlight coronary, mesenteric, renal, carotid, or cerebral atherosclerotic insufficiency. Adequate IV fluid administration should be provided to ensure adequate renal perfusion in an attempt to limit tubular damage. Alkalinizing the urine may also be of benefit. Cardiovascular compromise seen early in any case of hemolysis suggests a severe hemolytic event demanding close observation on the part of the clinician. Blood transfusion should be avoided unless significant sequelae of anemia are encountered. Prevention should always be encouraged. Discussion with the patient and family regarding the disease and its managment is essential. Patients should be supplied with a list of agents to avoid. In select cases, splenectomy has proven helpful in managing patients with severe chronic hemolytic anemia.

CASE SUMMARY Confirmation of the G6PD deficiency was carried out by laboratory methods. This patient did well over a 3-day hospital course and was sent home with a list of provocating medications and foodstuffs to avoid.

• •

BIBLIOGRAPHY

Arese P, DeFlora A: Pathophysiology of hemolysis in glucose-6-phosphate dehydrogenase deficiency, *Semin Hematol* 27:1, 1990.

Dessypris EN: Abnormal hematocrit. In Stien JH, ed: *Internal medicine*, St Louis, 1993, Mosby.

Kellermeyer RW: General principles of the evaluation and therapy of anemias, *Med Clin North Am* 68:533, 1984.

Sokol RJ, Hewitt S: Autoimmune hemolysis a critical review, *Crit Rev Oncol Hematol* 4:125, 1985.

Valentine WN, Tanaka KR, Paglia DE: Hemolytic anemias and erythrocyte enzymopathies, *Ann Intern Med* 103:245, 1985.

C A S E

8

Stephen C. Schwartz
Walter Fried

....

A 33-year-old man with no significant medical history came to emergency services, offering complaints of bleeding gums and a skin rash that has progressively worsened over a 2-day period. This patient has been in his stable state of excellent health until approximately 1 month ago, when he was involved in a motor vehicle accident. At that time the patient was seen in the emergency room for neck and back pain and was diagnosed with a C-spine flexion extension injury. A soft collar was provided, nonsteroidals given for pain, and a muscle relaxant administered for relief of spasms. The patient did well over 1 week until he noted modest bleeding from his gums after brushing his teeth. He also noted a diffuse skin eruption over his trunk and upper and lower extremities. The lower extremities were most prominently involved. The patient's neck and back pain had diminished by this time, and he discontinued his NSAIDs and muscle relaxants. The bleeding gums and eruption subsequently resolved over a 5-day period.

Two weeks later he reinjured his neck and back during an athletic event, and subsequently restarted the muscle relaxants and pain medications. Four days later the skin eruption and bleeding gums returned. Both problems were now more pronounced. In the emergency room, the patient was found to have stable vital signs. A nonblanching, nonpalpable petechial rash was distributed over his trunk and upper and lower extremities. Also noted were palatal petechiae and gingiva with oozing and dried blood. The remainder of his physical examination was unremarkable. The patient offered no history of a familial bleeding disorder or a propensity for prolonged bleeding or easy bruisability. The patient offered no recent history of upper respiratory tract infection and denied any and all gastrointestinal complaints.

QUESTION 1 What is the approach to patients with new skin lesions?

A thorough history and physical examination are essential to the assessment of new alterations in the skin. Skin lesions may represent a primary dermatologic entity or be the manifestation of a specific systemic disease. In generating a differential diagnosis, the physician must evaluate the patient profile, inspect and categorize the type of lesions present, and finally process this information with the remainder of the history and physical examination. The use of the INDOCIN model (infection, neoplasia, drug effect, occupation, connective tissue or cardiovascular disease, idiopathic, noninfectious/granulomatous) works well when formulating a differential diagnosis for a new skin lesion. Historical information to be gleaned from the patient should include (1) the presence of other symptoms such as fever, arthralgia, or fatigue; (2) current or newly initiated medications; (3) the presence of pruritis, burning, or pain; (4) a history of allergies or photosensitivities; (5) what relieves and what exacerbates lesions and/or symptoms; and (6) concurrent medical illnesses.

Patients should be examined while completely disrobed in adequate lighting. Physicians should first view patients from 1 to 2 meters, allowing for accurate assessment of general skin appearance and patterns of distribution. Lesions should be assessed for distribution, type of primary lesion, size, and pattern. The presence of blanching should be determined. Assessment of a lesion's proclivity to cross the midline or to involve mucosa should also be made.

A multitude of descriptive terms exist for characterizing dermatologic lesions. These terms should be mastered for their importance in generating a differential diagnosis. Common terms include macule, patch, papule, nodule, plaque, vesicle, bulla, cyst, wheal, telangiectasia, tumor, and pustule. A *macule* represents a flat, nonraised colored lesion less than 2 cm in diameter. A *patch* has the same attributes, but it is greater than 2 cm in size. *Papules* are solid lesions less than 1 cm in diameter raised above surrounding skin. A *nodule* resembles a papule but is between 1 to 5 cm in diameter. A *tumor* is greater than 5 cm. *Plaques* are flat, often raised lesions greater than 1 cm whose edges may be distinct or merge with the surrounding skin. *Vesicles* and *pustules* are raised, fluid-filled lesions, the former being less than 1 cm while the latter is filled with leukocytes. *Bullae* are fluid-filled translucent lesions greater than 1 cm in diameter. *Cysts* are soft and raised lesions with semisolid or liquid contents. *Wheals* are circular erythematous plaques or papules that are ephemeral and represent dermal edema. *Telangiectasias* are dilated superficial vessels. Lesions may be described as *lichenified*, thickened skin demonstrating increased skin fold markings, or *crusting* representing the dried exudate of bodily fluids. Hyperkeratotic lesions have an increased amount of pigment from high numbers of keratinocytes in the basal layer of the dermis. *Purpura* and *petechia* are nonblanching lesions caused by the extravasation of red blood cells into the dermis. They may be palpable or nonpalpable. Petechia are less than 2 mm, purpura greater than 3 mm. Common causes of nonpalpable purpura include trauma, solar purpura, thrombocytopenia, thrombasthenia, capillary fragility disorders, TTP, DIC, and cholesterol emboli. Palpable purpura are grouped into embolic and vasculitic categories. The latter group encompasses leukocytoclastic vasculitis, Henoch-Schönlein purpura, and periarteritis nodosa. Embolic purpura may be resultant to septic emboli with gram-positive or gram-negative organisms. Most noteworthy are meningococcus- and gonococcus-induced emboli. *Pseudomonas* and *Klebsiella* may also produce purpura in either localized or disseminated disease. *Candida* and *Aspergillus* species may produce petechia and purpura in the immunocompromised patient.

Evaluation of skin lesions also involves laboratory investigation. Pathologic assessment of new lesions is easily accomplished by excisional or punch biopsy. If an infectious source is sought, gram stain of extravasated contents, KOH prep, Tzanck smear, or Wood's lamp may be helpful. If a hypersensitivity reaction is suspected, a patch test may be undertaken to disclose the offending agent.

QUESTION 2 Routine laboratory analysis in the emergency room was remarkable for a platelet count of 15,000. The hemoglobin was 15 and the hematocrit 42. All other routine chemistries were within normal limits. Both the prothrombin and partial thromboplastin time were within normal parameters. Describe the role of platelets in normal hemostasis? What are the abnormalities seen in hemostasis when abnormal platelet number or function is present?

Platelets are the anuclear end products of the megakaryocytic cell line after fragmentation in the bone marrow. Subsequent to megakaryocytic fragmentation, platelets enter the circulation with a lifespan of 7 to 10 days. Upwards of 30% of the total platelet population will be sequestered in the spleen at any given time. In concert with the intrinsic and extrinsic arms of the coagulation cascade, platelets represent a principal component in the maintenance of adequate hemostasis. Platelets are the key component of primary hemostasis. In a receptor-mediated fashion, platelets bind to denuded collagen fibers of damaged vasculature. The primary hemostatic plug requires normal platelet interaction with the vessel wall (denuded subendothelial collagen), von-Willebrand's factor (responsible for the anchoring of platelets to the subendothelium), factor XIII (used to cross-link fibrin strands stabilizing the fibrin plug), thromboxane A_2 (a powerful platelet activator and vasoconstrictant), and fibrinogen. Physical findings accompanying a dysfunctional platelet population or an absolute decrement in platelet count include mucosal hemorrhage, easy bruisability, purpura, and petechia. Evaluation of the interaction between the platelet and the vessel wall is via the bleeding time. Prolongation of the bleeding time suggests thrombocytopenia or abnormal platelet function. Hemostatic abnormalities seen with platelet dysfunction include immediate bleeding after trauma or surgery. Disorders of platelet receptive binding as may occur in von Willebrand's disease may give rise to a clinically significant bleeding diathesis.

QUESTION 3 Define both thrombocytosis and thrombocytopenia.

Thrombocytosis is an absolute increase in the platelet count greater than 450,000 per µl. The platelet count may vary within normal physiologic parameters. Platelet count elevation is often found following ovulation and subsequently falls before the onset of menses. A reactive thrombocytosis is commonly seen in such clinical settings as infection, hemorrhage, malignancy, and other inflammatory disorders. This reactive thrombocytosis represents a benign condition. Thrombocytosis that accompanies the myeloproliferative disorders may give rise to pathologic hemorrhage or thrombosis resulting from the presence of high numbers of abnormally functioning platelets. Thrombocytosis is also seen in patients who have recently undergone splenectomy.

Thrombocytopenia, an absolute decrement in the platelet count to less than 150,000 per microliter, is a common clinical entity. Platelet counts may also rise and fall depending upon the nutritional status of the patient. Patients deprived of iron, B_{12}, or folate may have impaired platelet production by the bone marrow. The physician must guard against the presence of pseudothrombocytopenia. This entity occurs when platelets clump in a collection tube filled with EDTA or in

the presence of low levels of cold-agglutinins. In these scenarios platelet number is underestimated by mechanized counters.

QUESTION 4 What are the mechanisms of thrombocytopenia?

Mechanisms that produce thrombocytopenia fall into one of three broad categories. First, decrements in platelet number may be due to inadequate bone marrow production. Second, accelerated destruction may result from both nonimmune and immunologically mediated processes. Third, splenic sequestration brought about by passive congestion or active splenic infiltration as in malignancy may decrease platelet count.

Thrombocytopenia may result from direct insults to bone marrow progenitor cells. Infiltration of the marrow, known as a myelophthisic process, occurs when malignant or abnormal cells replace actively dividing marrow cells. Leukemias, lymphomas, and metastases from distant malignancies may infiltrate the marrow, producing pancytopenia. This process gives rise to a decrement in platelet production. Leukopenia and anemia often accompany thrombocytopenia in this setting as all cell lines are often equally involved. Direct toxins affecting bone marrow include numerous and varied chemotherapeutic agents, ethanol, radiation, chemicals, and assorted drugs including thiazide diuretics and estrogens. A congenital disorder that may produce a marrow devoid of the megakaryocytic cell line is congenital megakaryocytic hypoplasia and the thrombocytopenia found with toxic radii syndrome or TAR. A definitive diagnosis for the majority of cases is made by examination of the bone marrow, in which case an aspirate and biopsy are usually required. The results of this examination interpreted in the correct clinical context usually suggest a primary marrow production failure. A decrement of megakaryocytes in the marrow often suggests a primary production abnormality.

Thrombocytopenia may be the result of accelerated platelet destruction. Destruction may be mediated by nonimmunologic or immunologic mechanisms. Nonimmunologic mechanisms include consumptive processes such as DIC, HUS, or TTP, as well as a number of the vasculitides. Prosthetic heart valves, intravascular grafts, and intraaortic balloon pumps in the critical care setting also impart trauma to the platelet. Other nonimmunologically mediated mechanisms of platelet destruction include extracorporeal circulation in the form of dialysis, hypoxemia, fat emboli, extensive burns, acute glomerulonephritis, and direct infection by bacteria and viruses.

Immunologically mediated mechanisms of platelet destruction are often based on the generation of antibodies directed at platelet membrane proteins de novo or to various immunogens whose antibody cross reacts with platelet moieties. These platelets are subsequently removed by the monocyte-macrophage system in spleen and liver. A classic example of the former mechanism is that typified by idiopathic thrombocytopenic purpura (ITP). A multitude of drugs may act to transform platelet membranes, generating neoantigen and a subsequent immune response in the form of IgG. Platelet destruction is the end result through the activation of the terminal attack complex of complement. Drug-antibody immune complexes may interact with the FAB component in the platelet membrane activating complement-mediated platelet destruction. An example is the thrombocytopenia associated with heparin use.

Thrombocytopenia is associated with HIV infection and is largely immunologic. Indeed, thrombocytopenia may be an initial presentation of HIV infection. Mechanisms thought to mediate thrombocytopenia in this setting include nonspecific deposition of immune complex and complement onto platelet surface and specific IgG directed against platelet surface membrane proteins. The demonstration of increased numbers of megakaryocytes in the bone marrow help establish the diagnosis of an immunologically mediated thrombocytopenia. Specific tests for the detection of platelet directed antibody are also available for

routine use and are helpful in confirming the diagnosis.

Sequestration of platelets in the spleen is a common etiology of mild-to-moderate thrombocytopenia. Severe thrombocytopenia leading to a clinically significant bleeding diathesis is a rare occurrence. Splenic sequestration, or pooling, is said to exist when an increased percentage of the total platelet mass is held within the spleen. This pooling is thought to result from any of a number of underlying mechanisms including (1) a decreased velocity of platelet passage through splenic sinusoids, (2) increased interaction/cohesion between platelet, macrophage, and endothelial cells, or (3) a combination of the above mechanisms. Splenic sequestration is a common manifestation of those disorders that lead to passive splenic congestion. These include congestive heart failure, amyloidosis, hemochromatosis, glycogen or lipid storage disorders, lymphoproliferative and myeloproliferative malignancies, and severe portal hypertension from hepatic vein thrombosis or accompanying end-stage liver disease. Physical examination may reveal signs of liver or heart failure. An enlarged spleen is detectable in the majority of cases when sequestration is seriously considered. Ultrasonography may also be useful in confirming the existence of splenomegaly. (See Fig. 7-8-1 on p. 419.)

QUESTION 5 What is the goal of therapy for thrombocytopenia? What is the treatment for thrombocytopenia for the above mentioned etiologies?

Traditionally, therapy for thrombocytopenia has been directed toward maintaining a platelet count of greater than 20,000 platelets per microliter or a level above which active bleeding is aborted. Recent data confirm the safety of maintaining a platelet count greater than 10,000. Platelet counts of less than 10,000 are associated with a higher incidence of spontaneous hemorrhage in the central nervous system.

The use of platelet transfusion should be reserved for those patients who cannot maintain a platelet count greater than 10,000 or in those patients with life-threatening hemorrhage. Platelet transfusion is indicated in the thrombocytopenic patient before invasive procedures such as lumbar puncture and arterial or central venous catheter placement. Platelet transfusion can be administered in the form of (1) pooled random donor platelet fractions, (2) single donor fractions, or (3) HLA-matched platelets. Patients receiving multiple pooled random donor or single donor platelets may produce platelet-directed antibodies leading to a decrement in platelet transfusion responsiveness. Furthermore, since these products are made from the contributions of many people, the risk of transmitted infection is therefore greater (i.e., HIV and hepatitis B and C). HLA-matched transfusions ideally do not provoke an immune response and are therefore useful in treating those patients not responsive to random or single donor platelets.

Treatment of patients whose thrombocytopenia is resultant to a decreased marrow production revolves around regeneration of an active marrow. To this end, the discontinuation of a marrow-toxic agent may be sufficient in restoring a normal platelet count. One should not overlook nutritional deficiencies as an etiology of thrombocytopenia with a simple solution. Patients who have infiltrated marrows present special problems, as they will often require chemotherapy or radiotherapy for their underlying disease process. This will have the effect of prolonging and/or worsening the degree of thrombocytopenia. Those patients will require platelet transfusion to maintain adequate platelet levels until bone marrow recovery. Recently the discovery of thrombopoietin, an endogenous colony stimulating factor specific for the megakaryocytic cell line, has met with much acclaim. It is hoped that the eventual production of large quantities of recombinant thrombopoietin will obviate the need for repeated transfusions in cancer patients receiving marrow toxic chemotherapy. This drug may also be of benefit in patients with such disorders as ITP where its use

may augment platelet production, shifting the balance away from consumption to production with the subsequent maintenance of higher, safer platelet levels.

Patients with accelerated platelet destruction of nonimmunologic etiology related to prosthetic valves or balloon pumps seldom have a clinically significant bleeding diathesis. Removal of the hardware in the case of the intraaortic balloon pump will often restore normal platelet levels. Consumptive processes such as DIC or TTP require treatment aimed at the appropriate underlying process often requiring hospital admission and treatment. In the latter plasmapheresis and prednisone at 1 mg/kg/day has been shown to decrease mortality in several small trials and remains first-line therapy. In the former, low dose heparin and fresh frozen plasma transfusions with the goal of maintaining fibrinogen levels greater than 200 have been advocated.

Immune-mediated processes of platelet destruction such as idiopathic thrombocytopenic purpura in its pure form or antibody mediated platelet destruction related to malignancies may respond to corticosteroids. Although of unproven benefit in changing outcome, the use of corticosteriods is considered important first-line therapy. Steroids serve to down-regulate the avidity of Fc receptors on macrophages active in immune-mediated removal of platelets from the circulation. They also stabilize microvasculature, diminishing a tendency toward spontaneous hemorrhage. The use of intravenous gamma-globulin to saturate receptors on macrophages, limiting the uptake and destruction of antibody-coated platelets, has also been advocated. Splenectomy should be considered a viable treatment option in refractory or severe cases. Long-term benefit may be gained; however, only temporary improvement from this particular intervention is the norm. The use of immunosuppressive agents such as azathioprine or vincristine alone or in combination with systemic corticosteroids may be required in severe cases of thrombocytopenia. Platelet transfusion may be required in refractory cases where platelet counts are below 10,000 and where hemorrhage remains a significant problem. Immunologically mediated thrombocytopenia related to drug administration is usually treated by prompt removal of the offending agent. The discontinuation of any antiplatelet medication (i.e., aspirin, NSAIDs, and omega-3 fatty acids) should always be stressed. Platelet counts often return to normal within days. In severe cases the use of corticosteroids may be helpful. In 70% to 90% of HIV associated thrombocytopenia, systemic corticosteriods produce a favorable response and are well tolerated by the patient. Danazol, a synthetic androgen agent, has proven helpful in HIV induced thrombocytopenia as well as that produced by ITP. Splenectomy, as well as the use of intravenous gammaglobulin, has also been efficacious in this setting. Within days of the administration of AZT, platelet counts are found to rise to significant levels.

Patients with splenic sequestration rarely have clinically significant thrombocytopenia, and therefore splenectomy is seldom indicated. Treatment of the underlying condition, whether it be a shunt procedure to relieve portal hypertension, or chemotherapy to reduce tumor burden in the spleen, usually ameliorates the condition. When splenomegaly and thrombocytopenia are profound, splenectomy may be required. In chronic lymphocytic leukemia where spleen size is very large and immune-mediated and marrow production mechanisms of thrombocytopenia are at work, splenectomy may be required.

The functional capacity of the platelet must also be considered when selecting a suitable serum platelet level to maintain. In general, dysfunctional or *thromboasthenic* platelets are often found in systemic disease such as uremia and liver failure. Dysfunctional platelets are also found in congenital disorders. Primary platelet disorders may result from abnormal intracellular granules or release reaction (elaboration of ADP and fibrinogen) or abnormalities in the components of the primary hemostatic plug as seen in von-Willebrand's disease and Glanzmann's thrombas-

thenia (an abnormality in platelet clumping). These disorders require higher platelet counts to maintain the same degree of hemostasis. For treatment of the hemostatic abnormality of renal failure, use of desmopressin (DDAVP), a synthetic analog of vasopressin, can normalize the bleeding time. This agent works by stimulating endothelial cell production of von Willebrand's factor to help overcome a lack of platelet adhesion. Use of conjugated estrogens has a more prolonged effect than DDAVP. In uremia, transfusion of cryoprecipitate, a concentration of factor VIII and fibrinogen, has been found to be useful.

QUESTION 6 Should patients with thrombocytosis be treated? If so, how are they managed?

Patients with platelet counts greater than 1 million per cubic milliliter are at high risk for thrombotic events, although many patients live for years with counts this high without incident. Patients at risk for thrombosis from other causes (malignancy,) who have concomitant thrombocytosis with platelet counts over 1 million should be treated. There are several measures that may be helpful in avoiding thrombotic complications of thrombocytosis. Treatment of the underlying etiology of the thrombocytosis often suffices in bringing platelet numbers down below 1 million. Low doses of aspirin taken daily serve to irreversibly inhibit platelet function. The use of the drug anegralide has been recently evaluated for its capacity to reduce platelet counts. Results are encouraging.

QUESTION 7 What is the etiology of this patient's thrombocytopenia? How should he be managed?

The case described herein demonstrates a classic drug-induced thrombocytopenia. This patient's prescribed muscle relaxant, Robaxisol, has indeed been associated with such phenomena. The concomitant use of nonsteroidal antiinflammatory agents may have led to potentiation of the

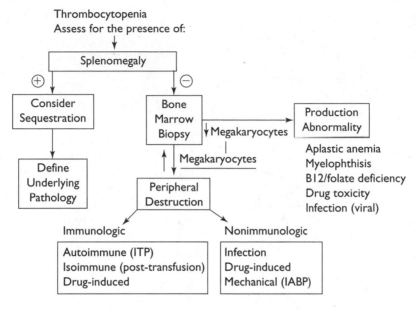

7-8-1 Thrombocytopenia decision tree.

effect. The recrudescence of the physical findings shortly after restarting this medication lends support to the diagnosis. Management should consist of an immediate discontinuation of the offending agent, Robaxisol, and the patient's nonsteroidal agent. A bone marrow aspirate and biopsy, as well as an HIV test, should be obtained to rule out other etiologies. He should be admitted for observation and considered for IV steroids. Platelet transfusions are not indicated in this case with platelet counts over 10,000 and minimal bleeding at the time of admission.

CASE FOLLOW-UP With a platelet count of 12,000 the patient was admitted to the hospital for observation, strict bed rest, and high-dose intravenous corticosteroids. The offending medications were immediately dispensed with. The patient did well over a 3-day hospital course, with his platelet count increasing to 65,000 by day 4. A marrow aspirate and biopsy demonstrated a reactive marrow with increased megakaryocytes. An HIV drawn on admission was negative by ELISA.

• •

BIBLIOGRAPHY

Berchtold P, McMillan R: Therapy of chronic idiopathic thrombocytopenia purpura in adults, *Blood* 74:2309, 1989.

Bolognia J, Braverman IM: Skin manifestations in internal disease. In Harrison's *Principles of Internal Medicine* 59:322-338, 1991.

Eisenstaedt R: Blood component therapy in the treatment of platelet disorders, *Semin Hematol* 23:1, 1986.

Karpatkin S: HIV-1 related thrombocytopenia, *Hematol Oncol Clin North Am* 4:193, 1990.

Kelton JG: Advances in the diagnosis and managment of ITP, *Hosp Pract* 20:95, 1985.

Rook A, et al, eds: *Textbook of dermatology*, ed 4, Oxford, 1986, Blackwell Scientific.

Williams WJ, et al, eds: *Hematology*, ed 4, New York, 1990, McGraw-Hill.

CASE

9

Stephen C. Schwartz
Walter Fried

• • • • • • • • • •

A 68-year-old woman with a medical history remarkable for multiple myeloma presented to emergency services after developing a productive cough, dyspnea, and fever to 104° F over a 3-day course.

She was found to have blood pressure of 60/40 mm Hg, pulse of 130 bpm, respiratory rate 35/min, and temperature of 104° F rectally. She was lethargic but responsive to commands. Cursory physical examination was remarkable for decreased breath sounds and rales at the (R) base. A grade II/VI systolic murmur was auscultated at the left lower sternal border radiating to the carotids. The abdomen was normal. The skin was cool and capillary refill poor. Prominent ecchymoses were noted on both upper and lower extremities. Petechiae were present on examination of the palate and mucous membranes. Central venous access was established, and the patient's blood pressure increased to 70/50 mm Hg with a 300 cc normal saline fluid challenge. A dopamine infusion was initiated and was titrated to a systolic pressure of 90.

QUESTION I Fever, cough, and dyspnea are suggestive of pneumonia. What are the most likely pathogens in this patient presenting from home?

The diagnostic approach to the patient with pneumonia should include a methodical assessment of (1) *the host,* including the patient profile (age, concomitant illness, and immune status: compromised versus noncompromised) and (2) *the area of acquisition* (community versus hospital versus nursing home). Patients may also be grouped into *typical* versus *atypical* pneumonias. Different age cohorts are prone to develop par-

ticular types of pneumonia. Although not absolute, individuals under the age of 40 are more likely to suffer from community acquired atypical pneumonias. This group of atypical pneumonias include viral, mycoplasma, chlaymidial, and protozoan pathogens. Atypical refers not only to the type of organism responsible for the infection but also the clinical presentation. Atypical pneumonias often present with a prodrome of myalgias, malaise, fever, and headache. Subsequent to this, a nonproductive cough ensues. Dyspnea and respiratory distress may be apparent in severe cases.

Older patients more commonly develop typical pneumonias. Pathogens included in this group are *Streptococcus pneumoniae, Staphylococcus aureus, Haemophilus influenza,* and *Klebsiella pneumoniae.* Older patients are also more apt to develop legionellosis and pneumonias caused by group B strep species. Presentations of typical pneumonia include the abrupt onset of shaking chills, a cough productive of rusty sputum, fever, and pleuritic chest pain.

Concomitant illnesses often predispose to a particular pathogen. *H. influenza* and *B. catarrhalis* are common pathogens in patients with COPD, while *Klebsiella* and anaerobic bacteria are common offenders in alcoholics. *S. aureus* and *S. pneumoniae* often develop as a superinfection following initial infection with influenza A or B virus. Disorders of immune regulation may result in a host susceptible not only to typical and atypical agents but to pathogens that ordinarily do not possess a high degree of virulence. Dysregulated cell-mediated immunity, such as that occurring in acquired immunodeficiency, may give rise to pulmonary infections with such agents as

Pneumocystis carinii. In the bone marrow transplant setting, CMV pneumonia develops in a well-defined number of these profoundly immunocompromised patients. Patients possessing impaired humoral immunity may have heightened susceptibility to infections with encapsulated organisms such as *S. pneumoniae* and *K. pneumoniae*. Patients who are anatomically or functionally asplenic and those with plasma cell dyscrasias are two examples of patients falling into this category.

Chest x-ray will be helpful in diagnosing a pneumonia; it is, however, less likely to define a pathogen. Studies have demonstrated the roentgenographic examination's lack of specificity in distinguishing typical from atypical pneumonias. The CXR is even less specific in defining a causative agent.

Ultimately diagnosis will rest on the ability of the physician to identify a possible organism on gram stain and isolate it in sputum or blood culture. Immunologic techniques have also been developed for the identification of various organisms (i.e., titers for mycoplasma and legionella). Given this patient's age and history of multiple myeloma, a pulmonary infection with an encapsulated organism found in the community is highly likely and should direct subsequent workup and initial therapy.

QUESTION 2 A chest x-ray demonstrated complete right lower lobe consolidation. The patient was pancultured and started on an antibiotic regimen consisting of vancomycin and ceftazidime for treatment of presumed pneumonia and sepsis. On subsequent transfer to the intensive care unit she was found to be extravasating copious amounts of serosanguineous fluid from both arterial and venipuncture sites.

Initial ABGs on room air returned as follows: Ph 7.30, $Paco_2$ 20 mm Hg, and a Pao_2 55 mm Hg. A repeat on 50% O_2 improved to pH of 7.32, $Paco_2$ 24 mm Hg, and Pao_2 of 65 mm Hg. The WBC was 30,000 with 70% segs, 20% bands, Hgb 7.5 g/dl, and HCT 25.8%, PLT count 25,000. Na was 138 mEq/L, K 5.4 mEq/L, CL 105 mEq/L, HCO_3 14 mEq/L, BUN 32 mEq/L, and Cr 2.1 g/dl.

Based on the patient's presentation with prominent ecchymotic lesions and palatal/mucous membrane petechiae, what initial coagulation studies would you order?

In the initial evaluation of a possible coagulopathy the most important tests that may yield diagnostic information include platelet count, prothrombin time (PT), activated partial thromboplastin time (APTT), and fibrinogen level. The PT is a measure of the extrinsic coagulation system, whereas the APTT is a measure of the intrinsic coagulation system. The former requires the exposure of blood to tissue thromboplastin, while the latter constitutes surface activation of coagulation proteins. Both the PT and PTT assess the adequacy of the final common hemostatic pathway. This represents the conversion of fibrinogen to fibrin by thrombin. Elevations in PT and/or PTT may suggest diminished concentrations of coagulation factors or functional limitations of these same proteins. These values may be elevated in instances where the enzymatic processes that oppose coagulation are inhibited (i.e., heparin as an agonist of antithrombin III). Platelets, important to the adequacy of the primary hemostasis, may be diminished secondary to a lack of production in the bone marrow, sequestration in the liver and spleen, or increased consumption by immune and nonimmune mechanisms. Fibrinogen is synthesized in the liver. It is ultimately converted to fibrin by thrombin for use in secondary hemostasis. Low levels of fibrinogen may be the result of diminished synthetic output or increased consumption. Abnormalities of fibrinogen or dysfibrogenemias may lead to dysfunctional fibrinogen with no corresponding lowering of the fibrinogen level.

QUESTION 3 A coagulation profile was drawn revealing a PT of 15% (16 sec) and a PTT of 60 sec. The fibrinogen level was 60 mg/dl. What is the differential diagnosis of the coagulopathy in this patient? What additional studies should be ordered to help confirm the diagnosis?

Disorders of coagulation are classified into two broad categories: congenital and acquired. *Congenital* disorders reflect abnormalities in or the absence of single coagulation factors. Most common are the deficiencies of factor VIII, known as hemophilia A, and factor IX, known as hemophilia B. *Acquired* disorders of coagulation occur with greater frequency and manifest as deficiencies in any of several coagulation proteins. As the case presented provides no history of a congenital disorder, discussion will be limited to examination of the differential diagnosis of an acquired coagulopathy, which includes: (1) vitamin K deficiency, (2) hepatic dysfunction, (3) use of vitamin K antagonists, (4) spurious laboratory values or pseudocoagulopathy, (5) transfusion washout, (6) immunologically mediated factor depletion, and (7) disseminated intravascular coagulation.

Vitamin K serves as an essential cofactor in the hepatic synthesis of coagulation proteins II, VII, IX, X, protein C, and protein S. In the absence of vitamin K, specific glutamic acid residues of coagulation factors are unable to undergo gamma-carboxylation. The factor is unable to appropriately bind calcium and phospholipid and participate in clot production. Vitamin K is a fat-soluble vitamin derived from dietary sources that include most green leafy vegetables. It is also synthesized by bacteria in the GI tract. Whether this represents a significant bioavailable source in humans remains unclear. The absence of vitamin K in the diet, problems with its bioassimilation, the administration of broad-spectrum antibiotics, and the presence of vitamin K antagonists may result in a wide spectrum of coagulation abnormalities. These range from laboratory prolongation of the PT and PTT to a frank hemorrhagic diathesis.

Pertinent physical findings may include easy bruisability and ecchymosis. Vitamin K stores may become depleted in the healthy patient within 1 to 2 weeks. In the critically ill patient being maintained NPO and receiving broad-spectrum antimicrobial therapy, the onset of vitamin K deficiency is hastened by a decreased nutritional intake and destruction of vitamin K-producing gut flora by antibiotic therapy. Treatment is reple-tion of vitamin K stores in either oral or intravenous formulations depending upon the presence or absence of a functional GI tract.

The liver serves a primary role in synthetic function related to vitamin K dependent coagulation factors. A modest reduction in serum levels of factors II, V, VII, and X leads to prolongation of the PT and PTT. This may be secondary to (1) a decrease in synthetic capacity secondary to parenchymal destruction, (2) vitamin K deficiency due to malabsorption produced by intrahepatic and/or extrahepatic cholestasis, or (3) vitamin K deficiency derived from nutritional inadequacies (i.e., hepatic failure and poor caloric balance). Bleeding is exacerbated by abnormalities in coagulation and platelet dysfunction. Patients with liver disease are at increased risk for hemorrhagic episodes resulting from structural lesions associated with parenchymal liver disease such as esophageal and gastric varices. The etiology of hepatic failure is often multifactorial in patients who present with cirrhotic liver disease. It is critical that the clinician distinguish between a coagulopathy produced by hepatic dysfunction versus one related to nutritional vitamin K deficiency because the latter is reversible with vitamin K administration. The administration of parenteral vitamin K assures that problems in assimilation related to cholestasis or GI mucosal absorption are bypassed. Failure to improve parameters by parenteral vitamin K administration in doses approaching 10 mg over a 24-hour period suggests a coagulation disorder related to synthetic dysfunction.

The treatment of choice for coagulopathy as a result of hepatic synthetic dysfunction is the use of fresh frozen plasma or cryoprecipitate (a richer supply of factor VIII and fibrinogen). In this manner, factors achieve adequate repletion. These supplements can be given with serial measurement of the PT and PTT until corrected.

Warfarin sodium is an oral anticoagulant often used in the treatment and prophylaxis of thromboembolic disease. Warfarin antagonizes vitamin K dependent carboxylation of coagulation factors required for adequate function. Clinical use is fraught with problems related to over anticoagu-

TABLE 7-9-1 Increased Sensitivity to Warfarin

Vitamin K deficiency	Synergism with Warfarin
Malabsorption syndromes	Vitamin E
Broad spectrum antibiotics	Anabolic steroids
Liquid paraffin	Danazol
Clofibrate	Decreased Warfarin metabolism
Displacement from albumin	Dilantin
Phenylbutazone	Chloramphenicol
Aspirin	Clofibrate
Indomethacin	Tricyclic antidepressants
Sulindac	Erythromycin
Mefenamic acid	Cimetidine
Tolemtin	Bactrim
Ibuprofen	Sulfinpyrazone
Naproxen	Unknown mechanism
Fenoprofen	Quinine
Dilantin	Quinidine
Oral hypoglycemic agents	Phenothiazines
Nalidixic acid	Disulfiram
Estrogen	Sulfisoxazole
Miconazole	Amiodarone

(From Wyngaarden JB, Smith L: *Cecil's textbook of medicine,* ed 18, vol 1, Philadelphia, 1988, WB Saunders.)

TABLE 7-9-2 Increased Resistance to Warfarin

Hereditary Warfarin Resistance	Increased Warfarin Metabolism
Increase in vitamin K	Barbiturates
Reduced drug absorption	Primidone
Malabsorption syndromes	Carbamazepine
Liquid paraffin laxatives	Ethchlorvynol
Cholestyramine resin	Glutethimide
Magnesium trisilicate	Meprobamate
	Griseofulvin
	Rifampin
	Nafcillin

(From Wyngaarden JB, Smith L: *Cecil's textbook of medicine,* ed 18, vol 1, Philadelphia, 1988, WB Saunders.)

lation and subsequent hemorrhage. In the setting of an acquired coagulopathy the clinician must remain vigilant. A thorough drug history must be elicited as coumadin is commonly prescribed, may be accidentally ingested, or used surreptitiously for secondary gain. Additionally, some drug interactions exist that increase the sensitivity to coumadin. These include aspirin, ibuprofen, Dilantin, oral hypoglycemic agents, estrogen, anabolic steroids, erythromycin, cimetidine, Bactrim, and others listed in Table 7-9-1. Other drug interactions increase resistance to Warfarin and are listed in Table 7-9-2.

The appropriate collection of laboratory specimens is necessary for the correct interpretation of coagulation studies. Both PT and PTT are sensitive to heparin contamination. Elevations in these parameters are likely to occur when specimens are drawn from central venous access sites with heparinized ports. An inadequate volume of specimen, as well as a hematocrit greater than 55%, will decrease the plasm:citrate-collection-tube anticoagulant ratio, thereby artificially prolonging both PT and PTT.

The transfusion of large quantities of blood products devoid of clotting factors may result in clinically significant coagulopathy. This washout phenomenon most commonly presents in patients requiring vigorous volume resuscitation secondary to GI bleed, trauma, or cardiopulmonary bypass. The coagulopathy itself results from a relative lack of coagulation factors and may be potentiated by dysfunctional or absent platelets and decreased calcium concentrations found in banked blood. Management of transfusion washout is generally supportive and includes the administration of FFP and platelets. A clinical rule of thumb advocates transfusing 1 unit of FFP and 4 units of platelets for every 5 units of packed red cells given.

Immunologically mediated factor depletion may arise from the production of (1) factor specific immunoglobulins referred to as circulating anticoagulants or (2) nonspecific "lupus-like" inhibitors directed against phospholipid. The latter may manifest as thrombotic episodes with a contradictory laboratory profile. Differentiating between the presence of a circulating anticoagulant versus a component deficiency rests in the performance of the plasma inhibitor dilution test. In this test equal parts of patient and normal serum are mixed. Plasma from patients with specific inhibitors will inactivate the coagulation factors of the admixed serum. Failure of an abnormal PT or PTT to correct is suggestive of the presence of inhibitor, while normalization of parameters points toward a factor deficiency. Nonspecific inhibitors prolong both PT and PTT in vitro. This effect may be overcome by the addition of or change in the type of phospholipid added or by further diluting the abnormal plasma.

Circulating anticoagulants to factor VIII are commonly seen in hemophiliacs who have received factor replacement and subsequently direct an immune response to this foreign antigen. Other specific circulating anticoagulants may be seen in entities such as systemic lupus erythematosis, rheumatoid arthritis, multiple myeloma, and Waldenstrom's macroglobulinemia. Exposure to various medications may also give rise to an immune response that produces circulating anticoagulants. Therapy for patients with immunologically mediated factor depletion may include (1) plasma factor concentrate or activated prothrombin complex transfusion, (2) plasmapheresis or exchange transfusion to lower antibody titers, (3) immunosuppression (corticosteroids) in instances of acquired factor VIII antibodies in nonhemophiliac patients used to both inhibit antibody production and down-regulate reticuloendothelial Fc-receptor uptake of immune complexes, (4) chemotherapy directed against plasma cell dyscrasias producing immunologically mediated factor depletion. This approach has eliminated circulatory anticoagulants in a number of case reports, and (5) use of factor eight inhibitor bypass activity (FEIBA) complex in cases where a specific inhibitor has developed to factor VIII.

Disseminated intravascular coagulation is a clinicopathologic syndrome whose sine qua non is the simultaneous generation of thrombin and plasmin representing activation of thrombogenic and fibrinolytic pathways. This entity may complicate such diverse disease processes as bacterial infection, sepsis, malignancy, trauma, ARDS, and obstetrical complications such as abruptio placentae. Given the elevated PT, PTT, and the decreased fibrinogen and platelet count, a consumptive process may be at work. However, this picture could also be seen in hepatic failure with limited synthetic function. Additional studies required to clarify the picture might include fibrin split products, D-dimers, and factor VIIIc. (See Fig. 7-9-1.)

QUESTION 4   One hour after her admission to the intensive care unit, the patient's coagulation profile returned as follows: PT 12%, PTT 67 sec, fibrinogen 40 mg/dl, fibrin split products >40, and factor VIIIc 24%. Given this coagulation profile, what is the specific diagnosis, pathophysiology, and treatment?

The diagnosis based on clinical grounds and the above coagulation parameters is disseminated intravascular coagulation (DIC). DIC may present in an acute hemorrhagic form or less commonly a subacute or chronic form. The acute form may have an initial thrombotic phase with shortened PT and PTT that quickly moves toward a bleeding diathesis and lengthened PT and PTT. This progression reflects continued activation of thrombin and plasmin, the production of fibrin thrombi, and the consumption of clotting factors and platelets that eventually produce a hemorrhagic state. Subacute or chronic DIC manifests either as clinically insignificant laboratory abnormality or in venous thrombosis. DIC represents an uncommon feature of certain malignancies, connective tissue disorders, hemangiomas, and retained fetal material.

For each underlying disease process a putative "trigger" mechanism has been postulated to activate both thrombin and plasmin. DIC may be imitated by the introduction of thrombogenic or procoagulant materials into the circulation. Neoplasms, both solid and hematologic, may secrete tissue thromboplastin, lysosomal granules, or a number of cytokines that have procoagulant effects. Obstetrical complications, severe trauma, snake venom, and various infections are known to act similarly in producing DIC.

Patients presenting in fulminant DIC are acutely ill from both the underlying primary pathology and the DIC itself. Physical findings on presentation usually reflect profound disturbances in primary and secondary hemostasis. This may include widely distributed ecchymosis, oozing from venipuncture sites, and petechiae on mucous membranes. Only seldom do patients present with thrombotic manifestations of the disorder. Laboratory abnormalities in DIC include (1) prolongation of both PT and PTT, (2) hypofibrinogenemia, and (3) thrombocytopenia. In the appropriate clinical setting alteration in these parameters will usually establish the diagnosis of DIC. Confirmatory tests to detect the presence of fibrin split products and D-dimers are beneficial in distinguishing DIC from hepatic dysfunction. Although the former is 100% sensitive and 56% specific, only the latter reflects simultaneous activation of thrombin and plasmin, endowing it with a 97% specificity. Combining the two tests gives a predictive accuracy of 96% for recognizing DIC. Also important in distinguishing DIC from hepatic failure is the presence of a diminished factor VIIIc concentration. As factor VIIIc is synthesized in endothelial cells of vessels, its production would not be affected in liver failure as it would in DIC.

Effective therapy in acute DIC should address correction of the underlying disease process and control of bleeding. Patients should receive FFP to correct coagulation factor depletion if hemorrhage is present. Fresh frozen plasma may be administered in an attempt to maintain fibrinogen levels at approximately 200 mg/dl. Platelet concentrates should be given to correct thrombocytopenia. Concentrates of antithrombin III are now available and may have efficacy in DIC. Heparin infusion has been advocated to decrease thrombin generation, ultimately preventing further factor consumption. Heparin should be reserved for those patients with thrombotic complications. Subacute DIC responds best to treatment of the underlying disorder, although prophylactic anticoagulation is advocated for those patients with thrombotic complications.

QUESTION 5 What is the etiology of this patient's DIC?

The patient described in this case presents with clinical pneumonia and sepsis. In gram-negative septicemia, the most common cause of DIC, endotoxin activates the coagulation cascade and alters the dynamic properties of vascular endothelium. This alteration establishes a microenvironment with increased procoagulant activity. The endotoxin-generated induction of tissue factor activity on leukocytes has been demonstrated and is also thought to incite mechanisms responsible for DIC. The medical history is remarkable for multiple myeloma that bestows upon this patient heightened susceptibility to infection by encapsulated organisms.

QUESTION 6 What is the most efficacious form of therapy for this patient?

The first line of therapy is to treat the underlying disease process. In this case it is treatment of the patient's pneumonia and sepsis. During this period vigilant monitoring of the patient's coagulation status is important to avoid hemorrhagic and thrombotic complications. The use of heparin as mentioned above is controversial. While it is accepted that heparin should be used for the treatment of major thrombotic episodes, other indications are uncertain. Replacement of clotting factors with FFP and cryoprecipitate to maintain fibrinogen levels within the normal range and the PT/PTT as near normal as possible is also important. There should always be secure IV access and a supply of matched blood products in the blood bank for transfusion if severe hemorrhage occurs.

Specific areas that are difficult to examine that may sequester large amounts of blood are the retroperitoneal space, the hip, and the brain. Therefore, one should maintain a high index of suspicion when changes in the hemoglobin concentration occur without an obvious source of blood loss.

CASE SUMMARY Empiric broad spectrum antimicrobial therapy was instituted early on with

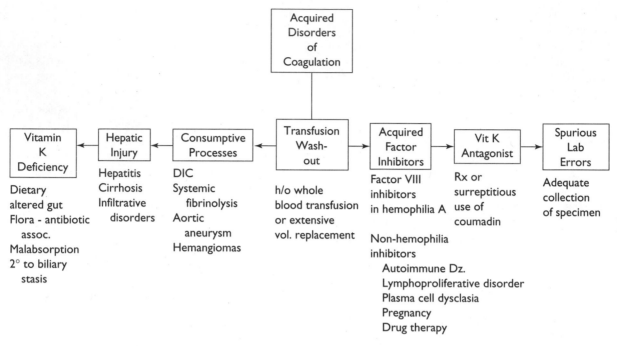

7-9-1   Diagnostic algorithm for acquired coagulopathy.

vancomycin and ceftazidime. Cultures from both blood and sputum were positive for *Streptococcus pneumoniae*.

The patient's clinical bleeding and coagulation profile did not improve after initially receiving FFP and platelets. She was subsequently transfused 4 more units of FFP and 2 units of platelets and cryoprecipitate. An FFP drip was started at 40 cc/hour with the goal of maintaining a fibrinogen level of greater than 200 mg/dl. A low-dose heparin drip was also started at 200 units/hour without an initial bolus. The patient remained on heparin and FFP drips on hospital days 1 through 3 although oozing stopped on day 2. On the fourth hospital day both heparin and FFP were stopped as the patient's coagulation profile stabilized. She improved clinically over a 1-week period and was discharged home after a 14-day course of intravenous antibiotics.

● ●

BIBLIOGRAPHY

Carr JM, McKinney M, McDonagh J: Diagnosis of disseminated intravascular coagulation, *Am J Clin Path* 91:280, 1989.

Donaldson GWK, Davis SH, Darg A, Richmond J: Coagulation factors in chronic liver disease, *J Clin Pathol* 22:199, 1969.

Glueck HI, Hong R: A circulating anticoagulant in VA multiple myeloma, *J Clin Invest* 44:1866, 1965.

Handin RI: Disorders of coagulation and thrombosis. In *Harrison's principles of internal medicine*, 1505-1511, 1991.

Kofar JC: Prediction of hemorrhage during long term/coumarin anticoagulation by excessive prothrombin ration, *Am Heart J* 103:445, 1982.

Ratnoff OD: Hemostatic mechanisms in liver disease, *Med Clin North Am* 47:721, 1963.

Robboy SJ, Lewis EJ, Schuv PH, Colman RW: Circulating anticoagulants to factor VIII, *Am J Med* 49:742, 1970.

Russell JE, Kumar R, Deykin: The spectrum of vitamin K deficiency, *JAMA* 5:40, 1977.

Schleider MA, Nachman RI, Jaffe EA, Coleman M: A clinical study of the lupus anticoagulant, *Blood* 48:499, 1976.

C A S E

10

Stephen C. Schwartz

A 22-year-old man presented to his family physician with complaints of painful oral ulcers and attendant low grade fevers over a 2-week period. During this same time he experienced gingival bleeding while brushing his teeth. He denied any intercurrent illnesses although he complained of modest lethargy. His mother, who accompanied him, commented upon his pale complexion. He presented no significant past medical history, was not sexually active, and did not use alcohol, tobacco, or drugs.

Physical examination revealed a well-nourished and well-developed, pale-appearing young male. The patient was tachycardic with a pulse of 120 bpm. The blood pressure was 116/80 mm Hg, respirations 18/min, and temperature 38.3°C. Examination of the oral cavity revealed necrotic herpetiform ulcerations distributed on the gingiva and mucous membranes. Areas of raised white plaques consistent with oral candidiasis appeared on the mucous membranes which were also noted to be pale. The neck and axillae were free of any significant lymphadenopathy. The chest was clear and the heart regular, tachycardic with an appreciable flow murmur. The abdomen was soft and non-tender with no demonstrable hepatosplenomegaly. The extremities were unremarkable and the neurologic examination was non-focal.

QUESTION 1 Discuss commonly encountered oral lesions in the practice of internal medicine. Which lesions are associated with systemic disease?

Assessment of the oral cavity is an important part of the physical examination in all patients. Primary oral-pharyngeal disease may be discov-

ered, and concomitant morbidity lessened, if appropriate therapy is instituted. Perhaps more importantly, systemic manifestations of disease may be uncovered, leading to early diagnosis and treatment of a variety of disorders. Physicians should direct their attention to the condition of the dentition, the appearance of periodontal tissue (gingiva), and abnormalities of the soft tissues and oral mucosa. Visual inspection of the oral cavity should be complemented by gloved bimanual palpation.

Pathology in the oral cavity may reflect infectious, neoplastic, dermatologic, or auto-immune processes. Oral lesions may also arise from nutritional inadequacies or immunosuppression. Dental caries is one of the most common of human diseases. This entity, which ultimately leads to the destruction of the hard tissues of the teeth, is the consequence of infection with *Streptococcus mutans* and other bacteria that inhabit the oral cavity. The use of fluoridated drinking water in the United States has lessened the incidence of caries significantly. Populations at risk for caries include those patients with poor oral hygiene, diabetes mellitus, xerostomia secondary to Sjögren's syndrome, and patients undergoing chemotherapy. Older populations, by virtue of their longevity and retained dentition are at higher risk for root caries. Patients with the eating disorder bulimia often present with profoundly deteriorated dentition secondary to gastric acid exposure.

Treatment will rely on extirpation of the infected hard tissue and the sealing of the dentine by an appropriate amalgam. Should dental caries progress, the pulp of the tooth may become infected producing acute pulpitis. A root canal or extraction may be necessary lest infection spread beyond the apex of the tooth to the periodontal ligament. Should this occur a periapical abscess may form. From here infection may spread through the alveolar bone to the soft tissues producing a cellulitis and possible bacteremia. *Ludwig's angina* is a severe form of cellulitis which arises from a mandibular molar. This infection may tract through the soft tissues of the submandibular space and the floor of the mouth. Dysphagia may be present with elevation of the tongue. Patients may have difficulty breathing. Airway compromise has been reported in this circumstance.

The teeth and oral cavity may themselves give rise to systemic infection. Examples of this include anaerobic lung abscesses, which arise when oral secretions are aspirated in an unprotected airway (the unconscious alcoholic with poor dentition is the most classic example). Bacterial endocarditis may also develop from the translocation of mouth flora. This may occur during dental procedures and is most commonly seen in the setting of native valvular disease or valvular prosthesis.

Periodontal disease encompasses a spectrum of conditions that ultimately lead to the deposition of bacterial plaque. This plaque may in fact mineralize. The most common form of periodontal disease is gingivitis. Gingivitis begins as an inflammation of the marginal gingiva. Ultimately this process may involve the periodontal ligament and alveolar bone. As these structures are compromised, abscess formation may occur. Tooth loss may follow after alveolar bone resorption, chronic abscess formation, and increased tooth mobility. Multiple organisms have been documented in periodontal disease, including *Bacteroides gingivalis, Eikenell corrodens, Capnocytophaga* and *Actinobacillus actinomycetem comitans. Bacteroides intermedius* has been associated with acute necrotizing ulcerative gingivitis (ANUG). This entity presents with painful necrotic gingiva, tissue sloughing, and halitosis and may be seen in patients with HIV or frank AIDS. Patients with diabetes mellitus and Down syndrome often have severe periodontal disease, whereas those with IgA deficiency and agammaglobulinemia develop this disease less

commonly. Appropriate therapy rests on extirpation of the bacterial plaque and improved oral hygiene.

Gingival hyperplasia may result from various medications including; phenytoin and nifedipine. Fibrous hypertrophy may be so great as to interfere with mastication. A heritable form of the disease exists. Discontinuation of the offending medication should allow for regression of the hypertrophy. Surgery is suggested for the heritable form of the condition.

The appearance of the oral mucous membranes often provides the physician with essential information. Pale mucous membranes are often associated with anemia while dry mucous membranes may represent dehydration. Oral candidiasis may signal immunocompromise or prior antimicrobial therapy. Lesions of the oral mucosa are most often associated with microorganisms; however, neoplastic, dermatologic and pigmented lesions also are recognized.

Viral infections of the mouth and oral mucosa are common in the general population. Primary and recurrent herpetic gingivo-stomatitis presents as vesicular lesions involving the lip, oral mucosa, gingiva, and palate. The offending agent is herpes virus type 1 and rarely type 2. The primary form is most often seen in children and young adults with concomitant fever, malaise, lymphadenopathy, and acute gingivitis. These lesions, which are extremely painful, heal within 14 days. The lesions in the recurrent form heal within 7 days. Recurrent aphthous ulcers or the ulcers seen in Behcet syndrome may mirror herpetic gingivostomatitis with regard to the morphology of the lesion. Other viruses including varicella-zoster, Epstein-Barr, coxsackievirus A and B, and HIV may develop vesicular lesions in the appropriate clinical setting.

Bacterial infections of the oral mucosa include primary, secondary, and tertiary syphilis as well as gonorrhea. The oral lesion of primary syphilis is a small papule progressing into a painless ulcer with an indurated border. Secondary syphilitic oral lesions are described as maculopapular covered by a grayish membrane. Sore throat is a common accompaniment. Oral lesions of tertiary syphilis arise from gummatous infiltration of the mucosa followed by ulceration and fibrosis.

The lesions in gonorrhea are usually limited to the site of inoculation, however, hematogenous spread from a primary focus has also been reported. Patients present early on with dry, burning, or itchy mouths. Some patients describe a sensation of heat in the mouth followed by severe pain. Tissues of the pharynx and tonsils are most often involved; however, the oral mucosa may be diffusely inflamed or ulcerated. Other bacterial pathogens with a proclivity to invade the oral cavity include actinomycosis and *Mycobacterium tuberculosis.*

Oral lesions related to fungal pathogens may abound in debilitated patients, those on glucocorticoids or antibiotics, and those with AIDS. Candidiasis (moniliasis) has several morphological variants and may be seen in any area of the mouth. The *pseudomembranous* type presents as creamy white curd-like patches underneath which a friable mucosa exists. The *erythematous* type develops as a red and flat lesion, while *candidal leukoplakia* is an unremovable white thickening of the tongue. *Angular cheilitis* is also a candidial infection presenting as sore fissures at the corner of the mouth. This type of lesion may also be seen in vitamin B_{12} deficiency.

Hairy leukoplakia may resemble pseudomembranous candidiasis in morphology. This entity, thought due to infection by the Epstein-Barr virus, usually is seen laterally on the tongue. These lesions range from small and flat to extensive and hairy. On rare occasions it is demonstrated on other areas of the oral mucosa. This entity is most often associated with HIV infection. Other white lesions mimicking candidiasis include lichen planus, white sponge nevus, smoker's leukoplakia, nicotinic stomatitis and chemical burns.

Dermatologic disorders may manifest in the oral cavity. Mucous membrane pemphigoid, pemphigus vulgaris, and lichen planus are entities with a predisposition for mucous membranes of the oral cavity. Erythema multiforme is believed to be an immune complex-mediated reaction following exposure to a drug (most commonly sulfonimides and penicillin), which results in an inflammatory response of the skin and mucous membranes. The iris or target lesion is pathognomonic for the process. When fever, toxicity, and mucous membrane reaction is present it is referred to as Stevens-Johnson syndrome.

Pigmented lesions, primary neoplastic lesions and those resulting from neoplastic processes have been described in the oral cavity. Melanotic macules, melanin pigmentation, melanotic nevi and malignant melanoma may all have similar presentations and morphologic features (brown to black pigmentation). Other pigmented lesions include those seen in syndromes such as Peutz-Jegher's and Addison's disease, as well as drug and heavy metal ingestion. Squamous cell carcinomas may arise from anywhere in the oral cavity. These lesions may be ulcerated and raised with indurated borders. The natural history is one of a persistent non-healing lesion. Both lymphoma and leukemia may present with ulcerative and necrotic lesions in the oral cavity (most commonly gingival tissue). At times these ulcers are complicated by secondary bacterial infection. Gingival swelling and infiltration with leukemic cells may arise in all leukemias; however, it is most common to leukemias with monocytic features.

A spincrit performed in the physician's office revealed a hemoglobin of 7.0. The patient was sent to the emergency room for further evaluation. In the emergency room a CBC was performed revealing a WBC of 70,000, HgB of 6.8, HcT of 19.2 and platelets of 43,000. A hematology consult was requested, admission labs were ordered, and a bone marrow aspirate and biopsy were performed. Bone marrow was sent for cytogenetics, immunohistochemistry, and flow cytometry. The patient was subsequently admitted to the hospital.

QUESTION 2 What is in the differential diagnosis of leukocytosis?

Leukocytosis denotes an elevation in the number of white blood cells in the peripheral blood.

Since most cases of leukocytosis are due to neutrophilia, this discussion will be restricted to those processes which produce leukocytosis by increasing neutrophil counts. Normal hematopoietic physiology is such that a significant number of neutrophils are loosely adherent to vascular endothelium. Many neutrophils are also distributed throughout the microcirculation. With the proper stimulus (i.e., stress, corticosteroids, or infection), these cells demarginate and enter the circulating pool of neutrophils (increasing the WBC). The bone marrow itself contains a neutrophil reserve that again under appropriate conditions releases neutrophils into the circulation. Under more profound conditions bone marrow production is increased and early neutrophil progenitor forms (bands and metamyleocytes) are released. This is commonly referred to as a left shift. Cytokines that promote demargination and neutrophil reserve release include G-CSF, GM-CSF, M-CSF, and interleukins-1,3,5,6. Potential etiologies of leukocytosis include physiologic, infectious, drug induced, inflammatory, metabolic dysfunction, hemorrhage, myeloproliferative, and idiopathic disorders. Exercise, stress, and the release of epinephrine transiently increase the WBC. The WBC ultimately returns to normal after the event. Infection with mainly bacterial pathogens gives rise to leukocytosis, viruses, and fungi less so. Inflammatory states such as tissue necrosis (myocardial and pulmonary infarction), extensive thermal injury and hypersensitivity states may generate a leukocytosis. Metabolic disorders (acidosis and renal failure) and drugs (glucocorticoids and lithium) are known to increase the WBC as well. Metastatic disease may not uncommonly produce leukocytosis. Most forms of leukemia and myeloproliferative disorders can be associated with an increase in the white count. An idiopathic form of leukocytosis has also been described.

In situations where an inciting event (infection) is profound, leukocyte counts may reach the 50,000 mark. This is referred to as a leukemoid reaction. Given this patient's profound elevation in WBC and accompanying cytopenias (anemia and thrombocytopenia) the diagnosis of acute leukemia should be strongly considered.

Review of the bone marrow aspirate and biopsy revealed a hypercellular, monotonous marrow replaced with large myeloid-appearing blasts. These blasts were granular and modestly differentiated. Auer rods were identified and a diminished number of megakaryocytes were present. The peripheral smear was remarkable for circulating blast forms. A presumptive diagnosis of acute myelogenous leukemia was made pending the return of marker studies, flow cytometry, and cytogenetics.

QUESTION 3 What are the different morphologic subtypes of acute myelogenous leukemia?

Acute leukemias are clonal hematologic malignancies separated into myelogenous and lymphoblastic forms, reflecting their cellular lineage. Eight distinct morphologic subtypes exist for acute myelogenous leukemia. The classification schema as adopted by the French-American-British (FAB) cooperative group recognizes FAB types M_0 through M_7 for AML. These subtypes are based on morphology of cells in the bone marrow as documented by light microscopy. If 30% of the cells in the bone marrow are blasts, the diagnosis of leukemia is made. To help confirm and appropriately subclassify the diagnosis of AML, special stains and immunohistochemical studies have been developed to complement light microscopy. Stains important in the diagnosis of AML include myeloperoxidase and chloroacetate esterase. If 3% of the blast cells stain positive for myeloperoxidase, a diagnosis of AML is made. If less than 3% of cells stain for myeloperoxidase but are positive for terminal deoxynucleotidyl transferase (TdT) the diagnosis of ALL should be considered. Batteries of monoclonal antibodies have been raised that react with various surface antigens on cell membranes. Myeloid surface antigens useful in the diagnosis of AML include CD11, CD13, CD14, CD33, CD41, CD42, and HLA-DR. For acute lymphoblastic leukemias of B-cell lineage CD19, CD20, and CD22 are often positive. For pre-B cell leukemias CD10 (CALLA) may be diagnostic. Surface immunoglobulin may be present in mature B cell leukemias such as Burkitt type ALL, whereas CD1, CD2, CD3, CD4, CD7, and CD8 are found in T cell ALL. T cell receptor gene rearrangements may also be found in ALL. It is also important to note that approximately 20% of myeloid malignancies express lymphoid markers.

The AML M_0 subtype is characterized by its lack of maturation and the absence of myeloperoxidase staining on light microscopy. These cells do stain for myeloperoxidase when observed by electron microscopy. This subgroup possesses myeloid surface markers as documented by immunohistochemistry and flow cytometry. Cells of the M_1 variant again show only minimal differentiation, fine azurophilic granules, and a paucity of auer rods (dense rod-like bodies located in the cytoplasm composed of lysosomal granules), while M_2 subtypes are more granular, have abundant cytoplasm with auer rods, and are more differentiated. Blasts in acute promyelocytic leukemia or FAB M_3 possess a densely granulated morphology akin to promyelocytes. Bundles of auer rods and bilobed nuclei are classic features. The M_4 (myelomonocytic) variety of AML is defined as having at least 20% non-erythroid cells being comprised of the monocytic series. In acute monocytic leukemia or FAB M_5, granulocytic precursors comprise less than 20% of the cell population. FAB M_6 or erythroleukemia is characterized by less than 30 percent granulocytic or monocytic precursors while more than 50% are erythroid precursors. FAB M_7 is also referred to as acute megakaryocytic leukemia. This entity is associated with a high degree of marrow fibrosis, micro- megakaryocytes and megakaryoblasts. Germ cell tumors arising with FAB M_7 have also been reported.

Approximately 30% of patients with AML have the FAB M_2 phenotype while 20% possess FAB M_1. FAB M_4 may also represent 15% to 20% of all cases of AML. The remainder of the subtypes occur only rarely.

Staining and immunochemistry revealed that 30% of the cell population was positive for my-

eloperoxidase and chloroacetate esterase. CD13, CD14, and CD33 were also positive. This cell population did not stain for TdT. Given the morphology, staining, and immunohistochemistry the diagnosis of AML FAB M_2 was confirmed.

QUESTION 4 What is the natural course of the disease? What are the most common presentations?

In AML, the expansion of the clonal leukemic cell population profoundly interferes with normal hematopoiesis. Leukemic cells are not rapidly proliferating but are continually accumulating in the bone marrow and other organs. S-phase (synthesis) analysis suggests that the number of leukemic cells in this phase of the cell cycle is indeed less than that of a normal cell population. The subsequent suppression of erythropoiesis, myelopoiesis, and thrombopoiesis ultimately leads to the presenting signs and symptoms of leukemia. Symptoms related to anemia such as fatigue and dyspnea are classic presentations. The development of fever in this patient population usually stems from absent or dysfunctional myeloid elements and may herald the onset of infection or a systemic inflammatory response. Infections of the upper respiratory tract and pneumonia are common. Flu-like symptoms are also noted in many cases. As leukemic clones expand in the marrow, megakaryoctes are diminished and those that are present are often dysfunctional. As a result patients become prone to easy bruising and mucosal hemorrhage. The FAB M_3 subtype may give rise to disseminated intravascular coagulation as a consequence of procoagulant release. Patients with FAB M_4 and M_5 can present with skin and gum infiltration.

Patients may present acutely ill and toxic or appear chronically ill. Up to 25% of AML patients demonstrate a myelodysplastic syndrome prior to developing frank leukemia. This pre-leukemic state involves the expansion of an unregulated clonal population of cells which produce various cytopenias. Clonal evolution ultimately produces a more malignant phenotype, eventually giving rise to AML. Untreated, AML has a mortality rate of 90% within 1 year.

QUESTION 5 On the floor, the patient's parents were understandably distressed over the recent diagnosis. Questions were raised as to how and why this happened to their son. How would you answer the parent's questions? How does leukemia arise? Are there risk factors for its development?

Etiologies of acute leukemia presently remain unclear. Both genetic and environmental determinants appear to play roles in the pathogenesis of this disease. Familial predispositions have been identified; however, this association plays a role in a minority of cases. Observations of familial clusters have found that siblings of patients with leukemia are only twice as likely to develop leukemia themselves. Age and ethnicity may also be important. Relative risks for the development of leukemia rise with age. White populations are more prone to develop this disease than are black populations. The incidence of this disease is higher for those from higher socioeconomic backgrounds and individuals of semitic extraction.

A number of hereditary disorders and chromosomal abnormalities predispose patients to leukemogenesis. Down syndrome patients with trisomy 21 are 20 times as likely to develop leukemia as those in the general population. Other disorders with increased incidence of leukemia development include Bloom's syndrome and Fanconi's anemia, both disorders associated with chromosomal breakage. Inherited immunodeficiency diseases such as Bruton agammaglobulinemia, hereditary ataxia-telangiectasia, severe combined immunodeficiency, congenital agammaglobulinemia, and Wiskott-Aldrich syndrome all show increased rates of AML.

Exposure to radiation and chemicals have been associated with AML. Individuals exposed to the atomic bomb blasts of Hiroshima and Nagasaki are up to 15 times more likely to develop leukemia as compared to those who were not exposed. Patients treated with ionizing radiation for ankylosing spondylitis, thymic enlargement, and men-

orrhagia all have an increased incidence of leukemia. Benzene is a well-recognized chemical associated with increased rates of leukemia in those exposed. Cigarette smoking may also predispose individuals with existing risk factors (cytogenetic abnormalities) to leukemia.

The retrovirus HTLV-1 has been linked to the development of adult T cell leukemia-lymphoma. Genomic sequences of HTLV-1 have been recovered from the genetic material of adult T cell leukemia-lymphoma cells. Although this links viruses with leukemogenesis, no association has been found between viruses and AML.

Patients treated with chemotherapeutic agents for other malignancies run the risk of developing a secondary leukemia. Treatments for Hodgkin's disease, breast cancer, nonHodgkin's lymphoma, ovarian cancer, and myeloma all have potentially leukemogenic cytotoxic agents in their various regimens. Therapies that incorporate alkylating agents are most often associated with the development of leukemia. These patients may initially present with a myelodysplastic syndrome. Time from exposure/treatment to the diagnosis is on the average 4 to 5 years. Those patients who develop secondary leukemias have unique chromosomal abnormalities which include complete or partial losses of chromosomes 5 or 7. Secondary leukemias are, in general, more refractory to treatment than other leukemias. Patients with limited karyotypic abnormalities have the best prognosis of those individuals who eventually develop a secondary leukemia. It remains essential for clinicians to follow at-risk patients closely for any change in hematologic status. This patient's parents should be reassured and made clearly aware that their son's illness is not inherited in the lay sense, and that this disease developed through no fault of their own. It is important that a thorough exposure history be taken. This may lessen the risk of exposure to other members of the household.

QUESTION 6 The consultants on hematology recommended initial therapy with Ara-c and daunorubicin. They estimated that the patient would be hospitalized from 4 to 6 weeks. The parents sought a second opinion regarding their son's condition and his potential therapy. Describe standard induction therapy for AML? What are the complications?

Therapy for AML is divided into two phases: induction and post-remission or consolidation. The aim in the induction phase of therapy is to deliver a high dose of chemotherapy, thereby eliminating several logs of leukemic cells. Accomplishing this allows for a more rapid expansion of normal stem cells. This should allow for the growth of all normal cell lines, ultimately lessening the presenting cytopenias. If evidence of a leukemic population in the marrow is lacking after chemotherapy, the patient is said to be in a clinical remission. The development of the drug ara-C in the late 1960s was critical in moving AML into the realm of curability. Combinations of ara-C and anthracycline agents such as daunorubicin, idarubicin, and mitoxantrone are now considered standard induction regimens. Combinations of ara-C and daunorubicin have enjoyed a great deal of success and are used routinely in many centers. Ara-C is given as a continuous infusion for 7 days at a dose of 100 mg/m^2 with an initial 25 mg/m^2 bolus loading dose. Daunorubicin is given as a bolus on days 1 to 3 at a dose of 45 mg/m^2. The use of idarubicin is also gaining in popularity. In a study by Berman et al., this drug, when given in combination with ara-C, produced significantly higher rates of remission than did the combination of ara-C and daunorubicin. Two other studies have also suggested an advantage to this combination. At Memorial Sloan-Kettering Cancer Center, the combination of idarubicin and ara-C is considered the standard induction regimen. Most recently, all trans retinoic acid (ATRA), a vitamin A derivative, has become the induction agent of choice in FAB M$_3$. This drug is believed to act by terminally differentiating malignant clones. Recent studies have demonstrated a molecular mechanism of action on the basis of a t(15,17) translocation that brings the retinoic acid receptor-alpha into proximity with a gene denoted as PML. The fusion product codes for a receptor that is exquisitely sensitive to ATRA as a ligand. It is unquestionably the altered receptor and a naturally occurring ligand with limited activity, which allows for initial cellular dysregulation leading to the malignant phenotype. Induction agents are not without their toxicities. Intense chemotherapy such as Idarubicin/Ara-c combinations will render bone marrow hypoplastic for periods approaching 4 weeks. This myelosupression will leave the patient susceptible to infection secondary to neutropenia and hemorrhage as a result of thrombocytopenia. Because of this extended period of myelosuppression, between 10% to 20% of patients succumb to the aforementioned complications of overwhelming infection and hemorrhage during induction therapy. Advances in antimicrobial therapy has lessened the risk of death by infection during induction. Patients are at most risk from auto-infection. The gut and respiratory tract are the two most common portals of entry. Bacterial pathogens dominate early and therapeutic strategies call for the use of broad spectrum antibiotics in the setting of neutropenia and fever. Those patients who are nadir for greater than 1 week are always at risk for fungal infections. Those patients persistently febrile after broad spectrum antibiotic coverage should be given a trial of amphotericin. Attention should always be focused on naturally occurring protective barriers such as the skin, which may be compromised by central venous access devices. The concept of *locus minoris resistencei* or area of least resistance, should help guide efforts in the search for pathogens in neutropenic fever.

Patients are also at risk for hemorrhage as a result of thrombocytopenia. In all likelihood, induction therapy will render the patient platelet transfusion dependent for several weeks. In the past, patients with less than 20,000 platelets/µl were routinely transfused. New guidelines have established 10,000/µl as a safe cutoff. Cerebral, pulmonary, and GI hemorrhage carry a great deal of morbidity and all may result in the setting of thrombocytopenia. Anemia will also be persistent, requiring multiple transfusions during the period of myelosupression. At MSKCC, all patients with hemoglobins less than 7.0 will receive a transfusion. Symptomatic patients or those with coronary insufficiency will require transfusion support sufficient to allow for optimal oxygen carrying capacity.

Some patients whose white blood counts are over 100,000 will present with leukostasis. This may result in infiltration of vital organs such as brain, lungs, liver, and kidney. Mental status changes, hypoxemia, altered hepatic function, hemorrhage and renal insufficiency have all been reported. Treatment for leukostasis revolves around early administration of chemotherapy. Leukapheresis has also found a role in lessening the leukemic burden in patients with profoundly elevated counts. Metabolic abnormalities resulting from high cell turnover include hyperuricemia, hyperkalemia, hypokalemia and hypocalcemia. The tumor lysis syndrome with its attendant life threatening hypokalemia, hyperuricemia, hyperphosphatemia and hypocalcemia is a not uncommon accompaniment of AML. This syndrome usually arises in patients undergoing induction therapy who possess significantly elevated counts. Vigorous hydration, allopurinol and careful observation of electrolyte status are the cornerstones of management. Patients with the FAB M_3 or acute promyelocytic leukemia (APL) may present with or develop disseminated intravascular coagulation with initial induction. The incidence of DIC has decreased with the addition of ATRA as a primary induction agent specifically for APL. Treatment-related toxicities with ATRA do exist. The retinoic acid syndrome is a life-threatening syndrome of fever and respiratory compromise similar to a capillary leak syndrome which may be attenuated by administration of corticosteroids. Intrinsic drug toxicities are also important in AML. Ara-C has neurotoxic properties while anthracycline agents are cardiotoxic. Early diagnosis of drug toxicity by frequent neurologic assessment may lessen morbidity. Pre-chemotherapy evaluation of cardiac function and ongoing assessment through the duration of therapy is warranted.

Those patients not achieving a post-induction remission are said to have primary refractory AML. Those who achieve an initial remission but do not maintain it have relapsed AML. At MSKCC bone marrow biopsies and aspirates are performed on day 14 after chemotherapy to confirm a hypoplastic marrow. A bone marrow is also obtained after the patient's counts have recovered to assess for remission. Patients with primary refractory or relapsed disease have a generally poor prognosis. Approximately 65% of patients will achieve a remission after induction therapy.

The patient received a standard induction regimen with Ara-C and daunorubicin. Intravenous acyclovir was started prophylactically on hospital day 1. He developed neutropenic fever on hospital day 8, at which time broad spectrum antibiotics (Timentin and Gentamycin) were administered. The patient remained febrile through day 13. Vancomycin was added to the regimen on day 12 with subsequent resolution of the fever. No organisms were cultured from any site during this time. A bone marrow performed on hospital day 15 demonstrated an empty marrow. On hospital day 16 the patient again became febrile. Amphotericin was added at a dose of 1 mg/kg. The patient's fever curve trended downward for the next 4 days, and the patient was afebrile on hospital day 20. Cultures remained negative throughout the admission. The patient's neutrophil count reached 1000 on hospital day 22. A marrow performed on hospital day 32 was read as a regenerating marrow without evidence of leukemia. The patient remained platelet and pRBC transfusion dependent during his hospital stay and required platelet transfusion up to 38 days post-chemotherapy. The patient was discharged home on hospital day 33 in good condition.

QUESTION 7 What further therapy should be administered to this patient given his present hematologic remission? What is the likelihood of cure for patients treated with present regimens? With bone marrow transplantation?

Post-remission or consolidation therapy has proven invaluable in the treatment of AML. Its value is derived from further log reduction of leukemic cell burden. Standard approaches to consolidation therapy have taken the form of 1 to 2 cycles of an ara-C/anthracycline regimen 30 to 45 days after remission is achieved by induction. This presupposes that the patient has recovered fully from the initial induction. As in induction, the consolidation phase of treatment will produce significant myelosuppression. Although 65% of patients with AML will achieve a remission, only 25% will maintain it after completion of consolidation. Because of this many investigators have attempted to improve on present modes of consolidation by dose intensifying regimens, extending the duration of therapy and by administering non–cross-resistant drugs not administered in the induction phase. Of these methods, dose intensification with higher doses of ara-C appears most promising. A report by Mayer et al. suggests that consolidation with high dose ara-C (3 g/m^2) may increase the duration of remission and overall survival for patients less than 65 years of age who are treated in this manner. Autologous transplantation has also been explored as an intensification method for patients achieving an initial remission. In this technique, bone marrow is harvested from the patient after a first remission (induction +2 cycles of consolidation) has been achieved. The bone marrow is then purged by immunologic (monoclonal antibodies) or cytotoxic means (2-HC) to further lessen the leukemic cell burden. Patients are then given intensive chemotherapy and/or radiation therapy with subsequent reinfusion of their marrow. Other investigators have shifted their focus to the harvesting of autologous stem cells. These CD33 positive cells can be subjected to columns with monoclonal antibodies, which are specific for CD33. The cells are collected and reinfused into the patient after intensive chemotherapy with or without radiation therapy. The advantage to this technique is the smaller (but not non-existent) leukemic cell population reinfused and an earlier engraftment. As this technique is perfected, non-leukemic stem cells may someday be grown ex vivo and subsequently reinfused as normal marrow elements into the patient after intensive chemotherapy/radiation therapy. This will obviate the reinfusion of a "contaminated" leukemic marrow as in autologous transplant and eliminate any need for allogeneic transplant with its concomitant morbidity of graft versus host disease (GVHD).

The use of allogeneic bone marrow transplantation for AML in first remission (after induction and consolidation) has become widespread. Long-term survival for good risk patients has been reported to be in the 40% to 50% range. For allogeneic transplant, bone marrow is harvested from an HLA-compatible donor. Six out of six HLA-loci are optimal for the procedure. Siblings are the most likely candidates with a 25% chance of producing a match. Transplants from related donors with 5/6 HLA matched loci have also been performed. This approach is limited by the morbidity of GVHD. This entity, which is present to some degree in all allogeneic transplants, is the result of donor T cell activation against the recipients tissues. Involvement of the skin and GI tract are common although other organs can be involved. Currently patients with GVHD are treated with cyclosporine and corticosteroids. Anti-thymocyte globulin may also be given early in the transplant to lessen the number of donor T cells. As GVHD has limited the success rates and overall survival of transplant recipients, new methods have evolved to circumvent this problem. The use of T cell-depleted transplants has lessened the severity of GVHD in those patients treated with this method. As donor T cells have an anti-leukemia effect (graft vs. leukemia), patients with T cell-depleted marrows have higher relapse rates when compared to non-T cell-depleted transplants. The use of donor T cell reinfusion has recently received a great deal of attention. This technique reinfuses donor T cells into transplant patients who have relapsed. This maneuver has placed chronic myelogenous leukemia (CML) patients back into remission in a high percentage of cases. Patients who benefit from this may possess chimeric bone marrows. As the leukemic population

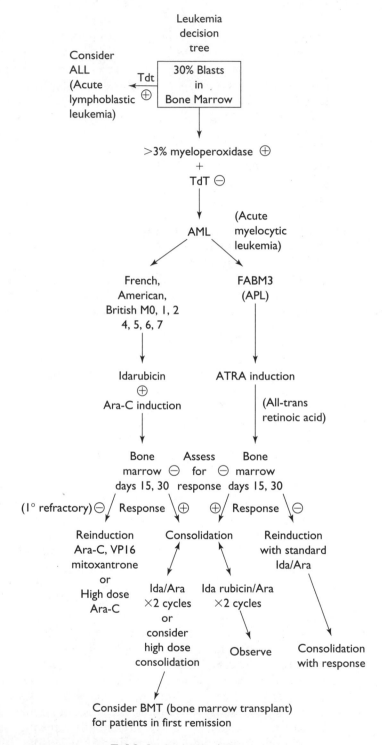

7-10-1 Leukemia decision tree.

grows, a point is reached where the leukemic population becomes dominant. The selective re-infusion of donor T cells shifts this balance back in favor of the transplanted marrow. In the future all allogeneic transplants for AML may be T cell-depleted with subsequent donor T cell transfusions at appropriate times.

The patient completed two cycles of consolidation with daunorubicin and ara-C and has remained in remission for approximately 6 months. He has one sibling who is HLA-compatible. He is now considering the option of bone marrow transplantation. A diagnostic algorithm for leukemia can be found in Fig. 7-10-1.

BIBLIOGRAPHY

Anderson M: The epidemiology of leukemia, *Adv Cancer Res* 31:1, 1980.

Arthur DC, Berger R, Golomb HM, et al: The clinical significance of karyotype in acute leukemias, *Oncology* 4:23, 1990.

Berman E: Chemotherapy in acute myelogenous leukemia: higher dose, higher expectations? *J Clin Oncol* 13(1):1-4, 1995.

Berman E, Heller G, Santrosaj S, et al: Results of a randomized trial comparing idarubicin and cytosine arabinoside with daunorubicin and cytosine arabinoside in adult patients with newly diagnosed acute myelogenous leukemia, *Blood* 77:1666, 1991.

Bennett JM, Catovsky D, Danial MT, et al: Proposals for the classification of acute leukemia, *Br J Haematol* 33:451, 1976.

Hug V, Keating MJ, McCredie KB, et al: Clinical course and response to treatment of patients with acute myelogenous leukemia presenting with a high white cell count, *Cancer* 53:773, 1983.

Keating MJ, Estey E, Kantarjian H: Acute leukemia. In Rosenberg SA, et al, eds: *Cancer: principles and Practice of Oncology,* Philadelphia, 1994, Lippincott.

Mayer RJ, Davis RB, Frei E, et al: Intensive post remission chemotherapy in adults with acute myeloid leukemia, *N Engl J Med* 331(14):896, 1994.

Warrell RP Jr, Frankel SR, Dmitrovsky E, et al: Differentiation therapy of acute promyelocytic leukemia with tretinoin (ATRA), *N Engl J Med* 324:1385, 1991.

Weil M, Glidewell OJ, et al: Daunorubicin in the therapy of acute granulocytic leukemia, *Cancer Res* 33:921, 1973.

INFECTIOUS DISEASE

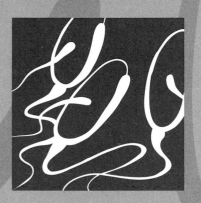

STACI FISCHER (CASES 1 TO 11)
KENT SEPKOWITZ (CASES 12
AND 13)
SECTION EDITORS

CASE

Staci Fischer
Jeffrey Lisowski

*T*he patient is a 26-year-old white man without prior medical problems who comes to the emergency room with complaints of sore throat and fever. He states that he felt well until 2 weeks before admission, when he developed low-grade fevers and a sore throat. He was evaluated on the third day of his illness by a local physician, who prescribed erythromycin for 7 days. He noted a partial improvement in his sore throat. He now presents with worsening odynophagia, myalgias, and subjective fever for 3 days. He denies cough or headache, but has had 3 to 4 loose stools per day for several days.

He is taking acetaminophen as needed for pain and fever control. He reports an allergy to penicillin, which results in a diffuse rash. The patient is employed as a television repairman and denies alcohol or intravenous drug abuse and smoking. He is married but occasionally has unprotected sexual contact with other women, the last of which occurred approximately 2 months ago. No family members or fellow workers are currently ill.

Physical examination reveals an acutely ill-appearing male with a temperature of 102.4°F, pulse of 110 bpm, blood pressure of 122/76 mm Hg, and respiratory rate of 22/min. He has marked bilateral tonsillar swelling and pharyngeal erythema with a thick white exudate bilaterally. Several shallow ulcers, 1 to 2 mm in diameter, are noted on the posterior pharynx. Bilateral tender cervical adenopathy is present. A faint erythematous macular eruption is present on the anterior chest and abdomen. The spleen is not enlarged, and no joint inflammation is present.

QUESTION 1 What is the differential diagnosis at this point?

The patient presents with fever and exudative pharyngitis despite a 1-week course of erythromycin. While the initial clinical suspicion was pharyngitis due to group A *Streptococcus*, failure of his symptoms to resolve after appropriate antibiotic therapy suggests that another pathogen may be responsible.

Less frequent bacterial causes of acute pharyngitis include *Neisseria gonorrhoeae*, *Corynebacterium diphtheriae* and *Arcanobacterium (Corynebacterium) hemolyticum*, all of which are generally sensitive to erythromycin. *Mycoplasma pneumoniae* should also be considered, but the patient's toxic appearance and lack of response to the drug of choice for this infection argue against a mycoplasmal etiology.

The patient's presentation is typical of infectious mononucleosis, a self-limited syndrome marked by fever, exudative pharyngitis, cervical lymphadenopathy, and fatigue, lasting 2 to 3 weeks on average. *Epstein-Barr virus (EBV)* is most commonly implicated.

QUESTION 2 Laboratory studies reveal the following: WBC count 3400/μl with 56% segs, 5% bands, 36% lymphocytes, and 3% monocytes, with 18% atypical lymphocytes. The hemoglobin and hematocrit are 13.0 g/dl and 38%, respectively, with a platelet count of 90,000/μl. The chemistry profile reveals an SGOT (AST) of 62 units/L and SGPT (ALT) of 58 units/L, an LDH of 280 units/L, an alkaline phosphatase of 190 IU/L, and total bilirubin of 0.8 mg/dl. The Monospot (heterophile agglutinin) test is negative. How have the laboratory studies narrowed the differential diagnosis?

The absence of leukocytosis and a left shift again argue against bacterial pathogens. The presence of atypical lymphocytes and mild elevation of transaminases is typical of infectious mononucleosis, but the negative Monospot test is unusual in acute EBV infections in adults (occurring in <5% of cases).

More definitive testing for EBV may be performed, as depicted in Fig. 8-1-1. At the time of presentation with infectious mononucleosis, most adults have detectable IgM and IgG antibodies to viral capsid antigen (VCA). The IgM fraction persists for several months following acute infection, but IgG is detectable throughout life. In addition, IgG antibodies to early antigens (EA) are usually detectable at presentation and persist for several months following the resolution of symptoms. The presence of antibodies to Epstein-Barr nuclear antigens (EBNA) indicates prior infection, as these antibodies are first detected 1 to 2 months following acute symptoms and persist throughout life.

QUESTION 3 Specific EBV serologies are drawn, with the available results at 24 hours as follows: VCA-IgM negative and VCA-IgG 1:40. What further diagnoses should be considered?

Acute EBV is now unlikely, so that the diagnostic considerations turn to causes of heterophile-negative mononucleosis: cytomegalovirus (CMV), viral hepatitis, toxoplasmosis, rubella, human herpesvirus-6 (HHV-6), and acute human immunodeficiency virus (HIV) infection.

CMV, the most common cause of heterophile-negative infectious mononucleosis, is usually transmitted via transfusion of blood or blood products; pharyngitis and adenopathy are not prominent findings in most cases. *Acute viral hepatitis* may present with fever, adenopathy, malaise, and even atypical lymphocytes, but transaminases are usually substantially elevated at the time of presentation.

Acute toxoplasmosis most commonly presents with asymptomatic lymphadenopathy, especially in the cervical area. Patients may develop fever, arthralgias, sore throat, and atypical lymphocytes (usually <10%). Severe exudative pharyngitis is uncommon. Transmission is associated with ingestion of undercooked meat or exposure to infected cats or dogs. *Rubella* infection is generally subclinical, but patients may present with fever and malaise followed by cervical lymphadenopathy (especially involving the posterior auricular, posterior cervical, and suboccipital chains). An erythematous maculopapular eruption develops on the face and subsequently spreads to the trunk. Fever is generally transient, resolving within 1 day of the onset of rash.

HHV-6, the cause of exanthem subitum (roseola) in infants and an acute febrile illness in young children, has recently been implicated as a cause of heterophile-negative infectious mononucleosis in adults. The clinical presentation in adults is variable, but significant fever, pharyngitis, and rash appear uncommon.

The patient's history and presentation seem most consistent with *acute retroviral syndrome,* a mononucleosis-like illness that occurs in 50% to 90% of adults acutely infected with HIV. Most patients develop several of the symptoms and signs listed in the box, but the severity varies substantially, so that only a fraction of affected patients present to physicians for evaluation.

QUESTION 4 What are the common features of the acute retroviral syndrome?

Symptoms generally occur within 2 to 4 weeks of infection, but may begin as early as 5 days or as late as 3 months after exposure. Fever, pharyngitis, and oral aphthous ulcerations have been described in a number of patients. Lymphadenopathy may be generalized, but the cervical, occipital, and axillary nodes are most commonly involved. Rashes that have been described include nonpruritic erythematous macular or maculopapular eruptions, roseola-like exanthems, and vesicular or pustular exanthems and enanthems. Neurologic findings vary from mild headaches to frank meningoencephalitis. Brachial neuritis, Guillain-Barré syndrome, acute myelitis, and peripheral neuropathy have also been described. Uncommon findings in acute HIV infection include pneumonitis, esophagitis, rhabdomyolysis, and anemia.

CLINICAL AND LABORATORY FINDINGS IN ACUTE HIV INFECTION

CONSTITUTIONAL
- Fever
- Chills
- Night sweats
- Malaise
- Lethargy
- Myalgia
- Arthralgia
- Lymphadenopathy
- Anorexia

GASTROINTESTINAL
- Nausea
- Vomiting
- Diarrhea
- Odynophagia
- Abdominal pain
- Oral and esophageal ulcerations

RESPIRATORY/PHARYNGEAL
- Sore throat
- Pharyngitis
- Dry cough

HEMATOLOGIC
- Leukopenia
- Atypical lymphocytosis
- Thrombocytopenia

NEUROLOGIC
- Headache
- Retroorbital pain
- Photophobia
- Irritability
- Aseptic meningitis
- Meningoencephalitis
- Seizures
- Brachial neuritis
- Myelitis
- Guillain-Barré syndrome
- Encephalopathy
- Peripheral neuropathy

MISCELLANEOUS
- Alopecia
- Rash
- Elevated transaminases or alkaline phosphatase

Laboratory findings in acute infection include transient leukopenia and thrombocytopenia, atypical lymphocytosis, and mildly elevated transaminases and alkaline phosphatase. While symptoms usually occur before standard ELISA and Western blot testing for HIV antibody becomes positive, HIV antigenemia in these patients may be prominent, so that antigen studies (such as p24 antigen) on serum or CSF are frequently positive. CD4 lymphocyte counts are transiently decreased during acute infection, but rise to near baseline levels following the resolution of acute seroconversion symptoms.

Symptoms (including neurologic sequelae) are self-limited and generally resolve in 3 to 14 days. Treatment is generally symptomatic, although controversy exists as to whether antiretroviral therapy (e.g., AZT) is indicated. Some investigators believe that patients presenting with severe manifestations of acute HIV infection may have a more rapid progression to AIDS than those with subclinical seroconversions, and that early treatment is therefore indicated. A controlled, randomized trial is currently attempting to answer this question.

CASE FOLLOW-UP   The patient's HIV ELISA test was negative; p24 antigen was detected in his serum. His symptoms resolved without specific intervention over the next 2 to 3 days, and he was discharged to home to follow up as an outpatient.

BIBLIOGRAPHY

Akashi K, Eizuru Y, Sumiyoshi Y, et al: Brief report: severe infectious mononucleosis-like syndrome and primary human herpesvirus 6 infection in an adult, *N Engl J Med* 329(3):168-171, 1993.

Clark SJ, Saag MS, Decker WD, et al: High titers of cytopathic virus in plasma of patients with symptomatic primary HIV-1 infection, *N Engl J Med* 324(14):954-960, 1991.

Cooper DA, Gold J, Maclean P, et al: Acute AIDS retrovirus infection: definition of a clinical illness associated with seroconversion, *Lancet* 2:537-540, 1985.

Daar ES, Moudgil T, Meyer RD, Ho DD: Transient high levels of viremia in patients with primary human immunodeficiency virus type 1 infection, *N Engl J Med* 324(14):961-964, 1991.

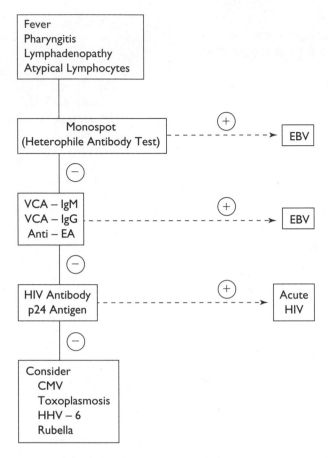

8-1-1 Evaluation of the patient with infectious mononucleosis syndrome. EBV, Epstein-Barr virus; VCA, viral capsid antigen; EA, early antigen; HIV, human immunodeficiency virus; CMV, cytomegalovirus.

Kessler HA, Blaauw B, Spear J, et al: Diagnosis of human immunodeficiency virus infection in seronegative homosexuals presenting with an acute viral syndrome, *JAMA* 258(9): 1196-1199, 1987.

Kinloch-de Loes S, DeSaussure P, Saurat JH, et al: Symptomatic primary infection due to human immunodeficiency virus type 1: review of 31 cases, *Clin Infect Dis* 17:59-65, 1993.

Niederman JC, Liu CR, Kaplan MH, Brown NA: Clinical and serological features of human herpesvirus-6 infection in three adults, *Lancet* 2:817-819, 1988.

Oren I, Sobel JD: Human herpesvirus type 6: review, *Clin Infect Dis* 14:741-746, 1992.

Rabeneck L, Popovic M, Gartner S, et al: Acute HIV infection presenting with painful swallowing and esophageal ulcers, *JAMA* 263(17):2318-2322, 1990.

Steeper TA, Horwitz CA, Ablashi DV, et al: The spectrum of clinical and laboratory findings resulting from human herpesvirus-6 (HHV-6) in patients with mononucleosis-like illnesses not resulting from Epstein-Barr virus or cytomegalovirus, *Am J Clin Path* 93(6):776-783, 1990.

Strauss SE, Cohen JI, Tosato G, Meier J: Epstein-Barr virus infections: biology, pathogenesis, and management, *Ann Intern Med* 118(1):45-58, 1993.

Tindall B, Barker S, Donovan B, et al: Characterization of the acute clinical illness associated with human immunodeficiency virus infection, *Arch Intern Med* 148: 945-949, 1988.

Tindall B, Cooper DA: Primary HIV infection: host responses and intervention strategies, *AIDS* 5:1-14, 1991.

CASE

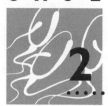

2

Staci Fischer
Jeffrey Lisowski

A *32-year-old woman presented to a Chicago emergency room in August with complaints of fever and diarrhea for 18 hours. A resident of Alabama, she was attending a real estate convention. On her second day in Chicago she noted the abrupt onset of watery stools and abdominal cramping, associated with mild nausea and chills. She passed six large watery stools in a 12-hour period and presented for further evaluation when subjective fever began.*

She denied significant prior diarrheal episodes and the presence of blood or mucus in stools. Her medical history included a history of mitral valve prolapse with intermittent palpitations and situational anxiety. She had no history of heart murmur. She took oral contraceptives regularly but was otherwise on no medications. There was no known family history of inflammatory bowel disease, and she denied alcohol or illicit drug usage.

In the emergency room, she was alert, anxious, and acutely ill-appearing, with an oral temperature of 102.2°F, a pulse of 100 bpm, and blood pressure of 100/60 mm Hg with orthostatic changes. Her abdominal examination revealed hyperactive bowel sounds throughout, with no masses or hepatosplenomegaly noted. Diffuse tenderness without guarding or rebound was present. The rest of the examination was unremarkable.

QUESTION 1 What is the definition of diarrhea? What are the usual electrolyte abnormalities expected in patients with diarrhea? What diagnostic and therapeutic interventions should be implemented in the emergency room?

Diarrhea is defined as the passing of three or more stools in 24 hours, or more than 200 g of stool per day, with >80% water content. With severe diarrhea, patients may lose large amounts of fluid and electrolytes including potassium, sodium, magnesium, and chloride. A hypochloremic metabolic acidosis and significant dehydration with orthostasis may result.

The presence of orthostasis in this patient indicates severe dehydration, so that fluid replacement should be initiated and electrolytes measured. Normal saline with the addition of potassium if necessary is the fluid of choice.

The presence of fever and toxicity suggests an infectious etiology for her diarrhea, the differential diagnosis of which is extensive (see the box). Further history is necessary, with an emphasis on recent travel, foods ingested, and antibiotic usage, all of which are potential risk factors for infectious diarrhea.

Intravenous fluids were administered and a detailed history obtained, which was unrevealing.

Stool evaluation for leukocytes is also indicated, to determine whether an invasive pathogen is involved.

Stool for methylene blue examination was submitted to the laboratory; the results are pending.

While the presence of dysentery (blood and mucus in stools, associated with fever, tenesmus, and abdominal pain) is characteristic of infection with invasive bacteria such as *Shigella, Campylobacter,* and certain *E. coli* strains, watery stools with leukocytes may be the initial clinical picture.

QUESTION 2 What are the major risk factors for infectious diarrhea?

CAUSES OF ACUTE DIARRHEA IN THE IMMUNOCOMPETENT HOST

INFECTIOUS ETIOLOGIES
Viral
- Rotavirus
- Norwalk agent/Norwalk-like viruses
- Adenoviruses
- Calciviruses
- Astroviruses

Bacterial
- *Campylobacter jejuni*
- *Salmonella* species
- *Shigella* species
- *Yersinia enterocolitica*
- *Clostridium difficile*
- *Aeromonas hydrophila*
- *Plesiomonas shigelloides*
- *Vibrio cholerae, V. parahaemolyticus*
- Enterotoxigenic *E. coli* (ETEC)
- Other *E. coli*
  - *E. coli* 0157:H7
  - enteroinvasive *E. coli* (EIEC)
  - enteropathogenic *E. coli* (EPEC)
- *Clostridium perfringens*
- *Staphylococcus aureus*
- *Bacillus cereus*
- *Clostridium botulinum*
- *Listeria monocytogenes*

Parasitic/Protozoal
- *Cryptosporidium*
- *Giardia lamblia*
- *Entamoeba histolytica*
- *Blastocystis hominis*

Helminthic
- *Strongyloides stercoralis*
- *Trichinella spiralis*
- *Capillaria philippinensis*
- *Schistosoma* species
- *Anisakis* species

Miscellaneous
- *Cyclospora*
- Ciguatera poisoning
- Paralytic shellfish poisoning
- Scombroid poisoning

NONINFECTIOUS ETIOLOGIES
- Irritable bowel syndrome
- Carbohydrate malabsorption (e.g., lactose intolerance)
- Fecal impaction
- Inflammatory bowel disease
- Colonic polyp/villous adenoma
- Colonic neoplasm
- Intestinal ischemia
- Zollinger-Ellison syndrome
- Ileal resection (bile-acid induced)
- Carconoid syndrome
- VIPoma

Drug-induced
- Laxatives
- Antacids (Mg-containing)
- Neomycin
- Antimetabolites
- Colchicine
- Alcohol
- Digitalis
- Quinidine
- Sorbitol

Risk factors for the development of infectious diarrhea include travel, close contact with an infected person (especially in homes with small children), HIV infection, and antibiotic usage.

Travel to areas with inadequate sewerage and water treatment systems predisposes to diarrheal infections, most commonly enterotoxigenic *E. coli* (ETEC). Traveler's diarrhea is produced by ingestion of contaminated food or water, and usually begins within the first 2 weeks of stay in an endemic area. However, it should be noted that patients may develop diarrhea acquired during travel even after returning home.

Outbreaks of disease due to *Giardia, Shigella, Salmonella,* and rotavirus have been described in institutions such as day care centers and nursing homes. Contact with a resident or staff member may predispose to the development of diarrhea.

HIV-infected patients are at particular risk for infection with numerous pathogens including *Cryptosporidium, Isospora belli,* microsporidium, *Giardia lamblia,* and cytomegalovirus. Discussion of the spectrum of diarrheal disease in this population is beyond the scope of this section; the reader is referred to the references for further information.

Recent antibiotic exposure (generally within 6 weeks of diarrhea onset) or hospitalization predisposes to infection with *Clostridium difficile.*

QUESTION 3   Methylene blue staining of stool smears revealed the presence of leukocytes. With this information and the epidemiologic data above, what further studies and interventions should be done in this patient?

The presence of leukocytes suggests involvement with an invasive pathogen. Common foodborne bacterial pathogens known to invade the colonic mucosa include *Salmonella, Shigella,* and *Campylobacter* and should be strongly considered in the patient with fever and stool leukocytes. In addition, any patient with recent antibiotic exposure or hospitalization should have a *C. difficile* toxin assay submitted.

Stool cultures for enteric pathogens were submitted.

QUESTION 4   The attending emergency room physician noted over the next 8 to 12 hours that three additional patients presented with diarrhea; each was attending the same convention and reported the abrupt onset of fever and watery stools within 24 hours of presentation. What further diagnostic evaluation should now be undertaken?

TABLE 8-2-1   Common Food Vehicles for Infectious Diarrhea

Food/Source	Pathogen/Disease
Water	*Giardia lamblia*
	Norwalk agent/Norwalk-like viruses
	Campylobacter species
	Cryptosporidium
	Cyclospora
	Vibrio species
	Aeromonas hydrophilia
Shellfish	*Vibrio* species
	Norwalk agent
	Plesiomonas shigelloides
	Neurotoxic shellfish poisoning
	Paralytic shellfish poisoning
Fish	Scombroid (tuna, mahi-mahi, mackerel)
	Ciguatera poisoning (grouper, amberjack, snapper)
	Anisakis (sushi)
Chicken	*Salmonella* species
	Campylobacter species
Eggs	*Salmonella* species
Milk	*Salmonella* species
	Campylobacter species
	Yersinia enterocolitica
Fried rice	*Bacillus cereus*
Beef, gravy	*Salmonella* species
	Campylobacter species
	Clostridium perfringens
Cheese, dairy products	*Listeria monocytogenes*

The occurrence of multiple cases of diarrhea in a group raises the possibility of a common source or foodborne outbreak. A detailed food history on each patient is necessary in hopes of identifying a potential source. Table 8-2-1 provides a list of common food vehicles for infectious diarrhea.

Further questioning revealed that all four patients had eaten at a large banquet on the evening before presentation to the emergency room. Each had enjoyed Caesar salad, baked chicken, and bread pudding. None of the patients reported an unusual taste to the food. The local health department was notified, and over the next few days, 147 patients with similar symptoms were identified and interviewed.

QUESTION 5 What are the most common pathogens causing diarrhea? Discuss their epidemiology, symptoms, and diagnosis.

Viruses cause 30% to 40% of infectious diarrhea episodes in the United States. Rotavirus, the most common cause of severe diarrhea in infants and small children, occurs during winter and is marked by low-grade fever, emesis, and watery diarrhea lasting 5 to 7 days. Adults caring for affected infants may acquire disease, which may be diagnosed by ELISA or latex agglutination detection of antigen or antibody in serum. Norwalk agent and associated Norwalk-like viruses are year-round causes of epidemics of gastroenteritis and have been linked to the intake of contaminated clams, oysters, salads, cake frosting, and drinking water. Disease is characterized by nausea, vomiting, and watery diarrhea, which last 24 to 48 hours. Older children and adults are commonly affected. Outbreaks in schools and restaurants and on cruise ships have been described.

ETEC is the most common cause of traveler's diarrhea. Infection occurs predominantly in the rainy summer seasons in tropical areas. Elaboration of either the heat stable or labile toxin causes watery diarrhea associated with nausea and bloating. While symptoms usually resolve within several days with symptomatic treatment alone, antibiotic therapy and bismuth subsalicylate have been shown to shorten the duration of symptoms when administered early.

Campylobacter jejuni, the most common bacterial pathogen isolated from patients with infectious diarrhea, occurs in all age groups, with peaks in children and young adults. Infection has been linked to ingestion of raw milk, poultry, and untreated water. Patients may present with abdominal pain mimicking appendicitis, often associated with mesenteric adenitis. Complications include bacteremia, a reactive arthritis in HLA-B27 positive patients, and Guillain-Barré syndrome.

Salmonella, the estimated cause of over 1 million cases of diarrhea in the United States yearly, is implicated in both sporadic and outbreak-associated disease. Infection is most common in infants and the elderly and occurs most frequently in the summer or fall. Disease has been frequently traced to infected eggs, poultry, and pet turtles. Symptoms include fever, headache, abdominal pain, and diarrhea, occurring after an incubation period of 5 to 72 hours. Fecal leukocytes may be seen, and disease may be complicated by bacteremia and metastatic infection, especially in immunocompromised hosts such as HIV-infected patients.

Shigella has been reported to cause infection in a number of summer and fall outbreaks in the United States, with *Shigella sonnei* comprising the majority of cases. Fever and watery stools develop 24 to 72 hours following exposure; subsequently, mucoid and bloody stools develop, often associated with tenesmus or rectal urgency. Symptoms typically last less than 7 days.

A recent pandemic of *Vibrio cholerae* infection has been reported from South America, associated with ingestion of contaminated food and river water. Disease is characterized by loose "rice-water" stools, altered mental status, and vomiting, beginning 1 to 4 days after ingestion of contaminated water or food. Sporadic cases have been reported from the Gulf Coast area in recent years, and treatment is generally supportive. Antimicrobial therapy with tetracycline is recommended.

E. coli O157:H7 has caused outbreaks of hemorrhagic colitis associated with ingestion of unpasteurized milk, undercooked ground beef, and contaminated drinking water, as well as with swimming in stagnant waters. Disease may be complicated by the development of a postinfectious hemolytic-uremic syndrome. Diagnosis is by stool culture and requires growth in specialized media.

Yersinia enterocolitica infection usually occurs secondary to the ingestion of contaminated water, dairy products, or foods. Most commonly the infection is self-limited, with diarrhea lasting up to 2 weeks. Mesenteric adenitis or terminal ileitis may occur, often in patients without diarrhea, frequently resulting in laparotomies for suspected appendicitis. Post-infectious reactive arthritis and ankylosing spondylitis may be seen in individuals who express HLA-B27; other sequelae include Reiter's syndrome and erythema nodosum.

Clostridium difficile causes diarrhea via the production of an enterotoxin, toxin A. Seen most commonly in those receiving recent antibiotic therapy, it is the most common nosocomial cause of diarrhea as well. Spores of this organism may persist in the environment as fomites and have been implicated in several outbreaks of disease in hospitalized patients. Disease may be complicated by the development of toxic megacolon, at times presenting without concurrent diarrhea. Diagnosis is made by the identification of toxin production in stool; cultures may be positive in those who are asymptomatic carriers, requiring no therapy. Treatment is with oral metronidazole or oral vancomycin, and relapses are common.

Giardia lamblia is the most common parasitic cause of diarrhea in the United States, causing waterborne and day care center outbreaks as well as sporadic disease. Endemic areas include the Rocky Mountains, New York City, St. Petersburg, Russia, and Rome, Italy. One to 2 weeks following ingestion of protozoal cysts, patients develop nausea, flatulence, abdominal bloating, and foul-smelling stools, sometimes with malabsorption. Diagnosis may require repeated examinations of stool for cysts (which are often undetectable at the time of presentation). Other methods of diagnosis include the string test (to obtain duodenal or jejunal secretions for evaluation) or a small bowel aspirate and biopsy. In select patients, a therapeutic trial of metronidazole or quinacrine is reasonable.

Cryptosporidium, a protozoan, is a cause of acute watery diarrhea in normal hosts and severe, protracted diarrhea in patients with AIDS. It has been implicated in large waterborne outbreaks, including one in Milwaukee in 1993, which affected over 350,000 people. Diarrhea is typically watery and profuse, with no detectable leukocytes, and lasts an average of 10 days.

QUESTION 6   When should specific stool studies be obtained?

In many circumstances, diarrhea is self-limited and may have resolved by the time stool cultures are available. In general, the patient with prolonged diarrhea (>48 hours) or evidence of dysentery should have a workup for specific etiology initiated. Fig. 8-2-1 depicts an evaluation scheme. While the presence of fecal leukocytes may be suggestive of involvement with invasive pathogens, cultures help guide antimicrobial therapy. Routine enteric cultures in most medical centers detect *Campylobacter, Salmonella,* and *Shigella;* special requests are often necessary to alert the lab to attempt to identify *Yersinia, E. coli* O157:H7, *Vibrio,* and viral species. Examination for ova and parasites is particularly important in the evaluation of patients with diarrhea lasting more than 2 weeks. *C. difficile* toxin studies should be obtained in those patients with nosocomial diarrhea or antibiotic exposure within the preceding 6 weeks. The workup in patients with HIV infection should also include smears with modified acid-fast staining (for *Isospora* and *Cryptosporidium* detection) and trichrome staining or electron microscopy (to search for microsporidium). More invasive evaluation with sigmoidoscopy may be necessary in the undiagnosed patient with persistent diarrhea and/or microscopic or gross evidence of colitis. The evaluation of outbreaks of diarrheal disease should include bacterial cultures, as mentioned previously, and an aggressive search for possible food vehicles in order to possibly

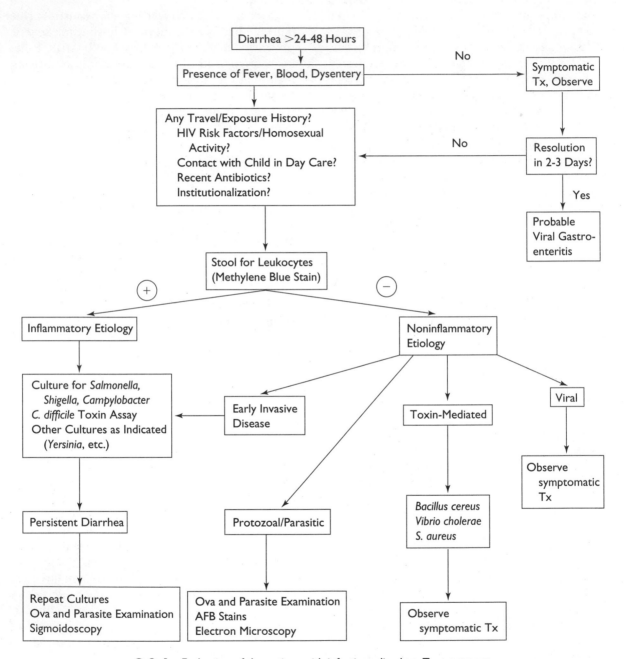

8-2-1 Evaluation of the patient with infectious diarrhea. Tx, treatment.

halt the spread of infection. Local health departments are useful in facilitating this evaluation.

Ciprofloxacin 500 mg orally twice daily for 5 days was prescribed because of the suspicion of a foodborne bacterial etiology to the patient's illness. Following hydration, she was able to tolerate oral liquids and was discharged from the emergency department. Her diarrhea and fever resolved over the next 2 to 3 days.

QUESTION 7 What are the major concepts governing the therapy of infectious diarrhea?

Treatment of infectious diarrhea consists of fluid and electrolyte replacement. If fever and dysenteric symptoms are absent, antiperistaltic drugs such as diphenoxylate or loperamide may be useful. The role of antimicrobials in the treatment of infectious diarrhea is based on pathogen susceptibility, impact on clinical disease course, and severity of illness. Even when susceptible bacteria are identified, antibiotics are frequently unnecessary because of the self-limiting nature of diarrheal disease. Antibiotics are indicated in the treatment of severe diarrheal illness resulting from a susceptible pathogen or in the compromised host. The use of antibiotics in mild to moderate disease should be evaluated on an individual basis.

While the agents responsible for acute infectious diarrhea are numerous, the approach to the patient with febrile gastroenteritis is straightforward. Knowledge of the epidemiology of these pathogens, the impact of host susceptibility, and appropriate strategies for diagnosis are paramount to the evaluation of such processes.

CASE FOLLOW-UP An extensive evaluation by the health department was undertaken; 690 of the estimated 900 conventioneers present at the banquet were found to develop gastrointestinal symptoms, with a mean incubation period of 18.9 hours (range, 6 to 37 hours). *Salmonella enteritidis* was isolated from the stool of this patient and 17 of 20 other specimens submitted from the same emergency room. The ingestion of bread pudding (prepared with lightly heated raw eggs) was subsequently found to be highly associated with the development of diarrhea; the egg supplier's flock was found to be infected.*

• •

BIBLIOGRAPHY

Baird-Parker AC: Foodborne salmonellosis, *Lancet* 336:1231-1235, 1990.

Blacklow NR, Greenberg HB: Viral gastroenteritis, *N Engl J Med* 325(4):252-264, 1991.

Chalker RB, Blaser MJ: A review of human salmonellosis: III. Magnitude of *Salmonella* infection in the United States, *Rev Infect Dis* 10(1):111-124, 1988.

Cohen ML: The epidemiology of diarrheal disease in the United States, *Infect Dis Clin North Am* 2(3):557-570, 1988.

DuPont HL, Ericsson CD: Prevention and treatment of traveler's diarrhea, *N Engl J Med* 328(25):1821-1827, 1991.

Ericsson CD, DuPont HL: Traveler's diarrhea: approaches to prevention and treatment, *Clin Infect Dis* 16:616-614, 1993.

Fan K, Morris AJ, Reller LB: Application of rejection criteria for stool cultures for bacterial enteric pathogens, *J Clin Microbiol* 31(8):2233-2235, 1993.

Genta RM: Diarrhea in helminthic infections, *Clin Infect Dis* 16(suppl 2):S122-S129, 1993.

Goodman LJ: Diagnosis, management, and prevention of diarrheal diseases, *Current Opinion Infect Dis* 6:88-93, 1993.

Goodman LJ, Lisowski JM, Harris AA, et al: Evaluation of an outbreak of foodborne illness initiated in the emergency department, *Ann Emerg Med* 22(8):1291-1294, 1993.

Goodman LJ, Trenholme GM, Kaplan RL, et al: Empiric antimicrobial therapy of domestically acquired acute diarrhea in urban adults, *Arch Intern Med* 150:541-546, 1990.

Guerrant RL, Bobak DA: Bacterial and protozoal gastroenteritis, *N Engl J Med* 325(5):327-340, 1991.

Guerrant RL, Shields DS, Thorson SM, et al: Evaluation and diagnosis of acute infectious diarrhea, *Am J Med* 78(suppl 6B):91-98, 1985.

Holmberg SD, Schell WL, Fanning GR, et al: *Aeromonas* intestinal infections in the United States, *Ann Intern Med* 105:683-689, 1986.

Holmberg SD, Wachsmuth IK, Hickman-Brenner FW, et al: *Plesiomonas* enteric infections in the United States, *Ann Intern Med* 105:690-694, 1986.

Hughes JM, Merson MH: Fish and shellfish poisoning, *N Engl J Med* 295(20):1117-1120, 1976.

Kapikian AZ: Viral gastroenteritis, *JAMA* 269(5):627-630, 1993.

---

*From Goodman LJ, et al: Evaluation of an outbreak of foodborne illness initiated in the emergency department, *Ann Emerg Med* 22(8): 1291-1294, 1993.

Knoop FC, Owens M, Crocker IC: *Clostridium difficile:* clinical disease and diagnosis, *Clin Microbiol Rev* 6(3):251-265, 1993.

Levine WC, Smart JF, Archer DL, et al: Foodborne disease outbreaks in nursing homes, 1975 through 1987, *JAMA* 266(15):2105-2109, 1991.

Lew JF, Glass RI, Gangarosa RE, et al: Diarrheal deaths in the United States, 1979 through 1987: a special problem for the elderly, *JAMA* 265(24):3280-3284, 1991.

Reed SL: Amebiasis: an update, *Clin Infect Dis* 14:385-393, 1992.

Ryan CA, Tauxe RV, Hosek GW, et al: *Escherichia coli* O157:H7 diarrhea in a nursing home: clinical, epidemiological, and pathologic findings, *J Infect Dis* 154(4):631-638, 1986.

Smith PD, Quinn TC, Strober W, et al: Gastrointestinal infections in AIDS, *Ann Intern Med* 116(1):63-77, 1992.

Swerdlow DL, Woodruff BA, Brady RC, et al: A waterborne outbreak in Missouri of *Escherichia coli* O157:H7 associated with bloody diarrhea and death, *Ann Intern Med* 117(10): 812-819, 1992.

Thorne GM: Diagnosis of infectious diarrheal diseases, *Infect Dis Clin North Am* 2(3):747-774, 1988.

Todd E: Epidemiology of foodborne illness: North America, *Lancet* 336:788-790, 1990.

CASE

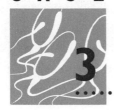

3

Deborah Schiappa
Gordon Trenholme

The patient is a 73-year-old woman who was in her usual state of health until 2 weeks prior to presentation when she developed daily fevers to 101°F, malaise, weakness, and poor appetite. She denied any localizing symptoms such as shortness of breath, cough, chest pain, headache, photophobia, nausea, vomiting, abdominal pain, dysuria, diarrhea, or joint pain. Her symptoms persisted. Since she was unable to continue functioning independently and perform her activities of daily living, she was admitted to the hospital for further evaluation. The patient took no medications and had a past history only of B-thalassemia trait and mitral valve prolapse (MVP).

Examination revealed a T 101.5°F, P 100 bpm, BP 120/78 mm Hg, RR 12/min. She was alert and oriented to person, place, and time. Head, ears, eyes, nose, and throat (HEENT) examination was unremarkable. There were no conjunctival or retinal hemorrhages. The patient was edentulous and had upper and lower dentures in place. Cardiac examination revealed a 3/6 systolic murmur at the left sternal border. The pulmonary examination was significant for diminished breath sounds at both bases but was otherwise clear. The abdomen was soft and nontender with normo-active bowel sounds present in all four quadrants. A spleen tip was palpable below the left costal margin. Extremities were without evidence of clubbing or edema. There were no skin lesions or rash noted. The neurologic examination was nonfocal.

QUESTION I You are the senior medical officer on call. The admitting resident remarks to you, after completing his evaluation, that the patient's clinical presentation suggests an infectious process. Furthermore, he is concerned with the presence of a heart murmur. Based on the patient's presenting medical history, what major infectious process should be considered at this point, and what are the associated physical findings?

The most important entity to consider is infectious endocarditis (IE). Although in theory the diagnosis of IE should be straightforward, in practice it is often difficult to establish with certainty. Some of the difficulty arises from the variable and often nonspecific clinical presentation, and the occurrence of culture negative endocarditis. New criteria are being developed that include results from transesophageal echocardiography and may prove to be more sensitive and specific. Although not pathognomonic, the combination of fever, vague constitutional symptoms, heart murmur, and splenomegaly strongly suggest the presence of IE.

The signs and symptoms of IE vary widely and may involve any organ symptom. The majority of patients present with fever (90%) and a heart murmur (>85%). In addition, cardiac infection may be accompanied by classic physical findings (embolic or immune-complex mediated) in up to 50% of patients. Embolic phenomena may include conjunctival or mucous membrane petechiae or hemorrhages. Septic emboli may occur on the extremities and are called Janeway lesions (painless lesions found on the palms and fingers). Splinter hemorrhages may be found in the proximal subungual area appearing as hemorrhagic slivers. Left upper quadrant pain may be due to splenic infarction. Ischemic colitis may result from superior mesenteric or inferior mesenteric occlusion and presents as abdominal tenderness. The central nervous system is also susceptible to embolic infarction. Patients may develop focal neurologic deficits. Cardiac manifestations include congestive heart failure from valvular dysfunction, heart block, arrhythmias, and pericarditis. Immune complex mediated manifestations include Osler's nodes (painful fingertip lesions) and renal involvement (microscopic hematuria).

QUESTION 2 Since the patient did not appear toxic, intravenous antibiotics were not begun initially. Blood was drawn for admission laboratory testing, and three sets (six bottles) of blood cultures were obtained. The following laboratories were soon available: WBC count 19,000 with 56% neutrophils and 17% band forms. Hemoglobin was 8.3 with a normal MCV. The platelet count was 80,000. The rheumatoid factor was positive, the erythrocyte sedimentation rate (ESR) was elevated to 65. How do these values support or refute the diagnosis of IE?

The laboratory findings are often varied and nonspecific. It is not uncommon to see a normocytic, normochromic anemia, leukocytosis, leukopenia, or thrombocytopenia. Other nonspecific findings include an elevated ESR, the presence of rheumatoid factor or circulating immune complexes, and decreased serum complement levels reflecting the immune response to endocarditis. Ultimately, the laboratory diagnosis of IE depends on isolation of the organism from blood cultures.

If the patient has not received prior antibiotics, the initial blood cultures obtained will yield the etiology most of the time. The yield will decrease by 50% if prior antibiotics have been given in the preceding 2 weeks. The best microbiologic yield is obtained from three sets of blood cultures drawn from different sites over time.

QUESTION 3 The following morning the microbiology lab informs you that 6/6 blood culture bottles are positive for gram-positive cocci in chains. How does this impact on your differential

diagnosis? What are the risk factors for the development of IE? What other diagnostic tests would you consider at this point?

The single most important test is the blood culture. Multiple positive blood cultures for the same organism prove the presence of constant bacteremia and an endovascular infection, independent of the height of the temperature spike. Bacteria are the most common cause. Other agents, including fungi, rickettsia, chlamydia, and possibly viruses, may be involved.

The factors placing an individual at increased risk for endocarditis include preexisting valvular lesions and exposure to events producing bacteremia or disruption of the endovascular integrity. Advanced age is a predisposing factor for the development of valvular calcific degeneration. Underlying cardiac lesions, such as mitral valve prolapse, idiopathic hypertrophic subacute stenosis (IHSS), and prosthetic heart valves, are implicated more frequently today than rheumatic heart disease. Conditions leading to the development of a bacteremic state include dental manipulations, gastrointestinal or genitourinary instrumentation, and intravenous drug use. Events causing disruption of the endovascular endothelium lead to the development of a nonbacterial thrombotic platelet/fibrin mesh. As bacteremia occurs, the microorganisms are trapped in this mesh that functions as a protective sheath against host defense mechanisms. Thus, the microorganisms are allowed to grow, multiply, and form a vegetation. Endothelial microtrauma, induced by central venous access catheters, hyperalimentation lines, pacemakers, or implanted prosthesis, are potential contributors to the pathogenesis of nosocomial endocarditis.

The patient should undergo further diagnostic evaluation with echocardiography. Transthoracic echocardiography can be helpful to visualize vegetations on the valve or chordae tendinae and to delineate the extent of involvement. Several studies reviewed echocardiographic results from cases in which endocarditis was pathologically confirmed and determined that the sensitivity of transthoracic echocardiogram ranged from 58% to 63%. In cases where transthoracic studies are inconclusive or of poor quality, a transesophageal echocardiogram can improve the sensitivity from 90% to 100%. In addition to higher detection rates for vegetations than transthoracic imaging, transesophageal echocardiography is more sensitive for detecting cardiac abscess, aneurysm, and other complications. The reliability of echocardiography to predict major clinical events and to determine the need for valve replacement, however, has not been completely evaluated.

Two caveats must be kept in mind when using echocardiography as a diagnostic modality. A negative study does not exclude the diagnosis, and a study that reveals a vegetation does not make the diagnosis of endocarditis. The result should always be interpreted in light of the current clinical circumstances. Transesophageal echo should be done in any high-risk patient when a normal or suboptimal transthoracic study is obtained or if there is concern about a perivalvular leak, presence of an abscess, native or prosthetic valve dysfunction, or fistula formation.

Diagnostic suspicion can be supported by the demonstration of splenic or hepatic infarcts as detected by ultrasound, or the presence of microscopic or gross hematuria, or multiple peripheral abscesses.

QUESTION 4 What is the appropriate medical therapy for IE?

Medical treatment includes intravenous antibiotics for up to 4 to 6 weeks. The gram-positive organisms associated with endocarditis include penicillin-susceptible streptococci, (such as *S. viridans* or *S. bovis*), relatively resistant or tolerant viridans strep (with MICS between 0.1 and 0.5 mg of penicillin/ml), and methicillin resistant staphylococci or enterococci. Antimicrobial agents should be selected that are bactericidal, unless otherwise contraindicated. A combination of penicillin G plus an aminoglycoside, such as streptomycin or gentamicin, for the first 2 weeks would be adequate treatment for uncomplicated pen-

icillin-susceptible viridans strep and *S. bovis* endocarditis. Alternatives include penicillin G for 4 weeks, once daily ceftriaxone for 4 weeks, or vancomycin if the patient is severely penicillin allergic.

Treatment of enterococcal endocarditis should consist of a combination of penicillin G plus an aminoglycoside (streptomycin or gentamicin), for a total of 4 to 6 weeks. The combination of a B-lactam and an aminoglycoside provides synergism. Vancomycin may be substituted for penicillin in the allergic patient. Special treatment regimens are required for relatively resistant or tolerant viridans streptococci, as well as for enterococci resistant to aminoglycosides and vancomycin. The final identification and susceptibility pattern of recovered blood isolates should always be taken into account, and antibiotic therapy individualized accordingly.

Recently, outpatient parenteral therapy for carefully selected patients with non-enterococcal penicillin-susceptible streptococcal endocarditis has been recommended as a cost-savings measure in several studies. However, further trials are necessary to evaluate the efficacy of these regimens. Long-term suppressive therapy may be necessary in patients in whom clearance of the infection is not possible and for whom valve replacement is not an option.

QUESTION 5 Transthoracic echocardiography is done, and the results are negative. However, a transesophageal study demonstrates a 10-mm vegetation on the mitral valve with moderate mitral regurgitation. The patient begins to improve clinically. However, 4 days later her hospital course is complicated by an exacerbation of congestive heart failure. What clinical concerns should be addressed at this point?

The clinician must evaluate the patient daily for evidence of possible complications of endocarditis and ensure that the blood cultures are sterilized. The patient has developed a common complication, that is, congestive heart failure (CHF), and needs to be treated aggressively. Causes of CHF include valvular incompetence or rupture of the interventricular septum. Transthoracic or transesophageal echocardiogram could detect the presence of a possible ruptured chordae tendinae with flail leaflet or a perforated valve cusp. Other potential cardiac complications arising in any patient with IE include myocardial abscess, involvement of the cardiac conduction system (secondary to extension of the infection from the perivalvular area leading to heart block or arrhythmias), myocardial infarction (secondary to embolization of the vegetation to the coronary arteries or coronary artery thrombosis), and purulent pericarditis. Potential extracardiac complications may include peripheral emboli, formation of a mycotic aneurysm, metastatic infections, and acute neurologic deficits.

QUESTION 6 The patient responded well to treatment with diuretics and after load reducers. What are the indications for valve surgery before completion of a standard course of antibiotics?

The most common indications for surgery include uncontrolled congestive heart failure (acute valvular dysfunction), repeated emboli, uncontrollable infections with persistently positive blood cultures in spite of appropriate antimicrobial therapy, myocardial or valve ring abscess, and fungal endocarditis. When the tricuspid valve is involved, persistent bacteremia and intractable congestive heart failure are indications for surgery. While other serious complications of tricuspid endocarditis may occur (i.e., large vegetations, septic pulmonary emboli and persistent fever), these are not independent indications for surgery.

The alternatives for valve replacement depend on which valve is infected, the patient's stability, and the extent of perivalvular involvement. Options may include valve replacement, valvulectomy/valvuloplasty, or vegetectomy.

QUESTION 7 The microbiology laboratory calls to tell you that no further blood cultures are positive for this organism, but the isolate recovered from the initial blood culture was identified as Strep bovis. What should be done?

Isolation of this organism from the blood should alert the physician to search for underlying GI pathology, specifically a colonic tumor or polyp. Therefore, the patient should undergo a colonoscopy. Strep bovis endocarditis may precede the development of colon cancer in some patients by years. Therefore, a negative colonoscopy should be followed up with repeated exams.

QUESTION 8 The colonoscopy revealed a benign polyp in the right colon. The patient responds quickly to treatment and completes her course of IV antibiotics. Because of her history of mitral valve prolapse, she was counseled on the need for future antibiotic prophylaxis. What is the appropriate antibiotic prophylaxis for this patient?

The trend, with regard to antibiotic prophylaxis, is toward simple regimens to encourage patient compliance and decrease costs, without sacrificing efficacy. Antibiotic prophylaxis, as recommended by the American Heart Association, can be divided into bacteremia prone procedures and the presence of vascular lesions, implanted devices, and other conditions. Predisposing cardiac conditions include the presence of a prosthetic valve, a prior history of endocarditis, congenital cardiac malformations, rheumatic and other acquired valvular dysfunction, hypertrophic cardiomyopathy, and mitral valve prolapse with valvular regurgitation. These conditions set the stage for the development of infection when bacteremia is encountered. Procedures that commonly produce bacteremia and require prophylaxis include any dental procedure known to induce gingival or mucosal bleeding, surgery of the upper respiratory tract, procedures involving the gastrointestinal or genitourinary tract, bronchoscopy with a rigid bronchoscope, obstetric infections, and any surgery involving infected tissue. The recommended standard oral prophylactic regimen for dental, oral, or upper respiratory procedures includes 3 g of amoxicillin orally, 1 hour before the procedure, then 1.5 g 6 hours after the initial dose. In the penicillin-allergic patient erythromycin or clindamycin may be substituted. Patients unable to take oral antibiotics

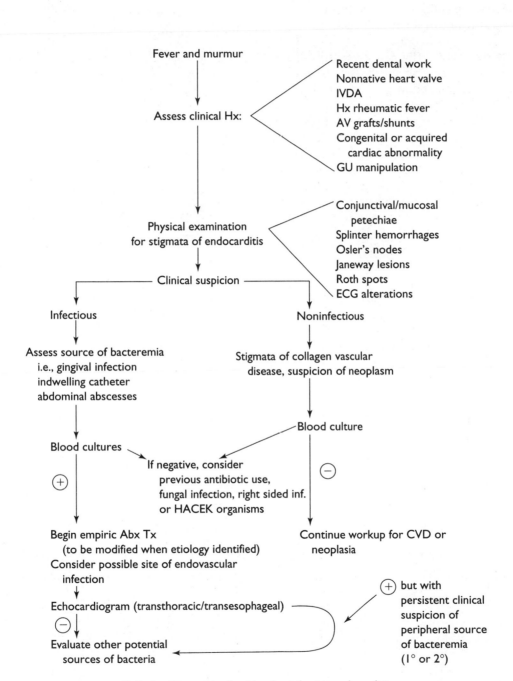

8-3-1   Diagnostic algorithm for infective endocarditis.

can receive ampicillin or clindamycin intravenously or vancomycin if penicillin-allergic.

CASE SUMMARY This case demonstrates several important points about IE. First is that the diagnosis hinges on obtaining blood cultures in the event of suspected persistent bacteremia. Echocardiographic results should be interpreted in light of the clinical circumstances. Secondly, be aware of the risk factors for the development of IE. This includes anything that causes bacteremia (dental manipulations, etc.) or anything that compromises the integrity of the endovascular endothelium (intravascular trauma, preexisting valvular lesions). The current trend is away from rheumatic heart disease as the primary cause of endocarditis and toward lesions of degenerative heart disease or preexisting anatomic abnormalities (i.e., MVP). Third, treatment is based on intravenous bactericidal antibiotics with modifications based on the identification and susceptibility of the organism. Fourth, as this case illustrates, the specific organism may be a clue for the origin of an occult malignancy. Fig. 8-3-1 shows a diagnostic algorithm for infective endocarditis.

• •

BIBLIOGRAPHY

Bayer AS: Infective endocarditis, *Clin Infect Dis* 17:313-322, 1993.

Baddour LM: Polymicrobial infective endocarditis in the 1980's, *Rev Infect Dis* 13:963-970, 1991.

Churchill MA, Geraci JE: Musculoskeletal manifestations of bacterial endocarditis, *Ann Intern Med* 87(6):754-759, 1977.

Coleman DL, Horwotz RI: Association between serum inhibitory and bactericidal concentrations and therapeutic outcome in bacterial endocarditis, *Am J Med* 73:260-267, 1982.

Dinubile MJ: Surgery in active endocarditis, *Ann Intern Med* 96:650-659, 1982.

Dojani A, Bisno AL: Prevention of bacterial endocarditis, *JAMA* 264(22):2919-2922, 1990.

Dreyfus G, Serraf A: Valve repair in acute endocarditis, *Ann Thorac Surg* 49:706-713, 1990.

Erbel R, Rohmann S, Drexler M, et al: Improved diagnostic value of echocardiography in patients with infective endocarditis by transesophageal approach, a prospective study, *European Heart J* 9:43-53, 1988.

Fang G, Keys TF: Prosthetic valve endocarditis resulting from nosocomial bacteremia: a prospective, multicenter trial, *Ann Intern Med* 119(7):560-567, 1993.

Harkonen M: Severe backache as a presenting sign of bacterial endocarditis, *Acta Med Scand* 210:329-331, 1981.

Lerner PI: Infective endocarditis: a review of selected topics, *Med Clin North Am* 58(3):605-622, 1974.

Mansur AJ, Grinberg M: The complications of infective endocarditis, *Arch Intern Med* 152:2428-2432, 1992.

Megran DW: Enterococcal endocarditis, *Clin Infect Dis* 15:63-71, 1992.

Mugge, Daniel, Frank, et al: Echocardiography in infective endocarditis: reassessment of prognostic implications of vegetation size determined by the transthoracic and transesophageal approach, *J Am Coll Cardiol* 14(3):631-638, 1989.

Nunley DL, Perlman PE: Endocarditis: changing trends in epidemiology, clinical and microbiologic spectrum, *Postgrad Med* 93:5, 1993.

Pesanti EL, Smith IM: Infective endocarditis with negative blood cultures, *Am J Med* 66:43-66, 1979.

Shapiro S, Bayer AS: Transesophageal and doppler echocardiography in the diagnosis and management of infective endocarditis, *Chest* 100:4, 1991.

Thompson PJ, Richsmuller M: Rheumatic manifestations of infective endocarditis, *Rheumatol Int* 12:61-63, 1992.

Tirone DE: Heart valve operations in patients with active infective endocarditis, *Ann Thorac Surg* 49:701-705, 1990.

Van Scoy RE: Culture-negative endocarditis, *Mayo Clin Proc* 57:149-154, 1982.

Watanakunakorn C: Infective endocarditis at a large community teaching hospital 1980-1990, *Medicine* 72(2):90-102, 1993.

Weinstein MP: Stratton CW: Multicenter collaborative evaluation of a standardized serum bactericidal test as a prognostic indicator in infective endocarditis, *Am J Med* 78:262-269, 1985.

C A S E

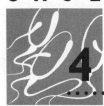

4

Deborah Schiappa
Gordon Trenholme

The patient is a 52-year-old female neonatologist who was referred to the infectious disease clinic for evaluation of fever for 24 days. She was in excellent health until the onset of symptoms that included headache, fatigue, and evening temperature elevations to 101.5°F. She denied other symptoms including cough, shortness of breath, chest pain, neck stiffness, photophobia, sore throat, rhinorrhea, dysuria, skin rashes, abdominal or back pain.

The physical examination revealed the following. Vital signs were T 98.6°F, P 100 bpm, RR 12/min, and BP 120/80 mm Hg. She was alert and oriented to person, place, and time. Her skin was warm and dry, and there were no lesions or rashes noted. HEENT examination was unremarkable. Her neck was supple with a palpable thyroid and no adenopathy. Cardiac examination was significant for a murmur of mitral valve prolapse. Her lungs were clear. Both abdominal and neurologic examinations were normal. Initial laboratory results revealed a normal complete blood count, chemistry profile, liver function tests, urinalysis, chest x-ray, and negative blood and urine cultures. No definite diagnosis had been reached after several visits to her primary physician.

QUESTION I Does this patient fulfill the criteria for a fever of unknown origin (FUO)? What parts of the history and physical examination are specifically important in evaluating this patient?

Petersdorf and Beeson in 1961 defined FUO as a temperature higher than 38.3°C (101°F) on several occasions for more than 3 weeks' duration and uncertain diagnosis after 1 week of in-hospital study. Because of changing medical practices, this definition has been modified to reflect the trend toward shorter hospital stays (3 days of in-patient evaluation) and more outpatient investigation for subacute and chronic illnesses (at least 3 visits). Additionally, FUOs have been subdivided into classic, nosocomial, neutropenic, and HIV-associated forms to account for differences in their duration, etiology, treatment, and outcome. This patient meets the criteria because she had nightly fevers to 101.5°F for more than 3 weeks without a definite diagnosis after investigations conducted on more than 3 outpatient visits.

The workup of this patient should begin with a complete history and physical examination. Questions regarding localizing symptoms, recent travel, contact with other ill persons, animals or insect bites, drug or toxin exposures, HIV risk factors, and immunization history should be sought. Physical examination should carefully seek areas for further evaluation, such as abdominal masses, hepatic or splenic enlargement, and presence of periumbilical lymph nodes. Skin, joints, and muscles should be assessed for the presence of swelling, lesions, or tenderness. The heart should be auscultated for murmur. Pelvic, rectal, and temporal artery examination for tenderness, swelling, or nodularity should be included. Several follow-up historical inquiries and physical examinations may be necessary to provide additional clues and to detect changes in clinical status. The physician should use these opportunities to clarify historical points, to discover new elements or changes on physical examination, such as a new heart murmur, and to look for improvement of symptoms after beginning intervention.

She had a history of a positive purified protein

derivative (PPD) tuberculin skin test as a child in India. She never received Bacillus Calmette-Guérin vaccination nor any form of prophylaxis or treatment. Since then she has had multiple work-related exposures to tuberculosis. She was taking no medications and had no known allergies. The patient sustained nightly fever up to 101.5° F, returning to normal for the rest of the day.

QUESTION 2   How is the fever curve useful as a clue to diagnosis?

Although not pathognomonic, the fever curve itself may be a useful clue to the etiology. Continuous fevers may occur in cases of brucellosis, typhoid fever, tularemia, psittacosis, pneumococcal pneumonia, and ricketsial infections. Intermittent fevers, involving wide temperature fluctuations and at least one normal temperature in a 24-hour period, are commonly seen in cases of pyogenic abscess or with irregular use of antipyretics. Relapsing fevers involve cyclical alternating periods of fever and normal temperature. These may be seen in lymphoma, rat-bite fever, borreliosis, and dengue fever. A pulse-temperature deficit may suggest leptospirosis, legionella, or typhoid. Temperature spikes higher than 102° F are more common in infections, lymphomas, or vasculitides. Prolonged fevers most commonly involve neoplasm or noninfectious processes such as granulomatous hepatitis. Drug fevers may demonstrate any pattern but frequently manifest a sustained pattern. The most specific temperature pattern in a patient with FUO is the double quotidian fever that consists of 2 spikes within a 24-hour period not induced by antipyretics. It may be seen in adult Still's disease, Leishmaniasis, malaria, and miliary tuberculosis.

She had no history of travel since moving from India to the United States at 8 years old. Her source of infectious exposures included contact with ill children at the hospital where she practiced. She denied the use of illicit drugs or any over-the-counter medications. Her physical examination was significant for a heart rate of 100 bpm, a cardiac murmur consistent with mitral valve prolapse, and a palpable thyroid.

QUESTION 3   What broad categories should be considered in the differential diagnosis? What further tests should be considered to help narrow the diagnosis?

Infection accounts for approximately 30% to 40% of all cases of classical FUO. Examples include abscesses, endocarditis, tuberculosis, viral infections including HIV, parasitic and fungal infections. With the exception of culture negative endocarditis, bacterial endocarditis is a rare cause of FUO due to improved blood culture techniques and efforts to prophylax patients with the underlying cardiac lesions. More common causes include tuberculosis, CMV, and several "newer" infectious causes such as Lyme disease and chlamydia/TWAR.

Neoplasm accounts for 20% to 30% of FUO. The most common is lymphoma of which non-Hodgkin lymphoma is most important. Hypernephroma is the most common localized, solid tumor. Other neoplastic causes include leukemia, atrial myxomas, and metastatic disease of the lungs, pancreas, and stomach.

Multisystem disease accounts for more than 15% of cases. Both rheumatoid arthritis and SLE are less frequent causes of FUO because of the development of more specific tests. Adult onset Still's disease, however, is not an uncommon cause of FUO. Perhaps the most important cause of FUO is temporal arteritis. This illness occurs in elderly patients (55 years or more) and has as its notable feature an erythrocyte sedimentation rate (ESR) in excess of 100 mm/hr. A temporal artery biopsy is necessary for definitive diagnosis. The biopsy should be done bilaterally (because of patchy involvement), if the artery is not abnormal on examination. If visual impairment is present, steroid therapy should be started early to avoid irresevible blindness. In appropriate population groups, sarcoidosis and granulomatous hepatitis are important considerations as potential etiologies of FUO.

Other causes include drug-related and factitious fevers. Commonly implicated medications include dilantin, heparin, aldomet, capoten, procainamide, and allopurinol. Factitious fevers, due to thermometer manipulation or deliberate intravenous injections of foreign material or bacterial inocula, are common in health professionals.

Miscellaneous causes range from pulmonary emboli, periodic disease (Familial Mediterranean fever), inflammatory bowel disease, and Whipple's disease to various "itises" such as pericarditis, thyroiditis, and relapsing polychondritis. Diagnosis may not be established in approximately 10% of cases.

Since the initial laboratory results were nonrevealing, additional tests to consider in this patient include a PPD skin test with anergy profile, an ESR, and an echocardiogram. If clinical suspicion for endocarditis were still high despite negative transthoracic echocardiogram results, a transesophageal echocardiogram and repeat blood cultures for fastidious organisms could be done.

The PPD skin test was markedly positive, but her chest radiograph remained normal. A transthoracic echocardiogram revealed mitral valve prolapse without regurgitation and no vegetations. An ESR was elevated at 107 mm Hg. Other tests of autoimmunity including rheumatoid factor, ANA, and complement levels were normal. Test of immune function including immune globulin level, CD4 counts, and HIV antibody tests were normal.

QUESTION 4 How does this information impact on your differential diagnosis? What diagnostic procedures should be considered?

In view of these findings and a normal chest x-ray the diagnosis of active tuberculosis appears less likely. Since blood cultures and transthoracic echocardiogram were negative and there was no evidence of peripheral stigmata, endocarditis is less likely. The elevated ESR suggests an occult inflammatory process or underlying malignancy. A gallium or indium scan could be done to locate this focus. Other imaging studies in selected cases include CT of the abdomen, GI series, or a bone scan.

More invasive procedures would include angiography to rule out vasculitis or aortitis and biopsy of the temporal artery, bone marrow, skin,

muscle, liver, or lung. As a concluding step in the workup of selected cases and to further clarify scanning abnormalities or to perform biopsies or drainage, an exploratory laparotomy may be considered. Although generally discouraged, a therapeutic trial with antituberculous agents, Naprosyn, salicylates, or, rarely, steroids may be considered for cases without an etiology after an extensive workup has been done. However, if there is no clinical response in several weeks, the therapy should be discontinued, and the patient reevaluated.

CASE SUMMARY The patient's gallium scan demonstrated increased uptake in the thyroid gland consistent with an inflammatory process (Fig. 8-4-1). Thyroid function test results were significant for a low TSH at 0.3 MIU/ml (0.38-6.5 MIU/ml) and an elevated T4 at 15.0. Radioactive iodine uptake was low, consistent with the acute phase of thyroiditis (Fig. 8-4-2). Microsomal and thyroglobulin antibodies were negative. Mycobacterial blood cultures remained negative. A clinical diagnosis of subacute thyroiditis was made. Subsequently, she developed thyroid tenderness. The patient was treated with nonsteroidal anti-inflammatory agents and responded. Thyroid function tests returned to normal within 2 months.

This case illustrates several important points regarding the evaluation and management of a FUO. First, it is important to establish whether the patient does, indeed, have a true FUO and to ensure that common infections or other common causes of fever have been ruled out. It is important to keep in mind that most cases represent unusual manifestations of common diseases (that are treatable or curable), and not rare diseases. Second, for most cases it is best to avoid empiric treatment that may change the temperature curve or partially treat an underlying infection. Third, essential parts in the evaluation of the patient with a true FUO include a careful history and a complete physical examination. Repeated examinations and requestioning may be necessary. Fourth, basic laboratory screens, including CBC, blood and urine cultures, urinalysis, chest x-rays, and stool examinations are indicated as well as review of the patient's medications to exclude

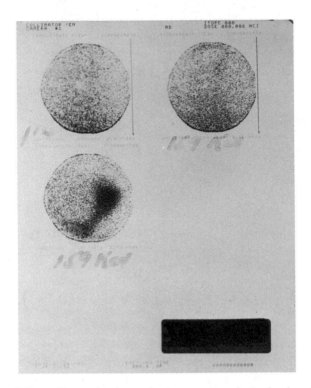

8-4-1   Gallium-67 scan demonstrating increased uptake in the thyroid gland.

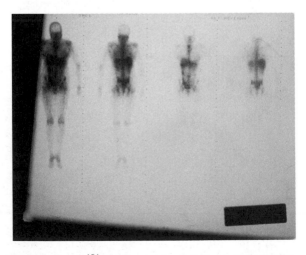

8-4-2   Low I^{131} uptake consistent with acute thyroiditis.

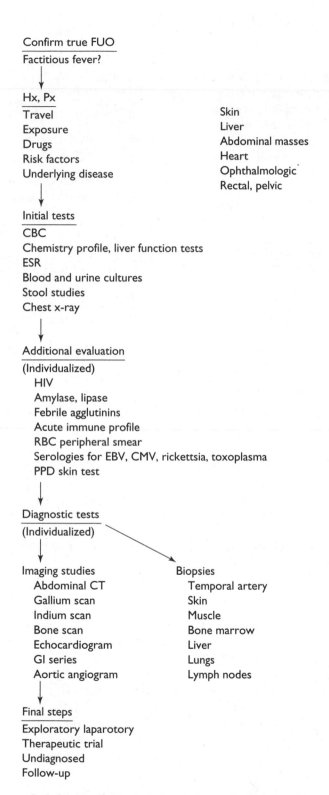

Confirm true FUO
Factitious fever?

Hx, Px

Travel
Exposure
Drugs
Risk factors
Underlying disease

Skin
Liver
Abdominal masses
Heart
Ophthalmologic
Rectal, pelvic

Initial tests
CBC
Chemistry profile, liver function tests
ESR
Blood and urine cultures
Stool studies
Chest x-ray

Additional evaluation
(Individualized)
  HIV
  Amylase, lipase
  Febrile agglutinins
  Acute immune profile
  RBC peripheral smear
  Serologies for EBV, CMV, rickettsia, toxoplasma
  PPD skin test

Diagnostic tests
(Individualized)

Imaging studies
  Abdominal CT
  Gallium scan
  Indium scan
  Bone scan
  Echocardiogram
  GI series
  Aortic angiogram

Biopsies
  Temporal artery
  Skin
  Muscle
  Bone marrow
  Liver
  Lungs
  Lymph nodes

Final steps
Exploratory laparotory
Therapeutic trial
Undiagnosed
Follow-up

8-4-3   Diagnostic algorithm for fever of unknown origin.

drug fever. Additional testing should be individualized and directed by the clinical presentation and the patient's immunologic status and the specific organ system involved. Exploratory laparotomy should be pursued for cases in which no definite diagnosis can be made despite extensive evaluation. Therapeutic trials may be appropriate for cases in which a diagnosis is strongly suspected. Finally, the more prolonged the FUO, the more likely that it is due to a neoplasm or noninfectious cause; while fevers higher than 102° F usually suggest an infectious process, lymphoma, or vasculitis. Fig. 8-4-3 shows a diagnostic algorithm for FUO.

• •

BIBLIOGRAPHY

Chang J, Gross H: Utility of naproxen in the differential diagnosis of fever of undetermined origin in patients with cancer, *Am J Med* 76:597, 1984.

Cronin R: Renal cell carcinoma: unusual systemic manifestations, *Medicine* 55(4):291, 1976.

Cunha B: Approach to the patient with fever of unknown origin. In Gorbach SL, Bartlett JG, Blacklow NR, eds: *Infectious diseases*, edition, Philadelphia, 1992, WB Saunders.

Dinarello C: Fever of unknown origin. In Mandell GL, Douglas R, Bennett JE, eds: *Principles and practice of infectious diseases*, ed 3, New York, 1990, Churchill, Livingstone.

DiNubile M: Acute fevers of unknown origin. A plea for restraint, *Arch Intern Med* 153:2525, 1993.

Duracle DT, Street AC: Fever of unknown origin: reexamined and redefined. In Remington JS, Swartz M, eds: *Current clinical topics in infectious diseases,* Boston, 1991; Blackwell Scientific Publications.

Esposito A, Glechman R: A diagnostic approach to the adult with fever of unknown origin, *Arch Intern Med* 139:575, 1979.

Fincher R: Clinical significance of extreme elevation of the erythrocyte sedimentation rate, *Arch Intern Med* 146:1581, 1986.

Goetz M: Fever of unknown origin in the elderly, *Infect Dis Clin Pract* 2 (5):377, 1993.

Hilson AJ, Maisey MN: Gallium - 67 scanning in pyrexia of unknown origin, *Br Med J* 2 (6201):1330, 1979.

Jacoby G, Swartz M: Fever of undetermined origin, *N Engl J Med* 289(26):1407, 1973.

Kazanjiam P: Fever of unknown origin: revised of 86 patients treated in community hospitals, *Clin Infect Dis* 15:968, 1992.

Klein I, Levey G: Silent thyrotoxic thyroiditis, *Ann Intern Med* 96(2):242, 1952.

Knockaert D, Vanneste L: Fever of unknown origin in the 1950's. An update of the diagnostic spectrum, *Arch Intern Med* 152:51, 1992.

Larson E: Adult Still's disease. Evaluation of clinical syndrome and diagnosis, treatment, and follow-up of 17 patients, *Medicine* 63(2):82, 1984.

Larson E, Featherstone N: Fever of undetermined origin: diagnosis and follow-up of 105 cases, 1970-1980, *Medicine* 61(5):269, 1983.

Petersdorf R: Fever of unknown origin. An old friend revised (editorial), *Arch Intern Med* 152:21, 1992.

Petersdorf RG, Beeson PB: Fever of unexplained origin. Report on 100 cases, *Medicine* 40:1-30, 1961.

Speck E, Murray H: Fever and fever of unknown etiology. In Reese R, Betts R, eds: *A practical approach to infectious disease,* ed 3, Boston, 1991, Little, Brown, pp 1-18.

Vickery D, Quinnell R: Fever of unknown origin - an algorithmic approach, *JAMA* 238 (20):2183, 1977.

Weinstein L: Clinically benign fever of unknown origin: a personal retrospective, *Rev Inf Dis* 7(5):692-699, 1985.

Wolff S, Fauci A: Unusual etiology of fever and their evaluation, *Ann Rev Med*:277, 1975.

CASE

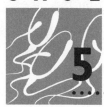

5

Neringa Zadeikis
Patricia Herrera

A 76-year-old diabetic female nursing home resident is admitted to the hospital with a 1-day history of fever to 101°F. An area of erythema measuring 4 cm by 4 cm is noted on the right calf extending to the popliteal area.

QUESTION 1 What is the differential diagnosis for the above presentation?

Possible etiologies include trauma, deep vein thrombosis, ruptured Baker's cyst, and infections such as cellulitis, erysipelas, or fasciitis.

Over the next hour, the patient's temperature rises to 102.5°F. The involved area has become more erythematous and is now also warm and tender. An ultrasound of the area is obtained. Thrombosis and popliteal cyst are ruled out.

Cellulitis, which is an infection of the skin and subcutaneous tissue, becomes the prime consideration. On occasion, a simple cellulitis will spontaneously resolve. Most, however, require antibiotic therapy. If left untreated, a cellulitis may predispose a patient, especially one at the extremes of age, to bacteremia.

QUESTION 2 The patient denies any history of trauma. This is corroborated by calling the nursing home and speaking to the patient's nurse. Blood cultures are obtained and antimicrobial therapy is initiated. How do you decide what the likely organisms are in order to initiate appropriate empiric antibiotic therapy?

Possible etiologic organisms include normal skin colonizers such as group A streptococci, group C and G streptococci, *Proprionibacterium acnes* and, less commonly, *Staphylococcus epidermidis* or *Staphylococcus aureus*.

The patient is an elderly diabetic likely to have both neuropathy and vascular insufficiency. Neuropathy precludes the sensation of pain even in the presence of significant inflammation. Such a patient would be at risk for sustaining trauma and developing a cellulitis and yet not be cognizant of these events. Furthermore, the peripheral vascular compromise would delay healing in the ischemic or necrotic tissue. Diabetic foot infections are characteristically polymicrobial. They contain organisms such as *S. aureus*, enterococci, Enterobacteriaceae, and anaerobes such as *Peptostreptococcus* species and *Bacteroides* species.

The etiologic agent of cellulitis may be recovered from blood cultures or from material aspirated from the subcutaneous tissue under the leading edge of the erythema. Yield from aspiration is quite low, however. Swab cultures from superficial surfaces are not useful because the skin may be colonized with organisms other than the true pathogen. Deep tissue cultures, which are most effectively obtained at the time of open surgical debridement, are of considerable value in identifying the pathogenic organisms.

QUESTION 3 If the anatomic region involved were the face, what other soft tissue infections might be considered?

Erysipelas, characterized by fever, chills, and an erythematous, indurated and raised advancing edge, is caused by a group A streptococcus or *S. aureus*. Besides the face, the lower extremities are a common area of involvement.

Buccal cellulitis in children is likely to be caused by *Haemophilus influenzae*. Preseptal cellulitis, which is eyelid cellulitis, is usually caused by *S. aureus* or beta-hemolytic streptococci. Orbital cellulitis involves the ocular structures with limited extraocular mobility, proptosis, and possible visual loss. When orbital cellulitis is suspected, CT scanning may help evaluate the extent of involvement. Whether the etiology is a foreign body, intraocular, dental, or sinus source is helpful as to narrowing the differential of possible pathogens.

Malignant external otitis may be described as cellulitis of the external ear canal that usually occurs in elderly diabetics. *Pseudomonas aeruginosa* is the etiologic agent. Malignant refers to the predilection for penetration into cartilage, bone, and brain.

Folliculitis describes a superficial infection that involves the hair follicles. *S. aureus* is the usual cause, and a common area of involvement is the beard. Topical therapy may be sufficient. A furuncle is a subcutaneous *Staphylococcus aureus* abscess that may have initially started as folliculitis. Topical therapy may suffice. More commonly, however, systemic antibiotics and even incision and drainage are necessary. Drainage and systemic antibiotics are recommended for carbuncles, which are collections of furuncles.

QUESTION 4 What would be your approach if the cellulitis were related to a bite wound?

Although most animal bites are minor, complications do occur in about one quarter of patients. Puncture wounds are of most concern in that a deep inoculation occurs and is inaccessible to cleansing. Dog and cat bites are the most common. Staphylococcal species, *Pasteurella multocida*, anaerobes and, in dogs, *Capnocytophaga canimorsus*, formerly DF2, may cause infection. *Pasteurella* is resistant to dicloxacillin and first generation cephalosporins commonly used in soft tissue infections. A combination of amoxicillin and clavulanate potassium is the preferred therapy, but second/third generation cephalosporins or doxycycline may be used. The specific circumstances surrounding the bite incident should be investigated in order to determine the need for rabies prophylaxis.

Human bites are also of concern. A common

scenario is a closed-fist punch with laceration of the metacarpophalangeal region on the other's teeth. In addition to staphylococcal and streptococcal organisms, *Bacteroides* species, and *Eikenella corrodens* may be involved. *Eikenella* is sensitive to penicillin but resistant to both oxacillin and clindamycin. Therefore, amoxicillin and clavulanate potassium remain the therapy of choice in bite wounds. As with any other wounds, immediate irrigation and cleansing is necessary. All clenched-fist injuries should be evaluated to exclude tendon or joint capsule involvement.

All patients should be evaluated for their current immunity status to tetanus. Tetanus immunization is recommended to be completed as a series of four immunizations during infancy and a booster at 4 to 6 years of age. After that, a booster should be administered every 10 years.

When a patient presents with a wound, proper cleansing, debridement, and antibiotic therapy will reduce the chance of developing tetanus. Attention is then turned to the individual patient's immunization history and wound appearance. If the patient has had a booster within the past 5 years, no booster is necessary. If the last immunization was in the past 5 to 10 years and the wound is a clean one, no additional prophylaxis is necessary. However, if the wound is grossly contaminated, an additional booster is to be administered.

If the last tetanus booster was more than 10 years ago, any type of wound warrants a booster. In the case where either primary immunization was never completed or if this information is unknown, a clean wound requires a booster, while a dirty one requires a booster and tetanus immune globulin.

QUESTION 5 On the next day you see the patient, she is more lethargic and the involved area is now 16 cm × 5 cm. She complains of severe pain. When you palpate the region, you detect a few regions of anesthesia. A hemorrhagic bullous lesion appears in the center, exuding a foul odor. A stat x-ray is done. The initial blood cultures did not grow any pathogens. What is the purpose of the x-ray?

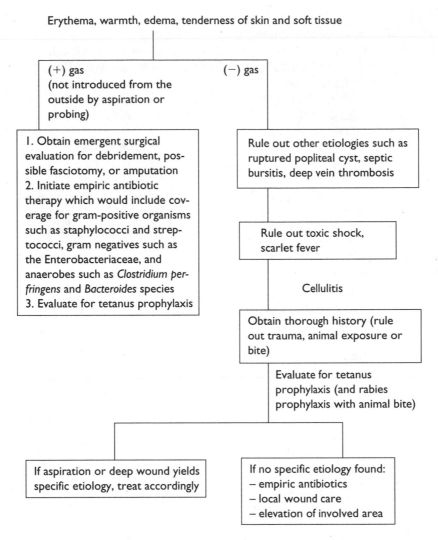

Erythema, warmth, edema, tenderness of skin and soft tissue

(+) gas
(not introduced from the
outside by aspiration or
probing)

(−) gas

1. Obtain emergent surgical
evaluation for debridement, possible fasciotomy, or amputation
2. Initiate empiric antibiotic
therapy which would include coverage for gram-positive organisms
such as staphylococci and streptococci, gram negatives such as
the Enterobacteriaceae, and
anaerobes such as *Clostridium perfringens* and *Bacteroides* species
3. Evaluate for tetanus prophylaxis

Rule out other etiologies such as
ruptured popliteal cyst, septic
bursitis, deep vein thrombosis

Rule out toxic shock,
scarlet fever

Cellulitis

Obtain thorough history (rule
out trauma, animal exposure or
bite)

Evaluate for tetanus
prophylaxis (and rabies
prophylaxis with animal bite)

If aspiration or deep wound yields
specific etiology, treat accordingly

If no specific etiology found:
– empiric antibiotics
– local wound care
– elevation of involved area

8-5-1   The approach to a patient with a soft tissue infection.

Although gas on the x-ray in such a situation may simply have been introduced by probing, anaerobes and some gram-negative organisms such as *Klebsiella* species and *Escherichia coli* do produce gas. This may be a clue to the diagnosis. The management of patients with this clinical presentation may be found in Fig. 8-5-1.

QUESTION 6   The x-ray does show gas between the posterior calf muscles. What diagnosis should you now consider, and who should be consulted?

The findings described previously are classic for necrotizing fasciitis. The antibiotic coverage should be broadened to a combination such as a penicillinase-resistant penicillin, an aminoglycoside and clindamycin or metronidazole. A surgeon should be consulted to obtain deep wound cultures and to debride all necrotic tissue immediately.

Necrotizing fasciitis is an acute infection that usually occurs in patients with diabetes, compromised circulation, or intravenous drug use. The extremities are usually involved, and the gangrene spreads along the superficial fascial planes, facilitated by enzymatic destruction of tissue. The deep fascia and muscle are not involved. Gas is seen on x-ray between the muscle layers.

Fournier's gangrene is a type of necrotizing fasciitis that involves the genitals and perineum with possible spread to the abdominal wall and thighs. Most cases involve men with the additional risk factors of diabetes, steroids, and surgical or traumatic genital injury.

The organisms implicated include anaerobes such as *Bacteroides, Peptostreptococcus,* gram negatives such as *E. coli, Klebsiella,* the Enterobacteriaceae, and also group A *Streptococcus.* Polymicrobial infections are the norm.

Necrotizing fasciitis is a clinical diagnosis made by finding skin and subcutaneous tissue with necrosis that produces severe deep pain. Areas of superficial anesthesia are present once neural destruction occurs. The skin initially appears normal or erythematous, but then necroses once the supplying vessels thrombose. Crepitance may be present. "Dishwater pus" may be released on exploration of the wound. A full-thickness skin biopsy may be of use if the diagnosis is still uncertain. This will distinguish between necrotizing fasciitis and a condition known as clostridial myonecrosis or gas gangrene (associated with trauma, septic abortions, or occurring spontaneously in patients with cancer or diabetes). *Clostridium perfringens* or *Clostridium septicum* are the two most common pathogens. Unlike necrotizing fasciitis, gas gangrene involves the muscle itself. The pale ischemic muscle does not bleed when incised. Debridement of all necrotic material is of paramount importance in this condition as well.

QUESTION 7 What are the concepts of therapy for such patients?

Surgical debridement is of vital importance in necrotizing fasciitis, as well as antibiotic therapy as described above. Hyperbaric oxygen may play a role by promoting neutrophil activity and by producing an inhospitable environment for anaerobes. Mortality remains high at approximately one quarter of patients.

CASE FOLLOW-UP When the patient returns from the operating room, her blood pressure is stable. Over the next few weeks, after completing a course of antibiotics, she has an uneventful recovery.

• •

BIBLIOGRAPHY

Canoso JJ, Barza M: Soft tissue infections, *Rheumatic Dis Clin North Am* 19(2):293-309, 1993.

Efem SE: Recent advances in the management of Fournier's gangrene: preliminary observations, *Surgery* 13(2):200-204, 1993.

File TM, Tan JS: Ticarcillin–clavulanate therapy for bacterial skin and soft tissue infections, *Rev Infect Dis* 13(suppl 9):S733-736, 1991.

Herr RD, Murdock RT, Davis RK: Serious soft tissue infections of the head and neck, *Am Fam Phys* 44(3):878-888, 1991.

Kahn RM, Goldstein EJC: Common bacterial skin infections, *Postgrad Med* 93(6):175-182, 1993.

Kirchner JT: *Clostridium septicum* infection, *Postgrad Med* 90(5): 157-160, 1991.

Kolbeinsson ME, Holder WD, Aziz S: Recognition, management and prevention of *Clostridium septicum* abscess in immunosuppressed patients, *Arch Surg* 126:642-645, 1991.

Lessner A, Stern GA: Preseptal and orbital cellulitis, *Infect Dis Clin North Am* 6(4):933-952, 1992.

Lindsey D: Soft tissue infections, *Emerg Med Clin North Am* 10(4):737-751, 1992.

Lipsky BA, Pecoraro RE, Wheat LJ: The diabetic foot, *Infect Dis Clin North Am* 4(3):409-432, 1990.

Paty R, Smith AD: Gangrene and Fournier's gangrene, *Urol Clin North Am* 19(1):149-162, 1992.

Ray D, Cohle SD, Lamb P: Spontaneous clostridial myonecrosis, *J Forensic Sci* 37(5):1428-1432, 1992.

Stephens BJ, Lathrop JC, Rice WT, et al: Fournier's gangrene: historic (1764-1978) versus contemporary (1979-1988) differences in etiology and clinical importance, *Am Surgeon* 59:149-154, 1993.

C A S E

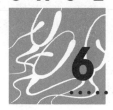

6

Neringa Zadeikis
John C. Pottage, Jr.

A *52-year-old man presents to the office complaining of cough occasionally productive of yellow sputum, mild dyspnea on exertion, and low-grade fever for 5 days. He has a long history of cigarette smoking. The patient denies chills, hemoptysis, and pleuritic chest pain. He has no history of prior hospitalizations, no drug allergies, and does not take any medications.*

QUESTION I   What is the differential diagnosis at this point?

The patient's symptoms are consistent with several respiratory infections including bronchitis, sinusitis, or pneumonia.

Acute bronchitis is an inflammatory upper respiratory tract condition commonly caused by viruses such as adenovirus, influenza, parainfluenza, rhinovirus, or coronavirus and much less commonly bacterial causes, such as *Bordetella pertussis* or *Mycoplasma pneumoniae*. The upper airway becomes edematous and produces abundant secretions. The symptoms are usually self-limited, and only symptomatic therapy is necessary. If, however, *B. pertussis* or *M. pneumoniae* is thought to be the cause, treatment should be initiated with erythromycin.

Sinusitis describes an infection of the paranasal sinuses by viral, bacterial, or fungal pathogens. Most causes of acute sinusitis begin as viral infections causing inflammation, which may then become secondarily infected by bacteria. The usual viral etiologies include rhinovirus, adenovirus, and influenza virus. Bacterial causes are *Streptococcus pneumoniae* and *Haemophilus influenzae* most commonly, but also gram-negative rods,

anaerobes, *Staphylococcus aureus*, and *Moraxella catarrhalis*.

Risk factors include anatomic abnormalities leading to ineffective drainage of secretions, obstructing foreign bodies such as nasogastric tubes, odontogenic infections, or barotrauma from diving.

The clinical presentation of sinusitis involves tenderness or swelling over the sinuses, headache, purulent nasal drainage, and fever, as well as diminished light transmission with attempted transillumination. However, sinusitis may present as fever with a productive cough only.

In most cases the diagnosis may be secured by the clinical criteria described above; however, sinus radiographs or CT scanning may be used for confirmation if any doubt remains. Antibiotic therapy to cover likely agents should be continued for 2 to 4 weeks.

Pneumonia is an infection of the lung parenchyma that occurs by inhalation of infectious particles, aspiration of oral or gastric contents into the tracheobronchial tree, or much less frequently, by hematogenous spread.

After inhalation into the upper airway, the nostril hairs and the branching tracheobronchial tree deflect the larger particles. Ciliary action then helps move the mucus-enveloped smaller particles up to areas where they may be expelled by coughing. When defense mechanisms are altered by smoking for example, which destroys the cilia, it becomes easier for infection to develop. Once these mechanisms are evaded, it is up to the alveolar macrophages to phagocytize the organisms in the lower respiratory tract.

Aspiration of minute amounts of oral contents

occurs in normal healthy adults during sleep. Persons at higher risk for aspiration include those with anatomic or neurologic abnormalities involving swallowing such as that complicating stroke or in Parkinson's disease. Also at higher risk are those with altered consciousness such as alcoholics and those with seizures or dementia.

The diagnosis of pneumonia is usually made clinically with the history of fever, cough, and purulent sputum, along with signs of consolidation on physical examination. The most reliable sign of pneumonia in the elderly, and sometimes the only sign, is an increased respiratory rate. A summary of the approach to a patient with pneumonia is provided in Fig. 8-6-1 on p. 474.

QUESTION 2 On physical examination the patient's temperature is 100.8° F, respiratory rate is 18/min, and blood pressure is 130/70 mm Hg. He is resting comfortably. There is no sinus tenderness, and transillumination of the sinuses is within normal limits. The lung examination is significant for a few right lower lobe rales. The remainder of the examination is normal. How does this information change or narrow the differential diagnosis?

The additional information obtained now is more consistent with a lower respiratory tract involvement (i.e., pneumonia).

Etiologic agents of community acquired pneumonia include *S. pneumoniae, M. pneumoniae, Chlamydia pneumoniae, H. influenzae, M. catarrhalis, Legionella* species, *S. aureus,* adenovirus, influenza, aerobic gram-negative rods, anaerobes, *Mycobacterium tuberculosis, Pneumocystis carinii,* and others.

All patients should be asked about exposure to *M. tuberculosis.* Tuberculosis is a significant public health concern and therefore needs special consideration. Also, patients should be questioned about their risk for HIV infection. *Pneumocystis carinii* pneumonia can be a presenting infection in an HIV-infected individual.

QUESTION 3 The patient is married, works as a waiter, and resides in Chicago. Of note is that he is

a recovering alcoholic. He adamantly denies having consumed any alcohol for several years. The patient denies any HIV risk factors, travel history outside of Chicago, exposure to tuberculosis, or animal exposure. He has not had an influenza vaccine this year nor a polyvalent pneumococcal vaccine. How may a patient's social and occupational history expand the differential diagnosis?

Besides the above-mentioned risk factors, other co-morbid conditions such as smoking put the patient at risk for *S. pneumoniae, H. influenzae,* and *M. catarrhalis* pneumonia. A history of alcoholism or seizures may lead to aspiration pneumonia. Having had a recent viral upper respiratory infection puts one at risk for secondary bacterial pneumonias with *S. aureus* or *S. pneumoniae.* A history of splenectomy or multiple myeloma puts one at risk for developing pneumonia caused by encapsulated organisms such as *S. pneumoniae* and *H. influenzae.* Immunocompromised patients, in addition to the usual bacterial pathogens, are at increased risk of infection with a myriad of other pathogens because of prolonged neutropenia and/or impaired cell-mediated immunity. Among them are cytomegalovirus, *M. tuberculosis, P. carinii,* and fungal pathogens such as *Cryptococcus neoformans, Histoplasma capsulatum,* and *Blastomyces dermatiditis.*

The above information is summarized in the box.

QUESTION 4 The patient is unable to provide a sputum specimen at this time. Blood cultures are drawn, oral cefuroxime is prescribed, and the patient is sent home. Is this an appropriate approach?

The patient has no coexisting chronic diseases that would make one consider him a poor risk for outpatient therapy. He has stable vital signs, no evidence of need for supplementary oxygen, and is judged to be compliant with his prescribed therapy.

Erythromycin is a useful empiric antibiotic in younger patients without any comorbid medical

CLUES TO ETIOLOGY OF PNEUMONIA FROM SOCIAL HISTORY

ANIMAL EXPOSURES

Bacterial
- *Bacillus anthracis* - sheep
- *Brucella* species - cattle, goats, pigs
- *Chlamydia psittaci* - parakeets, canaries, pigeons, ducks
- *Francisella tularensis* - rabbits, squirrels
- *Pasturella multocida* - cats, dogs, cattle, sheep
- *Yersinia pestis* - prairie dogs, squirrels

Viral
- Hantavirus - rodents

Rickettsial
- *Coxiella burnetii* - cattle, sheep, goats, cats

Fungal
- *Histoplasma capsulatum* - bats, pigeons, chickens, starlings, blackbirds
- *Blastomyces dermatitidis* - beaver dams and along river banks

GEOGRAPHICAL LOCATION CLUES

Bacterial
- Southwest U.S. - *Y. pestis*
- Southeast Asia - *Pseudomonas pseudomallei*
- Variety of locations (contaminated aerosolized water) - *Legionella* species

Viral
- Southwest U.S. - Hantavirus

Fungal
- Southeast and southcentral U.S. - *Blastomyces dermatitidis*
- Southcentral and eastcentral U.S. - *H. capsulatum*
- Southwest U.S. - *C. immitis*

Mycobacterial
- Southeast Asia, India, urban U.S. - *Mycobacterium tuberculosis*
- Variety of locations - atypical mycobacteria

UNIMMUNIZED PATIENTS
- Viral - influenza, rubeola
- Bacterial - *S. pneumoniae*

POSTINFLUENZA BACTERIAL PNEUMONIAS
- *S. aureus; S. pneumoniae*

SMOKER/COPD
- *S. pneumoniae; H. influenzae; M. catarrhalis*

POSTTRANSPLANT PATIENTS
- *S. pneumoniae*
- *H. influenzae*
- *Legionella* species
- CMV
- PCP
- *Strongyloides stercoralis*

HIV
- *S. pneumoniae*
- *H. influenzae*
- *M. tuberculosis*
- PCP
- *Cryptococcus neoformans*
- *H. capsulatum*

MISCELLANEOUS CLUES
- *S. pneumoniae/H. influenzae*
- Anaerobes
- Group A *Streptococcus*
- Elderly, splenectomy, multiple myeloma, alcoholism
- Risk of aspiration (e.g., alcoholics, stroke, dementia, seizures, drugs, emesis)
- Rapidly developing pleural effusion

conditions. They are more likely to have *S. pneumoniae, M. pneumoniae, C. pneumoniae,* or a viral etiology. Older patients, such as our subject, are at a greater risk of acquiring *S. pneumoniae, H. influenzae, M. catarrhalis,* and gram-negative pathogens. These patients are generally treated with second generation cephalosporins, unless *Legionella* is a strong consideration.

Sputum gram stain and culture may demonstrate the presumed pathogen. An acceptable sputum specimen contains fewer than 10 epithelial cells and greater than 25 white blood cells. Besides gram staining, stains for mycobacterial organisms and direct fluorescent antibody (DFA) staining for *Legionella* are available. If the patient is unable to produce an adequate sputum specimen, is severely ill from his pneumonia, or is not appropriately responding to empiric antibiotics, proceeding with an invasive procedure may be necessary. Transtracheal aspiration is no longer done in an attempt to isolate a lower respiratory tract specimen because of the high complication rate. Thoracentesis is a useful procedure if a patient has a free-flowing pleural effusion, and the diagnosis is not otherwise secured. Bronchoscopy with washings, brushings, and possibly, transbronchial biopsy is not usually performed when looking for routine bacterial pathogens. Even with the use of a protected brush catheter, wherein the specimen brush is protected from upper airway contamination, this technique is better reserved for the diagnosis of *Pneumocystis carinii*, mycobacterial, or fungal pathogens.

Blood cultures are important to obtain in the workup of a pneumonia, because they may be positive in up to one third of cases.

QUESTION 5   The patient is brought back to the office 2 days later by his wife who is worried that he is not improving. He now admits to drinking and having blacked out recently. The patient complains of foul-smelling sputum and is febrile to 102.4°F. Physical examination is otherwise unchanged.

An adequate sputum specimen is now available. Gram stain demonstrates abundant white blood cells, moderate gram-negative rods, and few gram-positive cocci. The previously drawn blood cultures do not yet demonstrate any growth. A chest x-ray is obtained that demonstrates a right lower lobe infiltrate.

The patient's therapy is broadened to clindamycin and cefuroxime. Arrangements are made for substance abuse counseling. Why were the above changes made, and what is the final diagnosis?

With the additional clue of putrid sputum in the setting of altered consciousness, an anaerobic aspiration pneumonia becomes more likely.

When aspiration of gastric contents occurs, the acidity causes an intense inflammatory reaction. Afterwards, atelectasis rapidly develops. The injured lung is then susceptible to bacterial infection. Common oral colonizing bacteria such as *Eikenella corrodens*, *Haemophilus* species, aerobic streptococci, *Peptostreptococcus* species, *Bacteroides* species, and *Fusobacterium* species are the usual pathogens. Most aspiration pneumonias are polymicrobial.

Aspirating only minute amounts usually does not have clinical sequelae. Conditions that allow a greater number of organisms or a larger volume of material to be aspirated increase the chance of pneumonia developing. This may occur with periodontal disease, which fosters the growth of a plethora of anaerobic bacteria, or emesis, which may result in a large volume aspiration.

If aspiration pneumonia is suspected, empiric therapy with an antibiotic combination such as a second-generation cephalosporin and clindamycin, penicillin and metronidazole, amoxicillin/clavulanate, ampicillin/sulbactam, ticarcillin/clavulanate, or piperacillin/tazobactam should be initiated.

There is an increased incidence of beta-lactamase producing *Bacteroides* and *Fusobacterium* species. This should be considered when prescribing therapy. *E. corrodens* is a unique organism because it is resistant to both clindamycin and metronidazole but sensitive to penicillin, ampicillin, and second- and third-generation cephalosporins.

QUESTION 6   Is the radiologic appearance of the chest x-ray in pneumonia helpful?

Chest x-ray findings may be quite variable. A particular pattern may be suggestive of an etiology, but is by no means specific (see box).

In aspiration pneumonia the more common lobes to be involved are the superior segments of the lower lobes and the posterior segments of the

CXR PATTERN CLUES TO PNEUMONIA

BRONCHOPNEUMONIA PATTERN
- S. pneumoniae
- C. pneumoniae
- M. pneumoniae
- H. influenzae
- Legionella spp.
- P. multocida
- C. psittaci
- S. aureus
- B. dermatitidis

INTERSTITIAL PATTERN
- C. pneumoniae
- M. pneumoniae
- C. psittaci
- C. burnetii
- Legionella spp.
- Varicella
- Influenza
- Rubeola
- P. carinii
- H. capsulatum
- C. immitis
- B. dermatitidis

CAVITARY PNEUMONIA
- Legionella spp.
- Brucella spp.
- Nocardia spp.
- Gram-negative rods
- P. pseudomallei
- P. carinii
- H. capsulatum
- C. neoformans
- B. dermatitidis

ASSOCIATED MEDIASTINAL LYMPHADENOPATHY
- C. psittaci
- M. pneumoniae
- F. tularensis
- Y. pestis
- M. tuberculosis
- C. immitis
- H. capsulatum
- B. dermatitidis

upper lobes. Right-sided involvement is more prevalent because of the more direct vertical route of the right mainstem bronchus down to the lungs.

Radiologic resolution lags behind clinical improvement. Most pneumonias should have resolved within 1 month; however, older patients or those with chronic obstructive lung disease may take up to 2 to 3 months for radiologic clearing. With a non-resolving infiltrate, an obstructive lesion should be excluded. However, in a young nonsmoker who is clinically well at follow-up, a repeat x-ray is not usually necessary.

QUESTION 7   What are possible complications of aspiration pneumonia, as well as other pneumonias?

Aspiration pneumonia may be complicated by the development of a lung abscess. This would be seen as a cavity developing 1 to 2 weeks after the aspiration episode. However, the abscess may not be detected for weeks or months until the patient presents with continued fever, malaise, or weight loss.

Other complications, which occur less frequently in aspiration pneumonia but are seen in other types of pneumonia, include pleural effusion and empyema. Up to one third to one half of all patients with pneumonia have noninfected parapneumonic effusions. Only a small percentage of these become infected and are then termed *empyemas*. These two entities may be differentiated by fluid analysis. An empyema has a thicker consistency, lower pH, and higher fluid-to-serum lactate dehydrogenase and protein ratios than a simple parapneumonic effusion. Because empyemas are purulent, drainage either by thoracentesis, chest tube thoracostomy, or surgical drainage is necessary for resolution.

CASE FOLLOW-UP   The patient completes 2 weeks of therapy with cefuroxime and clindamycin and improves clinically. Blood cultures remain negative. A chest x-ray is repeated in 1 month that demonstrates resolution of the infiltrate.

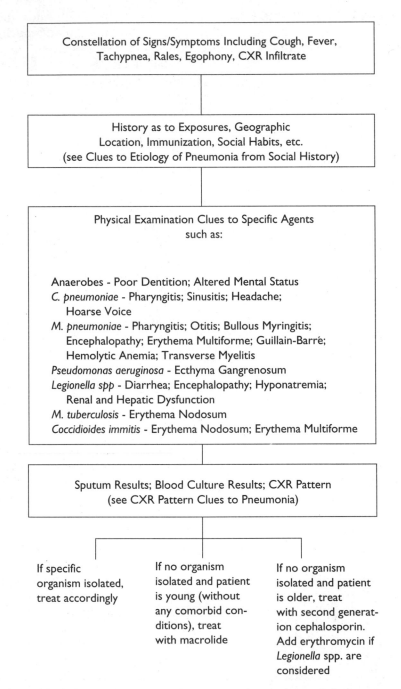

8-6-1   The approach to the patient with a respiratory infection.

BIBLIOGRAPHY

Bartlett JG: Anaerobic bacterial infections of the lung and pleural space, *Clin Infect Dis* 16(suppl 4):S248-255, 1993.

Batra P: Pulmonary coccidioidomycosis, *J Thorac Imaging* 7(4): 29-38, 1992.

Esposito AL: Pulmonary infections acquired in the work place, *Clin Chest Med* 13(2):355-365, 1992.

File TM, Tan JS: Community-acquired pneumonia, *Postgrad Med* 92(8):197-214, 1992.

Goodman LR, Goren RA, Teplick SK: The radiographic evaluation of pulmonary infection, *Med Clin North Am* 64(3):553-572, 1980.

Grayston JT: Chlamydia pneumoniae, strain TWAR, *Chest* 95(3):664-669, 1989.

Groskin SA, Panicek DM, et al: Bacterial lung abscess: a review of the radiographic and clinical features of 50 cases, *J Thorac Imaging* 6(3):62-67, 1991.

Ha HK, Kang MW, et al: Lung abscess: percutaneous catheter therapy, *Acta Radiologica* 34(4):362-365, 1993.

Hill MK, Sanders CV: Anaerobic disease of the lung, *Infect Dis Clin North Am* 5(3):453-466, 1991.

Johnson DH, Cunha BA: Atypical pneumonias, *Postgrad Med* 93(7):69-82, 1993.

Kayser FH: Changes in the spectrum of organisms causing respiratory tract infections: a review, *Postgrad Med* 68(suppl 3):S17-23, 1992.

LaForce FM: Antibacterial therapy for lower respiratory tract infections in adults: a review, *Clin Infect Dis* 14(suppl 2):S233-237, 1992.

Lambiase RE, Deyoe L, et al: Percutaneous drainage of 335 consecutive abscesses: results of primary drainage with 1 year follow-up, *Interventional Radiol* 184:167-179, 1992.

Lubitz RM: Resolution of lung abscesses due to *Pseudomonas aeruginosa* with oral ciprofloxacin: case report, *Rev Infect Dis* 12(5):757-759, 1992.

Marrie TJ: Community-acquired pneumonia, *Clin Infect Dis* 18:501-515, 1994.

Niederman MS, Bass JB, et al: Guidelines for the initial management of adults with community-acquired pneumonia: diagnosis, assessment of severity, and initial antimicrobial therapy, *Am Rev Respir Dis* 148:1418-1426, 1993.

Potgieter PD, Hammond JM: Surgical drainage of lung abscess complicating acute community acquired pneumonia, *Chest* 99:1280-1282, 1991.

Ruben FL: Viral pneumonias, *Postgrad Med* 93(7):57-64, 1993.

Wisinger D: Bacterial pneumonia, *Postgrad Med* 93(7):43-52, 1993.

CASE

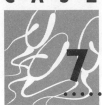

7

Deborah Schiappa
David Schwartz

The patient is a 24-year-old sexually active black man who is known to be HIV positive for the past 2 years. He has been taking AZT, and his latest CD4 lymphocyte count is 320. He denies a prior history of opportunistic infections and now presents with complaints of malaise, temperature to 99.9°F, myalgias, and a nonpruritic maculopapular eruption on his palms and soles. He also remembers developing a painless penile ulcer approximately 3 to 4 weeks earlier accompanied by bilaterally swollen areas near his groin. He admits to recent unprotected sexual relations with several new partners within the last 2 months, but cannot remember if they were "sick."

On physical examination his vital signs are T 99.9°F, P 76 bpm, RR 20/min and BP 140/80 mm Hg. He was alert and oriented to person, place, and time. HEENT examination was significant for normal pupillary responses and grayish patches on the roof of his mouth and tongue (Fig. 8-7-1). His neck was supple, and there was no palpable cervical adenopathy. Cardiac and pulmonary examination were normal. Abdominal examination was benign. There were bilaterally enlarged, nontender, inguinal lymph nodes present. No genital ulcerations or urethral discharge were noted. Rectal examination was significant for a 1 cm pearly gray, hypertrophic, wartlike lesion in the perineum. Patchy areas of hair loss were noted on his scalp. A generalized maculopapular rash, including the palms and soles, was noted (Fig. 8-7-2). The neurologic examination was nonfocal. Screening laboratories including a complete blood count and serum chemistry profile were within normal limits.

QUESTION 1 What relevant diagnoses should be considered in the differential diagnosis at this point?

The patient's history and presentation suggest a sexually transmitted disease. Evaluation should focus on the dermatologic findings including the maculopapular skin rash, genital ulcer, regional adenopathy, mucous patches, and wartlike perirectal lesion. The diagnostic considerations are listed in Table 8-7-1.

Of the possibilities listed, the most compatible diagnosis in a young, sexually active male with a history of a painless genital ulcer, inguinal lymph nodes, a palmar and plantar rash, mucous patches, and condyloma lata is syphilis. None of the other processes present with this constellation of findings.

QUESTION 2 What serologic testing should be done to confirm the diagnosis? How does the history of being HIV-infected impact on diagnostic testing?

If present, scrapings from the genital ulcer for immunofluorescent (DFA-TP) or darkfield microscopy could be done to demonstrate the spirochetes. Specimens collected from the oral mucosal lesions may lead to misdiagnosis as saprophytic spirochetes may be part of the normal oral flora.

Serologic tests include nontreponemal and treponemal tests. The nontreponemal tests, rapid plasma reagin (RPR) and venereal disease research laboratory (VDRL), detect IgG and IgM immunoglobulin directed against a lipoidal antigen. This test may be negative in the early stages of syphilis. False-positive reactions may also occur

TABLE 8-7-1 **Skin Manifestations of Some Sexually Transmitted Diseases with Differential Diagnoses**

Finding	Differential Diagnosis
Maculopapular skin rash	Pityriasis rosea
	Tinea corporis
	Psoriasis
	Syphilis
	Drug eruption
	Viral exanthem
Genital ulcer/adenopathy	Herpes simplex virus
	Chancroid
	Syphilis
	Lymphogranuloma venereum
	Granuloma inguinale
Mucous patches	Syphilis
	Herpes simplex virus
	Aphthous ulcer
Wartlike anorectal lesion	Condyloma lata
	Condyloma acuminata

in various conditions such as pregnancy, collagen vascular diseases, leprosy, and acute viral illnesses. The test is usually quantitated and reported as a titer to reflect disease activity and response to treatment. Confirmatory treponemal tests, including the fluorescent treponemal antibody-absorption (FTA-ABS) and microhem-agglutination-*Treponema pallidum* test (MHA-TP), use *T. pallidum* as the antigen and are considered more sensitive and specific. During the early stages of syphilis, the FTA-ABS may become positive before the RPR. A positive test will usually remain so for many years, despite adequate treatment.

Serologic tests may be difficult to interpret in patients coinfected with HIV. All patients with known HIV infection should be screened for possible untreated syphilis infection, and all pa-

tients with syphilis should be tested for HIV. Sexually transmitted diseases that cause genital ulcerations may be cofactors for acquiring HIV infection. The diagnosis of syphilis may be more complicated in HIV-infected patients because of atypical clinical presentations or unusual serologic test results. HIV-infected patients with syphilis may demonstrate unusual serologic responses including higher than expected titers, delayed seroreactivity, or falsely-negative results. False-negative readings as a result of the prozone phenomenon, in which antibody excess prohibits detection of antigen-antibody complexes, may be overcome by diluting the patient's serum before testing. When serology is not helpful, direct detection of the organism from ulcers by repeat darkfield microscopy or fluorescent and silver stains on lymph node biopsy samples may be necessary to confirm the diagnosis.

QUESTION 3 The patient's RPR was reactive at a titer of 1:512, and the FTA-ABS was also reactive. What are the salient points concerning syphilis?

Syphilis is a chronic, systemic infection with a variable presentation caused by the organism *Treponema pallidum*. It is acquired through sexual contact with an infected lesion or perinatally. The organism penetrates the skin or mucous membranes and spreads to the local lymphatics. From there, the organism disseminates hematogenously. The incubation period ranges from 3 to 90 days. The organism pathologically causes an obliterative end-arteritis, which may affect any tissue or organ system.

Both the clinical manifestations and laboratory results may be used to make the diagnosis. The clinical presentation begins with the *primary stage* at which time a painless chancre develops at the inoculation site. The chancre is accompanied by regional lymphadenopathy. The lesion may spontaneously heal within 3 to 6 weeks. The lymphadenopathy may persist. The *secondary stage* begins 2 to 8 weeks after the appearance of the chancre and occurs as a result of local multiplication and systemic dissemination. This stage of syphilis has

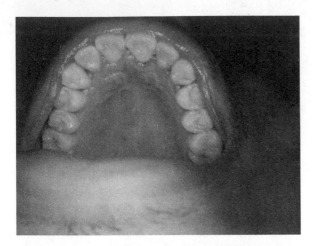

8-7-1   Grayish patches on roof of mouth and tongue.

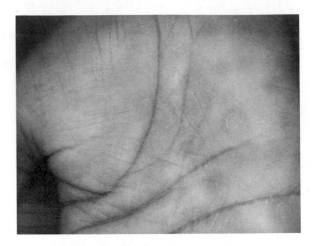

8-7-2   Palmar maculopapular rash.

been referred to as the "great imitator" because the clinical manifestation may be so diverse. Manifestations may include skin rash, condylomata lata, chancres, mucous patches, constitutional and neurologic symptoms or, rarely, renal, hepatic, or musculoskeletal involvement.

The *latent stage* is characterized by the absence of clinical manifestations but positive specific treponomal antibody tests, and is divided into early and late forms. The *early latent phase* occurs 1 to 4 years after infection. Relapses are common. The *late latent phase* is associated with relative resistance to relapse or reinfection. *Late, or tertiary, syphilis* may occur years after the initial infection and can affect any organ system. Manifestations include asymptomatic neurosyphilis, stroke complex, general paresis, tabes dorsalis, Argyll Robertson pupils, delusions, hallucinations, and memory loss. Other manifestations of late syphilis include otitis, uveitis, aortitis, and a granulomatous, inflammatory form characterized by gummas.

QUESTION 4   The patient complains of worsening headache and eye pain. What medical intervention is necessary at this point?

A cerebrospinal fluid (CSF) examination should be done on any HIV-infected patient with

neurologic signs or symptoms to rule out neurosyphilis. Characteristic abnormalities in the CSF include elevated leukocyte count and protein and a positive CSF-VDRL. The patient should be treated for neurosyphilis if the clinical manifestations and CSF changes are consistent, or if the patient is in the late latent phase (SBP >1 year) and CSF examination is not possible. The recommended treatment is 10 to 14 days of intravenous penicillin.

CNS disease may occur during any stage of syphilis in HIV-infected patients and may follow an accelerated course. A CSF examination should be done on any seropositive patient with unexplained behavioral changes, psychologic dysfunction, ocular, auditory, or neurologic signs and symptoms. Close follow-up of HIV-infected patients is important. Repeat CSF examinations should be done if serologic titers do not decrease with treatment because some patients may not respond to standard therapy.

QUESTION 5   What is the correct therapy of syphilis in both the non–HIV-infected patient and the HIV-infected patient?

The drug of choice for treatment of syphilis is penicillin. To maintain adequate blood levels for 7 days to attempt cure of early syphilis, benzathine

Assess risk for STDs

Multiple partners/partner of known STD case
Young age
Unprotected intercourse
Co-infection with HIV
Prostitution/IVDU

High risk group

Categorize into:
  a) Genital ulcer/lymphadenopathy - chancroid, HSV, LGV, syphilis, granuloma
     inguinale
  b) Vaginitis/cervicitis - GC, chlamydia, (NGU), HSV, mycoplasma
  c) Vaginal discharge - Trichomonas, bacterial vaginosis, Candida
  d) Pelvic inflammatory disease - GC, Chlamydia, mixed anaerobe infection
  e) Epididymitis - Chlamydia, GC

Miscellaneous
  f) Genital warts - condyloma lata (syphilis)
                   - condyloma acuminata (HPV)
                      (cervical cancer screen necessary)
  g) Proctitis - HSV, GC, Chlamydia, syphilis
  h) Hepatitis B
  i) Ectoparasite - P. pubis
                  - scabies
  j) HIV
         ↓
Diagnostic testing – use appropriate tests

Cultures/smears/scrapings/darkfield microscopy
Serology
Tissue biopsy
         ↓
Treatment

Based on specific diagnosis
         ↓
Follow-up

Clinical evaluation
Repeat serologies
Cultures for test of cure
         ↓
Retreatment

For reinfection, relapse,
treatment failures
         ↓
Prevention/screening

Education
Treatment of sexual partners

8-7-3   Diagnostic algorithm for STDs.

penicillin is recommended. Alternative antibiotics for treatment of early syphilis include tetracycline, erythromycin, and the cephalosporins. The dosage and length of treatment depend on the stage and clinical manifestations.

Neurosyphilis should be treated with intravenous penicillin G 2 to 4 million units q 4 hr for 10 to 14 days. This ensures reaching a therapeutic level in the CSF more rapidly. A penicillin-allergic patient with neurosyphilis or a pregnant woman with history of penicillin allergy should be considered for desensitization.

The Jarisch-Herxheimer reaction may occur within 1 to 2 hours after initiating any therapy for syphilis. This is a systemic reaction related to the release of organism components after lysis by antibiotics. Symptoms may include fever, chills, headache, and myalgias. There are no proven methods for preventing the reaction, although antipyretics may give symptomatic relief.

According to CDC guidelines, sexual partners exposed to a documented case within 90 days may be infected but seronegative and, therefore, must be treated presumptively. Sexual partners exposed to a patient with primary, secondary, or early latent syphilis >90 days before examination should also be presumptively treated if serologic test results are not immediately available and follow-up is uncertain. Pretreatment time periods used to identify at-risk sexual partners are 3 months plus symptom duration for primary syphilis, 6 months for secondary, and 1 year for latent syphilis.

Treated patients should be followed clinically and serologically at 3, 6, and 12 months intervals to catch treatment failures or reinfections. Re-evaluation is important in HIV-infected patients to ensure response to treatment.

CASE DISCUSSION This case illustrates several important points. The first is that all patients with known HIV infection should be screened for possible untreated syphilis, and all patients with syphilis should be tested for HIV. Sexually transmitted diseases causing genital ulcerations can be cofactors for acquiring HIV infection. Second, the diagnosis of syphilis may be more complicated in HIV-infected patients because of atypical clinical presentations or unusual serologic test results. Other diagnostic tests may be necessary to confirm the diagnosis, such as biopsies, darkfield examinations, and fluorescent stains. Third, central nervous system disease may occur during any stage of syphilis in HIV-infected patients. A cerebrospinal fluid examination should be done on any HIV-positive patient with unexplained behavioral changes, psychological dysfunction, ocular, auditory, or neurologic signs or symptoms. Finally, close follow-up of these patients is important and should include repeat CSF examinations if serologic titers do not decrease with treatment. Fig. 8-7-3 shows a diagnostic algorithm for sexually transmitted diseases.

• •

CASE FOLLOW-UP A lumbar puncture was done and revealed a WBC count of 42 cells/mm3 and an elevated protein of 74 mg/dl. The CSF VDRL was reactive to 4 dilutions. The patient denied a history of allergic reaction to penicillin and was started on 4 million units IV PEN G every 4 hours to complete a 14-day course.

• •

BIBLIOGRAPHY

Bolan G: Management of syphilis in HIV-infected persons. In Sande M, Volberdine P, eds: *The medical management of AIDS,* Philadelphia, 1990, WB Saunders.

Centers for Disease Control: Sexually transmitted disease treatment guidelines, *MMWR* 42:27, 1993.

Chambers C: Sexually transmitted diseases, *Primary Care* 17(4):833, 1990.

Clotez C: Sexually transmitted diseases and human immunodeficiency virus. Epidemiologic synergy? *Infect Dis Clin North Am* 7(4):753, 1993.

Csonka G, Oates J: Syphilis. In Csonka G, Oates J, eds: *Sexually transmitted diseases,* Philadelphia, 1990, WB Saunders.

Hutchinson C: Syphilis in adults, *Med Clin North Am* 74(6): 1389, 1990.

Melvin S: Syphilis: resurgence of an old disease, *Primary Care* 17(1):47, 1990.

Musher D, Baughn R: Syphilis. In Bradu S, Merican T, Bolognesi D, eds: *Textbook of AIDS medicine,* Baltimore, 1994, Williams & Wilkins.

Rein M: Sexually transmitted diseases. In Reese R, Betts R, eds: *A practical approach to infectious diseases,* ed 3, Boston, 1991, Little, Brown.

C A S E

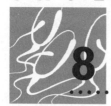

8 Vishnu Chundi
Patricia Herrera

A 61-year-old Polish man is admitted to the hospital for evaluation of a 3-day history of shaking chills, low back pain, and anorexia. The family states that he has not been disoriented or confused but has been complaining of weakness and increasing discomfort. There is no history of trauma, diabetes mellitus, or hypertension. He has not experienced similar symptoms before this episode. As the patient is being examined, he becomes combative and restless and requires restraints to prevent injury to himself. There is no history of either exposure to or active tuberculosis.

The patient was born in Poland. He is married and has two grown children. The patient emigrated to the United States 10 years ago. He worked as a coal miner in Poland for 30 years, is a nonsmoker, and drinks 1 to 2 six packs of beer a day.

On admission his vital signs are T 99.6°F, P 100 bpm, RR 28/min, and BP 130/80 mm Hg. He is a moderately obese man, alert but agitated, and is oriented only to self. His pupils are equally reactive to light and accommodate normally. Lungs are clear to auscultation. The heart sounds are normal. He has a soft ejection systolic murmur in the apical area without radiation. The abdomen is soft with normal bowel sounds and no organomegaly. He has no cranial nerve abnormalities. His muscle tone is normal. He is moving all four extremities and has symmetrical deep tendon reflexes. Gait cannot be tested because of the patient's lack of cooperation. Skull and spine examination reveal minimal tenderness over the lower lumbar vertebrae.

QUESTION I What is your presumptive diagnosis and your course of action at this point?

We are presented with a patient with an acute confusional state and 3 days of shaking chills with back pain. The differential diagnosis is very broad and should include infectious as well as noninfectious etiologies. The infectious diseases to consider include a primary CNS infection such as meningitis, meningoencephalitis, or encephalitis. Parameningeal foci must also be considered including osteomyelitis, paraspinal abscess, Pott's disease, and metastatic infections to the spine. Since this category includes disease processes with the highest morbidity and mortality, it is important to place them at the top of your differential list. Sepsis may also present in a similar manner.

Noninfectious causes in a patient with alcohol intake must include alcohol withdrawal. Metabolic derangements secondary to such processes as diabetes mellitus, hyperparathyroidism, hepatic dysfunction, and hypoxemia should be investigated and excluded. A more complete discussion of the metabolic etiologies of mental status alteration can be found in Neurology Case 2. Head trauma leading to concussion or a postconcussive syndrome should be ruled out.

If the suspicion of acute bacterial meningitis is high, intravenous antibiotics should be given as soon as possible. Lumbar puncture should be done if there are no contraindications. CT scan of the head should be done before lumbar puncture if there is papilledema or if focal neurologic signs are present. Appropriate evaluation would include a determination of serum chemistries including serum glucose, arterial blood gases, complete blood count to detect neutrophilia, toxicology screen, and a chest radiograph. Screening for thyroid and parathyroid dysfunction should be done. Blood and urine cultures should be done even in the absence of fever because in many abnormal hosts (including alcohol abuse as in this case) infection may not reliably present with the typical syndrome. A delay in instituting therapy for bacterial meningitis will likely increase mortality.

In an alcoholic, nutritional deficiency is an important consideration. In addition, patients are frequently given intravenous fluids upon arrival to an emergency room. It is important to remember that administration of dextrose-containing fluids may exacerbate a thiamine deficiency leading to further deterioration in the level of consciousness. Therefore, thiamine should be administered to this patient before a dextrose solution is administered. Similarly, knowledge of the serum sodium is also important. A patient from a nursing home with mental status changes resulting from hypernatremia requires a relatively hypotonic solution for therapy, whereas a markedly hyponatremic patient will require a different approach to fluid therapy based on the specific etiology.

In this patient, fever and chills are cardinal signs of infection. Localization of the infectious process is the next goal. His mental status changes may be due to either a systemic process or primary infection of the central nervous system. Therefore, since the morbidity and mortality of a primary CNS infection is greater, this becomes the chief concern in the diagnostic evaluation.

QUESTION 2 What are the signs and symptoms of infectious meningitis?

Integral to the diagnosis of infectious meningitis are the usual signs of infection including fever, chills, lethargy, and leukocytosis. Nuchal rigidity is an important finding on physical examination. Kernig's sign is demonstrated by placing the patient supine and flexing the knees. Encountering passive resistance to movement is interpreted as a positive test. Brudzinski's sign is the response to neck flexion by involuntary knee flexion when supine.

A physical examination should be carried out, with particular attention to evaluation of the

sinuses, middle ear, mastoids, spine, and paraspinal areas as potential sources of meningeal seeding. Additional physical findings to look for include those that contraindicate lumbar puncture including papilledema or focal neurologic deficits. An important visual clue is the presence of skin rash or mucous membrane petechiae, which may be associated with meningococcal meningitis.

QUESTION 3 The lab data are as follows: WBC 11,200/mm^3 with 68% segs, 2% bands, 27% lymphs, 3% monos; Hgb 10.1 gm%, HCT 34, platelets 114,000/mm^3; sodium 133 mEq/L, K 3.1 mEq/L, Cl 94 mEq/L, CO$_2$ 27 mEq/L; BUN 26 mg/dl, creatinine 1.4 mg/dl, Ca 9.4 mg/dl, glucose 140 mg/dl, SGOT 252 U/L, SGPT 10 U/L, LDH 531 IU/L; prothrombin time 12.5 sec (control 12.0), PTT 22 sec (control 23 sec). The toxicology screen is negative. CT scan of the head does not reveal any intracranial lesions, blood or mass effect, and the CXR is normal. The lumbar puncture opening pressure is 18 cm H$_2$O with a leukocyte count of 170/mm^3 and differential cell count of 85% polys, 3% bands, 7% lymphs, 5% monos with 490 RBC. The glucose is 21 mg %/dl and protein 1090 mg %/dl; the gram stain reveals many WBCs, with no microorganisms. Latex agglutination tests for streptococcal, *Haemophilus*, and meningococcal species are negative; the cryptococcal antigen test is negative, and blood and urine cultures are sent. Interpret the cerebrospinal fluid data. What is the differential diagnosis of this spinal fluid? What is the significance of the spinal fluid protein level? What therapeutic interventions would you proceed with at this point?

The CSF reveals a moderate neutrophilic pleocytosis, hypoglycorrhachia (low CSF glucose), and xanthochromia. The findings of neutrophilia and hypoglycorrhachia are compatible with infectious meningitis. While the differential remains broad, the number of white blood cells can help narrow the possibilities. A count >2000/cc usually suggests a bacterial process. The differential count usually has a neutrophilic predominance in bacterial meningitis but 10% may have a lymphocytic predominance. Conversely, one third of viral or tuberculous cases may have a predominance of PMNs. Thus, a physician is rarely justified in excluding bacterial meningitis based solely on CSF cell count, protein or glucose concentration. Furthermore, the specificity of the absolute glucose level in separating a bacterial from a viral process is low.

The markedly elevated protein with xanthochromia is an especially important clue. A protein level greater than 220 mg %/dl is a strong predictor of bacterial meningitis compared to viral meningitis. A protein of >1000 mg %/dl should prompt one to consider a CSF block or paraspinal process as an etiology. Thus, the CSF in this case is consistent with a bacterial meningitis complicated by a block or a parameningeal source for infection.

Specific etiologic diagnoses are usually determined by gram stain and culture. A gram stain of the centrifuged sediment is important as it is positive in 80% to 90% of cases with a positive culture. Prior antimicrobial therapy decreases this rate to approximately 60%. These tests both carry a high sensitivity and specificity. Both counterimmunoelectrophoresis and latex agglutination tests also are highly specific but have only moderate sensitivity.

In bacterial meningitis, the pleocytosis is usually neutrophilic; however, this can be mimicked by an early viral process. In such a situation, the clinical presentation of the patient must be used to further direct the evaluation. Cultures for bacteria, AFB, and fungi should not be overlooked. Other tests that may be necessary include AFB smear, cryptococcal antigen test, and latex agglutination tests for bacterial cell wall antigens.

In the bacterial group the most common agents include *Streptococcus pneumoniae*, *Neisseria meningitidis*, *Haemophilus influenzae*, and *Listeria monocytogenes*. Additional entities include spirochetal infection (Lyme disease and syphilis), tuberculosis, and fungi including *Cryptococcus*. Recurrent neisserial infections are predisposed to by deficiency of the terminal components of the complement cascade, the membrane attack complex (complement components C5-C9).

Neurosyphilis presents with a lymphocytic pleocytosis. The diagnosis of neurosyphilis may be difficult to confirm definitively. In the asymptomatic patient the combination of a positive serum specific treponemal test (MHA-TP or FTA-ABS) in conjunction with an elevated CSF VDRL or an elevated CSF immunoglobulin level supports the diagnosis. In asymptomatic HIV-negative patients, lumbar puncture may not be necessary with a positive serum test. Treatment can be an IM injection of benzathine penicillin G (2.4 million units × 3 doses over 3 weeks). In a patient with symptoms thought to be secondary to syphilis, lumbar puncture is necessary to determine the need for intravenous therapy to assure spirochetocidal levels of penicillin in the CSF.

Fungal and tuberculous meningitides may also present with a lymphocytic CSF profile. In cases of fungal or tuberculous meningitis, the CSF leukocyte count will be elevated nonspecifically; however, the CSF glucose level may be lower in cases of tuberculous meningitis. *Cryptococcus* can be identified by India ink smear, the only direct organism identifying test, with a sensitivity of 36% to 53% when tapped repeatedly. It is important to order this test in the correct clinical setting when suspicion is high. Acid fast smears of the CSF have been reported to be positive in up to 80% of tuberculous meningitis cases when large volumes are assayed, but in clinical practice, the AFB smear has poor sensitivity. Cultures are positive in 75% of cases.

Nonbacterial processes are commonly termed aseptic. However, this does not mean that every process in this category is noninfectious. This differential diagnosis includes viral agents such as echoviruses 3 and 9, mumps, and the lymphocytic choriomeningitis (LCM) virus. An important clue to remember is that both the mumps and LCM viruses can produce a CSF leukocytosis in the range that mimics a bacterial process.

It is also important to consider extraaxial processes such as a paraspinal abscess, sinusitis, brain abscess, or osteomyelitis if pain and other symptoms persist despite adequate antibiotic therapy.

In contrast to most other infectious processes, suspicion of bacterial meningitis is a direct and immediate indication for antibiotic therapy. Prompt institution of appropriate antibiotics should include coverage for *S. pneumoniae, N. meningitidis, Listeria,* and other streptococci. Empiric therapy could include high-dose penicillin and/or a third generation cephalosporin if there is a suspicion of *H. influenzae.* This patient should also undergo further imaging studies with particular attention to the lumbar spine, as he complains of backache. See Question 6 for further specific information concerning therapy.

QUESTION 4 What is the impact of epidemiology, age, and comorbidity on the differential diagnosis of the specific agent involved in meningitis?

Certain historical data are important in suggesting specific etiologic agents. Age is an important criterion in the decision process. Neonates have a propensity to be infected with *E. coli,* group B streptococci, *Listeria,* and herpes simplex virus (HSV-2). Infants less than 2 months of age have an increased incidence of group B streptococci, *Listeria,* and *E. coli,* whereas children less than 10 years old frequently have viruses, *H. influenzae, S. pneumoniae,* and *N. meningitidis* as their etiologic agent. Young adults are more frequently infected with viruses and meningococci. Adults and the elderly have pneumococci as their predominant organism although the elderly have gram-negative bacilli and *Listeria* in increasing frequency. When *H. influenzae* causes meningitis in older patients, it is usually associated with CSF leaks or immunodeficiency. While *Listeria* is one of the most common causes of bacterial meningitis in patients with hematologic malignancies, it is also seen in normal hosts and is implicated in outbreaks associated with food products. Meningococcal and *H. influenzae* infections are seen when a sibling or other close contact has concurrent meningitis. Meningococcal meningitis is unique in that a large percentage of patients present with a characteristic rash consisting of lower extremity or mucous membrane petechiae or purpura.

Underlying illness is an important factor as diabetes mellitus is associated with an increased incidence of *S. pneumoniae,* gram-negative bacilli, streptococci, *Cryptococcus,* and the fungal agents of mucormycosis. *S. pneumoniae* is a common bacterium seen in alcoholics. A history of tuberculosis should be sought in all patients. Tuberculous meningitis may present in a subacute manner or in an acute fashion with a rapidly progressive course. Mortality is high at either extreme of age and in patients with extensive neurologic deficits. Handling of hamsters or mice has been associated with LCM and contact with water used by rodents or domestic animals, with leptospirosis. Amebic meningitis occurs after swimming in fresh water lakes. Seasonal variation may be an important clue as viruses generally occur in the summer and fall but rarely in winter.

QUESTION 5 The patient is started on ceftriaxone. Blood cultures as well as CSF cultures subsequently grow *Staphylococcus aureus.* The patient's antibiotic is changed to vancomycin. What is the significance of a *S. aureus* meningitis, and how would you proceed in the management of this patient?

S. aureus meningitis is a rare entity and is most often seen in patients with underlying illnesses, premature or low birth weight infants, and following neurosurgic procedures. Hematogenous seeding of the meninges by *S. aureus* is mainly seen in older patients, although the incidence is low. Predisposing underlying diseases in patients without prior CNS illness include diabetes mellitus, alcoholism, chronic renal failure requiring hemodialysis, and malignancy.

S. aureus meningitis is a rare entity that is frequently seen after neurosurgic procedures. Occult *S. aureus* meningitis appears to be related to either direct inoculation of the organism into the CSF via an intracranial foreign body or via bacteremic spread from other sources. Increased mortality with *S. aureus* meningitis is associated with diabetes mellitus, age greater than 60, obtundation or coma on presentation, bacteremia, and

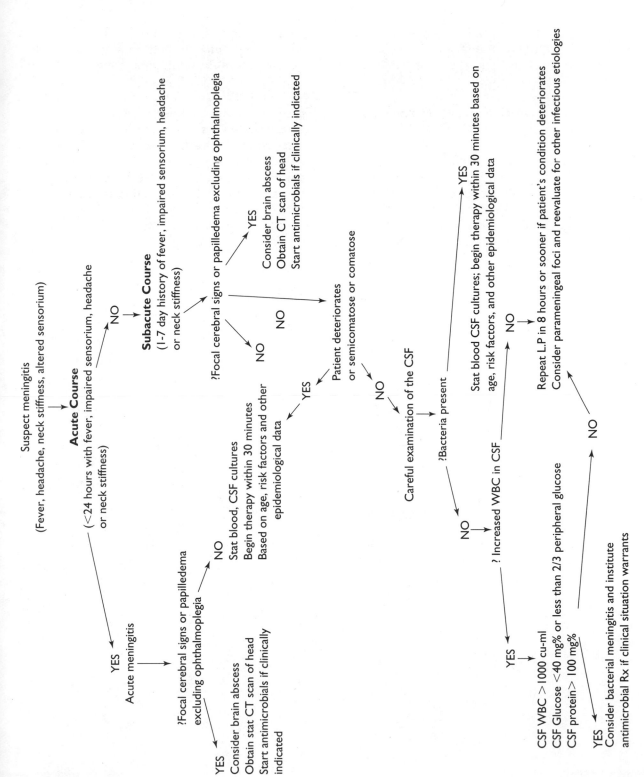

8-8-1 Evaluation of the patient with suspected meningitis.

DIC. Management of this patient should include a search for a source of bacteremia with an echocardiogram, CT of spine, and surveillance blood cultures.

QUESTION 6 What is the treatment of suspected meningitis?

Meningitis is a medical emergency that requires rapid diagnosis and early intervention to prevent serious neurologic sequelae or death. In the evaluation of a patient with suspected meningitis, initial management is often empiric and based on analysis of the CSF. While a CT scan is often done, treatment should be started as soon as possible (see Fig. 8-8-1).

Irrespective of age, meningitis without predisposing factors is treated similarly. Use of high-dose penicillin or ampicillin or a third-generation cephalosporin (cefotaxime/ceftriaxone/ceftazidime) is an appropriate choice. When contamination of the CSF is related to breach of the skin, gram-positive organisms become a more likely etiology, and vancomycin should be included in the initial regimen. When infection involves a ventriculoperitoneal shunt, the device should be removed. When meningitis is thought to be secondary to a brain or parameningeal abscess, anaerobic coverage with metronidazole is an important treatment modality. In addition, consideration should be given to drainage of a collection of purulence.

The use of corticosteroids as adjunctive agents has been shown to decrease the incidence of postmeningitic deafness in the pediatric population with *H. influenzae* infection. However, there have been no outcome data to support use of corticosteroids in the adult population.

CASE FOLLOW-UP An echocardiography of the patient's heart is performed, which does not reveal vegetations. A CT scan of his lower thoracolumbar area reveals a large epidural collection of fluid from L2 to S1. Neurosurgic consultation is obtained, and the fluid is drained. The patient's blood cultures become negative after institution of appropriate antibiotic therapy.

• •

BIBLIOGRAPHY

Comella CL, Bleck TP: The technique of lumbar puncture: steps that ensure a successful tap; how to interpret results, *J Crit Illness*, 3(9):61-66, 1988.

Conly JM, Ronald AR: Cerbebrospinal fluid as a diagnostic body fluid, *Am J Med* 102-108, 1983.

Durand ML, et al: Acute bacterial meningitis in adults, *N Engl J Med* 328:21-28, 1993.

Jensen AG, et al: *Staphylococcus aureus* meningitis, *Arch Intern Med* 153:1902-1908, 1993.

Mandell G, Douglas RG, Bennett JE: *Principles and practice of infectious diseases*, New York, 1990, Churchill Livingstone.

Marton KI, Gean AD: The spinal tap: a new look at an old test, *Ann Intern Med* 104:840-848, 1986.

Merritt HH, Fremont-Smith F.: *The cerebrospinal fluid*, Philadelphia, 1938, WB Saunders.

Ratzan KR: Viral meningitis, *Med Clin North Am* 69(2):399-412, 1985.

Schlesinger LS, Ross SC, Schaberg DR: *Staphylococcus aureus* meningitis: a broad based epidemiologic study, *Medicine* 66:148-156, 1987.

Spanos A, Harrell F, Durack D: Differential diagnosis of acute meningitis, *JAMA* 262:2700-2707, 1989.

C A S E

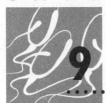

Jessica S. Khan

A 37-year-old bus driver from Chicago presents with intermittent fever, nonproductive cough, night sweats, 20-lb weight loss, and neck pain for the last 6 months. He has smoked 1 pack per day for the last 10 years and is a heavy alcohol drinker, but denies illicit intravenous drug use. He is heterosexual, lives with his wife and two children, and has not traveled out of state in the last 5 years.

On physical examination, he has the following vital signs: T 101°F, HR 100 bpm, RR 24/min, and BP 130/70 mm Hg. Mouth opening is limited to 3 cm because of neck pain. Point tenderness is present on percussion at the posterior midcervical region. He has multiple lymph nodes (5 mm in diameter) in both posterior cervical triangles, which are movable and nontender. Chest examination is significant for decreased breath sounds at the left lung base with egophony. Cardiovascular and abdominal examinations are unremarkable. CNS examination is normal.

QUESTION I What is your impression of this case?

This patient has a chronic respiratory syndrome of cough, fever, night sweats, and signs of consolidation at the left lung base. The neck pain and weight loss may or may not be related to his lung condition.

His problem is most likely infectious in etiology although noninfectious conditions should be kept in mind. Among the noninfectious causes, an endobronchial malignancy with resulting postobstructive pneumonia is a possibility and will certainly explain his respiratory complaints. He is,

however, rather young for a malignancy of this nature despite a 10 pack-year smoking history.

Another malignancy, more common in his age group, would be lymphoma with extrinsic compression of a bronchus, thereby causing a postobstructive pneumonia. His weight loss, fever, and night sweats might represent B symptoms.

Sarcoid is another condition that can present with a chronic cough, fever, night sweats, and weight loss. Consolidation is a rare sequela. Further, when it affects the bones, the spine is not a common site.

Yet another noninfectious possibility is a syndrome of primary neck pathology with a component of pulmonary involvement. Rheumatoid arthritis can affect the cervical vertebrae, causing chronic neck pain and limitation of motion, and is known to have distinct pulmonary manifestations. However, point tenderness is not a feature of this disease, and lung consolidation is not typical of its pulmonary involvement. Another form of arthritis that has a predilection to the spine is ankylosing spondylitis. Major areas of involvement are the lumbar, thoracic, and sacroiliac regions. It can also affect the cervical spine but rarely does so without prior involvement of the lower spine. Pulmonary consolidation is not seen with this condition.

Complaints of cough, fever, night sweats, and weight loss are nonspecific but, taken together with the prolonged duration, suggest tuberculosis (TB). In this age group, pulmonary tuberculosis is generally a reactivation process with the disease usually in the apical to midlung zones. It is much less common to present as a lower lobe consolidation. The two instances in which it presents as a lower lobe disease are (1) primary infection with rapid progression to a lower lobe pneumonia commonly encountered in the elderly and in immunocompromised patients, and (2) an endo-bronchial lesion with subsequent collapse and consolidation of the affected lobe. Unlike the former, this latter entity has no predilection for the immunocompromised host. This process is often difficult to diagnose and may require bronchoscopy in order to examine the airways directly and distinguish between the two.

Neck pain, consistent with this scenario, may represent extrapulmonary tuberculosis. Although it is a more common occurrence in the immunocompromised patient, up to 10% of tuberculosis is extrapulmonary in the immunocompetent host. Tuberculous vertebral osteomyelitis, Pott's disease, is not very common and accounts for about 1% of all cases of tuberculosis. It commonly involves the lower spinal areas with roughly 50% of cases in the lumbar and thoracic regions; only one third of cases involve the cervical spine. The neurologic presentation can range from a normal CNS examination to paralysis depending on the presence and location of cord involvement. Additional findings on physical examination may be related to development of a paraspinal abscess. An abscess may develop as an extension of bony necrosis to the surrounding soft tissues. It is also noteworthy that Pott's disease coexists with an active pulmonary focus in 50% of patients at the time of presentation. Thus, this patient's presentation is consistent with tuberculosis but is by no means a clear cut case.

The differential also includes blastomycosis, caused by the dimorphic fungus *Blastomyces dermatitidis*. This fungus is endemic in the Midwest and can cause a pulmonary syndrome similar to tuberculosis. The initial infection is caused by inhalation and can result in an acute infection that usually passes unnoticed. Some patients experience an influenza-like syndrome of cough, myalgia, and arthralgia with a radiologic picture of a lobar or segmental consolidation mostly in the lower lobes. The initial infection resolves spontaneously in the majority of cases, but may progress to a more indolent chronic phase with long-standing cough, pleuritic chest pain, weight loss, and occasional episodes of hemoptysis. Fever and night sweats are not very prominent features but may occur. Radiologic and pulmonary findings at this stage are generally in the upper lobes similar to tuberculosis, although lower lobe consolidation has been reported. Extrapulmonary disease is seen and most commonly involves the skin with lesions presenting as nonhealing ulcers. Skeletal involvement may also occur, commonly affecting the long bones, vertebrae, and ribs. Vertebral osteomyelitis caused by blastomycosis mimics that of tuberculosis both in clinical and radiographic presentation. Blastomycosis may also cause paraspinal abscesses. Differentiation is made by direct visualization and growth of the organism from aspirated fluid or biopsy material. This patient may have blastomycosis based on his clinical presentation.

Another entity that should be considered in this case is nocardiosis, caused by the actinomycete *Nocardia brasiliensis*. Its mode of infection is also pulmonary and may present as an acute, subacute, or chronic pulmonary process. Symptoms are nonspecific and include productive cough, weight loss, dyspnea, and pleuritic chest pain. It can occur acutely and resolve spontaneously or progress into a chronic form if left untreated. It can also present in the chronic stage without a prior acute episode. Lower lobe involvement is more common than apical disease and can range from bronchopneumonia to consolidation to cavitation and pulmonary abscess formation. Extrapulmonary manifestations include brain involvement and, less commonly, vertebral osteomyelitis. Similar to tuberculosis, this organism causes a more severe disease in the immunocompromised host. Again, this patient's presentation is not characteristic, but some aspects (such as cough, weight loss, lower lobe consolidation, and the chronicity of symptoms) make it suspicious for nocardiosis.

The fourth item on the infectious differential diagnosis is bacterial infective endocarditis causing septic embolization to the lungs, resulting in a pneumonia, and to the spine, leading to osteomyelitis or a paraspinal abscess. This postulate would mean that vegetations are present on both sides of the heart or that a right-to-left shunt is present with a paradoxical embolus. Another scenario includes the presence of vertebral osteomyelitis secondary to transient bacteremia from a currently unknown source. This then could serve as a reservoir for continuous bacteremia with seeding of the heart valves and subsequent embolization to the pulmonary bed resulting in pneumonia. The most common organism in this setting is *Staphylococcus aureus*. In either case, the presentation is usually more acute. Although a heart murmur is not imperative in the diagnosis, it is helpful when present. The pneumonia caused by the septic embolization to the lung presents the same as any bacterial pneumonia—acutely, with productive cough, fever, and shortness of breath as more prominent features. Hemoptysis may be more common than in typical pneumonias.

The patient's immune status may have important consequences for the manifestations of an infectious disease. For example, HIV disease or immunosuppressive medications may change the clinical presentation of different infections. We are not told of any medication that he is taking before his admission—we will assume he is not on any. He denies HIV risk factors. Imaging and laboratory testing will be needed to further elucidate this case.

QUESTION 2 The patient's chest x-ray shows an infiltrate in the left lower lobe. He also has an MRI of the cervical spine that demonstrates low signal intensity at the bodies of C2, C3, and C4 suggestive of osteomyelitis, along with a large epidural collection of purulent material from the clivus to C4 (Fig. 8-9-1 on p. 494). A CT of the neck and chest shows erosion of the anterior portion of the 1st through 4th cervical vertebral bodies and multiple lucencies in the neck, posterior cervical triangle, retropharyngeal space, upper thoracic paraspinal areas, and mediastinum suggestive of abscesses (Fig. 8-9-2 on p. 494). Laboratory tests reveal a Hb of 6.3 mg/dl, WBC of 5.6 K with 89% neutrophils and 10% lymphocytes. PPD testing is positive with 15 mm of

induration at 48 hours, and HIV testing is negative. How does this additional information help in the diagnosis?

The chest x-ray confirms what we already know by physical examination. The MRI and CT scan of the cervical spine showing changes consistent with osteomyelitis of C2-4 and extensive paraspinal soft tissue abscesses support our initial suspicion of an infectious process causing this patient's problems.

The positive PPD skin test tilts the balance towards tuberculosis as the most likely culprit.

QUESTION 3 What additional workup is necessary at this point?

Gram stain and AFB smear and culture of the sputum are needed as well as routine blood cultures. A definitive diagnosis has not yet been established and bacterial causes, most notably gram-positive organisms such as *Staphylococcus* and *Streptococcus,* as well as anaerobes, must be ruled out as these are common causes of soft tissue abscesses.

Aspiration of one of the more accessible fluid collections can prove to be diagnostic. Bronchoscopy will be the next step if the aspiration is not helpful in finding the answer to this patient's problems.

QUESTION 4 What therapy is indicated at this point?

Once initial cultures are obtained, empiric antibiotic coverage is indicated. Antibiotics should have a broad spectrum of activity with particular concern for gram-positive organisms and anaerobes as mentioned above.

Empiric antituberculous medications may be started on admission without significant impact on a diagnosis if diagnostic tests are performed promptly. Medications and CDC guidelines for therapy are listed in Tables 8-9-1 and 8-9-2. Major side effects and toxicities of these medications are listed in Table 8-9-3 on p. 492. Respiratory isola-

TABLE 8-9-1   Options for the Initial Treatment of TB Among Children and Adults

A. TB Without HIV

	Part A	Part B	Part C
OPTION 1*	Daily INH, RIF, PZA for 8 weeks (should include EMB or SM until susceptibility to INH and RIF is demonstrated)	Daily INH and RIF to complete at least 6 months and 3 months beyond culture conversion (can be given 2x/wk or 3x/wk as DOT in areas where the INH resistance rate is not documented to be <4%)	N/A
OPTION 2*	Daily INH, RIF, PZA, and SM or EMB for 2 weeks	All drugs at 2x/wk schedule as DOT for 6 weeks	INH & RIF 2x/wk as DOT for 16 weeks
OPTION 3*	INH, RIF, PZA, SM or EMB at 3x/wk schedule as DOT for 6 months	N/A	N/A

B. TB With HIV
   Options 1, 2, or 3 to complete 9 months total duration and at least 6 months beyond culture conversion.

C. Extrapulmonary TB
   Similar options and treatment duration apply as in the above table. It is recommended that duration is extended to 9 months for disseminated disease, bone and joint disease, or tuberculous lymphadenitis.

*Consult a TB specialist if patient is symptomatic or smear or culture positive after 3 months.
INH = isoniazid, RIF = rifampin, PZA = pyrazinamide, SM = streptomycin, EMB = ethambutol, DOT = directly observed therapy
(Adapted from Advisory Committee for Elimination of Tuberculosis: Tuberculosis in the era of multidrug resistance, *MMWR* 42(RR-7):1-8, 1993.)

tion should be considered in any patient suspected of having pulmonary tuberculosis. This patient should be placed in a respiratory isolation room until he has three sputum samples tested negative for acid fast bacilli (AFB) to prevent possible contagion. Sputum smears positive for AFB correlate well with infectiousness of the patient.

Antifungal drugs may be delayed until further diagnostic procedures are performed, especially in light of the significant toxicity associated with amphotericin B therapy. Should the patient's condition deteriorate on antibacterial and antituberculous therapy, the addition of antifungal coverage should be considered.

QUESTION 5 The patient is placed in isolation and is empirically started on ampicillin-sulbactam and four antituberculous drugs. A CT-guided aspiration of the thoracic paraspinal abscess is per-

formed, demonstrating numerous WBCs and acid fast bacilli on Ziehl-Neelsen (AFB) stain. Several weeks later culture of the material grows *Mycobacterium tuberculosis* susceptible to all of the first-line drugs. Sputum studies are negative for any organism on gram stain, culture, and AFB stain. Thus, respiratory isolation is discontinued. Blood cultures are all negative for growth. Ampicillin-sulbactam is stopped once blood culture results are negative. He defervesces 1 week after TB medications are started. What is the appropriate management of his contacts, namely his wife and 2 daughters, ages 6 years and 3 months?

They need to be screened for symptoms and have a Mantoux test using the PPD antigen. If positive, they must have a CXR to determine whether they have active pulmonary disease. Infection is defined as a positive Mantoux reaction in a close contact of an infected patient, (PPD

TABLE 8-9-2   Dosage Recommendations for the Initial Treatment of TB

Children (< = 12 Years)	Adults
A. Daily	
INH 10-20 mg/kg (max 300 mg)	5 mg/kg (max 300 mg)
RIF 10-20 mg/kg (max 600 mg)	10 mg/kg (max 600 mg)
PZA 15-30 mg/kg (max 2 gm)	15-30 mg/kg (max 2 gm)
EMB* 15-25 mg/kg (max 2.5 gm)	5-25 mg/kg (max 2.5 gm)
SM 20-30 mg/kg (max 1 gm)	15 mg/kg (max 1 gm)
B. 2x/week	
INH 20-40 mg/kg (max 900 mg)	15 mg/kg (max 900 mg)
RIF 10-20 mg/kg (max 600 mg)	10 mg/kg (max 600 mg)
PZA 50-70 mg/kg (max 4 gm)	50-70 mg/kg (max 4 gm)
EMB* 50 mg/kg (max 2.5 gm)	50 mg/kg (max 2.5 gm)
SM 25-30 mg/kg (max 1.5 gm)	25-30 mg/kg (max 1.5 gm)
C. 3x/week	
INH 20-40 mg/kg (max 900 mg)	15 mg/kg (max 900 mg)
RIF 10-20 mg/kg (max 600 mg)	10 mg/kg (max 600 mg)
PZA 50-70 mg/kg (max 3 gm)	50-70 mg/kg (max 3 gm)
EMB* 25-30 mg/kg (max 2.5 gm)	25 mg/kg (max 2.5 gm)
SM 25-30 mg/kg (max 1 gm)	25-30 mg/kg (max 1 gm)

*EMB is generally not recommended for children whose visual acuity cannot be monitored (<6 years old). It should be considered, however, for all children with organisms resistant to other drugs, when susceptibility to EMB is likely or demonstrated.
(Adapted from Advisory Committee for Elimination of Tuberculosis: Tuberculosis in the era of multidrug resistance, MMWR 42(RR-7):1-8, 1993.)

positive is ≥5 mm in duration at 48 to 72 hours) with a normal CXR. This implies that a person has been exposed and is harboring the organism in his or her body in quantities too small to cause organ damage. In contrast, disease is a positive reaction with symptoms and an abnormal CXR. Guidelines for interpreting PPD results for different patient populations are presented in the box.

If his wife and 6-year-old child are PPD (−), no further test or treatment is indicated. If they are PPD (+) with no symptoms and a normal chest x-ray, they can be started on chemoprophylaxis as stated in the guidelines issued by the CDC, summarized in the box. If his wife happens to be

CRITERIA FOR PREVENTIVE THERAPY FOR PERSONS WITH POSITIVE MANTOUX REACTION TO 5 TU OF PURIFIED PROTEIN DERIVATIVE (PPD)

A. WITH RISK FACTORS*
- Treat at all ages if PPD reaction is ≥10 mm (consider ≥5 mm as positive if patient is recent contact, HIV infected, or has radiographic evidence of old TB)

B. NO RISK FACTOR/HIGH INCIDENCE GROUP†
- Treat if PPD reaction is ≥10 mm and age <35 years
- No treatment if age is ≥35 years

C. NO RISK FACTOR/LOW INCIDENCE GROUP
- Treat if PPD reaction is ≥15 mm and age <35 years
- No treatment if age is ≥35 years

Use INH at 10 mg/kg for children and 300 mg/day for adults; may also use 15 mg/kg (max 900 mg) 2×/wk as DOT. Duration of treatment is 6 months except for (a) HIV-positive and (b) stable abnormal chest x-ray consistent with old TB, for which 12 months should be given.
*RISK FACTORS
1. HIV positive (PPD positive ≥5 mm)
2. Recent contact with newly diagnosed infectious tuberculosis case (positive PPD ≥5 mm). PPD negative (<5 mm) children and adolescents who are close contacts of infectious person (smear positive) in the last 3 months need prophylaxis for 3 months, then repeat PPD testing; if still PPD negative, may stop the treatment
3. Recent converters: PPD >10 mm increase within 2 years for age <35 years; PPD >15 mm increase within 2 years for age >35 years
4. Abnormal chest x-ray representing old healed TB (positive PPD ≥5 mm)
5. Intravenous drug user, HIV negative (positive PPD >10 mm)
6. Medical conditions reported to increase the risk of developing tuberculosis: silicosis, diabetes mellitus, chronic renal failure, gastrectomy or jejunoileal bypass, malnutrition, prolonged use of steroids or other immunosuppressive drugs, leukemia, lymphoma, other malignancies
†High incidence groups
1. Foreign born from high prevalence countries
2. Low-income populations and ethnic minorities (Afro-American, Hispanic, native American)
3. Residents of long-term care facilities (nursing homes, mental institutions, correctional institutions)
(Adapted from Advisory Committee for Elimination of Tuberculosis: The use of preventive therapy for tuberculosis infection in the United States, MMWR 39 [RR-8]:9-12, 1990.)

TABLE 8-9-3   **Toxicities and Side Effects of Commonly Used Drugs for the Treatment of Tuberculosis**

Drugs	Side Effects	Comments
Isoniazid (INH)	Hepatotoxicity	More common in the elderly, patients with liver disease, daily alcohol consumption, and concomitant therapy with INH
	Peripheral neuropathy	Related to interference with B_6 metabolism; concomitant B_6 administration can prevent or decrease its severity and is highly recommended for patients with increased incidence of neuropathy (DM, uremia, alcoholism, malnutrition)
	Optic neuritis, seizures	Also related to interference in B_6 metabolism; may be prevented or decreased in severity with concomitant B_6 administration
	Fever, rash, purpura, urticaria	Hypersensitivity reactions
	Drug interactions with	
	Phenytoin	Increases concentration of both drugs; need to monitor serum level of phenytoin and adjust doses accordingly
	Antacids (aluminum containing)	Decrease absorption of INH
Rifampin (RIF)	Gastrointestinal disturbance	Most common adverse reaction
	Body fluid becomes orange-colored	Need to warn patients; may cause permanent discoloration of soft contact lenses
	Hepatitis	Most serious adverse effect; increased incidence in the elderly, patients with liver disease and concomitant use of INH; toxicity occurs earlier than INH hepatotoxicity
	Anemia Thrombocytopenia Influenza-like syndrome	Associated with intermittent administration of RIF at doses >10 mg/kg; presumed immune reaction
	Drug interactions with Methadone Coumarin Glucocorticoids Oral hypoglycemic agents Estrogen preparations Digoxin Antiarrhythmics (quinidine, verapamil, mexilitine) Theophylline Anticonvulsants Ketoconazole Cyclosporine	Drug levels are decreased with concomitant RIF use because of accelerated drug clearance with induction of hepatic microsomal enzymes
Pyrazinamide (PZA)	Hepatitis	No added hepatotoxicity with concomitant use of INH and/or RIF
	Hyperuricemia	Results from decreased excretion of urate; acute gout attack uncommon
	Arthralgia	Responds to salicylates
	Gastrointestinal upset	
	Skin rash	

Continued.

TABLE 8-9-3   Toxicities and Side Effects of Commonly Used Drugs for the Treatment of Tuberculosis—cont'd.

Drugs	Side Effects	Comments
Ethambutol (EMB)	Retrobulbar neuritis	Dose-related; symptoms include blurred vision, central scotoma and red-green color blindness; color blindness is earliest symptom; may be reversible if the drug is stopped promptly
	Hyperuricemia	Caused by decreased clearance of urates
	Rash	
Streptomycin (SM)	Ototoxicity	Worse with age; vertigo more common than hearing loss; vertigo may be reversible but hearing loss often permanent if present; related to cumulative dose and peak serum concentration
	Nephrotoxicity	Less than other aminoglycosides; worse with age; related to both cumulative dose and peak serum concentration
	Neuromuscular blockade	Dose related; uncommon

TREATMENT OF TB DURING PREGNANCY

- Minimum of 9 months of therapy is recommended.
- The preferred initial treatment regimen is INH, RIF and EMB.
- SM is the only licensed anti-TB drug documented to have harmful effects to the fetus (i.e., congenital deafness).
- Routine use of PZA is not recommended because the risk of teratogenicity has not been determined. However, if resistance to other drugs is likely and susceptibility to PZA is also likely, the use of PZA should be considered, and the risks and benefits of the drug carefully weighed.
- Breastfeeding should not be discouraged because the small concentrations of anti-TB drugs in the breast milk do not produce toxicity in the nursing newborn.

pregnant, PPD (+), with no symptoms, chemoprophylaxis may be delayed until the third trimester or postpartum period. If she happens to be pregnant, PPD (+), and symptomatic with disease, treatment should be initiated according to the guidelines in the box.

The 3-month-old baby needs to be started on INH and pyridoxine (vitamin B_6) regardless of the PPD status since an infant's cellular immunity (that arm responsible for the delayed hypersensitivity to the Mantoux reaction) will not be developed until 6 months of age, and thus she may not be able to respond to the PPD antigen challenge. She needs to continue the INH and vitamin B_6 until she is 6 months of age, and then be retested with PPD again. If the result continues to be negative, then the drug may be discontinued provided no active disease exists in other family members.

CASE FOLLOW-UP   His wife is found to be PPD^+ with a normal CXR and is given INH and B_6 for 6 months. Both of his daughters are PPD−. The 3-month-old baby is given INH and B_6 for 3 months, at the end of which PPD retesting is again per-

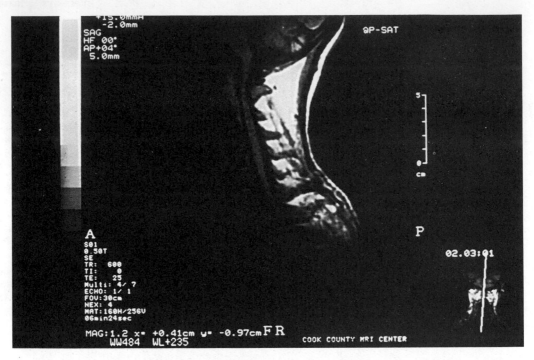

8-9-1 MRI of the cervical spine demonstrating low signal intensity in the bodies of C$_2$, C$_3$, and C$_4$, with a large epidural fluid collection.

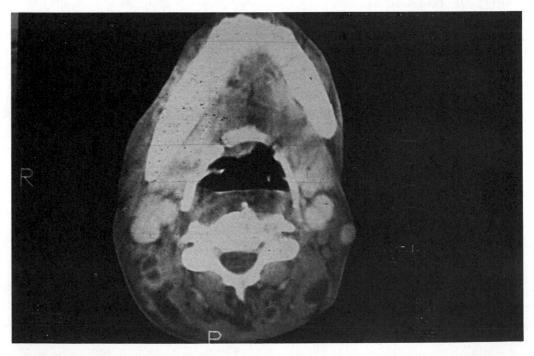

8-9-2 CT scan of the neck demonstrating erosion of the anterior vertebral body and soft tissue lucency suggestive of abscess.

formed. The result is again negative, and the drugs are discontinued.

• •

BIBLIOGRAPHY

Advisory Committee for Elimination of Tuberculosis: Screening for tuberculosis and tuberculous infection in the high risk populations, *MMWR* 39(RR-8):1-7, 1990.

Advisory Committee for Elimination of Tuberculosis: The use of preventive therapy for tuberculous infection in the united states, *MMWR* 39(RR-8):9-12, 1990.

Advisory Committee for Elimination of Tuberculosis: Tuberculosis in the era of multidrug resistance, *MMWR* 42 (RR-7):1-8, 1993.

American Thoracic Society: Treatment of tuberculosis and tuberculosis infection in adults and children, *Am J Respir Crit Care Med* 149:1359-1374, 1994.

Mandell GL, Douglas RG, Bennett JE, eds: *Principles and practices of infectious diseases,* ed 3, New York, 1990, Churchill Livingston.

Van Scoy RE, Wilkowski CJ: Antituberculous agents, *Mayo Clin Proc* 67:179-187, 1992.

Wilson JD, Braunwald E, Isselbacher KJ, et al, eds: *Harrison's principles of internal medicine,* ed 12, New York, 1994, McGraw-Hill.

Wurtz R, Quader Z, Simon D, Langer B: Cervical tuberculous vertebral osteomyelitis: case report and discussion of the literature, *CID* 16:806-808, 1993.

CASE

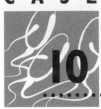

10

Vishnu Chundi
Gordon Trenholme

A *44-year-old Tanzanian man is seen in the emergency room with a chief complaint of fever accompanied by severe chills and rigors for 5 days. He returned 1 week ago after a 1-month visit to Tanzania. His fever is intermittent with severe myalgias and did not follow any pattern recognizable to the patient. While in Tanzania, he experienced similar symptoms that resolved with a course of chloroquine. He remembers numerous insect bites throughout his vacation. He did not take malarial prophylaxis.*

The vital signs revealed a temperature of 103°F with a respiratory rate of 22/min and a pulse rate of 110 bpm. He appears moderately ill but has an unremarkable physical examination. The heart, lungs, and abdomen are normal. The central nervous system examination is nonfocal.

QUESTION I Because of his recent travel to east Africa, you are concerned that he may have become infected while out of the United States. Based on this concern, what are your diagnostic considerations, and which laboratory tests would be appropriate?

The differential diagnosis includes many diseases with similar presentations. These include yellow fever and other hemorrhagic fevers, dengue, typhoid fever, leptospirosis, trypanosomiasis, leishmaniasis, schistosomiasis, plague, and typhus; however, the response to chloroquine would immediately narrow the differential considerations.

Of special importance in a febrile patient with recent travel to east Africa is the diagnosis of *malaria*. Much like the above-mentioned diseases, the presentation may be nonspecific. However, malaria should be included in the differential diagnosis because of the potential morbidity associated with delayed treatment.

Appropriate laboratory tests to order should include CBC with differential, blood cultures, urinalysis, electrolytes including BUN and creatinine, liver function tests, and malarial smears. In almost all patients, the diagnosis will be evident from careful examination of a thin smear. A thick smear should be done if repeated thin smears are negative. Speciation cannot be done with a thick smear.

QUESTION 2 The laboratory data are available and reveal a WBC count of 3500 per mm^3 with 49% granulocytes, 44% lymphocytes, and 7% monocytes. The platelet count is 138,000 per mm^3 with a hemoglobin of 13.4 g%. Liver function tests, electrolytes, and renal function are normal. Urinalysis reveals moderate protein. The peripheral smear demonstrates an intraerythrocytic parasitization rate of 3%. What are the likely pathogens?

The finding of erythrocytic parasites generates a limited differential diagnosis. The two most common organisms are *Plasmodium* and *Babesia*. *Babesiosis* is a tick-borne malaria-like organism that undergoes asexual reproduction within erythrocytes. It can be endemically acquired in the United States and is very uncommon in travelers. The tick species can be variable: it is usually a hard body tick and may be *Ixodes dammini* that feeds on deer, mice, and voles. It is not uncommon to see transmission of both *Babesia microti* and Lyme disease concomitantly as this tick is also the vector for *Borrelia burgdorferi*.

QUESTION 3 The technologist believes that the organism is of a *Plasmodia* genus but is unsure of the species. The patient defervesces in the emergency room and wants to go home. What are the typical findings on presentation and physical examination in cases of malaria?

The clinical presentation of malaria may be protean and include symptoms of abdominal pain, joint pain, or a flulike illness with a headache. Examination may reveal enlargement of the liver and spleen, signs of anemia, orthostatic blood pressure changes, and tachycardia. Hemolysis may result in jaundice with scleral or mucous membrane icterus. Development of microvascular congestion may result in pulmonary crackles or focal neurologic defects in cases of cerebral malaria. Paroxysms of fever may be associated with changes of sensorium or personality that resolve as the fever abates.

Laboratory abnormalities may include normochromic normocytic anemia, thrombocytopenia, and leukopenia. Proteinuria may be secondary to the high fever. Hyponatremia can be seen due to the elaboration of ADH and aldosterone as a response to hypoxemic vasodilatation in the renal microvasculature. Indirect hyperbilirubinemia may be a consequence of hemolysis. If the alkaline phosphatase or transaminase level is elevated, one should be suspicious for the development of centrilobular necrosis that may occur because of hypoxemia of the portal triad.

QUESTION 4 Upon further examination of the thin smear with Wright-Giemsa staining, the chief technologist and an infectious disease specialist concur that the organism is a *Plasmodium*. What are the species that cause malaria in man, and what other historical data would help in diagnosis?

The four species that cause malaria in man are *Plasmodium falciparum, Plasmodium vivax, Plasmodium ovale,* and *Plasmodium malariae.* The species can be surmised before smear examination by asking some simple questions (see Fig. 8-10-1).

First, it is important to ask the patient in what

area of the world he was traveling. Of the 2,548 cases of *P. falciparum* among U.S. civilians reported to the CDC from 1980-1992, 2096 (82%) were acquired in sub-Saharan Africa; 191 (8%) were acquired in Asia; 129 (5%) were acquired in the Caribbean and South America; and 132 (5%) were acquired in other parts of the world.* Most of the cases of *P. vivax* occur in the Indian subcontinent. *P. ovale* is virtually restricted to West Africa.

The next question concerns the periodicity of symptoms. Symptoms of malaria are due to its life cycle in the human. The human phase begins when an infected female *Anopheles* mosquito bites the host and injects sporozoites from her salivary glands. The sporozoites enter the host's circulation and rapidly reach the liver where they invade the cells. They replicate asexually in the liver cells and develop into primary tissue **schizonts,** the primary exoerythrocytic forms, and mature into tissue **merozoites.** The length of this time, called the **prepatent period,** lasts between 8 and 21 days, and varies depending on the species of *Plasmodium:* for *P. falciparum* it is 10 days; for *P. vivax* 12 days; for *P. ovale* it is 14 days; and for *P. malariae* 21 days. During the prepatent period the patient is asymptomatic.

At the end of the prepatent period, merozoites enter the blood stream, invade red cells, and begin intraerythrocytic development. *P. vivax* and *P. ovale* persist in the liver cells producing secondary exoerythrocytic forms; this does not occur with *P. falciparum* and *P. malariae.* The intraerythrocytic cycle ends when infected red cells rupture, releasing parasites, along with red cell debris and pigment, and infect other red cells.

The classic clinical signs of malaria include paroxysms of chills, fever, and sweating, in association with constitutional symptoms such as headache, myalgias, nausea, and vomiting. The fever, which can be up to 105°F, correlates with the time of schizont rupture. The classic periodicity of fever is due to synchronization of the

---

*CDC: *Health Information for International Travel,* 1994, pp. 105-108.

erythrocytic phase, the cycles being 48 hours (tertian malaria) for *P. falciparum, P. vivax,* and *P. ovale,* and 72 hours (quartan malaria) for *P. malariae.* There is a remarkable contrast between the deathly–ill-appearing patient during the paroxysm of symptoms and the well, sometimes euphoric, patient after the attack. In nonimmune individuals synchronization may not occur until several attacks have occurred, and in falciparum malaria, it may not happen at all. The life cycle is completed when some of the merozoites become microgametocytes or macrogametocytes. The gametocytes are infective to the mosquito and thus complete the life cycle.

The severity of the patient's symptoms may shed light on the specific organism involved. Severe illness is almost always due to *P. falciparum* species, with the exception being immunosuppressed individuals and splenectomized patients with *P. vivax.* Milder infection is usually caused by *P. vivax* or *P. malariae.* This phenomenon is due to infection of all ages of red cells by *P. falciparum. P. vivax* and *P. malariae* parasitize young and old red cells, respectively.

The time interval between the patient's leaving the endemic area or stopping prophylaxis and the appearance of symptoms may be specific. If it is less than 10 days, the species is usually *P. falciparum.* If it is between 10 days and 2 months, *P. falciparum, P. vivax,* or *P. malariae* may be present. If it is between 60 days and 1 year, *P. falciparum* is unlikely, and *P. vivax* or *P. malariae* is more likely.

Parasitization of red cells has both diagnostic and prognostic implications. Infection with *P. falciparum* is strongly suggested by the presence of more than 2% to 3% infected red cells. Higher levels of parasitemia (SBA >5%) are associated with more severe illness.

QUESTION 5 What is the appropriate management of this patient? What are some of the complications that may occur?

This patient traveled to east Africa, did not take prophylaxis, and symptoms appeared within 7 days of departure from the endemic area. He did not appear severely ill and had 3% malarial parasitization of red cells. Therefore, the most likely species of plasmodia is *P. falciparum.* The lack of clinical findings on examination and moderate levels of parasitemia should not be the sole basis for therapeutic decisions in falciparum malaria, as falciparum periodicity is 48 hours, and parasitization proceeds in a logarithmic manner. Therefore, erythrocyte infection increases rapidly, and it is possible to catch the patient during a relatively asymptomatic period and underestimate the true severity of illness. Peripheral smears should be examined twice daily to monitor response. When only moderately ill, patients with falciparum malaria should receive quinine 2 capsules q8h plus doxycycline 100 mg orally q8h if able to take oral medications. In a more severely ill patient, quinine gluconate or quinidine should be given intravenously for 3 days and be followed by a 7-day course of oral tetracycline.

QUESTION 6 The patient proved to have *P. falciparum.* He was treated with IV quinidine and doxycycline and improved. What is the appropriate prophylaxis for a traveler to east Africa?

Important elements of therapy are prevention and chemoprophylaxis. Wearing of appropriate clothing, use of effective insect repellent at night and "knock down" chemicals, and use of window screens and bednetting are non-specific measures one can take to reduce mosquito exposure.

The appropriate regimen of prophylaxis is based on the risk of acquisition of malaria and the prevalence of chloroquine resistance in the area of travel. Malarial transmission occurs in large areas of Central and South America, sub-Saharan Africa, the Indian subcontinent, southeast Asia, the Middle East, Oceania, and to a limited extent, in the Caribbean. The only chloroquine-sensitive areas remaining are in Central America and parts of the Middle East. Therefore a traveler to this area should receive chloroquine sulfate in doses of 500 mg/wk for 1 week before traveling through 4 weeks after traveling. Side effects of chloroquine most commonly are nausea/vomiting, abdominal

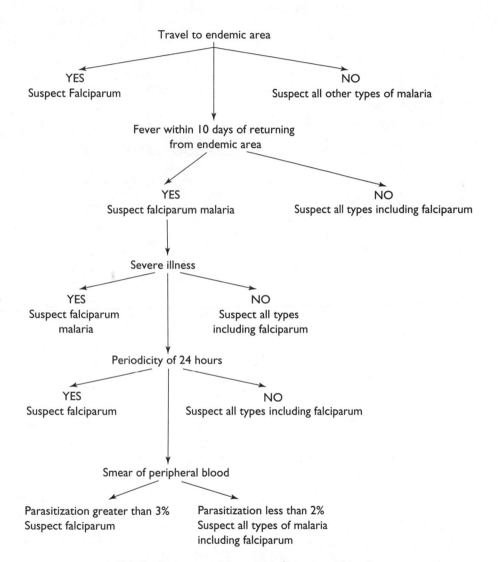

8-10-1 Evaluation of the patient with suspected malaria.

pain, dizziness, pruritus, hemolysis and cytopenias, and with long-term use, retinopathy. The alternative agent for use is the combination of pyrimethamine and dapsone.

Because of the increased prevalence of chloroquine resistance in other areas, a traveler to east Africa should receive mefloquine 250 mg/week starting 1 week before departure and continuing for 4 weeks after departure from the endemic area. Mefloquine should be avoided in patients on beta-blockers, calcium antagonists, or in situations of abnormal cardiac conduction. In addition, mefloquine is contraindicated in pregnant women. Patients intolerant of mefloquine should receive doxycycline 100 mg/day. If unable to take either mefloquine or doxycycline, pyrimethamine/sulfadoxine (Fansidar) may be used, although resistance has been reported. The traveler should be armed with a treatment dose of Fansidar to be taken three tablets at once at the onset of a febrile illness (in addition to the prophylactic medication being taken) if medical care is not readily available.

An important concept about malaria, namely the relapse that may occur after return from travel, dictates that primaquine be prescribed for patients who have had a long exposure to malarious areas. This treatment is aimed at extinguishing carriage of the *P. ovale* and *P. vivax* organisms in the liver. Patients should be screened for glucose-6-phosphate dehydrogenase deficiency before starting therapy.

A malaria hotline at the CDC may be contacted for detailed recommendations at (404) 332-4555.

BIBLIOGRAPHY

Centers for Disease Control: *Health information for international travel,* 1994, p 105-108.
Currier J, Maguire JH: Problems in management of falciparum malaria, *Rev Infect Dis* 11(6):988-995, 1989.
Strickland TG: *Hunter's tropical medicine,* ed 7, Philadelphia, 1991, WB Saunders.
Trenholme GM, Carson PE: Update on malaria, *Clin Microbiol Newsl* 2(15):1980.
Wyler DA: Malaria chemoprophylaxis for travelers, *N Engl J Med* 329:31-37, 1993.
Wyler DA: Malaria overview and update, *Clin Infect Dis* 16:449-458, 1993.

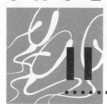

C A S E

Jessica S. Khan
Godofredo Carandang

A *22-year-old male student, previously healthy, presented with a 3-week history of progressive shortness of breath and dyspnea on exertion, nonproductive cough, and intermittent low-grade fever. He had taken antihistamines and antipyretics without any significant relief of symptoms. He denied smoking, drinking alcohol, or using illicit intravenous drugs. He admitted having homosexual activities with more than one partner but used condoms regularly in the last 2 years. He had not traveled in the last 4 years. He had no pets at home.*

On physical examination, he had a temperature of 102°F, heart rate of 104 bpm, respiratory rate of 32/min, and a blood pressure of 130/80 mm Hg. He had copious whitish plaques all over the hard and soft palate that scraped easily. There were no cervical, axillary, or supraclavicular lymph nodes appreciated. Lung sounds were clear with no rales or wheezes. There were no intercostal muscle retractions. Cardiovascular, abdominal, and neurologic examinations were unremarkable.

QUESTION 1 What is your impression of this case?

We have here a young patient with a subacute course of progressive respiratory symptoms, fever, mild respiratory distress, oral thrush, and no significant lung findings, who admits to high-risk behavior for acquiring HIV disease. The syndrome of a subacute course of cough, shortness of breath, and fever in a young person points to an atypical pneumonia rather than the typical pneumonia caused by the more classic pathogens of pneumonia such as *Streptococcus pneumoniae*. The latter

generally has a more acute course of illness, usually a 3-day symptom of cough productive of yellowish sputum, high-grade fever associated with rigors, and pleuritic chest pain. The agents of the syndrome called atypical pneumonia, so-named because it differs in presentation from the classic one just described, include *Mycoplasma pneumoniae*, *Legionella pneumophila*, *Chlamydia pneumoniae*, and viral pathogens. These organisms afflict both immunocompetent and immunocompromised hosts alike. All of these pathogens can give rise to a clinical picture such as seen in this patient. Slight variations in the pathogens' radiologic picture and laboratory findings may help in differentiating one from the other.

The presence of thrush in the absence of recent antibiotic use or intake of steroids reflects a defect in the patient's immune system, raising further the suspicion that he is infected with HIV. Thus, opportunistic infections are important to consider in this patient.

Of the opportunistic pathogens, *Pneumocystis carinii* tops the list, being the most common pulmonary infection encountered in HIV-infected patients. It has an incidence of 50% in the United States as the initial AIDS-defining illness in newly diagnosed HIV-infected patients. An HIV-infected patient has a 70% lifetime risk of developing *P. carinii* pneumonia (PCP) in the absence of preventive measures. The onset is usually insidious, starting as a dry cough associated with shortness of breath during heavy exertion. The respiratory symptoms are progressive to the point that it limits the patient's activities. Fever, usually low grade, is also a feature of the disease. Lung findings on physical examination range from normal to diffuse crepitations.

Tuberculosis is another possibility. Though it is not strictly an opportunistic pathogen, afflicting both immunocompetent and immunocompromised hosts alike, its incidence in the HIV-infected population is markedly higher than in the normal host. Its presentation is also altered in patients who are significantly immunosuppressed. The usual adult presentation of pulmonary tuberculosis is a reactivation of previously acquired infection. Although this is also commonly seen in HIV-infected patients, this group may present with primary or newly acquired pulmonary tuberculosis as well. The signs and symptoms are nonspecific and can range from a subacute nonproductive cough with minimal lung findings to a systemically ill patient with evidence of lung consolidation and/or pleural effusion. For all intents and purposes, an immunocompromised patient presenting with chronic pulmonary symptoms is suspect and should be screened for pulmonary tuberculosis.

Other opportunistic infections worth mentioning in the differential diagnosis include cryptococcal pneumonia as part of disseminated cryptococcal disease, chronic *Histoplasma* pulmonary infection, and CMV pneumonia. Patients with these conditions tend to appear more systemically ill than this patient, with more symptoms and findings on physical examination to direct suspicion to one pathogen or another.

QUESTION 2 What additional information would you like to obtain that may be pertinent to the case?

Additional historical accounts of exposure to animals or presence of a similar condition in household members or contacts will be helpful. Chlamydial infection may be associated with exposure to animals in 50% of cases. Similar symptoms in other household members or contacts is a soft clue for viral as well as mycoplasmal infections.

Laboratory examinations include a CBC, blood chemistries, arterial blood gas, serology for *Mycoplasma* and respiratory viral pathogens (influenza, adenovirus, respiratory syncytial virus), sputum for gram stain, routine culture, stain for AFB (at least 3 samples), fungal stain and culture, and *Legionella* probe and DFA studies, and blood cultures. HIV testing should be offered and highly encouraged in this patient as should immunophenotyping studies. A serum cryptococcal antigen, RPR, and hepatitis screen test should also be done. The routine baseline tests such as the CBC, blood chemistries, and arterial blood gas may not discriminate one pathogen from another but will be important in making decisions regarding this patient's therapy (such as the need for in-hospital treatment and empiric medications). The serum cryptococcal antigen would screen for cryptococcal disease. Any patient suspected of having a sexually transmitted disease, such as HIV infection, warrants screening for other sexually transmitted diseases such as syphilis and hepatitis B. Chest x-ray and placement of a PPD with controls are also necessary.

Bronchoscopically obtained lavage sample, biopsy, or an ultrasonically induced sputum are the appropriate materials necessary to diagnose PCP. The latter is only used in centers with a laboratory that has adequate experience in handling such specimens and has a good record of positive yield from these samples. There are very few centers able to accomplish this. For most institutions bronchioalveolar lavage and transbronchial biopsy are the only samples that can be used to make the diagnosis.

Initial laboratory findings showed a WBC count of $4.5 \times 10^9/mm^3$, with neutrophils of 78%. The Hb, Hct, platelet count, and blood chemistries were all within normal limits; the arterial blood gas had a pH of 7.35, Po_2 68 mm Hg, Pco_2 22 mm Hg, HCO_3 19.5, and O_2 saturation 91%. Sputum gram stain showed numerous WBC, few epithelial cells, and no organisms; sputum AFB stain was negative as was the sputum fungal stain and DFA study for *Legionella*.

Chest x-ray showed diffuse interstitial infiltrates. PPD was negative with positive reaction to controls (*Candida,* mumps, and tetanus antigens).

HIV testing was offered to the patient, which he declined, stating that he had been tested 1 month earlier at a private clinic and recently learned that the result was positive. He denied any exposure to birds or other animals. None of his household or other contacts suffered from a similar condition.

QUESTION 3 How does this additional information help in the diagnosis of this patient's condition?

The recently acquired information about the result of his HIV testing confirms the original concern about his immune status and strengthens the case for an opportunistic pathogen causing his problem.

The WBC count does not help in distinguishing any of the pulmonary pathogens in consideration since most, if not all, of them have normal WBC count or mild leukocytosis with slight left shift. The chest radiograph revealing diffuse interstitial infiltrates does not differentiate one from the other either since all of the pathogens currently in the differential diagnosis can have a diffuse interstitial picture, some more commonly than others. For example, pneumonia secondary to *Legionella pneumophila* typically has a patchy, multifocal alveolar infiltrate; however, it is also known to cause a diffuse interstitial pattern. Therefore, one pathogen cannot be selected out on the basis of this test alone. The arterial blood gas showing significant hypoxemia with an alveolar-to-arterial oxygenation gradient of 54 mm Hg reflects impairment of the gas exchange mechanism of the lung, commonly seen in interstitial lung disease. Any pulmonary infection can give rise to some degree of hypoxemia and impairment in diffusion mechanism of the lung. However, *P. carinii* is the most notorious pathogen to cause this degree of hypoxemia and diffusion impairment despite relatively benign symptomatology and clinical findings in HIV-infected patients. These findings are highly supportive of the diagnosis of PCP but do not clearly distinguish this organism from the other pulmonary pathogens in the differential.

The negative PPD with positive controls is helpful. A negative PPD reaction alone may indicate that he either has not been exposed to *Mycobacterium tuberculosis* or that his cellular immunity has been sufficiently impaired so that he cannot mount a delayed hypersensitivity reaction (Type IV immunologic reaction) despite a previous exposure. A control panel including mumps, *Candida* and tetanus antigens are used in conjunction with PPD testing to test the state of his cellular immunity. Thus, in his case, the negative result indicates that he has not been exposed to the organism and makes tuberculosis a less likely cause of his problem. This information also helps in eliminating the other opportunistic pathogens in consideration, namely, cryptococcal pneumonia and CMV pneumonia. Both of the pathogens occur in far advanced HIV infection, when the cellular immunity is sufficiently impaired so as not to be able to mount any delayed hypersensitivity reaction.

Exposure to birds and animals, as was previously mentioned, makes chlamydial disease a more likely possibility, but absence of exposure is not helpful. A similar respiratory illness present in the other people the patient has had contact with may be helpful, but its absence does not help. An algorithm of the steps needed to arrive at a diagnosis for patients presenting with symptoms similar to the ones this young man has is presented in Fig. 8-11-1 on p. 507.

QUESTION 4 Is empiric therapy indicated at this point? If so, what agents would be indicated?

Empiric treatment directed against PCP is indicated at this point because of the patient's clinical picture. Although he had been ill for a considerable amount of time with good tolerance, he is fast approaching the critical point. His oxygenation is still adequate for his metabolic demands, but he is obviously achieving it with considerable effort as evidenced by his respiratory distress. Thus, more urgent intervention is warranted even before a definitive diagnosis.

There are currently a number of agents available for treatment of PCP. Trimethoprim-sulfamethoxazole is the most effective agent available for acute therapy of PCP with a cure rate of close to 90%. It is given at a dose of 15 to 20 mg/kg/day of the trimethoprim component in four divided doses. In general, therapy is started intravenously in the hospitalized patient and subsequently switched to an oral formulation of the drug at an equivalent dose when the patient improves and is able to tolerate oral medications. Acute therapy of PCP requires 21 days of treatment to lessen the chance of recrudescence. Toxicity or adverse events to monitor are bone marrow suppression reflected by a falling WBC and/or platelet count, allergic reactions such as development of a rash, and GI intolerance marked by nausea and vomiting. The latter two are usually amenable to symptomatic therapy with antihistamines and antiemetics. It should be kept in mind, however, that severe skin reactions such as Stevens-Johnson syndrome have been reported in HIV-infected patients treated with trimethoprim-sulfamethoxazole. If severe allergic reactions occur or symptoms are not alleviated by symptomatic treatment, alternative agents are indicated.

Pentamidine isethionate is the second-line drug available if the patient is intolerant of trimethoprim-sulfamethoxazole, with a cure rate of 75%. It is given at a dose of 4 mg/kg/day as a once-a-day intravenous infusion administered over 1 hour. Therapy should also be completed for 21 days. There are no oral formulations available for this medication. However, alternative oral drugs may be substituted once the patient has significantly improved and can finish therapy on an outpatient basis. The toxicities and adverse events to monitor for this drug include hypoglycemia, hypotension, neutropenia, thrombocytopenia, and renal dysfunction. It can also cause acute pancreatitis and prolongation of the Q-T interval. Thus, patients should have blood glucoses monitored every 6 to 12 hours and CBC and renal function tests (blood urea nitrogen and serum creatinine) daily or every other day. They should be watched closely for the development of signs and symptoms of acute pancreatitis such as abdominal pain, nausea, and vomiting.

Other alternative regimens of proven value include combination therapy using clindamycin and primaquine, dapsone and trimethoprim, and individual agent therapy using trimetrexate or atovaquone. The clindamycin-primaquine combination has been shown to be as effective as trimethoprim-sulfamethoxazole for mild to moderate disease. However, in severe PCP with significant amount of hypoxemia, the methemoglobinemia associated with use of primaquine may aggravate the already impaired tissue oxygenation. If this combination is used for moderate to severe disease with marginal oxygenation, methemoglobin concentrations should be measured frequently. Clindamycin is given at a dose of 450 to 900 mg q8h orally or intravenously, and primaquine is given at a dose of 15 to 30 mg base/day orally. It has no intravenous formulation. Use of this combination has a success rate near 80% in mild to moderate disease. Toxicities to watch for include skin rash and diarrhea.

Trimethoprim-dapsone is another combination that appears to equal trimethoprim-sulfamethoxazole in efficacy for mild to moderate disease, based on few comparative studies. It is used as an alternative in patients intolerant of sulfa drugs but not of trimethoprim. The dose of trimethoprim is the same, 20 mg/kg/day in 4 divided doses, and dapsone is given as 100 mg/day. Both can be given orally, but only trimethoprim can be given intravenously. Patients should be screened for G-6-PD deficiency as dapsone can cause hemolytic anemia in deficient patients. The most notable adverse effects are skin rash, nausea, and vomiting.

Trimetrexate is another drug that is available for use in moderate to severe PCP. However, experience with this agent is limited because of its significant toxicity. It should always be given with leucovorin to counteract its toxic effect on mammalian cells. It is given at a dose of 45 mg/m^2 as a single daily infusion with leucovorin at 20 mg/m^2 q6h orally or intravenously. The major toxicity to monitor is bone marrow suppression as reflected by neutropenia and thrombocytopenia. Thus, it is only recommended as a salvage therapy for patients who have failed treatment using the other available agents.

Atovaquone is yet another option for mild to moderate disease. It is available only in oral form and is given at a dose of 750 mg q8h. A high fat meal before intake of the drug is necessary to ensure adequate absorption. Inadequate blood levels are achieved in patients with diarrhea or malabsorption disorders.

Adjunctive therapy currently recommended for treatment of presumed or proven PCP is the administration of corticosteroids within 72 hours of starting an anti-PCP regimen for patients with moderate to severe disease. The criteria for instituting steroids are a Po_2 <70 mm Hg and/or an alveolar-arterial gradient of >35 mm Hg. The recommended doses and schedule are as follows:
1. Prednisone 40 mg PO q12h for days 1 to 5 of treatment
2. Prednisone 40 mg PO once a day for days 6 to 10 of treatment
3. Prednisone 20 mg PO once a day for days 11 to 21 of treatment, then discontinue the drug

Intravenous steroid formulations equivalent to the above doses may be used for patients who cannot tolerate oral medications. Steroids should be used with caution in patients with presumed PCP since other diseases in which steroid use can be detrimental to the patient (e.g., mycobacterial and fungal infections) often mimic the clinical picture of PCP, emphasizing the need for prompt diagnosis. If bronchoscopy or induced sputum are not readily available, options include delaying initiation of steroids until definitive diagnosis of PCP is reached within the 72-hour window of benefit, or starting steroids with the anti-PCP agent if definitive diagnosis can be established within 48 to 72 hours. Steroids should be discontinued promptly if the condition is proven not to be due to PCP.

For this patient, trimethoprim-sulfamethoxazole is the best agent to initiate therapy, being the most effective agent and having the highest chance to achieve cure. It also has a broad spectrum of antibacterial activity and provides coverage against some gram-positive (e.g., streptococci) and some gram-negative (e.g., *Haemophilus*, *Klebsiella*) organisms.

Based on his arterial blood gas result, he should receive adjunctive steroid therapy. It is less worrisome to start steroid treatment in this patient because the likelihood that his disease is due to a mycobacterial pathogen is low. Although a fungal pathogen has not been entirely ruled out, steroids can be started provided he will get a bronchoscopic examination for definitive diagnosis in a day or two.

Therapy directed to other community-acquired pneumonia pathogens, particularly *Mycoplasma*, is also indicated for this patient, as these cannot be sufficiently ruled out with the available information. Erythromycin 500 to 1000 mg every 6 hours orally or intravenously should be added until further diagnostic information is available.

The patient was started on trimethoprim-sulfamethoxazole at 5 mg/kg of trimethoprim every 6 hours intravenously, prednisone 40 mg every 12 hours orally, and erythromycin 500 mg every 6 hours intravenously. He had a bronchoalveolar lavage done on his second hospital day that was smear positive for *Pneumocystis carinii* and negative for other pathogens. Erythromycin was discontinued, and he completed 21 days of therapy without significant toxic reactions.

QUESTION 5 This patient responded well to this treatment. For patients who do not do as well, what are the indications for changing treatment regimens?

The two main indications for changing treatment regimen are lack of efficacy or intolerable toxicity. Lack of efficacy is generally reflected as failure to improve or deterioration of clinical status despite the therapy instituted. This can be measured by monitoring arterial blood gas and the patient's symptomatology. Response or improvement is expected by day 5 of treatment. If the patient has not shown improvement at this point, altering the treatment regimen is justified provided the etiology is proven to be PCP. If the therapy is empiric, definitive diagnostic tests, as well as search for other potential pathogens, should be actively pursued.

Toxicity or intolerable adverse effect of the medication (as discussed previously) are grounds for switching therapy.

QUESTION 6 What are the options available for prophylactic therapy now that he has completed acute treatment, and when should it be started?

Prophylaxis for PCP can be divided into two classifications—primary and secondary. Primary prophylaxis is directed to patients known to be HIV-infected who have not had a previous bout of PCP. It is indicated in patients with (a) CD4 counts $<200/mm^3$, (b) thrush, or (c) unexplained fever of 2 or more weeks' duration, regardless of the CD4 count. Prophylactic therapy after a bout of PCP is termed secondary prophylaxis. The regimens available for both types as well as the doses are identical. The three main drugs available are trimethoprim-sulfamethoxazole, dapsone, and aerosolized pentamidine. Of the three, trimethoprim-sulfamethoxazole provides the highest protection with a relapse rate of 3% to 5% per year for secondary prophylaxis and close to complete protection for primary prophylaxis. The recommended dose is 160 mg of trimethoprim (equivalent to 1 double-strength tablet) once daily. This regimen has the additional advantage of providing some protection against other opportunistic infections including infection due to *Streptococcus pneumoniae, Hemophilus influenzae, Salmonella,* and *Toxoplasma,* to name a few. The major limitation of this regimen is adverse reactions to the drug, mainly rash and bone marrow suppression, occurring in about 20% to 40% of patients. For unexplained reasons, HIV-infected patients appear to be more prone to these reactions than normal hosts. The rash can be severe enough to be intolerable and necessitate discontinuation of the drug. For bone marrow suppression as reflected by neutropenia, the dose can be modified to one double-strength tablet 3 times/week provided the neutrophil depression is not severe (absolute neutrophil count $=/<1000/mm^3$).

Another oral option is dapsone at a dose of 50 to 100 mg/day orally. It has a relapse rate estimated at 5% to 20% per year. Dapsone can be used in patients allergic to sulfa drugs. A screen for G-6-PD deficiency is advised before initiation of use to avoid precipitating hemolytic anemia in these patients. However, with prolonged use, even nondeficient patients can develop hemolysis. The most common adverse reactions are rash and nausea, occurring in up to 20% to 40% of users.

The third option is aerosolized pentamidine. It has a relapse rate of 15% to 25% per year and a rate of breakthrough PCP on primary prophylaxis of 11%. Its main advantages are little systemic toxicity and ease of administration because it is only given once a month. Cough is the predominant adverse event. Its disadvantages include (1) high cost as a result of the additional expense of the mode of delivery, (2) lack of additional protection against other pathogens, and (3) predisposition to atypical (extrapulmonary) presentations of PCP due to lack of systemic effect. In addition, the noncompliant patient who misses one treatment session will be left unprotected for 2 months until the next session. The patient should be screened for pulmonary tuberculosis before initiation of treatment since bouts of coughing may promote production of aerosolized particles. The treatment is delivered using a Respigard II machine at a dose of 300 mg every month.

Options other than these three have been used by practitioners, but experience has mostly been anecdotal.

This patient should be started on trimethoprim-sulfamethoxazole at a dose of one double-strength tablet daily because he tolerated the drug well during the acute therapy and it confers the best protection among the choices. He should also

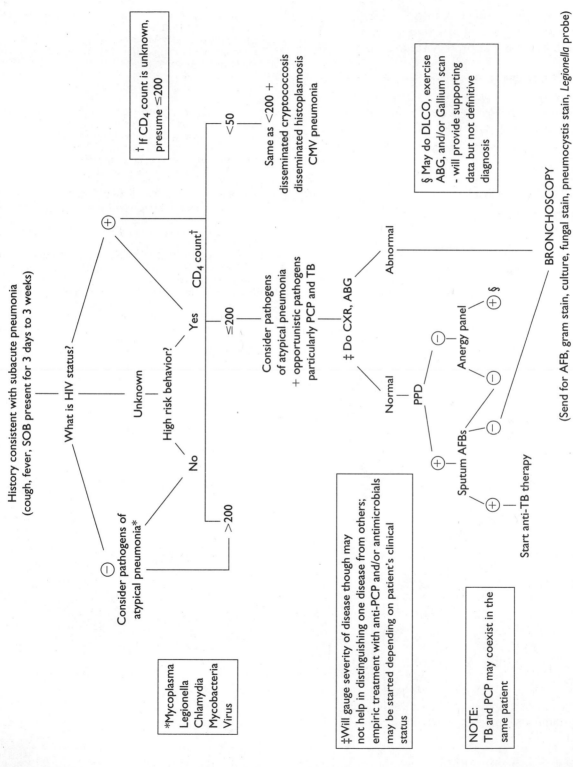

8-11-1   Approach to the HIV-infected patient with subacute respiratory symptoms.

be referred for routine HIV infection care, so that other issues regarding his therapy can be addressed, including antiretroviral treatment.

CASE FOLLOW-UP The patient was discharged on oral trimethoprim-sulfamethoxazole one double-strength tablet daily. He was followed up in a clinic that handles care for HIV-infected patients.

• •

BIBLIOGRAPHY

Barlett JG: The Johns Hopkins hospital guide to medical care of patients with HIV infection, ed 4, Baltimore, 1994, Williams & Wilkins.

Black JR, Feinberg, J, Murphy RL, et al: Clindamycin and primaquine as primary treatment for mild and moderately severe *Pneumocystis carinii* pneumonia in patients with AIDS, *Eur J Clin Microbiol Infect Dis* 10:204-207, 1991.

Gorbach SL, Bartlett JG, Blacklow NR, eds: *Infectious disease*, Philadelphia, 1992, WB Saunders.

Hopewell PC: *Pneumocystis carinii* pneumonia. Current concepts. In Sande MA, Volberding PA, eds: *The medical management of AIDS*, ed 3, Philadelphia, 1992, WB Saunders.

Hughes W, Leoung G, Kramer F, et al: Comparison of atovaquone (566C80) with trimethoprim-sulfamethoxazole to treat *Pneumocystis carinii* pneumonia in patients with AIDS. *N Engl J Med* 328:1521-1527, 1993.

Leoung GS, Mills J, Hopewell PC, et al: Dapsone-trimethoprim for *Pneumocystis carinii* pneumonia in the acquired immunodeficiency syndrome, *Ann Intern Med* 105:45-48, 1986.

Mandell GL, Douglas RG, Bennett JE, eds: *Principles and practices of infectious diseases*, ed 3, New York, 1990, Churchill Livingston.

Masur H, Meier P, McCutchan JA, et al: Consensus statement on the use of corticosteroids as adjunctive therapy for *Pneumocystis carinii* pneumonia in the acquired immunodeficiency syndrome. The National Institute of Health-University of California Expert Panel for Corticosteroids as Adjunctive Therapy for Pneumocystis Pneumonia, *N Engl J Med* 323:1500-1504, 1990.

Medina I, Mills J, Leoung G, et al: Oral therapy for *Pneumocystis carinii* pneumonia in the acquired immunodeficiency syndrome. A controlled trial of trimethoprim-sulfamethoxazole versus trimethoprim-dapsone, *N Engl J Med* 323: 776-782, 1990.

Sattler FR, Cowan R, Nielson DM, Ruskin J: Trimethoprim-sulfamethoxazole compared with pentamidine for treatment of *Pneumocystis carinii* pneumonia in the acquired immunodeficiency syndrome: a prospective noncrossover study, *Ann Intern Med* 109:280-287, 1988.

Sattler FR, Frame P, Davis R, et al: Trimetrexate with leucovorin versus trimethoprim-sulfamethoxazole for moderate to severe episodes of *Pneumocystis carinii* pneumonia in patients with AIDS: a prospective, controlled, multi-center investigation of the AIDS clinical trials group protocol 029/031, *J Infect Dis* 170:165-172, 1994.

Toma E, Fournier S, Poisson M, et al: Clindamycin with primaquine for *Pneumocystis carinii* pneumonia, *Lancet* i:1046-1048, 1989.

CASE

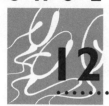

12 Conrad Fischer
Kent Sepkowitz

A 27-year-old man came to his internist in the spring of this year with fatigue and epistaxis. A complete blood count reveals pancytopenia, and a bone marrow biopsy and aspiration the following week reveals abnormalities consistent with acute myelogenous leukemia with 74% blasts. The patient is admitted to the hospital for induction chemotherapy with Idarubicin and ara-C. Seven days after chemotherapy the patient feels somewhat weak but generally well, and the white blood cell count drops to 1800/ml with an absolute neutrophil count (ANC) of 1400/ml. Three days later the ANC has dropped to 700/ml, and the following day it is 300/ml. The patient is afebrile and still feels generally well.

QUESTION I What is the approach to the patient at this time and what are the mandatory diagnostic tests and treatments?

The most common complication of hematologic malignancies is infection. Acute myelogenous leukemia predisposes patients to a large number of infections, primarily through either a decreased total number of neutrophils or a worsening of their function. The total number of white blood cells is not as important as determining the total number of neutrophils. The ANC also does not include immature cells such as blasts because they are presumed to be either nonfunctional or of profoundly limited function. Immature cells do not have the secondary granules necessary for these white cells to perform their functions of phagocytosis and oxidative killing. Therefore in discussing patients with leukopenia from either hematologic malignancy or from cytotoxic che-

motherapy, it is more appropriate to use the ANC to predict risk of infection from bacteria and the majority of fungal organisms. The risk of infection is inversely proportional to the ANC. There is no significant risk of infection when the ANC is above 1000/ml. There is clear risk when the count is below 500/ml, and an even greater risk when the count drops to 100/ml or less.

The majority of chemotherapeutic regimens for cancer are associated with suppression of bone marrow activity. Most of these agents kill rapidly dividing cells such as cancer cells, the basis of their therapeutic effect. Unfortunately, they also kill other rapidly dividing cells such as those in the bone marrow, the lining of the gastrointestinal system, and the hair follicles. The neutrophil counts generally start to drop 2 to 14 days after the start of the chemotherapy.

This patient began to be at risk of infection when his ANC dropped below 1000/ml. At an ANC of 300/ml there is a clear risk of infection, particularly from bacterial organisms. However, because the patient is generally comfortable and is afebrile, there is no indication for further diagnostic testing at this time, and no specific treatment is required in the absence of another identifiable sign or symptom. Although the patient is neutropenic, the American Society of Hematology recommends that cytokines such as G-CSF and GM-CSF **not** be given to patients with acute myelogenous leukemia. Cytokines should not be used because of the possibility that they may stimulate the production of blasts and other neoplastic cells.

There is no clear evidence that the prophylaxis of bacterial infection is effective in reducing mortality and long-term morbidity in an afebrile neutropenic patient. Hence, antibacterials such as oral quinolones or trimethoprim-sulfamethoxazole are not recommended because of a questionable efficacy and the possibility that they may predispose to increased bacterial resistance to antibiotics.

QUESTION 2 Two days later (12 days total after the start of chemotherapy), the patient's total WBC count is 200, and the ANC is 0.0. He is still without specific complaint, is afebrile, and has a normal physical examination. How would this affect your management?

Although the risk of infection increases as the neutrophil count drops, this patient is still afebrile and without any symptoms or physical examination signs of infection. Even though the ANC is 0.0/ml, this is not an indication for any specific diagnostic test or new treatment in the absence of a fever. Fever is generally defined as a single oral temperature of >100.9°F or several temperatures of >100.4°F over the course of a day.

QUESTION 3 The following day the patient's temperature rises to 102.6°F orally. There are no associated symptoms. What is the most important initial action to take in this febrile, neutropenic patient?

The most urgent action in a febrile neutropenic patient is the institution of broad-spectrum intravenous antibiotics. After appropriate cultures are obtained, the neutropenic patient who becomes febrile has a >60% chance of having an identifiable infection. Of patients with an ANC <100/ml, 20% are bacteremic. It is important to perform a thorough physical examination and laboratory evaluation, including two sets of blood cultures, before the start of antibiotics to more appropriately choose the right antibiotics. Physical examination should be particularly directed to the most common clinically evident sites of infection in neutropenic patients, which are the oral cavity, lung, skin, and perineum.

These evaluations must be expeditious and in

no way delay the delivery of antibiotics. Although an appropriate laboratory evaluation would include at least two sets of blood cultures for bacteria and fungi, urine culture, and possibly sputum and stool culture, there is absolutely no necessity to delay the start of antibiotics until the results of these studies are known. Other cultures may be appropriate depending upon the characteristics of an individual patient. If a central venous catheter is present, blood cultures should be drawn simultaneously through the catheter, as well as peripherally. Routine examination of cerebrospinal fluid is not indicated in the absence of specific signs or symptoms, although frank meningismus is rare. Chest x-ray must be done even in the absence of symptoms, since signs may be subtle (see Fig. 8-12-1).

QUESTION 4 What are the most likely organisms to cause bacterial infection in febrile neutropenic patients?

The spectrum of bacterial organisms in febrile neutropenic patients varies somewhat among different patient care settings. The most certain choice of empiric antibiotics is ultimately based on the most common organisms found in a given institution. In many institutions the most common organisms have been aerobic gram-negative bacilli. The majority of these have comprised *Escherichia coli, Klebsiella pneumoniae,* and *Pseudomonas aeruginosa.* Other less common gram-negative organisms have been *Enterobacter* spp. and *Proteus* spp. Gram-positive organisms have been *Staphylococcus aureus,* coagulase-negative staphylococci (*S. epidermidis* and others), and alpha-hemolytic streptococci, in particular the viridans group. Anaerobes are an uncommon cause of infection in this group of patients and account for <5% of infections.

The relative frequency of these organisms has changed somewhat over the past several decades. Through the 1960s and the early part of the 1970s Gram-negative organisms were more common. From the end of the 1970s through the 1980s Gram-positive organisms became more common as the use of central venous catheters became more routine. There is evidence that this trend may again be reversing in favor of Gram-negative organisms, although the reasons for these changes remain obscure.

QUESTION 5 What antibiotics would comprise an appropriate empiric choice in this setting?

An extremely broad range of antibiotics have been studied in empiric use in febrile neutropenic patients. These drugs have been used in combination and as monotherapy. We favor combination therapy over monotherapy for broader spectrum and less emergence of resistance. In particular, induction of beta-lactamases in a number of organisms such as *Enterobacter* or *Serratia* has been seen with monotherapy. An acceptable empiric regimen is one that combines an aminoglycoside (gentamicin/tobramycin/amikacin) with a third-generation cephalosporin (ceftazidime, cefoperazone) or an antipseudomonal penicillin (piperacillin, ticarcillin, azlocillin, or mezlocillin). Aminoglycosides should not be used alone. Double beta-lactam coverage alone such as ticarcillin/ceftazidime, piperacillin/cefoperazone is unlikely to offer an advantage over monotherapy and may result in emergence of enterococcal infection. Newer beta-lactam agents such as the carbapenems (imipenem) and monobactams (aztreonam) are also effective but should be used in combination with an aminoglycoside. These agents may be a useful alternative for patients allergic to penicillin.

Given the increasing number of gram-positive cocci causing infection in these patients, there has been prolonged debate on the empiric use of vancomycin. Many coagulase-negative staphylococci are sensitive only to vancomycin; however, coagulase-negative staphylococci tend to be of low virulence, suggesting that a delay of 3 to 4 days may not affect morbidity and mortality rates. In studies in which the addition of vancomycin on a selective basis to patients who grew these organisms while on the original antipseudomonal beta-lactam/aminoglycoside combination, the survival overall was not significantly different. Hence most experts feel that vancomycin does not need to be included with the original empiric regimen. In addition, there is profound concern that frequent and indiscriminate use of vancomycin will increase even more the growing incidence of resistance among gram-positive organisms, in particular the enterococci. Vancomycin can be selectively added later in the hospital course to those patients who grow a gram-positive organism or to those who remain persistently febrile despite 3 to 4 days of an appropriate beta-lactam/aminoglycoside combination. Greater gram-positive coverage can be achieved without the use of vancomycin by using the ticarcillin-clavulanic acid agent in combination with an aminoglycoside (see Fig. 8-12-1).

QUESTION 6 This patient was placed on ticarcillin-clavulanic acid in combination with gentamicin. The following day, the blood cultures drawn before the start of antibiotics grew gram-negative bacilli that were identified the following day as Pseudomonas aeruginosa. The patient's ANC remains 0.0/ml and his temperature begins to drop. The antibiotics are now changed to ceftazidime and tobramycin, which are narrower in spectrum but more specifically antipseudomonal. The patient defervesces over the next day and remains afebrile for the next several days.

Seven days after the start of antibiotics the patient develops a new fever to 103.8°F.

The patient has now been neutropenic for a total of 20 days.

What action would you take at this time, and what infectious organisms is the patient at risk for after this long a period of neutropenia?

The evaluation of the patient with a new fever while already on broad-spectrum antibacterial coverage would be similar to the initial evaluation when the patient first became febrile. An expeditious and thorough physical examination, blood cultures, and cultures of other sites as directed by the patient's symptoms and physical examination would be appropriate. With a more prolonged

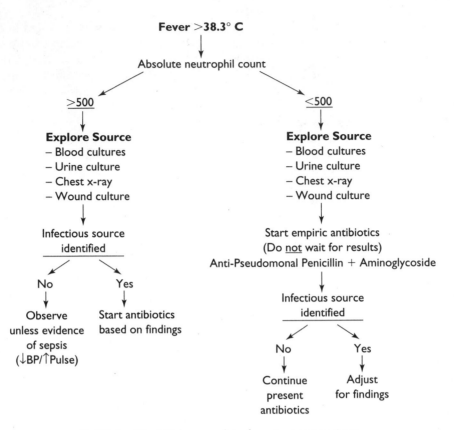

Fever >38.3° C
↓
Absolute neutrophil count

≥500 ← → **≤500**

↓

Explore Source
– Blood cultures
– Urine culture
– Chest x-ray
– Wound culture

↓

Infectious source
identified

No ← → Yes

↓   ↓

Observe   Start antibiotics
unless evidence   based on findings
of sepsis
(↓BP/↑Pulse)

↓

Explore Source
– Blood cultures
– Urine culture
– Chest x-ray
– Wound culture

↓

Start empiric antibiotics
(Do <u>not</u> wait for results)
Anti-Pseudomonal Penicillin + Aminoglycoside

↓

Infectious source
identified

No ← → Yes

↓   ↓

Continue   Adjust
present   for findings
antibiotics

8-12-1 The initial approach to fever in cancer patients.

period of neutropenia, while on appropriate antibacterials, the patient is at risk of a fungal infection. *Candida* species and aspergillus are the most common fungi causing infection in this setting. The most common *Candida* species are *C. albicans, C. tropicalis, C. parapsilosis,* and *C. glabrata.* (*Candida glabrata* is also known as *Torulopsis glabrata.*) The most common clinically encountered *Aspergillus* species are *A. fumigatus, flavus,* and *niger.* Amphotericin B should be given to any neutropenic patient who remains febrile after 7 days of appropriate antibacterial coverage or who develops a new fever after an initial response. The amphotericin should be given intravenously at a dose of 1 mg/kg of weight immediately after a test dose is tolerated. Lower doses of 0.5 to 0.7 mg/kg and the incremental increase in dosing over several days is not appropriate in this setting.

Fungemia in neutropenic cancer patients has been associated with a 50% to 90% mortality in the past, depending on the species identified, and even under optimal conditions still results in a 50% to 60% mortality. Amphotericin B must not be withheld while waiting for a microbiologically confirmed diagnosis since autopsy studies show that only approximately 50% of disseminated fungal infections are diagnosed antemortem despite appropriate premortem cultures. Azole antifungal agents such as fluconazole should not be used until controlled studies comparing them to Amphotericin B are completed.

QUESTION 7 The patient was started on amphotericin at a dose of 1 mg/kg after he tolerated the 1-mg test dose. The ceftazidime and tobramycin were continued, and levels of the tobramycin were checked for appropriateness. The patient continued to have a temperature of 101.8°F. A previous chest radiograph had been normal but was repeated because of persistence of the fever. The new x-ray revealed a left upper lobe infiltrate. The same antibiotics were continued, and 2 days later the patient remained febrile to 102.2°F. All blood, urine, and sputum cultures were unrevealing. A cough developed, and a new chest x-ray showed slight enlargement of the left upper lobe lesion with the possibility of slight cavitation developing. What diagnostic tests are most appropriate in this setting?

Although a CT scan of the chest may help better define the extent of the lesion, as well as the possibility of cavitation, this will not help obtain a specific microbiologic diagnosis and will not alter therapy. Bronchoscopy with lavage is most appropriate in this setting. Biopsy is most often not advisable because of the common presence of thrombocytopenia and the chance of bleeding even with platelet transfusion. Open lung biopsy will be more sensitive in detection of the underlying cause, but because of thrombocytopenia may be difficult.

CASE FOLLOW-UP   The patient has septate hyphae seen on lavage fluid that later grows a mold identified as *Aspergillus fumigatus*. The patient remains febrile, with an ANC of 0.0/ml and is now becoming dyspneic with worsening of the infiltrate on chest x-ray. The dose of amphotericin was increased to 1.25 mg/kg. Over the course of the next several days the patient's neutrophil count rose above 1000/ml, and the fever and dyspnea slowly resolved. Bacterial antibiotics were continued for 2 days after resolution of fever and neutropenia. Amphotericin was continued for 1 week after cessation of fever and neutropenia, and the chest x-ray started to improve as the neutropenia resolved. The addition of rifampin to acute treatment was considered as was the use of itraconozole for maintenance therapy.

· ·

BIBLIOGRAPHY

Armstrong D: Treatment of opportunistic fungal infections, *Clin Infect Dis* 16:1-9, 1993.

Gerson SL, Talbot GH, Hurwitz S, et al: Discriminant scorecard for diagnosis of invasive pulmonary aspergillosis in patients with acute leukemia, *Am J Med* 79:57-64, 1986.

Gibson J, Johnson L, Snowdon L, et al: Trends in bacterial infections in febrile neutropenic patients: 1986-1992, *Aust NZ J Med* 24:374-377, 1994.

Horn R, Wong B, Kiehn TE, Armstrong D: Fungemia in a cancer hospital: changing frequency, earlier onset, and results of therapy, *Rev Infec Dis* 7:646-655, 1985.

Hughes WT, Armstrong D, Bodey GP, et al: Guidelines for the use of antimicrobial agents in neutropenic patients with unexplained fever, *J Infect Dis* 161:381-396, 1990.

Pizzo PA: Management of fever in patients with cancer and treatment-induced neutropenia, *N Engl J Med* 328:1323-1332, 1993.

Pizzo PA, Robichaud KJ, Gill FA, Witebsky FG: Empiric antibiotic and antifungal therapy for cancer patients with prolonged fever and granulocytopenia, *Am J Med* 72:101-111, 1982.

Ramphal R, Bolger M, Oblon DJ, et al: Vancomycin is not an essential component of the initial empiric treatment regimen for febrile neutropenic patients receiving ceftazidime: a randomized prospective study, *Antimicrob Agents Chemo* 36:1062-1067, 1992.

Rubin M, Hathorn JW, Marshall D, et al: Gram positive infection and the use of vancomycin in 550 episodes of fever and neutropenia, *Ann Intern Med* 108:30-35, 1988.

Saral R: Candida and aspergillus infections in immunocompromised patients: an overview, *Rev Infect Dis* 13:487-92, 1991.

Whimbey E, Kiehn TE, Brannon P, et al: Bacteremia and fungemia in patients with neoplastic disease, *Am J Med* 82:723-730, 1987.

Yu VL, Muder RR, Poorsattar A: Significance of isolation of aspergillus from the respiratory tract in diagnosis of invasive pulmonary aspergillosis, *Am J Med* 81:249-254, 1986.

C A S E

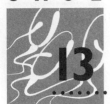

13

Conrad Fischer
Kent Sepkowitz

A 29-year-old female dancer with no significant medical history comes to your office with several days of urinary frequency, burning, and urgency. In addition, she notes a cloudy discoloration of her urine. She uses no medications, has no allergies, and has not seen a physician for several years.

QUESTION 1 What is your initial approach to this patient, and how would you use the history and physical examination to help you localize the infection?

Urinary tract infection (UTI) is one of the most common reasons for a visit to a physician's office, accounting for up to 6 million visits a year in the United States. UTI is particularly common in females, presumably because the female urethra is shorter than that of men, resulting in a higher risk of fecal flora contaminating the bladder. The history is important in trying to identify an underlying predisposition for an infection and in trying to identify any potentially correctable cause. The patient should be asked about a history of diabetes, urinary tract stones, congenital abnormalities, strictures, previous instrumentation and catheterization, or a history of previous infections. A sexual history is important as well because sexual intercourse predisposes to cystitis in women. In addition, several other sexually transmitted diseases such as herpes simplex, Chlamydia, and Trichomonas can also cause similar symptoms.

The physical examination is central in helping to localize the site of the infection (see Fig. 8-13-1 on p. 517). Complaints of dysuria such as pain, burning, frequency, and urgency can occur with an infection at any level of the urinary system: urethra, bladder, or kidney. Temperatures above 102.2°F, nausea, vomiting, chills, and other systemic symptoms are more suggestive of pyelonephritis, although this is not specific. Pyelonephritis characteristically gives back pain and tenderness to palpation at the costovertebral angle. Cystitis often results in suprapubic pain and tenderness. Urethritis can give a urethral discharge that can be clear, white, or yellow. The clinical distinction between cystitis and urethritis is seldom possible on the basis of symptoms and physical examination alone. A patient is considered to have urethritis if there are isolated symptoms of dysuria present in the absence of systemic symptoms with a negative urine culture.

QUESTION 2 On physical examination this patient had a temperature of (100.4°F) and suprapubic tenderness. There was no back or costovertebral angle tenderness, and there was no discharge noted from the urethra. On the basis of this presentation what laboratory studies would you use to help you confirm the diagnosis?

A urinalysis is the best initial test for any of the causes of dysuria described above. The leukocyte esterase test on a urine dipstick is a sensitive and rapid method of confirming the presence of white blood cells in the urine. The dipstick also contains strips for the detection of red blood cells, protein, glucose, nitrates, and pH. UTI is rare in the absence of white blood cells. Microscopic examination of the urine is also essential. A single white cell visible on a high power field is suggestive of infection. Gram staining of urine can also be helpful. A single bacterium visible on an unspun urine specimen viewed on a high power field correlates to growth on a culture of >100,000 bacteria/milliliter (ml) of urine. A urine culture growing >100,000 bacteria/ml of an organism from voided urine is strongly associated with the diagnosis of UTI. On a catheterized specimen, >100 bacteria per ml is considered positive, and any growth from a percutaneous aspiration of the bladder (suprapubic tap) is considered abnormal.

Imaging studies such as an ultrasound, intravenous pyelogram, CT scan, or retrograde urography are not a part of the routine evaluation of a patient presenting with symptoms of UTI. These studies are reserved for patients who fail initial treatment or to evaluate the possibility of a stone, stricture, tumor, or other anatomic abnormality that may have led to the infection.

QUESTION 3 This patient had a urinalysis that was strongly positive for white blood cells and mildly positive for red blood cells and protein. A urine culture was deferred because the patient's income was not sufficient for health insurance, and she wished to defer the cost of a urine culture. Given the clear history of several days of dysuria with low-grade fever, suprapubic tenderness, the absence of costovertebral angle tenderness, or urethral discharge, and the positive urine dipstick for WBCs, RBCs, and protein, the patient was diagnosed as having cystitis. What would be your approach to the treatment of such a patient? (See Fig. 8-13-1.)

The optimal treatment of any infection is determined by identifying the specific pathogen. By far the most common organism is *E. coli*, which accounts for at least 80% of cases. Other common causes are gram-negative rods in the family Enterobacteriaceae, such as *Proteus, Klebsiella*, and *Enterobacter* spp. *Pseudomonas* is an occasional cause, most often in diabetics. *Staphylococcus saprophyticus* may be anticipated in young, sexually active females. Patients on long-term antibiotics or with indwelling catheters are prone to fungal superinfection, particularly with Candida and Torulopsis.

In an uncomplicated lower UTI single-dose therapy is effective in 80% to 90% of cases. This is particularly useful in patients where the cost of medications is an important factor. Two double-strength trimethoprim/sulfamethoxazole tablets, Norfloxacin 800 mg, or tetracycline 2 g have often been effective as a single dose. Amoxacillin 3 g had been widely used previously but is not predictably effective because of increasing resistance to this agent among the Enterobacteriaceae. Although single-dose therapy has a higher relapse rate than treatment for 3 days, it has the advantage of greater compliance and less cost.

When cost and compliance are not an issue, optimal therapy for an uncomplicated lower UTI is for 3 days. Seven to ten days of treatment are not routinely required except in patients with underlying conditions such as diabetes, or pregnancy, or in the elderly. Other antimicrobial agents that are equally efficacious in this setting include ciprofloxacin, norfloxacin, and amoxacillin/clavulanic acid.

QUESTION 4 This patient is treated with two double-strength trimethoprim/sulfamethoxazole tablets. She leaves the following morning for a series of dance performances along the eastern coast of the United States and does not return to her home for 6 weeks. The day following her return she calls your office for an urgent appointment because she has been having fever and dysuria for the past several days as well as nausea and vomiting. In your office you find a very ill-appearing woman with a temperature of 102.9°F with marked costovertebral angle tenderness. What is your assessment of this patient's current diagnosis, and what would you do to evaluate and treat her at this point?

Given the persistence of her dysuria combined with new signs and symptoms of systemic disease such as high fever, vomiting, and costovertebral angle tenderness, this patient now seems to have developed pyelonephritis. Although single-dose treatments are often highly effective in an uncomplicated lower UTI, they should generally be given in a setting where good follow-up care is possible.

In this patient who was seen only once and then leaves to travel for a prolonged period of time without any form of medical care readily available, complications such as pyelopnephritis may develop unobserved. She represents one of the 10% to 15% of patients who will not be adequately treated by single-dose therapy.

The most prudent management of this case at this time is to admit the patient to the hospital and obtain a urinalysis, urine culture, and blood cultures. In addition, she will need intravenous antibiotics because of both the severity of symptoms and the nausea and vomiting, making her unable to tolerate oral medications.

QUESTION 5 What would be your choice for intravenous antibiotics at this time, and on what do you base the choice?

Initially, the choice of antibiotics is largely empiric because a urine culture will take at least 24 hours to yield any growth and an additional 24 hours to speciate the organism and obtain sensitivities. The choice can be guided somewhat by a knowledge of the most common bacteriology described above as well as a gram stain of the urine. Although it will not give the specific species, a gram stain will allow you to differentiate the gram-negative bacilli such as *E. coli* and *Klebsiella* from gram-positive cocci such as enterococcus and *S. saprophyticus*.

A urinalysis reveals 100 WBCs per HPF, 2+ protein, and 2+ blood. Gram stain of this patient's urine reveals gram-negative rods.

Many agents are active against gram-negative bacilli: third-generation cephalosporins (e.g., ceftazidime, cefotaxime, or ceftriaxone), ciprofloxacin, extended spectrum penicillins (e.g., ticarcillin, piperacillin, or mezlocillin), ticarcillin/clavulanate, or aztreonam would all likely be effective. Second-generation cephalosporins would also likely be adequate.

Trimethoprim/sulfamethoxazole intravenously is often an appropriate choice as well. However, it would be wiser to avoid trimethoprim/sulfamethoxazole in this patient with the history of breakthrough after use of the oral form and the possibility that the organism causing this woman's pyelonephritis is resistent to this agent.

The addition of an aminoglycoside in combination with any of the agents listed above is appropriate in those cases where a concomitant bacteremia, a very severe infection, or possibly a resistant organism is suspected.

QUESTION 6 The patient was placed on ceftazidime 1 g every 8 hours. The urine culture grew >100,000 bacteria/ml of *E. coli*, which was sensitive to ceftazidime and trimethoprim/sulfamethoxazole (TMP/SMZ). The blood cultures did not grow. The antibiotics were changed to TMP/SMZ.

Five days after the start of antibiotics the patient remains persistently febrile to 103.1°F with no change in her symptoms of flank and abdominal pain. What is a possible explanation of the persistence of this patient's fever and symptoms despite 5 days of adequate antibiotic coverage, and what tests would you choose to evaluate it?

Symptoms of pyelonephritis that have been appropriately treated should begin to resolve several days after the start of appropiate antibiotics. Ceftazidime, as a third-generation cephalosporin, represents an excellent choice for pyelonephritis, which is predominantly caused by gram-negative bacilli. In this case the organism is known to be *E. coli*. Another possibility could be resistance to the antibiotic on the part of the organism; however in this case we have sensitivity testing that shows that the organism is sensitive. Another possibility is the development of a perinephric abscess. Renal abscesses predominantly develop as a result of a previous pyelonephritis, most often in association with a kidney stone. The organisms that cause them are predominantly the same gram-negative bacilli that cause pyelonephritis. An exception to this are cortical medullary abcesses that are spread hematogenously and are caused by *S. aureus*. Renal abscesses present nonspecifically as persistence of fever, flank, and abdominal pain in a patient with pyelonephritis who has been placed on appropriate antibiotics.

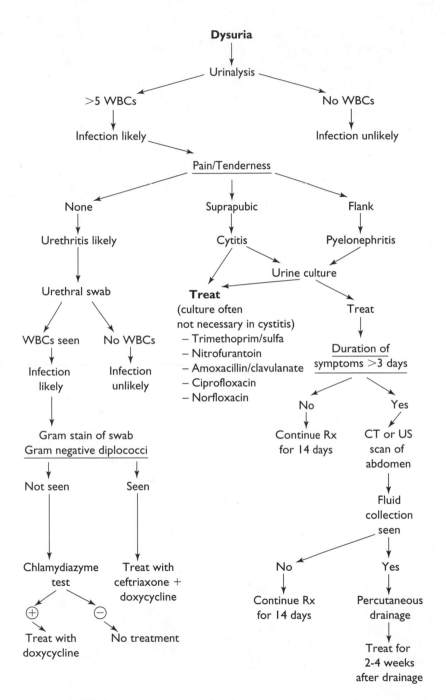

8-13-1   The approach to dysuria and urinary tract infections.

Although gallium and indium scans will show an abnormality in the region of the abscess, the most appropriate tests are ultrasound and CT scan. The ultrasound is often adequate to determine the presence of the abscess in the perinephric space. Infected material usually breaks through into the region of the perinephric fat and remains contained within Gerota's fascia. The CT scan may offer slightly better resolution in defining the extent of the abscess.

QUESTION 7 This patient initially has an abdominal ultrasound that reveals a collection of fluid around her right kidney. A CT scan done the following day further defines the collection as being contiguous to her kidney, penetrating the perinephric fat but contained within Gerota's fascia. What would you do differently in the management of this case given this new finding?

Intravenous antibiotics alone are inadequate in the treatment of perinephric abscess. In the past open incision and drainage with debridement and placement of drains was required. However, the percutaneous placement of drainage catheters by CT or ultrasound guidance in combination with antibiotics has proven adequate in an increasing number of cases.

CASE FOLLOW-UP This patient had percutaneous placement of a drainage catheter by CT guidance. A small volume of purulent material was recovered that subsequently grew an identical strain of *E. coli* to that obtained on the original urine culture. The drain was left in place for 7 days and was removed when the amount of drainage had become negligible, and the patient had become afebrile. Antibiotics were continued for 2 weeks after the removal of the catheter. The patient was discharged and seen in follow-up every several months for the next year with no recurrence of symptoms.

• •

BIBLIOGRAPHY

Gerzof SG, Gale ME: Computed tomography and ultrasonography for diagnosis and treatment of renal and retroperitoneal abscess, *Urol Clin North Am* 9:185, 1982.

Hooton TM, Stamm WE: Management of acute uncomplicated urinary tract infection in adults, *Med Clin North Am* 75:339, 1991.

Johnson JR, Stamm WE: Urinary tract infections in women: diagnosis and treatment, *Ann Intern Med* 111:906, 1989.

Patterson JE, Andriole VT: Renal and perinephric abscesses, *Infect Dis Clin North Am* 1:907, 1987.

Piccirillo M, Rigsby C, Rosenfeld AT: Contemporary imaging of renal inflammatory disease, *Infect Dis Clin North Am* 1:927, 1987.

Sheinfeld J, Eturk E, Spataro RD, et al: Perinephric abscess: current concepts, *J Urol* 137:191, 1987.

NEPHROLOGY

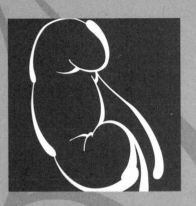

ROGER A. RODBY

SECTION EDITOR

CASE

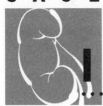

Roger A. Rodby
....

A 61-year-old male construction worker was taken to the emergency room after a witnessed seizure in a restaurant. His wife revealed that he had complained about fatigue, malaise, a mild headache, and a poor appetite over the last week. He had no significant past medical history except for an 80 pack-year history of cigarette smoking. There was no history of seizures, alcohol abuse, head trauma, or neurologic disorders.

The physical examination demonstrated a BP of 120/80 mm Hg, RR 24/min, and a temperature of 98.6°F. He was arousable but inattentive. The lungs were clear, the cardiac examination was normal, and there was no peripheral edema. The neurologic examination was nonfocal. Laboratory values revealed the following: sodium 105 mEq/L, potassium 4.0 mEq/L, chloride 70 mEq/L, bicarbonate 23 mEq/L, BUN 6 mg/dl, creatinine 0.6 mg/dl, uric acid 1.5 mg/dl (nl 3.5 to 5.0), and glucose 90 mg/dl.

QUESTION I The patient is markedly hyponatremic. What are the mechanisms by which salt and water homeostasis is maintained?

True hyponatremia (that associated with plasma hypoosmolality) is usually a result of water retention (or water and sodium retention: water > sodium) and therefore may be considered dilutional. Sodium loss by itself is rarely a cause of hyponatremia since the sodium concentration of the fluid that is lost would have to be higher than that of the serum. This is rarely the case, and therefore when hyponatremia is associated with sodium loss, it is usually also accompanied by water retention.

The key to understanding the development of hyponatremia depends on a knowledge of the normal mechanisms that maintain plasma osmolality and intravascular volume. Alterations in plasma osmolality are sensed by osmoreceptors located in the hypothalamus. These receptors are directly involved in water balance by controlling (1) water intake through the regulation of thirst and (2) water excretion through the regulation of urine osmolality by antidiuretic hormone (ADH). In response to a water load there is a decrease in plasma sodium and plasma osmolality. This results in the suppression of ADH release, thereby decreasing water reabsorption in the collecting duct. This allows excretion of the water load by creating a dilute urine. The kidney's handling of sodium is essentially unaffected by this mechanism. Therefore, hyponatremia is created by the kidney's handling of water, not by its handling of sodium, and hyponatremia may be seen with states of excess, normal, and depleted total body sodium. The key to understanding hyponatremia is to understand why sufficient amounts of water are not being excreted by the kidney. As will be discussed, the mechanisms leading to water retention often reflect volume-mediated ADH release, and the physical examination is critical in determining a patient's volume status. As is demonstrated in Fig. 9-1-1 on p. 526 the excretion of a water load depends upon (1) an adequate glomerular filtration rate (GFR), (2) normal proximal tubule handling of filtrate, (3) subsequent distal delivery of filtrate (steps 1 to 3 are critical since fluid must be delivered to the diluting segment), (4) dilution of filtrate through the resorption of sodium without water, and finally, (5) suppression of ADH release to prevent water reabsorption as a dilute filtrate passes through the collecting duct.

The inability to suppress volume-mediated ADH release is the most common cause of water retention and, therefore, hyponatremia. ADH secretion is controlled by osmoreceptors located in the hypothalamus and baroreceptors located in the vascular tree. These later receptors respond to any decrease in circulating volume by sending impulses to the brain to release ADH; this results in urinary concentration and water retention. If this water retention results in hyponatremia, osmoreceptor mediated ADH release will be suppressed. Nevertheless, water retention has preceded secondary to volume-mediated ADH release. Thus, plasma volume homeostasis always takes precedence over plasma tonicity homeostasis.

Volume depletion secondary to fluid loss from the body is a potent stimulator of ADH release. If these losses are replaced with more water than sodium, the ADH-mediated retention of water will lead to hyponatremia. On the other hand, total body fluid volume can be elevated, and ADH will not necessarily be suppressed if the fluid is either not in the vascular tree (edema or ascites) or if it does not adequately reach the tissues (congestive heart failure). Therefore, the term *effective circulating volume* has been used to refer to the actual volume of fluid that reaches tissue beds. It is similar to the cardiac output, except in the presence of tissue shunting where tissue perfusion may be compromised despite a normal or high cardiac output (e.g., cirrhosis). Therefore, a normal effective circulating volume ultimately depends on adequate tissue perfusion. This requires normal intravascular volume, cardiac function, and vascular tone. A defect in any of these factors may lead to a decrease in effective circulating volume and the subsequent release of ADH and water retention. Indeed, the most common causes of hyponatremia are related to ADH release (e.g., cardiac failure, cirrhosis, and nephrosis associated with a decrease in effective circulating volume).

Conditions associated with volume depletion (either real or "effective") not only result in ADH release and water retention, but in the stimulation of the renin-aldosterone axis and sodium reabsorption. When the effective circulating volume is decreased, the continued retention of both sodium and water will eventually produce edema. Therefore, edema may serve as a clue to the presence of volume-mediated ADH release. This may be confirmed by the finding of low concentrations of sodium in the urine, usually <20 mEq/L, unless diuretics are being used. As is demonstrated in Fig. 9-1-2 on p. 527, water excretion is further impaired in these conditions by the adverse effects of volume depletion on distal delivery of filtrate.

QUESTION 2 Additional labs reveal that the plasma osmolality is 219 mosm/L, urine osmolality 600 mosm/L, urine sodium 78 mEq/L. A chest x-ray revealed a right superior mediastinal mass. What is the differential diagnosis of hyponatremia?

Because sodium is the major extracellular osmotically active particle, hyponatremia usually reflects a decrease in serum osmolality. If another osmotically active solute that is predominantly extracellular is present, water will leave the intracellular space to the extracellular space so that osmolar equilibration will occur. This is the basis for hyponatremia that is seen with hyperglycemia. Although it is true hyponatremia, it is not true hypoosmolality, and the measured serum osmolality should be elevated. This laboratory test is usually not necessary since an elevated blood glucose should indicate the etiology, and a simple estimation can be made of the expected reduction in sodium compared to the increase in blood glucose. The serum sodium concentration will decrease by about 1.6 mEq/L for each 100 mg/dl increase in blood glucose above 100 mg/dl. Plasma sodium dilution can be similarly seen when high doses of mannitol are administered intravenously.

As was discussed, the most common causes of hyponatremia are those associated with the edematous states of cardiac, hepatic, and renal diseases. This diagnosis can usually be made at the bedside when edema is present and requires little if any further laboratory testing. Water retention in the edematous conditions may seem inappropriate because it occurs despite plasma dilution, but is only inappropriate from an osmotic standpoint. ADH release is considered inappropriate, that is, the syndrome of inappropriate ADH release (SIADH), only when there lacks both an osmotic and volume-mediated stimulus for its release. Therefore, the patient with SIADH appears euvolemic and should not have edema. The urine sodium will reflect the patient's volume status, which, unless the patient is volume depleted, will be >20 mEq/L. The urine osmolality need not be greater than the serum osmolality. As most normal individuals can dilute their urine to <100 mosm/L after a water load, any urine osmolality greater than this could be considered "inappropriate" (but only if a volume-mediated stimulus for ADH release is lacking).

The steps in the pathogenesis of the urinary biochemical findings in SIADH are demonstrated in Fig. 9-1-3 on p. 528. As water is retained related to an inappropriate release of ADH, mild volume expansion occurs. As water retention is the primary defect in this condition, water cannot be excreted to alleviate this volume expanded state. On the other hand, ADH has essentially no effect on sodium excretion, and therefore sodium is handled normally. A mild natriuresis can therefore occur to decrease the volume overloaded state. This natriuresis is secondary to inhibition of the renin-aldosterone axis in addition to the release of atrial natriuretic factor. Also associated with the volume expansion is a decrease in the proximal tubular reabsorption of sodium, thereby increasing distal sodium delivery. The increase in distal sodium delivery, in the setting of water reabsorption without proximal or distal sodium reabsorption in the collecting duct, leads to a urine with a high sodium concentration. The urine sodium can exceed the plasma sodium. Because sodium is handled normally, edema does not occur. This volume expansion leads to a high GFR that is reflected in a "low" BUN and creatinine. The uric acid is often below normal values as well. This may be related to the high GFR, although

other mechanisms may be involved. Because the urine sodium tends to be high, patients with SIADH have greater reductions in the serum sodium than patients with hyponatremia and edematous states where sodium retention accompanies water retention. As a result, cases of severe hyponatremia are more likely to be secondary to SIADH than one of the edematous states.

SIADH has many causes but usually relates to either a paraneoplastic process, pulmonary or cerebral pathology, or a pharmaceutical agent. Since normal thyroid and adrenocortical hormone levels must be present to appropriately suppress ADH, hypothyroidism and adrenal insufficiency should be ruled out before a diagnosis of SIADH can be made.

Hyponatremia can result from excessive water intake in patients with normally functioning kidneys, psychogenic polydipsia, only when extremely large quantities of water are ingested. The urine can be diluted to 50 mosm/L in normal individuals when ADH is totally suppressed. An average daily osmotic load is about 600 mosm/day and consists mostly of urea, sodium, potassium, hydrogen ions, and their associated anions. These 600 mosm can be excreted in any number of urine osmolalities, depending upon water intake. Under water depletion, they are excreted into a concentrated urine. When water intake is abundant, they are excreted into a dilute urine. Given a maximally dilute urine of 50 mosm/L, 12 L of urine will excrete the daily osmotic load of 600 mosm. Therefore with a daily solute output of 600 mosm/day, a daily water intake in excess of 12 L will result in hyponatremia. Most patients with psychogenic polydipsia have psychiatric histories, take a number of psychotropic agents, and are frequent smokers, all of which are associated with the release of ADH. This superimposed SIADH prevents them from being able to dilute their urine maximally, and this decreases the amount of fluid intake necessary before hyponatremia occurs. Even a small change in maximally dilute urine from the normal of 50 mosm/L to 100 mosm/L reduces the allowable water intake by one half from 12 to 6 L/day (600 mosm/day = 6 L of 100 mosm/L urine). In addition, psychotropic agents often have the anticholinergic side effect of creating a dry mouth. This may exacerbate water intake and hyponatremia.

If the osmotic load is greater, as would be the case on a high salt or high protein diet, water intake would have to increase before hyponatremia would ensue (800 mosm/day = 16 L of 50 mosm/L urine). Also, if the osmotic load is very low, which is the case in people who consume only beer or tea and toast (both diets consist mostly of water and carbohydrate that are free of osmotic solutes that need to be excreted), water intake need not be as excessive before water retention occurs. This is the basis for "beer drinkers hyponatremia" and "tea and toast hyponatremia." Given a daily osmotic load of only 100 mosm/day, despite a maximally dilute urine of 50 mosm/L, the ingestion of over 2 L of fluid may result in water retention and hyponatremia (100 mosm/day = 2 L of 50 mosm/L urine). Psychogenic polydipsia, beer drinkers hyponatremia, and tea and toast hyponatremia are distinguished from the other forms of hyponatremia by the fact that urinary dilution is intact, as demonstrated by a urine osmolality of <100 mosm/L.

Diuretic usage is often associated with hyponatremia. It must be appreciated that diuretics are often used in conditions associated with hyponatremia (i.e., the edematous states), and hyponatremia seen with diuretic usage may reflect the primary sodium and water retention state and not a primary effect of the diuretic. Nevertheless, by effecting urinary dilution (Fig. 9-1-1, step 4), they may impair water excretion, and if water intake is excessive, will result in hyponatremia. Also, by producing hypokalemia, an intracellular to extracellular potassium shift is accompanied by an extracellular to intracellular shift of sodium to maintain cellular electrical neutrality. This movement of sodium out of the extracellular compartment will lower the serum sodium. Finally, if diuretic usage results in intravascular volume depletion, ADH will be appropriately released. These three mechanisms make hyponatremia a

common sequela of diuretic usage. Loop diuretics affect not only the ability to dilute the urine but the ability to concentrate it as well. This concentration defect decreases the kidney's ability to retain water, and therefore hyponatremia is less common and less severe with the loop diuretics than when seen with thiazide diuretics that effect only urinary dilution.

Renal failure is a common cause of hyponatremia. Of course, if renal failure is severe and no urine is produced, and water intake is greater than sodium intake, plasma dilution must occur. Hyponatremia can also be seen in patients with less severe reductions in GFR. As nephrons are lost, secondary to any chronic renal disease, the remaining glomeruli increase their filtered load. This excessive solute excretion per nephron has essentially the same effect on the nephron as an osmotic diuretic. This impairs the diluting segment and limits the kidney's ability to excrete a water load.

Up to this point, all causes of hyponatremia represent "true hyponatremia," although not all of the situations are associated with hypoosmolality. "Pseudohyponatremia," on the other hand, is not true hyponatremia but relates to how sodium is measured with some techniques. Serum consists of an aqueous component (water) and a nonaqueous or solid component (proteins and lipids). These, by volume represent 93% and 7%, respectively, of serum. Therefore, a liter of serum can be considered to consist of 930 ml of a liquid phase and 70 ml of a solid phase. Sodium is found only in the liquid phase, and when its concentration is measured in that phase alone, it is approximately 154 mEq/L. Since there is only 930 ml of this liquid phase, the total number of mEq of sodium is 143 (154 mEq/L × 0.93 L = 143 mEq). If the solids are then added, the new volume is 1 L. The total sodium content stays the same but with the new volume of 1 L, the sodium concentration is 143 mEq/L. If the solid phase of the blood is significantly increased, as is the case in severe hyperproteinemia (multiple myeloma, Waldenstrom's macroglobulinemia) and severe hyperlipidemia, the effect of this phenomena is amplified. Although uncommon, pseudohyponatremia should be suspected when serum is grossly lipemic or obviously hyperviscous. The diagnosis requires demonstration of hyponatremia in the presence of measured normal plasma osmolality, usually by freeze point depression.

The first step in the workup of the patient with hyponatremia is an examination of the patient's volume status. If edema is present, sodium retention has occurred in addition to water retention, and the patient either has a decrease in effective circulating volume or renal failure. If the patient shows signs of intravascular volume depletion without edema, the hyponatremia is similarly related to volume-mediated ADH release. If the patient appears euvolemic and hyperglycemia is not responsible for the hyponatremia, measurement of the serum and urine osmolality and the urine sodium may help distinguish the etiology. A simplified approach to the differential diagnosis of hyponatremia is presented in Fig. 9-1-4 on p. 529.

QUESTION 3 The patient presented chiefly with changes in mental status. What is the pathophysiology by which hyponatremia leads to symptoms?

As water is retained and the plasma sodium and osmolality decrease, an osmotic gradient is created across all cell membranes. This leads to water movement from the extracellular space into virtually every cell in the body. Because the volume of the cranial cavity is strictly limited, even a small increase in brain cell water could lead to a marked increase in intracranial pressure. The brain therefore requires a mechanism to maintain cellular volume despite otherwise deleterious changes in extracellular osmolality. When this process is inadequate, cerebral edema occurs and is responsible for the presenting signs and symptoms of hyponatremia. Both the rate of development and the severity of hyponatremia are important factors in the pathogenesis of these neurologic changes. If hyponatremia develops acutely, the onset of neurologic symptoms is more rapid at any

given decrease in plasma sodium since adaptation by brain cells is not immediate.

In chronic hyponatremia, patients develop fewer and less severe symptoms because of the brain's ability to adapt to a hypoosmolar environment. As the osmolalities between the extracellular and intracellular compartments must equilibrate as water is retained, this can occur only through one of two processes. Water may move from the extracellular space into the intracellular space and is what occurs in the majority of the cells of the body. As this process occurs in the brain, cerebral swelling is limited by the finite size of the cranial vault and would result in an increase in intracranial pressure, which could have a disastrous outcome. The only other means by which equalization of osmolalities could occur is through the removal of solute, without water, from the cell. This process similarly achieves osmotic equilibrium, but without the need for cellular swelling. This mechanism occurs in the brain and appears to be fairly unique to that organ. Brain cells pump intracellular solutes, primarily potassium and organic osmolytes such as free amino acids, out of the cell. Water does not follow these solutes, thus leading to an equalization of extracellular and intracellular osmolalities. This results in a near normalization of brain water, size, and intracranial pressure. This process is not immediate, and therefore acute reductions in the serum sodium may result in cerebral edema and symptomatic hyponatremia. In addition, this mechanism cannot completely protect the brain at all levels of serum sodium. Although the likelihood of hyponatremia being symptomatic depends on the rate of drop of serum sodium, severe reductions, even over a prolonged period, may be too great for this process to protect the brain.

As a general rule it is uncommon to see symptomatic hyponatremia with serum sodium levels >125 mEq/L although the rate of decrease appears to be as important as the degree of decrease. Below 120 mEq/L, patients may develop headache, disorientation, gait disturbances, muscle cramps, hiccups, lethargy, and obtundation. Sei-

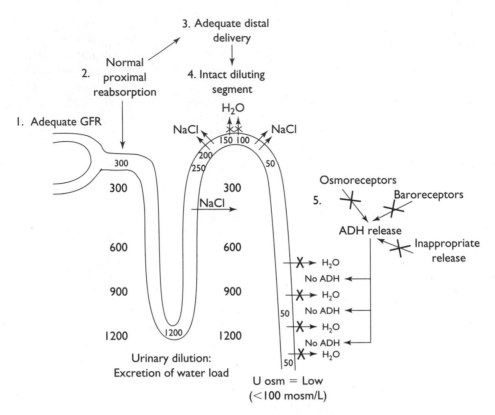

9-1-1 Excretion of a water load depends on 5 factors: (1) formation of a filtrate at the glomerulus, (2 and 3) delivery of filtrate to a "diluting segment," (4) formation of a dilute urine by removing sodium without water, and finally (5) suppression of ADH.

zures and coma may appear when the sodium concentration approaches 110 mEq/L. Still, severe hyponatremia, with serum sodium levels <110 mEq/L, can be asymptomatic if developed over a long enough period of time.

QUESTION 4   What is the treatment of hyponatremia, and what are the considerations for the patient with asymptomatic as opposed to symptomatic hyponatremia?

Since true hyponatremia is secondary to water retention, simple water restriction must accompany the treatment of all of these conditions. As long as the intake if fluid is less than the body's insensible losses of water, eventually this maneuver alone will correct the serum sodium. Treat-

ment beyond that is directed at the physiologic process that led to water retention. In most cases this includes an attempt to suppress ADH release. In the total body sodium depleted patient, repletion of sodium through the administration of intravenous saline will result in suppression of the volume-mediated response of ADH, and the patient will excrete a dilute urine. In the edematous patient, suppression of ADH may not be as easily achieved. Improvement of cardiac function with inotropes and afterload reduction may result in a decrease in ADH release and a more dilute urine in the patient with cardiac failure. Chronic water restriction is difficult to comply to and may not be an effective option by itself. Loop diuretics (in conjunction with water restriction) are often necessary as an additional treatment modality in the

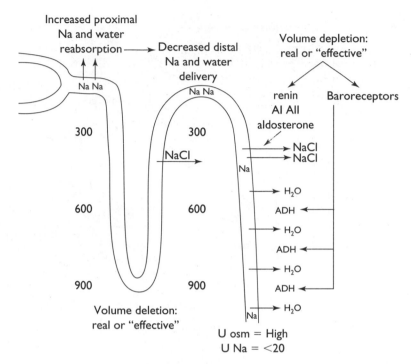

Increased proximal
Na and water
reabsorption ──────→ Decreased distal
Na and water
delivery

Volume depletion:
real or "effective"

Na Na   Na Na

renin
AI AII
aldosterone

Baroreceptors

300   300

NaCl ─────→

→ NaCl
→ NaCl

Na

→ H₂O

600   600   ADH ←

→ H₂O

ADH ←

→ H₂O

900   900   ADH ←

→ H₂O

Na

Volume deletion:
real or "effective"

U osm = High
U Na = <20

9-1-2 Urinary dilution is impaired in states associated with either a true or "effective"
decrease in circulation volume. This inability to dilute is related to effects of a decrease
in distal delivery of filtrate to diluting segment and stimulation of ADH release. Urine
is not only concentrated but is relatively sodium free, in an attempt to replete volume.

edematous patient. This may seem contraindicated since diuretics can cause hyponatremia, but
the effect that diuretics have on the serum sodium
is a function of the water intake. Since loop
diuretics inhibit both concentration and dilution,
the water loaded patient will retain water and
lower the serum sodium concentration, and the
water restricted patient will lose water and raise
the serum sodium. By "poisoning" the ascending
loop of Henle, loop diuretics decrease the osmolality of the medullary interstitium. Therefore,
even if ADH cannot be suppressed, the effects of
this hormone will be attenuated by the use of a
loop diuretic, and the urine will become more
dilute. Finally, there may be a therapeutic advantage to the sodium loss that is achieved with
diuretic usage in the edematous patient.

Patients with psychogenic polydipsia should be
easy to treat because mild water restriction alone
prevents the development of hyponatremia. This
"restriction" is only relative since the patient with
normal urinary dilution can still ingest several
liters of water per day without the development of
hyponatremia. Nevertheless, this is often difficult
because the delusions that frequently accompany
the psychiatric disease often involve water ingestion. Diuretics should be avoided in this condition
since urinary dilution is normal. Their usage
would exacerbate the hyponatremia if excessive
fluid intake remains constant.

The low solute intake-related hyponatremias
("tea and toast" and "beer drinkers") are rare but
are easily treated with an increase in solute
(sodium and protein) and a decrease in water
intake. Diuretics should similarly be avoided as
urinary dilution is also intact in these conditions.

Since the primary defect with the SIADH is
ADH release, ADH suppression may not be easily

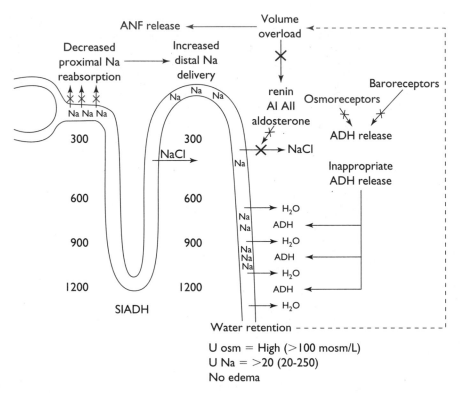

9-1-3 Because sodium is handled normally in SIADH, sodium excretion in urine reflects the volume status of patient. Because this tends to be high as water is retained, the urine sodium reflects this and is elevated. This natriuresis prevents edema formation.

accomplished unless related to a drug that can be discontinued. Treatment is aimed at water restriction in addition to decreasing the effects of ADH. The latter can be easily achieved with a loop diuretic. Lithium and high dose demeclocycline (1200 mg/day) have been used as they have the ability to directly block the effects of ADH on the collecting duct, but toxicity (lithium) and cost (demeclocycline) may limit their usage. If loop diuretics and fluid restriction alone are unsuccessful in maintaining the patient's serum sodium, the patient with chronic SIADH may benefit from an increased solute diet, high in dietary sodium and protein. This will allow a greater daily water intake. This can be achieved with salt tablets (17.4 g NaCl/day = 600 mosm/day) and/or oral administration of urea (36 g/day = 600 mosm/day). By increasing the daily osmotic load from 600 mosm/

day to 1200 mosm/day, the patient would be able to increase his or her daily intake of fluid by 100%. Most patients with SIADH can be adequately managed with a loop diuretic, a high sodium diet, and modest fluid restriction.

Severe hyponatremia, no matter what the cause, may require acute intervention. If the patient is asymptomatic, the brain's defense mechanisms have been successful in preventing cellular swelling, and fluid restriction alone should be sufficient. If the patient has symptomatic hyponatremia, either as a result of too rapid a fall or too severe a reduction in the serum sodium to avoid cellular swelling, treatment is aimed at rapidly reducing brain water. This can be achieved with hypertonic saline, usually accompanied by a loop diuretic to assist in urinary dilution. An increase in the serum sodium of 5 to 10 mEq/L (10

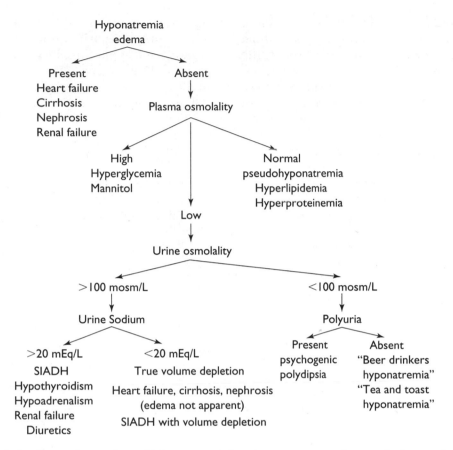

9-1-4 Approach to patient with hyponatremia based on presence or absence of edema and values of plasma and urine chemistries.

to 20 mosm/L) will decrease brain water significantly and should be attempted immediately in the symptomatic patient. After this increase has been achieved or after the patient becomes asymptomatic, whichever comes first, the patient is placed on fluid restriction alone to allow a slower correction. Increases in the serum sodium greater than 12 mEq/day are discouraged as this has been associated with the later development of central pontine myelinolysis (CPM), from which the patient may never recover. The clinical features of CPM include motor abnormalities that may insidiously progress to flaccid quadriplegia, respiratory paralysis, pseudobulbar palsy, and alterations in mental status with coma. This sequela appears to be more common in women, especially

those who are postoperative. Too rapid a correction in the extracellular osmolality may actually lead to brain cell dehydration and may be the pathophysiologic explanation for CPM. Because of the concerns of the development of this dreaded condition, patients with symptomatic hyponatremia need to be treated very carefully. Those that are asymptomatic should not be treated aggressively, and fluid restriction alone should suffice. Special care must be taken in treating symptomatic SIADH patients with intravenous fluids. Although normal saline has a sodium concentration of 154 mEq/L and would be expected to raise a patient's serum sodium when administered, it can actually result in a worsening of hyponatremia. This is the result of the kidney's continued retention of water in the face of sodium excretion. In other words, the kidney can extract the water out of the normal saline and excrete the sodium, thereby further lowering the serum sodium concentration. It is in this situation that the urine sodium concentration can exceed that of the serum. If normal saline is administered with a loop diuretic, this phenomenon will not occur since urinary concentration will be impaired. Therefore, if normal saline is being used as a therapy for the symptomatic patient with SIADH, a loop diuretic must be administered simultaneously for this treatment to be effective. This is not necessary when using 3% saline since the kidney cannot concentrate beyond the 3% being administered. Patients with symptomatic hyponatremia secondary to psychogenic polydipsia should be able to correct themselves fairly rapidly, with fluid restriction alone.

QUESTION 5 What are the pertinent positives of this case, and what is your treatment guideline?

The patient presents with symptomatic hyponatremia. He appears euvolemic and has no edema. His blood chemistries demonstrate a low serum osmolality, creatinine, uric acid, and a normal blood glucose. The urine is concentrated with a "high" sodium content. These findings are all consistent with SIADH (Fig. 9-1-4) and is most likely secondary to a paraneoplastic process related to his lung mass. Thyroid and adrenal function should be evaluated.

Because he is symptomatic, he should immediately receive hypertonic saline with a loop diuretic to decrease cerebral edema. His serum sodium should be followed every hour or two, and when it approaches 115 mEq/L, the hypertonic saline and diuretic should be discontinued, and he should be put on fluid restriction alone to minimize the risk of the later development of CPM. Chronic therapy will require fluid restriction with the possible addition of a loop diuretic and a high salt diet. If his urine osmolality remains constant at 600 mosm/L, he will be "allowed" an intake of 1L fluid/day if he has an osmotic output of 600 mosm/day. A loop diuretic, by poisoning the ascending loop of Henle, will decrease the medullary osmotic gradient. This would result in a urine concentration that is closer to 300 mosm/L. This maneuver by itself would allow an increase in the daily fluid intake to 2L if the daily solute intake remains at 600 mosm/day (2 L/day of 300 mosm/L urine = 600 mosm/day). Other therapies may be necessary if these are not sufficient.

BIBLIOGRAPHY

Berl T: Treating hyponatremia: damned if we do and damned if we don't, *Kidney Int* 37:1006-1018, 1990.

Chung H, Kluge R, Schrier RW, Anderson RJ: Clinical assessment of extracellular fluid volume in hyponatremia, *Am J Med* 83:905-908, 1987.

Cogan E, Debieve M, Pepersack T, Abramow M: Natriuresis and atrial natriuretic factor secretion during inappropriate antidiuresis, *Am J Med* 84:409-418, 1988.

Decaux G, Genette F: Urea for the long-term treatment of syndrome of inappropriate secretion of antidiuretic hormone, *Brit Med J* 283:1081-1083, 1981.

DeFronzo RA, Thier SO: Pathophysiologic approach to hyponatremia, *Arch Intern Med* 140:897-902, 1980.

Goldman MB, Luchins DL, Robertson GL: Mechanisms of altered water metabolism in psychotic patients with polydipsia and hyponatremia, *N Engl J Med* 318:397-403, 1988.

Jamison RL, Oliver RE: Disorders of urinary concentration and dilution, *Am J Med* 72:308-321, 1982.

Robertson GL, Aycinena P, Zerbe RL: Neurogenic disorders of osmoregulation, *Am J Med* 72:339-353, 1982.

Rose BD: Diuretics, *Kidney Int* 39:336-352, 1991.

Rose BD: New approach to disturbances in the plasma sodium concentration, *Am J Med* 81:1033-1040, 1986.

Schrier RW: Pathogenesis of sodium and water retention in high-output and low-output cardiac failure, nephrotic syndrome, cirrhosis and pregnancy, *N Engl J Med* 319:1065-1072, 1988.

Weisberg LS: Pseudohyponatremia: a reappraisal, *Am J Med* 86:315-318, 1989.

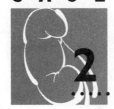
A *20-year-old man was admitted to the hospital complaining of polyuria and increased thirst. He also noted a craving for ice water. He estimated a daily urine volume in excess of 9 to 10 L/day. There was no history of head trauma, headache, visual changes, diabetes, or psychiatric disease. Upon admission, his physical and neurologic examinations were normal.*

The laboratory examination revealed: sodium 145 mEq/L, potassium 4.1 mEq/L, chloride 110 mEq/L, bicarbonate 23 mEq/L, BUN 8 mg/dl, creatinine 0.8 mg/dl, and blood glucose 96 mg/dl. The urinalysis revealed a specific gravity of 1.002; no glycosuria was present. His weight was 80 kg. The plasma osmolality was 290 mosm/L, and the urine osmolality was 60 mosm/L.

QUESTION I Define polyuria and what are the physiologic mechanisms that determine the daily urine output and allow for day-to-day changes in fluid intake?

Polyuria must be first distinguished from urgency and frequency resulting from lesions of the lower urinary tract. Since this may be difficult in some patients, a 24-hour urine volume measurement may be necessary to allow this distinction. It is difficult to define a normal urine flow in a 24-hour period. However, an understanding of the determinants of urine volume allow us to give a range of "normal" daily urine volumes. Under normal conditions, nitrogenous end-products (urea) and dietary electrolytes, when excreted into the urine, provide a daily solute load of approximately 600 mosm. The minimum amount of urine required to excrete this daily solute load depends on maximal urinary concentrating abil-ity. Under optimal conditions the urine can be maximally concentrated to 1200 mosm/L. This would require only 500 ml of urine to excrete the daily 600 mosm solute load (0.5 L × 1200 mosm/L = 600 mosm). Assuming no insensible losses (for ease of calculation, as will be the case for this entire chapter), this would require a 500 ml water intake to maintain a steady state. Regular dietary habits usually exceed 500 ml water intake per day, and therefore the solute load is excreted in a less than maximally concentrated urine. One liter of water intake per day, (and therefore 1 L of urine output/day) would require that the urine be concentrated to 600 mosm/L to excrete the daily 600 mosm solute load; 2 L oral intake = 2 L of 300 mosm/L urine, 3 L intake = 3 L of 200 mosm/L urine, 6 L intake = 6 L of 100 mosm/L urine and 12 L of intake would produce 12 L of 50 mosm/L urine. Therefore, in persons whose urinary concentrating and diluting ability is intact, fluid intake determines urine output. Since an average intake of fluid is usually less than or equal to 3 L/day, polyuria is often defined by daily urine volumes that exceed 3 L.

In situations where renal concentration is impaired, the minimum urine output required to excrete a daily solute load increases. For example, if the maximum urinary osmolality obtainable is 300 mosm/L, 2 L/day of urine are required to excrete the daily 600 mosm solute load. Although this appears to represent a relatively severe inability to concentrate urine (normal being 1200 mosm/L), the patient with this condition is usually asymptomatic since a 2 L/day urine output would not appear excessive to most people. As urinary concentration becomes more impaired, urine output increases significantly, and symptomatic polyuria is more likely to be seen. A patient with a maximum urinary osmolality (maximum Uosm) of 200 mosm/L would require 3 L/day to excrete the 600 mosm/day solute load; with a max Uosm of 100 mosm/L, 6 L of urine are required and with severe concentration defect of a maximum Uosm of 50 mosm/L, 12 L of urine/day are required. To avoid water depletion, the patient with a significant urine concentration defect must therefore replace urinary losses through oral intake of equal amounts of water.

If the daily solute load is increased, the urine output must increase for any given maximum Uosm. For example, if the daily osmotic load is increased from 600 to 800 mosm/day and the maximum Uosm is 100 mosm/L, the urine output must increase from 6 to 8 L/day to excrete this increased daily solute load. Therefore, when urinary concentration is impaired, urine output determines fluid intake, and urine output is a function of the daily solute load and the maximum Uosm obtainable.

QUESTION 2 Characterize primary as opposed to secondary polyuria, and what is a differential diagnosis of the polyuric state?

Polyuria can exist either as a primary response to "excessive" water intake or as a secondary response to a defect in urinary concentration. The key to understanding polyuria depends on the ability to distinguish an appropriate polyuria from one related to a defect in urinary concentration.

Polyuria secondary to excessive water intake is referred to as psychogenic polydipsia, and the reader should refer to Nephrology Case 1 for a discussion of the topic. As is demonstrated in that discussion, if urinary dilution is intact while undergoing a water load, water retention and plasma hypoosmolality (hyponatremia) are not seen unless water volumes in excess of 12 L/day are ingested. Water intake values less than this will still demonstrate significant polyuria, but hyponatremia should not be seen as long as urinary dilution is intact. When plasma hypoosmolality accompanies polyuria, it can usually be assumed that excessive water intake is driving the polyuria. Plasma hypoosmolality is easily detected by demonstrating hyponatremia, unless the hyponatremia is secondary to an intracellular to extracellular shift of water (secondary to an osmotically active substance that is being excluded from the intracellular space, i.e., glucose, mannitol). Thus, hyponatremia in the setting of polyuria and normoglycemia is usually indicative of psychogenic polydipsia.

Polyuria can also be caused by defects in urinary concentration related to the inadequate release of or response to antidiuretic hormone (ADH). ADH acts on the kidney to regulate the volume and osmolality of urine. When plasma levels of ADH are high, water reabsorption occurs in the collecting duct. As a result the urine becomes concentrated, and the urine flow decreases. Since about 10% of the glomerular filtrate reaches the collecting duct, in a normal person with a normal glomerular filtration rate of about 140 L/day, this results in the delivery of about 14 L of filtrate/day to the collecting duct. Since reabsorption from the collecting duct is predominantly dependent on ADH, a defect in this can lead to volumes of urine >10 L/day. Conditions that have defects in ADH mediated water reabsorption are termed *diabetes insipidus (DI)*. Central DI is due to the failure of synthesis or release of ADH usually related to hypothalamic or pituitary disease. It may be idiopathic, although in adults it is more commonly secondary to a destructive process in the ADH producing cells of the hypothalamus. This is usually related to head trauma, hypophyseal surgery, primary craniopharyngioma, metastatic brain tumors, sarcoidosis, tuberculosis, or histiocytosis. Patients with DI have polyuria with a hypotonic urine. Because they are always excreting a dilute urine, they often have a plasma osmolality (serum sodium) that is mildly elevated. For reasons that are unknown, the craving for ice and cold fluids is common to central DI. If water intake is adequate, plasma osmolality (serum sodium) can be maintained in the normal range. Despite the persistent loss of water and the tendency towards plasma hyperosmolality, as long as the patient has an intact thirst mechanism, is conscious, and has access to water, normal water intake will replete urinary water losses and prevent plasma concentration. Thus, the persistent polyuria and polydipsia are more of an inconvenience than a threat. When patients with this condition are either unconscious, lose their thirst mechanism, or are unable to obtain water, then the condition becomes life threatening as severe hypernatremia will rapidly develop.

Nephrogenic DI is secondary to a collecting duct unresponsiveness to ADH and can be acquired or congenital. The congenital form is a rare hereditary disorder that usually only manifests in males. It appears to be caused by a metabolic defect in the cyclic AMP-mediated increase in collecting duct permeability to water in response to ADH. Acquired nephrogenic diabetes insipidus, on the other hand, can be caused by a variety of diseases. Multiple myeloma, amyloidosis, sickle cell disease, hypercalcemia, hypokalemia, lithium carbonate, demeclocycline, methoxyflurane, and amphotericin B have all been invoked as causes of nephrogenic DI. There are other conditions in which urinary concentration does not increase despite the presence of adequate levels of ADH and therefore could technically be classified as causes of nephrogenic DI, but these are related to an abnormally low maximum medullary osmotic gradient (≤ 350 mosm/L), not an unresponsiveness to ADH. This is commonly seen in chronic renal disease. Sickle cell anemia can result in renal medullary infarction and present with a similar concentrating defect. Since these latter conditions are only associated with relatively mild impairments in urinary concentration, polyuria is not usually noted unless the solute load is significantly increased.

A solute or osmotic diuresis, usually related to excessive excretion of urea, glucose, or sodium, causes polyuria by two mechanisms: (1) an increase in the solute load and (2) a decrease in urinary concentrating ability. Although an increase in daily solute load will increase the minimum urine output even when urinary concentration is normal (1200 mosm/day solute load $\times$ 1200 mosm/L maximum Uosm = 1 L/day minimum urine output), this will not result in polyuria unless urine osmolality is affected as well. For example, if the solute load is increased from 600 to 1200 mosm/day and the max Uosm is decreased from 1200 mosm/L to 300 mosm/L, the minimum urine required to excrete this daily solute load increases to 4 L and would present as polyuria. In fact, a defect in urinary concentration is common in disorders associated with a solute or osmotic diuresis. This is a result of two factors. When large amounts of a nonreabsorbed solute (glucose, urea, or sodium in the sodium loaded patient) are present in the urine, an increase in medullary blood flow occurs and results in a medullary "washout" of the osmotic gradient. Also, if large amounts of hypotonic fluid accompany the solute load, ADH becomes chronically suppressed. As ADH is partially responsible for creating the medullary gradient through the recycling of urea, its chronic suppression results in a decrease in the medullary osmotic gradient and therefore the ability to concentrate the urine. This process will only affect the ability to create a medullary concentration gradient above that of serum. Thus, although urinary concentration is impaired, the patient with a solute or osmotic diuresis will have a urinary osmolality that is at least isosmotic (i.e., ≥ 300 mosm/L).

A solute diuresis from glucosuria is usually related to hyperglycemia and is easily diagnosed. A urea solute diuresis is usually secondary to excessive oral or intravenous (total parenteral nutrition) protein feeding. If there is a question about this diagnosis, one can measure the 24-hour urine urea nitrogen. When translated into mg/day, and divided by 28, one can estimate the daily osmotic load in mosm/day that is being produced as a result of protein catabolism. Overjudicious administration of sodium-containing intravenous fluids may also result in a sodium solute diuresis. This diagnosis is confirmed by demonstrating a decrease in urine output following a decrease in the fluid administration rate.

QUESTION 3 Within 6 hours of a fluid deprivation test, the patient's body weight decreased to 78 kg, the plasma osmolality rose to 303 mosm/L, and the urine osmolality rose to 150 mosm/L. Five units of aqueous pitressin (vasopressin) were given subcutaneously, and the urine osmolality rose to 500 mosm/L. What is the water deprivation test, and how does it help in the differentiation of polyuria?

From the above discussion it would appear easy to classify the causes of polyuria based on the serum and urine osmolality. The patient with primary polydipsia should have a plasma osmolality (serum sodium) on the low side of normal in addition to a dilute urine (<250 mosm/L). The patient with diabetes insipidus should have a plasma osmolality (serum sodium) on the high side of normal and a dilute urine (<250 mosm/L). The patient with a solute or osmotic diuresis should have a urine osmolality close to plasma (isosthenuria). In addition, certain clinical clues may help direct one's attention to a specific diagnosis. For example, a polyuric patient with a psychiatric history and episodic polyuria is suggestive of psychogenic polydipsia. A history of head trauma or neoplasm associated with the sudden onset of unrelenting polyuria, often accompanied by the craving for ice water, suggests central DI as the underlying disorder.

The most effective way to delineate between the disorders associated with a dilute urine, and to differentiate central from nephrogenic DI, is to perform a water deprivation test. Since the patient with psychogenic polydipsia will often go to great surreptitious lengths to obtain water, the water deprivation test may need to be done under constant supervision if this diagnosis is being entertained. Although the water deprivation test can be initiated as an outpatient, with fluid restriction overnight before arrival at the clinician's office, a severely polyuric patient with DI could become severely water depleted over this time.

This may put the patient at risk. Therefore, we recommend that the test be performed under observed conditions. The patient with psychogenic polydipsia will, when fluid restricted, demonstrate an appropriate decrease in urine flow and a significant increase in urine osmolality. The patient with DI will continue to be polyuric with water deprivation. The urine osmolality may increase mildly in the DI patient after fluid restriction as volume depletion occurs and distal tubular and collecting duct urine flow rates slow, allowing ADH-independent water reabsorption to occur. This may allow the urine osmolality to increase, but usually not greater than 250 mosm/L.

During the water deprivation test, patients should not be allowed to lose >3% to 5% of their body weight. Hourly weights and measurements of urine and plasma osmolality are obtained. When the plasma osmolality reaches 300 mosm/L, 5 units of aqueous vasopressin are administered subcutaneously. Hourly urine and plasma osmolality measurements are continued. An even mildly elevated plasma osmolality of 300 mosm/L will maximally stimulate ADH release in a normal individual, therefore values above this are not required before the administration of ADH. Patients with central DI respond with an increase in urine osmolality and a decrease in urine output, while those with nephrogenic DI do not. Fig. 9-2-1 demonstrates the various patterns of response in urine output and urine osmolality to this test. As demonstrated, "partial" nephrogenic and partial central DI may be difficult to distinguish from psychogenic polydipsia. Patients with "partial diabetes insipidus" have incomplete defects, and although cannot maximally concentrate their urine, usually are able to achieve a max Uosm of close to 300 mosm/L. This is a mild concentrating defect and rarely causes significant polyuria under conditions of a normal solute load. Therefore, the need to distinguish these partial DI disorders from psychogenic polydipsia is uncommon.

The water deprivation test is therefore useful in distinguishing the two forms of diabetes insipidus

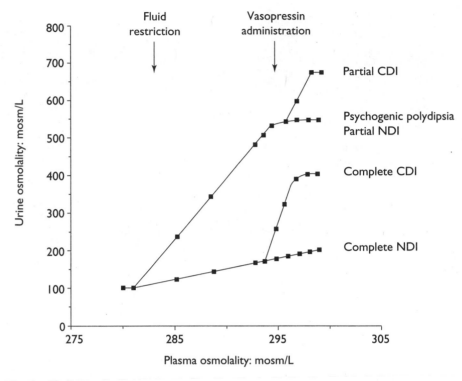

9-2-1 Different response patterns of urine osmolality to water deprivation test. Response in patients with "partial" diabetes insipidus disorders may be confused with psychogenic polydipsia although the need for this distinction is uncommon (see text).

from psychogenic polydipsia. These conditions are associated with a hypotonic urine. The patient with an osmotic or solute diuresis is easily distinguished from the former diagnoses by the demonstration of an isosmotic or slightly hypertonic urine, ≥300 mosm/L. Fig. 9-2-2 summarizes the approach to the polyuric patient, using the baseline urinary osmolality and the water deprivation test.

QUESTION 4 What is the appropriate mode of therapy for the polyuric patient?

The treatment of the various disorders associated with polyuria is fairly straightforward. If a solute diuresis is diagnosed, one simply has to decrease the solute load. Glycosuria is managed through improved diabetic control. A urea solute diuresis should respond to a decrease in protein intake. A saline diuresis should respond to a decrease in the intravenous fluid administration rate.

Central DI responds to ADH replacement, but it should be stressed that the goal in treating this disorder is to decrease, not normalize, daily urine output. Attempts at trying to normalize urine output risk inappropriate water retention and hyponatremia, if excessive ADH is administered and water intake continues. This would, if it occurred, be considered an iatrogenic form of SIADH. A nasal spray preparation of a long-acting vasopressin analog, DDAVP, is now commercially available and is both effective and convenient. Patients with mild central DI may require this therapy only at bedtime to prevent or minimize nocturia. Since urine output is a function of solute

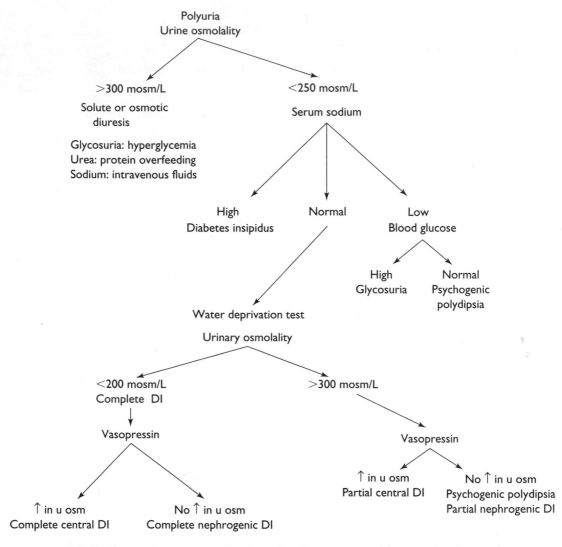

9-2-2 Approach to patient with polyuria based on urine osmolality, serum sodium, and response to water deprivation test.

intake in patients with concentrating disorders, patients with DI should avoid high solute (sodium) diets.

Patients with nephrogenic DI do not respond to ADH replacement. As long as patients maintain an intact thirst mechanism, polyuria may be the only complaint. This can be decreased by a pharmacologic regimen aimed at moderately reducing ex-tracellular fluid volume. Thiazide diuretics and salt restriction produce a mild volume depleted state. As a result, less filtrate is delivered to the collecting duct where the defect exists, and polyuria lessens. Loop diuretics may result in the same sodium depleted state but should be avoided because of the adverse effects on urinary concentration, which do not exist with thiazide diuretics.

CASE SUMMARY A 20-year-old man presents with a history of severe polyuria. Upon further questioning he can pinpoint the exact date on which his urine output increased. He also claims to crave very cold fluids. These aspects of his history are highly suggestive of central DI. His serum sodium is on the high side of normal, which makes psychogenic polydipsia unlikely. His urine is dilute despite this increase in plasma osmolality, indicating a urinary concentration defect. The patient undergoes a water restriction test, and his urine osmolality increases minimally, further ruling out psychogenic polydipsia. He has an excellent response to ADH that confirms the diagnosis of central DI. He should receive treatment with intranasal DDAVP to achieve a daily urine output of no less than 3 L/day. A computed tomography scan of his head demonstrated a craniopharyngioma. The patient underwent successful surgical removal but unfortunately continues to have central DI and will be maintained on intranasal DDAVP.

• •

BIBLIOGRAPHY

Boylan JW, Kramer K, Deetjen P: *Physiology of the kidney and water balance,* New York, 1992, Springer-Verlag.

Bricher NS, Kirschenbaum MA: *The kidney, diagnosis and management,* New York, 1984, John Wiley & Sons.

Gonick HC. *Current nephrology,* vol 7, New York, 1984, John Wiley & Sons.

Klahr S: *Renal and electrolyte disorders, differential diagnosis,* ed 2, Norwalk, Conn, Arco Diagnosis Series, Appleton-Century-Crafts.

Koeppen BM, Stanton BA: *Renal physiology,* St Louis, 1992, Mosby.

Rose BD: *Clinical Physiology of acid-base and electrolyte disorders,* ed 3, New York, 1989, McGraw Hill.

Seldin DW, Giebisch G: *The kidney: physiology and pathophysiology,* ed 2, vol 2, New York, 1992, Raven Press.

Wyngaarden JB, Smith LH, Bennett JC: *(Cecil's) textbook of medicine* ed 19, Philadelphia, 1992, WB Saunders.

CASE

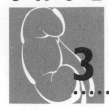

Roger A. Rodby

A 35-year-old man comes to the emergency room with a chief complaint of several days of abdominal pain and vomiting, secondary to chronic pancreatitis related to a long history of alcohol abuse. This condition has also caused chronic diarrhea from malabsorption and diabetes mellitus from insulin deficiency. He has been prescribed insulin, but admits to noncompliance. He denies intake of alcohol for several days.

On physical examination he was an ill-appearing, mildly confused male who was breathing heavily. The BP was 80/60 mm Hg, and the pulse was 100 bpm. There was an orthostatic drop of the systolic blood pressure to 60 mm Hg with an increase of the pulse to 120 bpm. The respiration rate was 24/min, and the temperature was 97.0°F. Diffuse abdominal pain was present without guarding or rebound; bowel sounds were absent. The cardiopulmonary examination was normal. He had no edema. The stool guaiac was negative.

Laboratory values revealed sodium 136 mEq/L, potassium 4.8 mEq/L, chloride 90 mEq/L, and bicarbonate 18 mEq/L. The blood glucose was 360 mg/dl, blood urea nitrogen (BUN) 11 mg/dl, and the creatinine 0.8 mg/dl. The amylase and lipase were both three times normal levels. An arterial blood gas demonstrated a pH of 7.44, $Paco_2$ 27 mm Hg, Pao_2 98 mm Hg, and HCO_3 18 mEq/L. A serum osmolality by freeze point depression was 306 mosm/kg. Ethanol was undetectable in his blood. The blood lactate level was not elevated. The urinalysis was normal except for the presence of a large amount of ketones.

The primary objective of this chapter is to present a systematic approach to the evaluation of acid-base disorders that should allow the reader to quickly and easily determine a patient's acid-base status. This is done with the aid of multiple examples based on fundamental physiologic principles. This chapter will not list all of the causes or treatments of each metabolic or respiratory disorder, to do so would triple its length and limit its usefulness. Metabolic acidosis will be discussed to a disproportionate degree because it appears to be more common and puts the patient at a greater risk than the other acid-base disorders.

QUESTION I What is the relationship of the HCO_3 and $Paco_2$ to the pH?

The pH of the blood is maintained within relatively narrow limits in the human body. This is necessary for the optimal function of most of our enzymatic systems. The pH of the blood can be estimated from the following equation where HCO_3 is in mEq/L and $Paco_2$ is in mm Hg:

• $pH = 6.10 + \log (HCO_3 / 0.03\ Paco_2)$

The utility of this equation is limited by the need for transforming the quantity ($HCO_3 / 0.03\ Paco_2$) into its logarithm. For purposes of examples and calculations, this equation can be converted to the simplified form where H^+ is in nanoequivalents/L, HCO_3 is in mEq/L, and $Paco_2$ is in mm Hg:

• $H^+ = 24\ Paco_2 / HCO_3$

By definition, the pH is the negative logarithm of the hydrogen ion concentration $[H^+]$. Therefore this equation also requires a familiarity with, and access to, logarithms. However, since there are a finite number of $[H^+]$ values compatible with life,

TABLE 9-3-1   pH Values that Correspond to H$^+$ in Nanoequivalents/L

pH	H$^+$	pH	H$^+$	pH	H$^+$	pH	H$^+$
8.00	10	7.64	23	7.29	51	6.94	115
7.99	10	7.63	23	7.28	52	6.93	117
7.98	10	7.62	24	7.27	54	6.92	120
7.97	11	7.61	25	7.26	55	6.91	123
7.96	11	7.60	25	7.25	56	6.90	126
7.95	11	7.59	26	7.24	58	6.89	129
7.94	11	7.58	26	7.23	59	6.88	132
7.93	12	7.57	27	7.22	60	6.87	135
7.92	12	7.56	28	7.21	62	6.86	138
7.91	12	7.55	28	7.20	63	6.85	141
7.90	13	7.54	29	7.19	65	6.84	145
7.89	13	7.53	30	7.18	66	6.83	148
7.88	13	7.52	30	7.17	68	6.82	151
7.87	13	7.51	31	7.16	69	6.81	155
7.86	14	7.50	32	7.15	71	6.80	159
7.85	14	7.49	32	7.14	72	6.79	162
7.84	14	7.48	33	7.13	74	6.78	166
7.83	15	7.47	34	7.12	76	6.77	170
7.82	15	7.46	35	7.11	78	6.76	174
7.81	15	7.45	35	7.10	79	6.75	178
7.80	16	7.44	36	7.09	81	6.74	182
7.79	16	7.43	37	7.08	83	6.73	186
7.78	17	7.42	38	7.07	85	6.72	191
7.77	17	7.41	39	7.06	87	6.71	196
7.76	17	7.40	40	7.05	89	6.70	200
7.75	18	7.39	41	7.04	91	6.69	204
7.74	18	7.38	42	7.03	93	6.68	209
7.73	19	7.37	43	7.02	95	6.67	214
7.72	19	7.36	44	7.01	98	6.66	219
7.70	20	7.35	45	7.00	100	6.65	224
7.69	20	7.34	46	6.99	102	6.64	229
7.68	21	7.33	47	6.98	105	6.63	234
7.67	21	7.32	48	6.97	107	6.62	240
7.66	22	7.31	49	7.96	110	6.61	245
7.65	22	7.30	50	7.95	112	6.60	251

these can be presented with their corresponding pH values in a table (Table 9-3-1) that allows the easy determination of pH from $[H^+]$. Using this table and the equation: $[H^+] = 24\ Paco_2\ /\ [HCO_3]$, one can predict the pH that would result from various levels of $Paco_2$ and HCO_3 in the blood and can be used to see how the pH would be affected by a change in either or both of these values.

The unit of H^+ measurement that is determined from this equation is nanoequivalents/L, or 10^{-9} equivalents/L. This is about one hundred thousandth the concentration of potassium in our blood, which is in mEq/L (10^{-3})! The normal $Paco_2$ of blood is 40 mm Hg, and the normal HCO_3 is 24 mEq/L. Therefore the normal $H^+ = 24 \times 40/24 = 40\ (\times 10^{-9})$. This value of the H^+, at 40×10^{-9} is equal to 4×10^{-8}. This number, 4×10^{-8}, is between 1×10^{-7} and 1×10^{-8}. The negative log (pH) of 10^{-7} is 7.0 and that of 10^{-8} is 8.0. Therefore, the negative log (pH) of the normal H^+ at 40×10^{-9} represents a pH between 7.0 and 8.0. Table 9-3-1 demonstrates that a H^+ of 40 nanoequivalents/L corresponds to a pH of 7.40.

QUESTION 2 What are the mechanisms by which the body maintains acid base homeostasis?

The body must be able to perform 3 "tasks" to maintain normal HCO_3 and $Paco_2$ concentrations, and therefore a normal pH.

Task #1
As the kidney filters the blood, it must be able to reabsorb all of the filtered HCO_3 (bicarbonate) as Task #1. With a normal HCO_3 concentration of 24 mEq/L, and a normal glomerular filtration rate of 120 ml/min (173 L/day), the kidney filters over 4000 mEq of HCO_3/day. It must reabsorb all of this filtered bicarbonate to avoid a metabolic acidosis. This is done by the proximal tubule, by secreting hydrogen ions into the urine and thereby generating bicarbonate ions that enter the blood at the same rate that they are being filtered (>4000 mEq/day). If a defect in this ability to maximally reabsorb HCO_3 is present, bicarbonate will spill into the urine, the urine will be alkalotic, the serum HCO_3 will drop, and the filtered load of

HCO_3 will decrease. For example, if an inadequate proximal reabsorption of HCO_3 causes the HCO_3 concentration to decrease to 18 mEq/L, then the daily filtered load becomes 18 mEq/L $\times$ 173 L/day = 3114 mEq/day. This is a 25% reduction in the filtered load, and the kidney may now be able to reabsorb all of the HCO_3 at this lower serum HCO_3 level. A new steady state is reached, and there is no bicarbonate spillage into the urine. The urine pH is no longer alkaline and should be acidic as the distal tubule performs its normal function of urinary acidification (see Task #2). This is the basis for a proximal renal tubular acidosis (RTA). The proximal tubule cannot maximally reabsorb HCO_3, and the HCO_3 level falls until a new steady state at the lower HCO_3 level is reached. The urine pH should be <5.5 under most circumstances. The anion gap is normal (discussion to follow). Hypokalemia usually accompanies this nonanion gap acidosis. Other proximal tubular defects may coexist: phosphate wasting, glycosuria with a normal serum glucose, hypouricemia, and aminoaciduria. When present this is termed *Fanconi's kidney.*

Task #2
In the metabolism of proteins (cationic and sulphur-containing amino acids), phospholipids and phosphoproteins (that yield phosphoric acid when hydrolyzed), hydrogen ions are produced. This does not occur with the metabolism of carbohydrates and other fats since they yield only CO_2 and H_2O, (see Task #3). For example, the metabolism by the liver of sulphur-containing amino acids results in the production of sulfuric acid (H_2SO_4), a very strong acid. The total amount of daily H^+ produced as a result of metabolism of these substances approximates 1 mEq/kg body weight/day. For a 70 kg person this is equal to 70 mEq of H^+ ions/day. The bicarbonate buffer system in our blood prevents these strong acids from changing the blood pH significantly. For example, if a buffer system were not available, the addition of 70 mEq of a strong acid to the 42 L of body water in a 70 kg person (70 kg $\times$ 60% body water = 42 L) would result in a new H^+ of 1.7 mEq/L (70/42 = 1.7). A H^+ of 1.7×10^{-3} represents a pH

between 2.0 and 3.0! Therefore, without a buffer system, our pH would drop to lethal levels within minutes, just related to normal daily metabolism and the production of H^+ as a byproduct. The bicarbonate system prevents this strong acid from releasing its hydrogen ions by the following buffer reaction:

- Strong acid (HA) + $NaHCO_3 \rightarrow NaA + H_2CO_3$

For each mEq of acid that is produced and buffered, 1 mEq of $NaHCO_3$ is utilized, 1 mEq of the salt of that acid is formed (NaA), and 1 mEq of carbonic acid (H_2CO_3 is formed. The NaA is easily filtered and excreted by the kidney. The carbonic acid breaks down into CO_2 and H_2O ($H_2CO_3 \rightarrow H_2O + CO_2$), and the CO_2 is rapidly excreted through the lungs. It is the job of the distal tubule to regenerate the HCO_3 that has been utilized in this reaction and represents the role of Task #2.

A buffer works best at a pH that it is close to its pKa. The pKa of the bicarbonate buffer system is 6.1, not very close to our physiologic pH of 7.4. This would limit the effectiveness of this buffer system. It is the ability to rapidly excrete the CO_2 produced (as a result of the buffering of acids) that allows this buffer system to work so well. For example, let us determine the pH that would result from the addition of the 70 mEq of daily acid to a hypothetical 70 kg patient if the CO_2 that is produced as a result of this reaction were not excreted. The addition of this acid utilizes 70 mEq of HCO_3. Using the total body water as the volume of distribution of HCO_3, 70 mEq of acid/42 L of total body water would add 1.7 mEq/L of acid to the body. Since each mEq of hydrogen ions utilizes 1 mEq of HCO_3, the serum HCO_3 would decrease by 1.7 mEq/L. This would create a new HCO_3 of 22.3 mEq/L ($24 - 1.7 = 22.3$). At the same time this reaction leads to the production of CO_2 via the reaction:

- $HA + NaHCO_3 \rightarrow NaA + H_2CO_3 \rightarrow H_2O + CO_2$,

which would increase the $Paco_2$ to 97 mm Hg (see Appendix 1). The new H^+ would now reflect the lowered HCO_3 and the raised Pco_2:

- $H^+ = 24 \, Paco_2/HCO_3 = 24 \times 97/22.3 = 104$

This corresponds to a pH of 6.98 (from Table 9-3-1).

This new pH is certainly better than the pH 2.0 to 3.0 predicted if we did not have the bicarbonate buffer system, yet still would be at a life-threatening level within a day. However, the CO_2 produced as a result of the buffering reaction is not retained since it is easily and rapidly excreted by the lungs. The $Paco_2$ therefore remains at 40 mm Hg, and the actual H^+ would be:

- $H^+ = 24 \, Paco_2/HCO_3 = 24 \times 40/22.3 = 43$

This corresponds to a pH of 7.37 (from Table 9-3-1).

The ability to excrete the CO_2 produced from the reaction:

- $HA + NaHCO_3 \rightarrow NaA + H_2CO_3 \rightarrow H_2O + CO_2$

allows the bicarbonate buffer system to be so effective despite working at a pH significantly different from its pKa. This buffer system allows us to metabolize cationic amino acids, sulphur containing amino acids and phospholipids without becoming profoundly acidotic in a relatively short time. It also helps us tolerate a lactic acidosis from normal physiologic processes such as anaerobic physical exertion, in addition to pathologic acidotic conditions such as ketoacidosis.

In the above example, 70 mEq of HCO_3 were utilized in 1 day as a result of normal metabolic processes. This resulted in the HCO_3 decreasing from 24 mEq/L to 22.3 mEq/L in that same time period. In actuality, this does not occur since the kidney is regenerating the HCO_3 at the same rate that it is being used. If this lost bicarbonate were not regenerated, we would eventually deplete our bicarbonate stores and become profoundly acidotic, just from the acid load of daily living. It is the role of the distal tubule to regenerate HCO_3, and represents Task #2. The distal tubule must be able to excrete approximately 1 mEq/kg body weight/day of hydrogen ions, thereby regenerating the same amount of HCO_3 to the blood, to maintain normal acid-base status.

About one third of the hydrogen ions that are secreted into the distal tubule combine with filtered inorganic acids and are termed *titratable acids*. The other hydrogen ions are excreted as ammonium (NH_4^+), and it is this system that can be increased or decreased depending on the acid load of the individual. The renal tubular cells create ammonia (NH_3), which diffuses freely into the tubular lumen. Hydrogen ions are secreted by the distal tubule and combine with the NH_3 in the tubular lumen to form NH_4^+. This charged molecule of NH_4^+ is lipid insoluble and becomes "trapped" in the urine, and therefore excreted. If the daily acid load increases (e.g., as a result of a high protein diet or ketoacidosis), NH_4^+ excretion increases. With each mEq of H^+ that gets excreted either as titratable acid or NH_4^+, 1 milliequivalent of HCO_3 reenters the blood.

In the presence of an acidemia, the distal tubule should maximally acidify the urine to a pH of 4.5 to 5.3. In a distal RTA, distal urinary acidification is impaired as indicated by the inability to create a urine with a pH of less than 5.5. The patient is in a positive net hydrogen ion balance since the HCO_3 that is utilized for daily metabolic needs is not being generated at the same rate that it is being utilized. This will eventually result in a severe metabolic acidosis. A distal RTA is diagnosed in the acidemic patient in which the urine pH is greater than or equal to 5.5. This condition is usually accompanied by hypokalemia and a normal anion gap.

Task #3

As was pointed out in Task #2, the lungs must be able to excrete large amounts of CO_2 to maintain a normal systemic pH. This is the role of Task #3. In the example in Task #2, the daily CO_2 production from the buffering of metabolically produced acids would result in the production of 70 mmol of CO_2. The ability to excrete that CO_2 was the difference between a pH of 6.98 and 7.37. Carbon dioxide is also produced as a result of the metabolism of fats and carbohydrates. The amount of CO_2 that is produced through this mechanism (15,000 mmol/day) is vastly greater than that from the metabolism of proteins. This CO_2 has the potential of becoming an acid load because it can combine with H_2O to form carbonic acid (H_2CO_3). Therefore, the lungs are a crucial organ in maintaining acid-base balance. Pulmonary disorders may result in an increase in the steady state $Paco_2$ and the potential for an acidemia, and when present is termed *a respiratory acidosis*.

QUESTION 3 How do alterations in the HCO_3 and $Paco_2$ produce and compensate for acid-base disorders?

From the equation $H^+ = 24\ Paco_2\ /\ HCO_3$, it can be seen that an increase in the $Paco_2$ or a decrease in the HCO_3 will increase the H^+ and decrease the pH. Similarly, a decrease in the $Paco_2$ or an increase in the HCO_3 will decrease the H^+, and increase the pH. Confusion can arise in terminology of acid-base disorders if strict rules are not followed. The final acid-base status of the blood should be termed *acidotic* if an acidemia is present (pH <7.38), and *alkalotic* if an alkalemia is present (pH >7.42), or *normal* when the pH is in the normal range (pH 7.38 to 7.42). When the terms *metabolic* and *respiratory* precede *acidosis* or *alkalosis*, it refers only to the level of HCO_3 and $Paco_2$ and not to the presence of an acidemia or alkalemia. For instance, a metabolic acidosis can be present with an acidemia or an alkalemia, depending on the level of $Paco_2$. Metabolic acidosis can also be called hypobicarbonatemia; metabolic alkalosis: hyperbicarbonatemia; respiratory alkalosis: hypocapnia; and respiratory acidosis: hypercapnia. When defining the acid-base status of a patient, one has to first determine whether or not an acidemia or alkalemia is present, and if so, what combination of metabolic or respiratory acidoses or alkaloses are responsible for the abnormal pH. The abnormalities in pH, $Paco_2$, and HCO_3 that determine each of the four primary acid-base disorders are presented in Table 9-3-2.

The relationship of pH to both the $Paco_2$ and HCO_3 allows the regulation of pH through two mechanisms, the kidney's regulation of HCO_3 and the brain/lung's regulation of $Paco_2$. Therefore, if a primary disorder occurs that increases or decreases one of these parameters, the other parameter can be altered in an attempt to "compensate," and thereby limit the change in pH. For instance, if the HCO_3 is lowered by a metabolic acidosis, the brain will sense this acidosis and send messages to the lungs (diaphragm) to increase ventilation, thereby decreasing the $Paco_2$ and attenuating the decrease in pH. This is the basis for compensation:

TABLE 9-3-2   The Primary Acid Base Disorders

Primary Disorder	pH	Primary Alteration	Compensatory Response
Metabolic acidosis	↓	Decrease in HCO_3	Decrease in $Paco_2$: Hyperventilation
Metabolic alkalosis	↑	Increase in HCO_3	Increase in $Paco_2$: Hypoventilation
Respiratory acidosis	↓	Increase in $Paco_2$	Increase in HCO_3 through an increase in renal H^+ excretion and increase in renal HCO_3 reabsorption
Respiratory alkalosis	↑	Decrease in $Paco_2$	Decrease in HCO_3 through a decrease in renal HCO_3 reabsorption and suppression of H^+ excretion

- For any primary process that changes either the $Paco_2$ or the HCO_3, the normal response is to compensate by changing the other parameter in the *same direction*, to limit the change in pH that would occur by the primary acid-base abnormality alone.

Compensation for the metabolic acid-base disorders occurs almost rapidly since the level of $Paco_2$ can be easily increased (metabolic alkalosis) or decreased (metabolic acidosis) by changing minute ventilation. Since it takes only minutes to increase or decrease the $Paco_2$, the only lag time in compensation for the metabolic disorders is in the time it takes for the brain's pH to change. As the systemic pH changes, the H^+ of the cerebral interstitial fluid is similarly affected, leading to the previously described changes in ventilation. However, this may take several hours since HCO_3 does not cross the blood brain barrier easily, and changes in the systemic HCO_3 are not immediately reflected in the HCO_3 concentration of the brain. Compensation for the respiratory acid-base disorders is less rapid since they require either a loss of HCO_3 (respiratory alkalosis) or generation of new HCO_3 (respiratory acidosis), processes that may take days to completely accomplish.

QUESTION 4 What degree of compensation is appropriate for each of the primary acid-base disorders?

The compensatory responses for each of the primary acid-base disorders are summarized in Table 9-3-3. A metabolic acidosis is defined by a low HCO_3 concentration (≤22 mEq/L) in the blood. This does not mean that all patients with a metabolic acidosis will be acidemic; that is determined by the patient's systemic pH. However, in patients with a decreased serum HCO_3 level and an acidemic pH (<7.38), the normal compensatory response is to lower the $Paco_2$ by increasing ventilation, and this should occur within hours of the development of the metabolic acidosis. For instance, if a patient has a metabolic acidosis with a HCO_3 10 mEq/L with a $Paco_2$ remaining at 40 mm Hg, the pH would be $H^+ = 24 \times 40/10 = 96 = $ pH 7.02 (Table 9-3-1). If on the other hand, ventilation increased, and the $Paco_2$ were lowered to 26 mm Hg, the pH would not be as depressed: $H^+ = 24 \times 26/10 = 62.4 = $ pH 7.21.

For a metabolic acidosis, the expected respiratory compensatory response can be quickly and easily calculated. For every 1.0 mEq/L decrease in the level of HCO_3 (from the normal value of 24 mEq/L), there is an expected decrease in the $Paco_2$ of 1.0 mm Hg (from the normal value of 40 mm Hg), although the range of 1.0 to 1.4 is more accurate (Table 9-3-3). In the above example, the metabolic acidosis reduced the HCO_3 by 14 to 10 mEq/L from a normal level of 24 ($24 - 14 = 10$). The expected reduction in $Paco_2$ would also be 14, and therefore a normal compensatory response would result in a $Paco_2$ of 26 mm Hg ($40 - 14 = 26$), which is what was present in the example. This one to one change in HCO_3 and $Paco_2$ demonstrates that an appropriate compensation has occurred. If the $Paco_2$ were lowered to a much greater degree, then it

TABLE 9-3-3   **Expected Compensatory Responses to Acid Base Disorders**

Disorder	Compensatory Response*
Metabolic acidosis	$\Delta\,Pa_{CO_2} = 1.0\text{-}1.4 \times \Delta\,HCO_3$
Metabolic alkalosis	$\Delta\,Pa_{CO_2} = 0.7 \times \Delta\,HCO_3$
Acute respiratory acidosis	$\Delta\,HCO_3 = 0.1 \times \Delta\,Pa_{CO_2}$
Chronic respiratory acidosis	$\Delta\,HCO_3 = 0.4 \times \Delta\,Pa_{CO_2}$
Acute respiratory alkalosis	$\Delta\,HCO_3 = 0.2 \times \Delta\,Pa_{CO_2}$
Chronic respiratory alkalosis	$\Delta\,HCO_3 = 0.5 \times \Delta\,Pa_{CO_2}$

*Pa_{CO_2} in mm Hg and HCO_3 in mEq/L.

must be secondary to a process other than, and independent from, the metabolic acidosis. For instance in the same patient, if the Pa_{CO_2} were reduced by 24 to 16 mm Hg ($40 - 24 = 16$), the pH would be $H^+ = 24 \times 16/10 = 38.4 = pH\ 7.42$. This degree of compensation is beyond what would normally occur from the metabolic acidosis alone (a decrease of 24 in the Pa_{CO_2} being well beyond the 14 mEq decrease in HCO_3). Although the pH is normal, this case represents a *primary* respiratory alkalosis in addition to the primary metabolic acidosis. An example of this may be the patient with a salicylate overdose, where a primary metabolic acidosis is accompanied by central stimulation of the ventilatory center. Therefore, a simple clue to the presence of two primary disorders is the presence of a normal or near normal pH, since:

- Compensation is meant to limit changes in pH but never provides a normalization of pH, and a normal pH in the presence of an abnormal HCO_3 or Pa_{CO_2} always indicates two primary acid-base disorders.

Similarly, in metabolic acidosis the Pa_{CO_2} may not be decreased enough for the level of HCO_3, resulting in an inadequate or incomplete compensation. For example, if the Pa_{CO_2} in the above metabolic acidosis were to compensate by only 4, to 36 ($40 - 4 = 36$), the resultant pH would be $H^+ = 24 \times 36/10 = 86.4 = pH\ 7.06$. This is only mildly better than the totally uncompensated pH

of 7.02 that we saw when the Pa_{CO_2} remained at 40. This may occur, for example, in a patient with a metabolic acidosis from diarrhea and an inadequate ventilatory response from narcotics. Finally, a patient with a metabolic acidosis may have an elevated Pa_{CO_2}. This may occur, for example, in a patient with chronic obstructive pulmonary disease (COPD) and lactic acidosis. If the same metabolic acidosis were accompanied by CO_2 retention (a primary respiratory acidosis) and a Pa_{CO_2} of 50 mm Hg, the pH would be $H^+ = 24 \times 50/10 = 120 = pH\ 6.92$. This indicates that:

- Acidemia and alkalemia are most severe when two primary disorders, that are both either acidotic or alkalotic, exist at the same time.

These examples are meant to demonstrate that the direction and the degree of change of the compensatory response are equally important when evaluating an acid-base disorder.

In a metabolic alkalosis, a decrease in the minute ventilation will attenuate changes in pH by increasing the Pa_{CO_2}. In a metabolic alkalosis, the Pa_{CO_2} should increase by 0.7 mm Hg (from the normal 40 mm Hg) for every 1.0 mEq/L increase in the HCO_3 (from the normal value of 24 mEq/L). For example, if a patient developed a metabolic alkalosis with the HCO_3 increasing by 10 mEq/L to 34 mEq/L, and no compensation were to occur, the pH would be $H^+ = 24 \times 40/34 = 28.2 = pH\ 7.56$. On the other hand, CO_2 retention will occur within hours, and the appropriate Pa_{CO_2} should be 47 mm Hg ($10 \times .7 = 7$, $40 + 7 = 47$). The appropriately compensated pH will be considerably lower at $H^+ = 24 \times 47/34 = 7.48$.

The compensation for each of the respiratory disorders involves two steps, one dependent and one independent of kidney function. The independent response is an immediate reaction that occurs within minutes of a change in Pa_{CO_2}. In acute respiratory acidosis, immediately after an increase in the Pa_{CO_2}, the reaction:

- $H_2O + CO_2 \longleftrightarrow H_2CO_3 \longleftrightarrow H^+ + HCO_3^-$

results in an enhanced production of H^+ and HCO_3. The H^+ produced in this reaction can be buffered by cellular proteins, leaving the HCO_3 to increase in the blood. This acute compensation does not increase the HCO_3 significantly, raising it by only 0.1 mEq/L for every 1.0 mm Hg increase in the $Paco_2$. For instance, if the $Paco_2$ were to acutely rise by 20 mm Hg from 40 to 60, the HCO_3 would acutely increase by 2 mEq/L. The resultant pH would be $H^+ = 24 \times 60/26 = 55.3 = pH\ 7.26$. This pH is only slightly less acidic than if this process did not occur and the HCO_3 remained at 24 mEq/L: $H^+ = 24 \times 60/24 = 60 = pH\ 7.22$.

The compensation for chronic respiratory acidosis is performed by the kidney. This involves an increase in NH_4^+ excretion (Task #2), which results in formation of new HCO_3 that enters the blood. There is also an enhancement of HCO_3 reabsorption (Task #1). This response is usually complete by 4 days and results in an increase in the HCO_3 of 0.4 mEq/L for every 1.0 mm Hg increase in the $Paco_2$. Therefore, in the patient with a chronic CO_2 retention to 60 mm Hg, renal compensation will increase the HCO_3 by 8 mEq/L to 32, and the new steady-state pH would be $H^+ = 24 \times 60/32 = 45 = pH\ 7.35$, a marked improvement over the uncompensated pH of 7.22 and the acutely compensated pH of 7.26 (above).

The acute compensation for a respiratory alkalosis also results from a renal-independent mechanism, but in this case produces a reduction in the HCO_3. This process will immediately decrease the HCO_3 by 0.2 mEq/L for every 1.0 mm Hg decrease in the $Paco_2$. Similar to the compensation for an acute respiratory acidosis, this has a minimal influence on pH. The mechanism of this response is secondary to the release of H^+ from nonbicarbonate buffers and is essentially the opposite of that which occurs in the reaction that is responsible for the acute change in pH for acute respiratory acidosis (see above).

In a chronic respiratory alkalosis, the HCO_3 will decrease by 0.5 mEq/L for every 1.0 mm Hg decrease in the $Paco_2$. This response is secondary to a decrease in the renal tubular reabsorption of HCO_3 and a decrease in the renal tubular excretion of NH_4^+. This compensation is usually complete within 3 days of the onset of the respiratory alkalosis. The response to this reduction in the HCO_3 results in a less alkalotic pH. For instance, if

a primary respiratory alkalosis were to lower the $Paco_2$ to 20 mm Hg from the normal of 40 mm Hg, the expected chronic compensation would lower the HCO_3 by 10 mEq/L from its normal level of 24 to 14. This would produce a pH of $H^+ = 24 \times 20/14 = 34.2 = pH\ 7.47$. This is considerably lower than if the HCO_3 remained at 24 mEq/L: $H^+ = 24 \times 20/24 = 20 = pH\ 7.70$.

QUESTION 5 What are the causes of a metabolic acidosis, and what is the usefulness of the anion gap in the differential diagnosis?

A metabolic acidosis can develop when the rate of an acid load (that utilized HCO_3), or the actual loss of HCO_3 from the body (from renal or gastrointestinal disease), is greater than the renal rate of HCO_3 generation. We should not develop a metabolic acidosis from daily metabolic processes since the distal tubule regenerates the HCO_3 that is utilized in normal metabolism at the same rate that it is consumed (unless a distal RTA is present). Although increases in dietary protein intake and catabolic states can increase the daily production of hydrogen ions several fold, this is not sufficient to cause an acidosis in the presence of intact kidney function. Therefore, it usually takes a greater and more acute acid load than that seen with normal metabolic processes to see a reduction in the HCO_3 concentration. This is usually the result of either a lactic acidosis, a ketoacidosis, or the production of an acid as the result of ingestion of a toxin.

A metabolic acidosis can also occur with a loss of bicarbonate from the body. If the HCO_3 loss is secondary to a proximal RTA, then the primary problem is renal, and the kidney cannot correct this condition. If the bicarbonate loss is from the gastrointestinal tract, the kidney can help by increasing HCO_3 generation. Therefore, for gastrointestinal bicarbonate loss to cause a metabolic acidosis, the rate of loss must exceed the kidney's ability to generate HCO_3.

Depending on the process that is responsible for the metabolic acidosis, an increase in the anion gap: $Na - (Cl + HCO_3)$ (normal = 12) may or may not be present. The anion gap is a useful tool in distinguishing the etiology of a metabolic acidosis. Electrical neutrality exists in our blood; all positive charges are accompanied by negative charges. If we measured all charged particles in the blood, there would be no anion gap. An anion gap (AG) exists because the normal amount of the cation that is used in the equation, sodium, is in a greater concentration than the addition of the anions that we use, chloride and bicarbonate. If we add the cations potassium, calcium and immunoglobulins to the equation, the anion gap increases. On the other hand, if we add the anions albumin, phosphates and sulfates, the anion gap decreases or may even be negative (a "cation gap"). The usefulness of the anion gap is that it allows the estimation of the level of nonchloride and nonbicarbonate anions, that if elevated may indicate the presence of the products of a metabolic acidosis. For instance, if a patient develops a lactic acidosis, the lactic acid is buffered by the following reaction:

• Lactic acid + $NaHCO_3 \rightarrow$ Na-lactate + H_2CO_3

From this reaction it can be seen that for each mEq of lactic acid/L produced, the HCO_3 will decrease 1 mEq/L. The Na stays the same since it is still there as Na lactate; the chloride is also unaffected by this reaction. Since the Na and Cl are unchanged, and the HCO_3 decreases by one, the anion gap must increase by one. If the patient makes 10 mEq/L of lactic acid, the HCO_3 will fall by 10 mEq/L (from 24 to 14), and the anion gap will increase by 10 (from 12 to 22). Therefore, an elevated anion gap may indicate the presence of nonchloride and nonbicarbonate anions that are responsible for a metabolic acidosis. These are usually the result of the reaction of $NaHCO_3$ with either lactic acid, beta-hydroxybutyric acid, acetoacetic acid, formic acid, or oxalic acid, etc. The increased portion of the anion gap therefore represents the sodium salt of the acid (e.g., sodium lactate, sodium acetoacetate, sodium betahydroxybutyrate). Although this reaction is not universally one to one, a good rule of thumb is:

• In an anion gap acidosis, the change (decrease) in the HCO_3 concentration (ΔHCO_3) should approximate the change (increase) in the anion gap (ΔAG),

where:

(The ΔHCO_3) = (24 – the patient's HCO_3), and

(the ΔAG) = (the patient's AG – 12)

In a severe metabolic acidosis, some of the hydrogen ions may be buffered by intracellular nonbicarbonate buffers. The use of these nonbicarbonate buffers will spare some of the HCO_3, and the HCO_3 will not decrease as low as it would without this process. The acids that are utilizing these buffers are still present, and therefore the degree of elevation in the anion gap (ΔAG) will not change. However, when this occurs, the ΔAG will be greater than the ΔHCO_3.

A metabolic alkalosis can coexist with a metabolic acidosis. Although this concept is often difficult to grasp, consider the following scenario. A patient develops a metabolic acidosis secondary to vomiting caused by a gastric ulcer. The patient has an alkalemic pH (7.50) and an increase in the HCO_3 concentration to 34 mEq/L. The patient also has a respiratory compensation with a Pa_{CO_2} elevation to 45 mm Hg: $H^+ = 24 \times 45/34 = 32 = pH$ 7.50. The patient's sodium is 140 mEq/L, the chloride is 94 mEq/L, and the bicarbonate 34 mEq/L giving a normal anion gap of 12. The patient then develops an acute upper gastrointestinal bleed, goes into shock, and develops an acute lactic acidosis, producing 10 mEq/L of lactic acid. The lactic acid is buffered by the patient's $NaHCO_3$, 1 mEq of lactate utilizing 1 mEq of $NaHCO_3$. But instead of starting with a normal HCO_3 concentration of 24 mEq/L, this patient starts with a HCO_3 of 34 mEq/L. Therefore the HCO_3 does not drop from 24 to 14 (24 – 10 = 14); it drops from 34 to 24 (34 – 10 = 24). The two metabolic disorders have essentially canceled each other out. The patient no longer has an elevated HCO_3, and therefore the Pa_{CO_2} returns to a normal level (40 mm Hg). The patient's acid-base status is now $H^+ = 24 \times 40/24 = 40 = pH$ 7.40. The pH, HCO_3, and the Pa_{CO_2} are all within normal limits and would suggest that there are no acid-base abnormalities, yet the patient is quite ill with a severe lactic acidosis. Since the HCO_3 concentration fell by 10 mEq/L by the production of 10 mEq/L of lactic acid, the anion gap should increase by 10 to 22. With the patient's sodium remaining at 140 mEq/L, the chloride at 94 mEq/L, and the bicarbonate decreasing to 24 mEq/L, the anion gap is 22. The only clue to the presence of the metabolic acidosis is this elevation in the anion gap. Therefore:

- A simultaneous metabolic acidosis and metabolic alkalosis can occur which can result in a normal-appearing blood gas. To completely rule out an acid-base abnormality, the patient must have a normal blood gas, HCO_3, $Paco_2$, and a normal anion gap.

In the previous example, the degree of the primary metabolic acidosis was created to cancel out the primary metabolic alkalosis, resulting in a normal pH. The severity of each of these two simultaneous primary disorders may not be equal, and therefore the pH may not be normal. In fact, any degree of primary metabolic alkalosis may coexist with any degree of primary metabolic acidosis, resulting in an acidemic, alkalotic, or normal pH. For instance, in the above example the patient produced 10 mEq/L of lactic acid, reducing the HCO_3 from 34 to 24 mEq/L. If the patient had produced only 6 mEq/L of lactic acid, the HCO_3 would have dropped from 34 to 28 mEq/L, and the patient would still have an alkalemic pH despite the presence of the metabolic acidosis. On the other hand, the patient could have produced 14 mEq/L of lactic acid, which would have reduced the HCO_3 from 34 to 20 mEq/L, and the patient would become acidemic (despite the presence of the metabolic alkalosis). All three of these examples (lactic acid production of 6, 10, and 14 mEq/L in the presence of a patient with a primary metabolic alkalosis) represent simultaneous primary metabolic acidosis and alkalosis, although one is alkalemic, one acidemic, and one has a normal pH. This becomes tricky to evaluate. However, the presence of the two simultaneous disorders can be determined by comparing the degree of elevation in the anion gap (Δ AG) to the degree of the reduction in the level of HCO_3 (ΔHCO_3). If a metabolic alkalosis is present at the time of the development of the anion gap metabolic acidosis, the HCO_3 will not be as low as would be predicted from the degree of elevation in the anion gap. This will reflect in a change in the anion gap from a normal value of 12 (Δ AG) that

is greater than the change in the HCO_3 from the normal value of 24 mEq/L (ΔHCO_3). Since this can also occur as a result of some of an acid load being buffered by intracellular buffers (see above), a Δ AG that is greater than the ΔHCO_3 does not always indicate a simultaneous metabolic acidosis and metabolic alkalosis. However, if this discrepancy is large, with the Δ AG $\geq 1.5 \times \Delta HCO_3$, this may be a clue that these two metabolic primary disorders are simultaneously present:

- A Δ AG that is $>1.5 \times$ the ΔHCO_3 indicates a simultaneous metabolic acidosis and metabolic alkalosis, where:
  (The ΔHCO_3 = (24 − the patient's HCO_3), and
  (the Δ AG) = (the patient's AG − 12)

If the final HCO_3 is acidotic (<24 mEq/L), the patient has a hidden primary metabolic alkalosis, and if the final HCO_3 is alkalotic (>24 mEq/L), the patient has a hidden primary metabolic acidosis. When a metabolic acidosis and alkalosis coexist, the expected respiratory response depends on the final HCO_3 concentration, just as though only one primary disorder were present. If the net effect of the two disorders results in an abnormally high level of HCO_3 (>24 mEq/L), the $Paco_2$ should compensate by an appropriate elevation. If the net effect of these two disorders results in a depressed level of HCO_3 (<24 mEq/L), the $Paco_2$ should be depressed. The degree of the respiratory compensatory response is the same whether or not one or two primary metabolic disorders are present and is determined by the final HCO_3 concentration by the amounts provided in Table 9-3-3.

When the respiratory compensation is not close to what would be predicted, a primary respiratory acid-base disorder is also present, and these are termed *triple acid base disorders*. These occur when a simultaneous metabolic acidosis and alkalosis are accompanied by either a primary respiratory acidosis or alkalosis. For instance, consider the above example of the vomiting alkalemic patient who develops a gastrointestinal bleed, shock, and lactic acidosis, where the lactic acidosis at 10 mEq/L exactly cancels out the alkalosis (final HCO_3 of 24 mEq/L). If that patient hyperventilates because of being in shock and acquires a $Paco_2$ of 30 mm Hg, the final pH would be $H^+ = 24 \times 30/24 = 30 =$ pH 7.52. This patient has the triple acid-base disorder of a metabolic acidosis, metabolic alkalosis, and a respiratory alkalosis. The arterial blood gas by itself would demonstrate only an uncompensated respiratory alkalosis. The presence of the Δ AG (10) being greater than the ΔHCO_3 (0) indicates the presence of the other two primary metabolic disorders.

The determination of a simultaneous metabolic acidosis and metabolic alkalosis requires an increased anion gap. It is possible to have a simultaneous metabolic alkalosis and nonanion gap acidosis, but it cannot be diagnosed by any of these laboratory values since they will all be normal. Since a respiratory acidosis and alkalosis cannot also coexist, quadruple acid-base disorders are impossible.

The major causes of an increased anion gap acidosis are listed in the box. In practice, the majority of the cases are due to either lactic acidosis, ketoacidosis, or renal failure. Much less common are the acidoses related to the ingestion of a substance that result in the production of large quantities of an acid (e.g., salicylate intoxication) and methanol or ethylene glycol ingestion. These latter three acidoses should not occur in the hospital setting and therefore are diagnoses that are more likely to be encountered in the emergency room. Methanol and ethylene glycol ingestion should always be considered in the alcoholic patient with an elevated anion gap acidosis, although that patient is also at risk for lactic acidosis and alcoholic ketoacidosis. Methanol and ethylene glycol blood levels are not usually readily available, and therefore the emergency room physician must have a high index of suspicion for these disorders since delay in diagnosis can have grave consequences. A clue to the ingestion of ethylene glycol is the presence of oxalate crystals in the urine, since this is a final breakdown product of this toxin.

Another clue to the ingestion of these substances is the presence of an elevated osmolal gap. The patient's serum osmolality can be estimated (ESO) using the following equation: ESO = (Na $\times$ 2) + ([BUN, in mg/dl]/2.8) + ([blood glu-

CAUSES OF ANION GAP AND NONANION GAP METABOLIC ACIDOSES

ANION GAP INCREASED
- Lactic acidosis
- Ketoacidosis
  - Diabetic
  - Alcoholic
  - Starvation
- Methyl alcohol ingestion
- Ethylene glycol ingestion
- Salicylate intoxication
- Renal failure

ANION GAP NORMAL
- Bicarbonate loss
  - Gastrointestinal losses
    - Diarrhea
    - Pancreatic, biliary, or intestinal fistulae
    - Ileal conduit
  - Proximal RT
- Distal RTA
- Administration of hydrochloric acid
  - HCl
  - Ammonium chloride

cose in mg/dl]/18). The patient's serum osmolality can be easily measured (MSO) by the laboratory, and should be done by the method of freeze point depression to determine the presence of any alcohols. The osmolal gap is equal to [MSO − ESO]. An elevation in the osmolal gap indicates the presence of large amounts of an unaccounted osmotically active molecule. In the presence of an elevated anion gap acidosis, an elevated osmolal gap of greater than 25 serves as a clue to the presence of an ingestion-related metabolic acidosis (methanol or ethylene glycol).

- An osmolal gap should be determined in patients presenting to the emergency room setting with an increased anion gap acidosis where another cause is not immediately apparent.

The most common cause of an elevation in the osmolal gap is the ingestion of ethanol, and therefore an ethanol level should accompany the determination of the serum osmolality. In addition, an elevation in the osmolal gap has been reported in renal failure, lactic acidosis, and ketoacidosis. Since these acidoses are also associated with an elevated anion gap, this would seem to limit the usefulness of the osmolal gap in the differential diagnosis of an increased anion gap acidosis. However, these conditions should not raise the osmolal gap above 25. Therefore, if one uses this cut off level, the osmolal gap can be a useful screen for methanol and ethylene glycol intoxications.

The other major subset of metabolic acidoses are those accompanied by a normal anion gap, also called "nonanion gap metabolic acidoses." The causes of these disorders are relatively straightforward. The most common cause is secondary to loss of HCO_3 from the body through either renal or gastrointestinal losses. The renal loss of HCO_3 secondary to a proximal RTA was discussed in Task #1. Administration of the carbonic anhydrase inhibitor acetazolamide essentially induces an iatrogenic proximal RTA and will produce a nonanion gap acidosis. Gastrointestinal losses of HCO_3 can result in a metabolic acidosis if the degree of loss is greater than the kidney's ability to increase HCO_3 generation. In both of the situations of gastrointestinal and renal loss of HCO_3, there is not an increase in the production of acid, and since the acid related anions, NaA, that are produced in the reaction: $HA + NaHCO_3 \rightarrow NaA + H_2CO_3$, are easily excreted, the anion gap does not increase. In a distal RTA, bicarbonate is not lost from the body, but the level of $[HCO_3]$ falls progressively since regeneration does not keep up with utilization. Again, the NaA-related anions are not retained in patients with a distal RTA, and the anion gap remains normal.

The loss of bicarbonate can occur at many levels of the gastrointestinal tract including small intestinal, pancreatic, and biliary drainage. In addition, if urine is diverted into the bowel through either a fistula or a surgically created ileal conduit, the chloride of the urine is exchanged for HCO_3 by the intestinal mucosa and is excreted in the "stool" (in the presence of a fistula) or in the urine (in the presence of a conduit).

Finally, a rare cause of nonanion gap acidosis is the ingestion of either hydrochloric acid or ammonium hydrochloride (the latter being the metabolic equivalent of hydrochloric acid). In both of these conditions the hydrochloric acid is buffered by $NaHCO_3$:

- $HCl + NaHCO_3 \rightarrow NaCl$ and H_2CO_3

Since the anion of the acid is chloride, and since it is still present and measured, the anion gap does not increase. The nonanion gap acidoses are summarized in the box.

An anion gap acidosis and a nonanion gap acidosis can also occur simultaneously. This could be the case in a patient with diarrhea and diabetic ketoacidosis. For example, with the HCO_3 loss associated with diarrhea, the HCO_3 could fall to 16 mEq/L, a ΔHCO_3 of 8 ($24 - 16 = 8$), but with a normal anion gap of 12. If the patient then develops diabetic ketoacidosis and produces 8 mEq/L of acetoacetic acid, the HCO_3 decreases another 8 mEq/L to 8 ($16 - 8 = 8$) with an increase in the anion gap by 8 to 20 ($12 + 8 = 20$). The patient now has a severe acidosis and has an elevated anion gap. However, the 16 mEq/L fall in the level of HCO_3 ($\Delta HCO_3 = 24 - 8 = 16$) is twice the increase of 8 in the anion gap ($\Delta AG = 20 - 12 = 8$). Therefore:

- A ΔHCO_3 that is greater than the ΔAG indicates a simultaneous anion gap and nonanion gap metabolic acidosis, where:
  (the ΔHCO_3 = (24 – the patient's HCO_3), and
  (the ΔAG) = (the patient's AG – 12)

QUESTION 6 What is an approach to the determination of a patient's acid-base status?

This is best accomplished by a set of rules. Most patients will have a simple primary acid-base disorder with an appropriate compensatory response. The evaluation of these disorders should be relatively straightforward. However, many patients will have 2 or 3 primary acid-base disorders.

These cases can be very confusing if not approached systematically. It must be appreciated that the evaluation of a patient's acid-base status must include the pH, the HCO_3, the $PaCO_2$, and the anion gap. If any of these are left out, evaluation becomes incomplete. It is best to start with the pH. This method should identify most acid-base disorders. Although small (2 to 3) increases or decreases in the $PaCO_2$, HCO_3, or anion gap may represent a mild acid-base disorder, abnormalities of such a minor degree may be within the margin of error of the measurement of these factors. Therefore, caution must be taken not to overestimate the clinical significance of these mild abnormalities.

1. From the pH, determine if an acidemia or alkalemia exists.
   a. If the pH is abnormal, determine the primary disorder(s): Is an abnormal HCO_3 or Pa_{CO_2}, (or both) responsible for the abnormality in pH? If only one abnormality is responsible, define the disorder and go to #2. If two primary abnormalities are responsible, define them and skip to #3.
   b. If the pH is normal, look at the HCO_3 and the Pa_{CO_2}. Remember that a normal pH does not rule out an acid base-disorder if two primary disorders cancel each other out (e.g., a metabolic acidosis and a respiratory alkalosis or a metabolic alkalosis and a respiratory acidosis). If two primary disorders are found with a normal pH, skip to #3.
   c. If the pH, the HCO_3, and the Pa_{CO_2} are all normal, skip to #3.
2. Determine if an appropriate compensation is occurring.
   a. The direction of change in the Pa_{CO_2} to compensate for metabolic disorders and the direction of change in the HCO_3 to compensate for respiratory disorders should be in the same direction as the increase or decrease of the HCO_3 or Pa_{CO_2} of the primary disorder.
   b. Determine if the degree of compensation is appropriate for the disorder (Table 9-3-2).

3. Calculate the anion gap.
   a. If normal, no other acid base abnormalities exist.
   b. If elevated, a primary metabolic acidosis is usually present, even if the HCO_3 is not depressed.
   c. If elevated and the HCO_3 is elevated, a hidden primary metabolic acidosis is present in addition to the primary metabolic alkalosis.
   d. If elevated and the HCO_3 is normal, a hidden primary metabolic alkalosis and a hidden primary metabolic acidosis are present.
   e. If elevated and the HCO_3 is depressed, compare the ΔHCO_3 to the ΔAG:
   f. If the ΔAG is > $1.5 \Delta HCO_3$, a hidden primary metabolic alkalosis is present in addition to the primary metabolic acidosis. If the ΔHCO_3 is > the ΔAG, the metabolic acidosis is a mixed anion/nonanion gap acidosis.

This approach is summarized in Fig. 9-3-1 on p. 555.

QUESTION 7 How are these disorders treated?

Once an acid-base disorder is identified, treatment should be aimed at reversing the primary disease condition. The treatment of the numerous acid-base disorders is beyond the scope of this chapter. However, there are some general considerations for the treatment of metabolic acidosis that will be discussed.

The first relates to the primary disease process. For instance, when one uses the example of diabetic ketoacidosis, there are issues of volume replacement, insulin administration, potassium and phosphorus balance, in addition to evaluating the cause of the ketoacidosis (infection, etc.).

The second issue relates to an understanding of the fate of organic acids, such as the keto acids and lactic acid, after they have been buffered by $NaHCO_3$. Their potential effect on systemic pH is significantly attenuated by their reaction with $NaHCO_3$. Using lactic acidosis as an example:

- Lactic acid + $NaHCO_3 \rightarrow$ Na Lactate + H_2CO_3

As long as lactic acid continues to be produced, this equation will deplete the stores of $NaHCO_3$, and a metabolic acidosis will be present. If the process that caused the lactic acidosis ceases, the regeneration of $NaHCO_3$ can begin to replete the bicarbonate stores. This occurs by two mechanisms. First, the sodium lactate produced by this reaction can undergo oxidative metabolism to produce bicarbonate by the following reaction:

- Na lactate + 3 $O_2 \rightarrow$ 2 CO_2 + 2 H_2O + $NaHCO_3$

If sodium lactate is not lost in the urine, then the HCO_3 stores can be completely repleted just by this conversion of sodium lactate back to HCO_3. This is the case in a seizure, where an acute and finite lactic acidosis will result in a rapid anion gap metabolic acidosis, which can reverse within minutes of the end of the seizure. Therefore, if $NaHCO_3$ were administered to that patient, the patient would eventually have an excess of HCO_3 and develop a metabolic alkalosis after the complete oxidative metabolism of the sodium lactate. Most lactic acidosis states do not reverse as rapidly as does a seizure, and therefore an extremely low pH may mandate the administration of $NaHCO_3$. If these patients recover and had received large amounts of $NaHCO_3$, they are at risk of developing a metabolic alkalosis.

The regeneration of HCO_3 by oxidative metabolism also occurs with the metabolic end-products of other organic acidoses, including ketoacidosis. Therefore, the metabolism of each mEq of Na-acetoacetate and Na-betahydroxybutyrate can also yield 1 mEq of $NaHCO_3$. These oxidative reactions occur very quickly and can result in rapid repletions of the HCO_3 to normal levels. In diabetic ketoacidosis, this can only occur after the production of the acids has slowed or ceased, which can be expected with appropriate insulin therapy. The degree to which the HCO_3 level can be increased by this process depends entirely upon the available amount of Na-acetoacetate and Na-betahydroxybutyrate. This in turn depends upon the amount of these anions that has been lost in the urine, and since high

intravenous fluid rates are often recommended as an integral part of the therapy of diabetic ketoacidosis, urinary losses of these anions can be substantial. This has led to the recommendation that intravenous fluid rates should be dictated by a patient's volume status as opposed to a preset "cookbook" rate, since patients receiving less fluid during the course of treatment have a more rapid rise in their HCO_3 levels than those receiving higher rates.

The other means by which $NaHCO_3$ is regenerated after an acid load is through the kidney. In the setting of a metabolic acidosis with acidemia, the distal tubule will increase its excretion of NH_4^+, resulting in HCO_3 regeneration to the blood (see Task #2). This is a relatively slow process, and it may take days to completely replenish a significantly depleted HCO_3 pool. In the setting of renal failure, this process may be severely limited, and an exogenous source of HCO_3 is even more likely to be necessary. This alkali therapy could be through the direct administration of $NaHCO_3$, or through an indirect source that results in the production of $NaHCO_3$ (e.g., Na citrate, Na acetate, or Na lactate).

The third issue in the treatment of a patient with an acid-base disorder relates to whether or not the pH needs to be acutely treated with sodium bicarbonate or another source of base. As was just presented, some patients may be able to correct their acidosis fairly rapidly by the oxidative metabolism of their anions and therefore do not need any exogenous source of base. Except in the case of a seizure, this may be difficult to predict in a given patient. Since severe acidemia may result in impaired myocardial function and vasodilatation, hypotension may occur. Patients are also at increased risk of cardiac arrhythmias. Therefore, certain patients may benefit from a maneuver that will rapidly increase the systemic pH. These deleterious effects of severe acidosis are most prominent when the pH falls below 7.20, and this level of pH may serve as a reasonable therapeutic end point. However, there is controversy about the efficacy and safety of giving

NaHCO$_3$ to patients with various metabolic acidoses. Because of the reaction:

$$\bullet \; HA + NaHCO_3 \rightarrow NaA + H_2CO_3 \rightarrow H_2O + CO_2$$

whenever an acid load is acutely buffered by NaHCO$_3$, CO$_2$ production acutely increases. As long as pulmonary function is intact, the lungs will rapidly excrete the CO$_2$, and the Pa$_{CO_2}$ does not necessarily increase. Nevertheless, an increase in the Pa$_{CO_2}$ is a risk of the treatment with NaHCO$_3$.

Also related to this acute increase in the Pa$_{CO_2}$ is the risk of paradoxically decreasing the pH of the central nervous system. When NaHCO$_3$ is administered, the systemic HCO$_3$ and pH both increase. There is a lag time for the HCO$_3$ to cross the blood-brain barrier, and therefore the central nervous system pH does not increase as rapidly. Also after the administration of NaHCO$_3$, some of the CO$_2$ produced diffuses easily into the cerebral spinal fluid. This acute increase in central nervous system CO$_2$ and lag in the increase in HCO$_3$ increases the ratio of CO$_2$ to HCO$_3$ and may lead to a paradoxical decrease in central nervous system pH, (despite a maneuver that was meant to increase it). A decrease in sensorium has been reported in patients after receiving NaHCO$_3$ for severe metabolic acidosis, but these reports are rare.

Ventilation, from an acid-base standpoint, is driven by the pH of the central nervous system. Since there is a lag time for the HCO$_3$ to cross the blood brain barrier after a NaHCO$_3$ load, the patient may continue to hyperventilate for several hours after the systemic HCO$_3$ and pH have increased. The persistently lowered Pa$_{CO_2}$ from this continued hyperventilation, in conjunction with an increased HCO$_3$, puts the patient at risk for an alkalemia. This overshoot alkalosis is yet another argument against the administration of NaHCO$_3$ to the acidotic patient.

The patient with a severe metabolic acidosis may require large quantities of NaHCO$_3$. Most intravenous preparations of NaHCO$_3$ are produced at a concentration of 1.0 mEq/ml. This solution has a sodium concentration of 1000 mEq/L and an osmolarity of 2000 mosm/L. Administration of large amounts of these solutions can therefore lead to hypernatremia and fluid overload, and patients must be followed carefully for the development of these complications.

Finally, there appears to be a negative feedback mechanism with the level of HCO$_3$ and the production of lactic and keto acids with acidemia slowing the production of these acids. Therefore, alkali loading could actually increase their production and perpetuate the acidosis.

These arguments against the use of NaHCO$_3$ in the severely acidotic patient (pH < 7.2) cannot be considered without an appreciation of the untoward effects of severe acidemia. Most of these concerns, although related to predictable biochemical and physiologic events, have been exaggerated as a cause of patient morbidity. Therefore it is the opinion of this author, that in most circumstances, the benefits of the judicious use of exogenous alkali for patients with severe metabolic acidemia greatly outweigh the potential risks.

The decision of whether or not to administer NaHCO$_3$ should be determined by the pH, although not all equivalent pH values carry the same risk to the patient. For instance, a pH of 7.20 can accompany a number of combinations of HCO$_3$ and Pa$_{CO_2}$:

pH	HCO$_3$	Pa$_{CO_2}$
7.20	20	53
7.20	15	39
7.20	10	26
7.20	5	13

Now let us assume that the HCO$_3$ falls, in each case, by another 2 meq/L, and that the Pa$_{CO_2}$ cannot be lowered further:

pH	HCO$_3$	Pa$_{CO_2}$	Δ pH
7.15	18	53	0.05
7.14	13	39	0.06
7.11	8	26	0.09
6.98	3	13	0.22

The patient with the lower initial HCO$_3$ is going to have a greater reduction in pH (Δ pH) given the same acid load than the patient with the higher initial HCO$_3$, despite having the same pH at the time of the acid load.

The same is true of small increases in the Pa$_{CO_2}$.

Let us assume that a patient begins to tire and cannot maintain his/her minute ventilation which results in an increase in the $Paco_2$ of 5 mm Hg. Although the HCO_3 would increase by 0.5 mEq/L as a direct result of the acute increase in $Paco_2$ (Table 9-3-3), this is negligible, and for the example we will maintain the HCO_3 at the prior levels:

pH	HCO_3	$Paco_2$	Δ pH
7.16	20	58	0.04
7.16	15	44	0.04
7.13	10	31	0.07
7.06	5	18	0.14

This indicates that the patient with the lower initial $Paco_2$ is going to have a greater reduction in pH given any CO_2 retention than the patient with the higher initial $Paco_2$, despite having the same initial pH.

Finally, let us look at what happens to the patient if both a 2 mEq/L decrease in the HCO_3 and a 5 mm Hg increase in the $Paco_2$ occur simultaneously:

pH	HCO_3	$Paco_2$	Δ pH
7.12	18	58	0.08
7.09	13	44	0.11
7.03	8	31	0.17
6.84	3	18	0.36

These examples are meant to demonstrate that it is not just the pH that should be considered when making a decision on treating an acidemia with $NaHCO_3$. Acidemic patients at the extremes of reductions in HCO_3 and $Paco_2$ are at great risk of severe depressions in pH with only mild further changes in these values. In addition, these examples can be reversed to see that it would take only a small increase in the HCO_3 to markedly increase the pH in the patients with the lowest HCO_3. Therefore, in the patient in whom the greatest need for $NaHCO_3$ therapy is present, the amount needed to improve the pH is the least.

QUESTION 8 How much $NaHCO_3$ needs to be given to correct an acidemia?

In the setting of a severe metabolic acidosis with a pH < 7.20, alkali therapy with $NaHCO_3$ may be advisable. In a patient with normal respiratory compensation, this level of acidemia (pH < 7.20) will not occur unless the HCO_3 is < 10 mEq/L. As was pointed out in the above examples, when the HCO_3 falls below 10 mEq/L, small further decreases in the HCO_3 will result in large reductions in the pH. On the other hand, small increases in the HCO_3 can improve the pH considerably. This may require an increase in the HCO_3 of only 2 to 4 mEq/L, and may serve as a general goal in the acidemic patient with a HCO_3 < 10 mEq/L. It would be undesirable to increase the HCO_3 to a normal level since an overshoot alkalosis is likely to occur.

By using Table 9-3-1 and the equation $H^+ = 24\ Paco_2/HCO_3$, a simple calculation can be made to determine the level of HCO_3 that will produce a safer level of pH. The $\Delta\ HCO_3$ is the patient's actual HCO_3 subtracted from the higher desired HCO_3. When the desired $\Delta\ HCO_3$ (in mEq/L) is multiplied by the volume of distribution of HCO_3 (in liters), the milliequivalent amount of $NaHCO_3$ needed to achieve the $\Delta\ HCO_3$ is obtained. The volume of distribution of HCO_3 has been estimated to be as low as 40% of the body weight in patients with a mild metabolic acidosis, to 80% of the total body weight in patients with severe metabolic acidosis. A reasonable guide is to use 60% of the body weight, which also approximates the total body water.

For example, let us assume that a 70 kg patient has a metabolic acidosis with a pH of 7.06 ($H^+ = 87$), a HCO_3 of 6 mEq/L, and a $Paco_2$ of 22 mm Hg. If we wanted to increase the pH to the safer level of 7.24, the new H^+ associated with this pH would be 58 (see Table 9-3-1). If we assume that the $Paco_2$ remains constant, the HCO_3 associated with this improved pH would be: $H^+ = 24\ Paco_2/HCO_3$, $58 = 24 \times 22/HCO_3 = 9$ meq/L, or an increase in the HCO_3 of 3 mEq/L ($9 - 6 = 3$). The patient has an estimated volume of distribution of HCO_3 of 42 liters ($70 \times 0.6 = 42$). Therefore, 3 mEq/L $\times$ 42 L = 126 mEq of $NaHCO_3$, and this amount of $NaHCO_3$ would be expected to raise this patient's pH from 7.06 to 7.24. The $Paco_2$ may acutely rise as a result of the $NaHCO_3$ load.

This should not persist, but this transient elevation in $Paco_2$ will lower pH somewhat, and a greater amount of $NaHCO_3$ may be necessary to achieve the desired increase in pH. In addition, severely acidotic patients may have a volume of distribution of HCO_3 that is greater than 60% body weight and may similarly not have the expected response in pH. Nevertheless, this method can serve as a guide in the acidemic patient to estimate the quantity of $NaHCO_3$ that needs to be administered to achieve an expected increase in the HCO_3 and pH.

CASE DISCUSSION This case is meant to illustrate how important it is to fully explore a patient for hidden acid-base disorders. The history suggests many possibilities. The vomiting could lead to a metabolic alkalosis. The diarrhea could produce a nonanion gap acidosis. There are a number of potential anion gap acidoses. The patient is hypotensive and may have a lactic acidosis. The diabetes could produce a ketoacidosis. The history of alcoholism should make one consider alcoholic ketoacidosis and alcoholic lactic acidosis, in addition to the possibility of an ingestion of either methanol or ethylene glycol.

The pH is only mildly abnormal and by itself does not suggest the extent of the patient's illness. The pH at 7.44 defines a mild alkalemia. The next step is to find the cause of the elevated pH. The $Paco_2$ is depressed, and therefore this is a respiratory alkalosis. The next step is to see if a compensatory response is present and if so, is it at an appropriate level. The HCO_3 is depressed, representing the expected compensatory response. The actual level of HCO_3 is 18 mEq/L, a decrease from normal of 6 ($24 - 18 = 6$). For a respiratory alkalosis, the HCO_3 should decrease by a range of 0.2 mEq/L (acutely) to 0.5 mEq/L (chronically) for every 1.0 mm Hg decrease in the $Paco_2$. The $Paco_2$ in this case is 27, a decrease of 13 mm Hg from normal ($40 - 27 = 13$). Therefore, the expected range of decrease in the HCO_3 would be 0.2 to 0.5×13, or 2.6 to 6.5 mEq/L. The actual decrease in HCO_3 was 6.0 mEq/L, and therefore this appears to be a normal metabolic compensation to a chronic respiratory alkalosis, and this acid-base disorder would be defined as a simple primary respiratory alkalosis. Respiratory alkalosis can be seen in patients that are in severe pain, as is the case here.

However, the evaluation of an acid-base disorder does not end with the pH, HCO_3, $Paco_2$, and Table 9-3-3. The next step is to calculate the anion gap, and if elevated, to see if the amount of elevation (Δ AG) corresponds to the degree of depression in the level of HCO_3 (ΔHCO_3). The anion gap in this case is elevated at 28, ($136 - 90 - 18) = 28$. The elevated anion gap indicates that the depression in the HCO_3 at 18 mEq/L is not simply a compensation for the respiratory alkalosis. Its presence indicates that a *primary* metabolic acidosis is present in addition to the *primary* respiratory alkalosis. Because of the patient's alcoholic history and the possibility of ingestion of methanol or ethylene glycol, the serum osmolality was measured (306 mosm/kg). The estimated serum osmolality was 296 ($[136 \times 2] + [360/18] + [11/2.8]$). The osmolal gap therefore is only 10 ($306 - 296 = 10$) and made significant ingestions of these substances unlikely. The lactate level was normal. The patient was found to have an elevated level of beta-hydroxybutyric and acetoacetic acid in his blood, and therefore his primary metabolic acidosis was secondary to either diabetic or alcoholic ketoacidosis.

The normal anion gap is 12, and the patient's anion gap is 28, representing a Δ AG of 16. The patient's HCO_3 is 18 mEq/L, a reduction from normal (ΔHCO_3) of 6 ($24 - 18 = 6$). The Δ AG of 16 is considerably greater than the ΔHCO_3 of 6; this indicates that there is also a hidden *primary* metabolic alkalosis. This was caused by the patient's vomiting. The two primary metabolic disorders have essentially canceled each other out. The final acid-base diagnosis is a triple acid-base disorder, a primary respiratory alkalosis, a primary metabolic acidosis, and a primary metabolic alkalosis. The latter two would not have been appreciated if not for evaluation of the anion gap.

Since the pH in this case is not markedly abnormal, treatment should be directed at the primary disease states, and maneuvers that would result in acute changes in either the HCO_3 or the $Paco_2$ are not necessary.

• •

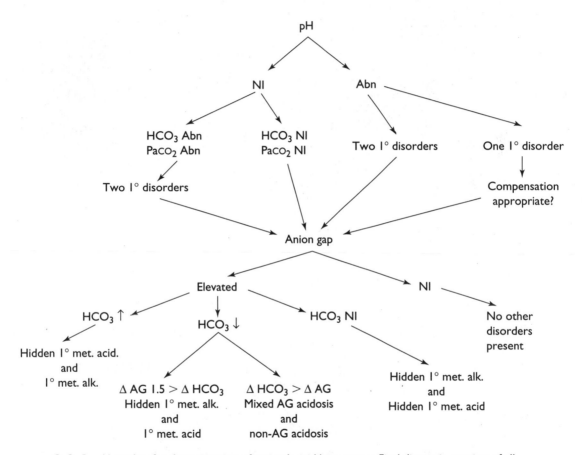

9-3-1   Algorithm for determination of patient's acid base status. Final diagnosis consists of all primary disorders determined as algorithm is completed. Abn, abnormal; NI, normal; 1°, primary; AG, anion gap.

APPENDIX I

The law of mass action:

- $H^+ = 24\ Pa_{CO_2}/HCO_3$

uses the partial pressure of carbon dioxide, the $PaCO_2$. The concentration of carbon dioxide can also be expressed as the concentration in its aqueous phase, or the amount that is dissolved in the blood, the CO_{2dis}. The two measurements are related by the equation:

- $[CO_2]_{dis} = 0.03 \times Pa_{CO_2}$.

Therefore, a variation of the law of mass action, using the CO_{2dis} is:

- $H^+ = 800\ CO_{2dis}/HCO_3$

From the equation:

- $HA + NaHCO_3 \rightarrow NaA + H_2CO_3 \rightarrow H_2O + CO_2$

the addition of 70 mEq of hydrogen ions to 42 L of total body water would decrease the HCO_3 by 1.7 meq/L (70/42 = 1.7). It would also increase the aqueous phase of CO_2, (CO_{2dis}), by 1.7 mmol/L.

From the equation:

- $CO_{2dis} = 0.03 \times Pa_{CO_2}$

a CO_{2dis} of 1.7 mmol/L is equal to a Pa_{CO_2} of 57 mm Hg (1.7/0.03 = 56.6). This, when added to the baseline Pa_{CO_2} of 40 mm Hg (if the CO_2 produced in this reaction were not excreted by the lungs) gives us the new Pa_{CO_2} of 97 mm Hg (40 + 57 = 97).

BIBLIOGRAPHY

Adrogue HJ, Barrero J, Eknoyan G: Salutary effects of modest fluid replacement in the treatment of adults with diabetic ketoacidosis, *JAMA* 262:2108-2211, 1989.

Cohen JJ, Kassirer JP, eds: *Acid base*, Boston, 1982, Little Brown.

Narins RG, Jones ER, Dornfeld LP: Alkali therapy of the organic acidoses: a critical assessment of the data and the case for judicious use of sodium bicarbonate. In Narins RG, ed: *Controversies in nephrology and hypertension*, New York, 1984, Churchill Livingston.

Rose BD, ed: *Clinical physiology of acid-base and electrolyte disorders*, ed 3, New York, 1989, McGraw-Hill.

Schrier RW, ed: *Renal and electrolyte disorders*, ed 3, Boston, 1986, Little, Brown.

CASE

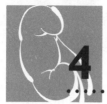

4

Roger A. Rodby
C. William Wester

. . . .

A previously healthy 27-year-old man came to the emergency room with a change in mental status and hyperthermia. The patient works in a foundry, and at quitting time he was found slumped over by a fellow worker.

In the emergency room, the physical examination revealed an obtunded patient with a temperature of 106°F, BP 70/50 mm Hg, P 48 bpm, RR 14/min. The lungs revealed bibasilar crackles, and the cardiovascular examination revealed bradycardia with occasional pauses; no pericardial rub was appreciated. The abdominal examination was unremarkable. The neurologic examination revealed a Glasgow Coma Scale of 8; no cranial nerve or focal motor and/or sensory deficits were elicited.

The patient received intravenous 50% dextrose, naloxone, and thiamine without improvement in his mental status. The initial arterial blood gas demonstrated a pH of 7.16, P_{CO_2} 28 mm Hg, P_{O_2} 40 mm Hg, and O_2 saturation of 76% on room air. The patient was intubated.

QUESTION I In an attempt to ascertain the underlying diagnosis for this patient's change in mental status, the laboratory analysis revealed a sodium of 150 mEq/L, potassium 6.9 mEq/L, chloride 114 mEq/L, bicarbonate 8 mEq/L, BUN 20 mg/dl, and serum creatinine of 4.8 mg/dl. The remainder of his laboratory data was remarkable for a serum calcium of 7.1 mg/dl, phosphorus 7.2 mg/dl, serum aspartate aminotransferase (SGOT) 420 U/L, lactate dehydrogenase (LDH) of 160 U/L, uric acid of 9.4 mg/dl, serum creatine kinase (CPK) of 55,000 U/L, and serum lactic acid (lactate) of 16.0 mmoles/L. The complete blood count (CBC) revealed a hemoglobin of 12.1 g/dl, white blood cell count of $7,600 \times 10^9$/L (with normal differential), and platelet count of $75,000 \times 10^9$/L. The urinalysis revealed 4+ blood and 30 mg/dl protein on dipstick with microscopic evaluation revealing 0-5 RBC/HPF. Multiple pigmented casts were visualized. The urinary chemistries demonstrated a sodium of 37 mEq/L and a creatinine of 74 mg/dl. What diagnosis is suggested by these labs and what are the potential ramifications of this disease process?

Acute renal failure (ARF) is a clinical syndrome of diverse etiologies characterized by an acute deterioration in renal function often, but not invariably, associated with oliguria. Any acute reduction in glomerular filtration will result in the accumulation of nitrogenous wastes (azotemia) that defines this syndrome.

Depending on the disease process and its reversibility, ARF may last anywhere from a few days to many weeks. If recovery is delayed, dialysis may be necessary until renal function recovers. When renal function is lost (either acutely [ARF], or chronically [CRF]), the body becomes a "closed system," unable to excrete fluid, electrolytes, and toxins. As a result these substances are retained, and changes in the composition of the body's intracellular and extracellular fluid occur. Potassium retention leads to hyperkalemia, which has deleterious effects on the heart. Hydrogen ion retention produces a metabolic acidosis. Sodium retention leads to edema, hypertension, and pulmonary congestion. Water retention causes hyponatremia. The inability to excrete the by-products of protein metabolism leads to accumulation of urea in the blood: azotemia. Urea, and other nitrogen-containing breakdown products produced as a result of protein catabolism, in high concentrations, produce a number of symptoms referred to as the uremic syndrome, including nausea, vomiting, pruritus, pericarditis, lethargy, coma.

Because there are causes of hyperkalemia, hyponatremia, and metabolic acidosis other than ARF, the clinical diagnosis of ARF rests on increases in the plasma levels of two final products of protein and muscle metabolism that are eliminated by the kidney through glomerular filtration: urea and creatinine. The blood urea nitrogen (BUN) is easily measured and is used as a determination of the level of protein breakdown products in the blood. Its level correlates fairly well with the level of the severity of the clinical syndrome of uremia. Creatinine is measured because it is freely filtered, neither reabsorbed nor secreted (for all practical purposes), and is produced on a constant basis, therefore serving as a measure of GFR. Depending on the severity of the reduction in GFR and the muscle mass of the patient, the serum creatinine increases by 0.5 to 2.0 mg/dl/day in patients with ARF (typical increase is approximately 1 mg/dl/day). Muscle injury will result in an increase in creatinine production, and the serum creatinine may rise at a faster rate (2 to 4 mg/dl/day). Urea accumulation rates vary considerably depending on the protein catabolic rate but average 10 to 20 mg/dl/day. ARF is often oliguric (<400 ml/day of urine). Nonoliguric ARF is usually associated with less injury and a less severe reduction in GFR. Its prognosis is better than oliguric ARF because of the propensity for an earlier recovery and because hypervolemia and hyperkalemia are less common.

QUESTION 2 How do you categorize the types of ARF? What are the major differential diagnoses for each type?

The disease processes that cause ARF can be separated into 3 major categories:

1. Prerenal ARF: A decrease in glomerular filtration rate (GFR) secondary to inadequate renal plasma flow to functionally and structurally intact kidneys

2. Intrinsic ARF: A decrease in GFR secondary to diseases of the renal parenchyma
3. Postrenal ARF: A decrease in GFR secondary to obstruction to the outflow of urine

The understanding of ARF depends upon an understanding of the factors that produce normal glomerular filtration. There are 4 major steps involved in the urinary elimination of nitrogenous waste:

1. Delivery of plasma to the glomerular capillaries via an adequate renal blood flow
2. Formation of a filtrate of the plasma through the glomerulus
3. Normal tubular handling of the ultrafiltrate
4. Excretion of final urine through a nonobstructed urinary tract

An interruption in any of these processes may precipitate ARF. Diseases that affect step #1 are considered "prerenal ARF"; the kidney is functionally and structurally intact but cannot perform its function because of inadequate renal perfusion. The kidney accommodates in two ways to maintain GFR in these situations. First, as renal perfusion pressure decreases, renal plasma flow may be maintained via the normal autoregulatory response of arterial vasodilatation (common to all organs). As this mechanism may be inadequate to maintain sufficient renal plasma flow to avoid a decrease in GFR, a second mechanism, unique to the kidney, is available. Afferent arteriolar dilatation (prostaglandin-mediated) and efferent arteriolar constriction (angiotensin II-mediated) occur. The combination of these two microvascular hemodynamic changes increases both the glomerular capillary hydrostatic pressure and filtration fraction; where GFR = renal plasma flow × filtration fraction. This helps to maintain GFR despite the decrease in renal plasma flow that is seen in prerenal states: [lower renal plasma flow] × [greater filtration fraction] = [maintained GFR]. If renal blood flow is further compromised, these mechanisms may not be able to maintain GFR, and acute renal failure occurs. Any condition that leads to a reduction in renal blood flow may cause prerenal azotemia.

Intravascular volume depletion from any cause

may result in a reduced cardiac output, lowered renal plasma flow, and the possibility of ARF if severe enough. Given the same amount of fluid loss, fluids with higher sodium concentrations are more likely to cause a reduction of GFR than those with a lower sodium concentration since the former will represent a greater amount of extracellular (as opposed to intracellular) and therefore intravascular volume loss. This intravascular fluid loss does not have to be associated with a loss of weight if third spacing occurs as can be seen with edema, ascites, pleural effusions, burns, etc.

Any cardiac disease associated with a reduced cardiac output may impair renal perfusion and result in prerenal ARF. These conditions include valvular, pericardial, and myocardial diseases. States of peripheral vasodilatation, on the other hand, are associated with a high cardiac output state. If shunting of blood is present, renal perfusion may nevertheless be compromised and produce ARF. This may be seen in patients with severe liver failure, septic shock, or the sepsis syndrome.

Finally, systemic hemodynamics may be normal, but if vasoconstriction of the renal vascular bed is present, an impairment in renal blood flow can cause prerenal ARF. This may be seen in patients receiving cyclosporine, amphotericin B, and nonsteroidal antiinflammatory agents (NSAIAs), especially if renal blood flow is already impaired for any reason before the administration of these agents. Severe hypercalcemia may also precipitate ARF through renal vasoconstriction. Since there may be no specific signs and symptoms of primary renal vasoconstriction, the diagnosis may depend on the history of exposure to one of these predisposing factors in addition to information gained from the urinary chemistries.

The degree of GFR reduction in prerenal azotemia is usually not as severe as that seen in other forms of ARF. Oliguria is common. The BUN may rise disproportionately to the creatinine since urea reabsorption increases as a result of passive diffusion secondary to the increased sodium and water reabsorption seen in all prerenal states. As a result, the BUN:creatinine ratio often exceeds 20:1. The BUN is also affected by the protein catabolic rate, and care must be taken not to include or exclude the diagnosis of prerenal ARF on the basis of the BUN:creatinine ratio alone. The diagnosis of prerenal azotemia is often suggested by the physical examination when signs of volume depletion, heart disease, or an edematous state are present. Because the kidney itself is not responsible for the reduction in GFR, and because it interprets low renal perfusion as volume depletion, the kidney will attempt to retain both sodium and water. Therefore the chemical composition of the urine can be extremely useful in evaluating and confirming prerenal states.

Diseases that affect step #4 of glomerular filtration, diseases that cause obstruction to the outflow of urine, are classified under "postrenal ARF." Approximately 15% of all ARF is secondary to obstruction, and all patients with ARF should have this ruled out with a renal ultrasound unless another cause of ARF is immediately apparent. Obstruction may occur at any level of the urogenital tract and may be secondary to stones, tumors (intrinsic or extrinsic), an enlarged prostate, blood clots, or sloughed renal papillae. Obstruction of a single ureter will not cause ARF if two functional kidneys are present since functional reserve of a healthy contralateral kidney is enough to prevent a significant reduction in GFR. Therefore obstruction must be bilateral or distal to the urinary bladder to result in ARF. Obstruction at any site will cause ARF in the patient with a structurally or functionally solitary kidney.

Obstruction may be accompanied by (1) anuria <50 ml/day (total obstruction), (2) oliguria, (3) a normal urine output, or (4) polyuria; the latter three associated with partial obstruction. Anuria is suggestive of obstruction, but there are conditions other than obstruction that are associated with anuria. Since obstruction can be associated with the complete range of urine outputs, the urine flow rate should not be a strong factor in whether obstruction is considered in the patient with ARF. Even partial obstruction can be associated with severe reductions in GFR as the glomerular capillary pressure is negated by pressure in Bowman's space. Polyuria may occur as a result of damage to the collecting duct secondary to the high intratubular pressures that accompany obstruction. In this situation the collecting duct no longer responds normally to antidiuretic hormone, and nephrogenic diabetes insipidus with large dilute urine volumes may occur. Similar damage to the distal tubule may affect potassium secretion and urine acidification, resulting in hyperkalemia and acidosis.

The renal collecting system dilates rapidly proximal to an obstruction. This can be seen with ultrasound visualization of the kidney, ureters, and bladder. Rarely, obstruction can occur without dilatation as seen if the obstruction is caused by a process that encases the kidney and ureter. This is termed *non-dilated obstruction* and must be considered in those patients at risk for ureteral encasement (e.g., abdominal carcinomatosis, prostatic or cervical cancer, lymphoma, or a history of methysergide usage [retroperitoneal fibrosis]). The clinician must maintain a high index of suspicion for these conditions because they will not be diagnosed with the usual means of evaluating for obstruction (renal ultrasound). If a nondilated obstruction is suspected, patients require cystoscopy with retrograde pyelography to determine patency of the ureteral drainage system.

Disease processes that affect steps #2 and #3 represent injury to renal parenchyma itself and are classified under "intrinsic ARF." These include diseases of the largest (renal artery and vein) to the smallest (glomerular capillaries) blood vessels of the kidney, in addition to diseases of the renal tubules.

Arterial occlusion may result from thromboses, emboli, or dissection of the thoracic aorta or renal arteries. Renal vein involvement is usually the result of thrombosis. ARF will only occur if these processes are bilateral or if the patient has a functionally or structurally solitary kidney. Complete obstruction to renal blood flow leads to anuria. If renal infarction has occurred, patients will usually have flank pain and hematuria (if not anuric). The serum level of LDH will also increase markedly when a large amount or renal tissue has infarcted, since this enzyme is abundant in the kidney (isoenzyme 1).

There are a number of conditions that affect the smaller blood vessels of the kidney that may produce ARF. Included in this category are diseases of the capillaries of the kidney (the glomerulus). The injury may be due to an immunologic inflammatory response (glomerulonephritis and vasculitis), intravascular thrombi formation (microangiopathic syndromes), or to direct barotrauma (malignant hypertension). These disorders are suggested by an abnormal urinary sediment that includes proteinuria, RBCs ± RBC casts. If the microvascular disease is entirely preglomerular, which can occasionally be seen in some of the larger vessel vasculitides, the urinary sediment may be normal. Many of the glomerular and vasculitic diseases that are associated with ARF are associated with a systemic disease with other organ system involvement that direct the differential diagnosis. In addition there are a number of serologic tests that may be useful in the diagnosis (see Fig. 9-5-1 in Nephrology Case #5 and Table 9-6-1 in Nephrology Case #6).

Most of the glomerulopathies and vasculitides do not cause ARF unless severe, and when they do are termed rapidly progressive (RPGN). Glomerular damage in RPGN is often accompanied by crescents (crescentic GN). On the other hand, the microangiopathic syndromes are frequently associated with severe ARF. Common to the microangiopathic diseases is injury to endothelium with vascular thrombosis of the arterioles and/or glomerular capillaries. As a result, actual infarction may occur in areas of the cortex. This is termed *cortical necrosis* and may be seen in patients with the hemolytic uremic syndrome (HUS), thrombotic thrombocytopenic purpura (TTP), disseminated intravascular coagulation (DIC), and preeclampsia. Patients with cortical necrosis are often anuric. The initiating endothelial damage may be the result of an infection (HUS), or any cause of DIC (e.g., endotoxemia, amniotic fluid embolism, and retained dead fetus). The hallmark of the diagnosis of a microangiopathic process is the presence of hemolysis associated with schistocytes on the peripheral smear, usually accompanied by thrombocytopenia. Unlike most other causes of ARF including acute tubular necrosis, recovery from cortical necrosis is often incomplete. This seems to be a result of actual loss of renal mass secondary to the patchy infarction.

Finally, the small blood vessels of the kidney may be affected by atheroemboli, small plaques of cholesterol that embolize to the kidney. This is usually seen only in patients with severe atherosclerotic disease of the aorta and large arteries, and when present, usually follows a major intravascular procedure such as arteriography. Many patients will have stigmata of peripheral embolization (e.g., blue toes and ischemic central nervous system events), which may be confused with systemic vasculitis. The reason for renal failure in this condition is not clear since only a small percentage of the renal blood vessels become occluded. Infarction is not always apparent. Other factors may be responsible. An elevated erythrocyte sedimentation rate with peripheral eosinophilia is often present and suggests that an allergic mechanism may be involved. The eye grounds are a particularly sensitive area to look for cholesterol clefts (Hollenhorst plaques). This disorder is usually nonoliguric, and the urine is benign. The diagnosis often requires a renal biopsy.

Allergic interstitial nephritis encompasses a large group of disorders that include many mechanisms. Usually though, there appears to be a reduction in GFR as a result of a reaction to a toxin, usually a drug. The hypersensitivity response to drugs is often, but not invariably, accompanied by a generalized allergic reaction consisting of fever, rash, and peripheral eosinophilia. This condition was originally described with methicillin, although a number of other drugs (e.g., antibiotics, diuretics, sulfa-containing medications), have been shown to produce a similar response. Although interstitial infiltrates and tubular cell damage is present, the reason for the acute reduction in GFR is not clear. Mechanisms similar to that in acute tubular necrosis (to follow) may be involved. Discontinuation of the respon-

sible agent is usually all that is required to result in renal recovery, although glucocorticoids have been used in severe cases. Patients are usually nonoliguric and will often have WBCs, WBC casts, or epithelial cell casts in their urine. Other signs of tubular damage may be present and include renal tubular acidosis and glycosuria in the presence of a normal serum glucose concentration.

ARF can be seen as a result of tubular obstruction from very high filtered load of urate, usually produced as a result of massive breakdown of cells following chemotherapy for lymphoma or leukemia. Tumor lysis is more likely to occur in patients with extreme elevations in their LDH before chemotherapy. ARF may be avoided by aggressive hydration, allopurinol, and alkalinization of the urine. ARF from tubular obstruction may also be seen with precipitated filtered myeloma proteins in patients with multiple myeloma. Drugs that may cause a similar tubular obstruction include acyclovir, certain relatively insoluble sulfonamides, and methotrexate.

QUESTION 3   What is acute tubular necrosis, and what is the pathophysiologic explanation for the reduction in GFR? What are the different stages of recovery?

The final and most common cause of intrinsic ARF is referred to as acute tubular necrosis (ATN). This syndrome is characterized by an abrupt and severe reduction in GFR, usually initiated by a clearly defined event. There are two categories: postischemic and nephrotoxic.

Although the kidney may be able to maintain renal blood flow through autoregulatory mechanisms in states of impaired cardiac output, this compensatory response may not be sufficient. If a severe enough reduction in renal blood flow occurs that results in renal ischemia and tubular cell injury, the patient may develop ARF. This is the basis for postischemic ATN. Similarly, certain nephrotoxic agents can cause renal tubular cell damage and ARF: nephrotoxic ATN. Both are associated with a similar pathologic description, clinical course, and pathophysiologic explanation for the severe reduction in GFR. In patients with ATN, the GFR is abruptly reduced from a normal level of over 100 ml/min to usually less than 5 ml/min. Reversal of the shock or removal of the nephrotoxic agent does not immediately restore the GFR.

Any situation with a severe prolonged impairment in renal perfusion may result in ischemic ATN. In addition to obvious states of shock, this includes all the causes of decreased renal perfusion mentioned in the section on prerenal ARF, when severe and prolonged.

There are a number of nephrotoxins that can cause tubular damage and nephrotoxic ATN. These include aminoglycoside antibiotics, certain heavy metals, halogenated hydrocarbons as well as many other medications and toxins. Myoglobin (released from damaged muscle) and hemoglobin (released with intravascular hemolysis) can be filtered and cause ARF when large amounts are released into the blood. By themselves they do not appear to be nephrotoxic but when accompanied by volume depletion may form intratubular casts with tubular cell damage. It is unclear if they are only toxic in settings of volume depletion or if other substances released as a result of muscle breakdown or hemolysis are responsible for the ATN. One of the more common causes of nephrotoxic ATN is iodide-containing radiocontrast. The exact mechanism for tubular cell damage in many forms of nephrotoxic ATN is yet to be determined.

There are several theories regarding the pathogenesis of the severe reduction in GFR that follows ATN, but the best understood is explained by changes in renal blood flow and glomerular hemodynamics. It appears that whatever the initiating event in the kidney, be it ischemic or nephrotoxic, decreased perfusion of the renal cortex secondary to afferent arteriolar vasoconstriction occurs. Agents that have been proposed as the mediator of this vasoconstriction include angiotensin II and adenosine. In addition, there appears to be a vasodilatation of the efferent arteriole. The combination of afferent vasoconstriction and efferent vasodilatation produces a low capillary hydrostatic pressure and filtration fraction in the glomerular capillary bed and is at least partially responsible for the severe impairment in GFR seen in ATN. This afferent and efferent arteriolar vascular tone relationship is the opposite of what is seen in prerenal states where the GFR is maximized for a given renal blood flow (high glomerular transcapillary hydrostatic pressure gradient and a maximized filtration fraction).

Pathologically, ATN is often associated with morphologic evidence of damage to the renal tubular cells. One may see atrophic changes in some cells, total destruction of other cells, and mitotic figures in some remaining viable tubular cells. It is for this reason that the lesion is referred to as *acute tubular necrosis (ATN)*. However, the morphologic abnormality is not necessarily noted in all cases and clinical examples of ATN with a profound depression of renal function with normal or relatively normal appearing renal tubular cells can be seen. This does not imply that the renal tubular cells are necessarily functioning normally. In these cases the damage is apparently not severe enough to be expressed morphologically.

The clinical course of the renal failure in ATN is usually self-limiting and often follows an oliguric, diuretic, and recovery phase. Whether the insult be ischemic or nephrotoxic, the initial phase of ARF is usually associated with a decrease in urine output. Generally, the urine volume is of the order of 10 to 20 mls per hour (oliguria), although some patients may be anuric. Because of the unresponsive nature of the lesion to attempts to reverse the condition, the urine volume does not significantly increase with the administration of agents that increase the blood volume, cardiac output, or renal plasma flow. Because of the low GFR, there is a poor response to diuretic agents. The glomerular filtration rate is usually only a few percent of normal. Eventual recovery is the rule if new tubular insults are avoided. This occurs spontaneously over a course of days to weeks. If recovery never occurs, consideration must be made that the patient had cortical necrosis over and above ATN.

The "diuretic phase" of ATN is often the first indication that the lesion is undergoing spontaneous recovery. In this instance the patient's urine volume progressively increases. The increased urine volume reflects a slowly increasing glomerular filtration rate. The patient's urine flow may increase to 50 to 200 ml/hr. Most of this "diuresis" is an appropriate response to volume expansion and solute retention that has accompanied the acute renal failure. Although improved, the GFR may still be markedly impaired, and it is therefore not surprising that the patient's BUN and creatinine may continue to rise (although less rapidly). This stage is a good prognostic indicator of recovery from ATN. The diuretic phase of ATN slowly blends with a "recovery phase" in which the glomerular filtration rate continues to rise concomitant with a peaking of the BUN and creatinine, followed by a decline in their serum levels until they normalize. The kidney also reaches a state in which the salt and water content of the urine are determined by physiologic mechanisms. That is, the urine content reflects the patient's intake of salt and water and the need for excretion of these substances.

The great majority of patients with ATN will ultimately regain normal renal function. Hence, while the lesion is not immediately reversible by providing factors that could improve renal perfusion such as returning a patient's blood volume to normal or removal of the nephrotoxin, the kidney is capable of spontaneously reversing this abnormal state over a period of days to weeks.

There is a suggestion that the profound decrease in GFR in ATN is actually a teleologic adaption to the tubular cell damage that occurs from ischemia or nephrotoxins. The normal kidney reabsorbs over 99% of the filtered sodium. Tubular cell damage leading to only a mild decrease in this ability to reabsorb sodium would lead to massive volume depletion because the filtered load with a normal GFR is so large. The "acute renal success" theory states that the acute reduction in GFR through hemodynamic mechanisms is actually protective by decreasing the filtered load of sodium and therefore avoiding the risk of volume depletion.

In summary, ATN secondary to either an ischemic event or the administration of a nephrotoxin leads to a clinicopathologic entity characterized by:

1. A profound decrease in the flow of blood to the renal cortex
2. A profound decrease in the filtration fraction and the glomerular filtration rate
3. Renal tubular cell dysfunction, which is sometimes associated with morphologic evidence of necrosis
4. Resistance of this lesion to immediate reversal by extrarenal factors such as restoration of renal blood flow or the withdrawal of the nephrotoxin
5. A tendency to spontaneous resolution to normal function over a period of days to weeks

QUESTION 4 An abdominal ultrasound demonstrated normal-sized kidneys without evidence of obstruction. The hyperkalemia and metabolic acidosis were treated appropriately. Additional supportive measures were administered, and the patient was transferred to the medical intensive care unit in guarded condition. The patient's blood pressure improved after the administration of several liters of normal saline, but he remained oliguric and his BUN and creatinine continued to rise. What are the diagnostic steps in the evaluation of ARF?

The first step in evaluating a patient with ARF is to distinguish among prerenal, postrenal, and intrinsic renal causes. This usually starts with a renal ultrasound. A careful history must be obtained, including exposure to hemodynamic insults and nephrotoxins. Both the history and physical examination must look for evidence of prerenal states, systemic diseases, and general vascular insufficiency. Evaluation of the urine is an important tool. Proteinuria and hematuria usually accompany the glomerulonephritides and vasculitides. Red blood cell casts are specific for glomerular inflammation (see Nephrology Case #6). A positive urine dipstick for blood in the absence of microscopic hematuria suggests the presence of hemoglobinuria or myoglobinuria. White blood cells, WBC casts, and tubular cell casts usually indicate tubulointerstitial disease (interstitial nephritis). Eosinophils in the urine suggest an allergic interstitial nephritis. Obstruction, atheroemboli, and prerenal azotemia are usually associated with a "bland" urine without significant protein, cells, or casts. This is also true of diseases of the larger renal vessels, if the glomeruli are spared inflammation. ATN will often have a urine displaying tubular cell casts, as well as numerous coarse granular casts consisting of tubular cell debris. Lastly, papillary necrosis, a diagnosis suspected in patients with diabetes mellitus, hemoglobinopathies, and chronic analgesic abuse is associated with a urine sediment containing many white blood cells in clumps or casts as well as, on occasion, an identifiable renal papilla.

The hematologic profile may be useful as well. Peripheral eosinophilia suggests allergic interstitial nephritis and atheroembolic disease. Schistocytosis suggests one of the microangiopathic diseases associated with cortical necrosis.

Urine chemical composition may be extremely helpful in determining the cause of ARF. The kidney is functionally intact in prerenal ARF, and it retains the ability to reabsorb sodium and water. Because the kidney detects volume depletion in these states, an attempt is made to preserve volume. As a result, the concentration of sodium in the urine (UNa) is usually low: <20 mEq/L. The tubular cell damage in ATN prevents this from being possible (independent of the patients volume status), and the UNa is usually >40 mEq/L. (UNa 20 to 40 are nondiagnostic.)

One of the problems with using the UNa to differentiate prerenal from intrinsic causes of ARF is that the UNa is affected by the degree of water as well as sodium reabsorption. Since water reabsorption is impaired in ATN (secondary to the loss of the osmotic gradient as a consequence of damage to tubular cells), the UNa will be reduced

by dilution. This lowering of the UNa in an ATN state may make it appear to be a prerenal condition. On the other hand, increased water reabsorption in prerenal states (secondary to volume-mediated antidiuretic hormone release) can raise the UNa above 20 mEq/L, even in the face of avid sodium retention. This may make the prerenal state appear to be an ATN condition. These effects of water transport can be overcome by measuring the fractional excretion of sodium (FE_{Na}) which is a direct measure of sodium excretion. The FE_{Na} represents the percent of the filtered sodium that is excreted =

$$\frac{\text{Urine sodium (mEq/l)} \times \text{Plasma creatinine (mg/dl)}}{\text{Plasma sodium (mEq/l)} \times \text{urine creatinine (mg/dl)}} \times 100$$

This is usually <1% in prerenal states and >1% in states associated with ATN. There is essentially no overlap between the FE_{Na} associated with prerenal states (<1%) and ATN (>1%). Therefore this measurement is the most useful of the urinary indices in evaluating patients with ARF. There are a few conditions, usually not considered prerenal, that may have a low FE_{Na} if evaluated very early in their course. These include early obstruction, early pigment nephropathy (hemoglobinuria and myoglobinuria), and early radiocontrast nephropathy. The sodium avidity is probably related to a vasoconstrictive phase that occurs before tubular cell damage. A low FE_{Na} can also be seen in patients with acute glomerulonephritis since tubular flow may be impaired with tubular function remaining intact.

For all practical purposes, creatinine is neither secreted nor reabsorbed by the renal tubules. Therefore the increase in concentration of creatinine in the tubular fluid relative to plasma is directly related to the amount of H_2O reabsorbed in the renal tubules. The urine to plasma (U/P) creatinine ratio becomes a quantitative index of total water absorption by the kidneys. Water absorption is high in prerenal states, and as a result, the U/P creatinine ratio increases. A U/P creatinine >40 is usually seen only with prerenal ARF. Urinary concentration (water reabsorption) is impaired in ATN syndromes, and the U/P creatinine will be lower than in prerenal states. ATN is usually associated with a U/P creatinine ratio <20. (Values between 20 and 40 are considered nondiagnostic.)

Urinary concentration depends upon intact tubular function. ATN is usually associated with isosthenuria, a urine osmolality equal to serum osmolality. Prerenal states usually demonstrate a urine that is concentrated compared to the serum. Urine concentration is dependent on an osmotic gradient in the renal medulla. This in turn depends on solute delivery to the loop of Henle. Because proximal reabsorption is enhanced in prerenal states, distal delivery is impaired, and solute delivery to the loop of Henle is reduced. As a result, in prerenal states, renal concentration may be less than would be otherwise expected. Therefore, overlap in urine osmolalities can be seen in patients with ATN and prerenal ARF (300 to 500 mosm/L). Still urine osmolalities >500 mosm/L are usually seen only in prerenal states.

For a summary of the diagnostic approach in dealing with ARF, refer to the algorithm displayed in Fig. 9-4-1.

QUESTION 5 For each of the pathophysiologic mechanisms of ARF, what are the correct modes of therapy?

Obstruction is usually treatable by either urologic or radiographic procedures. The degree of recovery will depend on how long the obstruction has been present. The renal failure of acute obstruction will usually totally reverse if it has not persisted longer than 1 to 2 weeks.

Patients with prerenal ARF should respond immediately to an improvement in renal circulation. Unfortunately, except for cases of pure volume depletion, most causes of an impairment in renal circulation are not immediately reversible.

Patients with ATN need time to recover. The most important factor is to try to avoid further tubular insults. This requires an attempt to maximize systemic hemodynamics, to avoid other ischemic events, and the avoidance of further nephrotoxic insults.

The proper management of all patients with ARF, regardless of the cause, demands close attention to many details of the patient's daily physical examination and blood chemistries. Since the body becomes a closed system, care must be taken to monitor the composition and amount of all intravenous fluids, medications, and dietary intakes. A patient with oliguric ARF may quickly and dangerously expand body fluid volume unless fluid intake is restricted. The best monitor of the adequacy of the fluid therapy is the daily clinical assessment of volume status and weights. Adequate caloric intake must be provided to the ARF patient so as to minimize endogenous catabolism.

Since infections remain the leading cause of death in ARF, constant vigilance in the maintenance of IV lines, pulmonary toilet, and avoidance of unnecessary indwelling urinary catheters is necessary. Acute gastrointestinal hemorrhage is a common comorbid factor.

Last, meticulous attention must be paid to metabolic derangements including hyperkalemia, hyponatremia, metabolic acidosis, hyperphosphatemia, and hypocalcemia. Serum electrolytes may need to be followed daily or more often. Absolute indications for dialysis include central nervous system and gastrointestinal disturbances, pericarditis, severe electrolyte abnormalities, and pulmonary congestion. The choice of dialytic method depends on the clinical situation.

CASE DISCUSSION Our patient is a young man presenting with ARF complicated by multiorgan system involvement. He suffers from many of the complications related to exertional heatstroke, which in this case caused nontraumatic rhabdomyolysis, myoglobinuria, and ARF. Rhabdomyolysis and its associated complications of hyperkalemia, hyperphosphatemia, hypocalcemia, hyperuricemia, and myoglobinuria are common findings in exertional heatstroke.

The patient was hypotensive when he presented and suggested a pure prerenal cause of his ARF. Volume resuscitation improved his systemic hemodynamics but did not improve his renal function. His

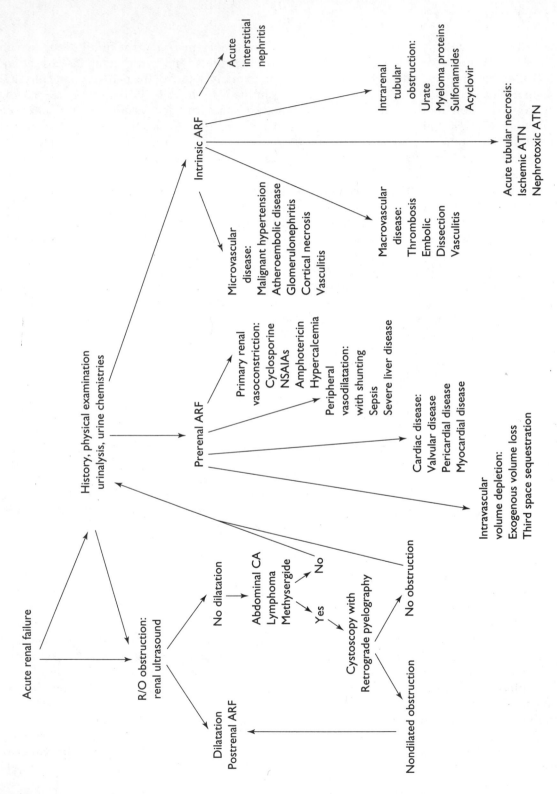

9-4-1 Approach to patient with acute renal failure based on radiographic, history, physical examination, and biochemical features.

urine chemistries suggested ATN (FE_{Na} 1.6%, U/P creatinine 15.4, urine Na 37). The diagnosis of myoglobinuric ARF is suggested by the marked rise in muscle enzymes in the presence of a dipstick indicating large amounts of blood in the urine without red blood cells on microscopic examination. In addition, the increase in creatinine out of proportion to the BUN suggests rapid muscle catabolism. This patient developed nephrotoxic ATN secondary to myoglobinuria and may have a component of ischemic ATN secondary to his transient hypotension. He will likely recover, but not until after an unpredictable period has elapsed that may require dialytic support.

• •

BIBLIOGRAPHY

Bricker NS, Kirschenbaum MA: *The kidney: diagnosis and management*, New York, 1984, Wiley Medical Publications.

Dewaredener HE: *The kidney: an outline of normal and abnormal function*, ed 5, New York, 1985, Churchill Livingstone.

Hamenbaum W, Hamburger R: *Nephrology: an approach to the patient with renal disease*, Philadelphia, 1982, JP Lippincott.

Llach F: *Papper's clinical nephrology*, ed 3, Boston, 1993, Little, Brown.

Marter HR, Martin KJ: Acute renal failure, *Postgrad Med* 72(6):175-197, 1982.

Massry SG, Glassode RJ: *Textbook of nephrology*, ed 2, vol 1, Baltimore, 1983, Williams & Wilkins.

Rose BD: *Pathophysiology of renal disease*, ed 2, New York, 1987, McGraw-Hill.

Seldin DW, Grebish G: *The kidney: physiology and pathophysiology*, ed 2, vol 3, New York, 1992, Raven Press.

CASE

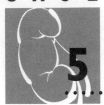

5

C. William Wester
Roger A. Rodby

A previously healthy 55-year-old man came to the emergency room with an acute onset of shortness of breath, tachycardia, and pleuritic chest pain. He denied fever, arthralgias, rash, or other upper respiratory tract-related complaints. His only medication was an over-the-counter multivitamin.

The physical examination was remarkable for a temperature of 98.4°F, BP 118/70 mm Hg, P 124 bpm, RR 28/min. There was wheezing in the right lung. Cardiovascular examination revealed a loud P2 but was otherwise normal. The lower extremities were without asymmetry or erythema but were noteworthy for 4+ pitting edema to the knees bilaterally.

The patient's laboratory results revealed a BUN of 22 mg/dl, creatinine 1 mg/dl, total protein of 6.1 g/dl, albumin of 2.0 g/dl, and cholesterol 355 mg/dl. The urinalysis was remarkable for 300 mg/dl of protein on dipstick, no cellular elements or cellular casts, and a few waxy casts. An arterial blood gas on room air demonstrated: pH 7.48, P_{CO_2} 30 mmHg, P_{O_2} 62 mm Hg, and Sao_2 86%.

QUESTION I Describe the anatomy of the glomerulus and the manner in which filtration occurs. What is the nature of immunologic glomerular damage?

The glomerulus is a tuft of branching capillaries interposed between two resistance vessels, the afferent and efferent arterioles. Normally, approximately 20% of the cardiac output passes through these capillaries and is fractionated as an initial ultrafiltrate (170 L/24 hr) into Bowman's space. The formation of this ultrafiltrate is made

possible by the unique architecture of the filtration unit, and is largely influenced by the interplay between the various cell types of the glomerulus and its extracellular matrices. The individual capillary tufts are arranged in lobules and supported by a stalk consisting of mesangial cells and their basement membrane-like extracellular matrix.

The capillary wall, through which the filtrate must pass, is made up of 3 layers: (1) the inner, fenestrated endothelial cell, (2) the glomerular basement membrane (GBM), and (3) the outer epithelial cell (which is attached to the basement membrane via direct cytoplasmic extensions, called foot processes or podocytes). The glomerular capillary wall is highly permeable to small solutes (sodium, urea) and water. The filtration of macromolecules, proteins as well as polysaccharides, is inversely proportional to the molecular weight (MW) and therefore size of the given substance. Molecules the size of inulin (MW 5200) are filtered freely, whereas larger MW substances such as albumin (MW 69000) are not filterable under normal conditions. Molecular charge is another important determinant governing filtration across the GBM. Cationic and neutral dextrans are filtered to a significantly greater degree than anionic dextrans of similar molecular sizes. This effect is mediated primarily by negatively charged sialoproteins and proteoglycans (such as heparin sulfate) located within the GBM, providing it with a net negative charge. This interferes with the filtration of anions (such as albumin) but facilitates the filtration of cations. Both experimental and clinical observations suggest that the loss of these anionic sites is partially responsible for the increased filtration of albumin seen in many of the glomerular disorders.

Nonimmune factors are important in certain clinical glomerulopathies (e.g., diabetes mellitus), but the vast majority of such disorders are thought to be immune mediated. Antigen-antibody lattices may form in the mesangium or in the glomerular capillary wall. This may occur by the reaction of circulating antibody to an antigen previously deposited in the GBM ("in-situ" immune complex formation). Immune complexes that form in the serum, "circulating" immune complexes, may also deposit in the glomerulus. A variety of antigens, both endogenous (i.e., DNA, tumor associated, thyroglobulin) and exogenous (hepatitis B, drugs, bacterial) have been implicated in the immune complex pathogenesis of many glomerular diseases.

QUESTION 2 Subsequent laboratory data revealed the following: A 24-hour urine collection contained 18 grams of protein. Tests for syphilis, hepatitis B surface antigen, antibodies to HIV and hepatitis C virus, serum cryoglobulins, rheumatoid factor, and antinuclear antibody were all negative. Immunoelectrophoresis of the serum and urine were normal as were serum complement levels. Later, in the course of the hospitalization, a renal biopsy was performed.

This patient presents with the clinical syndrome of marked edema, hypoalbuminemia, hyperlipidemia, and marked proteinuria. What do these elements characterize? What is the differential diagnosis of this disease?

The nephrotic syndrome (NS), although often thought of as an actual disease, is a clinical syndrome seen in patients with glomerular diseases that are characterized by a marked increase in capillary wall permeability to serum proteins. The primary abnormality in NS is the excretion of large quantities of protein in the urine (usually greater than 3.5 g per day). Other associated manifestations that may occur secondary to proteinuria include hypoalbuminemia, edema, hyperlipidemia, and lipiduria.

NS may be due to a number of primary glomerulopathies in addition to those associated with a systemic disease: secondary glomerulopathies. Differentiation is based on a number of clinical clues, serologic tests, and ultimately a renal biopsy in most cases.

The prototype idiopathic primary glomerulopathy associated with NS is minimal change disease (MCD), also referred to as nil disease or lipoid nephrosis. This is primarily a disease of children, and it is responsible for more than 80% of idiopathic NS in children and 10% of NS in adults. The median age of onset in children is 2.5 years with 80% of children afflicted being less than 6 years of age at time of diagnosis. Males are affected nearly twice as often as females, but in adults the sex ratios are close to unity. There appears to be a greater incidence of atopic diseases, particularly asthma, eczema, and hay fever in children with MCD than in matched controls. There is also an association with Hodgkin's disease and the use of nonsteroidal antiinflammatory agents. Patients with MCD typically present with the acute onset of edema, often involving the eyelids and scrotum. There is often a profound depression in the serum albumin as well as an extreme elevation of the serum cholesterol.

Pathologically, this clinical entity gets its name by having normal-appearing glomeruli on light microscopy with negative immunohistochemical staining for complement or immunoglobulins. Electron microscopy demonstrates the only histologic abnormality, with fusion of the epithelial foot processes. Patients with MCD have an excellent prognosis as the vast majority are steroid responsive. Renal failure and steroid unresponsiveness are uncommon and, when present, should alert the physician to the possibility that the patient has focal segmental glomerular sclerosis that was not apparent on original biopsy.

The clinicopathologic syndrome of proteinuria with the glomerular lesion of focal-segmental glomerulosclerosis (FSGS) is the second most common cause of NS in children and adults. Adults may present with either nephrotic or nonnephrotic proteinuria. In addition to the idiopathic variety, this lesion has been demonstrated in association with heroin abuse, chronic urinary reflux, and infection with the HIV virus. There is an increased incidence of FSGS in black hypertensive patients, although the hypertension is likely a result of the glomerulopathy instead of the reverse. Patients with FSGS often present with less edema and have a higher blood pressure than those with MCD. Serum creatinine levels may be elevated at the time of discovery of disease, especially in patients who present with massive proteinuria. In other patients, renal insufficiency develops months to years after diagnosis. The urinalysis may demonstrate hematuria and leukocyturia. Light microscopy reveals focal (not every glomerulus is involved) and segmental (only a part of each affected glomerulus being involved) collapse and sclerosis within the glomerulus. The sclerotic segments may contain lipid-laden foam cells and homogenous eosinophilic acid-schiff positive globules (hyalinosis) that appear red with the Masson trichrome stain. Immune complexes are uncommon. The pathogenesis of this disorder remains unknown. As with MCD, it is thought to be possibly humorally mediated, although serologic testing fails to demonstrate immune complexes, and serum complement levels are usually normal. This is supported by the fact that within hours of renal transplantation in the patient with FSGS, massive proteinuria from the previously normal transplanted kidney has been reported. FSGS is generally associated with progressive loss of renal function. The renal prognosis is dependent upon the response to immunosuppressive therapy, with those that go into remission during a course of steroid therapy having an improved prognosis compared to those who are "steroid resistant."

The most common form of idiopathic glomerulonephritis (GN) presenting with the nephrotic syndrome in adults is membranous glomerulonephritis (MGN). Most patients present in their third to sixth decade of life. Some patients come to clinical attention only by chance following the incidental asymptomatic detection of proteinuria on routine urinalysis. Microscopic hematuria is present in approximately 30% of patients but is usually mild. Renal function is usually normal at presentation. Serologic testing for immune complexes, paraproteins, and serum complements are normal as in primary MGN and FSGS.

Pathologically, the most significant change in MGN is a diffuse thickening of glomerular capillary walls, usually in the absence of hypercellularity of the cells in the glomerular tuft. The true hallmark of MGN is seen on electron microscopy, with the accumulation of discrete electron-dense deposits along the subepithelial border of the GBM. As these deposits enlarge, the glomerular cells respond by producing GBM matrix between the immune aggregates. This leads to the "spikes" seen on silver stain that typifies MGN. Immunofluorescent techniques reveal a preponderance of IgG in a beaded or granular appearance along the basement membranes of the capillary loops.

Research has centered on determining the actual pathogenesis of this unique clinical entity. Although it has been proposed that the pattern of granular subepithelial immune deposits characteristic of MGN indicate circulating immune complex trapping, experimental models of MGN have shown that immune deposits at this site aggregate locally because of the reaction of circulating antibody to antigens, either exogenous or endogenous, previously localized on the epithelial surface of the capillary wall.

Although most cases of MGN are idiopathic, a variety of antigens have been identified and are thought to be pathogenetic in the secondary forms of MGN. These include DNA in MGN associated with systemic lupus erythematosus, hepatitis B surface antigen, thyroglobulin, tumor antigens, and treponemal antigens.

Pharmacologically important agents in secondary MGN include gold salts and penicillamine. Important infectious etiologies include chronic hepatitis B, schistosomiasis, malaria, leprosy, and secondary syphilis. The most important clinical correlate is the association of MGN with solid tumors. The most commonly implicated tumors are carcinoma of the lung, colon, stomach, breast, thyroid, kidney, ovary, cervix, and skin. Therefore, when presented with a patient with biopsy proven MGN, one should perform a battery of solid tumor screening tests (e.g., chest x-ray, digital rectal exam, stool guiacs, xero-mammography, etc.) as the development of NS may precede clinical recognition of the tumor.

The natural history of MGN is quite variable as it relates more to the clinical features than it does to actual histological staging. Patients who present with asymptomatic proteinuria and never become nephrotic rarely develop renal failure. They may spontaneously remit or have persistent proteinuria. Patients with NS have a poorer prognosis. Spontaneous remission occurs in about one third of patients followed for 5 years. Another third will remain nephrotic without development of renal failure. Progressive deterioration of renal function occurs in the remaining one third.

Membranoproliferative glomerulonephritis (MPGN) is another disease classification causing idiopathic NS . Along with its distinct histologic appearance, certain clinical and laboratory parameters make this diagnosis unique as this is the only primary glomerular disease associated with abnormal complement profiles. There is an extensive list of secondary causes of MPGN such as systemic lupus erythematosus (SLE), cryoglobulinemia, bacterial endocarditis, infection with hepatitis C, partial lipodystrophy, and alpha-1 antitrypsin deficiency.

Histologically, MPGN often demonstrates a lobular appearance of the glomeruli. Immune deposits can be seen either in a sub-epithelial pattern (Type 1 MPGN) or in a continuous intramembranous pattern (Type 2 or "dense deposit disease"). The basement membrane is usually duplicated, giving it a "tram track" appearance.

Patients may present with either the nephrotic or nephritic syndrome. Hypertension is common. The pathogenesis of MPGN is unknown. Type 1 MPGN has serologic features of an immune-complex mediated disease with some patients having circulating immune complexes. A larger percentage have evidence of complement activation by the alternate, and occasionally the classic, pathway. This results in depressed levels of C3 in

the majority of cases. Clinical indicators of poor prognosis include nephrotic range proteinuria and hypertension. Steroid and cytotoxic responsiveness is variable. Primary MPGN is uncommon in adults, and the histologic picture of MPGN should alert the physician to look for diseases that may give a similar histologic picture (e.g., SLE, cryoglobulinemia, bacterial endocarditis, and chronic Hepatitis C infection).

Mesangial proliferative GN is characterized by glomerular mesangial hypercellularity, usually affecting all lobules to a certain degree. The incidence of this disorder is unknown, but it may account for between 5% and 10% of renal biopsies performed for a number of reasons including the workup of low-grade proteinuria, NS, and hematuria, microscopic to gross. Hypertension may be present in approximately 25% to 50% of patients. Serologic studies such as serum complements, anti-nuclear and anti-streptococcal antibodies are normal or negative in patients with the idiopathic variety. However, this morphologic lesion may be seen in other disorders including mesangial lupus GN, IgA nephropathy (Berger's disease), and Henoch-Schonlein purpura. The mesangial regions of the glomerulus are expanded and display varying degrees of increased cellularity, often with an associated increase in mesangial matrix. Mesangial immune deposits are common. The prognosis varies depending on the degree of inflammation. Patients with isolated microscopic hematuria maintain renal function for long periods of time. Patients with low-grade proteinuria with or without microscopic hematuria also have a favorable long-term prognosis. On the other hand, patients with heavy proteinuria and hypertension are more likely to develop renal insufficiency that may progress to end-stage renal disease.

Several systemic disease states are linked with the development of NS. Perhaps the most important multisystem disease causing NS is systemic lupus erythematosus (SLE). While many histopathologic patterns may be seen in nephrotic patients with SLE, membranous lupus and the severe proliferative lesions are more common in patients with NS. Membranous lupus appears similar to idiopathic membranous except that in membranous lupus, mesangial immune deposits are seen in addition to the subepithelial deposits.

Renal involvement occurs in approximately 75% of patients with primary and secondary forms of amyloidosis. In the past, renal amyloidosis often complicated the course of patients with chronic suppurative infections (e.g., tuberculosis and osteomyelitis). Today, with effective antibiotic regimens, renal amyloidosis is more commonly related to primary amyloidosis and multiple myeloma, although it may still be a complication of chronic inflammatory bowel disease and familial Mediterranean fever. The pathogenesis of the disorder remains controversial, but is thought to result from deposition of altered immunoglobulin fragments produced in excess by stimulated plasma cells. For the majority of patients with secondary renal amyloid, the only treatment is that relating to the underlying primary inflammatory disease.

Diabetic glomerulosclerosis is the most common cause of NS in the United States. Therefore, when confronted with diabetic patients with proteinuria, a renal biopsy is usually not performed unless there is historic, physical examination, or serologic evidence for a lesion other than diabetic nephropathy. This is one of the few conditions in the adult that NS does not require histopathologic confirmation. The absence of diabetic retinopathy by careful ophthalmologic examination may lead to the consideration for renal biopsy, as retinopathy occurs in 85% to 95% of patients with diabetic glomerulopathy.

The diagnostic approach to the patient with GN is demonstrated through the algorithm in Fig. 9-5-1, which includes glomerulopathies that present with either the nephrotic or nephritic syndrome. A renal biopsy is performed on most adults unless an obvious medication is felt to be causative, or the patient has diabetes with diabetic retinopathy and nothing else to suggest another disease process. A number of serologic tests may be useful in making a diagnosis, although not all of these tests may be appropriate for all patients before renal biopsy.

QUESTION 3 A chest x-ray was normal, and an electrocardiogram revealed an S1, Q3, T3 configuration with an incomplete right bundle branch block. A ventilation-perfusion lung scan was read as high probability for pulmonary embolus, and the patient was begun on heparin and oxygen by face mask. Apart from renal disease, what are the extrarenal manifestations of this disease?

Extrarenal manifestations of NS are of substantial significance. The "nephrotic syndrome" encompasses five clinical features: proteinuria, hypoalbuminemia, hyperlipidemia, lipiduria, and edema. The first, proteinuria, is the cardinal feature of the syndrome, without which the diagnosis cannot be made. Protein excretion of 3.5 g/24 hours is usually accepted as the minimal level for nephrotic-range proteinuria and leads consecutively and in varying degrees to the other four features. As proteinuria develops, hepatic synthesis of albumin is enhanced, but insufficient to cause the serum albumin concentration to return to normal.

Besides albumin, other proteins are lost in the urine of patients with NS. The urinary loss of antithrombin III has been associated with an increased thrombogenic tendency. Therefore, severely nephrotic patients may benefit from prophylactic anticoagulation. Increased excretion of various complement factors (such as factor B) with the resultant impairment of complement-mediated opsonization, in addition to the urinary loss of immunoglobulins, leaves the nephrotic patients at an increased risk for certain bacterial infections, specifically encapsulated organisms. The peculiar susceptibility of nephrotic children to infections with *Streptococcus pneumoniae* has long been a prominent feature of the NS. Another problem that was a significant cause of death in the preantibiotic era, was rapidly progressive soft tissue cellulitis. This infection commonly spread with terrifying rapidity in the edematous tissue of malnourished nephrotic patients.

Hyperlipidemia and the subsequent lipiduria occur because of an increase in lipoprotein synthesis, especially LDL and VLDL, with a corresponding rise in total serum cholesterol. Triglyceride levels are variably elevated, and HDL, due to enhanced urinary excretion, is often diminished. Naturally, these changes in circulating lipid concentrations have led to speculation that nephrotic patients are more susceptible to atherosclerotic vascular disease. Much of the current data, however, has been inconclusive. Patients with severe hypercholesterolemia may benefit from cholesterol-lowering agents.

The pathogenesis of edema in NS has generally been ascribed to the overall decrease in the plasma oncotic pressure associated with a low serum albumin concentration. Diminished plasma colloid osmotic pressure results in fluid transudation into the body's interstitial space. This resultant decrease in plasma volume leads to stimulation of the renin-aldosterone axis with secondary sodium retention. However, the plasma volume is often normal to increased in many nephrotic patients. Second, blood pressure is often normal or elevated in many patients with NS. Finally, renin and aldosterone levels are often decreased indicating primary rather than secondary renal salt retention. Therefore, the mechanisms leading to edema in nephrotic patients remains to be elucidated.

QUESTION 4 What is the therapeutic approach to a patient with NS?

There is no definitive approach for treatment of the respective causes of idiopathic NS. As a rule, MCD is very steroid responsive, and these patients are generally treated. Patients with FSGS are often treated with similar protocols, although the response rate is less than 50%. There is little justification for treating unselected patients with MGN, since the majority have a relatively good prognosis. If renal function deteriorates, evidence at present favors long-term treatment with an alkylating agent and steroids. Most secondary causes of NS necessitate treatment of the underlying systemic disease. NS associated with cancers will usually remit if the malignancy can be cured. When NS is caused by a drug, its discontinuation will similarly result in remission.

Aside from treating the actual glomerular lesion, certain guidelines apply to management of the complications associated with NS. Volume status needs to be continually addressed, and loop diuretic therapy with salt restriction is usually appropriate. Anticoagulation should be considered in the patient with massive proteinuria and severe hypoalbuminemia to prevent thrombosis. Cholesterol-lowering agents may be required in the severely hypercholesterolemic patient. The use of albumin infusions in the severely hypoalbuminemic patient may be efficacious in patients with evidence of intravascular volume depletion and may facilitate the response to diuretics. Angiotensin converting enzyme inhibitors may lower proteinuria, independent of their effects on blood pressure. As with all renal diseases, close attention to blood pressure may slow progression of renal failure.

CASE SUMMARY: This 55-year-old man presented with insidious lower extremity edema and proteinuria and suffered acutely from a pulmonary embolus. He was on no medications known to be associated with NS. With his age and sex, absence of a history of diabetes, normal serum complement levels and other negative serologic markers, and a benign urinary sediment, MGN would be the most likely diagnosis. This was confirmed on renal biopsy. Because of the association with solid tumors, the patient underwent routine screening which demonstrated blood in his stool. Colonoscopy was performed, and he was found to have adenocarcinoma of the colon. He underwent successful resection and was initially maintained on coumadin, furosemide, and lovastatin. Over the course of the next year the patient's NS resolved, and these medications were discontinued. A diagnostic algorithm for nephrotic range proteinuria is shown in Fig. 9-5-1.

• •

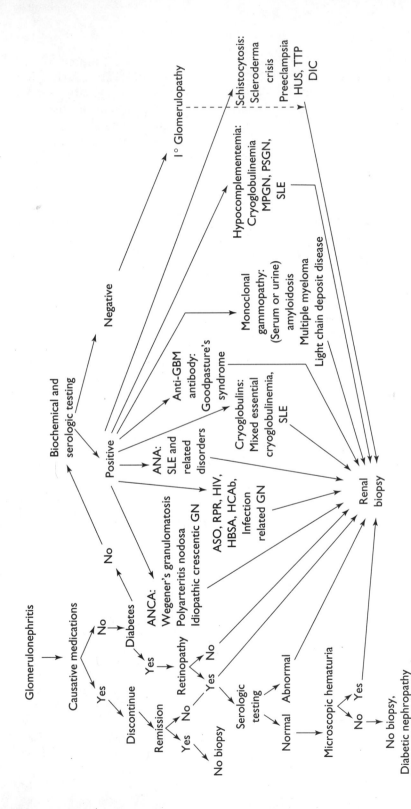

9-5-1 Algorithm for evaluation of patient with glomerulonephritis. Every one of these sero-logic tests may not be appropriate for every patient. ANCA: Anti-neutrophil cytoplasmic antibody; ASO: Anti-streptolysin-O antibody; VDRL: Venereal disease research labora-tory test; HIV: Human immunodeficiency virus antibody; HBSAg: Hepatitis B surface antigen; HCAb: Hepatitis C antibody; ANA: Anti-nuclear antibody; MPGN: Membrano-proliferative glomerulonephritis; PSGN: Post-streptococcal glomerulonephritis; HUS: Hemolytic uremic syndrome; TTP: Thrombotic thrombocytopenic purpura; DIC: Disseminated intravascular coagulation; Anti-GBM: Anti-glomerular basement membrane antibody; SLE: Systemic lupus erythematosus.

BIBLIOGRAPHY

Bernard DB: Extrarenal complications of the nephrotic syndrome, *Kidney Int*, 33:1184-1202, 1988.

Brenner BM, Stein JH: *Nephrotic syndrome. Contemporary issues in nephrology*, vol 9, New York, 1982, Churchill Livingstone.

Bruns FJ, Adler S, Fraley DS, Segel DP: Sustained remission of membranous glomerulonephritis after cyclophosphamide and prednisone, *Ann Intern Med*, 114:725-730, 1991.

Cameron JS, Glassock RJ: The nephrotic syndrome. In Lewis EJ, ed: *Management of the nephrotic syndrome in adults*, New York, 1988, Marcel Dekker.

Cameron JS: The nephrotic syndrome and its complications, *Am J Kidney Dis* X(3):157-171, 1987.

Cogan MG: Nephrotic syndrome, Medical Staff Conference, University of California, San Francisco, *West J Med*, 136: 411-417, 1982.

Falk RJ, Hogan SL, et al: Treatment of progressive membranous glomerulopathy, *Ann Intern Med*, 116:438-445, 1992.

Flamenbaum W, Hamburger RJ: *Nephrology: an approach to the patient wth renal disease*, Philadelphia, 1982, JB Lippincott.

Humes HD: *Pathophysiology of electrolyte and renal disorders*, New York, 1986, Churchill Livingstone.

Kanwer YS, Zheng ZL, Kashihara N, Waller EI: Current status of the structural and functional basis of glomerular filtration and proteinuria, *Semin Nephrology* 11(4):390-413, 1991.

Massry SG, Glassock RJ: *Textbook of nephrology*, vol 1, Baltimore, 1989, Williams & Wilkins.

Mathieson PW, Rees AJ: A critical review of treatment for membranous nephropathy. In Grünfeld, ed: *Advances in nephrology*, St Louis, 1991, Mosby.

Pei Y, Cattran D, et al: Evidence suggesting under-treatment in adults with idiopathic focal segmental glomerulosclerosis, *Am Med* 82:938-944, 1987.

Rose BD: *Pathophysiology of renal disease*, ed 2, New York, 1987, McGraw-Hill.

Wagoner RD: *The nephrotic syndrome: discussions in patient management*, New York, 1981, Medical Examination Publishing.

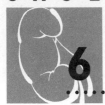

6

C. William Wester
Roger A. Rodby

A previously healthy 27-year-old man presented with gross hematuria, flank pain, and generalized malaise for 3 days. He had low-grade temperatures, a mild productive cough, and myalgias for approximately 4 days last week immediately preceding the acute onset of his genitourinary symptoms. The patient denied a previous history of gross hematuria but states that on two occasions in the past he was seen by emergency room physicians for sports related injuries and was told that he had blood in his urine. There were no arthralgias or episodes of hemoptysis.

The physical examination was remarkable for a temperature of 98.1°F, BP 140/92 mm Hg, P 84 bpm, and RR 14/min. The pulmonary and cardiovascular examinations were normal. The abdomen revealed normal bowel sounds with moderate right costovertebral angle tenderness. His extremities were without edema or rash.

The laboratory examination revealed BUN 18 mg/dl, creatinine 1.4 mg/dl, total protein 6.8 g/dl, albumin 3.8 g/dl, uric acid 7.0 mg/dl, and serum calcium 8.8 mg/dl. Serum complement levels were normal, and antinuclear antibody titers were not elevated. Hepatitis B surface antigen or antibodies to hepatitis C were not present. The urinalysis revealed 4+ blood and >300 mg/dl protein on dipstick with microscopic evaluation revealing > 100 rbc/hpf and 2 rbc casts. A 24-hour urine collection revealed 850 mg of protein. A renal biopsy was performed.

QUESTION I What is the profile of a patient with active glomerular inflammation? What are the important clues in the diagnosis of proteinuria and hematuria?

Acute glomerulonephritis (GN) refers to the abrupt onset of hematuria and proteinuria, often associated with an impairment in renal function, salt and water retention, edema, and hypertension. When severe and accompanied by fluid overload, this is often referred to as the "nephritic syndrome."

When glomerular inflammation is severe enough to cause hematuria and proteinuria, the glomerular filtration rate (GFR) is often diminished. This ranges from a minimal reduction in GFR with serum creatinine levels in the normal range, to acute renal failure (rapidly progressive glomerulonephritis [RPGN]). Depending on the degree of glomerular inflammation, patients may present with oliguria or anuria. Multiple factors may contribute to the reduction in GFR, including the effects of acute immune injury on glomerular pathology as well as the development of glomerular intracapillary thromboses, acute tubular necrosis, tubular obstruction by casts, and compression of the glomerular tuft by proliferating epithelial cells as they form crescents. Consequently, the return of normal renal function depends not only on cessation of the initial process, but also on the extent of underlying irreversible changes, represented pathologically as fibrosis.

Hypertension and pulmonary congestion are also common manifestations of acute GN and may be the sole presenting signs in older patients. Both are largely volume-mediated, reflecting extracellular fluid volume expansion due to the renal retention of sodium and water. The actual mechanisms of renal sodium retention are poorly understood but include a decreased filtered sodium load as well as increased sodium reabsorption in the distal nephron. Unlike edema associated with the nephrotic syndrome, the nephritic syndrome often manifests edema in nondependent areas, such as the eyelids, face, and hands.

Hematuria, microscopic or gross, is the hallmark of the nephritic syndrome. Hematuria associated with proteinuria and red blood cell casts reflects an underlying glomerular inflammatory process that has the potential for rapid decline in renal function. Red blood cells may originate from any location along the urinary tract, and urologic diseases must be distinguished from glomerular diseases. The majority of patients with hematuria will have urologic disease. These situations are usually associated with minimal proteinuria. As there is protein in blood, bleeding in the urinary tract may lead to proteinuria either by dipstick screening or through quantification with timed collections. This may be confused with glomerular damage. Nevertheless, nephrotic range proteinuria (>3.5 g/day) from blood in the urinary tract would require 50 ml/day of urologic bleeding. This amount of blood in urine will turn the urine extremely dark, and therefore urologic bleeding is a rare cause of significant proteinuria, unless the bleeding is extensive. Hematuria associated with clots is always extraglomerular in origin. Hematuria associated with red blood cell casts is always of glomerular origin.

QUESTION 2   What is the differential diagnosis of acute GN?

Glomerulopathies that cause the nephritic syndrome tend to have acute glomerular inflammation (e.g., endocapillary proliferation, necrosis, crescents, etc.). Glomerular lesions associated with the nephrotic syndrome tend to have less inflammation. This is reflected in the urinalysis with the proliferative lesions of the nephritic syndrome having more hematuria and often less proteinuria than that seen in the urine of the nephrotic patient. Certainly, overlap of these factors exists in a number of diseases. Still, there is some utility to the use of the terms nephritic and nephrotic since the clinical presentation of the patient's volume status, urinary sediment, and

renal function may serve as a guide to the glomerular pathology.

The prototypical model of a proliferative acute GN associated with hematuria and the nephritic syndrome is poststreptococcal glomerulonephritis (PSGN). Although certain other viral and bacterial infections have been linked to the development of postinfectious GN, it is classically described following infection of the pharynx or skin with a Group A beta-hemolytic *Streptococcus*. An increased incidence is known to be associated with certain streptococcal subtypes, especially type 12 and to a lesser extent types 1,2,3,4,18, and 25. Rheumatic fever follows only pharyngeal infection with group A strep, whereas nephritis may follow either skin or pharyngeal infection. PSGN is primarily a disease of children, and there is a male predominance. Upon presentation, patients may be entirely asymptomatic (with the incidental finding of hematuria on routine urinalysis) or may present in oliguric acute renal failure and signs of central volume expansion. In the classic form, the clinical onset is rather abrupt. The normal latent period averages approximately 10 days following the streptococcal infection. Another common presentation is gross hematuria with the urine taking on a smoky, rusty, or cola color, and this may be accompanied by oliguria. Some degree of hypertension and edema is found in greater than 75% of patients. Typically, the edema involves the face, eyelids, and hands and is notably worse upon first rising. Ascites and encephalopathy have been reported in children. In elderly patients, however, it is often the manifestations of cardiopulmonary congestion that dominates the clinical picture, although this can be seen in children as well.

Hematuria dominates the urinary sediment. Proteinuria is usually present but is less than 3.0 g/day in greater than 75% of cases. Glomerular filtration rate (GFR) and urinary sodium excretion are reduced with the fractional excretion of sodium often <1% during the acute phase. Throat or skin cultures will frequently demonstrate streptococcal infection. The magnitude of the antibody response to the extracellular products of streptococci have little role in providing protective immunity to patients. These antibody levels nevertheless serve as useful markers in the diagnosis of recent/present streptococcal infection. These include antibodies to antistreptolysin O (ASO), antihyaluronidase, and antidesoxyribonuclease. The ASO titers exceed 200 Todd units in approximately 70% of affected patients, with the elevation persisting for several months. Another common abnormal serologic finding includes hypocomplementemia with C3 being depressed and C4 remaining near normal, indicating activation of the alternate complement pathway.

Pathologically, one finds all glomeruli involved with diffuse proliferation and narrowing of the capillary loops. The hypercellularity results from the proliferation of mesangial and endothelial cells as well as from the accumulation of polymorphonuclear cells in the glomerular capillaries, giving this lesion the alternate name of a "suppurative glomerulonephritis." Immunofluorescent stains reveal bright, diffuse granular staining for both IgG and C3 along the glomerular basement membrane. The most characteristic finding is by electron microscopy demonstrating discrete large subepithelial electron-dense nodules called "humps."

Prominent features of this disease complex include the latent period between infection and onset of nephritis, hypocomplementemia, and the granular immune glomerular deposition. These imply that this process is analogous to the acute serum sickness model and is mediated solely by circulating immune-complex deposition; however, the exact etiologic mechanism remains unknown.

PSGN is usually benign, with over 95% of patients recovering normal renal function within two months. The disease is less aggressive in younger patients. Approximately 5% of patients have a crescentic lesion that may result in irreversible glomerular damage and the development of end-stage renal failure within months to years after diagnosis. Symptomatic and supportive therapy is usually all that is indicated. Only with evidence of persistent streptococcal infection does one employ antimicrobial therapy, although it is often used to prevent the spreading of nephritogenic strains to close contacts.

Occasionally a primary glomerulopathy can present as an acute GN. This is most often caused by IgA nephropathy or Berger's disease. In addition, it is the most common cause of asymptomatic hematuria with associated proteinuria. The entity is defined by the deposition of IgA in the glomerular mesangium. IgA nephropathy is more common in males. There is a reported increased incidence in populations with the HLA-Bw 35 and DR4 phenotypes. Patients often present with gross hematuria coincident with or immediately following an upper respiratory tract infection. Myalgias, malaise, low-grade fevers, dysuria, and loin pain are also common. The actual features of the nephritic syndrome, such as dependent edema and hypertension, are present in fewer than 50% of patients. In addition, fewer than 25% have impaired renal function during active disease with serum creatinine levels rarely exceeding 3 mg/dl. Predictors of poor prognosis include male gender, a prolonged clinical course, the development of hypertension or nephrotic range proteinuria, and the presence of extensive glomerulosclerosis on renal biopsy. Patients may also present with asymptomatic microscopic hematuria, normal blood pressure, and normal renal function found on a screening health examination. These patients generally have a good renal prognosis.

Because this disease often presents with gross hematuria following a sore throat, it is often confused with PSGN. Clinically, it is the absence of a latent period, as well as normal levels of complement and antistreptococcal antibodies (unless the patient has had a recent unrelated streptococcal infection) that distinguish this entity from PSGN. Pathologically, immune deposits are present in the mesangium of all glomeruli. IgA is the predominant immunoglobulin. Fifty to sixty percent of patients have a corresponding elevation in serum levels of IgA, but these levels do not correlate with the level of disease activity. No specific therapy has been demonstrated to provide consistent benefit. Treatment with steroids has not been uniformly satisfactory. Fortunately, the disease is mild and self-limiting in the majority of cases.

There are a number of systemic diseases that may have GN as a component of the disease presentation. These include the vasculitides and other autoimmune disorders, antiglomerular basement membrane antibody disease, the microangiopathic processes, and GN associated with infections. In addition, the primary glomerulopathy, membranoproliferative glomerulonephritis (MPGN), may present with the clinical picture of the nephritic syndrome. Each of these disorders may demonstrate mildly progressive renal insufficiency to rapidly progressive renal failure. The term rapidly progressive glomerulonephritis (RPGN) is used when a glomerular disease is associated with acute renal failure and pathologically usually associated with crescents. Patients with systemic disease-associated GN may present with the nephritic syndrome, or they may present with the symptoms of the systemic disease and are later found to have an abnormal urinary sediment or renal failure. Renal biopsy should be performed early in patients with renal insufficiency. Without appropriate therapy when available, these patients have a "rapidly progressive" course and can require dialysis within weeks to months of diagnosis. Examination of the urine reveals a "telescopic sediment" with many formed elements, including red blood cell casts, white blood cell casts, pyuria, and microscopic hematuria. Although abnormal quantities of protein are found in the urine, nephrotic range proteinuria is less common than in the glomerular diseases that are associated predominantly with the nephrotic syndrome.

This clinicopathologic picture of RPGN can be seen in PSGN and IgA nephropathy, but it is more commonly seen in one of three categories of diseases: (1) RPGN associated with a systemic disease (30%), (2) RPGN associated with antiglomerular basement membrane disease (20%), and (3) RPGN associated with idiopathic crescentic glomerulonephritis (50%).

QUESTION 3   What are the major systemic diseases that may lead to RPGN? What are the key elements of each process?

Vasculitic syndromes represent the majority of RPGN associated with systemic diseases and encompass a diverse group of clinicopathologic syndromes defined by inflammation and necrosis of blood vessels. Classic polyarteritis nodosa (PAN) is a necrotizing vasculitis of medium and small-sized muscular arteries. Most causes are idiopathic, although some have been reported in association with chronic infection with the hepatitis B virus. With active arteritis, there are local regions of fibrinoid necrosis with supervening infiltration of neutrophils and monocytes. Weakening of the arterial walls results in aneurysmal dilatations, typically at bifurcations. Manifestations of renal disease often occur in the setting of systemic illness characterized by fever, malaise, and weight loss. Involvement of other organ systems includes the GI tract, the cardiovascular and the nervous systems. Renal involvement usually presents as renal failure, severe accelerated hypertension, hematuria, and proteinuria. Interestingly, if only the large renal vessels are involved, renal biopsy may not be diagnostically helpful since the glomeruli may be intact. Abdominal angiography may be required to make the diagnosis. Overall, the prognosis remains poor in patients with major organ involvement. However, high dose steroids alone or in combination with cytotoxic agents have been shown to substantially improve survival.

Systemic necrotizing vasculitis of the small vessels usually affect the glomerulus and therefore may present with hematuria, proteinuria, and renal insufficiency. These include Wegener's granulomatosis, microscopic PAN, essential mixed cryoglobulinemia, and Henoch-Schonlein purpura.

Wegener's granulomatosis is a vasculitic syndrome characterized by upper and lower respiratory tract involvement as well as glomerulonephritis (GN). Upper respiratory symptoms such as rhinorrhea, epistaxis, and sinusitis are present in most patients and often precede other manifestations. Pulmonary involvement consists of cough, dyspnea, parenchymal infiltrates that may cavitate, and life-threatening pulmonary hemorrhage. Renal biopsy usually reveals a segmental necrotizing GN without immune deposits. Crescents may be present. This picture is similar to that found with other small vessel vasculitides and is not diagnostic unless necrotizing granulomas are present. Biopsy results may aid in the exclusion of other causes of a pulmonary-renal syndrome such as Goodpasture's syndrome and systemic lupus erythematosus. Circulating antineutrophil cytoplasmic antibodies (ANCA) are usually present and appear in a cytoplasmic distribution (C-ANCA). Cyclophosphamide in conjunction with steroids have been shown to significantly enhance disease survival.

Microscopic PAN is similar to Wegener's granulomatosis except that upper respiratory tract symptoms and pulmonary hemorrhage are less common. The glomerular lesion is also a segmental necrotizing GN. It is usually distinguished from Wegener's by the paucity of respiratory tract symptoms in addition to the pattern of ANCA, which in the case of microscopic PAN, is in a perinuclear (P-ANCA) pattern.

Essential mixed cryoglobulinemia is characterized by the clinical triad of weakness, arthralgia, and cutaneous vasculitis. The skin lesions most often involve the distal lower extremities and manifest as palpable purpura with frequent ulceration. Serologic evidence of chronic infection with hepatitis B or more recently hepatitis C has been associated with this disorder. Laboratory features include the presence of mixed serum cryoglobulins, an elevated rheumatoid factor, and depressed serum complement levels. Although no therapy is established, patients are often treated with steroids, immunosuppressive agents, and plasmapheresis.

Henoch-Schonlein purpura (HSP) is a syndrome characterized by cutaneous vasculitis, abdominal symptoms, and arthralgias. The skin lesions usually take the form of crops of palpable purpura on the lower limbs and buttocks. Ab-

dominal involvement is characterized by colicky pain and gastrointestinal bleeding. Joint involvement is usually mild and limited to the knees and ankles. Acute renal failure occurs in about one third of cases but usually resolves within a few weeks. However, 20% of these patients develop chronic renal failure over the course of several years. Renal biopsy reveals a focal or diffuse proliferative GN. Patients with significant renal failure at time of biopsy often display crescentic and necrotizing GN similar to a vasculitis. Granular deposits of IgA are found in the mesangium of all glomeruli. Because of this finding, its extrarenal symptoms, and since it often follows a URI infection, HSP is often referred to as the systemic disease form of IgA nephropathy. Like IgA nephropathy, no therapy is of proven benefit.

Systemic lupus erythematosus (SLE) is the most common nonvasculitic form of acute GN associated with a systemic disease. Circulating immune complexes, decreased serum complement levels, and auto-antibodies (particularly double stranded DNA) are often present and aid significantly in the diagnosis. It is primarily a disease of young and middle-aged females. The severity of renal disease in SLE does not always correlate with the severity of the extrarenal manifestations. Glomerular disease can be minimal with only a mild mesangial involvement to severe with diffuse endocapillary proliferation, crescents, and fibrinoid necrosis. Immune deposits may be seen in the mesangial, subepithelial, and subendothelial areas. Occasionally, few immunoglobulin deposits are seen in conjunction with segmental necrosis, suggesting a nonimmune complex-mediated vasculitic form. Treatment of the more severe forms of lupus nephritis consists of high-dose steroids, often with the addition of cytotoxic agents.

Other nonvasculitic causes of acute GN associated with systemic diseases include infectious related glomerulonephritides that are associated with chronic visceral abscesses, bacterial endocarditis, chronic ventriculoperitoneal shunt infection, and infection with the hepatitis B or C viruses.

The final category of systemic diseases associated with a RPGN presentation include the microangiopathic hemolytic processes. These include thrombotic thrombocytopenic purpura (TTP), hemolytic uremic syndrome (HUS), malignant hypertension, disseminated intravascular coagulation (DIC), scleroderma renal crisis, and preeclampsia. Usually there is evidence for one of these conditions at presentation. Glomerular microthrombosis predominates, and other signs of inflammation (proliferation and crescents) may be absent. The hallmark of these disorders is the presence of schistocytes on the peripheral blood smear. Other laboratory signs of intravascular hemolysis should be present, and thrombocytopenia is common.

Anti-glomerular basement membrane (anti-GBM) nephritis is caused by a circulating antibody directed against an antigen present in the glomerular basement membrane. In about two thirds of cases, renal involvement is associated with pulmonary hemorrhage: an entity called "Goodpasture's syndrome." In the remainder, the disease is localized to the kidney. Goodpasture's syndrome characteristically occurs in young males with a mean age of onset of 21 years. Patients usually present with hemoptysis, iron deficiency anemia, RPGN, and a linear pattern of antibody deposition on the glomerular basement membrane on renal biopsy. In most cases, the pulmonary manifestations appear first and vary from mild hemoptysis to life-threatening pulmonary hemorrhage. Renal involvement typically begins a few weeks after the onset of pulmonary symptoms and is usually evident on urinalysis as microscopic hematuria. A few cases of spontaneous recovery have been reported in patients with milder forms of renal involvement. However, the lesion is usually quite severe with the rapid development of RPGN associated with red blood cell casts, proteinuria, oliguria or anuria, and the potential for development of end-stage renal failure if treatment is delayed. Nephrotic range proteinuria is rare. Anti-GBM antibodies can be present in the circulation by indirect immunofluorescence in approximately 75% of patients. Complement levels are normal. Untreated, one third of patients with Goodpasture's syndrome die of pulmonary involvement, and most of the remainder progress to end-stage renal disease in an average of three to four months. Plasmapheresis combined with immunosuppressive therapy is effective if initiated early and is currently the treatment of choice.

Finally, the term *idiopathic RPGN* refers specifically to crescentic glomerulonephritis that is not mediated by anti-GBM antibody and not associated with any recognizable systemic illness. Similar to microscopic PAN and Wegener's granulomatosis, there are no glomerular immune deposits on immunofluorescence staining. The entity may in fact represent a form of small vessel vasculitis that is limited to the kidney. This is supported by the fact that the majority of these patients have circulating ANCA, usually in the perinuclear (P-ANCA) pattern. This disease may therefore represent a renal limited form of microscopic PAN. The disease is one of relatively older patients, with a mean age of onset of about 58 years (range 12 to 80). About one half of the reported patients are oliguric when first seen and have serum creatinine levels exceeding 6 mg/dl. Nonspecific signs/symptoms of renal failure are often present and include weakness, anorexia, nausea and vomiting, and weight loss. A history of recent flu-like illness with fever, myalgias, and polyarthralgia is common. Untreated, the vast majority of patients die or become hemodialysis dependent within two years. Although no controlled studies are available, because of the similarity to idiopathic vasculitis, treatment is usually similar and includes high dose intravenous steroids in combination with cyclophosphamide.

QUESTION 4 How does one differentiate between the above processes?

Because of the diverse nature of the diseases associated with hematuria, patients should have a complete history and physical examination. Close inspection of the urinary sediment is essential as red blood cell casts indicate that the hematuria is of glomerular origin and urologic evaluation may

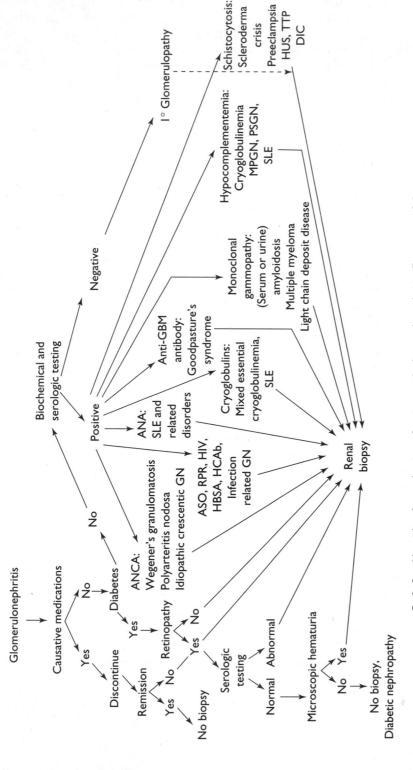

9-6-1 Algorithm for evaluation of patient with glomerulonephritis. Every one of these serologic tests may not be appropriate for every patient. ANCA: Anti-neutrophil cytoplasmic antibody; ASO: Anti-streptolysin-O antibody; VDRL: Venereal disease research laboratory test; HIV: Human immunodeficiency virus antibody; HBSAg: Hepatitis B surface antigen; HCAb: Hepatitis C antibody; ANA: Anti-nuclear antibody; MPGN: Membranoproliferative glomerulonephritis; PSGN: Post-streptococcal glomerulonephritis; HUS: Hemolytic uremic syndrome; TTP: Thrombotic thrombocytopenic purpura; DIC: Disseminated intravascular coagulation; Anti-GBM: Anti-glomerular basement membrane antibody; SLE: Systemic lupus erythematosus.

TABLE 9-6-I Clinical and Serologic Features of Glomerulopathies Associated with the Nephritic Syndrome

GN	Purpuric Rash	Pulmonary Hemorrhage	C3	ANA	Cryos	ANCA	AGBM	HBSA	HCVAb	RF	Schistocytes
PAN	+/–	+/–	nl	–	–	+P	–	+	+	–	+/–
Wegener's	+/–	++	nl	–	–	+C	–	–	–	–	+/–
HSP	++	–	nl	–	–	–	–	–	–	–	+/–
MEC	++	+/–	low	+	+	–	–	+	+	+	+/–
PSGN	–	–	low	–	–	–	–	–	–	+	–
SBE	+/–	+/–	low	+	+	–	–	–	–	+	–
SLE	+/–	+	low	++	+	–	–	–	–	+	+/–
Anti-GBM	–	++	nl	–	–	–	+	–	–	–	–
Idiopathic Crescentic	–	–	nl	–	–	+P	–	–	–	–	–
Microangiopathic Processes											
HUS, TTP, DIC	+/–	–	nl	–	–	–	–	–	–	–	++
Preeclampsia	–	–	nl	–	–	–	–	–	–	–	++
Scleroderma	–	–	nl	+	+/–	–	–	–	–	+	++

Legend: ++ (very commonly seen), + (commonly seen), +/– (not common but is reported), – (not present), nl (levels in normal range), low (levels in low range), P (perinuclear pattern), C (cytoplasmic pattern).

C3, third component of complement; ANA, anti-nuclear antibody; Cryos, cryoglobulins; ANCA, anti-neutrophil cytoplasmic antibody; Anti GBM, anti-glomerular basement membrane antibody; HBSA, hepatitis B surface antigen; HCAb, hepatitis C antibody; RF, rheumatoid factor.

GN, glomerulonephritis; PAN, Classic polyarteritis nodosa or microscopic polyateritis nodosa; HSP, Henoch-Scholein purpura; MEC, mixed essential cryoglobulinemia; PSGN, poststreptococcal glomerulonephritis; SBE, subacute bacterial endocarditis; SLE, systemic lupus erythematosus; Anti-GBM, anti glomerular basement antibody disease; HUS, hemolytic uremic syndrome; TTP, thrombotic thrombocytopenic purpura; DIC, disseminated intravascular coagulation.

be avoided. Twenty-four-hour urine collection for protein should be undertaken because the presence of significant proteinuria usually confirms that the hematuria is of glomerular origin. Elevation of the blood urea nitrogen (BUN) or creatinine indicate that evaluation should be immediate since delay in diagnosing an RPGN may lead to irreversible renal failure. All African-American patients with isolated hematuria should undergo evaluation for sickle cell trait to rule out sickle cell disease as this is a common cause of hematuria in the African-American population. Patients with symptoms of an upper respiratory tract infection preceding the hematuria, or with symptoms suggestive of a systemic disease, need the appropriate serologic studies. Depending on the symptoms, these serologic markers include ASO titers, ANA, ANCA, anti-GBM, serum complement levels, and cryoglobulins. The peripheral blood smear should be evaluated for the presence of schistocytes. Ultimately, a renal biopsy should be performed in most patients in whom acute glomerular disease is suspected. This includes patients presenting with glomerular hematuria, the nephritic syndrome, RPGN, or patients with systemic diseases known to be associated with renal pathology with features on urinalysis suggestive of glomerular involvement. Because of the overlap of the diseases that present as either the nephrotic syndrome or the nephritic syndrome, the algorithms for Nephrology Cases 5 and 6 are identical. Table 9-6-1 in this chapter lists the more common diseases associated with the nephritic syndrome and categorizes them by the presence or absence of certain historical, physical examination, and laboratory features (e.g., pulmonary hemorrhage; or on physical examination, e.g., purpuric rash and complement levels, etc.).

CASE SUMMARY: Our patient is a young male with a history of recurrent yet unevaluated microscopic hematuria who now presents with loin pain, gross hematuria, hypertension, and mild renal insufficiency immediately following an upper respiratory

infection. The red blood cell casts obviated the need for urologic work up. His laboratory values and serologic determinations, specifically ASO titers and complement levels, were normal and distinguished it from poststreptococcal glomerulonephritis. This is a common presentation for IgA nephropathy, and this was demonstrated on renal biopsy. Without treatment the gross hematuria resolved. At last follow-up he was without hypertension and edema and had normal kidney function with only trace amounts of blood and protein on urinalysis.

A diagnostic algorithm for glomerulonephritis is shown in Fig. 9-6-1.

Table 9-6-1 provides a listing of various forms of acute glomerulonephritis and findings which aid in diagnosis.

• •

BIBLIOGRAPHY

Abuelo JG: *Renal pathophsiology: the essentials,* Baltimore, 1989, Williams & Wilkins.

Brenner BM, Coe FL, Rector FC Jr: *Clinical nephrology,* Philadelphia, 1987, WB Saunders.

Brenner BM, Rector FC Jr: *The kidney,* ed 4, vol 1, Philadelphia, 1991, WB Saunders.

Bricker NS, Kirschenbaum MA: *The kidney: diagnosis and management,* New York, 1984, Wiley Medical Publications.

Briggs WA, Johnson JP, et al: Antiglomerular basement membrane antibody mediated glomerulonephritis and Goodpasture's syndrome, *Medicine* 58(5):348-360, 1979.

Flamenbaum W, Hamburger R: *Nephrology: an approach to the patient with renal disease,* Philadelphia, 1982, JB Lippincott.

Jacobson HR, Striker GE, Klahr S: *Principles and practice of nephrology,* Philadelphia, 1991, BC Decker.

Leatherman JW, Davies SF, Hoidal JR: Alveolar hemorrhage syndromes: diffuse microvascular lung hemmorhage in immune and idiopathic disorders, *Medicine* 63(6):343-360, 1984.

Salant DJ: Immunopathogen of crescentic glomerulonephritis and lung purpura, *Kidney Int* 32:408-425, 1987.

Seldin DW, Giebisch G: *The kidney: physiology and pathophysiology,* ed 2, vol 3, 1992, Raven Press.

Suki WN, Eknoyan G: *The kidney in systemic disease,* ed 2, Perspectives in Nephrology and Hypertension, New York, 1981, Wiley Medical Publications.

Wyngaarden JB, Smith LH, Bennett JC: *Cecil textbook of medicine,* ed 19, vol 2, Philadelphia, 1992, WB Saunders.

NEUROLOGY

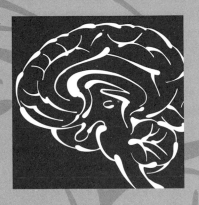

PHILIP GORELICK

SECTION EDITOR

CASE

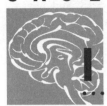

Christopher Hughes
Philip Gorelick

A *76-year-old white woman with a medical history of diabetes mellitus, hypertension, and stroke presents with left arm and leg weakness. These symptoms began approximately 2 hours earlier, at which time she was found by her family in bed, lethargic, not moving her left side, and unaware of her condition. On further questioning the patient states that she has been taking her medications (including insulin) as prescribed but has not been eating well for the past few days. She had fallen earlier that day but cannot remember if she hit her head or lost consciousness. Her blood pressure and serum glucose were well controlled at her last outpatient office visit, and she denies any recent febrile illness.*

Her medications include NPH insulin 20 units each morning and 10 units each evening, Inderal-LA 60 mg each morning, and Colace 1 capsule each day. Past medical history includes a stroke 8 months ago. The episode occurred shortly after awakening from sleep and caused left face, arm, and leg weakness. The weakness resolved after many months of physical therapy.

On physical examination the vital signs were BP 180/100 mm Hg, P 82 bpm, RR 20/min, T 98.6°F. There were no carotid bruits. Heart rate was irregularly irregular. S1 and S2 sounds were normal. On lung auscultation there were crackles at both bases. Neurologic examination revealed a lethargic but arousable patient who followed 1-step commands and had no language deficits. She had mild dysarthria and complained of a mild headache. Pupils were equal and reactive to light. A right gaze preference was noted, but the horizontal oculocephalic (doll's

eyes) reflex was normal. There was a left homonymous hemianopsia, a left lower facial droop, a flaccid left arm, and an externally rotated left leg (4 minus out of 5 motor power). Motor power was normal in the right arm and leg. Deep tendon reflexes were diminished in the left arm and absent in the legs. The Babinski sign was present on the left side. There was no response to deep pain in the left arm; slight acknowledgment of painful stimulus to the left leg; and normal pain sensation of the right arm and leg. Gait was not tested.

QUESTION I Given the above physical examination, localize the patient's neurologic findings, compare and contrast them to the patient's previous stroke deficit. What are the major accepted risk factors for cerebrovascular disease?

The patient's neurologic findings can be explained by dysfunction in the right or nondominant cerebral hemisphere in the territory of the middle cerebral artery (MCA). Lack of awareness of neurologic deficit may occur with a right or nondominant hemisphere lesion. Babinski coined the term *anosognosia* for unawareness of loss of motor power. The patient's previous stroke symptoms suggest a subcortical location. When stroke involves this region, it often causes weakness or sensory deficits in the face, arm, and leg in the absence of higher cortical dysfunction.

Lethargy may result when there is bilateral cerebral hemisphere dysfunction or involvement of the reticular activating system. In either case the underlying lesion can be a structural lesion as might occur with an infarct or tumor mass, or a physiologic lesion as might occur with toxic-metabolic disease (e.g., renal failure). In this case the lethargy resulted from a cortical mass lesion.

Right gaze preference can be caused by dysfunction of the right frontal gaze center. The ipsilateral frontal eye field controls conjugate eye movement to the contralateral side. As the right frontal gaze center becomes hypoactive, the normal functioning left frontal gaze center drives the eyes to the right. An active seizure focus causing hyperactivity of the left frontal gaze center could also cause conjugate eye deviation to the right. With a seizure, however, there may be nystagmus that manifests as "lightning" or fast beat movements in the direction of the conjugate eye deviation.

Left homonymous hemianopsia suggests postchiasmal dysfunction of the right optic radiation in the temporal and parietal lobe or occipital lobe. This finding is due to loss of the right nasal visual field and the left temporal visual field as, after the optic chiasm, these fibers run together in the right optic tract and hemisphere and can be damaged by a common lesion.

The motor examination findings can be explained by the cerebral vascular supply. The face and arm regions of the motor cortex (area 4) are supplied by the middle cerebral artery while the leg region is supplied by the anterior cerebral artery. In this case there was marked left faciobrachial weakness that may typify middle cerebral artery territory motor dysfunction.

It is also important to distinguish depressed reflexes from absent reflexes. Depression of the deep tendon reflexes can occur with an acute stroke in the cerebral cortex. Absence of the deep tendon reflexes in the legs are likely due to neuropathic dysfunction from diabetes mellitus.

Risk factors for cerebrovascular disease include age, male gender, coronary heart disease, atrial fibrillation, cigarette smoking, hypertension, diabetes mellitus, and heavy alcohol consumption. In young adults one must consider procoagulant states including the presence of the lupus anticoagulant, protein C or S deficiency, antithrombin III deficiency, and drug abuse (e.g., cocaine).

QUESTION 2   Discuss the differential diagnosis given the above neurologic history and physical examination. What are examples of specific stroke syndromes?

A right MCA territory ischemic stroke is the first differential diagnosis. This diagnosis is supported by the acute onset of focal neurologic findings consistent with cortical dysfunction in the anatomic area supplied by the MCA. High blood pressure upon presentation (180/100 mm Hg) is also commonly found in patients with acute stroke. It is important to consider a cardioembolic etiology. This may present as a sudden deficit in a patient with atrial fibrillation or other potential source (e.g., rheumatic heart disease, dilated cardiomyopathy, acute myocardial infarction). With exceedingly high blood pressure (e.g., 230/130 mm Hg), acute intracranial hemorrhage should be considered. When the source of an embolus is from either the left atrium or the systemic circulation via a patent foramen ovale or atrial septal defect, it is known as a paradoxical embolus.

Depending on the length of the patient's symptoms the diagnosis may be transient ischemic attack (TIA), reversible ischemic neurologic deficit (RIND), or stroke. In a TIA, the deficit is resolved within a 24-hour period. The RIND lasts up to 2 to 3 days before recovery. The deficit from a stroke may be indefinite.

An alternative diagnosis is Todd's paralysis. This is a transient focal neurologic deficit following a focal seizure. These deficits are thought to be caused by a relative hypofunctioning of the seizure focus and surround inhibition, a physiologic mechanism to prevent spread of the electrical seizure focus. Seizures can develop in the region of previous cortical strokes. They typically begin 6 to 18 months after the ischemic event but may also occur during the acute stroke period. Secondary generalization of a focal seizure can also cause postictal lethargy. If there is radiologic evidence that this patient's previous stroke was cortical in distribution, a postictal Todd's paralysis could explain her current neurologic findings.

The patient could also be suffering from a subdural hematoma as she is elderly and had a fall on the day of hospitalization. Therefore, acute subdural hematoma must be ruled out. Even without a clear history of head trauma, chronic subdural hematoma can develop in the elderly and cause focal neurologic deficits as well as an alteration in mental status. Classically, visual field defects are not observed with this condition. The presence of headache would also support the diagnosis.

Hypoglycemia is a metabolic derangement that can lead to mental status changes. The patient is an insulin-dependent diabetic who continued to use insulin despite eating poorly. Hypoglycemia can cause, accentuate, or unmask previous neurologic deficits. Other metabolic abnormalities such as hyponatremia, hypernatremia, uremia, or hepatic encephalopathy may precipitate mental status changes. As this patient had a previous stroke, hypoglycemia could be unmasking her previous deficits or could account for her mental status change and fall earlier in the day. Diaphoresis and other manifestations of hypoglycemia may be masked by her use of a beta-blocker medication.

Another etiology that must be considered is vasculitis. Small to medium size artery vasculitis may involve the brainstem, spinal cord, or meninges. The diagnosis rests on isolation of a systemic or primary nervous system illness that causes vasculitis and biopsy that reveals an inflammatory infiltrate in the vessel wall.

A stroke syndrome includes identification of the location of the anatomical lesion, the arterial territory involved, and evaluation of the associated neurologic deficits. An example of a stroke syndrome is the lateral medullary syndrome. This is usually the result of vertebral artery occlusion. The syndrome includes loss of ipsilateral facial sensory function (CN V palsy), contralateral loss of pain and temperature sensation (spinothalamic tract dysfunction), dysarthria and dysphagia (lateral brainstem dysfunction), ataxia (cerebellar infarction), and an ipsilateral Horner's syndrome (sympathetic fiber loss). MCA syndrome leads to contralateral hemiplegia and aphasia if the dominant hemisphere is involved. The posterior cerebral artery syndrome results in cranial nerve III palsy (ptosis) and contralateral hemiplegia as well as complex visual and behavioral deficits. Infarction of the territory of the anterior cerebral artery leads to contralateral lower extremity weakness and dysphasia because of supplementary motor area involvement on the dominant side. Lastly, basilar artery thrombosis may result in quadriplegia (bilateral corticospinal tract dysfunction), horizontal gaze palsy (paramedian pontine reticular formation involvement), altered level of consciousness (reticular activating system), and corticobulbar dysfunction.

QUESTION 3 The following laboratory data are now available: electrolytes are normal; serum glucose is 97 mg/dl, and CBC is normal. An ECG shows atrial fibrillation with a ventricular response of 80 bpm. A previous echocardiogram showed normal left ventricular function, normal valvular function, and a normal-sized left atrium. How does this laboratory information alter the differential diagnosis, and what test would be most helpful at this juncture?

The normal serum glucose level rules out hypoglycemia. The new onset atrial fibrillation lends support to the diagnosis of a cardioembolic infarct in the right MCA territory. The normal echocardiogram does not support the diagnosis of infective or thrombotic endocarditis though vegetations may be missed by this type of study. The echocardiogram can also be used to diagnose a patent foramen ovale (PFO) or atrial septal defect (ASD). This is done by injection of micro-bubbles into the venous circulation and noting their presence in the left heart chambers.

A CT scan of the brain should now be performed. This will help rule out subdural hematoma, right MCA stroke that has become hemorrhagic, and other mass lesions. Hemorrhagic conversion can occur with ischemic strokes caused by emboli.

QUESTION 4 The CT scan of the brain is performed and shows an old right subcortical infarct. Subdural hematoma, intracerebral hemorrhage, or other acute findings are not noted. What is the most likely diagnosis, and how should the patient be managed?

The prior stroke is subcortical and therefore is unlikely to be a cause of seizures or postictal paralysis. A CT scan with contrast (or an MRI of the brain with and without gadolinium) is required to rule out a brain neoplasm. However, plain CT scan findings and the lack of a history of systemic cancer make the latter diagnosis unlikely. The most likely diagnosis is an embolic stroke to the right middle cerebral artery territory that is secondary to atrial fibrillation (Fig. 10-1-1).

There are several important management issues regarding this case. Understanding the role of blood pressure and intracranial perfusion is essential to adequate management. Elevated blood pressure may be observed in the first weeks following acute stroke. A common mistake is to acutely lower the blood pressure to the normal range. In the presence of an occluded cerebral artery, cerebrovascular autoregulation is impaired. Lowering the blood pressure may decrease blood flow around the ischemic penumbra, making the stroke deficit worse. In ischemic stroke, blood pressure should be gently and gradually reduced or not reduced at all unless there is hypertensive encephalopathy or manifestations of malignant hypertension that requires emergent treatment.

Control of serum glucose control may be important. Hypoglycemia will increase cell death, especially when coupled with failing cerebral blood flow in acute ischemic stroke. Hyperglycemia will increase lactic acid production in the ischemic region as glucose is used in the absence of oxygen and will lead to acidosis. Experimental and clinical studies have shown that infarct size or associated neurologic deficit is greater when hyperglycemia is present. Elevation in serum glucose should be treated; however, one must avoid hypoglycemia during correction of serum glucose.

Another issue concerns anticoagulation. The patient has atrial fibrillation and a suspected cardioembolic stroke. Anticoagulation may reduce the risk of recurrence of cardioembolic stroke when there is nonvalvular atrial fibrillation, dilated cardiomyopathy, prosthetic heart valve disease, ventricular aneurysm, and recent MI. However, emboli that lodge in cerebral blood vessels and cause ischemia can lyse and lead to reperfusion of previously ischemic regions of cortex. If this occurs, bland infarctions may transform into hemorrhagic infarctions as blood leaks through the damaged blood vessel wall during reperfusion. The risk of hemorrhagic transformation is high early on after embolic stroke. In nonvalvular atrial fibrillation, anticoagulation is generally postponed for 48 hours at which time a repeat CT scan of the brain is performed. If the scan shows no evidence of hemorrhagic transformation, and an extensive CT or neurologic deficit is not present, anticoagulation is usually administered.

For mild noncardioembolic TIA or mild stroke, aspirin or ticlopidine may be used for secondary prevention. Most favor the use of aspirin based on risk-benefit studies. The optimal dose of aspirin for secondary stroke prevention is controversial (975 to 1300 mg versus ≤375 mg). Higher doses may be more effective in reducing primary outcome endpoints, but the safety profile (e.g., gastrointestinal hemorrhage) may be worse. Ticlopidine (250 mg bid) may be more effective in certain patient subgroups such as women, diabetics, and African-Americans, but is associated more frequently with such adverse effects as reversible neutropenia, skin rash, and diarrhea.

Data now exist that clarify the role of carotid endarterectomy in patients with ipsilateral hemispheric symptoms due to angiographically determined carotid stenosis of 70% to 99%. The North American Symptomatic Carotid Endarterectomy Trial (NASCET) and the European Carotid Surgery Trial found surgical repair to be superior to medical therapy in such cases.

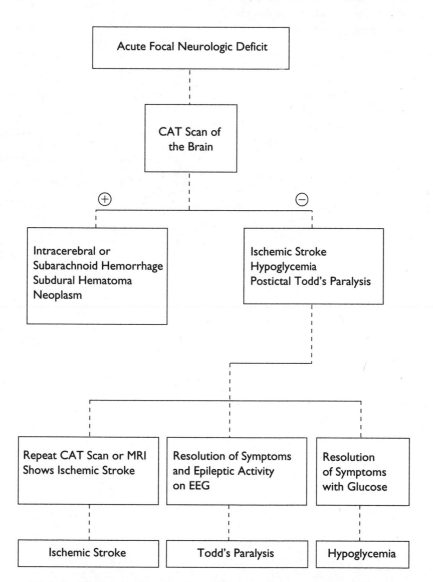

10-1-1   Diagnostic algorithm for middle cerebral artery (MCA) syndrome.

QUESTION 5 The patient is admitted to the hospital. Twelve hours later the patient's nurse informs you that the patient is unarousable and now has an unreactive pupil. Which pupil do you suspect is dysfunctional? What is the significance of this finding, and does this alter your management strategy?

The patient's lethargic state at presentation suggests a large cortical infarct. As swelling occurs within the fixed space of the cranium, intracranial pressure is increased and herniation can occur. With a large right MCA territory stroke the right cerebral hemisphere will swell and cause midline shift to the left side. The cortex can also press downward and/or medially and compress the third cranial nerve on the right side. The worsening mental status and unreactive pupil on the right side suggests cerebral herniation. Progression of this herniation will eventually lead to a complete third cranial nerve palsy. Steroid treatment has not been shown to be consistently effective in this situation. However, acute intervention to decrease intracranial pressure may include mannitol infusion (1 g/kg over 20 minutes) and elective intubation with hyperventilation. The goal of hyperventilation is to reduce the P_{CO_2} to 25 to 30 mm Hg. It is important to note that the ICP will stabilize after 24 to 48 hours with this therapy.

BIBLIOGRAPHY

Becker DP: Acute subdural hematomas. In Vigouroux RP, McLaurin RL, eds: *Extracerebral collections: advances in neurotraumatology,* New York, 1986, Springer-Verlag.

Brihaye J: Chronic subdural hematomas. In Vigouroux RP, McLaurin RL, eds: *Extracerebral collections: advances in neurotraumatology,* New York, 1986, Springer-Verlag.

Cerebral Embolism Task Force: Cardiogenic brain embolism: the second report of the Cerebral Embolism Task Force, *Arch Neurol* 46:727-743, 1989.

Gupta R: Postinfarction seizures: a clinical study, *Stroke* 19: 1477-1481, 1988.

Malouf R: Hypoglycemia: causes, neurological manifestations, and outcome, *Ann Neurol* 17:421-430, 1985.

Marsh EE: Circadian variation in onset of acute ischemic stroke, *Arch Neurol* 47:1178-1180, 1990.

Masdeu C: The localization of lesions affecting the cerebral hemispheres. In Brazis PW, ed: *Localization in Clinical Neurology,* Boston, 1990, Little, Brown.

Stroke Prevention in Atrial Fibrillation Study Group Investigators: Preliminary report of the stroke prevention in atrial fibrillation study, *N Engl J Med* 322:863-868, 1990.

Tinuper P: Prolonged ictal paralysis: electroencephalographic confirmation of its epileptic nature, *Clin Electroencephalogr* 18:12-14, 1987.

C A S E

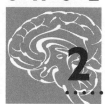

2

Christopher Hughes
Philip Gorelick
•••••••••

A 25-year-old white man with a medical history of Crohn's disease came to the emergency room with a 3-week history of daily diarrhea. He states that his Crohn's disease has been symptomatic for 3 years. The night prior to presentation he awoke with mild abdominal pain. Since that time, the waves of abdominal pain have increased in frequency and intensity. The patient now complains of continuous nausea and 3 episodes of emesis. Past medical history is remarkable only for Crohn's disease, which was diagnosed 5 years ago. No surgical therapy has been required; however, the patient has been hospitalized twice in the past for exacerbations. Currently, he takes no medications.

Physical examination shows mild orthostatic hypotension, hyperactive bowel sounds, and mild diffuse abdominal tenderness. There is no rebound tenderness. The patient is alert, oriented, and able to follow 3-step commands. Plain abdominal x-rays show dilated loops of small bowel. Blood drawn for electrolyte analysis revealed slight hypokalemia. The patient was admitted to the hospital and administered hydrocortisone 100 mg IV every 6 hours and Azulfidine suppositories. Five percent dextrose solution in 0.45 normal saline with supplementary potassium chloride was given intravenously to maintain hydration. Tigan suppositories were used to control nausea, and meperidine was ordered for pain. No oral feedings were given.

Over the next 24 hours the patient improved. There was less abdominal pain and diarrhea; however, nausea persisted. There was one episode of emesis. The next day the patient was found to be unsteady while walking in the hall. His blood pressure was normal, and he was

placed on bed rest. Later that evening the patient repeatedly attempted to leave his bed despite instructions from his nurse. He stated that he needed to clean the garage. He was not oriented to time or place. The nurse described him as globally confused. The physician on call was asked to evaluate the patient.

QUESTION I Discuss the differential diagnosis of confusion in this patient. What additional information would be helpful in determining the etiology of his symptoms?

Causes of mental confusion in this patient can be divided into the following categories: drug effect/withdrawal, metabolic, infectious, neurologic, and psychiatric (Table 10-2-1).

Effects of medications may be due to an adverse reaction or withdrawal (e.g., secondary to dependence). Narcotics (meperidine), steroids (hydrocortisone), and antihistamines (Tigan) may be associated with altered mental status. This is especially true in the elderly where marked mental status changes may occur with even small doses of these medications. Furthermore, given the present epidemic of drug abuse among young adults, one should consider illicit drug use or alcohol withdrawal. In the latter condition, symptoms of agitation, confusion, and tremor will begin 24 to 48 hours after abstinence. When alcohol withdrawal occurs, delirium tremens may occur. Autonomic hyperactivity (tremulousness, sweating, tachycardia, elevated blood pressure) and acute confusion are the hallmarks of this syndrome. Benzodiazepine withdrawal is a commonly encountered drug withdrawal syndrome. Blood and urine toxicol-

TABLE 10-2-1   Differential Diagnosis of Confusion in this Patient

Category	Cause	Investigations
Drugs/Drug Withdrawal	Steroids Anticholinergics Antihistamines Drug withdrawal	Vital signs, medication list, and urine/blood toxicology
Metabolic	Hyper/hyponatremia Hyper/hypocalcemia Hyper/hypoglycemia Liver failure Kidney failure	Blood chemistry profile
Infectious	Sepsis Peritonitis Meningitis	Vital signs, CBC, sedimentation rate, consider lumbar puncture
Psychiatric	Psychotic depression Schizophrenia Anxiety Mania	History and psychiatric evaluation

Neurologic	Mass lesion
	Brainstem compression
	Subdural hematoma
	Nutritional deficiency
	Postictal state
		Neurologic examination
		  Consider brain CAT scan
		  Consider lumbar puncture
		  Empiric thiamine infusion
		  Consider EEG

ogy screens help to establish the diagnosis of drug withdrawal.

Electrolyte abnormalities may be associated with confusion. Hyponatremia is of particular concern in this patient given the history of diarrhea. Patients with inflammatory bowel disease may be treated with long courses of corticosteroids on a long-term basis. Abrupt withdrawal of corticosteroids can lead to Addisonian crisis. Hyperglycemia should also be considered given the use of intravenous dextrose and steroid treatment. Abnormalities in calcium homeostasis can also cause altered mental status as may uremia, hepatic encephalopathy, folate deficiency, and B_{12} deficiency.

In a patient with fever and altered mental status, meningitis must be considered. Physical findings that may support this diagnosis are fever, nuchal rigidity, leukocytosis, and Kernig's or Brudzinski's sign (for more detail concerning meningitis see Infectious Disease Case 10). Systemic infections may also be associated with altered mental status, especially in the elderly.

Hospitalization may be an important stressor.

For example, patients with histories of psychiatric disease may decompensate during hospitalization. Bipolar disorder, agitated or psychotic depression, and schizophrenia should all be considered. Patients without past psychiatric disease may develop anxiety, agitation, or depression.

Possible neurologic causes of altered mental status in this patient include cerebral mass lesion, cerebellar infarction, or nutritional deficiencies associated with chronic diarrhea or gastrointestinal disturbance.

QUESTION 2 The house officer evaluating the patient noted the following information: blood pressure was 130/80 mm Hg, pulse rate 90 bpm, breathing rate 16/minute, and temperature 99.2° F. A chemistry profile drawn 2 hours earlier showed no significant abnormalities. CBC was unremarkable. No Tigan or meperidine had been administered for 6 hours. The last steroid dose was administered 5 hours earlier. Blood and urine toxicology screens were negative. The patient's wife confirmed the unusual nature of the patient's current behavior and the lack of a psychiatric

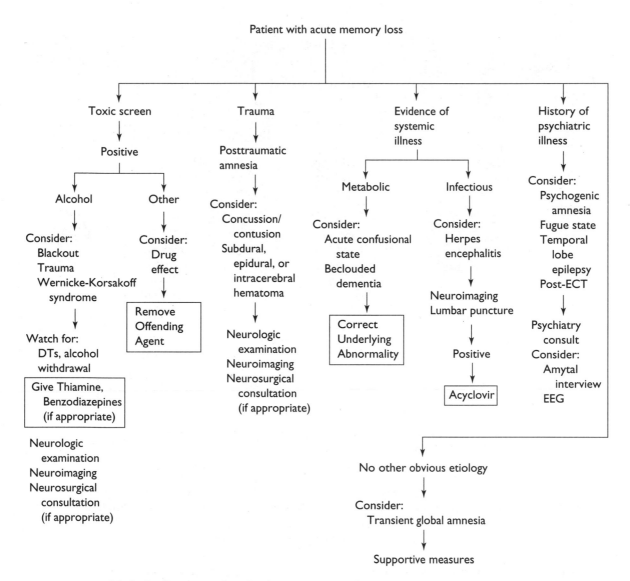

Patient with acute memory loss

Toxic screen

Positive

Alcohol

Consider:
Blackout
Trauma
Wernicke-Korsakoff
syndrome

Watch for:
DTs, alcohol
withdrawal

Give Thiamine,
Benzodiazepines
(if appropriate)

Neurologic
examination
Neuroimaging
Neurosurgical
consultation
(if appropriate)

Other

Consider:
Drug
effect

Remove
Offending
Agent

Trauma

Posttraumatic
amnesia

Consider:
Concussion/
contusion
Subdural,
epidural, or
intracerebral
hematoma

Neurologic
examination
Neuroimaging
Neurosurgical
consultation
(if appropriate)

**Evidence of
systemic
illness**

Metabolic

Consider:
Acute confusional
state
Beclouded
dementia

Correct
Underlying
Abnormality

Infectious

Consider:
Herpes
encephalitis

Neuroimaging
Lumbar puncture

Positive

Acyclovir

**History of
psychiatric
illness**

Consider:
Psychogenic
amnesia
Fugue state
Temporal
lobe
epilepsy
Post-ECT

Psychiatry
consult
Consider:
Amytal
interview
EEG

No other obvious etiology

Consider:
Transient global amnesia

Supportive measures

10-2-1 Diagnostic algorithm for acute memory loss.
(From Greene HL, Johnson WP, Maricic MJ: *Decision making in medicine,* St Louis, 1993, Mosby.)

history. How does this information help one focus on the differential diagnosis of confusion in this patient and what aspects of the physical examination should be emphasized?

The absence of metabolic abnormalities or drug toxicity on screening blood chemistry, urine, and other studies makes the diagnosis of toxic-metabolic disorder unlikely. Furthermore, no

therapeutic drugs have been given in the last 6 hours. Despite the lack of fever or change in the WBC, an infectious process such as peritonitis could be present. A detailed abdominal examination should be performed. Psychiatric disease is unlikely given the nature of the symptoms and the lack of a past history of psychiatric disease. A detailed neurologic examination should be performed at this juncture.

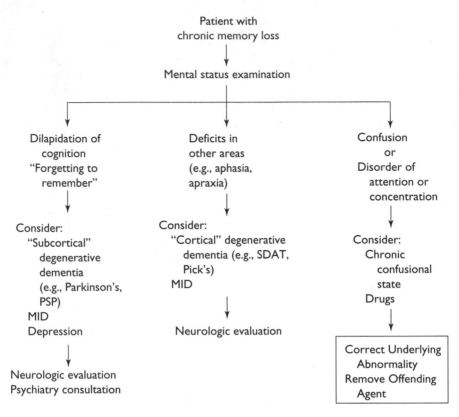

Patient with
chronic memory loss

↓

Mental status examination

| Dilapidation of cognition "Forgetting to remember" | Deficits in other areas (e.g., aphasia, apraxia) | Confusion or Disorder of attention or concentration |

↓

| Consider: "Subcortical" degenerative dementia (e.g., Parkinson's, PSP) MID Depression | Consider: "Cortical" degenerative dementia (e.g., SDAT, Pick's) MID | Consider: Chronic confusional state Drugs |

↓

| Neurologic evaluation Psychiatry consultation | Neurologic evaluation | Correct Underlying Abnormality Remove Offending Agent |

10-2-2 Diagnostic algorithm for chronic memory loss.
(From Greene HL, Johnson WP, Maricic MJ: *Decision making in medicine*, St Louis, 1993, Mosby.)

QUESTION 3 History and physical examination showed that the patient denied abdominal pain or headache. He did complain of intermittent blurred vision. Abdominal examination was unremarkable. He was oriented to person only and was able to follow one-step commands. There was global confusion and slight agitation. Recent memory was impaired, but long-term memory was intact. The patient complained of double vision on lateral gaze, and there was limitation of lateral eye movements bilaterally. Motor power was normal, and deep tendon reflexes were diminished in the legs. There was mild dysmetria on finger-to-nose testing and marked heel-to-shin ataxia. Gait was wide-based. What is the proper diagnosis and treatment?

Ataxia, global confusion, and ophthalmoplegia are hallmarks of Wernicke's encephalopathy, a condition associated with a deficiency of thiamine. In this case, thiamine deficiency was likely linked to chronic diarrhea and Crohn's disease. Thiamine is necessary for glucose metabolism. The condition was precipitated in this patient after intravenous dextrose infusion in the absence of adequate thiamine supplementation. Acute treatment of Wernicke's encephalopathy includes intravenous thiamine followed by oral thiamine. If the diagnosis is correct, ophthalmoplegia may resolve quickly, often within 30 minutes. Ataxia and confusion may resolve promptly with intravenous thiamine therapy but often persist for a longer period of time.

Wernicke's encephalopathy is traditionally a disease of alcoholics with poor nutritional intake. Wernicke's encephalopathy should be considered whenever confusion develops in a poorly nourished patient. This is an example of how even the most benign-appearing interventions may become problematic. As this case illustrates, frequent emesis or chronic diarrhea can also be associated with thiamine deficiency. This disorder has also been described in morbidly obese patients who have had gastroplasty.

In Wernicke's encephalopathy there is ataxia. Many types of ocular abnormalities can be present. The most common is bilateral horizontal nystagmus (85%). Bilateral sixth cranial nerve palsy is found in 54% of patients and conjugate gaze palsy in 45%. Less common findings include ptosis, anisocoria, and retinal hemorrhage. The mental confusion of Wernicke's encephalopathy is often characterized by apathy, spacial disorientation, and diminished short-term memory. Over 80% of these patients progress to exhibit Korsakoff's psychosis, which is characterized by retrograde and anterograde amnesia with confabulation. Approximately 25% of these patients will fail to recover.

At autopsy in patients with Wernicke's encephalopathy, lesions are often found in the mammillary bodies, cerebellum, hypothalamic nuclei, and in periaquaductal regions of the brainstem. Transketolase activity which is low in thiamine deficient states is a laboratory assay that may be useful in the diagnosis of Wernicke's encephalopathy.

Diagnostic algorithms for a patient with memory loss are shown in Figs. 10-2-1 and 10-2-2.

BIBLIOGRAPHY

Blass JP, Gibson GE: Abnormalities of a thiamine requiring enzyme in patients with Wernicke-Korsakoff syndrome, *N Engl J Med* 297:1367-1373, 1977.

Fried RT, et al: Wernicke's encephalopathy in the intensive care patient, *Crit Care Med* 18:779-780, 1990.

Gomez CA: Gasteroplasty in the surgical treatment of the morbid obesity, *Am J Clin Nutr* 33:406-410, 1980.

Harper C: The incidence of Wernicke's encephalopathy in Australia—a neuropathological study of 131 cases, *J Neurol Neurosurg Psychiatry* 46:593-601, 1983.

Torvik A, Lindboe CF, Rogde S: Brain lesions in alcoholics: a neuropathological study with clinical correlation, *J Neurol Sci* 56:233-240, 1982.

Victor M, Adams RD, Colins GH: *The Wernicke-Korsakoff Syndrome*, Philadelphia, 1971, FA Davis.

CASE

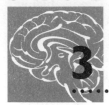

3

Christopher Hughes
Philip Gorelick
• • • • • • • • •

A 50-year-old man is brought to the emergency room by his family. He is in a stuporous state and unable to answer questions. His family members, who were all visiting from out of town, state that approximately 15 minutes ago they were preparing to go out to dinner. As they were about to leave, they heard a loud grunt followed by a loud crash. They returned to the living room and found the patient on the floor, stiff and breathing irregularly. This was followed by 60 seconds of rhythmic shaking of the arms and legs. One observer noted that during the event, the patient's head was turned to the left. After the shaking stopped, the family brought him to the hospital.

The patient had not eaten much that day but had consumed two bottles of beer just before the event. His past medical history includes myocardial infarction and congestive heart failure. The patient had an automobile accident 8 months earlier in which he hit the right side of his head on the windshield. He was hospitalized, but further details of the event are unknown. Additional medical history and currently prescribed medications are not known.

Physical examination reveals a stuporous patient. Vital signs are normal. There are coarse breath sounds, normal heart sounds, and a nontender abdomen. Neurologic examination reveals equal, reactive pupils, no gaze preference, normal tone in the arms and legs, and a withdrawal response to painful stimuli in the arms and legs.

QUESTION 1 What are the differential diagnoses of the patient's event and the cause of his mental status impairment?

Seizure and syncope are the major differential diagnoses in this patient. Since the patient has a clouded sensorium, it is imperative to interview an observer of the event. The description of the event is most consistent with a generalized tonic-clonic seizure. A single forceful grunt commonly occurs at the onset of a tonic-clonic seizure. This is caused by tonic contraction of the respiratory muscles that leads to forceful exhalation. The tonic phase is usually followed by 1 to 2 minutes of clonic, synchronous, jerking of the arms and legs. The emergency room presentation of lethargy and confusion is consistent with a postictal state.

Focal neurologic findings during or immediately after a seizure are extremely important since they may suggest the neuro-anatomic location of the seizure focus. In this case the family described head deviation to the left. This finding suggests a right hemispheric irritative focus. Eye deviation to the left would have also supported this conclusion. Head deviation, however, may not be a reliable sign of the cerebral origin of a seizure focus. Postictally, focal neurologic deficits (e.g., Todd's paralysis) suggest focality of seizure onset. If this patient had a seizure originating in the right frontal lobe, a left hemiparesis and right gaze preference, mimicking a right hemispheric stroke, might be observed during the immediate postictal period.

Syncope is the other major category of diagnosis to consider in this case. Given the patient's history of myocardial infarction and congestive heart failure, cardiac arrhythmia with cerebral hypoperfusion is possible. Orthostatic hypotension could also cause syncope in this patient.

Syncope can be confused with seizure since

there are some characteristics common to both conditions. Syncope may begin with lightheadedness, pallor, sweating, and dimming of vision. It may also be precipitated by emotional events. If syncope occurs while standing, the fall to the floor is oftentimes gradual ("syncopal slump") as opposed to a sudden crash that is commonly observed with seizures. Unconsciousness due to syncope may last 10 to 20 seconds after which alertness returns quickly. However, this depends on the cause of syncope. Thus, with syncope there is usually a rapid onset and termination of the event. Aphasias and other focal neurologic deficits commonly found after tonic-clonic seizures do not occur with syncope. Misdiagnosis of seizure may occur if during the unconsciousness of syncope or spell, the patient displays tonic extension of all four limbs. Patients may then have generalized or irregular myoclonic jerks that may be misinterpreted as tonic-clonic movements. For example, Lin documented such nonepileptic movements in 42% of subjects experiencing syncope during blood donation. Special forms of syncope also exist and are identified by their unique precipitants such as coughing (cough syncope) or micturition (micturition syncope).

QUESTION 2 What are the different types of seizures and the usual treatment for each type?

There are five major types of seizures. Absence seizures almost always begin in childhood and appear as "staring spells." These seizures may impair school performance or may go unnoticed for prolonged periods of time. The seizure can be artificially precipitated by hyperventilation. The classic EEG profile is a 3 cycle/second spike and wave pattern. Accepted therapy includes ethosuximide or valproic acid.

Complex partial seizures lead to impairment of consciousness without loss of consciousness. They may be preceded by automatisms such as lip smacking movements or temporal lobe symptoms including déjà vu, emotional outbursts, or olfactory hallucinations. Treatment is phenytoin or carbamazepine.

Generalized seizure may be a primary event or a product of generalization of a focal seizure. There is onset of rapid extension/flexion of the limbs alternately and loss of consciousness for up to 10 to 30 minutes. Postictally consciousness is clouded and returns to normal slowly. Care should be taken to avoid allowing the patient to injure herself, aspirate oropharyngeal contents, or injure her tongue. Treatment is phenytoin or carbamazepine.

Status epilepticus is sustained or successive seizure activity without interruption. The most immediate concern is assuring the patient's airway, breathing, blood pressure, and cessation of the electrical seizure activity. Arresting the motor symptoms without arresting the brain epileptic activity is inadequate. Immediate treatment is with the intravenous agents Valium or Ativan. Maintenance therapy with intravenous phenytoin should also be started immediately. If the seizure activity is refractory to these treatments, general anesthesia with an intravenous barbiturate is required. Fever, leukocytosis, and systemic acidosis are common laboratory findings.

QUESTION 3 What investigational tests would be helpful in determining the etiology of this patient's event?

Electrocardiography and cardiac enzymes are useful diagnostic tests. These tests help determine the presence of abnormalities of cardiac rhythm or conduction, a cardiac source of thromboemboli (e.g., myocardial infarction and regional wall motion abnormalities). A 24-hour cardiac monitor would be useful to rule out periodic arrhythmia as a source of hypoperfusion. Electrolyte assays are important to rule out hypocalcemia, uremia, elevation of ammonia, or hypokalemia as a precipitant of cardiac arrhythmia.

It may often be difficult to differentiate a true seizure from a pseudoseizure. A prolactin level, if drawn 15 to 20 minutes after a complex partial or generalized tonic-clonic seizure, is expected to be elevated compared to a baseline level with a true seizure as opposed to a pseudoseizure.

A CAT (or MRI) scan of the brain with and without intravenous contrast is an important diagnostic test. The CAT scan is the test of choice to rule out acute intraparenchymal or subarachnoid hemorrhage as well as to assess the bony cranial structures. The MRI is more sensitive for diagnosing infarcts, infectious lesions, demyelinating lesions, tumors, lesions at the craniocervical junction, and intracranial blood older than 24 hours. Some of these lesions may only be diagnosed after contrast infusion.

Hemorrhagic cerebral infarction may also be associated with seizures. Such lesions can also be diagnosed by CAT (or MRI) scan. These lesions may not be diagnosed acutely on CAT scan, but given this patient's history of congestive heart failure and myocardial infarction, cardiac source embolic stroke should be considered in the differential diagnosis. Cerebral infarct, however, is unlikely in this case given the nonfocal neurologic examination.

The lumbar puncture is essential in the diagnostic workup of this patient. Altered mental status, seizure, and signs of infection suggest the possibility of meningitis or encephalitis. Findings supportive of meningitis include CSF pleocytosis with a predominance of neutrophils, hypoglychorrachia, decreased protein, and abnormal gram stain and culture. Subarachnoid hemorrhage is diagnosed when there are red blood cells in the CSF and xanthochromia. A CSF pleocytosis may also be seen after a generalized seizure. However, the microbiologic tests should be negative. If the CAT or MRI brain scan shows no evidence of hemispheric swelling or mass effect, a patient presenting with fever and seizure should have a lumbar puncture. This patient had no signs of infection.

Though not commonly available for routine use in emergency rooms, the EEG may show focal slowing or epileptiform activity suggestive of seizure.

QUESTION 4 After 30 minutes, the patient was reexamined, and the following laboratory results were available: Cardiac monitoring showed no arrhythmia. ECG showed no acute ischemic changes and was unchanged from an ECG taken 8 months ago. CPK enzyme levels and serum electrolytes were normal. CAT scan of the brain showed no significant abnormalities; however, review of a CAT scan performed 8 months earlier, at the time of the automobile accident, showed a hemorrhagic contusion of the right frontal and temporal lobes. This abnormality was not seen on the current scan. Prolactin level drawn 22 minutes after the event was 72 (normal range 0 to 15). Physical examination showed normal vital signs, a nonfocal neurologic examination and significant improvement in the patient's mental status. What conclusions can be drawn from these findings, and how should the patient be managed?

The cardiac workup was unremarkable, and thus, provides no evidence for a cardiac cause of hypoperfusion syncope. The prolactin level is consistent with a seizure while the prior CAT scan of the brain suggests an underlying etiology for the ictal event. The right frontal-temporal location of the previous cerebral hemorrhage is consistent with the ictal observation that the patient's head deviated to the left.

There are no strict guidelines for management of this type of patient; however, the following approach is commonly recommended. The patient is admitted to the hospital for observation overnight, and an EEG is scheduled. Anticonvulsant treatment is administered because an etiology for the seizure (previous cerebral hematoma) was discovered. If the patient is stable and has no recurrent seizures, he may receive an oral loading dose of phenytoin (15 to 18 mg/kg) in 3 divided doses given 3 hours apart. After this loading dose the patient receives a maintenance dose of 300 mg of phenytoin each day. An alternative to loading the patient with oral phenytoin is to administer the entire loading dose intravenously at a rate no greater than 50 mg/min. This method of administration should be avoided in this case for two reasons. First, intravenous phenytoin has a very high pH and can cause significant inflammation of surrounding tissue if not infused into a large,

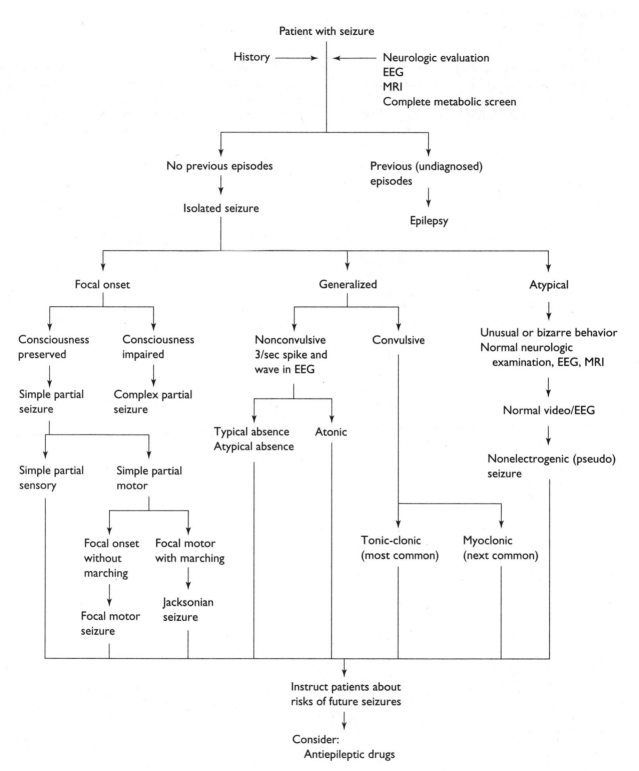

10-3-1 Diagnostic algorithm for seizures.
(From Greene HL, Johnson WP, Maricic MJ: *Decision making in medicine*, St Louis, 1993, Mosby.)

intact vein. Second, phenytoin can cause hypotension during infusion. Given this patient's history of congestive heart failure, this risk may not be warranted. If the oral route is not feasible, cardiac monitoring and frequent blood pressure checks during slow infusion can minimize the risks associated with intravenous administration. The only generally accepted indication for intravenous phenytoin is status epilepticus or impaired gastrointestinal absorption. If a patient has a second seizure during the oral phenytoin loading period, 2 mg of intravenous lorazepam may be administered to prevent further seizures until a therapeutic level of phenytoin is achieved.

This patient's posttraumatic seizure occurred 8 months after the episode of head trauma and presented as a secondary generalized tonic-clonic seizure. Generally, seizures after head injury occur immediately or within 7 days of the event. Delayed seizures usually present within 1 to 2 years after the trauma. This patient's previous cerebral contusion is the cause for the epileptic focus formation since residual iron from blood deposition is known to be associated with irritation of the cortex. This patient's inadequate food intake and consumption of alcohol may have lowered his seizure threshold and precipitated the event. Like many other types of seizures in patients of this age, anticonvulsants are usually prescribed and continued at least 2 years. During the first 6 to 12 months after the seizure patients are advised strongly not to drive motorized vehicles. This recommendation may vary by state or physician. If the patient remains seizure free for 2 years, has no neurologic deficit or CAT scan abnormality, and routine follow-up electroencephalograms show no epileptiform activity, anticonvulsant withdrawal can be considered.

A diagnostic algorithm for seizures is shown in Fig. 10-3-1.

BIBLIOGRAPHY

Isenstein D, Nasraway SA: Hypotension during slow phenytoin infusion in severe sepsis, *Crit Care Med* 18:1036-1038, 1990.

Kilaski D: Soft-tissue damage associated with intravenous phenytoin, *N Engl J Med* 311:1186-1192, 1984.

Lin JTY, et al: Convulsive syncope in blood donors, *Ann Neurol* 11:525-528, 1982.

Mattson RH, et al: Prolactin changes following temporal and extra temporal seizures of varying severity, *Epilepsia* 29:704-710, 1988.

Roa V: Extravasation injury to the hand by intravenous phenytoin, *J Neurosurg* 68:967-971, 1988.

C A S E

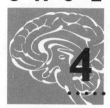

4

Christopher Hughes
Philip Gorelick
· · · · · · · · ·

A 35-year-old white woman presents with dizziness, mild headache, and intermittent double vision that began on awakening from sleep. The dizziness is constant, unrelated to head position, and is not associated with true vertigo or a "spinning" sensation. The headache is localized to the right temporal region and is described as a dull, constant pain. The double vision consists of side-by-side images most pronounced on right lateral gaze. Vertical gaze produces no symptoms. The patient currently denies numbness, weakness, nausea, or vomiting. No recent fevers or diaphoresis have been experienced, but she had an upper respiratory infection approximately 2 weeks ago. There have been no previous episodes of these symptoms.

The patient has no currently active medical conditions and does not take medications. Her first childbirth was normal. The second delivery was complicated by peripartum hypertension lasting 3 days and a 1 week episode of left eye pain that developed 3 months after the birth. Both resolved without sequelae. As a child she experienced infrequent headaches associated with nausea and emesis. These headaches remitted at the age of 16 and only recurred briefly during her first pregnancy.

The patient's mother is 62 years old, has a history of migraine headaches, and suffered a stroke at age 50. Her father is 64 years old and has coronary artery disease. A sister has a history of migraine headaches. The patient has smoked 1 pack of cigarettes/day for 15 years. She consumes alcohol infrequently.

On physical examination, vital signs were within normal limits, and there were no orthostatic blood pressure changes. General examina-tion was normal. There were no meningeal signs. Neurologic examination revealed full visual fields, a visual acuity of 20/20 in the right eye, and 20/50 in the left eye. Pupils were equal, round, and reactive to light; however, there was mild paradoxic dilation of the left pupil on the "swinging flashlight" test. Vertical gaze was normal. Horizontal gaze to the left was normal. On right lateral gaze, nonrotatory horizontal nystagmus was noted in the abducting (right) eye, and the adducting (left) eye failed to cross the midline. There was no ptosis, and the remaining cranial nerves functioned normally. Motor power and sensory examination were normal. Deep tendon reflexes were symmetric, but abdominal reflexes were absent. Cerebellar examination was normal, but gait was unsteady and slightly wide-based.

QUESTION 1 What is the name of the gaze abnormality exemplified in this case? Where is the lesion, and what is the pathophysiology causing the patient's double vision?

The ocular examination reveals an inter-nuclear ophthalmoplegia. The underlying lesion is in the medial longitudinal fasciculus (MLF) within the pons or midbrain. The MLF coordinates conjugate lateral gaze. The following example illustrates how the MLF coordinates gaze. Normally, when a patient attempts to look to the right, the left frontal cortex activates the right conjugate gaze center in the pons, a structure called the paramedian reticular formation (PPRF). The PPRF synapses with the ipsilateral abducens nerve nucleus (cranial nerve VI), which causes the ipsilateral eye to abduct via contraction of the lateral rectus muscle. Simultaneously, the contralateral eye adducts by signals from the PPRF that travel to the contralateral oculomotor nucleus (cranial nerve three) through the MLF. When a lesion occurs within the MLF, as in this case, the adducting eye fails to move medially because of the blocked signal, and the abducting eye develops nystagmus. The lesion is located in the MLF on the side of the adduction abnormality.

QUESTION 2 What is the "swinging flashlight" test and how does it relate to this case?

Pupillary constriction is controlled by a simple reflex arc. When light strikes the retina, it causes activation of the afferent optic pathway leading to the Edinger Westphal nucleus (EWN), a subnucleus of the third cranial nerve nuclear complex within the midbrain. Stimulation of the EWN causes bilateral pupillary constriction. If there is retinal or optic nerve damage, the amount of EWN activation from light presented to the affected eye will be less than the amount of activation from light presented to the normal, contralateral eye. The swinging flashlight test consists of first eliciting bilateral pupillary constriction by illuminating the normal eye. If the light source is then "swung" to the affected eye, the damaged nerve system will produce less activation of the EWN relative to the normal eye and therefore cause paradoxic dilation of the pupils. This condition can be simulated in a normal person by covering one eye with a sunglass lens. This finding is referred to as a Marcus Gunn pupil or an afferent pupillary defect. The condition is most commonly seen in optic neuritis and primary retinal disease.

QUESTION 3 How does one test for superficial abdominal reflexes, and what is the significance of this finding?

With the patient supine and the abdomen relaxed, the abdominal reflexes are elicited by lightly stroking a pin diagonally across the patient's abdomen in a diagonal manner. A normal response is contraction of the underlying abdominal muscles. Absence of this reflex is pathologic, particularly in young adults, and can be found in spinal cord or pyramidal tract disease.

QUESTION 4 What are the differential diagnoses of this patient's condition?

In this case, the patient has dizziness, pupillary abnormalities, and unsteady gait. Infectious meningitis must be ranked first on the list because of a compatible set of complaints and the morbidity and mortality associated with an undiagnosed and untreated case. This patient has a headache and brainstem dysfunction. Tuberculous meningitis and Listeria meningitis are both known to cause such symptoms. In the HIV+ population, fully 75% of patients with cryptococcal meningitis will not manifest symptoms classically associated with meningitis. Yet, an infectious meningitis is unlikely in this immunocompetent patient since there is no fever, meningeal signs, or cognitive changes.

Another possible diagnosis is that of an ophthalmoplegic migraine. The patient has a family history and past medical history of migraine headache. She now presents with headache and a form of ophthalmoplegia. Yet, ophthalmoplegic migraine typically affects pediatric patients, is rare, and usually develops during severe, protracted migrainous events. This patient presents with only a mild headache and has internuclear ophthalmoplegia as compared to oculomotor paresis, which is the ophthalmologic finding associated most commonly with migraine headaches.

Another possible diagnosis is vasculitis. This diagnosis sould be considered in any patient who presents with headache and focal neurologic deficits. Systemic vasculitis from Wegener's granulomatosis or polyarteritis nodosa rarely cause CNS symptoms without concurrent systemic manifestations. However, isolated vasculitis of the CNS (i.e., granulomatous angiitis) may present in this way. Behcet's disease can also cause CNS inflammation, with particular affinity for the cranial nerves. However, she does not have the typical clinical triad of relapsing oral or genital ulcers, uveitis, and meningoencephalitis commonly found in Behcet's disease. Patients with granulomatous angiitis restricted to the nervous system may present with focal cerebral signs of the hemisphere, brainstem, or cerebellum, and dementia and depressed consciousness are reported in all cases.

Sarcoidosis involves the central nervous system in 5% to 10% of cases. Intraparenchymal lesions can occur, but basal meningeal involvement is much more common and usually manifests as isolated cranial nerve dysfunction. Visual loss because of involvement of the optic nerves or chiasm and facial palsy are the more common CNS manifestations. This condition is more common in blacks than caucasians and has a peak incidence between 15 and 40 years of age.

Factors that might place this patient at increased risk for ischemic stroke include a family history of stroke and her use of cigarettes. Nonatherosclerotic stroke mechanisms such as vasculitis, coagulation disorders that lead to thrombosis (e.g., the presence of anticardiolipin antibodies), and unusual arteropathies (e.g., fibromuscular dysplasia, moya-moya disease) are to be considered in this patient.

However, in a patient with this presentation the most likely diagnosis is multiple sclerosis (MS). MS is the most common demyelinating disease of young adults and affects women more commonly than men. The prevalence of the disease is generally higher in geographic locations away from the equator. Neurologic deficits may be brought out by elevated body temperature such as in warm weather, during fever, and hot baths or showers. The finding of internuclear ophthalmoplegia (INO) in a young patient is most likely caused by MS. The MLF is one of the first fiber tracts to myelinate and is highly susceptible to demyelination in MS. INO in an older patient is more commonly caused by stroke. When MS causes acute demyelinization within the brainstem, the patient may experience mild headache and dizziness. Furthermore, the history of transient eye pain and the afferent pupillary defect found on physical examination suggest an optic nerve lesion and optic neuritis.

Absent abdominal reflexes suggest a third site of CNS dysfunction. Other neurologic signs and symptoms that may be seen in MS include diplopia, dysarthria, ataxia, bowel/bladder dysfunction, hemi/paraparesis, tremor, impotence, and sensory loss. The spinal form of MS with spastic paresis may slowly progress through life. Since the diagnosis of MS requires at least two separate episodes of neurologic dysfunction in two separate locations within the CNS (multiple lesions in time and space of the central white matter), this patient satisfies the clinical definition of this disease.

QUESTION 5 What laboratory tests would help determine the cause of this patient's condition?

Patients with sarcoidosis frequently have hilar adenopathy on chest x-ray, high serum calcium levels, and high ACE levels. A gallium scan might show preferential uptake of the radioactive tracer into the parotid glands or chest lymph nodes, signs often found in patients with sarcoid.

The Westergren erythrocyte sedimentation rate (WESR) is a nonspecific marker of inflammation and will be elevated in most infectious and inflammatory conditions. The notable exceptions pertinent to this case are primary CNS vasculitis and MS.

A brainstem hemorrhage is identified with the use of CAT scan. A vascular malformation might be diagnosed after CAT scan when intravenous contrast is used. If the patient's condition is caused by ischemic stroke or MS, the CAT scan may be normal in the acute phase. The MRI is more sensitive for areas of white matter disease.

Examination of the spinal fluid is indicated in this patient. Acute inflammatory cells (PMNs) are generally found in bacterial infections of the meninges while lymphocytes usually predominate in other conditions such as sarcoidosis and MS or vasculitis. In bacterial or mycobacterial meningitis, spinal fluid glucose levels are often low, and spinal fluid protein levels are high. Spinal

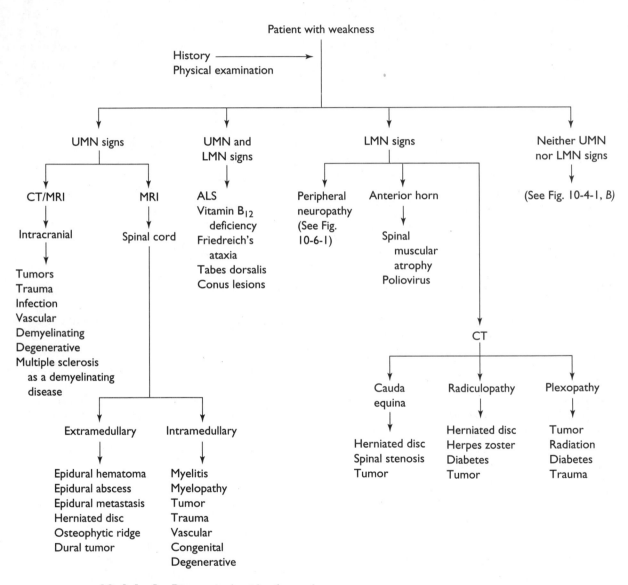

10-4-1, A Diagnostic algorithm for weakness.

(From Greene HL, Johnson WP, Maricic MJ: *Decision making in medicine*, St Louis, 1993, Mosby.)

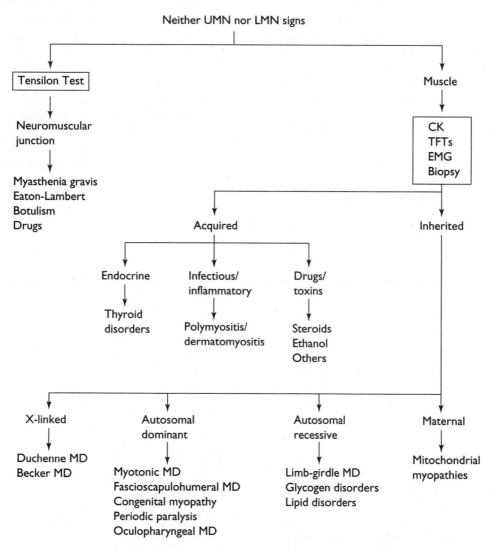

10-4-1, B   Diagnostic algorithm for weakness—Cont'd.

fluid lactate may help to differentiate bacterial/mycobacterial infections (high lactate) from viral and noninfectious (low lactate) conditions. Analysis of the spinal fluid protein can provide additional diagnostic information. IgG is usually elevated with inflammatory processes within the CNS. This would include sarcoid, infectious meningitis, vasculitis, and MS. Electrophoresis of the spinal fluid protein will frequently show a polyclonal or oligoclonal banding pattern. Oligoclonal bands are typically seen in MS. Furthermore, ACE levels may be elevated in the CSF of patients with sarcoid.

In this patient the following results were obtained: chest x-ray, serum calcium level, and ACE level were normal. WESR was 20 mm/hr, CAT scan of the brain was within normal limits, showing no hemorrhage or hypodensity within the brainstem. Lumbar puncture was performed and analysis of the spinal fluid showed the following: white blood cell count was 5, red blood cell count was 4, and glucose, lactate, and ACE levels were normal. Spinal fluid protein was elevated at 50 mg/dl. IgG to albumin ratio was elevated at 0.6. Electrophoresis showed an oligoclonal banding pattern.

CASE SUMMARY With this information, a clinical diagnosis of MS was made, and the patient was admitted to the hospital for further workup and treatment. The following day an MRI scan of the brain showed several small, periventricular foci of increased signal on the proton density scan. These abnormalities are commonly seen in MS. In addition, a focus of increased signal was seen within the pons, in the region of the MLF, on the T2 weighted scan. This finding is consistent with an inflammatory process within that region.

• •

A consensus regarding treatment of an acute exacerbation of MS with brainstem signs has yet to be reached. Many neurologists who specialize in the treatment of MS would recommend intravenous or intramuscular ACTH while others would recommend the use of intravenous methylprednisolone. While useful acutely, the impact on long-term prognosis is controversial.

During either treatment, gastric protection with antacids is recommended as both of the above agents are ulcerogenic. Additional therapy includes the use of Baclofen for muscle spasticity. Baclofen carries many neurologic side effects including drowsiness, confusion, weakness, fatigue, and seizure or hallucinations when withdrawn rapidly. Oxybutynin is used for spasmodic bladder dysfunction. Tegretol may be used to treat the neuritogenic pain resultant to demyelination.

A diagnostic algorithm for a patient presenting with weakness as a chief complaint is shown in Fig. 10-4-1.

BIBLIOGRAPHY

Breen LA: Gaze abnormalities. In Walsh TJ, ed: *Neuro-ophthalmology: clinical signs and symptoms,* Malverne, Pennsylvania, 1992, Lea and Febiger.

Fishman RA: CSF findings in diseases of the nervous system. In Fishman RA, ed: *Cerebral spinal fluid in diseases of the nervous system,* Philadelphia, 1992, WB Saunders.

Francis GS: Inflammatory demyelinating diseases of the central nervous system. In Bradley WG, Daroff RB, Fenichel GM, Marsden CD, eds: *Neurology in clinical practice,* Boston, 1991, Butterworth Heinemann.

Glaser JS: *Neuroophthalmology,* Philadelphia, 1990, JB Lippincott.

Scott TF: Diseases that mimic multiple sclerosis, *Postgrad Med* 89:187-191, 1991.

Silberberg DH: Sarcoidosis of the nervous system. In Aminoff MJ, ed: *Neurology and general medicine,* New York, 1989, Churchill Livingstone.

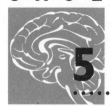
A 75-year-old woman came to the emergency room after an episode of complete left monocular visual loss. This visual loss began suddenly and was not associated with pain or other symptoms. After 5 minutes, her vision gradually returned to normal. The patient states that she has never experienced visual loss before and has no history of ocular disease. Her past medical history includes mild hypertension that has been treated for 20 years with a diuretic. She had migraine headaches as a teenager and young adult, has never required surgery, and has given birth to 2 healthy children.

There is a history of arthritis of the hands, hips, shoulders, and neck for the last 8 years. She usually feels stiff and sore in the mornings and has difficulty manipulating small objects with her hands. These symptoms have worsened over the last year. In fact, 3 days ago she dropped a cup of coffee. For a 10-minute period, her right hand seemed much less coordinated than usual. Furthermore, as the day continues her shoulders and hips begin to feel sore, making stair climbing and reaching for objects on high shelves difficult. Aspirin has been partially effective in relieving these symptoms.

Review of systems resulted in the following symptoms. Headaches develop approximately once per week for the past year. The patient believes that the headaches are caused by her neck arthritis and states that they occur during days when there is a great deal of head movement. Aspirin provides symptomatic relief. Epigastric pain occurs after meals and is relieved by antacids. This occurs 3 to 4 times per week and has been present for 3 years. Constipation has been a problem for approximately 2 years. The patient's internist prescribed metamucil, which has only partially relieved the symptoms. There is urinary incontinence when laughing and occasionally when walking. This symptom has been present for 5 months.

Physical examination shows normal vital signs. There is slight limitation of movement and tenderness of the shoulders bilaterally and limitation of neck movement and slight tenderness of all finger joints when testing hand grip strength bilaterally. Neurologic examination was normal. Ophthalmologic examination showed intact visual fields, normal fundi, and small reactive pupils.

QUESTION I What is the relevant differential diagnosis for transient monocular blindness in this patient? Cite information from the patient's history or review of systems that would support each diagnosis.

Temporal arteritis (TA) is an inflammatory arteritis commonly affecting the elderly and presents with headaches, jaw claudication and transient or permanent visual loss (the arteritic form of ischemic optic neuropathy). This patient's headaches may be due to TA and not degenerative neck "arthritis." This condition is often associated with polymyalgia rheumatica (PMR), a painful condition in which there is myalgia of the proximal extremity musculature of the upper extremities. The patient's complaints of "arthritis" could be consistent with PMR. Temporal headache, jaw claudication, visual loss, or decreased acuity may be associated symptoms. Rapid diagnosis of TA is imperative as progression of the disease can lead to bilateral visual loss.

Carotid artery stenosis can lead to transient monocular blindness because of an embolus from a carotid atheroma or low flow to the retina secondary to high-grade carotid stenosis. This is referred to as *amaurosis fugax*. This condition must always be considered when elderly patients develop transient monocular visual symptoms. Often patients will describe the onset of the visual loss as a shade being pulled down over their eye. There may be associated signs of cerebral dysfunction. This patient's description of transient right hand clumsiness may have been a transient central nervous system ischemic event from the same carotid disease rather than an "arthritic" attack. The two events could be due to left carotid artery disease. A left carotid bruit might be expected in this patient if carotid stenosis is the cause of her symptoms. However, with very high-grade carotid stenosis there is substantially reduced flow through the vessel, and a bruit may not be heard.

Migraine must also be considered as a cause of the symptoms as there is history of migraine headaches. Though the patient denied that headache was associated with the transient visual loss, patients with a history of migraine can have neurologic deficits develop as a migrainous aura without an associated headache (i.e., transient migrainous accompaniments of late life). Though rare, isolated retinal artery vasospasm has been noted in some patients with transient monocular blindness. Many patients have a personal history or family history of migraine.

QUESTION 2   What diagnostic tests are important in this patient?

Patients with TA commonly have elevated Westergren erythrocyte sedimentation rate (WESR). The level may often be greater than 90 mm/hr. If such a value is found in a patient with this clinical presentation, steroids should be administered quickly to prevent visual loss or other permanent neurologic deficits. Furthermore, bilateral temporal artery biopsy would be performed. It is important to obtain an adequate vessel sample as the disease may be patchy in its involvement of the artery.

Transient left monocular blindness and transient right hand dysfunction suggest possible left carotid occlusive disease. Physical examination may reveal a bruit. An excellent way to visualize blood flow in the carotid artery is duplex ultrasonography. If ultrasonography is performed and confirms high-grade carotid stenosis, cerebral angiography would be performed to validate the degree of stenosis if the patient is considered a candidate for carotid endarterectomy.

In the case of carotid stenosis causing a transient ischemic attack, a CAT scan or MRI should be performed to rule out radiologic evidence of previous stroke. Other disorders that could mimic transient cerebral ischemia such as cerebral hemorrhage, subdural hematoma, and brain neoplasm may also be diagnosed by these imaging techniques.

QUESTION 3   The patient's sedimentation rate was 10 mm/hr. Carotid ultrasonography showed a 90% stenosis of the left internal carotid artery and a normal right internal carotid artery. With these results, the diagnosis was amaurosis fugax secondary to high-grade carotid stenosis. CAT scan of the brain showed a small hypodense lesion in the region of the right internal capsule. A cerebral angiogram confirmed high-grade stenosis of the left carotid artery, and left carotid endarterectomy was performed. Postoperatively, the patient did well and was treated with aspirin. What are the current recommendations for carotid endarterectomy (CEA) for patients with atherosclerotic carotid arterial disease?

Recently the North American Symptomatic Carotid Endarterectomy Collaboration Group reported the results of their study comparing CEA plus aspirin to use of aspirin alone in patients with symptomatic carotid stenosis. The data showed that patients with stenosis of 70% to 99% had a better 2-year outcome if treated with surgery plus aspirin compared to aspirin alone. A similar study

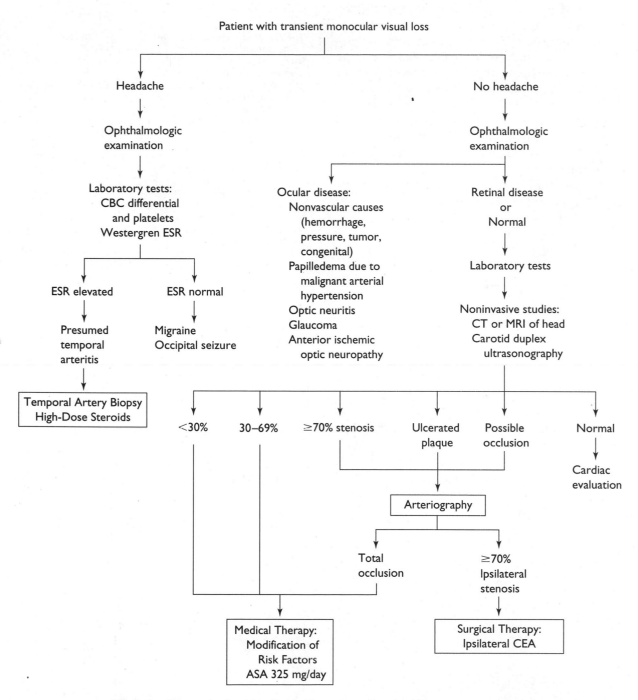

10-5-1 Diagnostic algorithm for transient monocular visual loss.
(From Greene HL, Johnson WP, Maricic MJ: *Decision making in medicine,* St Louis, 1993, Mosby.)

performed in Europe confirmed the results. Thus, patients with symptomatic carotid stenosis measuring 70% to 99% by angiographic criteria should be considered for CEA. Based on the European study patients with stenosis of less than 30% should be treated with antiplatelet therapy. Finally, the proper therapy for patients with symptomatic carotid stenosis of 30% to 69% and patients with asymptomatic carotid stenosis has yet to be answered. Studies are currently being performed to address these issues.

A diagnostic algorithm for a patient presenting with transient monocular vision loss is shown in Fig. 10-5-1.

BIBLIOGRAPHY

The Amaurosis Fugax Study Group: Current management of amaurosis fugax, *Stroke* 21:201-207, 1990.

Burger SK, et al: Transient monocular blindness caused by vasospasm, *N Engl J Med* 325:870-873, 1991.

The CASANOVA Study Group: carotid surgery versus medical therapy in asymptomatic carotid stenosis, *Stroke* 22:1229-1235, 1991.

Dyken, ML, Barnett HJM, et al: Low dose aspirin and stroke: "it ain't necessarily so," *Stroke* 10:1395-1399, 1992.

European Carotid Surgery Trialists' Collaborative Group: MRC European carotid surgery trial: interim results for symptomatic patients with severe (70-99%) or with mild (0-29%) carotid stenosis, *Lancet* 337:1235-1243, 1991.

Goodwin, JA, Gorelick, PB, Helgason CM: Symptoms of amaurosis fugax in atherosclerotic carotid artery disease, *Neurology* 37:829-832, 1987.

Meyer FB, et al: Carotid endarterectomy in elderly patients, *Mayo Clin Proc* 66:464-469, 1991.

North American Symptomatic Carotid Endarterectomy Trial Collaborators: Beneficial effect of carotid endarterectomy in symptomatic patients with high-grade carotid stenosis, *N Engl J Med* 325:445-453, 1991.

C A S E

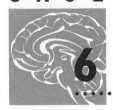

6 Christopher Hughes
Philip Gorelick

An 18-year-old man came to the emergency room with the complaint of difficulty walking. Six hours earlier, he awoke from sleep and noted a heaviness in his left leg. Within 2 hours there was a similar sensation in his right leg. He describes a feeling of tiredness and weakness of the legs while climbing stairs. The patient also complains of a dull backache. The pain is deep and nonradiating. There are no complaints of arm weakness, visual symptoms, headache, or shortness of breath. The patient has never experienced similar symptoms in the past.

The patient's past medical history includes right arm fracture suffered 2 years ago. He takes no medications. There is no family history of neurologic or endocrinologic disease. The patient does not smoke, drink alcohol, and denies illicit drug use. He had an upper respiratory infection 10 days ago and recently traveled to rural Canada.

QUESTION I What neurologic emergency should be considered in patients complaining of back pain and leg weakness? What further questions should be asked of the patient to substantiate this diagnosis, and what confirmatory signs might be found on physical examination?

For patients presenting with back pain and leg weakness, spinal cord compression must be ruled out. Spinal cord compression is commonly diagnosed in cancer patients with vertebral metastasis extending into the spinal canal but can also be caused by extraaxial spinal cord tumors or epidural abscesses. Associated symptoms include radicular pain, bowel incontinence, and urinary retention. Physical examination findings include absent or hyperactive deep tendon reflexes in the legs, the Babinski sign, decreased rectal tone, and a sensory level to pin prick. An infectious or demyelinating inflammatory process within the spinal cord, called transverse myelitis, can also present as a similar clinical syndrome. Acutely, deep tendon reflexes below the spinal level are depressed or absent, and the legs are flaccid. Later, hyperreflexia, spasticity, and bilateral Babinski signs occur.

QUESTION 2 What are other differential diagnoses, confirmatory history and physical examination findings and the appropriate diagnostic laboratory investigations?

Bilateral leg weakness may be caused by disease of the spinal cord, peripheral nerve, neuromuscular junction, muscle, or even the paramedian frontal lobes. The remaining differential diagnoses can be divided into acute, subacute, and chronic processes.

The Guillain-Barré syndrome (GBS) is also referred to as acute inflammatory demyelinating polyneuropathy (AIDP). This condition often presents with symmetric ascending muscle weakness, minor tingling sensations, variable loss of sensation, areflexia, and occasionally autonomic instability. These symptoms are caused by an immune-mediated demyelination of the fast large conducting peripheral nerves. Weakness can involve the respiratory muscles and lead to death. Bilateral facial weakness (facial diplegia) will frequently develop in this condition, but weakness may be asymmetric. Vague back or neck discomfort can also be present during the acute phase of the illness. The syndrome is commonly preceded by a viral illness but recently has also been linked to gastrointestinal infection with *Campylobacter jejuni*. CAT scan of the brain is usually normal. Spinal fluid analysis classically shows a high protein and normal white blood cell count (albumin-ocytologic dissociation). Nerve conduction studies are used to document the reduced speed of conduction caused by the demyelination and are useful for gauging prognosis.

Botulism is caused by ingestion of food contaminated with *Clostridium botulinum*. This bacteria produces a toxin that inhibits the release of acetylcholine at the neuromuscular junction. Approximately 24 hours after ingestion, the patient develops nausea, diarrhea, bradycardia, and diffuse weakness from neuromuscular blockade. Common neurologic signs include ophthalmoplegia, pupillary unreactivity, diffuse weakness, areflexia, and respiratory distress. Blood and stool samples should be taken to identify the toxin. Trivalent botulism antitoxin is used to treat the condition.

Tick paralysis is caused by a toxin produced by the *Dermacentor* or *Ixodes* species of tick. These ticks are most commonly found in the American northwest and Canada. They normally live on deer but will attach to hairy areas such as the scalp, axilla, or genital areas of unsuspecting individuals. There, the tick infuses the toxin into the bloodstream of the victim. Five to seven days after exposure to the tick the patient develops rapidly ascending, progressive, paralysis associated with areflexia and nystagmus. Facial paresthesias will also commonly occur and are significant since they are rare among other causes of diffuse paralysis. On physical examination the tick must be located, identified, and removed. Symptoms will then begin to resolve spontaneously. The site of action of the toxin has been postulated as being the terminal branches of the nerves.

Acute intermittent porphyria is the most common of the autosomal dominant porphyrias. Acute symptomatic episodes often begin during the third or fourth decade of life and are more common in women. These attacks can be precipi-tated by physiologic stressors such as dieting, alcohol consumption, or acute febrile illness or an assortment of drugs including barbiturates, analgesics, sulfonamides, and anticonvulsants. Clinical manifestations include abdominal pain, nausea, emesis, acute progressive peripheral neuropathy, and psychiatric symptoms. Neurologic dysfunctions include blood pressure instability from autonomic involvement and diffuse motor neuropathy that begins in the feet and legs or hands and arms. Cranial nerves are involved in the most severe cases. High levels of delta amino-levulinic acid and porphobilinogen are found in the urine during the attacks. Acute exposure to organophosphate toxins produces acute neuropathy as can systemic effects of diphtheria toxin.

Subacute presentations include HIV-associated neuropathy and metabolic processes. Patients who have HIV can develop an acute, subacute, or chronic polyradiculoneuropathy. When acute, this condition is very similar to GBS. Motor neuron dysfunction begins in the lower extremities and ascends to involve more proximal muscles. Sensory nerve fiber involvement is usually minimal. Like GBS, deep tendon reflexes are absent or diminished, but unlike GBS autonomic instability is rare. Spinal fluid analysis will show an elevated protein level in both of these diseases, but HIV infection leads to an increased spinal fluid white blood cell count, not found in GBS. Importantly, this condition may be found in HIV patients without symptoms of AIDS. Therefore, any patient presenting with ascending motor weakness and areflexia should be screened for HIV.

Hypokalemic periodic paralysis is an autosomal dominant condition with male predominance, which usually becomes symptomatic during the second decade of life. This patient's presentation of bilateral leg weakness and backache upon awakening from sleep is consistent with this condition. Often the attacks are precipitated by heavy exercise within the prior 24 hours or a meal high in carbohydrate. On physical examination, in addition to muscle weakness the affected muscles often feel firm and swollen. Respiratory muscles are usually minimally affected, and deep tendon reflexes may be reduced or absent. Serum electrolyte analysis can show potassium levels well below the normal range. Symptoms normally resolve with acute oral potassium administration and chronic acetazolamide treatment. There is also a form of hyperkalemic periodic paralysis and a less well-defined normokalemic variety.

Paraproteinemias can lead to subacute polyneuropathy. This may be evident in the POEMS (polyneuropathy, organomegaly, endocrinopathy, m-protein, and skin rash) syndrome seen in multiple myeloma. Amyloid protein deposition in nerve cells associated with plasma cell dyscrasias leads to a predominantly sensory neuropathy associated with autonomic insufficiency. Exposure to toxins including lead, hexane, and glue sniffing can also lead to subacute neuropathy.

The differential diagnosis also contains chronic processes. Though unlikely to present with such acute progressive symptoms, generalized myasthenia gravis without ocular symptoms can occur in persons of this age. As a postsynaptic, autoimmune disorder of the myoneural junction, myasthenia gravis classically presents with intermittent ptosis, diplopia, or limb weakness which typically worsens by the end of the day (diurnal variation). Affected muscles often become symptomatic or worse with exercise. Acetylcholine receptor antibodies are commonly found in patients with myasthenia gravis. Intravenous administration of the short acting acetylcholinesterase inhibitor endrophonium (Tensilon) will temporarily reverse the symptoms of the disease and can be used as a confirmatory diagnostic test. Given the high incidence of coexistent thymoma, a CAT scan of the mediastinum is recommended in patients with this disease.

Amyotropic lateral sclerosis (ALS) is a chronic disease that involves both upper and lower motor neurons. Thus, both limb and bulbar signs are present. Signs of lower motor neuron disease are weakness, fasciculations, and atrophy. Upper motor neuron disease leads to hyperreflexia and spasticity. Symptoms usually begin in mid to late adulthood. There is no curative treatment, and the disease is usually fatal within 5 years of onset.

Poliomyelitis must also be considered as a component of the differential diagnosis. It has largely been eradicated in this country and presents as muscle weakness which may be asymmetrical. A related condition is the Post-Polio syndrome. This is manifest as progressive weakness many years later in previously involved areas of the initial disease. This is thought to be related to secondary neuronal dropout over time.

On physical examination the patient is found to have a blood pressure of 140/100 mm Hg, a pulse of 100 bpm, a respiratory rate of 20/min, and a normal body temperature. Head and neck examination was normal. Oral and pharyngeal mucosa were not erythematous or discolored. Lungs were clear to auscultation. Heart sounds were normal. The abdomen was nontender with normal bowel sounds. Rectal examination was normal. Mild back tenderness to palpation was noted. There were no ticks or abnormal lesions on the skin.

On neurologic examination the patient was alert and oriented. Pupils reacted normally. Extraocular movements were intact without nystagmus. No ptosis was observed. Facial sensation was normal to light touch and pin prick. Facial asymmetry was noted with a complete left facial palsy. The tongue and palate moved normally. Motor examination revealed normal tone and bulk in the arm and leg muscles. No muscle tenderness was noted. There was a mild left arm drift and impairment of fine motor movements in the left hand. There was marked weakness of the legs. Deep tendon reflexes were reduced symmetrically in the arms and absent in the legs. Babinski responses were also unobtainable. Sensory examination was intact to light touch and pin prick. There was no sensory level to pin prick. Vibratory and proprioceptive sensation was significantly reduced in the legs bilaterally. The patient required assistance to walk and displayed a wide-based gait.

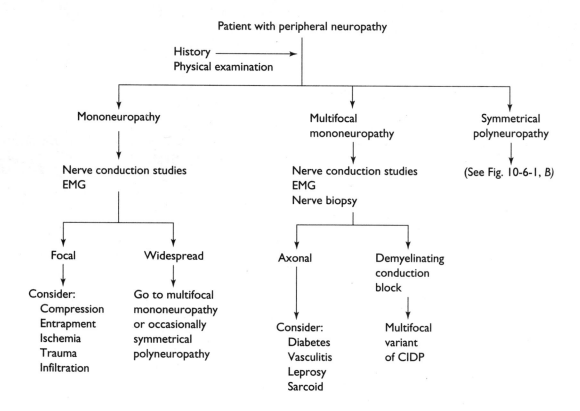

CIDP=Chronic inflammatory demyelinating
        polyradiculoneuropathy

10-6-1, A Diagnostic algorithm for peripheral neuropathy.
(From Greene HL, Johnson WP, Maricic MJ: *Decision making in medicine,* St Louis, 1993, Mosby.)

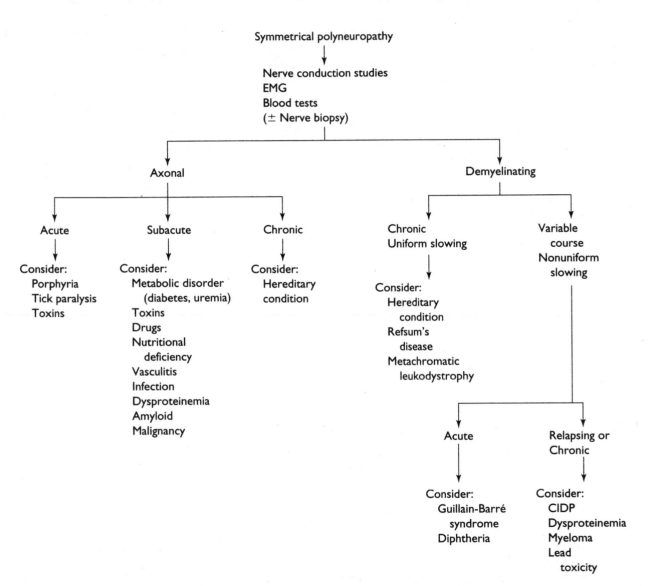

10-6-1, *B* Diagnostic algorithm for peripheral neuropathy—Cont'd.

QUESTION 3   Given the physical examination, what reassessment of the differential diagnosis and outline of the proper laboratory investigations can be made?

Leg and facial weakness, loss of vibratory and proprioceptive sensation along with areflexia are the most important elements of the physical examination. This is most consistent with Guillain-Barré syndrome. However, HIV polyradiculoneuropathy is still a possible diagnosis. Myasthenia gravis is less likely given the normal ocular examination and lack of fatigable muscle weakness. Spinal cord compression is also unlikely given the lack of a sensory level hyperreflexia, or Babinski sign. Tick paralysis will no longer be considered as the skin examination was unremarkable. Botulism is unlikely with normal ocular movements and the absence of abdominal symptoms, as is the diagnosis of porphyria.

An MRI of the spinal cord would be recommended at this point to rule out a spinal cord lesion. If no spinal cord compression was found, the next step would be to perform a lumbar puncture.

QUESTION 4   The MRI scan of the spinal cord showed no compression or intrinsic cord pathology. A lumbar puncture was performed, and there were two white blood cells, two red blood cells, a normal glucose level, and a protein of 94 mg/dl. Serum electrolytes including potassium level were normal. An HIV blood screen was negative. With these results, hypokalemic periodic paralysis and HIV polyradiculoneuropathy were excluded, and the diagnosis of post-viral GBS was made. What is the appropriate treatment for GBS?

Traditionally, severe cases of GBS have been treated with plasmapheresis. If instituted within the first 2 weeks of the illness, this treatment has been shown to improve the long-term prognosis. Recently, intravenous gamma globulin has been used as an alternative to plasmapheresis. Use of corticosteroids has not been shown to be effective.

Treatment of GBS primarily involves supportive care. Bedside physical therapy and subcutaneous heparin are recommended to help prevent complications of immobility. Cardiac monitoring allows early recognition of autonomic involvement and instability, which includes rapid and large scale fluctuations of heart rate and blood pressure. Frequent vital capacity measurements are suggested to closely assess respiratory function. If respiratory compromise develops (vital capacity approaching 1 L), elective intubation is often required.

The prognosis is dependent on the development of axonal damage. If this occurs, the patient is likely to have more residual neurologic deficits. In a high percentage of cases, patients are able to recover their previous level of function or attain near normal status.

A diagnostic algorithm for peripheral neuropathy is shown in Fig. 10-6-1.

BIBLIOGRAPHY

Cornblath DR, McArthur JC, Kennedy PG, et al: Inflammatory demyelinating peripheral neuropathies associated with HTLV-III infection, *Ann Neurol* 21:32, 1987.

Dutch Guillain-Barré Study Group: A randomized trial comparing intravenous immune globulin and plasma exchange in Guillain-Barré syndrome, *N Engl J Med* 326:1123-1129, 1992.

Guillain-Barré Syndrome Study Group: Plasmapheresis and acute Guillain-Barré syndrome, *Neurology* 35:1096, 1988.

Ropper AH: The Guillain-Barré syndrome, *N Engl J Med* 326:1130-1136, 1992.

Tenorio G, Ashkenasi A, Benton JW: Guillain-Barré syndrome. In WM Scheld, RJ Whitley, DT Durack, eds: *Infections of the central nervous system,* New York 1991, Raven Press.

CASE

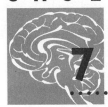

Christopher Hughes
Philip Gorelick

A 40-year-old woman was brought by ambulance to the emergency room. Upon arrival, her husband states that approximately 1 hour ago, while watching television, she screamed, grabbed her head, fell to the ground, and was unconscious. No tongue biting, urination, or tonic-clonic movements were observed. While in the ambulance she began to awaken. She now presents with lethargy and complains of severe headache. Further history from the husband reveals that she developed an intense headache 3 days ago that partially subsided but continued day and night to the present time. Earlier in the day the patient began to complain of blurred vision in her left eye. Her husband noted that her left eyelid was slightly lower than the right eyelid. She did not complain of nausea, emesis, scotomas, or other focal neurologic symptoms. The patient was not concerned about the headache since she believed it to be a migraine attack.

She has a history of classic migraine that began as a teenager and was treated prophylactically. At that time the headaches were associated with nausea and emesis. Over the past 5 years she has had approximately 1 migraine headache every 9 months. Her past medical history is otherwise unremarkable. She takes no medications other than aspirin for headache and has no allergies.

QUESTION 1 This patient presents with an acute episode of unconsciousness preceded by headache. What is the differential diagnosis?

This patient suffered a headache for 3 days which was followed by acute loss of consciousness. Typically, acute cerebral events are either due to seizure or cerebrovascular disease. The

lack of forced urination, tongue biting, tonic-clonic movements, or history of seizure disorder reduces the likelihood of the former diagnosis. Regarding vascular etiologies, the history is classic for aneurysmal subarachnoid hemorrhage (SAH). The prodrome, headache for 3 days, could be due to either a small, warning (sentinel) bleed or to aneurysmal dilation before rupture. The description of the patient's scream, head grabbing, and unconsciousness has been reported frequently by observers of patients with SAH. The bleed typically occurs quickly and with great force. The resulting acute rise in intracranial pressure (ICP) is thought to cause loss of consciousness.

Intracerebral hemorrhage could also present as headache. Patients with chronic hypertension may develop hemorrhage in the subcortical region (e.g., putamen, thalamus, caudate), but they do not usually have a 3-day prodrome of headache. Further, this patient did not have a history of hypertension. Intracerebral hemorrhage can also be caused by rupture of an arterial-venous malformation (AVM). Though not unusual at this patient's age, AVMs are commonly associated with seizures. Finally, a bacterial brain abscess can present as headache. An abscess can rupture into the adjacent ventricle leading to acute decompensation. Abscesses are rare in otherwise healthy persons but should be considered in the differential diagnosis.

Diagnostic algorithms for patients with headaches are shown in Figs. 10-7-1 on p. 622 and 10-7-2 on p. 623.

QUESTION 2 What physical examination findings will help confirm or rule out the various diagnoses discussed above?

Raised ICP, regardless of etiology, can often lead to elevated blood pressure (to maintain cerebral perfusion) and bradycardia. This triad is known as Cushing's reflex. Fever can accompany bacterial abscess but also can be found in patients with SAH. In the case of SAH, chemical meningitis leads to meningeal signs (nuchal rigidity, Kernig's sign, etc.). When patients present with fever, meningeal signs, and a decreased level of consciousness, one should also consider the diagnosis of bacterial meningitis. Furthermore, if a bacterial abscess were to rupture into the ipsilateral lateral ventricle, bacterial ventriculitis and meningitis can develop. Fortunately, the diagnostic workup of these two serious diseases is the same.

The patient's husband described ptosis of the left eyelid. This finding is usually caused by aneurysm at the junction of the internal carotid and posterior communicating arteries that compresses the ipsilateral third cranial nerve. With this information one could hypothesize that the history of blurred vision in the left eye was caused by eyelid ptosis or a dilated left pupil. Pupillary constriction is controlled by the third cranial nerve and is often rendered dysfunctional by aneurysmal compression of this nerve. Thus, the pupil is dilated and does not react to light. Complete third cranial nerve dysfunction from compression would result in impaired adduction and vertical movement of the left eye. The sixth cranial nerve controls the lateral rectus muscle of each eye and can become dysfunctional in states of raised ICP as the nerve is stretched. In this context, sixth nerve dysfunction is referred to as a "false" localizing sign because it signals a diffuse pathology (raised ICP) rather than pathology localized to the sixth cranial nerve or nucleus. If raised ICP is present, there may be papilledema. When SAH occurs, blood can extravasate into the retina causing subhyaloid hemorrhage. This finding may be bilateral.

All the physical examination findings discussed above are consistent with an extraaxial process or pathology outside of the brain tissue. Findings such as conjugate eye deviation, visual field defect, motor tone or strength asymmetries, reflex or Babinski sign asymmetries would suggest intraaxial (intraparenchymal) lesions such as tumor, abscess, brain hemorrhage, or ischemia.

QUESTION 3 On physical examination vital signs were BP 170/100 mm Hg, P 100 bpm, RR 16/min, T 100.8°F. The general physical examination was within normal limits. On neurologic examination the patient was lethargic and only able to follow one-step commands. She complained of severe headache, nausea, and stiff neck. Nuchal rigidity was present. Visual fields were intact. Funduscopic examination showed subhyaloid hemorrhage in the left eye. No papilledema was present. The left pupil was dilated and unreactive. Ptosis was present on the left. Extraocular movements were consistent with a left third cranial nerve palsy showing limited left eye upward, downward, and medial movement, and the left eye was deviated downward and outward. The remainder of the neurologic examination was unremarkable. The patient has a dilated, unreactive pupil. Is she suffering from temporal lobe (uncal) herniation?

There are four commonly encountered causes for a dilated, unreactive pupil. The first is anticholinergic medication. Eye drops containing anticholinergic medications, scopolamine patches, and even systemic atropine have all been known to cause (asymmetrical) dilated, unreactive pupils. These patients are alert and have no other neurologic findings. A second cause is the Holmes-Adie syndrome, which is believed to result from loss of parasympathetic neurons innervating the eye. This leads to unopposed sympathetic dilation of the affected pupil. Patients with this condition may complain of unilateral blurred vision and are often areflexic. Third cranial nerve compression leading to unilateral pupillary dilation, as discussed above, is most commonly associated with aneurysm and is often associated with oculomotor dysfunction and headache. Uncal herniation is usually associated with large temporal lobe mass lesions and is found in comatose patients. The fact that this patient is alert and able to follow commands indicates that uncal herniation is not the cause of her dilated pupil. Since SAH and uncal herniation both cause pupillary dilation by compression of the third cranial nerve, the patient's history as well as other physical findings and neuroimaging studies are used to differentiate between the two disease states.

QUESTION 4   The physical examination is most consistent with SAH. Yet, the low-grade fever may suggest early bacterial meningitis in the presence of nuchal rigidity and lethargy. Name three types of infectious meningitis that can cause focal cranial nerve signs. What is the proper diagnostic workup for this patient?

Listeria, tuberculous, and fungal meningitis can all cause focal cranial nerve dysfunction by affecting the basal meninges. Most infectious meningitides have a less dramatic onset than that found in this patient. Nevertheless, a lumbar puncture (LP) is needed to rule out meningitis. Before this procedure, the patient should have a noncontrast CAT scan of the brain. Brain abscess, intracerebral hemorrhage, and most cases of SAH are diagnosed by this imaging procedure. If CAT scan is not diagnostic and there is no contraindication to spinal puncture, lumbar puncture can be performed.

QUESTION 5   The CAT scan showed a concentric focus of increased density in the parapontine cistern. No cortical abnormalities were noted. The LP was then performed, and the following spinal fluid results were obtained: Tube 1: 9237 RBC, 12 WBC; Tube 4: 8214 RBC, 9 WBC. Both samples were red in color, but the supernatant was clear when centrifuged. Protein, glucose, and lactate levels were normal. What conclusions can be drawn from these results?

No intraparenchymal hemorrhage or abscess was seen. The focus of increased density in the parapontine cistern is most consistent with blood from an aneurysmal SAH. The spinal fluid analysis is also consistent with SAH. The RBC is elevated in both tubes 1 and 4. When bloody spinal

fluid is caused by a traumatic LP, the RBC usually falls significantly from tubes 1 to 4. The spinal fluid WBC is elevated, but this mild increase is explained by the bloody contamination alone. When spinal fluid contains blood, the spinal fluid WBC increases by one for approximately every 500 to 700 RBC found (assuming a normal WBC: RBC ratio in the peripheral blood). Furthermore, the spinal fluid protein, glucose, and lactate levels do not support an infectious process. Spinal fluid xanthochromia is usually found in SAH but is not found in this case. This discrepancy is due to the fact that xanthochromia usually takes 2 to 4 hours to develop. By history, this patient's event occurred approximately 1 hour before the LP.

QUESTION 6   What cardiac, pulmonary, and electrolyte abnormalities can develop as a consequence of subarachnoid hemorrhage?

SAH leads to a significant release of catecholamines that have a number of detrimental systemic effects. For example, cardiac arrhythmias may be observed in patients with SAH. These arrhythmias may be life-threatening. The electrocardiogram can also reflect cardiac abnormalities including ischemic ST segment and T wave changes, and changes in the QT interval. Despite a lack of coronary artery disease, focal, subendocardial hemorrhage, or focal necrosis has been found in patients with SAH. There may even be elevation of cardiac isoenzymes.

An uncommon pulmonary complication of SAH is neurogenic pulmonary edema. At autopsy the lungs are found to contain large amounts of extravascular water. Premorbidly, this condition leads to intrapulmonary shunting and hypoxia. Some authorities believe that it is caused by the direct effect of catecholamines on the lung tissue, while others believe that it is a manifestation of cardiac dysfunction.

Approximately one third of patients with SAH develop abnormalities of sodium and water homeostasis. Most common are hyponatremia and volume depletion. Originally the hyponatremia in SAH was attributed to inappropriate antidiuretic

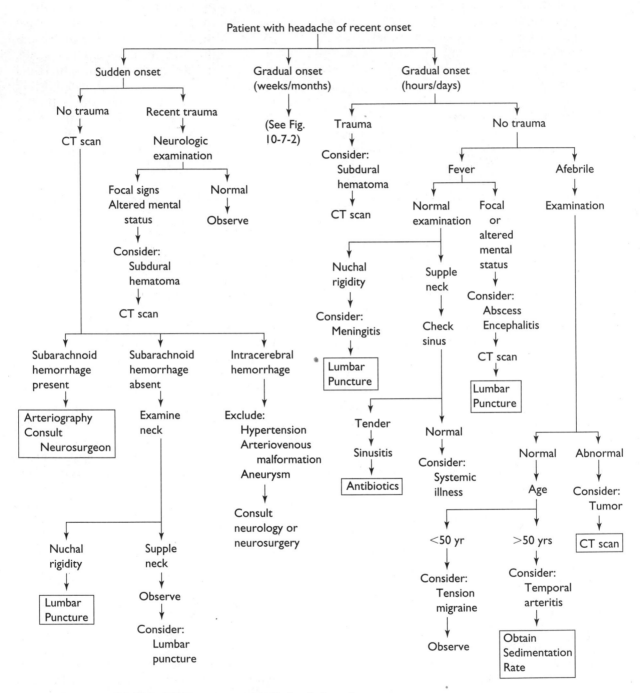

10-7-1 Diagnostic algorithm for headaches of recent onset.
(From Greene HL, Johnson WP, Maricic MJ: *Decision making in medicine*, St Louis, 1993, Mosby.)

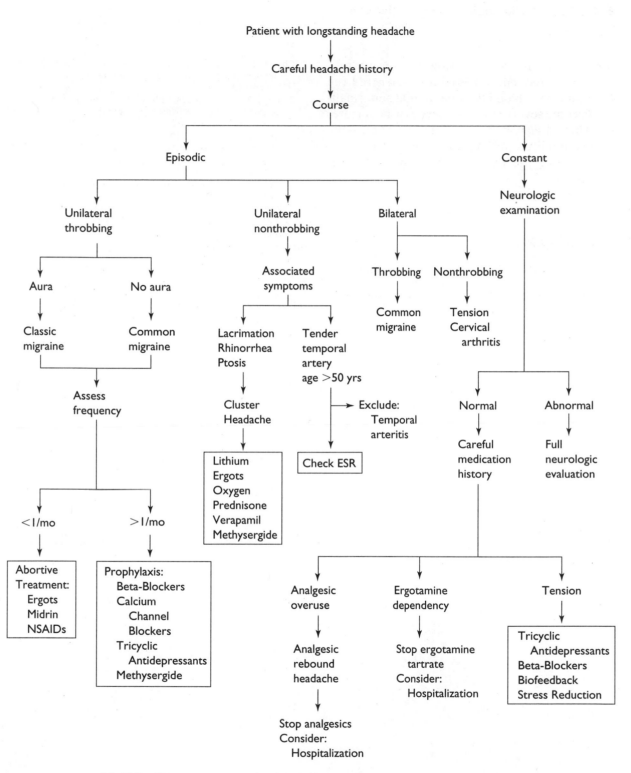

10-7-2 Diagnostic algorithm for longstanding headaches.
(From Greene HL, Johnson WP, Maricic MJ: *Decision making in medicine,* St Louis, 1993, Mosby.)

hormone release (SIADH). However, recent studies show a reduction in sodium, water, red cell mass, and total blood volume. If fluid abnormalities become severe enough, there may be seizures or an increased risk of ischemic stroke. These same studies implicate atrial natriuretic factor in this process, but the exact mechanism is still unknown.

BIBLIOGRAPHY

Adams HP: Clinical manifestations and diagnosis of subarachnoid hemorrhage, *Sem Neurol* 4:304, 1984.

Biller J, Gogersky JC, Adams HP: Management of aneurysmal subarachnoid hemorrhage, *Stroke* 19:63, 1988.

Chyatte D, Fode NC, Sundi TM: Early versus late intracranial aneurysm surgery in subarachnoid hemorrhage, *J Neurosurg* 69:326, 1988.

Disney L, Weir B, Grace M, Roberts P: Trends in blood pressure, osmolality and electrolytes after subarachnoid hemorrhage from aneurysms, *Can J Neurol Sci* 16:299, 1989.

Gorelick PB: Ischemic stroke and intracranial hematoma. In Olsen J, Tfelt-Hansen P, eds: *The headaches,* New York, 1993, Raven Press.

Rosenfeld JV, Barnett GH, Sila CA, et al: The effect of subarachnoid hemorrhage on blood and CSF atrial natriuretic factor, *J Neurosurg* 71:32, 1989.

Vermeuden M, Van Gijn J: The diagnosis of subarachnoid hemorrhage, *J Neurol Neurosurg Psychiatry* 53:365-372, 1990.

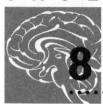

CASE

8

Christopher Hughes
Philip Gorelick

....

A 65-year-old man came to the emergency room complaining of severe right hip pain after a fall. The patient was getting dressed that morning and fell backward while putting on a sweater. There was slight dizziness before the fall, but he denies diaphoresis, nausea, or palpitations. There was no loss of consciousness or head trauma. He was unable to arise, and the paramedics were called.

The patient has a past medical history of Parkinson's disease, which was diagnosed 10 years ago. He is taking Sinemet (25/100), 1 tab 4 times a day, Permax 0.25 mg 3 times per day, and Eldepryl 5 mg twice a day. His symptoms of tremor and "slowness" are well controlled by these medications. He walks well but has had recent impairment of balance. Permax was added to treat this symptom. The patient takes no other medications and has no allergies. Review of systems reveals three recent episodes of transient dizziness upon standing. These episodes lasted approximately 30 seconds each and were associated with a slight blurring of vision.

On physical examination the right leg was externally rotated, and the hip area was tender when passively moved. Neurologic examination shows normal intellect and cranial nerves. Motor tone was increased in both arms with mild cogwheel rigidity. A slight resting tremor was noted in both hands. Deep tendon reflexes were within normal limits. The patient was unable to stand secondary to hip pain. A plain x-ray of the right hip confirmed a fracture. The orthopedic service was consulted and after evaluation, scheduled the patient for surgery.

QUESTION 1 What are the four major signs of Parkinson's disease?

In Parkinson's disease there is selective loss of dopaminergic neurons in the pars compacta of the substantia nigra. This leads to four classic signs. Rest tremor is most commonly found in the hands and is described as "pill rolling" because the hand appears to be rolling a pill between the thumb and first finger. The tremor is usually bilateral but may be asymmetric early in the disease. The second is bradykinesia or slowness of movement. Parkinson's disease patients have slowness and difficulty initiating movement. For example, they may have difficulty arising from a chair or initiating walking. They also complain of feeling "stiff and slow" as though they are walking through water. Rapid movements are difficult to perform. Third, there may be cogwheel rigidity. Increased tone is found in agonist and antagonist muscle groups of the extremities. With passive movement, a cogwheel (rachet-like) phenomenon is noted, especially across the elbow and wrist joints. Cogwheel rigidity is distinctly different from spasticity and the clasp-knife rigidity found in stroke patients. Finally, postural reflex instability is the fourth major manifestation of Parkinson's disease. Diminished postural reflexes cause a tendency to fall. Parkinson's patients are prone to fall backward as the retropulse or forward as the propulse.

QUESTION 2 What is the neurochemical mechanism of Parkinson's disease and what are the pharmocologic interventions that may be used?

The symptoms of Parkinson's disease are related to an imbalance of dopamine (DA) and acetylcholine (ACH) in the striatum. As dopaminergic neurons drop out, the DA/ACH ratio falls. Therefore, pharmacologic intervention is aimed at restoring the balance or loss of dopamine.

The patient presented in this case was on Sinemet. This is a combination medication containing levodopa, the precursor to dopamine, and carbidopa, which is an inhibitor of L-aromatic amino acid decarboxylase that prevents peripheral breakdown of dopamine before it enters the CNS and allows lower doses of dopamine to be administered. Levodopa crosses the blood brain barrier (BBB) and is converted into dopamine by presynaptic neurons in the substantia nigra. Sinemet is prescribed using the following formulations: 10/100, 25/100, and 25/250. The numerator indicates the number of milligrams of carbidopa, and the denominator indicates the number of milligrams of levodopa. A sustained release form, Sinemet CR 50/200, is also available.

Ergot agents, including bromocriptine and pergolide (Permax), act as direct dopamine receptor agonists. This mechanism normalizes receptor activity by directly stimulating postsynaptic dopamine receptors in the brain. Eldepryl is a selective monoamine oxidase (type B) inhibitor when administered in recommended doses. In the substantia nigra, inhibition of this enzyme leads to decreased catabolism of dopamine. The result is a general increase in the concentration of dopamine in this region of the brain. Eldepryl may increase dopamine activity by other mechanisms or could act as a protective agent that inhibits production of potentially damaging neuronal toxins that accumulate through the monoamine oxidase B metabolic pathway.

Use of anticholinergic agents is an alternative strategy. These may be effective early in the course of disease and in patients whose predominant symptom is tremor.

QUESTION 3 What are the two most likely reasons for the patient's fall?

The patient fell backward while putting on a sweater. To achieve this, he stood erect, retropulsed as he tugged on the sweater, and fell as he had poor postural reflex righting ability. This is a classic scenario for Parkinson's disease. Furthermore, the loss of visual information while the sweater was being pulled over his eyes potenti-

ated the tendency to fall. The second mechanism may be related to the patient's medications. Permax, a medication started just before the episode, was prescribed recently for postural instability. Since beginning this medication the patient has experienced episodes of "pre-syncope." He complained of dizziness upon standing associated with blurring of vision that was related to orthostatic hypotension, a well-known complication of anti-Parkinson's medications. Tolerance to the hypotensive effect of Permax may develop if the medication is started at low doses (0.05 mg twice a day) and gradually increased. This patient was started on a much higher dose of Permax, 0.25 mg 3 times per day.

Surgery was performed successfully, and the patient was eventually returned to his hospital room. His right leg was immobilized, intravenous hydration therapy was administered, and a regular schedule of injectable morphine was ordered for pain. The patient had normal bowel sounds, so a general diet was ordered, and his regular Parkinson's medications were continued at the usual doses. Later that night the surgery resident was called to evaluate the patient. The patient was agitated and thrashing about in bed. He was very distractable but denied significant pain. He also denied shortness of breath or chest discomfort. Despite reassurance he continued to be agitated. On neurologic examination he did not follow commands well and had no cranial nerve deficits. There were no motor deficits. The right leg was still immobilized. On closer examination his "thrashing" movements were involuntary, semirhythmical, and choreatic. These movements involved his entire body including neck, trunk, arms, and legs. A general physical examination, electrocardiogram, arterial blood gas, and chest x-ray were normal.

QUESTION 4 What is causing the patient's clinical syndrome?

This patient is displaying signs of sympathetic nervous system and catecholamine excess. The agitation and chorea suggest that dopamine receptors are being stimulated excessively. Ad-

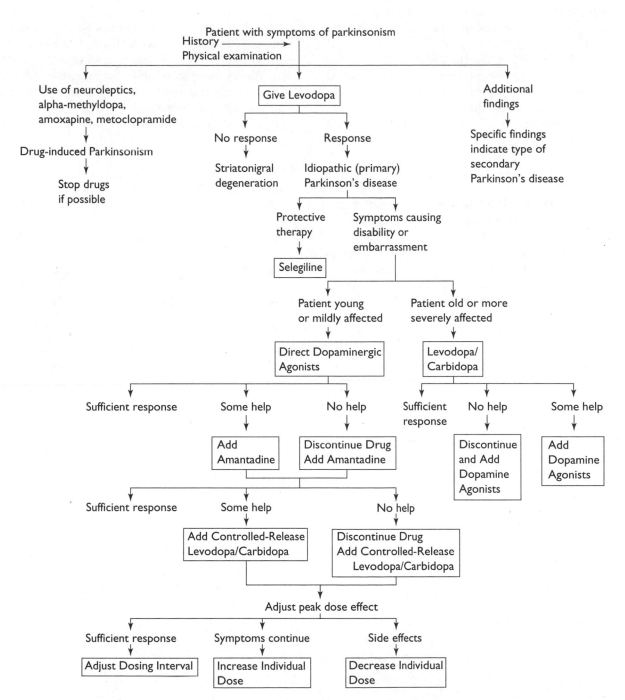

10-8-1   Approach to the patient with symptoms of parkinsonism.
(From Greene HL, Johnson WP, Maricic MJ: *Decision making in medicine*, St Louis, 1993, Mosby.)

vanced Parkinson's patients may be sensitive to changes in dopaminergic brain activity. When undermedicated, they often develop symptoms of their disease. When overmedicated, signs of dopamine excess can occur. In this case, the clinical manifestations were probably caused by catecholamine excess that resulted from use of morphine. In combination with his regular medications, a state of excessive dopaminergic stimulation was produced. When the morphine was discontinued, the patient's symptoms resolved.

QUESTION 5   The following day the patient appeared to be in no acute distress. However, he began to complain that there were children and small animals in his room. On physical examination the patient appeared calm and attentive. He insisted that the children and animals were observed but denied that they were threatening or frightening to him. He had no cognitive deficits and none of the signs of catecholamine excess witnessed the night before. He denied hearing voices or having intrusive thoughts. What is the explanation for the patient's problem?

The patient is describing hallucinations in Parkinson's disease. The exact cause for these hallucinations is unknown, but they often occur in patients with a long history of the disease and in those who have been overmedicated with dopaminergic compounds. The hallucinations may be of nonthreatening animals or children. The patient shows no signs of delirium or agitation but rather calmly experiences these visual phenomena. They occur momentarily and resolve without treatment. A reduction in anti-Parkinson's medication is usually recommended to prevent their recurrence.

An algorithm for approaching a patient with symptoms of Parkinsonism is shown in Fig. 10-8-1.

BIBLIOGRAPHY

Jankovic J, Marsden CD: Therapeutic strategies in Parkinson's Disease. In Jankovic J, Tolosa E, eds: *Parkinson's disease and movement disorders*, Baltimore, 1988, Urban and Schwarzenberg.

Parkinson's Study Group: Deprenyl and tocopherol antioxidant therapy of parkinsonism (DATATOP), *Acta Neurol Scand Suppl* 126:171-175, 1989.

Parkinson's Study Group: Effects of tocopherol and deprenyl on the progression of disability in early Parkinson's disease, *N Engl J Med* 328:176-183, 1993.

Weiner WJ, Lang AE: Parkinson's Disease. In Weiner WJ, Lang AE, eds: *Movement disorders, a comprehensive survey*, New York, 1989, Futura.

C A S E

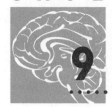

Christopher Hughes
Philip Gorelick

A 72-year-old man with a history of alcohol abuse is brought by his family to the doctor's office for evaluation. The wife and son of the patient state that he cannot remember names and is confused easily. They are worried that he may have Alzheimer's disease. On further questioning they state that he has trouble finding household objects and will often ask odd questions. He occasionally will say things that don't make sense and will answer questions with nonsensical phrases. He is still able to dress and eat independently but has not used the telephone or read a newspaper recently. They believe that this behavior began approximately 2 months ago. The patient has had no recent illnesses and has not complained of headache, double vision, or focal weakness. He generally sleeps well, has a good appetite, and has maintained his weight. He has a long history of alcohol abuse. Approximately once a week, he will consume enough beer and wine to become drunk and lose consciousness. He has never had alcohol withdrawal seizures or delirium tremens. He has smoked one pack of cigarettes per day for 40 years. There is no history of recent head trauma or change in diet.

Two years ago he was diagnosed with hypertension but has inconsistently taken the propranolol that was prescribed for this condition. His past medical history is otherwise unremarkable. His mother and father both died at the age of 74, but the cause of their deaths is unknown. He has two brothers who have no medical illnesses. There is no history of dementia in any family members. Review of systems is unremarkable.

QUESTION I The patient was brought to medical attention because of cognitive and behavioral problems. What are some of the different states of altered consciousness, and how do you characterize them? How would you characterize this patient's mental status?

Confusion describes a state of inattentiveness that is characterized by misinterperatation of sensory stimuli, faulty memory, bewilderment, and difficulty following commands. A subset of patients may demonstrate *disorientation,* the lack of awareness concerning usual surroundings and relationships (people, places, or time). *Delirium* refers to a floridly abnormal mental state characterized by disorientation, fear, irritability, and misperception of sensory stimuli. *Dementia* refers to a deterioration of intellectual function without diminution of arousal.

Stupor is a state where the level of consciousness is depressed but from which the patient can be aroused by vigorous and repeated stimuli. The *comatose* patient has a further depression of consciousness from which arousal cannot be accomplished (unarousable psychologic unresponsiveness).

By the above definitions, this patient appears to be demented. *Dementia* is a general term that refers to the progressive loss of previously acquired cognitive abilities. Generally, this term is applied when deterioration begins to impact on the patient's social and occupational function. Dementia causes impairment of higher cortical function including memory, language, executive function, calculation, attention, praxis, and orientation. When considering the diagnosis of dementia, impairment of arousal, depression, and delirium (from drugs, fever, sepsis, etc.) must be excluded.

An algorithm for approaching the patient with chronic behavior change is shown in Fig. 10-9-1.

QUESTION 2 What is the differential diagnosis of dementia?

Alzheimer's disease is the most common form of primary dementing illness. Typically this condition becomes symptomatic after the age of 50 and is characterized by progressive memory loss. Both the incidence and prevalence of the disease increases exponentially with age. Alzheimer neuropathologic changes occur with Down syndrome patients by age 40. Disturbances of executive function, language, praxis, orientation, calculation, and behavior are common. Memory loss is the cardinal manifestation. The time course of the disease is slowly progressive. The etiology is uncertain. Brain necropsy shows neurofibrillary tangles and senile plaques. Tacrine may have relatively short-term benefits for some patients; however this treatment is not curative.

Vascular dementia (VaD) is the second leading cause of irreversible dementia. VaD is usually caused by multiple cortical or subcortical infarctions. The disease usually manifests a stepwise progression. Since hypertension, diabetes mellitus, heart disease, cigarette smoking, and atrial fibrillation are common risk factors for stroke, patients with these diseases are at increased risk for this form of dementia. VaD patients have a high incidence of focal neurologic signs and symptoms because of cortical or subcortical ischemia.

Pick's disease, though often difficult to differentiate from Alzheimer's disease, is a condition referred to as a "frontal lobe" dementia because of prominent frontal lobe features. Patients can develop prominent personality changes and emotional alterations such as apathy, irritability, depression, and behavioral disinhibition. Gait difficulties and language dysfunction may also occur. Neuroimaging typically shows prominent atrophy of the frontal and temporal lobes. Progression of the disease usually results in death after 6 to 12 years. There is currently no effective treatment.

QUESTION 3 What is the differential diagnosis of reversible causes of dementia?

These medical conditions include hypothyroidism, nutritional deficiency (e.g., B_{12}, folate, thiamine), neurosyphilis, and hepatic dysfunction. Diagnosis can be confirmed by appropriate diagnostic blood studies and exclusion of other causes of dementia. However, establishing the diagnosis of neurosyphilis may be more complicated. Elderly patients with a history of dementia and a reactive serology for syphilis require a lumbar puncture to rule out neurosyphilis. The CSF profile in patients with dementia due to neurosyphilis include a reactive VDRL, increased protein and globulins, normal glucose, and an elevated cell count with a predominance of lymphocytes.

The major syndromes of neurosyphilis are syphilitic meningitis, gummas, meningovascular syphilis, tabes dorsalis, and general paresis. General paresis is accepted as the more common dementing form of syphilis. The patient presents with a syndrome of dementia, neuropsychiatric manifestations such as delusions, lightning-like pains, ataxia, areflexia, and a Romberg sign. In this disease the Argyll-Robertson (AR) pupil may be present. With an AR pupil there is impairment of the light reflex, but the pupils constrict to accommodation.

Treatment is intravenous penicillin. Reduction of the CSF pleocytosis, followed by serial lumbar puncture, is the goal. However, this may not return to normal immediately after treatment. Retest of the CSF in 6 months and at 1 to 2 years is essential to prove adequacy of treatment.

QUESTION 4 Physical examination demonstrated BP 170/110 mm Hg, P 65 bpm, RR 12/min, T 99.5°F. The cardiovascular, pulmonary, and gastrointestinal examinations were normal. No cardiac murmur or carotid bruit was present. On neurologic examination the patient was pleasant and his speech was fluent. He was able to close his eyes and stick out his tongue to command but could not follow any other verbal commands. He would often

respond to questions with nonsensical phrases that were not relevant. When presented with a spoon he could not name it but could show how it was used. He was able to state that he used it every day and "eats with it" but nothing more. Similar cognitive impairments were found when the patient was presented with a comb and a pencil. He was unable to write his name or read the word *dog* though the family states that he previously had the ability to read and write. Because the patient had such profound difficulty with naming, formal memory testing could not be performed. Throughout the cognitive testing the patient did not appear to be disturbed by his deficiencies.

Fundoscopic examination showed sharp disk margins. There was no obvious field defect. Cranial nerve function was within normal limits. There was no nystagmus. Motor system testing showed normal strength in the arms and legs. Sensory examination was normal for pin prick and vibratory testing. Cerebellar function was normal. The patient swayed during Romberg testing but did not fall. Gait was slightly wide-based. Heel to toe walking was slightly impaired. There were no frontal lobe release signs. What is aphasia? What are the common forms of this condition?

Aphasia refers to a disorder of language. The language centers of the brain are located in the perisylvian area of the dominant cerebral hemisphere. For the spoken word to be "comprehended" the posterior portion of the temporal lobe of the dominant hemisphere known as Wernicke's area must be intact. The motor or output portion of language is dependent on an area in the posterior portion of the inferior frontal gyrus referred to as Broca's area. These two centers are connected by a white-matter pathway known as the arcuate fasciculus and cortical-to-cortical connections. The ability to repeat a spoken phrase therefore requires "comprehension" (Wernicke's area), transmission along the arcuate fasciculus and cortical connections, verbal reproduction (Broca's area). All three components of the system must be intact for a patient to be able to repeat a phrase. The

forms of aphasia reviewed below correspond to dysfunction of each of these respective system components.

In Broca's aphasia, one can comprehend speech and follow commands. However, speech is nonfluent and telegraphic (connecting words are deleted and only substantiatives such as nouns and verbs are used). Because of its proximity to the motor cortex, patients with Broca's area dysfunction will often have contralateral faciobrachial weakness.

In Wernicke's aphasia speech production and fluency are preserved as Broca's area is intact. However, comprehension of language is abnormal and language oftentimes does not make sense, leading the uninitiated examiner to the erroneous conclusion that these patients are confused or in a state of delirium as there are paraphrasias.

Conduction aphasia refers to dysfunction of the arcuate fasciculus or the corresponding cortical connections. With both Broca's and Wernicke's areas unaffected, fluency and comprehension are generally preserved. The main deficit in this form of aphasia is an inability to repeat. Since each of the aforementioned components of the language system is required to repeat a spoken phrase, repetition will be impaired in each of these perisylvian aphasias.

This patient's history and physical examination are most consistent with a Wernicke's aphasia. His major deficit is language comprehension, since he is unable to read or follow most commands but speaks fluently. The acute onset of language dysfunction is most consistent with a focal cortical process, such as stroke, rather than a progressive dementing illness. Commonly, as Wernicke's aphasia improves, patients are left with residual difficulties naming objects (anomia) and understanding complex phrases. The ability to comprehend written words is variable. In contradistinction, in the early stages of Alzheimer's disease, the type of aphasia usually encountered is transcortical sensory aphasia (i.e., similar to Wernicke's aphasia except the ability to repeat is preserved).

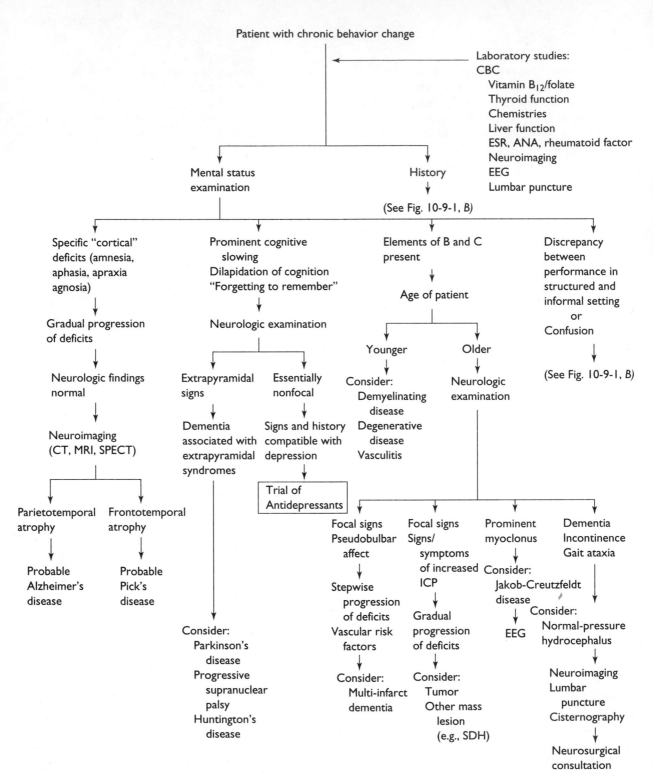

10-9-1, A Approach to the patient with chronic behavior change.

(From Greene HL, Johnson WP, Maricic MJ: *Decision making in medicine*, St Louis, 1993, Mosby.)

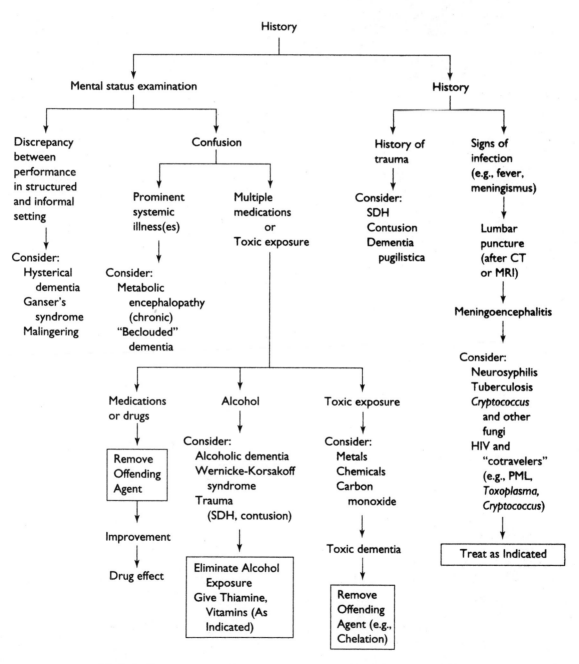

10-9-1, B Approach to the patient with chronic behavior change—Cont'd.

QUESTION 5   A CT scan of the brain was performed and showed an "old" cortical infarct in the left superior temporal lobe. An electrocardiogram demonstrated intermittent atrial fibrillation, and left atrial enlargement was diagnosed by echocardiography. Carotid doppler and blood analysis showed no significant abnormalities. Are these laboratory findings expected given the patient's history and physical examination findings?

The CT scan of the brain confirmed a stroke as the cause of the patient's aphasia. Many Wernicke's area strokes in the elderly are embolic in etiology. Atrial fibrillation is a known risk factor for cardio-embolic stroke. Furthermore, alcohol intoxication is associated with cardiac arrhythmias (e.g., the "Holiday Heart" syndrome), and heavy alcohol consumption is thought to be an independent risk factor for stroke. This combination of factors may have led to the stroke.

BIBLIOGRAPHY

Appell J, Kertesz A, Fisman M: A study of language functioning in Alzheimer patients, *Brain Lang* 17:73-91, 1982.

Arie T: Management of dementia: a review, *Brit Med Bull* 42:91-96, 1986.

Chui HC, Teng EL, Henderson VW: Clinical subtypes of dementia of the Alzheimer type, *Neurology* 35:1544-1550, 1985.

Cummings JL, Miller B, Hill MA: Neuropsychiatric aspects of multi-infarct dementia and dementia of the Alzheimer type, *Arch Neurol* 44:389-393, 1987.

Geschwind N, Quadfasel F, Segarra: Isolation of the speech area, *Neuropsychologia* 6:327-340, 1969.

Gorelick PB: Alcohol in stroke, *Stroke* 19:268-27, 1987.

Gorelick PB, Roman G, Mangone CA: Vascular dementia. In Gorelick PB, Alter M, eds: *Handbook of neuroepidemiology*, New York, 1994, Marcel Decker.

Kirshner HS, Casey PF, Henson J: Behaviourial features and lesion localization in Wernicke's aphasia, *Aphasiology* 3:169-176, 1989.

C A S E

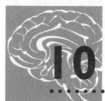

10

Christopher Hughes
Philip Gorelick

A 65-year-old woman with a history of hypertension was riding in the car with her husband. Suddenly, she made a strange sound and became unresponsive. Her husband immediately drove to the nearest hospital. Ten minutes elapsed before their arrival at the emergency room. Cardiac monitoring disclosed that the patient was in ventricular fibrillation with no recordable blood pressure. The acute cardiac life support (ACLS) protocol was initiated. Ten additional minutes passed before a sustained pulse and blood pressure were obtained. During this time the patient was intubated, an arterial line and central intravenous access were secured. The patient was then transferred to the cardiac intensive care unit.

The patient's past medical history included hypertension and treatment with propranolol. There was no history of cardiac disease. There was a family history of coronary artery disease and hypertension. The patient smoked over a pack of cigarettes per day for 40 years. Neurologic consultation was requested to assess neurologic status.

The patient was examined in the emergency room by the neurology service 1 hour after her acute event. The patient had been asystolic for approximately 20 minutes. At the time of evaluation she was intubated and received a continuous lidocaine infusion. Vital signs were T 98.8°F, P 110 bpm, RR 16/min, BP 125/75 mm Hg.

On neurologic examination the patient displayed no spontaneous movement. There was no response to verbal command. Doll's eyes (oculocephalic maneuver) were present and easily obtainable in both the vertical and horizontal planes. Fundoscopic examination showed sharp
disk margins bilaterally. Corneal reflexes were intact. On motor examination there was spasticity in the arms. The legs had increased extensor tone. Deep tendon reflexes were hyperactive. The Babinski sign was present bilaterally.

QUESTION 1 With manual eyelid elevation the pupils were 5 mm in diameter and unresponsive to light bilaterally. The eyes roved spontaneously from left to right in a cyclical manner. What is the likely cause for the patient's dilated, unresponsive pupils? Has she suffered bilateral temporal lobe (uncal) herniation?

Pupillary dilation in the presence of uncal herniation is due to compression of the third cranial nerve. This nerve also controls medial and vertical eye movement. Given the easily obtainable oculocephalic reflex, third cranial nerve dysfunction is unlikely. A review of the ACLS record shows that atropine was administered to this patient. The combination of excessive sympathetic discharge associated with cardiac arrest and administration of the anticholinergic, atropine, is the most likely cause for the dilated and unreactive pupils.

QUESTION 2 What is the cause of the roving eye movements? What is the oculocephalic reflex, and what is its significance?

Roving eye movement and the oculocephalic reflex are indicative of diffuse cortical dysfunction with preservation of the brainstem oculomotor pathway. As the cortex becomes dysfunctional, the brainstem/cerebellar neuronal circuits become disinhibited. The roving eye movements are probably a result of disinhibited brainstem activity. The oculocephalic reflex, a brainstem reflex, is heightened by cortical disinhibition. The oculocephalic reflex is tested by rotation of the patient's head from side to side or up and down with the eyelids held open. If brainstem function is intact, the eyes should move conjugately and completely in the direction contralateral to head turning. If the brainstem is not functioning normally, the eyes will not move or will show striking limitations of movement.

QUESTION 3 The arms were in a flexed posture while the legs were extended bilaterally. These limb postures were accentuated by painful stimulus, and no purposeful movements were seen. Of what significance is the patient's limb posture?

Bilateral flexion of the arms in combination with leg extension is known as decorticate posturing and is seen in comatose patients with bilateral cortical dysfunction. Decerebrate posturing consists of bilateral arm and leg extension and is indicative of dysfunction at the brainstem level (midbrain). Both postures may be accentuated by painful stimuli. Overall, the patient's neurologic examination was consistent with diffuse cortical injury and intact brainstem, cerebellar, and spinal cord function.

The patient was examined again 2 days later. At that time she was still intubated but breathing spontaneously. Vital signs remained stable, and she was afebrile. There was minimal spontaneous movement in the arms and legs. The patient opened her eyes to verbal command but required constant verbal stimulus to remain attentive. She could make a fist and showed two fingers to verbal command. Pupils were 2 mm in diameter and reactive bilaterally. Roving eye movements were no longer present. Extraocular movements were full as the patient spontaneously looked into all fields of vision. Yet, to verbal command the patient could not visually track the examiner's finger. The patient responded appropriately to visual threat, and further visual testing revealed intact visual fields. The remaining cra-

nial nerves were intact. The patient was unable to hold her arms above her head. Biceps, triceps, and distal arm strength was normal bilaterally. Even when the examiner assisted the patient to compensate for the proximal arm weakness, she was unable to reach for an object held in front of her.

QUESTION 4 What is the significance of this interval change in the patient's neurologic examination? What is critical watershed ischemia?

The patient's current examination indicates that some higher cortical function has returned. Roving eye movements are no longer present, and the patient now follows verbal commands.

There are three main cerebral arteries supplying the cerebral hemispheres: the anterior, middle, and posterior cerebral arteries. The cortical regions supplied by overlapping distal branches of these vessels are known as the watershed areas. During hypotensive events, watershed regions are prone to underperfusion. With prolonged hypotension the watershed areas are vulnerable to infarction.

QUESTION 5 Explain the patient's bilateral proximal arm weakness.

Branches of the anterior and middle cerebral arteries converge on the lateral aspect of the frontal and parietal lobes. This region is therefore considered a watershed region and somatopically corresponds to the shoulder region on the primary motor cortex homunculus. With hypotension this area can become ischemic with resultant weakness in the shoulder regions bilaterally. This bi-brachial paresis is referred to as the "man-in-the-barrel" syndrome because the bilateral proximal arm weakness makes the patient appear as though she has a barrel around her upper arms and chest that restricts movement of the arms proximally.

QUESTION 6 What is the cause of the patient's visual disturbance?

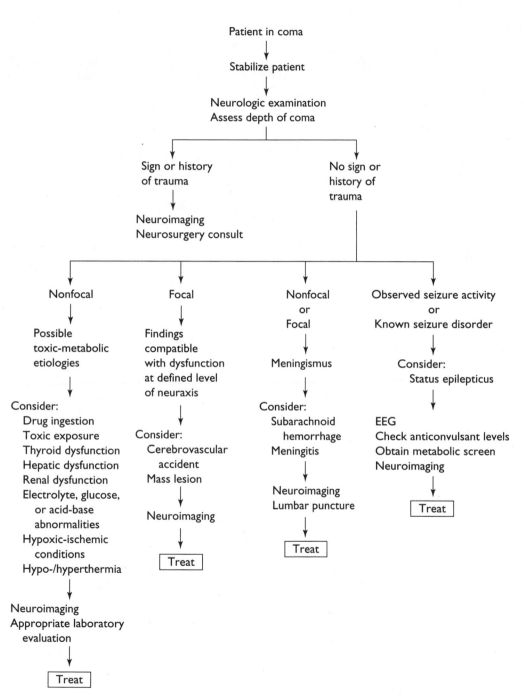

I0-I0-I   Approach to the patient in a coma.
(From Greene HL, Johnson WP, Maricic MJ: *Decision making in medicine*, St Louis, 1993, Mosby.)

Adequacy of the patient's primary vision was confirmed by bedside testing. Yet the patient could not visually track the examiner's finger. Smooth pursuit (tracking) of a visual object is functionally controlled by the parietal lobe. When this region of the brain becomes dysfunctional, smooth pursuit is no longer possible. Failure to look voluntarily into the peripheral field, despite full eye movements, is known as psychic paralysis or fixation of gaze. The inability to use visual information to coordinate limb movements is known as optic ataxia. In this case, the patient could not coordinate her arm movements to touch an object held in front of her. The combination of these findings and visual inattention is known as Balint's syndrome.

Both Balint's syndrome and bi-brachial paresis syndrome can be caused by watershed ischemia. Given the patient's prolonged asystole, watershed infarction is the most likely cause for her residual symptoms. An MRI of the brain was eventually performed and confirmed bilateral watershed ischemia. The patient continued to recover and after 3 weeks was discharged with moderate proximal arm weakness bilaterally.

QUESTION 7 What are the clinical predictors for neurologic recovery following cardiac arrest?

As this case illustrates, cardiac arrest can cause acute central nervous system dysfunction with variable recovery. Serial neurologic examinations are important because they can be used to predict neurologic outcome. A study by Bell and Hodgson (1974) found that full recovery was unusual in patients who were comatose for more than 3 days. A similar study performed by Longstreth (1983) also found that more than 3 days of coma was a poor prognostic sign. If brainstem reflexes (e.g., pupillary light reflex, corneal reflex, oculocephalic reflex) are impaired for more than 12 to 24 hours after the arrest, patients generally have poor outcomes.

An algorithm for approaching a patient in a coma is shown in Fig. 10-10-1.

BIBLIOGRAPHY

Bell JA, Hodgson HJF: Coma after cardiac arrest, *Brain* 97:361-372, 1972.

Gorelick PB, Kelly M: Neurologic complications of cardiac arrest. In Goetz C, Tanner C, Klawans H, eds: *Handbook of neurology,* New York, 1993, Elsevier Science Publications.

Howard R, Trend P, Russell RWR: Clinical features of ischemia in cerebral border zones, *Arch Neurol* 44:934-940, 1987.

Longstreth WT Jr, Inui TS, Cobb LA: Neurologic recovery after out-of-hospital cardiac arrest, *Ann Intern Med* 98:588-592, 1983.

Maiese K, Caronna J: Coma after cardiac arrest: clinical features, prognosis, and management. In Ropper AH, ed: *Neurologic and neurosurgical intensive care,* New York, 1993, Raven Press.

Plum F, Posner J: The diagnosis of stupor and coma, ed 3, Philadelphia, 1982, FA Davis.

PULMONARY

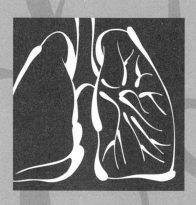

CHARLES J. GRODZIN
SECTION EDITOR

C A S E

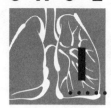

Charles J. Grodzin
James J. Herdegen

The patient is a 22-year-old black female college senior without significant past medical history who came to her university health clinic with complaints of wheezing and shortness of breath. She denies any use of cigarettes, marijuana, or other inhalational exposure. She recalls that her wheezing has been present intermittently over the past 6 months and seems to begin when she is around cigarette smoke or near animals but gradually clears when these exposures are removed. She has been markedly more symptomatic during a recent period of very cold weather. She recalls having had chicken pox and measles as a child and receiving shots because of allergies. This morning she awoke wheezing and while sitting in class this morning became gradually worse and felt it was necessary to seek medical attention.

QUESTION 1 What important points of the history help characterize the underlying disorder?

The patient presents with the clinical symptom of wheezing. Turbulent air flow, because of alteration of the airway lumen, results in vibration of the bronchial wall, heard as a wheeze. Alteration of luminal anatomy may be due to smooth muscle contraction or the accumulation of secretions or inflammatory fluid. Additionally, it is apparent that this patient suffers symptoms in specific circumstances. (She identifies cigarette smoke, animals, and cold air as triggers.) Importantly, she realizes that the wheezing abates when the triggers are removed. This signifies a component of reversibility.

The patient recalls having allergy shots as a child. This may mean that she has a propensity

toward atopy. Atopy is the immunophysiologic response to a specific allergen. Exposure leads to the production of specific IgE that becomes fixed to mast cell surfaces. Crosslinking of the IgE leads to mast cell degranulation with release of mediators of inflammation: histamine, slow reacting substance of anaphylaxis, cytokines, leukotrienes, thromboxanes, and serotonin. This cascade leads to smooth muscle contraction, cellular chemotaxis, and inflammatory fluid exudation into the airways.

QUESTION 2 On physical examination her vital signs are normal except for a respiratory rate of 20/min. Her lung examination reveals diffuse inspiratory and expiratory wheezes with a mild prolongation of the expiratory phase. The cardiovascular, abdominal, extremity, and neurologic examination were normal. The peak flow is 140 L/min. What is the differential diagnosis of the patient's wheezing at this point?

Entities that produce wheezing that are primary to the lung include chronic obstructive pulmonary disease (COPD) and asthma. Asthma is the consequence of bronchial hyperactivity that has a reversible component. Asthma often presents with wheezing and eosinophilia. In this case wheezing is diffuse and has come on gradually.

Some patients with COPD will manifest a bronchospastic component although the main abnormality is due to emphysema (parenchymal destruction) with scarring and airway collapsibility. As lung destruction continues over many years, airways become increasingly weakened, closing early during expiration, and leading to air trapping. This places the respiratory muscles at an increasing mechanical disadvantage. The patient becomes barrel chested with an increased anteroposterior diameter and diaphragmatic depression. Loss of parenchyma retards normal gas exchange with hypoxemia and hypercarbia. Patients with COPD are very sensitive to even mild bronchospasm as they have a large degree of air trapping as a baseline.

The differential diagnosis also includes systemic diseases that can produce wheezing. Congestive heart failure leads to airway edema as a result of increased pulmonary capillary wedge pressure. Pulmonary emboli can stimulate the release of bronchovasoactive mediators from lung injury. Upper airway obstruction can produce inspiratory stridor, and lower airway obstruction can produce a unilateral focal wheezing. The carcinoid syndrome (both gastrointestinal and bronchial) may produce bronchoconstrictive mediators or present as an endobronchial lesion and wheezing. In addition, wheezing can be a presenting symptom in cases of polyarteritis nodosa and hypersensitivity pneumonitis.

The combination of wheezing and eosinophilia can be seen in other diseases. These include Churg-Strauss angiitis, pulmonary infiltrate with eosinophilia, infection with *Strongyloides stercoralis,* and allergic bronchopulmonary aspergillosis (ABPA). ABPA is due to a hypersensitivity (type I and II) reaction to aspergillus antigens. Colonization of asthmatics is common. Diagnosis is suggested in a patient with recurrent sputum and serum eosinophilia with recurrent pulmonary infiltrates. Culture of aspergillus from nasal secretions is also supportive; however, this is not specific. Furthermore, diagnosis is suggested by presence of aspergillus precipitins, elevated IgE >1000 ng/ml, and central bronchiectasis. The treatment is steroids and must be started early to avoid irreversible bronchiectasis.

In addition to these cardiopulmonary etiologies, one must consider less common etiologies for wheezing. Exposure to insecticides with cholinergic properties, use of beta-blocking agents (i.e., eye drops) and paradoxic vocal cord movement may also lead to wheezing.

A diagnostic algorithm for a patient with wheezing is shown in Fig. 11-1-1 on p. 646.

QUESTION 3 Because of the patient's lack of preexisting medical history and characteristic presentation, you give her a diagnosis of asthma. What is the profile of a patient with an exacerbation of asthma? What findings may be present on physical examination, chest radiograph, and electrocardiogram? What are the acute changes found by pulmonary function testing?

The pathophysiologic changes manifest to the clinician with classic signs: the examiner will find a tachypneic patient with a hyperresonant chest, inspiratory and expiratory wheezes, and a prolonged expiratory phase. Evolution to the silent chest with overt accessory muscle use signifies a more dire situation.

Physical examination should concentrate on the lung examination to identify wheezing and to assess the degree of airway obstruction and respiratory distress. Upon questioning, the patient will be variably able to complete sentences depending on the degree of obstruction. Observation of accessory muscle use (intercostals, neck and abdominal muscles) can give valuable information about patient status. When diaphragmatic dysfunction occurs, the abdomen will move inward paradoxically. The patient will often assume an upright position to maximize muscle function. Cardiac examination may reveal a right ventricular heave, a split S2, tachycardia, and palpable PA pulsations.

When one is building a clinical suspicion, the chest x-ray can harbor vital information. A great majority of films are normal; however, the keen observer will find overinflation, manifest by flattened or everted diaphragms, increased sternal bowing, and an increased retrosternal airspace. The electrocardiogram changes because of lung hyperinflation revealing poor R wave progression across the precordial leads and decreased voltage in lead I. This is due to poor electrical conduction through the hyperinflated lung.

Alterations seen on pulmonary function testing include hyperinflation with increased total lung capacity, mild hypoxemia, and hypocapnia. Interestingly, the diffusion capacity (DLCO) may be increased due to the relative increase in capillary blood volume (especially in mild asthma). Evaluation of patients in the emergency room must often assess the severity of the attack. Advanced stages of asthma may include reduction of the $FEV_{1.0}$ and peak flow, pulsus paradoxus of greater than 10 mm Hg, disappearance of wheezing, and signs of right ventricular dysfunction.

QUESTION 4 What are the various types of asthma?

Bronchospasm can be related to multiple etiologies. The sine qua non, however, is the presence of nonspecific bronchial hyperreactivity. Bronchospasm related to gastroesophageal reflux disease (GERD) is characterized by symptoms that are nocturnal, positional, worsen after initiation with theophylline (due to the further incompetence of the lower esophageal sphincter), and otherwise refractory bronchospasm.

Exercise-induced asthma, more common in children, is presumably due to sensitivity of the airway to dry and cool air drawn deeper into the lung with stimulation of afferent nerve endings. In situations where air is cold but moist (i.e., swimming), bronchospasm is not encountered. Stimulation of alpha-adrenergic receptors may result directly in smooth muscle contraction.

Infection with viral pathogens and mycoplasmal agents, as opposed to bacterial infection, can lead to bronchospasm. Aspirin, Indomethacin, acetaminophen, and other agents that block metabolism of arachidonic acid can provoke bronchospasm. It is important to note that the sodium salicylate preparation does not produce bronchospasm, although acetylsalicylic acid may in the same patient. As a bronchodilator, PGE_2 may be elevated in asthmatics, which heightens reflex bronchospasm when this prostaglandin is acutely inhibited. Samter's triad (found in 10% of asthmatics) includes aspirin sensitivity, nasal polyps, and bronchospasm.

Inhalation of allergens leads to airway narrowing in a sensitized individual. This includes atmospheric pollens, fungal spores, and animal dander. Occupational asthma occurs when occupational exposures lead to reversible bronchospasm. Features of diagnosis include previously described changes on examination, airway obstruction on physiologic testing, an episodic nature of symptoms related to being at work, a history of atopy, positive skin testing to work-related antigens, elevated IgE levels, and response to bronchodilatory agents. Specifically, cotton dust, grain dust, tetrachloroplatinate exposure in the metal-refining industries, toluene diisocyanate from the production of polyurethane, tetrachlorophthalic anyhdride involved in the production of epoxy resins, vinyl chloride pyrolytic compounds from the heating of plastic used to wrap meat, and abietic primaric acids from solder materials all lead to exacerbations of bronchospasm in susceptible individuals.

Food additives can also have similar effects. These include sulfiting agents used to maintain color and crispness in fruits and vegetables, and yellow dye #5 and tartrazine dyes used as coloring agents.

Miscellaneous etiologies include alcohol-containing beverages (especially in Asians), exposure to monosodium glutamate, the premenstrual period, emotion, areas with high levels of sulfur dioxide, air pollution, hymenoptera venom, anaphylaxis, and ozone in the atmosphere.

QUESTION 5 What is the pathopysiology of airway obstruction in this disease?

Asthma can be categorized as extrinsic (elevated IgE, early onset, positive family history and a tendency to remit) or intrinsic (later onset, positive family history, more resistant disease, and an increased incidence of autoimmune disease). Both types can present with eosinophilia. Asthma can present with chronic cough in up to 45% of patients and may also be the sole complaint. It has been noted that a large percentage of asthmatics experience dips in peak expiratory flow rate in the morning with maximal wheezing occurring between 4:00 to 4:30 AM. Evaluation of the sputum will reveal Creola bodies (ciliated epithelial cells), Charcot-Leyden crystals (breakdown products of eosinophils), and Curschman spiral (strands of mucous).

Regardless of which etiology is operant, what follows is well established: bronchospasm, epithelial cell desquamation, mucosal edema, and mucous gland hyperplasia. The mucus is tenacious and viscid.

There is an early (1 to 2 hours after exposure) and a late (4 to 8 hours after exposure) phase airway response. The therapeutic impact of this response will be revisited in the discussion of therapy. A state of lung hyperinflation is produced because of airway obstruction. Hyperinflation leads to a state where pleural pressure is greater than airway pressure, resulting in early airway closure, and ventilation/perfusion mismatching. As mentioned, the inspiratory muscles are placed at a mechanical disadvantage because of their length-tension relationship. Diaphragmatic fatigue ensues and, as the diaphragm flattens, contributes paradoxically to chest closure rather than expansion. Due to increased airway resistance, exhalation time is decreased and fails to empty the lung to normal functional residual capacity. This "stacking of breaths" phenomenon leads to development of "auto" or "intrinsic" positive end-expiratory pressure (PEEP). Muscle fatigue ensues leading to worsening dyspnea and hypoventilation. This cycle may lead to respiratory failure unless therapy is begun.

QUESTION 6 What are the basic tenets of therapy for asthma?

Therapy of asthma is based on the known pathophysiology of airway edema, mucous gland hypersecretion, and smooth muscle contraction. The optimal regimen for asthma is planned avoidance of all known triggers. This requires that patients understand their specific triggers. Since this is practically impossible, a stepped-care approach has been developed. The success of home-based management depends on the patient's use of an inexpensive peak expiratory flow rate (PEFR) meter. With good technique the PEFR can accurately approximate the forced expiratory volume in 1 second ($FEV_{1.0}$). The patient should establish a personal range associated with good function. When flow rates drop to <80% of this range, therapy may need to be intensified. Symptoms or flow rates <50% signal the need for more aggressive treatment.

The step care approach identifies *Step one* as the use of inhaled bronchodilators as the first line of therapy. Proper technique is essential to success. Therefore, it is important to demonstrate correct metered dose inhaler technique to each patient. Some patients may need an Inspir-ease/aerochamber device or a roto-cap inhaler to inhale an adequate dose of the medication. Inhaled agents most commonly used include β-2 agonists that act by relaxing bronchial smooth muscle. Anticholinergic agents antagonize vagally mediated bronchial smooth muscle contraction.

Step two adds the use of prophylactic antiinflammatory agents. Inhaled corticosteroids may be used in an effort to reduce the later inflammatory component, potentiate β-2 sensitization, decrease capillary permeability, inhibit histamine, and stabilize lysosomal membranes. Unlike β-2 agonists, which offer immediate relief, education must support patient compliance.

Alternatively, cromolyn or nedocromil sodium can be used strictly as a prophylactic measure. These agents stabilize mast cell membranes inhibiting degranulation of inflammatory mediators. The newer agent, Nedocromil, also stabilizes atypical mucosal type mast cells and neutrophils. Preliminary studies have supported the usefulness of Nedocromil with inhaled steroids, oral theophylline, and inhaled or oral beta-agonists.

Step three includes the use of systemic corticosteroids. Study has shown that both oral and intravenous dosing have equal efficacy. The goal is to inhibit the late phase of bronchoconstriction. Patients can be maintained on doses of up to 1 mg/kg for several days followed by subsequent dose reduction as the exacerbation remits. The patient is then maintained on the lowest dose that prevents return of symptoms. Transition from systematic to inhaled steroids follows to prevent return of airway inflammation.

Exercise-induced asthma, exposure of the smaller airways to cool dry air, is a situation where the trigger is known before exposure. Inhaled cromolyn sodium and beta-agonists, when used prophylactically, can prevent bronchospasm.

QUESTION 7 What characteristic identifies a morbidity/mortality-prone asthmatic?

Several qualities are generally accepted to identify patients that are at higher risk for morbidity or fatality from an exacerbation of asthma. These include long-lasting disease in a young patient who has had a previous hospital admission or a life-threatening episode in the last year, frequent emergency room visits, and lack of compliance to follow-up and use of medication.

QUESTION 8 What is the approach to the patient who comes to the emergency room in status asthmaticus? What is the role of theophylline?

Oxygen is first-line therapy. Important effects are dilatation of bronchi and of the pulmonary artery. An initial PEFR should be measured, and β-2 agonists should then be administered in a nebulized form. Further dosing can be as frequent as every 20 to 30 minutes. Because of the likelihood of a late bronchospastic component, early steroid administration is important. In patients with severe airways obstruction, respiratory muscle fatigue may ensue. Sahn demonstrated that mechanical ventilation in asthmatics was associated with a worse prognosis. Therefore, intubation should be put off as long as possible. To avoid muscle exhaustion necessitating intubation, the following strategies can be used: position changes (sitting upright), maximal step-one and step-two therapy, avoiding metabolic alkalosis, and normalizing serum potassium, magnesium, and phosphorous.

The use of magnesium in the treatment of status asthmaticus is controversial. The onset of action is within 2 to 20 minutes with a short duration of action. Improvement of the forced vital capacity (FVC), $FEV_{1.0}$, and decreased airway resistance (Raw) is seen. Magnesium inhibits the movement of calcium into the sarcoplasmic reticulum, leading to muscle relaxation. Overdose can lead to paradoxical muscle paralysis.

Endotracheal intubation may become necessary. The decision to intubate is made by the care team when it is apparent that the patient is approaching ventilatory failure. Severe bronchospasm with elevation of airway pressures (dynamic or peak pressure) is a significant risk factor for barotrauma. Therefore, ventilator adjustments should be undertaken to minimize inspiratory pressures. Methods include neuromuscular blockade and reduction of respiratory rate, tidal volume (Vt), or reduction of the peak inspiratory flow rate and allowance of permissive hypercapnea. Reduction of Vt to as low as 5 cc/kg will lead to hypercarbia and respiratory acidosis (pH 7.0 to 7.2). Low pH is tolerated unless the patient experiences a consequence of acidosis.

Another problem is the development of autoor intrinsic PEEP. Because of airways obstruction, rapid respiratory rates can lead to inspiration before full expiration of the previous breath. This pattern furthers air trapping. Consequences may include decreased preload secondary to increased intrathoracic and pleural pressure and increased airway pressures. This may be alleviated by increasing inspiratory time by increasing inspiratory flow rates, as long as peak airway pressures remain acceptable (<40 cm H_2O), allowing a longer period for expiration. PEEP, at low levels, can be used to keep airways open to facilitate emptying. The exact level of PEEP to use is difficult to determine. An important, potential adverse effect is the exacerbation of intrinsic PEEP.

A newer modality under scrutiny is the use of helium. Helium is used as a substitute carrier for oxygen instead of nitrogen. By increasing the relative helium concentration of the inspired air mixture, greater laminar flow is produced leading

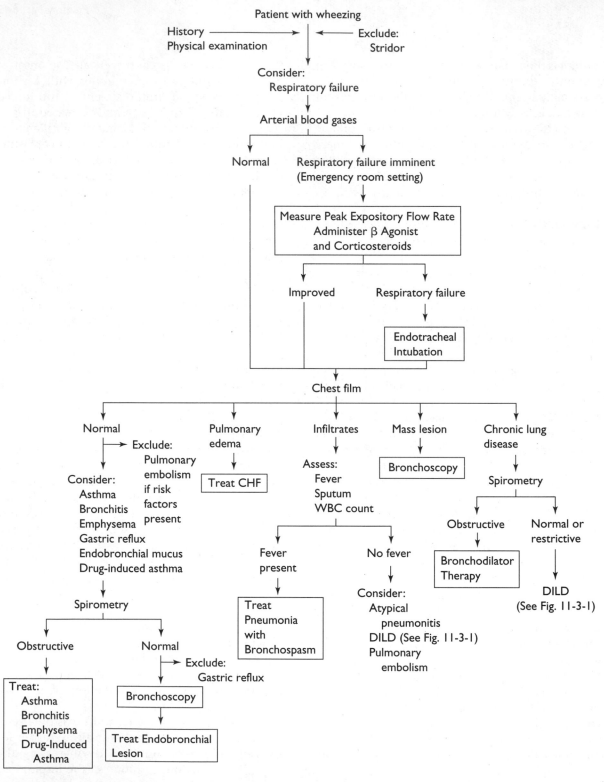

II-I-I Diagnostic algorithm for wheezing.

(From Greene HL, Johnson WP, Maricic MJ: *Decision making in medicine*, St Louis, 1993, Mosby.)

to decreased airway turbulence and patient work. This modality requires a ready supply of helium in the emergency room. While not a traditional therapy, Heli-ox may have a temporizing role for severe status asthmaticus.

The role of theophylline is controversial. Although the exact mechanism of action is unknown, there is good evidence to suggest that theophylline strengthens diaphragmatic contraction and can augment cardiac output. One limiting feature is the high rate of adverse reactions. The elimination rate of theophylline is reduced in severe liver disease, congestive heart failure, COPD, concomitant use of cimetidine, clonidine, digoxin, erythromycin, and quinolone antibiotics, obesity, oral contraceptives, and high carbohydrate/low protein diets. In these situations doses should be reduced carefully. Conversely, smoking increases the rate of clearance and warrants an increased dose. Cessation of smoking can lead to a rapid climb of theophylline levels necessitating rapid dose reduction.

BIBLIOGRAPHY

Bates DV: *Respiratory function in disease,* ed 3, Philadelphia, 1989, WB Saunders.

Bel EH, Timmers C: The long term effects of nedocromil sodium and beclomethasone diproprionate on bronchial responsiveness to methacholine in nonatopic asthmatic subjects, *Am Rev Respir Dis* 141:21-28, 1990.

Bone RC: Acute respiratory failure and chronic obstructive lung disease: recent advances, *Med Clin North Am* 65(3): 563-578, 1981.

Boyle JT: Mechanisms for the association of gastroesophageal reflux and bronchospasm, *Am Rev Respir Dis* (Suppl) 131(5): 516-520, 1985, Mosby.

Cherniak RA: Double-blinded multicenter group comparative study of the efficacy and safety of nedocromil sodium in the management of asthma. The North American Tialde Study Group, *Chest* 97:1299-1306, 1990.

Dunhill MS: The pathology of asthma with special reference to bronchial mucosa, *J Clin Pathol* 13:27-33, 1960.

Gluck EK: Helium-oxygen mixtures in intubated patients with status asthmaticus and respiratory acidosis, *Chest* 98:693-698, 1990.

Kikuchi Y, Okabe S: Chemosensitivity and perception of dyspnea in patients with a history of near fatal asthma, *N Engl J Med* 330:1329-1334, 1994.

Kunkel DB: The enigma of occupational asthma, *Emerg Med* 24(4):209-231, 1992.

Marini JJ: Occult positive end expiratory pressure in mechanically ventilated patients with airflow obstruction, *Am Rev Respir Dis* 126:166-170, 1982.

Molfino NA, Nannini LJ, Rebuck AS: The fatality prone asthmatic patient, *Chest* 101:3, 1992.

Nowak RM: Comparison of peak expiratory flow and FEV1.0 admission criteria for acute bronchial asthma, *Ann Emerg Med* 11(2):64-69, 1982.

Okayama H: Bronchodilatory effects of intravenous magnesium sulfate in bronchial astma, *JAMA* 257(8):1076-1078, 1987.

Ragg LR: Diurnal variation in peak expiratory flow in asthmatics, *European J Respir Dis* 61:298-302, 1980.

Rolla G: Acute effect of intravenous magnesium sulfate on airway obstruction of asthmatic patients, *Ann Allergy* 61: 388-391, 1988.

Tobin MJ: *Principles and practice of mechanical ventilation,* New York, 1994, McGraw-Hill.

C A S E

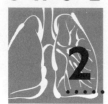

2

Charles J. Grodzin
James J. Herdegen

As the medical senior you are asked to evaluate a patient on the surgical service. The patient is a 57-year-old woman with no significant history who, earlier that day, underwent surgical stabilization for a femoral fracture suffered in a motor vehicle accident. The patient tolerated surgery well.

At about 2:45 AM she began to cough, producing small amounts of blood-tinged sputum. She gradually became more short of breath and eventually called the nurse because of increasing feelings of anxiety about her condition. Medications included ibuprofen and ASA. Her medical history was significant for osteoarthritis.

QUESTION I As a medical consultant you are asked to aid in the evaluation of this patient. As you are making your way to the patient's room, what are the key points about acute onset dyspnea that you must consider?

The complaint of acute dyspnea is primarily of cardiac or pulmonary origin. Pulmonary causes can be thought of as acute versus chronic. Causes of acute dyspnea, include pneumonia, thromboembolic disease, pneumothorax with or without a tension component, massive pleural effusion, upper airway obstruction (acute angioedema, aspiration of a foreign body, complication of a central access catheter, or trauma), and bronchospasm.

Thromboembolic disease may be suspected in patients with proximal lower extremity thrombosis or risk factors for thrombosis. Symptoms may include hemodynamic instability, cough/hemoptysis, pleuritic chest pain, ECG changes, new infiltrates on chest radiograph, and hypoxemia.

Local rales, egophony or pectoriloquy, purulent sputum, and fever suggest infection. Any change of mental status places the patient at risk for aspiration.

A unilateral hyperresonant chest to percussion with absent breath sounds and tracheal shift are the hallmarks of pneumothorax. The subsequent onset of hypotension signifies development of tension with mediastinal compression. Focal dullness to percussion, decreased breath sounds, and an elevated level of resonance may be due to the presence of fluid or an elevated hemidiaphragm. Atopic patients are at risk for acute airway closure when exposed to antigen. Stridorous breathing, heard over the larynx, will be present if upper airway edema or spasm develops as a result of allergy. The development of wheezing may be due to diffuse bronchospasm (status asthmaticus). When wheezing is localized, an endobronchial lesion should be suspected (i.e., tumor, foreign body, carcinoid, bronchial adenoma). This finding may be more easily audible by asking the patient to exhale forcefully from full inspiration.

Cardiogenic causes include left ventricular failure as a result of volume overload or ischemia, acute development of a pericardial effusion, dysrhythmia, or worsening cardiomyopathy. In the case of LV dysfunction, left-sided filling pressure (pulmonary capillary wedge pressure) is transmitted to the pulmonary capillary bed. Alteration of starling forces elevates hydrostatic pressure leading to interstitial edema and/or alveolar filling. This reduces pulmonary compliance and thickens the membrane through which gas must diffuse. The outcome is hypercapnia, hypoxemia, and the sensation of dyspnea.

Physical examination may reveal rales, S3, a cardiac murmur, an irregular rhythm, and the ECG may show an acute injury pattern (ST-segment elevation) if myocardial ischemia/infarction has occurred. Ischemia is usually accompanied by substernal/left-sided chest pain that may radiate to the neck, jaw or shoulder, precordial heaviness or tightness, dyspnea, nausea/vomiting, or diaphoresis. One must keep in mind that diabetics may not manifest pain as a major component because of autonomic dysfunction. The presenting symptoms of an elderly patient may be very nonspecific and should be approached with high suspicion. Findings that suggest the presence of a pericardial effusion are distant heart sounds, clear lungs, and jugular venous distension in the face of hypotension and dyspnea. Patients who report palpitations or rapid heart rates may be having arrhythmias that impair diastolic filling time and lead to pulmonary congestion. A history of hypertension, diabetes mellitus, myocardial infarction, congestive failure, or known ventricular dysfunction should raise the question of further decompensation.

In some cases of pharyngitis the patient may feel dyspneic due to extrinsic upper airway obstruction. When accompanied by throat pain and drooling, examination of the upper aerodigestive tract should be postponed until the epiglottis is successfully visualized on a lateral neck film. Epiglottitis can predispose to acute laryngospasm leading to airway occlusion, with even gentle examination of the oropharynx. Therefore, it is prudent to place materials for emergent tracheostomy at the bedside before beginning the examination. Pain or visual asymmetry may denote a peritonsillar or pharyngeal abscess encroaching on the airway.

QUESTION 2 What are the major risk factors, and what are the available means of prophylaxis for deep vein thrombosis (DVT)?

An important concept is that pulmonary embolism (PE) should be thought of as a complication of proximal lower extremity DVT. Predisposing factors for DVT include immobilization, surgery, malignancy, and systemic disease that leads to a hypercoagulable state (protein C and S deficiency, lupus anticoagulant/anticardiolipin antibody, anti-thrombin III deficiency, dysfibrinogenemia, disorders of plasminogen activation, homocystinuria). Use of oral contraceptives also places women at increased risk.

In hospitalized patients PE remains the most common acute pulmonary problem, yet remains underdiagnosed. Indeed, 70% of those dying with PE will never have the diagnosis made. Prophylactic measures include SQ heparin, adjusted dose hepatin, intravenous dextran, intermittent pneumatic compression (IPC), compressive elastic stockings (CES), warfarin, and IVC interruption.

Hyers and Hull reviewed the recommended regimen for prevention of venous thrombosis. They highlighted the efficacy of subcutaneous heparin at low dose in general surgical patients undergoing elective procedure, after acute MI, stroke, and for patients with respiratory failure. The standard regimen includes 5000 U subcutaneously every 8 to 12 hours. This has been substantiated in numerous clinical trials.

Another method of heparin administration is the adjusted dose schedule. In this scenario, the dose is adjusted to maintain the APTT at the upper limit of the normal range (e.g., 31 to 38 seconds). This approach has been used postoperatively in patients after knee or hip surgery.

Dextran is another agent that can be used for DVT prophylaxis. This is a polysaccharide polymer that increases blood viscosity, reduces the platelet-vessel interaction, and increases fibrinolysis. This agent must be administered intravenously and is limited because of significant volume expansion and allergy. It has been used most in surgical patients after hip or obstetric/gynecologic procedures.

An alternate method of nonpharmacologic prophylaxis is the combination of CES and IPC. This combination has proven better than the use of CES alone. In the neurosurgical patient with increased risk of intracranial hemorrhage, IPC is the treatment of choice.

Inferior vena caval interruption is reserved for individuals at major risk for PE who cannot undergo systemic anticoagulation or who have had previous bleeding, recurrent embolism on anticoagulation, when free-floating thrombus is present and as an adjunct to embolectomy. The presence of septic emboli after gynecologic procedures or in intravenous drug abusers is an important consideration and may also indicate caval interruption. Inferior vena caval interruption devices have not proven useful in the prevention of successive emboli. Large collaterals become patent almost immediately and allow entry of embolism into the central circulation. Greenfield followed 26 patients: there were no fatalities due to the procedure, and minor complications were rare. Of 99 patients at follow-up, 41 needed CES to control edema, 6 patients developed stasis ulceration, and recurrent PE was documented angiographically in 5. The long-term patency rate was 98%. Transient bacteremia from such an intravascular source makes surgical removal a consideration.

A diagnostic algorithm when deep venous thrombosis is suspected, is shown in Fig. 11-2-1.

QUESTION 3 The physical examination revealed vital signs: T 98°F, RR 22/min, HR 106 bpm, and BP 121/75 mm Hg. The patient is well developed, well nourished, sitting semi-upright in bed restricted by the traction device, unable to finish entire sentences without taking a breath. The lungs are clear; there are no cardiac murmurs. The right leg is elevated in traction, and removal of the dressing reveals postoperative changes. The abdomen is benign. ECG and CXR that morning were normal. What clinical findings are present in patients with PE? How are the results of a ventilation-perfusion scan interpreted? What is the definition of a normal/near normal, low, intermediate, and high probability lung scan? When is a pulmonary angiogram indicated?

Clinical suspicion is a powerful tool in the evaluation of patients with PE. Stein found that the presence of rales, a fourth heart sound, in-

creased component of the second heart sound on physical examination, and the findings of atelectasis or parenchymal abnormality, pleural effusion, a pleural-based opacity, decreased pulmonary vasculature, and pulmonary edema on chest radiograph were statistically significant for the presence of pulmonary embolism.

The decision to treat is simplified in cases of high clinical suspicion or positive noninvasive leg studies (NILS). Further testing is used to determine those patients in whom heparin therapy can be discontinued. Lung scanning is an important modality when combined with clinical suspicion. The Prospective Investigation of Pulmonary Embolism Diagnosis (PIOPED) study found that 98% of patients with PE fell into the combined high/intermediate/low probability category. This high sensitivity makes VQ scanning a good screening test. The finding of positive NILS identifies proximal DVT and provides ample reason for continuation of heparin therapy. When NILS are negative, a normal VQ scan is sufficient to discontinue therapy. The combination of low clinical suspicion and negative NILS raises the negative predictive value of the low probability and normal/near normal scan from 84% to 88% and 91% to 96%, respectively. Should the VQ scan (done when clinical suspicion is high and NILS are negative) be read as low or intermediate performance of a pulmonary angiogram is necessary to determine therapy. A high probability lung scan obviates the need for angiography and is an indication to begin or continue therapy.

The definition of normal/near normal, low, intermediate, and high probability results are summarized in the box.

QUESTION 4 What are the local features of pulmonary embolism? What are other embolic phenomena that must be considered in this patient, and what are the salient points about these syndromes?

PE is the most common acute pulmonary disease of hospitalized patients. The feeling of dys-

PIOPED CENTRAL SCAN INTERPRETATION CATEGORIES AND CRITERIA*

HIGH PROBABILITY

- ≥2 Large (>75% of a segment) segmental perfusion defects without corresponding ventilation or roentgenographic abnormalities or substantially larger than either matching ventilation or chest roentgenogram abnormalities
- ≥2 Moderate segmental (≥25% and ≤75% of a segment) perfusion defects without matching ventilation or chest roentgenogram abnormalities and 1 large mismatched segmental defect
- ≥4 Moderate segmental perfusion defects without ventilation or chest roentgenogram abnormalities

INTERMEDIATE PROBABILITY (INDETERMINATE)

- Not falling into normal, very-low-, low-, or high-probability categories
- Borderline high or borderline low
- Difficult to categorize as low or high

LOW PROBABILITY

- Nonsegmental perfusion defects (e.g., very small effusion causing blunting of the costophrenic angle, cardiomegaly, enlarged aorta, hila, and mediastinum, and elevated diaphragm)
- Single moderate mismatched segmental perfusion defect with normal chest roentgenogram
- Any perfusion defect with a substantially larger chest roentgenogram abnormality
- Large or moderate segmental perfusion defects involving no more than 4 segments in 1 lung and no more than 3 segments in 1 lung region with matching ventilation defects either equal to or larger in size and chest roentgenogram either normal or with abnormalities substantially smaller than perfusion defects
- >3 Small segmental perfusion defects (<25% of a segment) with a normal chest roentgenogram

VERY LOW PROBABILITY

- ≤3 Small segmental perfusion defects with a normal chest roentgenogram

NORMAL

- No perfusion defects present
- Perfusion outlines exactly the shape of the lungs as seen on the chest roentgenogram (hilar and aortic impressions may be seen, chest roentgenogram and/or ventilation study may be abnormal)

*PIOPED indicates Prospective Investigation of Pulmonary Embolism Diagnosis.
(From PIOPED Investigators: Value of the ventilation/perfusion scan in acute pulmonary embolism, JAMA 263(20):2753-2759, 1990.)

pnea accompanies PE in virtually all cases. Embolism abruptly increases dead space, requiring an increase in total ventilation. Pneumoconstriction is an attempt to restore ventilation/perfusion (V/Q) equality. There are other signs and symptoms that may add to the clinical suspicion. Surfactant is lost in 24 hours; atelectasis may follow. Infarct occurs in <10% of cases because of the rich vascular supply of the lung parenchyma. Since emboli are usually only partially occlusive, an occasional bruit is audible. The most common outcome in the vascular tree is arterial patency with <10% having perfusing defects present at 6 weeks. Cardiac sequelae include an RV lift and loud P2 as a result of increased pulmonary artery pressure. A fixed and split S2 is an ominous sign of RV decompensation. Additionally, a pleural rub or effusion, fever, cough, and hemoptysis may be found.

In this patient with a history of long bone fracture, the fat embolism syndrome must be considered. Found in virtually all of these cases are fever and a widened A-a gradient. Diffuse infiltrates (81%), delirium or coma (76%), and petechiae (71%) may also be found. The most common settings are motor vehicle accidents and femoral/tibial fractures.

If the patient had been undergoing an intra-vascular procedure, had been a victim of thoracic trauma or a penetrating chest wound, air embolism becomes a consideration. When ambient air pressure exceeds intravascular pressure, arterial or venous, air can enter the bloodstream down a pressure gradient. A pulmonary arterial embolus is trapped at the level of the arteriole; an embolus into the pulmonary venous system threatens the coronary arteries or other distal circulation. The most successful treatment is hyperbaric oxygen therapy, but this is rarely available. The increased pressure enhances the solubility of oxygen in plasma, evacuating retained air. Acutely, placing the patient in the left lateral decubitus position facilitates collection of bubbles in the superior right atrium.

QUESTION 5 What is the correct treatment for pulmonary embolism in this patient?

Therapy of acute PE is heparin. Heparin acts as an anti-thrombin III agonist inhibiting the activity of thrombin and allowing endogenous lytic mechanism to remove the thrombus. An initial bolus of 15,000 to 20,000 units is necessary to offset the release of vasoactive amines from platelets and to retard local platelet aggregation. The most important immediate goal is establishment of the partial thromboplastin time (PTT) to 1.5 times control. Coumadin acts by interfering with the cyclic interconversion of Vitamin K to its epoxide form which catalyzes gamma-carboxylation and activation of dependent clotting factors. The goal prothrombin time (PT) is 1.25 to 1.5 times control (INR of 1.5 to 2.3) for treatment of DVT and 1.6 to 2.0 times control for treatment of PE (INR of 2.5 to 3.5). (See Appendix)

Heparin therapy is discontinued when adequate prolongation of the PT by coumadin is achieved. Beginning coumadin therapy without previous heparinization may inhibit the procoagulant function of protein C and S and lead to a hypercoagulable state known as coumadin necrosis.

The length of pharmacologic therapy depends on the patient's risk of recurrent embolic phenomena. Clot organization requires 7 to 10 days determining the minimal amount of time that heparin anticoagulation is necessary. When risk factors remain, therapy is extended 3 to 6 months with either maintenance subcutaneous heparin or oral coumadin. Further courses are necessitated if further embolization takes place or follow-up perfusing lung scans reveal additional perfusion defects.

Lytic therapy for DVT maintains venous valve function, decrease chronic vascular dysfunction (leg pain, edema, and stasis ulceration), and avoids the postphlebitic syndrome due to rapid achievement of vascular patency. There has been no significant evidence that use of thrombolytic therapy in a patient with uncomplicated PE improves morbidity/mortality. However, in the case of massive embolism advantages of rapid lysis include rapid improvement of pulmonary perfusion, a shortened period of hypotension, and improved right ventricular dynamics. Important contraindications include high blood pressure, intracranial malignancy, recent head trauma, and recent CVA. An algorithm for anticoagulation is seen in Fig. 11-2-2.

APPENDIX 1:

The INR is a means of objectively comparing the degre of anticoagulation. The definition of INR is:

$$INR = \left(\frac{Patient\ Prothrombin\ Time}{Mean\ Prothrombin\ Time\ of\ Control} \right)^{ISI}$$

ISI = International Sensitivity Index. This is a factor dependent on the type of tissue thromboplastin used at each institution.

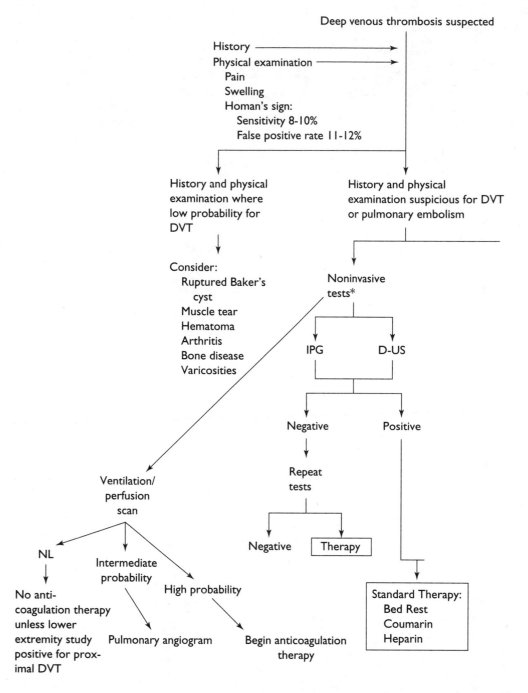

Deep venous thrombosis suspected

History ─────────────────→

Physical examination ────────→
    Pain
    Swelling
    Homan's sign:
        Sensitivity 8-10%
        False positive rate 11-12%

History and physical examination where low probability for DVT

History and physical examination suspicious for DVT or pulmonary embolism

Consider:
    Ruptured Baker's cyst
    Muscle tear
    Hematoma
    Arthritis
    Bone disease
    Varicosities

Noninvasive tests*

IPG   D-US

Negative   Positive

Repeat tests

Ventilation/ perfusion scan

Negative   Therapy

NL   Intermediate probability   High probability

No anti-coagulation therapy unless lower extremity study positive for proximal DVT

Pulmonary angiogram

Begin anticoagulation therapy

Standard Therapy:
    Bed Rest
    Coumarin
    Heparin

* Pursue LE studies and ventilation/perfusion scans simultaneously

11-2-1 Diagnostic algorithm for a thromboembolic episode.
(From Greene HL, Johnson WP, Maricic MJ: *Decision making in medicine*, St Louis, 1993, Mosby.)

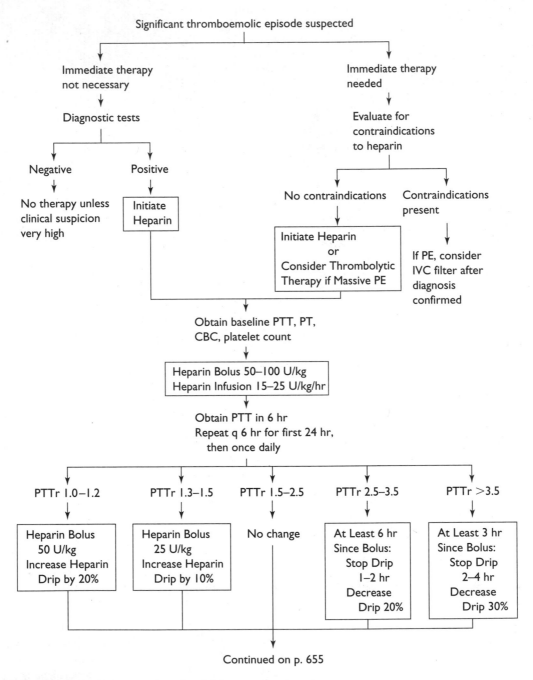

Significant thromboemolic episode suspected

Immediate therapy not necessary → Diagnostic tests

Negative → No therapy unless clinical suspicion very high

Positive → Initiate Heparin

Immediate therapy needed → Evaluate for contraindications to heparin

No contraindications → Initiate Heparin or Consider Thrombolytic Therapy if Massive PE

Contraindications present → If PE, consider IVC filter after diagnosis confirmed

Obtain baseline PTT, PT, CBC, platelet count

Heparin Bolus 50–100 U/kg
Heparin Infusion 15–25 U/kg/hr

Obtain PTT in 6 hr
Repeat q 6 hr for first 24 hr, then once daily

PTTr 1.0–1.2 → Heparin Bolus 50 U/kg Increase Heparin Drip by 20%

PTTr 1.3–1.5 → Heparin Bolus 25 U/kg Increase Heparin Drip by 10%

PTTr 1.5–2.5 → No change

PTTr 2.5–3.5 → At Least 6 hr Since Bolus: Stop Drip 1–2 hr Decrease Drip 20%

PTTr >3.5 → At Least 3 hr Since Bolus: Stop Drip 2–4 hr Decrease Drip 30%

Continued on p. 655

11-2-2 Diagnostic algorithm for deep venous thrombosis.
(From Greene HL, Johnson WP, Maricic MJ: *Decision making in medicine,* St Louis, 1993, Mosby.)

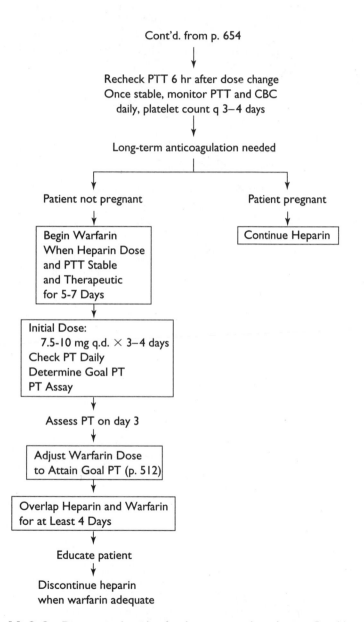

Cont'd. from p. 654

Recheck PTT 6 hr after dose change
Once stable, monitor PTT and CBC
daily, platelet count q 3–4 days

Long-term anticoagulation needed

Patient not pregnant

Patient pregnant

Begin Warfarin
When Heparin Dose
and PTT Stable
and Therapeutic
for 5-7 Days

Continue Heparin

Initial Dose:
  7.5-10 mg q.d. × 3–4 days
Check PT Daily
Determine Goal PT
PT Assay

Assess PT on day 3

Adjust Warfarin Dose
to Attain Goal PT (p. 512)

Overlap Heparin and Warfarin
for at Least 4 Days

Educate patient

Discontinue heparin
when warfarin adequate

11-2-2   Diagnostic algorithm for deep venous thrombosis—Cont'd.

BIBLIOGRAPHY

Chastre J: Bronchoalveolar lavage for rapid diagnosis of the fat embolism syndrome in trauma patients, *Ann Intern Med* 113(8):583-588, 1990.

Collins R, Scrimgeour A: Reduction in fatal pulmonary embolism and venous thrombosis by perioperative administration of subcutaneous heparin: overview of results of randomized trials in general, orthopedic and urologic surgery, *N Engl J Med* 318:1162-1173, 1988.

Counselman FC: Best tests for pulmonary embolism, *Emerg Med* 22(21):67-86, 1990.

Dines DE: The clinical and pathologic correlation of fat embolism syndrome, *Mayo Clinic Proc* 50(7):407-411, 1975.

Estrea AS: Systemic arterial air embolism in penetrating lung injury, *Ann Thorac Surg* 50(2):257-261, 1990.

Fulkerson WJ: Diagnosis of pulmonary embolism, *Arch Intern Med* 146:961-967, 1986.

Greenfield L: Vena caval interruption and pulmonary embolectomy, *Clin Chest Med* 5(3):495-504, 1984.

Grim PS, Gottlieb LJ: Hyperbaric oxygen therapy, *JAMA* 263(16):2216-2220, 1990.

Guenter CA: Fat embolism syndrome, *Chest* 79(2):143, 1981.

Hull R: Different intensities of oral anticoagulation therapy in the treatment of proximal vein thrombosis, *N Engl J Med* 30(27):1676-1681, 1982.

International Multicentre Trial: Prevention of postoperative pulmonary embolism by low doses of heparin, *Lancet* 2:45-51, 1975.

Kane G: Massive air embolism in an adult following positive pressure ventilation, *Chest* 93(4):874-876, 1988.

Kelley MA: Diagnosing pulmonary embolism: new facts and strategies, *Ann Intern Med* 114:300-306, 1991.

Levy D: The fat embolism syndrome—a review, *Clin Orthop* 261:281-286, 1990.

Mathur VS: Pulmonary angiography one to seven days after experimental pulmonary embolism, *Invest Radiol* 2(4):304-312, 1967.

Mohr DN: Recent advances in the management of venous thromboembolism, *Mayo Clin Proc* 63:281-290, 1988.

Moser KM: Thromboendarterectomy for chronic, major vessel thromboembolic pulmonary hypertension, *Ann Intern Med* 107:560-565, 1987.

Moylan JA: Diagnosis and treatment of fat embolism, *Am Rev Med* 28:85-90, 1977.

Parmley LF: Hemodynamic alterations of acute pulmonary thromboembolism, *Circ Res* 11:450-64, 1967.

Pioped Investigators: value of the ventilation/perfusion scan in acute pulmonary embolism, *JAMA* 263(20):2753-2759, 1990.

Presson RG, Jr: Fate of air emboli in the pulmonary circulation, *J Applied Physiol*, 67(5):1898–1902, 1989.

Roe BB: Trendelenburg position with air embolism [letter], *Ann Thorac Surg* 46(3):369-370, 1988.

Stein Paul D, et al: Clinical, laboratory, roentgenographic and electrocardiographic findings in patients with acute pulmonary embolism and no preexisting cardiac or pulmonary disease, *Chest* 100:598-603, 1991.

C A S E

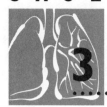

3

James J. Herdegen
Charles J. Grodzin
·············

The patient is a 26-year-old black man with a history of hypertension and mitral valve prolapse who presents to the emergency room with a 5-day history of fevers and chills, night sweats, generalized arthralgias, and bilateral knee swelling.

The patient states he has been in good general health until the past several weeks. Two weeks before admission he developed a sore throat treated with cefaclor for 1 week. Four days before admission he underwent a root canal procedure for which he was prophylaxed with amoxicillin. For the past week PTA he has noticed persistent intermittent fevers and chills, night sweats, and an 18-lb weight loss. His arthralgias developed soon afterward, initially of his lower extremities followed by progression to generalized arthralgias. One day before admission he developed tender, raised, erythematous nodules predominantly over the anterior portion of his LE. He denied shortness of breath, hemoptysis, or IV drug use. Admission medications included nifedipine, indapamide, KCl, and ibuprofen.

His past medical history was unremarkable. He admitted to smoking 1/2 pack per day for 8 years. He works in the office of a large steel mill, and previously lived in North Carolina and South Carolina until 4 years ago.

Physical examination revealed a well-developed male, T 101.6°F, P 100 bpm, BP 140/96 mm Hg. Several raised erythematous nodules were present over both LE, 2 to 3 cm in diameter, predominantly over the right pre-tibial region and were tender to palpation. He demonstrated shoddy bilateral cervicaladenopathy and normal cardiopulmonary examination.

QUESTION 1   This patient presents with a non-specific historical constellation of fever, chills, night sweats, and arthraligas. What is the skin disorder with which he also presents? What is the differential diagnosis of this disorder?

The patient presented with raised, erythematous, nodular lesions over his anterior pretibial area. Examination found these lesions to be 2 to 3 cm in size and to be tender to palpation. These lesions are classically characterized as erythema nodosum (EN). These lesions are the result of a hypersensitivity reaction leading to inflammation of the subcutaneous fat, a panniculitis. They are transient and do not ulcerate.

These lesions are seen in a number of conditions. These include reactions to certain drugs (e.g., penicillin, sulfonamides, oral contraceptives) pregnancy, inflammatory bowel disease, sarcoidosis, infection with streptococci, subacute bacterial endocarditis, tuberculosis, and *Yersinia enterocolitica*. Of these diagnoses, his presentation is most consistent with sarcoidosis.

EN occurs in about 8.2% of patients with sarcoidosis, most commonly associated with stage 1 disease (lymphadenopathy without pulmonary infiltrates). EN is the most common dermatologic form of sarcoid with a female:male ratio of 4:1.

Other types of skin involvement in sarcoidosis include granuloma formation and lupus pernio, the most common skin manifestation. This lesion consists of violaceous plaques on the face. It may involve the nasolabial and periorbital areas, and may result in disfiguring scarring.

QUESTION 2   The patient is admitted to your general medical floor. Six hours later the following lab values are received:

WBC 14.5 × 10⁹/L	Na 137 mEq/L	TPr 7.6 g/L
Differential	K 3.7 mEq/L	LDH 237 U/L
P-65, L-21,	Cl 99 mEq/L	SGOT 26U/L
M-13, E-1	HCO₃ 26 mmol/L	Alk Phos 81 U/L
Hb 14.2 g/dl	BUN 8 mg/dl	CPK 179 U/L
Hct 41%	Cr 1.3 mg/dl	ACE level 29 U/L
Plts 361 × 10⁹/L		(nl 8-52)
ESR 28 mm/hr		

Does the ACE (Angiotensin Converting Enzyme) level provide diagnostic information?

Angiotensin converting enzyme catalyzes the production of angiotensin 1 to angiotensin 2. It is produced in capillary endothelial cells in the lung. It is elevated in about 60% of patients with sarcoidosis but lacks specificity. Elevation can also be found in cases of Gaucher's disease, leprosy, coccidioidomycosis, *Mycobacterium avium-intracellulare* infection, inflammatory bowel disease, and diabetes mellitus.

Acute presentations of sarcoid tend to have lower ACE levels as ACE levels are thought to reflect the extent of granuloma formation.

QUESTION 3   The admitting chest x-ray (CXR) demonstrated multiple pulmonary nodules. Pulmonary function tests (PFTs) were within normal limits. What is the staging system for sarcoidosis based on radiographic findings, and what are the usual diagnostic modalities?

Staging of sarcoidosis is dependent on the degree of lymphadenopathy and parenchymal infiltrate or fibrosis. Some common radiographic findings of the CXR include hilar, mediastinal, and peritracheal lymphadenopathy that may show a pattern of eggshell calcification. Parenchymal infiltrates are usually diffuse. Stage zero disease is defined as a normal CXR. Stage I demonstrates bilateral symmetrical hilar adenopathy. Stage II disease combines both adenopathy and infiltrates. Stage III will have only infiltrates, and Stage IV

will reveal fibrotic parenchymal changes with/without cystic changes in the parenchyma. This particular patient demonstrated a nodular infiltrate on CXR. A large case series demonstrated 2% of 135 patients studied (Turlaf et al) and 4% of 180 patients studied (Sharma) to have this variant pattern. Pleural effusions are rare.

The chest x-ray, PTFs, and tissue sampling for microscopic analysis are the diagnostic tests of choice. Pulmonary function tests may reflect the degree of interstitial pulmonary disease. With more advanced disease, the most striking abnormalities include volume restriction and a decreased diffusing capacity.

Fiberoptic bronchoscopy can be used to perform bronchoalveolar lavage or transbronchial biopsy. In sarcoidosis, recovery of lavage fluid can show an increase in lymphocytes from 40% to 60% with a predominance of T cells. Transbronchial biopsy is the best means to obtain tissue for microscopic evaluation. In patients without radiographic evidence of disease, noncaseating granulomas can be recovered in about 60% of cases. With obvious parenchymal disease, recovery rates increase to 85% to 90%. The granulomas in sarcoid consist of whorls of epithelioid cells that may contain giant cells and inclusion bodies but that do not caseate. While not independently specific for sarcoid, the absence of organisms on culture and special stains and the presence of additional characteristic features supports the diagnosis of sarcoidosis.

An alternate approach for tissue sampling is biopsy of an easily reachable superficial lymph node or the conjunctiva in cases of eye involvement. The finding of noncaseating granulomas peripherally is as useful as lung findings in the correct clinical setting.

Fraser notes that elevation of the serum angiotensin converting enzyme (ACE) level is seen in between 33% to 88% of cases if not being treated with steroids when assayed. However, the specificity of an elevated level is low. ACE levels appear to mirror disease activity. Therefore, the use of ACE levels as a diagnostic tool is limited to a confirmational role in the correct clinical settings.

The ACE level may be more useful as a marker of disease activity for patients in whom correlation has been previously demonstrated clinically.

The gallium-67 scan is used as an indicator of inflammation in the lung. The sensitivity is approximately 80% to 90% with a somewhat lower specificity due to the wide spectrum of diseases that may produce lung inflammation (e.g., infection, malignancy, drug-induced pneumonitis). Gallium scanning has not been found to be a reliable indicator of disease activity.

QUESTION 4 The patient was given a presumptive clinical diagnosis of sarcoidosis. A medical student following this patient comes to you early the next morning to report that he discovered new onset blurred vision and a left facial palsy. What do these changes mean in light of this presumptive diagnosis?

This acute change in the patient's neurologic examination is consistent with nervous system involvement from sarcoidosis. Neurologic involvement occurs in approximately 5% of patients with sarcoidosis. Cranial neuropathy, including anosmia, decreased visual acuity, and peripheral neuropathy are the most common, seen in 48% to 73% of patients. Aseptic meningitis occurs with a cerebrospinal fluid profile demonstrating increased protein, pleocytosis, increased opening pressure, and hypoglycorrachia. The CSF has been found normal in 6% to 30% of patients. Hydrocephalus occurs in 9% to 17% of patients.

Cerebral parenchymal disease includes focal mass lesions (15% to 50%), encephalopathy and vasculopathy (4% to 48%), and seizures (18% to 22%). Myopathy can also be seen in up to 12% of patients.

QUESTION 5 What are other features of sarcoidosis that are important to look for in the workup of this patient?

Symptoms in sarcoidosis revolve around the metabolic activity or the physical presence of the granuloma. Fraser and Pare state that peripheral lymph nodes may be involved in approximately 73% of cases. They are most frequently palpable in the cervical area. Additionally, they note Kaplan's three forms of bone and joint involvement: (1) migratory arthritis associated with erythema nodosum, (2) poly/mono articular arthritis, and (3) persistent arthritis. The most common manifestation appears in the acute disease, involves large joints, and may last from days to weeks. While the heart and liver may be infiltrated with granulomas, function is rarely compromised.

Hypercalcemia can develop and require specific therapy. Macrophages within granulomas can activate vitamin D from the 25-OH vitamin D_2 to the 1,25-$(OH)_2$ vitamin D_2 form. This leads to increased calcium absorption, hypercalciuria, and potentially, nephrolithiasis.

Eye involvement may manifest as anterior uveitis, conjunctivitis, retinitis, or can involve the lacrimal glands. Eye symptoms can become severe enough to lead to blindness. The combination of uveitis with parotitis and facial nerve palsy is known as Heerfordt's syndrome. This combination also hearkens back to the classic name: uveoparotid fever. The combination of EN, uveitis, and arthritis is known as Loeffgren's syndrome.

QUESTION 6 Bronchoscopy with transbronchial biopsy demonstrated perivascular giant cells, an occluded bronchiole, and noncaseating granulomas. Because of the consistent features of the patient's presentation, a final diagnosis of sarcoidosis is established. What is the appropriate therapy for sarcoidosis?

An important aspect of treating sarcoidosis is that a relatively large number of patients with low stage disease will spontaneously remit. Up to 80% to 90% of patients with disease limited to hilar and mediastinal LAN will remit without therapy. Therefore, therapy is relegated to patients with symptoms secondary to vital organ dysfunction or hypercalcemia.

Corticosteroids are the treatment of choice. Prednisone is usually begun in doses of 30 to 40

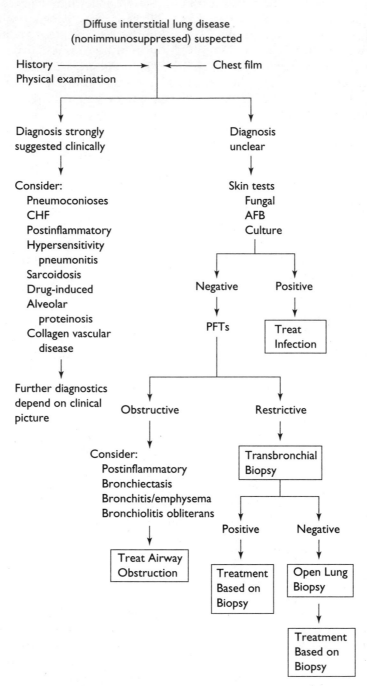

11-3-1   Diagnostic algorithm for sarcoidosis.
(From Greene HL, Johnson WP, Maricic MJ: *Decision making in medicine,* St Louis, 1993, Mosby.)

mg/day (0.5 to 1 mg/kg/day) or on an alternate day schedule at higher dose. A clinical response should be seen within 2 to 4 weeks, at which time the steroid level can be gradually tapered. The goal is to reach the lowest level of steroids that maintain an asymptomatic state.

It is important to bear in mind a prior history of tuberculous exposure as the steroid therapy may allow reactivation due to breakdown of granulomas originally formed to wall off tuberculous infection. A tuberculin skin test should be carried out to assess the patient's risk of reactivation of disease. Those with positive tests may require antituberculous prophylactic therapy.

It is important in each patient to identify a method of following the activity of disease. Accepted methods include clinical complaints, CXR, serum Ca level, gallium scanning, signs and symptoms of alveolitis. A diagnostic algorithm for sarcoidosis is shown in Fig. 11-3-1.

BIBLIOGRAPHY

Delaney P: Neurologic manifestations in sarcoidosis. Review of the literature, with a report of 23 cases, *Ann Intern Med* 87:336-345, 1977.

Fraser RG, Pare JA, Pare PD, et al: *Diagnosis of diseases of the chest,* ed 3, vol IV, Philadelphia, 1991, WB Saunders.

Ketonen L, Oksanen V, Kuuliala I: Preliminary experience of magnetic resonance imaging in neurosarcoidosis, *Neuroradiology* 29:127-129, 1987.

Onal E, Lopata M, Lourenco RV: Nodular pulmonary sarcoidosis, clinical, roentgenographic and physiologic course in five patients, *Chest* 72:296-300, 1977.

Sharma OP: Sarcoidosis: unusual pulmonary manifestations, *Postgrad Med* 61(3):67-73, 1977.

Stern BJ, Krumholz A, Johns C, et al: Sarcoidosis and its neurological manifestations, *Arch Neurol* 42:909-917, 1985.

CASE

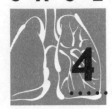

James J. Herdegen
Charles J. Grodzin

E.R. is a 62-year-old woman referred for symptoms of DOE and chest tightness. She described a several-year history of mild, chronic shortness of breath, recently progressive, now limiting her exercise activity. Two months before evaluation she had an acute onset of SOB and chest tightness prompting an emergency room visit where she was treated with a bronchodilator and eventually discharged. She has a distant history of TB exposure, never treated or prophylaxed, never smoked, and had a sister die from pulmonary hypertension. The patient's medical history is significant for hypertension, osteoarthritis of the L-S spine and right hip, gout, and an episode of cholecystitis and pancreatitis 3 years before presentation.

QUESTION I What is the true definition of dyspnea? What are the important historic and physical findings in the evaluation of a patient with chronic dyspnea?

Dyspnea is a subjective sensation experienced by a patient that signifies a sensation of being unable to breath. Essentially, there is an inequality of the delicate balance between neurologic respiratory drive and the mechanical means to carry out this task. This can be due to changes of lung compliance or airway resistance, increased respiratory drive, or sensations arising from stretch receptors (J-receptors) and other parenchymal reflexes. This can also be driven by hypercarbia, hypoxemia, and states of respiratory muscle mechanical disadvantage.

A complete history and physical examination are indispensable in pursuit of the etiology. Questions must probe the patient's environmental exposure, both at home and at work, as well as the surroundings for the presence of construction sites, area of ground turnover, pulling up of old carpeting at home, home rehabbing, new insulation at home, etc. This includes exposure to fumes, toxins, smoke, etc. A history of episodic remission of symptoms over the weekend or when away from work can help isolate a trigger.

The physical examination should concentrate first on the chest. Episodes of dyspnea following exertion or exposure to allergens associated with diffuse wheezing is suggestive of asthma. Productive cough with purulent sputum in a smoker or individual with frequent colds suggest chronic bronchitis. Findings that support lung hyperinflation with hyperresonance to percussion, depressed diphragms, soft vesicular breath sounds, increased AP diameter of the chest, and a history of smoking support a diagnosis of COPD/emphysema. The presence of a Horner's syndrome or brachial plexus dysfunction can be the symptom of an apical lung neoplasm.

The cardiac examination is also important. The presence of an S3 gallop, elevated neck veins, pitting lower extremity edema, enlarged heart and liver, and history of orthopnea, paroxysmal nocturnal dyspnea, lower extremity edema, right upper quadrant abdominal pain (tension on Glisson's capsule), or weight gain can be seen in heart failure. The findings of an opening snap, diastolic murmur, and history of rheumatic fever suggest mitral stenosis. A paradoxically split S2 and a palpable P2 can be found in pulmonary hypertension.

When the cardiopulmonary examination is normal, dyspnea reported mainly on exertion leads one to consider severe anemia, severe obesity, late pregnancy, ascites, and hyperthyroidism as etiologies. Physical examination can easily identify the presence of these diagnoses. Dyspnea reported mainly at rest suggests a psychogenic etiology. Deformity of the chest cavity, as in severe kyphoscoliosis, can lead to dyspnea. When the chest configuration is normal, one must consider pulmonary fibrosis and neuromuscular disease as possible etiologies. Both of these disorders can present with decreased lung capacity on pulmonary function testing.

In general, up to two thirds of patients with complaints of dyspnea that lasts more than 2 to 3 weeks will be due to either chronic obstructive pulmonary disease, asthma, interstitial lung disease, or cardiomyopathy.

QUESTION 2 What is the differential diagnosis of chronic dyspnea?

Chronic dyspnea has many potential etiologies. These include exposure to toxic drugs that may leave chronic scarring (bleomycin, amiodarone) or that may produce acute hypersensitivity reactions (methotrexate). Chronic exposure by patients to an unexpected antigen (i.e., pets, pigeon roosts) can produce subtle but persistent symptoms. Slowly progressive pleural effusions, tumor, or fibrosis will produce dyspnea. Vascular lesions including vasculitis and chronic thromboembolic disease must also be suspected. Abnormalities of the thoracic cage such as kyphscoliosis and abdominal loading including obesity, pregnancy, and ascites can produce dyspnea.

Neurologic lesions such as phrenic neuropathy, systemic neuromuscular disease, incoordination of the respiratory musculature, and severe deconditioning can all compromise the mechanics of breathing. Severe anemia should be considered as well.

QUESTION 3 The patient's current medications included Naprosyn, ranitidine, atenolol, premarin, and allopurinol. Physical examination revealed a moderately obese woman, weight 240 lbs. Vitals were normal. Physical examination was significant

for rare bilateral inspiratory crackles over the lower lung fields. Since this patient is moderately obese, in what way can this body habitus compromise respiratory function?

Important historic points when a patient is being considered for obesity-related dyspnea include excessive daytime sleepiness, snoring that can pose major inconvenience to bedmates, history of hypertension, a recent increase in weight, morning headaches, enuresis, and occasionally impotence. Obesity-related dyspnea has a male predominance, can be seen in patients who drink large amounts of alcohol, may accompany hypothyroidism or acromegaly, and may be seen in conjunction with the use of sedative-hypnotic medications.

Besides severe obesity, examination may reveal excessive redundant uvular/pharyngeal tissue and nasal obstruction, retrognathia, and a short thick neck.

A small subset will demonstrate the obesity hypoventilation syndrome (OHS) with polycythemia and CO_2 retention. This group will demonstrate hypercarbia and desaturation during sleep on continuous monitoring. Decreased lung compliance due to the abdominal fat pad, especially when recumbent, may exacerbate borderline respiratory function in this group. Evaluation should rule out both neuromuscular and parenchymal disease underlying a hypoventilation syndrome. Blood gas should reveal a well-compensated respiratory acidosis with hypercapnia.

This patient does not provide any of the previous historical elements or findings on physical examination. The arterial sample does not reveal hypercarbia. Another diagnosis should be sought for chronic dyspnea in this patient.

QUESTION 4 Laboratory findings included: WBC 7.2×10^9 cells/L, Hb 13.8 g/dl, Plts 249×10^9 cells/L, ESR 16 mm/hr, normal electrolytes with BUN 44 mg/dl, creatinine 1.8 mg/dl, LDH 347 U/L, AlkPhos 116 U/L, TProtein 6.9 g/L, SGOT 16. ACE level was 64 U/L (8 to 52 nl), ANA 1:640, RF <1:20. ABG was pH 7.43/Paco$_2$ 37 mm Hg/Pao$_2$ 52 mm Hg

(RA). Diagnostic studies included a CXR with pattern characterized as interstitial and alveolar, and normal IPG/Doppler studies. V/Q scan revealed extensive matching abnormalities in LL with perfusion slightly greater than ventilation. Initial PFTs included the following:

FVC	FEV$_1$	DLCO	TLC
1.84 (57%)	1.26 (54%)	51%	60%

Maximum inspiratory pressure = -48 cm H_2O
Maximum expiratory pressure = 86 cm H_2O

What is the correct interpretation of pulmonary function tests?

Pulmonary function tests are divided into lung volumes and airway flow as well as gas exchange capability. Lung volume analysis reveals a reduced total lung volume. Additionally, although both the FEV$_{1.0}$ and FVC are decreased, the FEV$_{1.0}$/FVC ratio is 0.74 (74%), meaning that the FEV$_{1.0}$ is reduced proportionally for lung capacity. This implicates a restrictive process. This is further supported by finding a reduced diffusing capacity (DLCO). The combination of a restrictive condition and decreased diffusion suggests an interstitial process. An interstitial process could also account for reduced oxygen diffusion as is evident by a Pao$_2$ of 52 mm Hg. The MIP (maximal inspiratory pressure) and MEP (maximal expiratory pressure) are measures of chest muscle strength. Values greater than 20 to 25 are normal. This patient does not manifest muscle weakness.

QUESTION 5 The patient has owned a parakeet for several years and frequently allows the bird to fly around the house outside of the cage. What impact does this have on the differential diagnosis?

This additional history supports a diagnosis of extrinsic allergic alveolitis also known as hypersensitivity pneumonitis. Hypersensitivity pneumonitis can present as an acute or chronic form with the chronic form resulting from exposure to smaller quantities of antigen and includes symptoms of cough, dyspnea, malaise, weakness, and weight loss in addition to dyspnea.

The classic association is farmer's lung (secondary to thermophilic actinomycetes) due to exposure to moldy hay or contaminated air with up to 1.6×10^9 actinomycete spores. About 90% of patients have antibodies to thermophilic actinomycetes. In a study of 200 pigeon breeders, 40% demonstrated precipitins without evidence of disease. The natural history includes a 30% 5-year rate of morbidity. Respiratory insufficiency is due to pulmonary fibrosis. The most common pulmonary function profile demonstrates lung restriction (72%) and diffusion abnormalities (100%); obstruction is far less commonly seen in only 27% of cases.

The prospect of improvement is excellent. This depends on the length of exposure. One series demonstrated recovery of function in 12 of 12 subjects with exposure less than 2 years; another demonstrated recovery in 6 of 10 when exposure was greater than 2 years. The mean time of normalization in function tests, once the exposure was eliminated, was 3.4 ± 2.43 months. An earlier study showed that PFTs normalized in 44% of patients 9 months after the exposure was removed.

QUESTION 6 Because of the severity of her respiratory insufficiency, the patient went to open lung biopsy. This procedure revealed patchy, chronic interstitial infiltrate composed predominantly of lymphocytes and a few plasma cells, associated scattered granulomas without necrosis, located predominantly in the peribronchial and periseptal areas. Does this description support the diagnosis of extrinsic allergic alveolitis?

Histologically, tissue samples demonstrate a combination of an inflammatory cell infiltrate, fibrosis, and granulomata. The inflammatory cell infiltrate, as opposed to that of sarcoidosis, reveals a relative increase in the proportion of T-suppressor cells. Lymphocytes are increased to about 70% as opposed to about 8% in normal tissue. In addition, immunofluorescent staining reveals an increase in the amount of immunoglobulin, particularly, IgG and IgM.

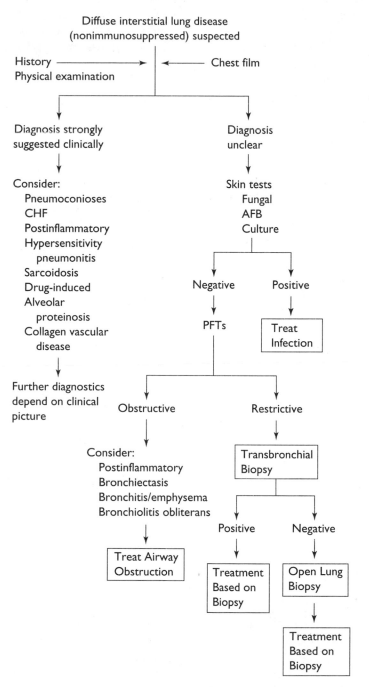

11-4-1   Diagnostic algorithm for sarcoidosis.
(From Greene HL, Johnson WP, Maricic MJ: *Decision making in medicine*, St Louis, 1993, Mosby.)

QUESTION 7 What is the appropriate mode of therapy for this patient?

The mainstay of therapy is avoidance of the inciting allergen. In mild to moderate disease, this may be all that is necessary. In the acute form of the disease it is wise to make a lifestyle behavior change or pursue changing the environment (i.e., changing work location or altering the home environment) to remove the allergen.

In the chronic form accompanied by altered pulmonary function or when exertion-limiting symptoms are present, a trial of corticosteroids may be useful. The dose and duration of use should be as minimal as possible to control symptoms due the potential adverse effects of this agent. When long-term steroids are considered, it may be wise to carry out a tuberculin skin test initially with the intent of prophylactic antituberculous therapy should the skin test be positive. It is generally accepted that systemic steroid therapy may alter the course of the acute process but has less impact on long-term pulmonary function.

BIBLIOGRAPHY

DeGracia J, Morell F, Bofill JM, et al: Time of exposure as a prognostic factor in avian hypersensitivity pneumonitis, *Respir Med* 83:139-143, 1989.
George RB, Light RW, Matthay M, Matthay R: *Chest Medicine: essentials of pulmonary and critical care medicine*, Baltimore, 1990, Williams & Wilkins.
Warren WP, Woolf CR: Avian-induced hypersensitivity pneumonitis, *Can Med Assoc J* 107:1196-1199, 1972.

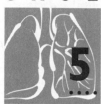

5

James J. Herdegen
Charles J. Grodzin

R.M. *is a 57-year-old white man with a 10-year history of chronic lymphocytic leukemia (CLL) presenting with an 8-month history of progressive shortness of breath (SOB) with recent severe dyspnea on exertion (DOE) and low grade fevers.*

The patient's medical history dates to 1983 when he was diagnosed with CLL. His symptoms progressed 1½ years later to fatigue and generalized lymphadenopathy (stage III), and he was treated with 6 cycles of vincristine and chlorambucil followed by daily prednisone. He first noticed SOB in March 1993 with progressive DOE and decreased work tolerance by June. He developed an episode of acute SOB September 3 with mildly productive cough and low-grade fever and a chest radiograph showing minimal changes by report. He was treated for bronchitis with 10 days of ciprofloxacin but continued to have low-grade fevers (99° to 100°F), fatigue, SOB, and DOE. Three weeks before admission he noticed worsening DOE with difficulty walking more than 2 to 3 blocks, difficulty concentrating, and a dull headache. His only medication at the time was prednisone 10 mg/day.

Physical examination at initial presentation demonstrated only diffuse bibasilar inspiratory crackles.

QUESTION I In what ways is this patient immunocompromised, and what is the differential diagnosis of pneumonia in the immunocompromised patient?

This patient is immunocompromised in two distinct ways. First, the patient has an underlying diagnosis of lymphocytic leukemia. In this disor-der, a clone of lymphocytes unable to undergo specific clonal proliferation to a specific immunogen are produced. Because of the attendant hypogammaglobulinemia and granulocytopenia the patient is predisposed to bacterial infections. As the disease progresses, cellular mediated immunocompetence wanes and risk for viral, fungal, and parasitic infection increases. In addition the patient has been on chronic systemic corticosteroids. Chiefly, prednisone blocks production of IL-1, a cytokine involved in mononuclear cell proliferation. One must watch for the development of side effects of chronic prednisone including: osteoporosis with fracture, hyperglycemia, ulcer development, cataracts, myopathy, and poor wound healing.

Multiple pathogens can be found to cause pneumonia in the immunocompromised patient. Common bacteria are often recovered. *Legionella pneumophila* causes the constellation of cough, diarrhea, headache, and mental status abnormalities. In particular, hyponatremia may be found. Diagnosis depends on recovery of the organism or a diagnostic change in acute and convalescent sera. Direct fluorescent antibody stain is most useful for immediate diagnosis and is found positive in about 50% of patients. A titer of at least 1:256 is presumptive evidence for diagnosis. Treatment includes intravenous erythromycin. *Nocardia asteroides* produces alveolar consolidation, abscess formation, and may cavitate. There is a higher tropism for patients with pulmonary alveolar proteinosis, lymphoreticular malignancies, and chronic steroid use. Metastatic infection can be found in brain, bone, skin, and soft tissue. The organism is weakly acid fast. Diagnosis is confirmed by culture. Community-acquired bacteria, including *Streptococcus pneumoniae, Haemophilus influenzae,* and Neisserial organisms, should also be considered.

Mycoplasma pneumoniae produces a milder illness with systemic symptoms and a dry cough. Rare clues to this diagnosis include bullous myringitis, hemolytic anemia, and the presence of cold agglutinins. This organism is seen less commonly in immunocompromised hosts. *Mycobacteria* produce a syndrome of fever, night sweats, weight loss, cough, and pulmonary infiltrates. Consideration should be given to reactivation disease in patients with a chronic immunosuppressing disease or in those patients on chronic steroids. *Mycobacterium avium-intracellulare* occurs in up to 50% of patients with AIDS. Skin testing can be negative in infected patients due to anergy. Recovery of the organism can be from expectorated sputum, blood cultures, samples from bronchoscopy, or inferred from the presence of caseating granulomas on tissue biopsy. The radiograph can show patchy apical infiltrates, cavitation, or a miliary pattern.

Fungi are also seen in this population. *Aspergillus* is the most common pulmonary pathogen. Disease can be either of a hypersensitivity form, noninvasive infection (aspergilloma), or invasive disease. Leukemia is the greatest risk factor. Clinical presentation of invasive disease is similar to the bacterial pathogens and may include hemoptysis. The fungus has a propensity to involve small blood vessels leading to tissue infarction. An aspergilloma may present with a "crescent sign" as the fungus ball grows in a preexisting cavity and is surrounded by a crescent of air. The organism appears as septate hyphae with acute branches when recovered by sputum sample or bronchoscopic washings or biopsy. Growth of the organism on culture is not diagnostic as evidence of tissue invasion is necessary. Serologic tests are fraught with a high level of false positivity.

Treatment for aspergillosis depends on the clinical situation. For invasive disease, amphotericin B is the mainstay of therapy. However, this agent is useless in the treatment of aspergillomas. Hemorrhage may complicate an aspergilloma, in which case, either direct instillation of amphotericin B into the cavity or surgical excision is necessary.

Mucormycosis has a profile similar to aspergillosis. The organism is identified by broad nonseptate hyphae branching at right angles. Culture negativity is the rule. Treatment for mucormycosis is amphotericin B. Histoplasmosis, blastomycosis, and coccidioidomycosis present similarly with diffuse reticulonodular infiltrates with potential hematogenous dissemination. Histoplasmosis is more common in the Missouri River Valley, blastomycosis in the Ohio River Valley, and coccidioidomycosis in the southwestern part of the country. *Pseudoellescheria boydii* presents as above also. Hematogenous dissemination to the thyroid, kidney, heart, and brain has been seen. Importantly, this fungus is more responsive to miconazole or ketoconazole. Candida infection is more common after use of broad spectrum antibiotics. Diagnosis depends on the demonstration of tissue invasion or when hyphal elements are seen and no other infectious agents are identified microscopically or by culture.

Cytomegalovirus (CMV) can produce bilateral diffuse infiltrates. CMV is a common coinfecting agent in the presence of *Pneumocystis carinii.* Diagnosis depends on positive culture, + CMV antigen serology or presence of CMV virions (intranuclear inclusion or "Owls Eyes") in tissue sample. The infection begins as multifocal lesions but eventually becomes homogeneous. Culture positivity depends on the finding of cytopathic effects but may require several weeks to become positive. Fluorescent antibody staining has sped up the process. Elevated IgM antibody titers can be helpful, although many immunocompromised individuals have chronically elevated titers without infection. Treatment is with gancyclovir. Pneumonia with *Herpes zoster* and *Herpes simplex* should also be suspected when other pathogens are not found.

The chief protozoan to cause infection is *Pneumocystis carinii.* Presentation includes dyspnea, fever, and hypoxia with a bilateral diffuse infiltrate. The chief risk factor is impaired cell-mediated immunity, use of corticosteroids, or after chemotherapy for hematologic malignancies. Toxoplasma is a less common pathogen. Diagnosis in immunocompetent patients depends on premorbid knowledge that the patient was seronegative. Serological tests are less helpful in immunosuppressed patients.

Pulmonary infiltrates can be due to processes other than infections. One should consider extension of the primary disease, reactions to chemotherapeutic drugs, parenchymal hemorrhage, radiation pneumonitis, and lymphangitic carcinomatosis.

An algorithm for the approach to a patient presenting with these symptoms is shown in Fig. 11-5-1.

QUESTION 2 Over the next several days his condition became progressively worse with chills/sweats, T 102°F, and persistent SOB. Admission labs included a WBC 72.5 × 10^9 cells/L (P-1, L-99), HgB 15.2 g/dl, Plts 208 × 10^9 cells/L, HCO$_3$ 22 mmol/L, Cr 1.2 mg/dl, LDH 334 U/L, SGOT 45 U/L, SGPT 40 U/L, ABG (RA) pH 7.48/Pa$_{CO_2}$ 31 mm Hg/Pa$_{O_2}$ 51 mm Hg. Chest radiograph revealed a diffuse bilateral multilobar infiltrate. What is the correct interpretation of the patient's arterial blood gas, and what is the impact of the chest radiograph on the initial differential diagnosis?

The arterial blood gas sample reveals a respiratory alkalosis and hypoxemia. This appears to be an acute process because the degree of alkalosis is matched by the degree of hypocarbia mathematically. Insight into the need to hyperventilate is derived from the depressed Pa$_{O_2}$. It is safe to figure that hypoxemia is the driving force behind the patient's hyperventilatory response. In some patients with chronic respiratory failure (COPD) one can see an elevated serum bicarbonate level, which is testimony to metabolic buffering necessitated by the respiratory acidosis of chronic pulmonary insufficiency. The normal serum bicarbonate in this case argues against a chronic process.

Unfortunately, the specificity of an infiltrate on chest x-ray is diminished in patients who are immunologically incompetent. For example, the usual apical infiltrate of tuberculosis may be seen less than the miliary form in this population of patients. Therefore, the differential diagnosis should remain wide and empiric therapy, if necessary, aimed at broad spectrum coverage until an organism is isolated.

QUESTION 3 *Pneumocystic carinii* is strongly suspected. What are the routine ways in which a definitive diagnosis may be reached in this patient?

Since there are no serologic tests for *Pneumocystis carinii*, diagnosis rests on demonstrating the organism in lung tissue or respiratory secretions. Fiberoptic bronchoscopy is well accepted as the diagnostic procedure of choice. Study by the National Heart, Lung and Blood Institute found that a diagnosis was established in 95% of patients. Transbronchial biopsy tissue touch prints and tissue specimens established diagnosis in 93%. Examination of bronchoalveolar lavage fluid was diagnostic for only 79% of patients.

A variety of noninvasive tests have been evaluated to heighten suspicion of pneumocystis infection. These include lung gallium scans, widened A-a gradient, decreased diffusing capacity, and arterial blood gas measurement. Although these tests may be highly sensitive, they are uniformly nonspecific.

It is important to bear in mind that the recovery of Pneumocystis organisms from a patient with a previous infection is of unknown significance. Organisms are still recoverable 3 to 6 weeks after a primary infection in 25% to 67% of patients. In such a scenario, it is important to consider pneumocystis infection as a diagnosis of exclusion. In the critically ill, empiric treatment can be started and discontinued if another organism is identified.

QUESTION 4 Sputum samples did not provide diagnostic information, and a bronchoscopy with bronchoalveolar lavage and transbronchial biopsy was carried out. Special stains included methenamine that revealed clusters of cystic organisms in foamy eosinophilic intraalveolar exudate. What is the significance of this discovery?

The finding of eosinophilic intraalveolar exudate that exhibits clusters of cystic organisms on methenamine silver stain is specific for *Pneumocystis carinii* (PC) pneumonia. There are multiple histologic findings found in sections of lung from PC infections. Typically there is interstitial edema with a lymphocytic infiltration and proliferation of type 2 pneumocytes. A frothy collection of intraalveolar exudate containing macrophages is present. This can be seen in specimens obtained via bronchoalveolar lavage. In addition, one may find multinucleated giant cells, interstitial and intraalveolar granulomas, interstitial fibrosis, and diffuse alveolar damage. Interstitial fibrosis can be focal or diffuse and can lead to a residual restrictive defect.

The cysts can be identified with routine H&E stain, Papanicolaou stain, Giemsa and Wright's stain, but are highlighted best by the Gomori's or Grocott's methenamine silver stain. Characteristically, there may be an intracystic black dot that corresponds to the cyst wall seen *en face*.

In this patient, the findings on bronchoscopy definitively confirm the diagnosis of PC pneumonia infection.

QUESTION 5 What is the specific therapy for PC pneumonia?

Antibiotic therapy has been most extensively studied in patients with the acquired immunodeficiency syndrome. First line therapy for *Pneumocystis carinii* pneumonia is Bactrim (trimethoprim-sulfamethoxazole (TMP-SMZ)) in a dose of 20 mg/kg TMP and 100 mg/kg SMZ q6h for 14 to 21 days. Studies by Murray and Haverkos demonstrated that about 45% of patients are unable to complete a full course. Adverse reactions include leukopenia, skin rash, drug fever, hepatotoxicity, and thrombocytopenia. Bactrim may be contraindicated in patients unable to tolerate a moderate

fluid load. Use of concomitant folic acid may help prevent leukopenia.

The second line agent of choice is *Pentamidine* in a dose of 4 mg/kg/day for 14 to 21 days. Adverse reactions include leukopenia, renal impairment, hepatic dysfunction, and alteration of glucose metabolism. Intravenous administration can produce hypotension if infused over less than one hour. It appears safe to switch from Bactrim to Pentamidine if patients become leukopenic.

Either agent should be allowed 4 days before considered a treatment failure. These agents are the only anti-pneumocystis agents to have been studied in controlled trials. Other agents awaiting evaluation include *alph-diflouromethylornithine (DFMO), pyremethamine-sulfadiazine,* and *Dapsone.*

Adjunctive therapy has become better understood lately. Studies have shown that early institution of corticosteroids (to be included in the initial regimen or within 72 hours of presentation) in HIV-infected patients with moderate to severe disease as determined by the presence of hypoxemia (Pao_2 <75 mm Hg) had beneficial effects. Adjunctive steroid therapy was seen to prevent respiratory failure, increase survival to discharge, decrease respiratory rate, improve Sao_2, and improve exercise tolerance at 30 days postdischarge. Although doses have been different, the largest study to support these findings used doses of prednisone at 40 mg bid for 5 days, followed by 40 mg/day for 5 days, and then 20 mg/day through the duration of antibiotic therapy. Tapering the dosing schedule appeared to decrease the rate of clinical relapse. Although this data was collected in HIV-infected patients, it appears applicable to other immunosuppressed populations. However, further controlled studies are required to fully substantiate benefit.

BIBLIOGRAPHY

Bleiweiss IJ, et al: Granulomatous *Pneumocystis carinii* pneumonia in three patients with the acquired immune deficiency syndrome, *Chest* 94:580-583, 1988.

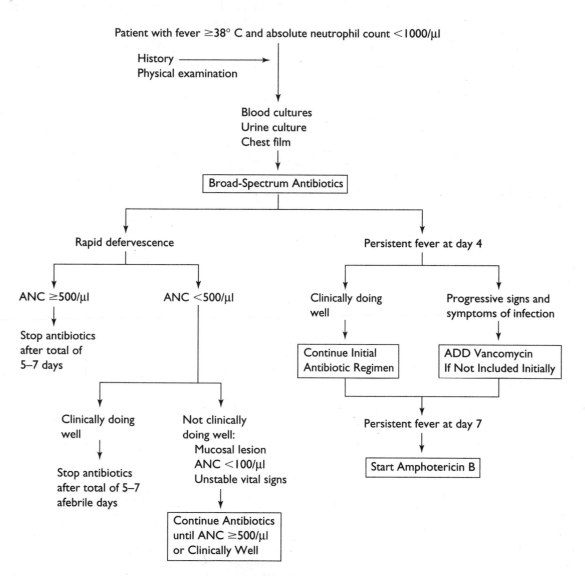

11-5-1 Approach to the patient with fever ≥38°C.
(From Greene HL, Johnson WP, Maricic MJ: *Decision making in medicine*, St Louis, 1993, Mosby.)

Bozette SA: The use of corticosteroids in *pneumocystis carinii* pneumonia, *J Infect Dis* 162:1365-1369, 1990.

Catterall JR, Potasman I, Remington JS: Pneumocystis carinii pneumonia in the patient with AIDS, *Chest* 88(5):758-762, 1985.

Cohn DL: Pulmonary infections in the acquired immune deficiency syndrome, *Semin Respir Med* 10(1):1-11, 1989.

Gagnon S, Boota AM, Fischl MA: Corticosteroids as adjunctive therapy for severe pneumocystis carinii pneumonia in the acquired immunodeficiency syndrome, *N Engl J Med* 323: 1444-1450, 1990.

Hartz JW, et al: Granulomatous pneumocystosis presenting as a solitary pulmonary nodule, *Arch Pathol Lab Med* 109:466-469, 1985.

Luna MA, Cleary KR: Spectrum of pathologic manifestations of *Pneumocystis carinii* pneumonia in patients with neoplastic diseases, *Semin Diagn Pathol* 6:262-272, 1989.

McCabe RE: Diagnosis of pulmonary infections in immunocompromised patients, *Med Clin North Am* 72(5):1067-1068, 1988.

Saldana MJ, Mones JM: Cavitation and other atypical manifestations of *Pneumocystis carinii* pneumonia, *Semin Diagn Pathol* 6:273-286, 1989.

Smith CB: Cytomegalovirus pneumonia: state of the Art. Aspen Lung Conference: Infections and the Lung, *Chest* 95(3)(suppl):1715-2425, 1989.

Travis WD, et al: Atypical pathologic manifestations of *Pneumocystis carinii* pneumonia in the acquired immune deficiency syndrome, *Am J Surg Pathol* 14:615-625, 1990.

C A S E

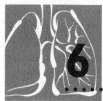

6

James J. Herdegen
Charles J. Grodzin

The patient is a 36-year-old man with a history of endocarditis requiring mitral valve replacement in 1988 now presenting with a 1-day history of hemoptysis and shortness of breath. The patient states that before the onset of these symptoms, he was in his usual state of health, denying recent fever, chills, chest pain, or weight loss. The patient has a history of mild hypertension for which he takes a beta-blocker.

QUESTION 1 Acute symptoms of hemoptysis associated with shortness of breath can be life-threatening. What are some potential causes for hemoptysis in this patient?

The primary etiologies for hemoptysis have slowly changed over the past 50 years. In the 1950s and 1960s, United States data indicated that bronchitis/bronchiectasis, lung cancer, and tuberculosis were the most common causes of hemoptysis.

Other causes for nonmassive hemoptysis include chronic necrotizing pneumonia (including lung abscess), congestive heart failure, mitral stenosis, lung cancer, pulmonary infarction, foreign body aspiration, trauma, aspergilloma, and vasculitis (i.e., Wegener's granulomatosis and systemic lupus erythematosus [SLE]). Arteriovenous malformations and bronchial adenomas, though not common, are important because of their tendency to bleed massively.

Less commonly, idiopathic pulmonary hemosiderosis, Goodpasture's syndrome, and bronchiololithiasis lead to hemoptysis.

A systemic bleeding diathesis should be suspected when bleeding is out of proportion to the severity of disease or recurs frequently with mild

underlying comorbidities. In a woman, bleeding may occur around the menses because of the presence of ectopic endometrial tissue in endometriosis.

The cause of hemoptysis can be differentiated, to some extent, on whether or not the bleeding is massive (defined in various series as more than 200 to 600 ml of blood in 24 hours). In one study, massive hemoptysis was most commonly associated with active pulmonary tuberculosis, bronchiectasis, and chronic necrotizing pneumonia.

QUESTION 2 The patient's chest film demonstrated diffuse hazy infiltrates predominantly distributed in the upper lung fields. A tuberculin skin test was placed. The patient states he has coughed up about 3 tablespoons of bright red blood within the past 3 to 4 hours. How does this new information impact on the differential diagnosis for this patient?

The chest film can harbor vital information as to the etiology of hemoptysis. If an abnormality is present on the x-ray of a smoker or a patient >50 years old, and infection is not suspected, one is obliged to perform endobronchial or transbronchial biopsy to rule out the presence of malignancy. When the chest x-ray is normal and no abnormality can be found on fiberoptic bronchoscopy, hemoptysis is likely to subside, and no cause will ever be identified.

In this patient, diffuse upper lobe infiltrates suggest etiologies such as atypical or fungal infections, congestive heart failure, and drug or inhalational lung injury. One would expect other organ system involvement in cases of SLE, Goodpasture's syndrome, and vasculitis. The history does not include trauma, and young age places malignancy lower on the list. The absence of signs of infection argues against lobar pneumonia, bronchitis, and tuberculosis. Hemoptysis from bronchitis or associated with infection will often be accompanied with purulent sputum. The x-ray pattern is not consistent with a pulmonary infarct (usually a nodular or wedge-shaped defect) or lung abscess (usually demonstrating an air-fluid level).

An algorithm for the approach to a patient with hemoptysis is shown in Fig. 11-6-1.

QUESTION 3 What are the important aspects of the pulmonary anatomy that impact on the evaluation of hemoptysis?

The goal of pulmonary blood flow is two-fold: to provide a thin film of blood to participate in gas exchange and to provide metabolic raw materials to the lung parenchyma. Ninety-five percent of pulmonary circulation originates from the right ventrical and pulmonary arterial tree; this is a low-pressure high-flow system. The remaining 5% of the circulation is from the arterial circulation, a low-flow high-pressure system. These vessels are branches of intercostal arteries under systemic arterial pressure.

Bronchial venous blood may drain to the heart via two pathways: the azygos/hemiazygos system to the right side of the heart or by anastomoses with pulmonary venules reaching the left side of the heart. This represents a normal physiologic right-to-left shunt known as a venous admixture.

The bronchial vessels are responsible for new vasculature for repair of lung tissue after injury. It is also chiefly the bronchial circulation that bleeds in cases of alveolar or airway bleeding. In long-standing disease (e.g., chronic bronchiectasis) the bronchial circulation expands. The left-to-right shunt may increase dramatically in volume. This may predispose to more profuse bleeding.

QUESTION 4 On the second hospital day, the tuberculin skin test (placed prior to admission) was read as negative. Serial blood cultures were also negative. In what circumstances is bronchoscopy or angiography a useful procedure? What are the immediate and definitive modes of treatment?

First, it is important to rule out hemoptysis as an epiphenomenon secondary to nasal, oral, or nasopharyngeal bleeding or from misinterpreted hematemesis. Asking the patient to blow his or her nose is an easy way of determining a nasal/nasopharyngeal source of bleeding.

There is a need to perform bronchoscopy early to localize the site of bleeding in cases of massive hemoptysis. Aortic angiography may reveal an aortic aneurysm, whereas pulmonary angiography may reveal a pulmonary embolism or arteriovenous malformation as etiologies of hemoptysis.

Treatment has several important goals. Foremost is the prevention of exsanguination. Therefore, one should evaluate clotting activity and take measures to treat any coagulopathy. Asphyxiation can be prevented by removal of blood from the lung. Coughing, unless bleeding is exacerbated, is a good way to clear blood. A maneuver using glottic closing before coughing will clear secretions more efficiently. Postural drainage may also be a helpful maneuver. Furthermore, one should attempt to prevent bronchial obstruction by blood clots. A clot located in a central airway can produce massive atelectasis and, by check valve action, lead to distal hyperinflation with possible barotrauma (an indication for bronchoscopy). If infection is thought to be present, spread of infection should be minimized both by control of bleeding and antibiotic therapy.

Hemodynamic stability is an immediate concern in the bleeding patient. The patient may need fluid or blood resuscitation, and these should not be withheld for fear of exacerbating bleeding. Immediate maneuvers in the bleeding patient include placing the patient in the decubitus position with the bleeding side down. This helps to keep blood on one side, leaving contralateral alveoli free. In extreme cases the contralateral

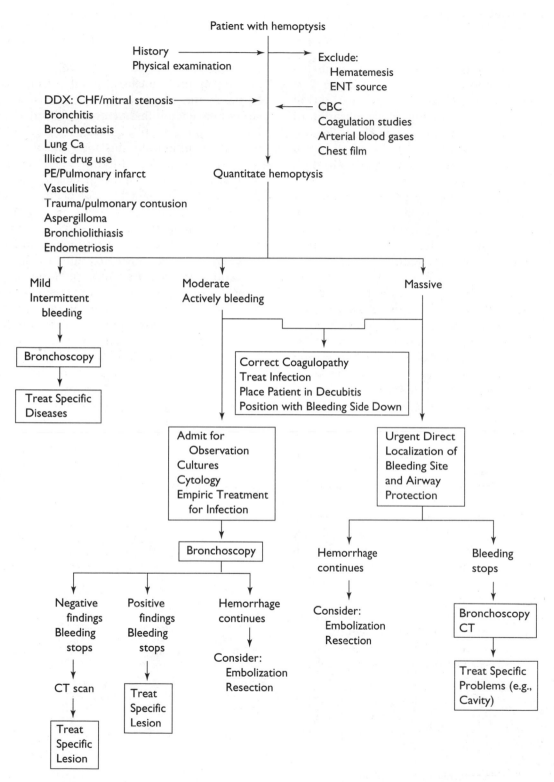

11-6-1 Approach to the patient with hemoptysis.
(From Greene HL, Johnson WP, Maricic MJ: *Decision making in medicine,* St Louis, 1993, Mosby.)

main stem bronchus may be selectively intubated with a cuffed endotracheal or double lumen tube to protect that side. More definitive methods of treatment include angiographic embolization of the bleeding vessel or local tamponade via Fogarty catheter once the site is known. Bleeding from a large central vessel may only respond to ligation or lung resection.

It is important to address the fears and anxiety of the patient. However, sedatives or agents that may compromise mental status are contraindicated. The best intervention includes reassurance from members of the care team.

QUESTION 5 Further history was pursued, and the patient reluctantly stated that about 5 minutes after cocaine inhalation he developed left upper back pain and hemoptysis with associated shortness of breath. His shortness of breath and hemoptysis persisted for several hours prompting him to be seen in the emergency room. What are some of the pulmonary complications associated with cocaine abuse?

A variety of pulmonary manifestations associated with cocaine use, specifically crack cocaine, are becoming increasingly recognized. These include the development of pulmonary edema which may result from either (1) the change in central adrenergic outflow, increasing pulmonary microvascular pressure, and vascular permeability or (2) an increase in systemic vascular resistance resulting in transient left ventricular dysfunction and alveolar flooding. A hypersensitivity pneumonitis has also been associated with cocaine abuse, possibly related to adulterants used in processing, such as lidocaine, benzocaine, or lactose. There is typically an associated peripheral eosinophilia and elevated IgE level. Clinical signs and symptoms include nasal ulceration or epistaxis and cough with hemoptysis. Autopsy studies have identified hemosiderin-laden alveolar macrophages. In an autopsy study, 27% of patients had hemosiderin-laden alveolar macrophages. In a study by Tashkin, 79% of 35 moderate crack users described pleuritic chest pain. The etiology of chest pain has not been fully elucidated. Pulmonary barotrauma, pneumothorax, or pneumomediastinum, has also been described and is believed to be the result of a prolonged Valsalva maneuver during cocaine inhalation.

Itkonen studied a small population of "freebase" cocaine users admitted to a chemical dependence center. He found that, of 19 consecutive patients, 10 demonstrated a decreased diffusion capacity to less than 70% of normal. Compared to the cocaine-using patients with a diffusion capacity greater than 70%, there was no difference in the average duration of cocaine use, age, cigarette smoking history, and pulmonary function test parameters including TLC, $FEV_{1.0}$, and FEF_{25-75}.

BIBLIOGRAPHY

Ettinger NA, Albin RJ: A review of the respiratory effects of smoking cocaine, *Am J Med* 87:664-668, 1989.
Forrester JM, Steele AW, Waldron JA, Parsons PE: Crack lung: an acute pulmonary syndrome with a spectrum of clinical and histopathologic findings, *Am Rev Respir Dis* 142:462-467, 1990.
Heffner JE, Harley RA, Schabel SI: Pulmonary reactions from illicit substance abuse, *Clin Chest Med* 11:151-162, 1990.
Itkonen J, Schnoll S: Pulmonary dysfunction in "freebase" cocaine users, *Arch Intern Med* 144:2195-2197, 1984.
Tashkin DP, Simmons MS: Respiratory effects of cocaine "freebasing" among habitual users of marijuana with or without tobacco, *Chest* 92:638-644, 1987.

C A S E

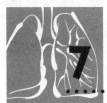

7

James J. Herdegen
Charles J. Grodzin

The patient is a 34-year-old woman with a history of asthma, obesity, and clinically mild heart failure who presented to a local hospital with complaints of increasing shortness of breath for 2 days and burning substernal chest pain radiating to the right arm. The patient was monitored in the CCU and was noted to have a room air arterial blood gas of pH 7.34, Pa_{CO_2} 58, and Pa_{O_2} 58. A myocardial infarction was ruled out, and she was treated with furosemide. Telemetry monitoring demonstrated variable nocturnal episodes of bradycardia and asystolic periods of up to 5 seconds associated with apneic periods of respiration. The patient was transferred to a tertiary care hospital for further evaluation.

QUESTION 1 One of the abnormalities on the emergency room arterial blood gas is an elevated Pa_{CO_2}. What disease processes could cause hypercapnia (an increased Pa_{CO_2}) in a 34-year-old?

Hypercapnia is a well-recognized consequence of a variety of diseases involving the lungs as well as the neural, muscular, chest wall, and circulatory components of the respiratory system. In most clinical settings, four factors contribute to hypercapnia: alterations in carbon dioxide production, disturbances in the gas exchanger (the lungs), abnormalities in the mechanical system (the respiratory "bellows"), and changes in the ventilatory control system.

Changes in the metabolic rate resulting from alterations in the level of activity, fever, or disease can have profound effects on the production of carbon dioxide. For example, carbon dioxide production increases by 13% for every increase in temperature of 1°C above normal. Lung disease contributes to the retention of carbon dioxide by reducing effective alveolar ventilation, even when total ventilation is maintained. This can occur because disease has affected ventilation and perfusion unequally, producing a mismatch, or by the absolute reduction of alveolar area (i.e., emphysema). Signals emanating from the medulla stimulate the contraction of the diaphragm and other muscles of the chest wall. If the respiratory muscles are weak or fatigued, if they are working ineffectively because of changes in resting length, or if they must overcome the increased workload posed by decreased compliance or increased resistance of the respiratory system, respiratory drive will not be translated effectively into adequate ventilation. The central respiratory control system, which activates the muscles of the respiratory pump, is a crucial determinant of respiratory drive and hence adequate ventilation and the elimination of carbon dioxide. Decreased drive correlates with carbon dioxide retention.

Thus, specific disease processes associated with hypercapnia include metabolic alkalosis and drug intoxication (e.g., narcotics) which inhibit central drive; hypothyroid myopathy and muscular dystrophies may lead to muscular weakness; an increased metabolic rate from illness (i.e., sepsis, burns, hyperthyroidism, etc.) increases CO_2 production; spinal-cord injury at or above C3, disease of the neuromuscular junction (e.g., myasthenia gravis), and peripheral neuropathy (e.g., Guillain-Barré syndrome) compromise muscle activation; obesity and kyphoscoliosis reduce chest wall compliance; upper-airway obstruction, asthma, chronic obstructive pulmonary disease, and congestive heart failure impair alveolar gas exchange. All of these mechanisms may decrease exchange of carbon dioxide and lead to hypercarbia.

QUESTION 2   What is your differential diagnosis for the patient's shortness of breath? How do you interpret the blood gas in a patient with hypercapnia?

Dyspnea is the sensation of an increased exertional component to breathing. The differential diagnosis of dyspnea includes lung disease, heart failure, neuromuscular disease, disorders that cause persistent hyperventilation, and severe anemia.

If dyspnea is caused by lung disease, there should be some demonstrable abnormality in respiratory function. While any abnormality can lead to increased efferent activity, most patients with dyspnea have reduced levels of $FEV_{1.0}$, maximal voluntary ventilation (MVV), and/or maximal inspiratory pressures. The degree of abnormality in these tests of respiratory function only roughly correlates with symptoms of dyspnea. Similarly, there is no obvious relationship between the degree of dyspnea and arterial blood gas tensions in patients with chronic lung disease.

Exercise testing may help in distinguishing pulmonary from nonpulmonary disease. The finding of a normal $Paco_2$ and relatively normal Pao_2 at rest is consistent with most of the above disease processes. Patients with airway obstruction or chest restriction, chronic heart failure, and mild to moderate neuromuscular disease often will have relatively normal blood gases at rest. However, during exertion, significant impairment in gas exchange, oxygen delivery, or respiratory muscle fatigue can lead to CO_2 retention and a fall in Pao_2. In obstructive sleep apnea only 10% to 15% of patients develop chronic hypercapnia and usually have normal daytime blood gases. Severe anemia would not be expected to alter the partial pressure of CO_2 or O_2 unless the patient's oxygen carrying capacity was severely compromised.

Correct blood gas evaluation in this patient is crucial. As mentioned, absolute gas tensions have little correlation with the presence of dyspnea in patients with underlying cardiopulmonary disease. The first consideration is evaluation of the patient on clinical grounds despite any blood gas results. Questions about respiratory rate, evidence of cyanosis, how easily is the patient conducting a conversation, or how much can he or she talk without having to take a breath are important pieces of information. No treatment should be instituted that is contradicted by the clinical status of the patient. The next consideration is the pH of the blood gas. As gas exchange is further compromised, patients lose their sensitivity to hypercapnia as the drive to breath. Gradual hypoxia and respiratory acidosis are buffered by an elevation of the serum bicarbonate with a resulting compensated respiratory acidosis. The pH usually levels off in the range of 7.30 to 7.35. Changes in patient status will be accompanied by changes in the pH as further metabolic compensation is a slow process. Because the Pao_2 and $Paco_2$ are abnormal to start, their use for directing therapy is limited. Therefore, administration of therapy should be based on changes of the pH.

The administration of oxygen can be problematic. Since patients depend on central hypoxemia as the main stimulus to breathe, removing this input by acutely increasing the Pao_2 will lead to hypoventilation and a markedly elevated $Paco_2$ with the risk of acute acidosis and CO_2 narcosis that can further inhibit breathing. Additionally, one may wipe out the compensatory renal retention of bicarbonate. The reestablishment of this compensatory alkalosis takes several days.

However, one should not be satisfied with extremes of hypoxemia. Oxygen should be administered to bring the Po_2 above 55 to 60 mm Hg or to a saturation greater than 90%. The low-flow nasal cannula system is a reliable means of delivering oxygen; however, one cannot estimate the exact concentration of oxygen delivered. The actual oxygen concentration provided varies from breath to breath depending on the respiratory flow rate generated by the patient. In situations of rapid breathing, significant room air entrainment has a major dilutional effect on the Fio_2. The high flow Venturi system is a more reliable method of providing oxygenation support. Usual flow rates are between 40 to 120 L/min as determined by the diameter of the hole on the Venturi adapter for each Fio_2 desired. Therefore, the patient's contribution to room air entrainment is minimized. The Fio_2 provided in a Venturi system can be measured more exactly. This system is the preferred oxygen delivery system for patients with hypercapnia.

QUESTION 3 Upon further questioning, the patient describes a several-year history of poor sleep, daytime somnolence, dyspnea on exertion, and nightmares. She describes a 60- to 80-lb weight increase over the past year with her present weight being 350 lbs. The patient's symptoms have been present greater than 1 year with difficulty walking more than 100 feet for the past year. Occasionally, she found herself falling asleep while driving her car. She describes progressive lower extremity edema over the past several months, worsening dyspnea on exertion, and admits to smoking 1 pack/day with a 40 to 50 pack-year smoking history. She feels that her dyspnea and poor sleep have gotten worse over the past year concurrent with her weight gain. Therefore, you are concerned about the diagnosis of sleep apnea. What are the features of obstructive and central sleep apnea, and what are some of the clinical and physiologic features and sequelae associated with sleep apnea?

Sleep apnea syndromes have an incidence of 1% to 4%. Many patients exhibit elements of both obstructive and central apnea syndromes. The obstructive type accounts for approximately 85% to 90% of cases.

The exact etiology of obstructive sleep apnea is not fully known. However, it is apparent that a combination of anatomic narrowing of the upper airway as well as a disorder of arousal work together. The abnormality of upper airway muscle tone maintenance during sleep allows obstruction to occur, and the delayed arousal response allows the apnea to persist.

The most common manifestations of obstructive sleep apnea are neuropsychiatric and behavioral, with excessive daytime sleepiness being the most common complaint. Initially, daytime sleepiness develops under passive conditions such as watching television and reading, but as the disorder progresses, sleepiness encroaches progressively into all daily activities and can become severely disabling and dangerous. The most common nocturnal symptom is loud snoring, indicative of upper airway narrowing. Chronic sleep deprivation leads to irritability, anxiety, poor concentration, and personality changes.

Nocturnal cardiac arrhythmias are common in these patients. However, in most patients a moderate bradycardia of 30 to 50 bpm during the apnea episodes alternate with a tachycardia of 90 to 120 bpm following resumption of breathing. Systemic blood pressure may rise transiently during obstructive apnea as a result of reflex vasoconstriction. Blood pressure generally falls toward baseline upon resumption of ventilation. Over 60% of patients with obstructive sleep apnea have systemic hypertension, the mechanism of which is not clear. Ten to fifteen percent of sleep apnea patients develop sustained pulmonary hypertension leading to right heart failure. Acute pulmonary vasoconstriction has been well documented during obstructive apnea, but pulmonary arterial pressure during wakefulness is typically normal. The development of sustained pulmonary hypertension appears to require the presence of daytime hypoxemia and hypercapnia in addition to severe nocturnal desaturation.

Ten to fifteen percent of patients with obstructive sleep apnea develop chronic hypercapnia. The development of chronic CO_2 retention appears to require the presence of obesity, mild to moderate diffuse airways obstruction, and reductions in ventilatory chemosensitivity and respiratory drive. The syndrome of right heart failure, obesity, and daytime sleepiness defines the Pickwickian or obesity-hypoventilation syndrome.

Central sleep apnea is defined as a cessation of breathing during sleep as a result of transient abolition of drive to the respiratory muscles. The definitive event in central sleep apnea is the withdrawal of effective central drive to the respiratory muscles. The resulting decrease in ventilation initiates a primary sequence of events similar to those that occur in the obstructive sleep apnea syndrome.

Three distinct underlying mechanisms have been identified to account for the cessation of central respiratory output during sleep. First, there are outright defects in the respiratory control system or in the respiratory neuromuscular apparatus. Such defects generally result in a chronic alveolar hypoventilation syndrome, manifested by some degree of daytime hypercapnia. However, the full impact of such defects usually becomes apparent only during sleep, when the stimulatory influence of behavioral, cortical, and reticular inputs to brainstem respiratory neurons is minimized, and breathing is now critically dependent on the defective metabolic respiratory control system.

Some central apneic disorders arise from transient fluctuations or instabilities in an otherwise intact respiratory control system. These instabilities typically occur only during drowsiness or light sleep, and because there is no defect in respiratory control or drive, $Paco_2$ levels during steady-state wakefulness or slow-wave sleep are normal or even low.

Even in the absence of hypoxia, hyperventilation of any cause, including CNS disease, predisposes to periodic breathing and central sleep apnea. Circulatory slowing by cardiac failure is thought to generate instability in the respiratory control system by prolonging the time lag between changes in blood gas values and detection of changes by the peripheral and central chemoreceptors. In animals, several well-described reflexes result in an inhibition of central respiratory drive and transient central apnea. These reflexes included the pulmonary inflation reflex and upper airway chemoreflexes and mechanoreflexes. The strength of these reflexes is often enhanced during sleep, resulting in more prolonged apnea episodes than occur during wakefulness.

QUESTION 4   Laboratory evaluation revealed a hemoglobin of 12.6 g and normal electrolytes but

for an elevated bicarbonate. Further workup included a MUGA scan with an LVEF of 70%. Echocardiogram estimated pulmonary systolic pressures of 35 to 45 mm Hg. A sleep study demonstrated severe primarily obstructive apnea episodes with Sao_2 ranging from 64% to 94%. The apnea/hypopnea index was 138.4 events/hour. What findings on physical examination would support the presence of an obstructive sleep apnea syndrome? When is a polysomnographic study indicated? What information from a sleep study would confirm obstructive sleep apnea?

The physical examination can help build suspicion that an obstructive process is present. Findings include a short, thick neck, redundant pharyngeal tissue and a large uvula, nasal obstruction, an enlarged tongue, and retrognathia. These findings are readily found on detailed examination of the head and neck.

A polysomnographic sleep study is indicated when excessive daytime sleepiness or unexplained cor pulmonale is present with a supportive clinical syndrome. Characteristic sleep study findings are cyclical fluctuations in heart rate and recurrent episodes of arterial oxygen desaturation as measured by ear oximetry. However, the accuracy of such screening tests in the diagnosis of obstructive sleep apnea has not yet been established. Therefore, the definitive diagnosis often requires a detailed polysomnographic study. In obstructive sleep apnea, the study demonstrates recurrent episodes of airflow cessation accompanied by continuing respiratory effort. Paradoxic movements of the rib cage and abdomen or continuation of negative esophageal pressure swings without displacement of air are also present. Alternatively, in central sleep apnea, there is arrest of breathing effort and airflow concurrently.

QUESTION 5   What treatment is useful for patients with obstructive sleep apnea?

Treatment options for obstructive sleep apnea are varied and somewhat controversial since there are few long-term outcome studies and the compliance with various therapies is often poor. Other approaches in current use can be considered to act either by increasing upper airway muscle tone during sleep, increasing the size of the oropharyngeal lumen, or by preventing the generation of a critical airway collapsing pressure during sleep. Patients with mild to moderate sleep apnea can often be managed effectively by avoidance of alcohol and other agents that depress upper airway muscle activity, modest degrees of weight reduction, and medical or surgical correction of nasal narrowing. Avoiding sleep in the supine position can also be effective in mild cases.

In patients with more severe sleep apnea, pharmacologic, surgical, and mechanical approaches have been tried. The tricyclic antidepressants such as protriptyline appear to increase tone of the upper airway muscles; however, long-term improvement has not been established.

The use of nocturnal oxygen should be reserved for a subgroup of patients. It appears that this modality is useful for the treatment of nocturnal arrhythmias and offsetting the development or worsening of pulmonary hypertension. However, daytime somnolence is not improved. Use of exogenous oxygen should be proven useful in a controlled sleep lab before being used at home.

At present, the most effective treatment is mechanical-nasal continuous positive airway pressure (nasal CPAP), which provides a pneumatic splint to the airway and prevents development of critical subatmospheric collapsing pressure.

Surgical approaches include uvulopalatopharyngoplasty, which is designed to increase the size of the oropharyngeal lumen by removing redundant soft tissue. Short-term improvement has been reported in about 50% of cases, but long-term benefits have not been established. In patients with severe obstructive sleep apnea in whom all other treatment approaches are ineffective or intolerable, tracheostomy is indicated and provides immediate relief by bypassing the site of oropharyngeal obstruction during sleep. In such cases, the tracheostomy needs to be opened only at night and can be plugged during waking hours.

QUESTION 6 If this patient were to have manifested elements of central sleep apnea, what would be the treatment of choice?

Acetazolamide, which produces a metabolic acidosis due to bicarbonate loss, is used as a central respiratory stimulant. The use of oxygen should be reserved for hypoxic patients who have not demonstrated CO_2 retention in the past. The goal of oxygen therapy is a Pao_2 >55 mm Hg. This may be accomplished by mild elevation of the $Paco_2$. Gradual metabolic compensation should follow to avoid significant acidosis. Commonly, a means of respiratory support is needed. This includes negative or positive pressure ventilation, tracheostomy, nasal mask, diaphragmatic pacing, or tracheostomy.

An algorithm for approaching the patient with sleep disturbance is shown in Fig. 11-7-1.

BIBLIOGRAPHY

Borowiecki B, et al: Indications for palatopharyngoplasty, *Arch Otolaryngol* 11:659-663, 1985.

Borowiecki B, Sassin JF: Surgical treatment of sleep apnea, *Arch Otolaryngol* 109:508-512, 1983.

Connaughton JJ, et al: Do sleep studies contribute to the management of patients with severe chronic obstructive pulmonary disease? *Am Rev Respir Dis* 138:341-344, 1988.

Conway W, et al: Uvulopalatopharyngoplasty: one year follow-up, *Chest* 88:385-387, 1985.

Douglas NJ, Flenley DC: Breathing during sleep in patients with obstructive lung disease, *Am Rev Respir Dis* 141:1055-1070, 1990.

Esclamado RM, et al: Perioperative complications and risk factors in the surgical treatment of obstructive sleep apnea syndrome, *Laryngoscope* 99:1125-1129, 1989.

Findley LJ, et al: Automobile accidents involving patients with obstructive sleep apnea, *Am Rev Respir Dis* 138:337-340, 1988.

Flenley DC: Sleep in chronic obstructive lung disease, *Clin Chest Med* 6:651-661, 1985.

Fletcher EC, et al: Nocturnal oxhemoglobin desaturation in COPD patients with arterial oxygen tensions above 60 mm Hg, *Chest* 92:604-608, 1987.

Fujita S, et al: Evaluation for the effectiveness of uvulopalatopharyngoplasty, *Laryngoscope* 95:70-74, 1985.

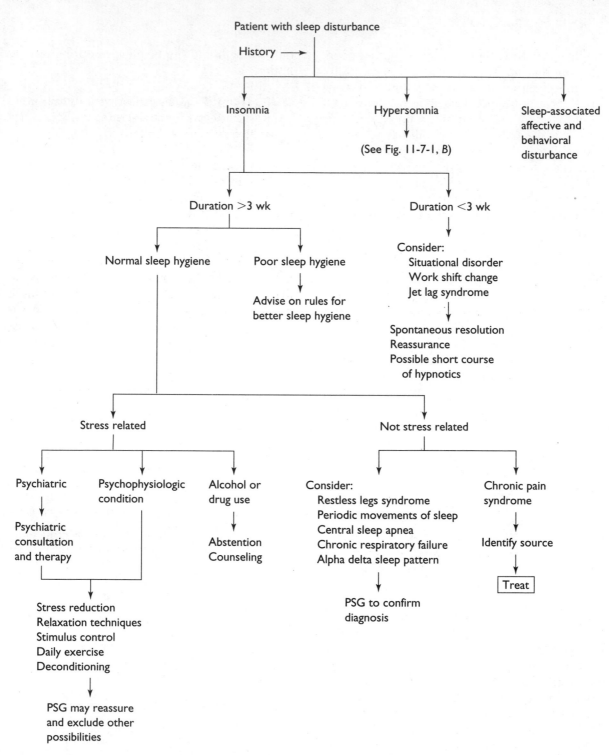

11-7-1, A Approach to the patient with sleep disturbance (PSG = Polysomnography, SDC = sleep disturbance clinic, MSLT = multiple sleep latency testing).
(From Greene HL, Johnson WP, Maricic MJ: *Decision making in medicine*, St Louis, 1993, Mosby.)

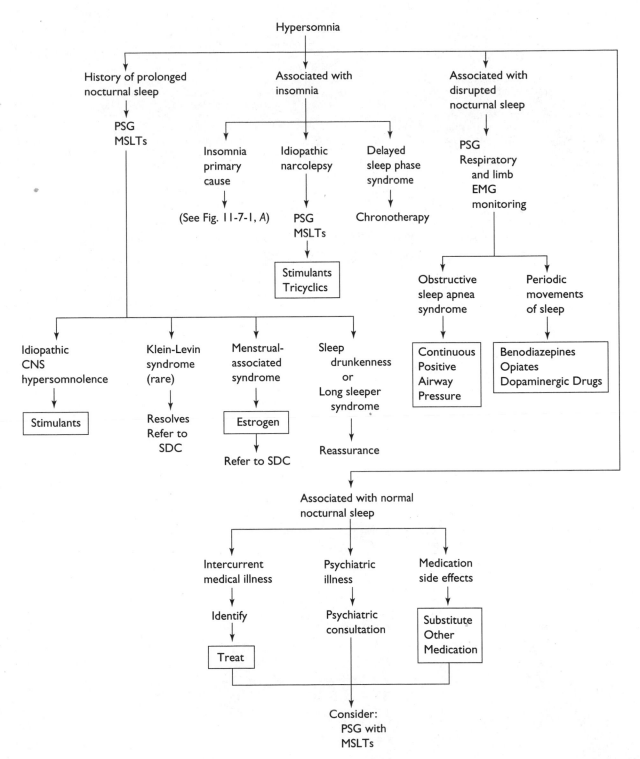

11-7-1, B Approach to the patient with sleep disturbance—Cont'd.

He J, et al: Mortality and apnea index in obstructive sleep apnea: experience in 385 male patients, *Chest* 94:9-14, 1988.

Johnson JT, Sanders MH: Breathing during sleep immediately after uvulopalatopharyngoplasty, *Laryngoscope* 96:1236-1238, 1986.

Katsantonis GP, et al: Further evaluation of uvulopalatopharyngoplasty in the treatment of obstructive sleep apnea syndrome, *Otolaryngol Head Neck Surg* 93:244-250, 1985.

Katsantonis GP, et al: Nasopharyngeal complications following uvulopalatopharyngoplasty, *Laryngoscope* 97:309-313, 1987.

Larsson SG, et al: Computed tomography of the oropharynx in obstructive sleep apnea, *Acta Radiologica* 29:401-405, 1988.

Moser RJ, Rajagopal KR: Obstructive sleep apnea in adults with tonsillar hypertrophy, *Arch Intern Med* 147:1265-1267, 1987.

Phillips B, et al: Sleep apnea: prevalence of risk factors in a general population, *South Med J* 82:1090-1092, 1989.

Rajagopal KR, et al: Effects of medroxyprogesterone acetate in obstructive sleep apnea, *Chest* 90:815-882, 1986.

Reimao R, et al: Obstructive sleep apnea treated with uvulopalatopharyngoplasty: a systemic follow-up study, *South Med J* 79:1064-1066, 1986.

Sanders MH, et al: Polysomnography early after uvulopalatopharyngoplasty as a predictor of late postoperative results, *Chest* 97:913-919, 1990.

Sullivan CE, Issa FG: Obstructive sleep apnea, *Clin Chest Med* 6:633-650, 1985.

Wetmore SJ, et al: Postoperative evaluation of sleep apnea after uvulopalatopharyngoplasty, *Laryngoscope* 96:738-741, 1986.

White DP: Central sleep apnea, *Clin Chest Med* 6:623-632, 1985.

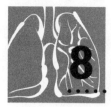
The patient is a 36-year-old white woman with a 1 to 2 year history of progressive dyspnea on exertion and weight loss. She is presenting via referral from an outside hospital for evaluation of an abnormal chest x-ray (CXR) and bronchoscopy report.

The patient states she was in her usual health until approximately 1 to 2 years before admission when she noticed progressive dyspnea on exertion, a 30-lb weight loss over 1 year, and an intermittent productive cough of yellow sputum. She denies a history of smoking.

QUESTION I This patient is clinically presenting with significant weight loss and symptoms consistent with a progressive chronic disease process. What lung disorders can lead to such a presentation?

Progressive dyspnea on exertion suggests a cardiac or primary lung disorder that is impairing effective oxygen delivery to tissue beds. This implies an ineffective cardiac output or chronic dysfunction of gas exchange leading to hypoxia.

Chronic lung disorders which present with clinical manifestations of progressive shortness of breath, weight loss, and decreased exercise tolerance are numerous and quite varied.

The classic chronic lung disorder is emphysema or chronic obstructive lung disease. One source of emphysema in a 36-year-old woman is a genetic predisposition to alpha-1 antitrypsin (A1AT) deficiency. This is a heritable disease wherein an imbalance develops between proteases and antiproteases. The primary antiprotease is A1AT. Deficiency leads to parenchymal matrix destruction of the lung and, in some cases, may affect the liver. Cigarette smoking magnifies this process 5 to 10 times by recruiting neutrophils to the lung and by inhibiting elastase inactivation by A1AT by 2000X. Levels of A1AT vary according to genotype. Levels greater than 11 microM remain protective against development of emphysema. Replacement therapy with synthetic A1AT is an accepted therapy for patients with antiprotease deficiency and symptomatic lung disease. In this case, there is no family history of emphysema, and it is unlikely that the extent of her smoking history would cause emphysema.

Interstitial lung diseases commonly present with chronic exertional dyspnea and incorporate a large number of disorders. This group of diseases can be separated into those associated with and without granulomas. Granulomas can be seen in sarcoidosis, histiocytosis X (HX), also known as eosinophilic granuloma (EG), granulomatous vasculitis including Wegener granulomatosis, lymphomatoid granulomatosis, and allergic granulomatosis of Churg-Strauss. Granulomas are not expected in cases of idiopathic pulmonary fibrosis (cryptogenic fibrosing alveolitis), pulmonary alveolar proteinosis, bronchiolitis obliterans-organizing pneumonia, diseases associated with collagen vascular disorders (rheumatoid arthritis, systemic lupus erythematosus, systemic sclerosis, dermatomyositis), hemosiderosis, Goodpasture's syndrome, ankylosing spondylitis, eosinophilic lung disease, and sequelae of radiation therapy. The pulmonary infiltrates with eosinophilia (PIE) syndromes include Loeffler's syndrome, tropical eosinophilia, ABPA, and chronic eosinophilic pneumonia.

Lymphangioleiomyomatosis (LAM) and tuberous sclerosis should also be kept in mind in the correct clinical situations.

Occupational lung disorders can present as an interstitial lung process. The more common occupations include mining (copper, iron, uranium) or quarrying (sand, sandstone, slate). Foundry, abrasive and ceramic work are also associated with risk for silicosis. Berylliosis and hypersensitivity pneumonitis should also be considered as occupational lung diseases.

Malignancy is always an important process to exclude when someone presents with weight loss, fatigue, and a significant smoking history. Lymphangitic spread of primary or secondary lesions can produce an interstitial pattern. Some of the more common extrapulmonary tumors which commonly metastasize to the lung include lymphomas, hypernephroma, breast, thyroid, melanoma, testicular, and choriocarcinoma. In bone marrow transplant patients the lung may be affected by both veno-occlusive disease and graft versus host disease.

Drug exposure is known to produce interstitial changes that may produce chronic dyspnea. Examples include methotrexate, which cause both acute/chronic hypersensitivity pneumonitis and a dose-related toxicity, bleomycin, gold, penicillamine, amiodarone, nitrofurantoin, cyclophosphamide, aspirin, sulfasalazine, dilantin, penicillin, and many others.

In the appropriate settings one should also consider heart failure as a cause of an interstitial infiltrate.

QUESTION 2 The patient had been working as a supervisor at a steel storage warehouse for the past 10 years, exposed to, but not directly involved in, the cutting of steel products. The patient admits to smoking 1½ packs of cigarettes per day for the past 10 to 15 years. How does this history impact upon the preceding differential diagnosis?

The patient's occupational history is not supportive of an exposure etiology. She is too young to strongly suspect a malignancy; however, a complete physical examination should be done (including a testicular examination in a man). There is no significant drug exposure. There was no finding of eosinophilia or travel history. The PIE syndromes are usually associated with drug use, filarial exposure in patients with asthmatic symptoms in an endemic area, a peripheral radiographic infiltrate, or an atopic history. HX, EG, and SLE characteristically present with pneumothorax. LAM is suggested by the finding of a chylothorax after ruling out lymphoma or chest trauma. The combination of lung-renal disease, especially with the presence of hemoptysis, supports Wegener's granulomatosis and Goodpasture's syndrome. Skin findings such as adenoma sebaceum and shagreen patches support tuberous sclerosis; erythema nodosum, erythema multiforme, and eye disease including uveitis and conjunctivitis suggest sarcoidosis (uveo-parotid fever). Myopathy is seen with polymyositis. Peripheral smear findings of plasmacytoid lymphocytes are evidence of lymphomatoid granulomatosis.

In relation to this patient, her history is not inclusive of any of the above findings. These characteristics comprise the panacea of questions in the historical interview of a patient with suspected interstitial lung disease and chronic respiratory failure.

QUESTION 3 Physical examination demonstrated a thin woman in minimal discomfort; extremities demonstrated bilateral clubbing of the fingers; lung exam demonstrated tubular breath sounds with rare bilateral basilar inspiratory crackles; no wheezing was present. What is clubbing, and what are some disease states associated with its development?

Clubbing of the digits was first described in the writings of Hippocrates and has been associated with a number of disease states. Clubbing is a component of the entity known as hypertrophic pulmonary osteoarthropathy along with proliferative periostitis and painful polyarthropathy of the distal long bones (i.e., ankles and wrists). Clubbing is defined as a distinctive change in the appearance of the nails, with some or all of the following characteristics: (1) softening and peri-ungual erythema of the nail beds such that they exhibit a floating rather than firm feel on palpation; (2) loss or reduction in the normal 15-degree angle the nail makes with its cuticle; (3) increased thickness of the terminal phalanx, sometimes with warmth and dusky erythema; and (4) increased convexity of the nail. It is important to ask the patient whether or not the nails have always been shaped as such or if there was a point at which the change occurred.

Disease states associated with clubbing include an idiopathic or familial variant of pulmonary fibrosis, bronchrectasis, bronchogenic cancers and mesothelioma, hepatomas, cyanotic congenital heart disease, or chronic hypoxia for other reasons, bacterial endocarditis, myxedema, and polyarteritis nodosa. It is important to recognize that clubbing is not a component of chronic bronchitis and emphysema.

QUESTION 4   The patient's admission laboratory data included a WBC 8.2×10^9 cells/L, HgB 18.9 g/dl, Hct 55.4%, total protein 6.6 g/dl, albumin 4 g/dl, SGOT 55 U/L, LDH 627 U/L, and an ABG on room air was pH 7.43, Pa_{CO_2} 36 mm Hg, Pa_{O_2} 40 mm Hg. An HIV test from referral hospital was reported as negative. The patient's CXR showed diffuse hazy bilateral infiltrates (see Fig. 11-8-1). Pulmonary function testing is reported below:

TEST	VALUES	% OF PREDICTED
Forced vital capacity (FVC)	3.23L	59
Forced expiratory volume in one second ($FEV_{1.0}$)	2.95L	66
Diffusion capacity corrected for alveolar volume (DL/VA)	1.71	30
Total lung capacity (TLC)	4.35L	60

What are the definitions of the PFT measurements above? How would you interpret the patient's pulmonary function tests?

Both the forced vital capacity (FVC) and forced expiratory volume in one second ($FEV_{1.0}$) are flow measurements. The FVC is a measure of the volume of gas that can be maximally exhaled. The $FEV_{1.0}$ is the volume of gas exhaled in one second. Both measures are decreased in restrictive and obstructive lung disease. These are differentiated by the finding of a reduced $FEV_{1.0}$/FVC ratio in obstructive lung diseases. The diffusing capacity is a measure of the diffusion of carbon monoxide. This will be reduced by loss of surface area, thickening of the alveolar membrane and changes of hemoglobin-oxygen affinity. As an example, the diffusing capacity is commonly reduced in emphysema as a result of loss of parenchyma. The total lung capacity (TLC) is one measure of volume. Increased TLC suggests hyperinflation because of obstruction to return of gas out of the lung during exhalation. This may be due to loss of airway tone and early airway collapse, trapping air in distal alveoli. Alternately, a restrictive defect will decrease lung volumes.

The patient's PFTs are consistent with a restrictive ventilatory defect as demonstrated by the decreased FVC, TLC, and diffusion capacity. Other findings supportive of chest restriction would include decreased lung compliance, chronic alveolar hyperventilation, and an increased (A-a) gradient.

QUESTION 5   The chest x-ray raised concern over a possible infectious etiology and prompted a diagnostic bronchoscopy. A PAS stain of a transbronchial biopsy specimen was made. The specimen showed relatively normal alveolar lining cells with a periodic acid-Schiff (PAS)-positive, amorphous, granular material deposited in the alveolar spaces. The lavage sample was markedly turbid secondary to this intraalveolar and intramacrophage material. How would you interpret these findings?

These findings are characteristic for pulmonary alveolar proteinosis, an idiopathic process resulting from the alveolar and bronchiolar deposition of an amorphous, insoluble, proteinaceous material rich in phospholipid. It is important to note that the findings on light microscopy may be sometimes confused with *Pneumocystis carinii*. In such situations, a methenamine silver stain

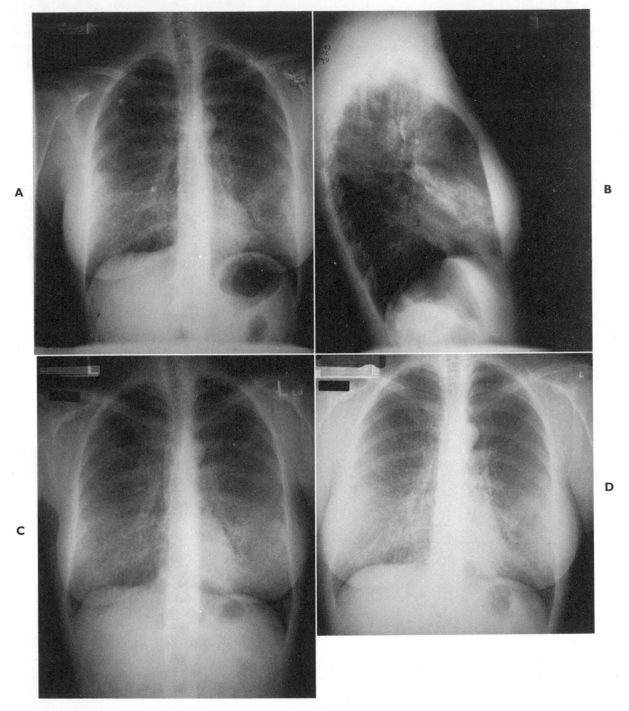

11-8-1 **A and B,** PA and L radiographs of active pulmonary alveolar proteinosis. **C,** The same patient after bilateral whole lung lavage. **D,** One year follow-up radiograph revealing intercurrent disease progression just prior to the next bilateral whole lung lavage.

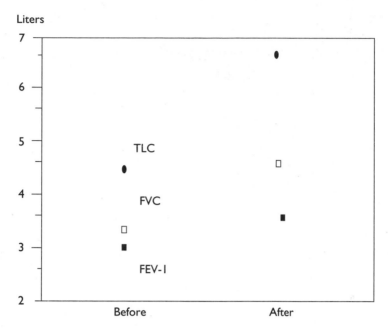

11-8-2 Pulmonary function tests before and after whole lung lavage.

should be done to demonstrate presence or absence of organisms.

This alveolar deposition results in impairment in oxygen transfer to the blood perfusing the involved alveoli and explains the patient's marked hypoxia and reduced diffusion capacity. A ventilation-perfusion mismatch develops as alveoli are filled with this material, but the perfusing capillaries remain patent. An attendant diffusing capacity decrease is seen. Commonly, dyspnea is precipitated by exertion, but later in the disease the patient is short of breath at rest. Fatigability and weight loss are common. As with other diseases with chronic hypoxia, polycythemia is common.

The chest radiograph demonstrates a patchy infiltrate, confluent in areas; usually bilateral and symmetrical.

Because macrophages phagocytose the alveolar material, their role as the principal cellular defense is compromised. The most frequent infecting agents include Nocardia, Cryptococcus, Aspergillus, and Mucorales.

QUESTION 6 How would you manage the patient based on the clinical and bronchoscopy findings?

Pulmonary alveolar proteinosis (PAP) remains an idiopathic disease process with little understanding of its natural history. However, with the introduction of whole lung lavage in 1965, the prognosis for PAP appears to have been improved. In brief the procedure involves using a double lumen endotracheal tube, such as a Carlen's tube, to separate both lungs. Deflation of one lung followed by drowning the lung with saline is done while providing gas exchange for the patient with the other lung. Typically, 20 or more liters of saline is used for each lung lavage with chest percussion being performed during the procedure. Patients treated with whole lung lavage usually do well although some require repeat lung lavage treatments at 6 to 12-month intervals until the disease process becomes quiescent.

The patient did undergo bilateral lung lavage on 2 separate days. The gradual clearing of lavage material was evident during the procedure, and

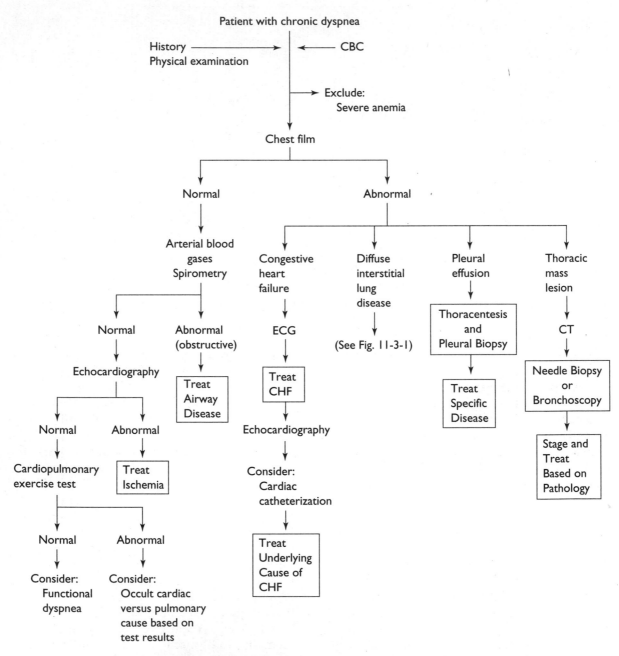

11-8-3   Diagnostic algorithm for chronic dyspnea.
(From Greene HL, Johnson WP, Maricic MJ: *Decision making in medicine,* St Louis, 1993, Mosby.)

the improvement in pulmonary function testing is demonstrated in Fig. 11-8-2.

A diagnostic algorithm for a patient with chronic dyspnea is shown in Fig. 11-8-3.

BIBLIOGRAPHY

Claypool WD, Rogers RM, Matuschak GM: Update on the clinical diagnosis, management, and pathogenesis of pulmonary alveolar proteinosis (phospholipidosis), *Chest* 85: 550-557, 1984.

Godwin JD, Muller NL, Takasugi JE: Pulmonary alveolar proteinosis: CT findings, *Radiology* 169:609-613, 1988.

Hoffman RM, Dauber JH, Rogers RM: Improvement in alveolar macrophage migration after therapeutic whole lung lavage in pulmonary alveolar proteinosis, *Am Rev Respir Dis* 139:1030-1032, 1989.

Kariman K, Kylstra JA, Spock A: Pulmonary alveolar proteinosis: prospective clinical experience in 23 patients for 15 Years, *Lung* 163:223-231, 1984.

Prakash UBS, Barham SS, Carpenter HA, et al: Pulmonary alveolar phospholipoproteinosis: experience with 34 cases and a review, *Mayo Clin Proc* 62:499-518, 1987.

Rogers RM, Levin DC, Gray BA, Moseley LW: Physiologic effects of bronchopulmonary lavage in alveolar proteinosis, *Am Rev Respir Dis* 118:255-264, 1978.

CASE

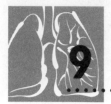

9

Amy Jenkins-Mangrum
James J. Herdegen

The patient is a 45-year-old man without significant medical history who presents to the emergency room with a 2-week history of shortness of breath and gradual onset chest pain. Initially dyspnea was present only with exercise but is now present at rest. He also notes a 3-day history of sharp, stabbing right-sided chest pain that is worsened with deep inspiration. He denied any complaints of palpitations, diaphoresis, nausea, vomiting, edema, orthopnea, hemoptysis, or paroxysmal nocturnal dyspnea. He denied any history of hypertension, myocardial infarction, or tuberculous exposure. Social history was negative for tobacco, alcohol, or intravenous drug usage.

QUESTION I What is your differential diagnosis of the patient's presenting symptoms?

Dyspnea can be defined as the uncomfortable awareness of breathing. Causes of dyspnea can be broadly categorized into cardiac and pulmonary etiologies. Cardiac causes of dyspnea include congestive heart failure (CHF), cardiomyopathy, and myocardial infarction, which may be accompanied by chest pain. Pulmonary causes for dyspnea can be generalized as acute or chronic. Acute episodes of dyspnea include acute exacerbation of asthma or chronic obstructive pulmonary disease (COPD), pneumothorax, bronchitis, pneumonia, foreign body aspiration, or pulmonary emboli. Chronic causes of dyspnea include COPD, chronic bronchitis and bronchiectasis, chronic thromboembolic disease, pneumonia, pleural effusions, collagen vascular disease, and neoplastic processes.

In this patient, acute myocardial infarction is unlikely. The patient's history is negative for cardiac risk factors. Ischemic pain is usually described as a deep, dull, relatively steady substernal pain unassociated with respiratory movements. There is a characteristic pattern of radiation to the left neck, shoulder, and arm. This patient described the quality and distribution of pain as being worse with deep breathing (i.e., pleuritic) without radiation. CHF can present as dyspnea that may progress until the patient is dyspneic at rest. This patient denied any history of orthopnea, paroxysmal nocturnal dyspnea, lower extremity edema, or pre-existing symptoms of CHF. He has no known history of cardiomyopathy. A cardiac process that may present with atypical chest pain with a positional or pleuritic component is pericarditis. Global and nonspecific electrocardiographic changes can be seen in cases of pericarditis. However, dyspnea may be due more to pain rather than congestive pathophysiology.

The patient denied a history of previous lung diseases or sputum production (purulent or clear), which may mark the presence of COPD, bronchitis/bronchiectasis, or pneumonia. Community acquired pneumonia can have an indolent presentation including upper respiratory symptoms, fatigue, lethargy, weakness, fevers and chills or present acutely with fever, hemoptysis, and a shaking chill. Recurrent pulmonary emboli can occur as episodes of dyspnea at rest and be accompanied by pleuritic chest pain. However, this patient's history is negative for hemoptysis, leg swelling, previous venous thrombosis, hypercoagulability, or fever. Pleural effusion can present with complaints of dyspnea and pleuritic chest pain. Further physical examination and testing will aid in narrowing the differential diagnosis.

QUESTION 2 The physical examination revealed normal vital signs. The cardiovascular examination had a regular rate and rhythm without a rub, murmur or gallop. There was no jugular venous distention. Lung examination revealed reduced tactile fremitus, dullness to percussion, and decreased breath sound over the left hemithorax. The right chest examination was normal. Abdominal examination was normal, and the extremities were normal without edema, erythema, calf tenderness, cords, or swelling. What is your impression of the physical examination, and how does it impact on the differential diagnosis?

The lung examination is composed of inspection, palpation and percussion, and auscultation. Inspection of a patient's breathing can reveal asymmetry of the hemithoraces as seen with a pneumothorax, paradoxic movements of the chest and abdomen as seen in diaphragmatic dysfunction, and use of accessory musculature. The shape of the chest may reveal hyperinflation as a sign of airways obstruction. Hoover's sign is found as a result of hyperinflation and represents paradoxical retraction of the lower chest wall because of contraction of a flattened diaphragm. This mechanical alteration may be palpated by placing the examiner's hands on the lower costal margins and asking the patient to inspire.

Palpation can also isolate pleural friction rubs, which feel like a "velcro" type of coarseness during air movement. Percussion is used to assess density of underlying structures. In cases of pneumothorax, the sound is resonant; whereas in cases of effusion, consolidation, or empyema the percussion note is dull.

Auscultation is another modality to examine the chest via sound transmission. The air-filled lung is a relatively poor conductor of sound. Liquid material in the pleural space will decrease sound transmission. When there is parenchymal consolidation, sound is transmitted better. Therefore, asking the patient to whisper while auscu-

latating an area of consolidation will increase the volume. This is known as "whispered pectoriloquy." Areas of consolidation will also demonstrate egophony such that vocalization of the letter *"e"* will sound like the letter *"a"* to auscultation. This maneuver works best if the stethoscope edge is applied to the chest wall so that the vocalization is audible via air conduction, and then applying the diaphragm while the patient continues to say "e", listening for change of the sound to "a". Tactile fremitus is present when vibration from vocalization is transmitted through an area of consolidation and is palpable focally on the chest wall.

The presenting physical examination is typical for a pleural effusion. Fluid in the pleural space separating the air-filled lung from the chest wall blocks the transmission of sound, resulting in the classic findings: decreased breath sounds, dullness to percussion, and decreased tactile fremitus.

QUESTION 3 What is the pathophysiology of pleural effusion and the mechanisms of pleural fluid collection and removal?

The pleura is a serous membrane that is divided into the parietal and visceral pleura. The visceral pleura covers the entire lung surface. The parietal pleura covers the inner surfaces of the thoracic cage, mediastinum, and diaphragm. The two leaves meet only at the lung root. The space created between the visceral and parietal pleura is the pleural space. This space is usually occupied by 10 to 15 ml of serous fluid.

The movement of liquid across the pleural membrane is governed by Starling's law of transcapillary exchange. High hydrostatic pressures "push" fluid out of the capillaries, whereas oncotic (osmotic) pressure tends to "pull" fluid back into the capillaries. There is a dynamic pressure gradient between hydrostatic and oncotic pressure in the pleural vessels that influences movement of liquid in and out of the pleural space.

The parietal pleura receives its blood supply from the systemic circulation, whereas the visceral pleura is supplied by the low pressure pulmonary circulation. Therefore, the hydrostatic pressure in the parietal pleural capillaries is greater than that of the visceral pleura. The oncotic pressure in both the parietal and visceral pleural capillaries are similar. Therefore, the major determinant of fluid accumulation within the pleural space is hydrostatic capillary pressure. Because of this pressure difference, movement of fluid is from the parietal surface into the pleural space.

Additionally, pressure in the pleural space is negative because of the opposite elastic recoil of the chest wall away from the lung. This negative hydrostatic pressure further assures that fluid will move from the parietal pleura into the pleural space.

Fluid that enters the pleural space may exit by two mechanisms. Eighty to ninety percent of fluid filtered from parietal capillaries is reabsorbed into the venous end of the visceral pleura capillaries. The remaining fluid, composed of protein and blood cells, is returned to the vascular space via the lymphatics. The lymphatic vessels in the parietal pleura are in direct communication with the pleural space by means of stomata. Stomata are round or slit like openings, 2 to 12 picometers in size and the only route through which cells and large particles leave the pleural space. The visceral pleura is also abundantly supplied with lymphatics but without direct communication with the pleural fluid.

It is the balance between formation and removal of fluid that keeps a thin layer of fluid in the pleural space. A pleural effusion develops only when the rate of formation exceeds the rate of removal.

Recently, another theory states that both transudates and exudates are due to systemic and local factors, respectively, that influence fluid accumulation. In studies of sheep, volume overload is followed by lung edema, engorgement of the interstitium, and the development of a transudative pleural effusion. This fluid has similar protein concentration as serum. A local process (i.e., pneumonia) leads to capillary leak and accumulation of exudative pleural effusion with an elevated protein concentration.

QUESTION 4 What are the categories of pleural effusion? What is the biochemical means by which each category is identified?

Pleural effusions can be divided into transudative and exudative effusions. Exudative pleural effusions meet at least one of the following criteria:
1. Pleural fluid/serum protein >0.5
2. Pleural fluid LDH/serum LDH >0.6
3. Pleural fluid LDH > two thirds of the upper limit of normal for serum

Lack of any of these qualities classifies the effusion as a transudate. Transudative effusions are due to abnormalities in the Starling hydrostatic or oncotic pressures. Exudative effusions are due to alterations of the pleural surfaces, allowing leakage of protein, sloughing of pleural cells, or lack of reabsorption. Six mechanisms are responsible for the accumulation of pleural fluid. Causes of transudates are:
1. Increase in hydrostatic pressure in the microvascular circulation (e.g., CHF).
2. Decrease in oncotic pressure in the microvascular circulation as in low protein states (e.g., nephrotic syndrome, malnutrition, cirrhosis).
3. Movement of fluid from the peritoneal space (ascites). Fluid can leak through defects in the diaphragm, the foramen of Morgagni or Bochdalek, or via lymphatics.

Causes of exudative pleural effusions are:
1. Increased permeability of the microvascular circulation in inflammatory conditions such as pneumonia or serositis wherein liquid and protein leak because of local inflammation.
2. Impaired lymphatic drainage from the pleural space. A blockage at any point in the lymphatic system will result in pleural fluid accumulation (i.e., chylothorax).
3. Decreased pressures in the pleural space. This occurs in states such as atelectasis or fibrosis where there is a more negative pleural pressure causing an even larger hydrostatic pressure gradient promoting fluid accumulation.

A chylothorax is characterized by a white milky effusion rich in lipid. The most common etiologies are ductal trauma (surgery or closed chest injury) and ductal obstruction as seen in lymphoma. Biochemically, the fluid is characterized by a triglyceride level >110 mg/dl as contrasted to pseudochylous effusions that are characterized by cholesterol level in excess of 1000 mg/dl. If these indices are nondiagnostic, differentiation can be done by isolation of chylomicrons in a true chylothorax. The thoracic duct can be indicated as the source of the effusion by the ingestion of food-colored butter that will stain the pleural fluid within several hours.

A diagnostic algorithm for the patient with pleural effusion is shown in Fig. 11-9-1.

QUESTION 5 The chest x-ray shows a large homogeneous density at the left lung base, decreased lung markings and obscuration of the left hemidiaphragm, and a meniscus at the left lateral chest wall. The rest of the lung fields appear normal. The cardiac size is normal. What information can be drawn from the CXR? What other radiographic studies may be useful?

When a patient is upright, fluid first accumulates between the inferior surface of the lower lobe and diaphragm. If the amount of fluid exceeds 75 ml, it will spill into the posterior costophrenic angle, causing blunting appreciated best in the lateral projection. As the fluid increases, blunting of the lateral costophrenic angle on the posteroanterior radiograph is seen. As more fluid accumulates, the entire outline of the diaphragm on the affected side is obscured because of the silhouette phenomena. Fluid will conform to the lateral chest wall, forming the typical meniscus shape.

Lateral decubitus films should be obtained when free pleural fluid is suspected. When a patient is placed in the lateral decubitus position, free fluid gravitates to the most dependent portion of the pleural space. Should this not happen, one must postulate loculation of a pleural effusion or the presence of an unanticipated pleural or parenchymal process.

Ultrasound is a valuable technique for visual-

ization of loculated pleural fluid or small fluid collections not clearly evident on conventional radiography. The detection of an echo-free space aids in collection of fluid via thoracentesis or drainage of complex loculations. Both the exact location and depth of fluid collections can be easily seen.

Computed tomographic scanning is able to delineate the parenchymal and pleural anatomy. Parenchymal consolidation, abscess, air-fluid levels, areas of atelectasis as well as irregularities of the pleural surface can be seen. Free-flowing fluid will accumulate in dependent areas as the patient is supine for the examination. Air and pleural fluid (both transduates and exudates) have characteristic appearances.

QUESTION 6 Upon further questioning, the patient reported working in the shipping industry for 15 years as a "grinder," forming molds for hot metal with a heavy exposure to asbestos. What are the indications for, procedure, and complications of thoracentesis?

A thoracentesis is indicated for diagnostic and therapeutic purposes. It is performed as a diagnostic tool in newly diagnosed pleural effusions, evaluation of an associated parenchymal lesion with concurrent fever, and to evaluate the presence of an empyema. This requires withdrawal of 30 to 60 ml of fluid with a small-bore needle. A therapeutic thoracentesis is indicated when a large pleural effusion is believed to be the cause of gas exchange abnormalities that contribute to the patient's dyspnea.

Pleural fluid can be sampled easily. After diligent sterilization and adequate local anesthesia to the skin, inferior rib periosteum and pleural membrane, a needle is introduced over the inferior rib with care to avoid the neurovascular bundle present on the inferior edge of the immediately superior rib. The needle is gradually advanced with suction until a flash of fluid returns into the syringe. The distance should be carefully noted so as to avoid potential trauma to the underlying lung.

Generally, no more than 1.5 L of pleural fluid should be collected at one time to prevent the complication of reexpansion pulmonary edema. A postthoracentesis CXR should be ordered to check for complications (i.e., pneumothorax, hemothorax) and to assess both the reduction of the effusion and to examine the now visible underlying lung.

QUESTION 7 A diagnostic thoracentesis was performed. During the thoracentesis, the resident noted a marked resistance to the needle entering the pleural space. The procedure went without apparent complications; 400 ml of pleural fluid was obtained. It was odorless, translucent, and reddish in color. Results are as follows: LDH 225 U/L (serum 98), protein 8 g/dl (serum 6). The WBC count was 4.5×10^9 cells/L with 75×10^3 RBC; gram stain was negative. Cytology was positive for atypical cells. What information can be obtained from the characteristics of the fluid?

The color of the fluid can be helpful in diagnosis. A bloody effusion in the absence of trauma is most likely due to malignancy; (2) a white or milky pleural effusion is due to either chyle, cholesterol, or empyema; (3) brown fluid results when an amebic liver abscess ruptures into the pleural space; (4) a yellow-green fluid may be seen in rheumatoid pleurisy; (5) a viscous effusion suggests a malignant mesothelioma due to increased levels of hyaluronic acid; (6) a putrid odor is diagnostic for the presence of purulence; and (7) food particles suggest esophageal rupture.

A few helpful tips for interpreting lab values follow. The demonstration of a reduced glucose level (<60 mg/dl) is most commonly seen in cases of a parapneumonic effusion (usually glucose <40 mg/dl), rheumatoid pleural effusion (glucose <30 mg/dl), malignancy, and an effusion due to tuberculosis.

The LDH level in the pleural fluid is an accurate indicator of the degree of inflammation in the pleural space. However, an elevated LDH is nonspecific. The LDH may be helpful in subsequent thoracentesis to evaluate activity of a particular disease process.

Polymorphonuclear leukocytes predominate in acute processes such as pneumonia, pulmonary embolism, tuberculosis, and pancreatitis. Greater than 50,000 WBC are found with parapneumonic effusions. Mononuclear cells are due to chronic inflammation in such cases as carcinoma, tuberculosis, and rheumatoid pleuritis. Eosinophilia can be seen in hemothorax, pneumothorax, previous thoracentesis, parasitic or fungal infections, asbestos exposure, and drug reactions.

Cytologic evaluation is useful in the evaluation of malignancies that involve the pleural surface as a primary or secondary pleural disease. Positive results are obtained in 50% to 90% of cases and may be increased with serial specimens.

Pleural pH (<7.30) may be an important clue. A low pH narrows the differential diagnosis to empyema, malignancy, rheumatoid, lupus, or tuberculous pleuritis and esophageal rupture. Only a sample collected anaerobically, immediately placed on ice, and analyzed rapidly will yield accurate pH.

QUESTION 8 A post-thoracentesis CXR revealed a 50% reduction of the pleural effusion. The underlying parenchyma was normal, but there were several areas of pleural thickening along the left lateral chest wall. The patient is very anxious to find out why he has this pleural effusion. After receiving the lab data, there is a high suspicion for a malignancy. What approach should be taken given the above clinical presentation and the patient's pleural fluid profile?

An undiagnosed exudative pleural effusion is the major indication for percutaneous pleural biopsy. Examples include malignant or tuberculous pleuritis when other diagnostic modalities have been inconclusive.

Contraindications to a pleural biopsy are an obliterated pleural space as a result of previous pleurodesis, radiation, chronic infection, an uncooperative patient, and anticoagulation or bleeding diathesis. The procedure is easier to carry out when there is substantial fluid in the pleural space. However, small amounts of fluid are not absolute contraindications to a pleural biopsy.

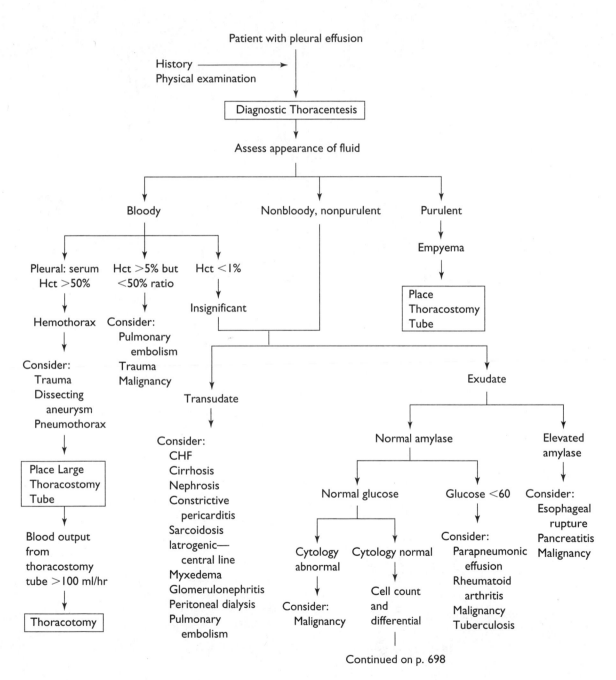

Patient with pleural effusion

History ⟶
Physical examination

Diagnostic Thoracentesis

Assess appearance of fluid

Bloody — **Nonbloody, nonpurulent** — **Purulent**

Purulent → Empyema → Place Thoracostomy Tube

Bloody:
- Pleural: serum Hct >50%
- Hct >5% but <50% ratio
- Hct <1%

Pleural: serum Hct >50% → Hemothorax → Consider: Trauma, Dissecting aneurysm, Pneumothorax → Place Large Thoracostomy Tube → Blood output from thoracostomy tube >100 ml/hr → Thoracotomy

Hct >5% but <50% ratio → Consider: Pulmonary embolism, Trauma, Malignancy

Hct <1% → Insignificant

Transudate → Consider:
CHF
Cirrhosis
Nephrosis
Constrictive pericarditis
Sarcoidosis
Iatrogenic—central line
Myxedema
Glomerulonephritis
Peritoneal dialysis
Pulmonary embolism

Exudate → Normal amylase / Elevated amylase

Normal amylase → Normal glucose / Glucose <60

Normal glucose → Cytology abnormal / Cytology normal

Cytology abnormal → Consider: Malignancy

Cytology normal → Cell count and differential

Glucose <60 → Consider: Parapneumonic effusion, Rheumatoid arthritis, Malignancy, Tuberculosis

Elevated amylase → Consider: Esophageal rupture, Pancreatitis, Malignancy

Continued on p. 698

11-9-1 Diagnostic algorithm for pleural effusion.
(From Greene HL, Johnson WP, Maricic MJ: *Decision making in medicine,* St Louis, 1993, Mosby.)

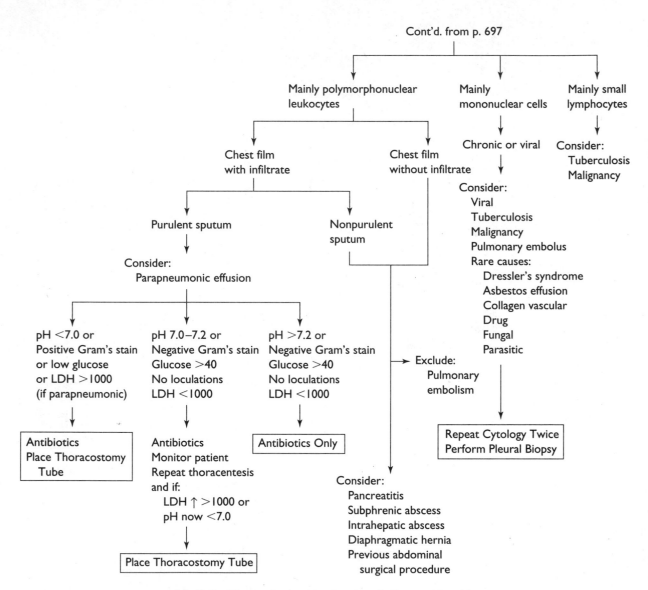

Cont'd. from p. 697

Mainly polymorphonuclear leukocytes

Mainly mononuclear cells

Mainly small lymphocytes

Chest film with infiltrate

Chest film without infiltrate

Chronic or viral

Consider:
Tuberculosis
Malignancy

Purulent sputum

Nonpurulent sputum

Consider:
Viral
Tuberculosis
Malignancy
Pulmonary embolus
Rare causes:
    Dressler's syndrome
    Asbestos effusion
    Collagen vascular
    Drug
    Fungal
    Parasitic

Consider:
Parapneumonic effusion

pH <7.0 or
Positive Gram's stain
or low glucose
or LDH >1000
(if parapneumonic)

pH 7.0–7.2 or
Negative Gram's stain
Glucose >40
No loculations
LDH <1000

pH >7.2 or
Negative Gram's stain
Glucose >40
No loculations
LDH <1000

Exclude:
Pulmonary
embolism

Antibiotics
Place Thoracostomy
Tube

Antibiotics
Monitor patient
Repeat thoracentesis
and if:
    LDH ↑ >1000 or
    pH now <7.0

Antibiotics Only

Repeat Cytology Twice
Perform Pleural Biopsy

Consider:
Pancreatitis
Subphrenic abscess
Intrahepatic abscess
Diaphragmatic hernia
Previous abdominal
    surgical procedure

Place Thoracostomy Tube

11-9-1   Diagnostic algorithm for pleural effusion—Cont'd.

Two major complications are pneumothorax and bleeding caused by inadvertent laceration of the intercostal vessels that course inferior to each costal margin. For these reasons, a postprocedure CXR is necessary.

QUESTION 9   A pleural biopsy was obtained and cytology revealed cells suspicious for malignant mesothelioma. Follow-up CXR revealed a small pneumothorax without mediastinal shift. What are the indications for chest tube placement?

Indications for chest tube placement include pneumothorax (with or without tension), persistent bronchopleural fistula, hemothorax, empyema, and recurrent malignant effusion for the purposes of pleurodesis.

The decision to place a chest tube depends on the degree of respiratory and hemodynamic compromise. Therefore, one should make note of the respiratory rate, blood pressure, presence of jugular venous distension, and serial chest radiographs to evaluate evolution of the pneumothorax. Alternatives to tube thoracostomy exist. These include placement of 16 to 18 gauge 20 cm catheters attached to a Heimlich valve for the removal of air. Another approach is the serial thoracentesis of air using a three-way stopcock and syringe. The presence of air in a hemithorax after pleural biopsy may also represent air that has been introduced into the pleural space from the biopsy needle. This may occur during inspiration with the generation of negative intrathoracic pressure.

CASE SUMMARY   In conclusion, the pleural effusion cytology was suspicious for malignant me-

sothelioma. The percutaneous pleural biopsy did not sample tissue adequate for definitive diagnosis. Therefore, the patient underwent a thoracotomy, which yielded tissue that firmly established the diagnosis of malignant mesothelioma. This diagnosis explained the marked resistance to the needle entering the pleural space (as in this case), and on CXR one can see pleural thickening.

Pleural effusions secondary to metastic disease are the second most common type of exudative pleural effusion, 30% being lung cancer, 25% breast cancer, and 20% lymphoma.

Pleural mesotheliomas are more common in males. The onset is usually manifested as chest pain.

• •

BIBLIOGRAPHY

Bone RC, Dantzker DR, George RC, et al: *Pulmonary and critical care medicine*, vol 2, sect O, 1994, St Louis, Mosby.

Bone RC, Petty TL: *Yearbook of pulmonary disease 1993*, 1993, St Louis, Mosby.

Broaddus VC, Light RW: What is the origin of pleural tranudates and exudates? *Chest* 102:658-659, 1992.

Iberti TJ, Stern PM: Chest Tube Thoracostomy, *Crit Care Clin* 8(4):879-896, 1992.

Light RW: *Pleural diseases*, 1990, Philadelphia, Lea and Febiger.

Murray JF, Nadel JA: *Respiratory medicine*, Philadelphia, 1988, WB Saunders.

Sahn SA: The differential diagnosis of pleural effusions, *West J Med* 137:99-108, 1982.

Sahn SA: The pleura, *Am Rev Respir Dis* 138:184-234, 1988.

Squire LF, Novelline RA: *Fundamentals of radiology*, ed 4, 1988, Boston, Harvard University Press.

Wiener-Kronish JP, Matthay MA, Callen PA, et al: Relationship of pleural effusions to pulmonary hemodynamics in patients with congestive heart failure, *Am Rev Respir Dis* 132:1253-1256, 1985.

C A S E

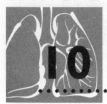

10

Robert Winn
James J. Herdegen

The patient is a 39-year-old ex-college basketball player without significant medical history who came to the emergency room with a 12-hour history of constant, sharp left-sided chest pain. He had been in his usual good state of health and denies recent fever, chills, night sweats, weight loss, or hemoptysis. He states that he awoke with acute onset of pain in his chest that radiated to his left shoulder. He also noted mild shortness of breath (SOB). The pain was exacerbated by deep breathing and caused him to cough. He denies any history of cardiopulmonary, renal, gastrointestinal, or genitourinary disease.

QUESTION I Acute syndromes that manifest chest pain can be life threatening. What are the most likely causes of chest pain in this patient?

Pleuritic pain is defined as pain related to respiratory movements and aggravated by cough and/or deep inspiration. It can also be brought on by swallowing. The differential diagnosis of acute pleuritic chest pain includes pneumothorax, pleural inflammation, pneumonia, pericarditis, pulmonary embolism, neoplasm, mediastinal disease, and abnormalities of the chest wall or musculoskeletal system. Clues in the patient's history can help to differentiate these varied etiologies.

Pneumothorax may present in adults with a male:female predominance of 6:1. Often, pneumothoraces occur while the patient is at rest. Patients with spontaneous pneumothorax are often tall and thin, have a family history of pneumothorax, and occur at a younger age in women compared to men. Pleural inflammation can be seen in rheumatic disorders (systemic lupus erythematosus and rheumatoid arthritis).

Alternatively, in the absence of physical and roentgenographic findings, pain may be due to epidemic pleurodynia (Bornholm's disease). While the pathology is not characterized with certainty, there is a relationship to coxsackie or echovirus infection, producing skeletal muscle swelling and tenderness. Patients experience severe stabbing, crushing, or viselike paroxysms of pain exacerbated by any movement. Patients may experience abdominal pain and have undergone laporotomy before the diagnosis is suspected. The patients usually fully recover, although relapses are common. Treatment is supportive.

The postpericardiotomy syndrome (Dressler's syndrome) is another process due to pleural inflammation. This syndrome presents as pleuro-pericarditis with pleural and pericardial effusion usually 6 weeks to 6 months after cardiac surgery. It results from pericardial trauma. There is a rapid response to treatment with nonsteroidal antiinflammatory agents or corticosteroids.

The presence of parenchymal disease on chest x-ray (CXR) and the physical signs of pleuritic chest pain with fever would suggest an infectious process such as acute bacterial pneumonia. Inflammation of the visceral pleura causes friction against the parietal pleura, which is the portion of the pleura containing nerves, leading to pain.

The pain of pericarditis is usually associated with a pleuritic or positional component. On auscultation, one hears a pericardial friction rub (a sound akin to crumpling a paper bag). Distinct diastolic and systolic components may be audible; however, the rub is usually transient and fleeting, may be audible only in specific areas, and may be positional. Pericarditic pain may be of two types:

an episodic discomfort associated with the respiratory cycle or a steady substernal pain that mimics angina. The pain associated with pericarditis is thought to be due to inflammation of the adjacent parietal pleura. It is frequently referred to the neck, mimicking angina pectoris, but typically pleuritic pain lasts longer. The mechanism of this steady substernal pain is not certain, but may arise from marked inflammation of the relatively sensitive inner parietal surface of the pericardium or from irritated afferent cardiac nerve fibers lying in the periadventitial layers of the superficial coronary arteries.

Pulmonary infarction secondary to pulmonary embolism may also cause inflammation of the pleural surface. Under these circumstances, hemoptysis may be a presenting feature. The pain resulting from pulmonary embolism may resemble that of acute myocardial infarction.

Pain associated with movement of the respiratory apparatus may be a product of the musculoskeletal system. Pain arising in the chest wall or upper extremity may develop as a result of muscle or ligament strain. Pain may come from the costochondral or chondrosternal junctions or the chest wall musculature. Other causes are osteoarthritis of the spine, a ruptured vertebral disc, vertebral body compression fracture, and thoracic nerve outlet compression. Pain in the left upper extremity and precordium may be due to compression of portions of the brachial plexus by a cervical rib or by spasm and shortening of the scalenus anticus muscle secondary to high fixation of the ribs and sternum. Pain arising in the chest wall or shoulder girdles or arm is reproducible to palpation, and there is a clear relationship between pain and motion. Deep breathing or movements of the chest and shoulder girdle may elicit and duplicate the pain.

In the patient under consideration, the denial of fever, chills, cough productive of purulent sputum, and signs of infection make pneumonia much less likely. Furthermore, since he does not have a recent history of trauma or musculoskeletal disease, these etiologies are lower in the differential diagnosis. He characterizes his pain as

constant and lacking a positional component such that pericarditis is less likely. He does not manifest risk factors for venous thrombosis or pulmonary embolism. Additionally, there is no history of rheumatic disease.

QUESTION 2 What are the important findings on physical examination that may suggest that pleuritic chest pain is due to pneumothorax?

Physical examination may reveal tachypnea, asymmetric expansion of the chest with decreased expansion on the affected side due to the outward recoil of the chest wall as the lung collapses, mediastinal shift with deviation of the trachea and apex beat toward the side of the pneumothorax, and hyperresonance to percussion with diminished breath sounds over the affected side. One may find decreased vocal fremitus and resonance on the side of the pneumothorax. The side of the chest with the pneumothorax will appear raised when the patient is supine as the counterforce opposing chest wall expansion is absent.

In a tension pneumothorax, due to the high intrapleural pressure, there is a pressure gradient that restricts venous return to the right side of the heart. This leads to increased central venous pressure, jugular venous distension, clear lung fields on the side of the pneumothorax, cyanosis, and hypotension. The pressure within the lungs, the alveolar pressure (palv), is 0 mm Hg (i.e., atmospheric pressure). The pressure in the intrapleural fluid surrounding the lungs, the intrapleural pressure (Pip), is approximately 4 mm Hg less than atmospheric pressure (i.e., −4 mm Hg). Therefore, there is a pressure difference of 4 mm Hg across the pleural surface. This is the force acting to hold the lungs open; there is an identical force, but opposite in direction, keeping the chest wall from moving outward. Water is highly indistensible, and as the lungs and chest wall move away from each other, the resulting infinitesimal expansion of the water-filled intrapleural space drops the intrapleural pressure below atmospheric pressure. Thus the elastic recoil of the lung and chest wall creates the subatmospheric intrapleural pressure that keeps them from moving any further apart. When the chest wall is pierced, atmospheric air rushes into the intrapleural space, the pressure difference across the lung wall is eliminated, and the stretched lung collapses.

QUESTION 3   The patient's chest roentgenogram demonstrated a radiolucent band along the left lateral chest wall without visible pulmonary markings between the lung edge and chest wall. An arterial blood gas revealed a pH of 7.46, $Paco_2$ of 30 torr, and a Pao_2 of 71 mm Hg. The electrocardiogram demonstrated sinus tachycardia but was otherwise normal. How does this new information impact on the differential diagnosis?

The chest roentgenogram mentioned above is quite characteristic of pneumothorax. Often expiratory films are necessary to reveal the edge of the collapsed lung. The reason for this is that the negative pleural pressure generated during inspiration will pull the visceral pleura against the parietal pleura obliterating the pleural space. In addition, in an expanded hemithorax the volume of pleural air compared to lung parenchymal air is relatively less. Conversely, during expiration, positive pleural pressure pushes the lung edge farther from the chest wall, making it visible on x-ray.

Upright films are more useful than supine films, because, in the upright position, air rises in the chest to the apex so that the apical pleura is parallel to the x-ray beam, rendering it visible. In supine films, air rises to the anterior chest wall, and the lung edge is perpendicular to the x-ray beam, making it invisible on radiography. If the patient cannot be positioned upright, a reasonable alternative is to place the patient in the decubitus position.

Hypoxemia and reduced oxygen saturation are commonly seen in the presence of a pneumothorax. This is due to the presence of ventilation-perfusion mismatching. Autoregulation of blood flow responds by vasoconstriction to poorly ventilated areas in an effort to better match ventilation and perfusion. Shunt physiology may be evident because of the lack of improvement of Pao_2 when given high concentrations of oxygen.

Sinus tachycardia is the most common electrocardiographic finding in the present of a pneumothorax. If the pneumothorax is on the left side a rightward frontal axis, precordial T wave inversion, and decreased R wave voltage simulating the presence of an anterior wall myocardial infarction may be seen on the ECG.

A diagnostic algorithm for pneumothorax is shown in Fig. 11-10-1 on p. 705.

QUESTION 4   What role do lung bullae play in the development of pneumothorax? What is the difference between a primary and secondary pneumothorax?

The presence of subpleural bullae is a risk factor for the development of pneumothorax. How bullous disease develops is still unclear. One hypothesis to explain the development of bullae is that underlying emphysema destroys alveoli adjacent to connective tissue septa or pleura, and small air bubbles may form in these areas. Should one or more rupture, a pneumothorax may ensue. Other ideas include:

1. Alveolar wall weakness predisposes to the formation of bullae.
2. Inflammatory disease of a bronchiole leads to progressive air trapping and distension of airspaces.
3. Collateral ventilation is responsible.
4. The same mechanisms responsible for generalized emphysema underlie the formation of bullae.

When rupture occurs, alveolar air is allowed to pass into the interstitium and dissect proximally along bronchovascular sheaths toward the pleural space. A primary spontaneous pneumothorax appears in otherwise healthy individuals, whereas a secondary spontaneous pneumothorax occurs in patients with underlying lung disease that predisposes to alveolar rupture (e.g., COPD or patients receiving positive pressure ventilation) (see the box).

UNDERLYING LUNG DISEASES ASSOCIATED WITH SECONDARY SPONTANEOUS PNEUMOTHORAX

INFECTION
- Pneumonia
- Staphylococcal septicemia
- Lung abscess
- Tuberculosis
- Coccidioidomycosis
- Hydatid disease

OBSTRUCTIVE AIRWAY DISEASE
- COPD
- Asthma

GRANULOMATOUS DISEASES
- Sarcoidosis
- Berylliosis

NEOPLASTIC DISEASE
- Cancer of lung
  - Primary
  - Secondary

CONNECTIVE TISSUE DISEASE
- Rheumatoid disease
  - Scleroderma
  - Systemic lupus erythematosus

IDIOPATHIC DISEASE
- Idiopathic pulmonary fibrosis
- Histiocytosis X/ Hand-Schüller Christian disease/ Letterer-Siwe disease
- Pulmonary alveolar proteinosis
- Idiopathic pulmonary hemosiderosis
- Marfan's syndrome

INTERSTITIAL LUNG DISEASE
- Cystic fibrosis
- Lymphangioleiomyomatosis

MISCELLANEOUS DISEASE
- Xanthomatosis
- Biliary cirrhosis
- Pulmonary infarction
- Nasal cocaine insufflation

Spontaneous pneumothoraces tend to occur when a subpleural bleb ruptures, usually apical, compromising the alveolar/pleural barrier and allowing air to escape into the interstitium. It is a common misconception that spontaneous pneumothoraces occur during strenuous activity; most occur at rest.

The major physiologic results are decreased vital capacity and hypoxemia as a result of ventilation–perfusion imbalance. Respiratory insufficiency is not likely unless there is a pre-existing pulmonary disease.

QUESTION 5 What is barotrauma and what role does mechanical ventilation play in the development of a pneumothorax? How does a tension pneumothorax occur?

Barotrauma means pressure-induced injury, but the culprit in mechanical ventilation may be overinflation of alveoli. When the airspaces rupture, air dissects along tissue planes along the bronchovascular bundles into the mediastinum and neck. This is known as *pneumomediastinum*.

Pneumomediastinum may also occur due to a tear in the esophagus, tracheobronchial tree, or from dissection of air from ruptured alveoli. Patients complain of sharp chest pain and dyspnea. On physical examination one may palpate subcutaneous crepitance. Hamman's sign may be noted with auscultation (i.e., a crunching sound is heard with the heartbeat). Usually a chest x-ray is diagnostic, and the treatment is observation for simple spontaneous pneumomediastinum and surgical intervention if severe.

If the air then breaks through the parietal pleura, entering the pleural space, pneumothorax occurs. The air can also rupture into the pericardium or enter the peritoneal cavity. Predisposing factors include excessive inflation volume and high peak and plateau airway pressures. In one study, the incidence of barotrauma was as high as 43% if the peak inflation pressure exceeded 70 cm H_2O. Steir et al. reviewed records of 74 patients who developed nontraumatic pneumothorax during ventilatory support. At the time of pneumothorax development, mean tidal volume averaged 18 ml/kg, and mean peak inspiratory pressure was 46 cm H_2O. Fourteen patients received PEEP, at a mean level of 12 cm H_2O. Seventeen percent of patients treated with PEEP developed pneumothorax.

Although inflation pressure is of clear pathogenetic significance, inhomogeneity of lung injury also plays an important role. Ventilator delivered volume distributes preferentially to compliant areas fed by low resistance pathways, augmenting the risk of local overdistention. Thickened secretion, blood clots, or foreign objects can also produce ball-valve airway obstruction and regional hyperinflation.

Mechanical ventilation is associated with a 3% to 5% incidence of barotrauma. Risk varies with the underlying lung disease and with the amount of positive pressure applied to the lung. High airway pressure is an important predisposition for pneumothorax. Measurement of airway pressures allows appropriate manipulation of ventilator parameters to lessen airway pressure and avoid barotrauma.

In patients on positive pressure ventilation, every pneumothorax should be considered a potential tension pneumothorax. If pressure inside the pneumothorax becomes greater than the atmospheric pressure, as might happen with a one-way leak into the pleural space ("ball—valve" leak), a tension pneumothorax is present. For this to occur, there must be an open airway through which air under positive pressure is being pushed, through a rent in the pleura without being allowed to escape. Transmission of intrathoracic pressure to the central vessels and heart can lead to marked obstruction to venous return, right ventricular filling, and hypotension.

Tension pneumopericardium is a condition hemodynamically similar to acute hemorrhagic cardiac tamponade. In adults it usually occurs as a result of esophageal rupture, penetrating chest trauma, carcinomatous bronchopericardial fistula, gas production from contiguous infection, and diagnostic procedures like sternal bone marrow aspiration. Clinical clues of pneumopericar-

dium are muffled heart sounds, bradycardia, and shifting tympany over the pericardium.

Hydropneumothorax is a collection of fluid and gas within the pleural cavity. When air is present, the air-fluid interface forms a horizontal air-fluid level. The continued absorption of intrapleural gas produces markedly subatmospheric pleural pressures that favor the formation and accumulation of a transudate. A hemothorax is the accumulation of blood within the thorax. It is usually a complication of thoracic trauma or iatrogenic-laceration of the intercostal vessels after thoracentesis. Movement of the heart and lung tend to defibrinate blood, preventing it from clotting in the pleural space. If the blood clots, it may organize to form "peels" on both the visceral and parietal surfaces. Persistent, organized clot can encase the lung and impair gas exchange. Decortication primarily focuses on removing the peel from the visceral pleura to free both lung and diaphragm.

QUESTION 6 What are the immediate and definitive modes of treatment?

There are multiple treatment modalities available. Depending on the size of the pneumothorax (<25% or less than 4 cm from the apex), the patient may be observed and evaluated with serial inspiratory and expiratory x-rays. Over a short time the pneumothorax may resolve on its own. The use of high concentrations of oxygen by face mask can help to speed reabsorption of gas in the pleural space. This works by decreasing the amount of nitrogen in the pleural space and increasing the rate of reabsorption of intrapleural oxygen that remains.

Larger pneumothoraces may require more definitive therapy. Tube thoracostomy is usually indicated for pneumothorax of greater than 25% of the lung, severe dyspnea, or tension pneumothorax. The tube is placed by making a small incision in the chest wall in the 4th-5th intercostal space in the mid-axillary line. One bluntly dissects down to the chest wall with a finger or a curved clamp and manually isolates the desired intercostal space. A curved clamp is attached to the tip of

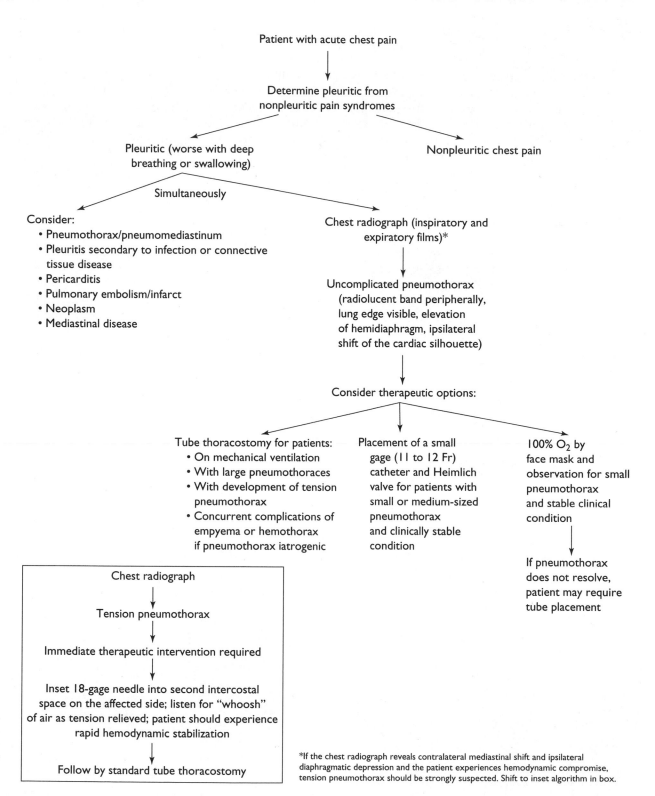

Patient with acute chest pain

↓

Determine pleuritic from nonpleuritic pain syndromes

Pleuritic (worse with deep breathing or swallowing)　　　　　　　　Nonpleuritic chest pain

Simultaneously

Consider:
- Pneumothorax/pneumomediastinum
- Pleuritis secondary to infection or connective tissue disease
- Pericarditis
- Pulmonary embolism/infarct
- Neoplasm
- Mediastinal disease

Chest radiograph (inspiratory and expiratory films)*

↓

Uncomplicated pneumothorax (radiolucent band peripherally, lung edge visible, elevation of hemidiaphragm, ipsilateral shift of the cardiac silhouette)

↓

Consider therapeutic options:

Tube thoracostomy for patients:
- On mechanical ventilation
- With large pneumothoraces
- With development of tension pneumothorax
- Concurrent complications of empyema or hemothorax if pneumothorax iatrogenic

Placement of a small gage (11 to 12 Fr) catheter and Heimlich valve for patients with small or medium-sized pneumothorax and clinically stable condition

100% O_2 by face mask and observation for small pneumothorax and stable clinical condition

↓

If pneumothorax does not resolve, patient may require tube placement

---

Chest radiograph

↓

Tension pneumothorax

↓

Immediate therapeutic intervention required

↓

Inset 18-gage needle into second intercostal space on the affected side; listen for "whoosh" of air as tension relieved; patient should experience rapid hemodynamic stabilization

↓

Follow by standard tube thoracostomy

---

*If the chest radiograph reveals contralateral mediastinal shift and ipsilateral diaphragmatic depression and the patient experiences hemodynamic compromise, tension pneumothorax should be strongly suspected. Shift to inset algorithm in box.

11-10-1 Diagnostic algorithm for patient with acute chest pain.

the chest tube and another to the distal end. Pressure is exerted on the parietal pleura until the tube pops into the pleural space. Often, fluid or air will rush back once the space is entered. A CXR is necessary to confirm the location of the tube. To evacuate air or fluid the tube is placed to suction.

In an emergent situation when there is hemodynamic compromise and suspicion of tension in the pleural space or when there is progressive shift of the mediastinum, placement of a 21-gauge needle in the second intercostal space on the suspected side to relieve pressure is necessary. A rush of air is universally heard upon insertion of the needle when tension is present. Hemodynamic instability usually disappears rapidly. In the case of an errant diagnosis, the needle should not be removed until chest tube thoracostomy can be carried out.

QUESTION 7 Further history revealed that the patient frequently smoked cocaine. Is there a relationship between crack cocaine use and pneumothorax?

Drug abuse has increasingly become a risk factor for pneumothorax. Patients who smoke cocaine are at increased risk of pneumothorax. This is thought related to toxic effects of cocaine smoke and the high negative pressure created during nasal insufflation and a forced Valsalva maneuver during drug inhalation.

BIBLIOGRAPHY

Braunwald E: *Heart disease: a textbook of cardiovascular medicine,* ed 4, Philadelphia, 1992, WB Saunders.
Fishman AP: *Pulmonary Disease and Disorders,* ed 2, New York, 1988, McGraw-Hill.
Kollef MH: Risk factors for the misdiagnosis of pneumothorax in the intensive care unit, *Crit Care Med* 19:906-910, 1991.
Petersen GW, Baier H: Incidence of pulmonary barotrauma in a medical ICU, *Crit Care Med,* 11:67-69, 1983.
Shesser R, Davis C, Eclelstein S: Pneumomediastinum and pneumothorax after inhaling alkaloidal cocaine, *Ann Emerg Med* 10:213-215, 1981.
Sternbach G, Raftery K: Presentation and management of spontaneous pneumothorax, *Hosp Phys* 30(5):18-23, 1994.
Vander AJ: *Human physiology: the mechanism of body function* ed 4, New York, 1985, McGraw-Hill.
Walston A, Brewer DL, Kitchens CS, et al: The electroradiographic manifestations of spontaneous pneumothorax, *Ann Intern Med* 80:375-379, 1974.

C A S E

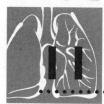

Francis P.A. Jamilla
James J. Herdegen

The patient is a 62-year-old man with a medical history significant for hypertension and chronic obstructive pulmonary disease presenting with increasing dyspnea and frequency of admissions for shortness of breath over the past year. He is referred to you for evaluation for possible lung transplantation.

He began smoking 1 to 2 packs of cigarettes a day at age 19. Initially, he complained of decreased exercise tolerance and a persistent minimally productive cough. Despite limiting himself to one half pack of cigarettes a day, his symptoms persisted and gradually worsened. He began to experience dyspnea walking one city block or climbing one flight of stairs. His cough increased in frequency with chronic production of yellow sputum.

QUESTION 1 The patient is very concerned about his future therapy. Specifically, he wants to know if he is a candidate for lung transplantation. Who are the patients who receive lung transplants?

The first successful lung transplant took place at the University of Toronto in 1983. Since then, 2330 patients have received single-lung transplants (as of January 1994). Idiopathic pulmonary fibrosis has been replaced by chronic obstructive pulmonary disease (COPD) as the most common indication for the procedure. Based on the St. Louis International Lung Transplant Registry, the most common diseases for which lung transplantation is undertaken are as follows: COPD (26.9%), idiopathic pulmonary fibrosis (16.4%), cystic fibrosis (14.9%), alpha-1 antitrypsin deficiency emphysema (13.4%), primary pulmonary hypertension (8.9%), and others (19.5%). In-

cluded in the latter category are infection, inflammatory, malignant, toxic, and environmental/occupational lung diseases.

QUESTION 2 He refused to seek medical advice until age 51, when he came to an emergency room and was found to have pneumonia, an elevated blood pressure, and stigmata of COPD. After appropriate therapy for pneumonia, pulmonary function tests revealed mild airway obstruction with an $FEV_{1.0}$ 41% of predicted, and an $FEV_{1.0}/FVC$ ratio of 66%. An exercise desaturation study on 2 L revealed desaturation to 87% after 3 minutes. He was treated with ipratoprium bromide and albuterol-metered dose inhalers with moderate improvement. Although he was able to stop smoking, his symptoms did not completely resolve. For the next 3 years, the frequency of hospital admissions increased. Inhaled steroids and oral theophylline were added with some relief, but admissions were necessary 2 to 3 times per year. Repeat exercise desaturation testing on room air revealed a saturation of 82% on room air after 1 ½ minutes of exercise and 85% on 2 L of oxygen. Subsequently, arterial blood gases revealed hypercapnia and hypoxemia, which initially resolved with therapy but worsened such that the patient was placed on home oxygen therapy. He was placed on oral steroids for each exacerbation but became increasingly difficult to wean, requiring varying doses of prednisone for the next 18 months. He has also noted intermittent bipedal edema. When should a patient be referred for a lung transplant evaluation?

The decision to refer a patient for evaluation is individualized and takes into consideration the underlying disease, the patient's rate of deterioration, and present level of function. Common indications for referral regardless of primary disease include an accelerated rate of deterioration, frequent hospitalizations, secondary pulmonary hypertension, resting hypoxemia (Pao$_2$ less than 60 mm Hg) or hypercapnia (Paco$_2$ greater than 50 mm Hg), and the postbronchodilator FEV$_{1.0}$ less than 30% of predicted.

Without the benefit of a formal laboratory workup the patient presented in this case has several reasons for transplant evaluation including a rapidly worsening clinical condition, resting hypoxemia, and evidence on physical examination of pulmonary hypertension (prominent S2, systolic murmur consistent with tricuspid regurgitation, and peripheral edema).

QUESTION 3 Physical examination revealed a mildly obese elderly man in no distress at rest, but notably short of breath with minimal exertion. He was on oxygen by nasal cannula. He was afebrile with a BP of 138/86 mm Hg, HR 88 bpm, RR 22/min. Head and neck examination was significant for JVD 4 cm above the sternal angle. There was a prolonged expiratory phase of breathing and with basilar rhonchi and scattered end-expiratory wheezes noted on auscultation. His family history is noncontributory. The patient was accepted for inpatient evaluation at the transplant center. How are lung transplant recipients selected?

The selection process involves two phases. The initial screening includes referral, wherein the patient is determined to have the appropriate clinical indications and is referred to a transplant center. This allows for the thorough review of the medical records and further physical examination. An important consideration is determination of any contraindications to transplant. Absolute contraindications include active or uncontrolled infection, systemic disease with nonpulmonary vital organ involvement, recent or active malignancy, significant left ventricular dysfunction or coronary disease, significant liver or kidney disease, recent or active smoking or substance abuse, and a history of medical noncompliance or psy-

chosocial disturbances. Relative contraindications are felt to be mechanical ventilation, prior cardiothoracic surgery or pleurodesis, severe osteoporosis, and current high-dose systemic corticosteroid use.

The second phase includes multiple laboratory tests and an extensive evaluation of cardiopulmonary function. These tests include ABO blood typing, HLA typing, and screening for viral titers (HIV, EBV, CMV, varicella-zoster, and hepatitis A, B, and C). Pulmonary testing involves arterial blood gases taken at rest and during exercise, pulmonary function tests, an exercise desaturation test, quantitative ventilation-perfusion lung scanning, and a CT scan of the chest. Evaluation of cardiac function is likewise extensive, being composed of radionuclide ventriculography, Doppler echocardiography, and right heart catheterization. If indicated, transesophageal echocardiography and left heart catheterization may be performed. Social, psychiatric, and nutritional consults may also be obtained.

The patient presented did not have any absolute contraindications. As far as his steroid requirement was concerned, it has been suggested that small doses (20 mg/day or less of prednisone) do not adversely affect outcome. Given that patients clinically stable on systemic steroids often deteriorate when these are withdrawn, titration to the lowest possible dose before transplant would be the ideal approach. The patient has also stopped smoking and appears to have a good mental outlook and stable social support.

As with all organ transplantation programs, donors are in short supply. Therefore, qualifications should include pulmonary disease not amenable to further medical or other surgical therapy and a limited life expectancy. This was formerly set at 1 year or less, but because of longer waiting periods, this has been changed to 18 months. The patient should be stable enough to survive the wait. Another result of the limited availability of donor organs is the philosophy of offering donor organs to the youngest patients and those most likely to survive the surgery. Age is accordingly a major factor with limits of 50 years or younger for heart-lung transplantation, 50 to 55 years for bilateral transplants, and 65 years for single-lung transplantation. Based on these criteria this patient would be eligible for only a single-lung transplantation.

An analysis of 211 patients referred to Washington University in St. Louis for lung transplant evaluation over a 12-month period beginning in April of 1988 showed that 50% were rejected after initial screening. Only 21% of these received full evaluation. The majority of remaining referrals were not pursued by either the physicians or the patients. Of those who underwent further assessment, only 7.6% of the original population eventually received transplants. The major reasons for rejection included age limits, systemic steroid use, cardiovascular disease (usually coronary artery disease), and other medical conditions. It must be emphasized, however, that since the time this study took place advances in surgical technique and further studies have eased the original strict selection criteria. For example, systemic corticosteroid therapy is no longer an absolute contraindication. The use of single-lung transplants for COPD as opposed to bilateral or heart-lung transplantation now allows older patients to be eligible for the procedure.

QUESTION 4 What are the types of lung transplantation, and what are the indications for each procedure?

Surgery may involve single-lung, bilateral lung, and heart-lung transplantation (SLT, BLT, and HLT, respectively). The choice between procedures is dependent on the underlying disease entity, patient age, and the presence or absence of chronic native lung infection and concomitant nonpulmonary medical conditions. With growing experience in this field, the indications for SLT and BLT have grown while those for HLT have decreased.

SLT was initially used for idiopathic pulmonary fibrosis. The relative success of the procedure was attributed to the preferential perfusion and ventilation of the allograft in the face of the high vascular resistance and low compliance of the native lung. SLT was less successful for COPD at the outset. However, it was found that SLT in this setting resulted in a relative increase in perfusion to the allograft combined with a relatively greater ventilation of the native lung as a result of lower compliance worsening the ventilation-perfusion mismatch. It was also thought that hyperinflation of the native lung would occur and cause compression of the allograft. Experience has shown these concerns to be erroneous and such problems attributable to avoidable complications that occurred in the allograft. SLT is now increasingly used in COPD with good results. More recent experience has shown SLT to have potential use in the setting of primary and secondary pulmonary hypertension, the traditional approach having been HLT.

BLT, once the procedure of choice in COPD, is now used in the presence of a chronic airway infection complicating the pulmonary disease. Examples include chronic bronchitis, cystic fibrosis, and bronchiectasis. The risk of a "spillover" infection from the native to the allograft lung precludes the use of SLT.

HLT is used less frequently because of the growing use of SLT combined with an increasing shortage of donors. There is also the added risk of complications affecting the transplanted heart, such as chronic rejection and accelerated coronary artery disease. HLT is thus indicated only in patients with pulmonary hypertension and congestive cardiomyopathy or irreparable cardiac defects.

QUESTION 5 What are the selection criteria for the donors?

At the University of Minnesota immunologic, functional, infectious, and anatomic criteria have been used. They required ABO matching between donor and recipient. Acceptable pulmonary function was demonstrated by a clear chest x-ray, a Pao_2 of 100 mm Hg or greater on an Fio_2 of 40%, and normal lung compliance (peak airway pressure of 30 mm Hg or less with normal tidal volume). There had to be no obvious pulmonary infection with secretions negative for gram-negative or fungal organisms on smear. Size matching was more critical in HLT and BLT with donor lungs having to be equal to or smaller in size compared to the recipient. A larger donor lung was tolerated in SLT.

The average waiting time for donors at this institution during this time (before 1991) naturally demonstrated a marked difference between heart-lung and lung-only transplants. In the former the wait was 384 ± 88 days, whereas it was 166 ± 39 days in the latter. The waiting time for SLT was 150 ± 42 days.

QUESTION 6 Initial screening at the transplant center revealed that his hypertension had been fairly well controlled on diltiazem. There was no evidence of hypercholesterolemia. For the past 9 months he had been on glyburide with good glycemic control. Other medications included albuterol, ipratopium bromide, triamcinolone-metered dose inhalers, and prednisone (15 mg/day). A dipyridamole-thallium study was performed 1 year ago for an episode of chest pain and was unremarkable. Further workup demonstrated a decline in the $FEV_{1.0}/FVC$ ratio to 28% with an $FEV_{1.0}$ of 0.45 L. A repeated exercise test was done with a marked reduction in exercise tolerance with marked worsening of abnormalities in ventilation and gas exchange responses compared to previous studies. Attempts to wean his steroids failed, and he had two hospital admissions for exacerbations of symptoms, each requiring mechanical ventilation. A quantitative perfusion scan of the right lung was 50.6% on the left and 49.4% on the right. Cardiac examination included an echocardiogram revealing pulmonary arterial hypertension and right ventricular hypertrophy and dilatation, confirmed by right heart catheterization. He had recurrence of atypical chest pain prompting a coronary angiogram that did not reveal significant coronary disease. He was accepted for lung transplantation, and after a 4-month wait, successfully underwent a SLT. He did well until the 9th postoperative day when he became febrile and dyspneic. He developed pro-gressive dyspnea, hypoxia, and new infiltrates in the allograft lung on chest radiographs. What might be the causes of his deterioration?

There are several possible causes including pulmonary edema resulting from reimplantation, hypervolemia, acute lung injury, pneumonia, acute allograft rejection, and airway complications.

Acute lung injury is the result of different processes including obstruction of the pulmonary venous anastomoses, poor allograft preservation, reperfusion injury, prolonged allograft ischemia, and unrecognized pneumonitis in the allograft. The incidence of acute injury varies between 8% and 20%, and treatment is primarily supportive with prolonged mechanical ventilation and extracorporeal membrane oxygenation.

Pneumonia is very common. Bacterial pneumonia develops in up to one third of patients during the first 2 weeks posttransplant. Gram-negative organisms and *S. aureus* are most common pathogens in bacterial infections, and empiric broad-spectrum perioperative antibiotic coverage is indicated, having been shown to significantly decrease early pneumonia. Cytomegalovirus pneumonitis is the most common infectious complication, with up to 70% of patients having histologic confirmation. Fungal infections are uncommon. Although *Candida* often colonizes the airway, invasive disease is rare. *Aspergillus* is a common agent for clinically significant pneumonia. Gancyclovir, effective in most cases of CMV pneumonia, is used in many institutions for prophylaxis, although such use is still controversial.

Acute rejection occurs in most patients commonly in the second posttransplant week. Histologic confirmation of the diagnosis by transbronchial biopsy reveals perivascular mononuclear infiltration as the characteristic findings. At the University of Pittsburgh, cyclosporine, azathioprine, and methylprednisolone are used as a perioperative immunosuppression protocol. Acute rejection is treated with a 3-day course of intravenous methylprednisolone. Recurrent or refractory episodes often require antithymocyte globulin. At the above institution, antithymocyte globulin, given as prophylaxis, was found to significantly reduce the frequency of acute rejection when compared to the standard immunosuppression regimen alone. All patients, however, suffered at least one episode of rejection, and there was no survival advantage noted. Another immunosuppressive agent, FK-506, is under investigation, and preliminary results suggest that it may reduce acute rejection and improve survival.

Posttransplantation airway abnormalities occur in about 25% of patients. They usually involve superficial mucosal necrosis distal to the anastomosis, which is of minor clinical significance. Dehiscence of the anastomosis with airway obstruction and atelectasis is less common and may require placement of an endobronchial stent.

The preceding discussion emphasizes the critical role of bronchoscopy and transbronchial biopsy in the immediate post-transplant period in the setting of clinical deterioration. A definite diagnosis must be made since the therapeutic approaches are very different. Transbronchial biopsy may even play a role in asymptomatic patients; in one study surveillance bronchoscopy and biopsy revealed an unsuspected diagnosis, usually acute rejection or CMV pneumonitis, in 57% of cases.

QUESTION 7   He was found to have acute rejection and responded to appropriate therapy. The remainder of his hospital stay was relatively uneventful.

Three months after discharge he reported a significantly improved sense of well being and improved exercise tolerance. Pulmonary function tests demonstrated a marked increase of his $FEV_{1.0}$ to 2.3 L (from 0.45 L) and the $FEV_{1.0}$/FVC ratio to 77% (from 28% predicted). He was also able to walk 1900 feet in an exercise test without desaturation.

What is the long-term prognosis for lung transplant patients, and what is the role of lung transplantation in the management of end-stage lung disease?

Pulmonary function, hemodynamics, and exercise capacity are criteria by which outcome is measured. Improvement can be seen in all of the above parameters. There is a decrease in pulmonary artery and right heart pressures and an increase in right ventricular ejection fraction. Patients with significant symptoms of congestive heart failure before transplant can improve their New York Heart Association functional class from III-IV to I-II.

A study involving a small number of patients compared the results of SLT and BLT for COPD. The immediate preoperative values for $FEV_{1.0}$ were 0.47 L and 0.49 L for SLT and BLT, respectively. At 12-weeks posttransplant, these had increased to 1.63 L for the SLT group and 3.44 L for the BLT group. The 6-minute walk test pretransplant and posttransplant distances were 780 and 1729 feet, respectively, for the SLT group. The corresponding figures for the BLT group were 829 and 2195 feet. It was speculated that some of the difference might be explained by a disparity in the average age of patients; the BLT group had an average age 15 years younger than those that received SLT. It is also unclear if these numbers translate into a significant difference in terms of the ability to perform activities of daily living or the quality of life.

Survival is another measure of outcome. According to the St. Louis International Transplant Registry, the overall 1- and 2-year survival up to 1992 was 68% and 69%, respectively, although individual centers reported better results. At the University of Pittsburgh, survival data showed similar outcomes for SLT and BLT that were better than those of HLT. Their data, accrued over 10 years (1982-1992), also revealed that patients who received transplants during the last year of that decade had a better 1-year survival rate (70%) than their predecessors (53%). The underlying disease also plays a role with the best outcomes seen in patients with emphysema. Those with cystic fibrosis complicated by multiple resistant organisms fare relatively poorly.

The causes of death vary depending on the duration since the transplant. Bleeding, technical

Chronic lung disease
    Accelerated rate of deterioration
    Frequent hospitalizations
    Secondary pulmonary arterial hypertension
    PaO_2 <60 mm Hg or $PaCO_2$ >50 mm Hg
    Postbronchial $FEV_{1.0}$ <30% predicted
    No improvement with maximal therapy

Consider lung transplantation
Primary evaluation

Relative contraindications
  Mechanical ventilation
  Previous cardiothoracic
    surgery or pleurodesis
  Severe osteoporosis
  High dose steroid use

Absolute contraindications
  Acute or uncontrolled infector
  Other systemic diseases
  Malignancy
  Significant LV dysfunction or coronary
    artery disease
  Hepatic or renal failure
  Recent or current smoking
  Medical noncompliance

Secondary evaluation
  Blood and HLA typing
  Viral serology
  Exercise and rest arterial blood gas determinations
  Pulmonary function testing
  Ventilation/perfusion scanning
  Chest CT
  Cardiac function evaluation
  Chest x-ray

Waiting period for SLT 150 ±42 days

Transplantation

Early deterioration
  Pulmonary edema (etiology—post-perfusion)
  Airway disease (mucosa, anastomosis)
  Acute lung injury
  Pneumonia (bacterial, viral)
  Acute rejection (requires biopsy)

Late deterioration
  Infection
  Chronic rejection (follow $FEV_{1.0}$)
  Bronchiolitis obliterans

11-11-1   Diagnostic approach to chronic lung disease.

difficulties, graft dysfunction, and infection are the major causes of death in the early post-transplant period. After the first year infection continues to be a problem, but chronic rejection becomes the major concern. Patients with chronic rejection may present with exertional dyspnea, fatigue, and cough. Pulmonary function tests reveal decreased airflow in the midvital capacity range of FEF_{25-75} consistent with small airways disease as the earliest abnormality. A decline in the $FEV_{1.0}$, $FEV_{1.0}/FVC$ ratio and TLC reflect more severe disease. The diagnosis is made by transbronchial biopsy and commonly reveals bronchiolitis obliterans. Therapy involves a combination of corticosteroids and antilymphocyte agents such as OKT-3 and antithymocyte globulin. The best approach is prevention and is dependent on adequate maintenance immunosuppressive regimen including prednisone, cyclosporine, and azathioprine.

Lung transplantation is no longer felt to be experimental and is a therapeutic option in the appropriate patient. Better surgical techniques and immunosuppression have been instrumental in the increasing success of lung transplants. Donor shortage, however, is a growing problem. Improved allograft preservation and expanded use of SLT may help alleviate the shortage. Acute and chronic rejection is still a concern, and the effectiveness of new agents such as FK 506 remains to be seen. The present environment of health care reform and cost containment will also limit the availability of lung transplantation for wider use. A diagnostic algorithm for chronic lung disease is shown in Fig. 11-1-1.

CASE FOLLOW-UP The patient now resides at home and participates in a pulmonary rehabilitation program. He is considering returning to work on a limited basis. The most recent pulmonary function tests are an $FEV_{1.0}$ of 2.57 L, FVC of 3.33 L, $FEV_{1.0}/FVC\%$ 77%, and a DLCO of 71%.

BIBLIOGRAPHY

Bolman RM, et al: Lung and heart transplantation: evolution and new applications, *Ann Surg* 214:456-470, 1991.

Calhoon JH, et al: Single lung transplantation: alternative indications and techniques, *J Thorac Cardiovasc Surg* 101:816-829, 1991.

Cooper JD: Lung transplantation for chronic obstructive lung disease, *Ann NY Acad Sci* 624:209-211, 1991.

Egan TM, et al: Analysis of referrals for lung transplantation, *Chest* 99:867-870, 1991.

Egan TM, et al: Isolated lung transplantation for end-stage lung disease: a viable theory, *Ann Thorac Surg* 144:433-451, 1992.

Emery RW, et al: Treatment of end-stage chronic obstructive pulmonary disease with double lung transplantation, *Chest* 3:533-537, 1991.

Ettinger NA, Cooper JD: Lung transplantation. In Baum BE, Wolinsky E, eds: *Textbook of pulmonary disease,* Boston, 1994, Little, Brown.

Ettinger NA, Trulock EP: Pulmonary considerations of organ transplantation, *Am Rev Respir Dis* 144:433-451, 1991.

Griffith BP, et al: A decade of lung transplantation, *Ann Surg* 218:310-320, 1993.

Mal H, et al: Unilateral lung transplantation in end-stage pulmonary emphysema, *Am Rev Respir Dis* 140:797-802, 1989.

Pasque MK, Trulock EP, et al: Single lung transplantation for pulmonary hypertension, *Circulation* 84:2275-2279, 1991.

Trulock EP, et al: The role of transbronchial biopsy in the treatment of lung transplant recipients, *Chest* 102:1049-1054, 1992.

Trulock EP, et al: The Washington University-Barnes Hospital experience with lung transplantation, *JAMA* 266:1943-1946, 1991.

C A S E

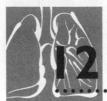

12
Charles J. Grodzin
James J. Herdegen
• • • • • • • • • •

It is your first day on the pulmonary consult service. After morning rounds you are informed that there is a patient in the emergency room to be evaluated. Upon arrival you find the patient to be a 71-year-old man who came to the emergency room with complaints of worsening shortness of breath over the last 5 days. His wife tells you that he has been more short of breath walking through the house, an activity that he is usually able to accomplish. Furthermore, you learn of a 70 pack-year smoking history and that the patient uses 2 L of oxygen by nasal cannula continuously at home. He has a chronic cough, but his sputum production has not changed in amount or character. He denies recent fever, chills, nausea, vomiting, night sweats, or leg edema.

QUESTION I From the patient's history of smoking, use of continuous oxygen, and chronic cough, you are concerned that he has chronic lung disease. What do the terms *chronic obstructive lung disease (COPD), chronic bronchitis, emphysema, bronchiectasis, bullae,* and *bleb* mean?

Chronic obstructive pulmonary disease is a category of chronic lung disease within which processes are characterized by the obstruction of airflow during exhalation and pulmonary hyperinflation. There are two predominant types: chronic bronchitis and emphysema. Although distinctly different, most patients manifest elements of both processes.

Chronic bronchitis is characterized by a history of chronic cough lasting for 3 weeks in 2 consecutive years. This disease process is most commonly a result of smoking. Patients manifest cough,

sputum production, and recurrent respiratory tract infections with *S. pneumoniae* and *H. influenzae*. These patients are described as "blue bloaters" because of their propensity to become cyanotic (blue) and develop lower extremity edema (bloater) as a result of right ventricular heart failure. Gas exchange is also impaired. Hypercapnia is invariably found, and hypoxemia may be present as a result of ventilation/perfusion mismatching.

Emphysema is characterized by the combination of parenchymal lung destruction and airflow obstruction. Smoking is the leading cause of emphysema. The primary insult is destruction of alveolar septae that decreases the lung's elastic recoil and surface area for diffusion. Patients are described as "pink puffers" because they rarely become hypoxemic (remain pink) and maintain a rapid respiratory rate (puffer). Patients complain more commonly of dyspnea and less of cough and sputum production. Since hypoxia is less common, patients do not develop pulmonary arterial hypertension and cor pulmonale.

There are three types of emphysema: panacinar, centriacinar, and distal acinar. **Panacinar** emphysema is characterized by loss of distinction between alveolar ducts and alveoli. **Centriacinar** emphysema is due to damage to the respiratory bronchiole and all distal structures. The lower lobes are predominantly involved. This is the type of emphysema associated with alpha-1-antitrypsin deficiency. **Distal acinar** emphysema is due to damage to the alveolar ducts and alveoli themselves. The subpleural location of this insult predisposes to a more significant risk of pneumothorax as compared to other types. The major differences between chronic bronchi-

TABLE 11-12-1   Chronic Obstructive Lung Disease: Characteristics

	Emphysema	Chronic Bronchitis
Age of onset	60+	50+
Dyspnea	Severe	Mild
Cough	After onset of dyspnea	Before onset of dyspnea
Sputum	Scanty	Copious
Infection	Infrequent	Frequent
Episodes of respiratory insufficiency	Progressive until terminal clinical status	Recurrent
Chest radiograph	Hyperinflation with bullous changes	Increased bronchovascular markings at bases
Pa_{CO_2} (mm Hg)	35-40	50-60
Pa_{O_2} (mm Hg)	65-75	45-60
Hematocrit (%)	35-40	50-55
Cor pulmonale	Less common until terminal decompensation	Common
Elastic recoil	Severe decrease	Normal
Airway resistance	Normal	High
Diffusion capacity	Decreased	Normal or slightly increased

tis and emphysema are summarized in Table 11-12-1.

Bronchiectasis refers to a fixed dilatation of bronchi with thickened walls resulting from chronic inflammation. This most commonly occurs secondary to recurrent infection. The most common associated diseases are cystic fibrosis, immunoglobulin deficiency, and those associated with abnormal ciliary function (dyskinetic cilia syndrome, yellow nail syndrome, Young's syndrome). Bronchiectasis may be classified as either cylindrical, saccular, or cystic. These airways are frequently colonized with bacteria leading to chronic foul-smelling purulent sputum. Clubbing, weight loss, fever, and hemoptysis are common symptoms. Thickened bronchial walls on longitudinal section may appear as parallel "tram tracks" on chest radiography. High resolution CT scanning is now the most popular modality to demonstrate thickened bronchial walls.

Bullae are emphysematous spaces greater than 10 mm in diameter. These spaces can enlarge and cause problems as a result of compression and obstruction of other airways or vessels. Blebs refer specifically to collections of air in layers of the pleura.

QUESTION 2 You have a strong suspicion, based on the history, that the patient may have COPD. What are the important epidemiologic facts about COPD?

Chronic bronchitis is the most common form of COPD, followed by asthma and emphysema. COPD ranks as the fifth most common cause of death (3.4% of deaths in 1985). Emphysema is a disproportionate cause of death in the elderly population (50.5/100,000 in 75- to 84-year-old age group). The frequency of chronic bronchitis is greater in women, while emphysema is more common in men. Chronic bronchitis is more prevalent in the western United States, whereas emphysema predominates in the southern United States.

QUESTION 3 The patient's medications included a Ventolin inhaler, prednisone 10 mg/day, xanax, and buspirone. On physical examination the patient is found sitting upright in bed. Vital signs are T 99.6°F, RR 20/min, HR 102 bpm, and BP 133/78 mm Hg. On inspection he was barrel-chested with retraction of the chest wall during inspiration. He had reduced breath sounds to auscultation without egophony and resonance to percussion. Inspection of the abdomen revealed inward movement during inspiration. There was no lower extremity tenderness or edema. The cardiac examination was normal. What are the physical examination signs of COPD? What changes are seen on chest x-ray and electrocardiogram?

The physical examination is an important part of the evaluation when COPD is suspected. Depending on the underlying disease process, the patient can be categorized as a "pink puffer" or "blue bloater" as described. Hyperinflation caused by airflow obstruction results in an increased AP diameter leading to a barrel-chested appearance. This leads to flattening of the diaphragm, decreased diaphragmatic excursion, and paradoxical inward retraction of the chest wall during inspiration (Hoover's sign).

Airway collapse leads to pursed lip breathing and a prolonged expiratory phase. Use of accessory muscles may be seen, chiefly the intercostals and scalenes. The tripod sign (patient leaning forward with hands on knees) is a posture that places the sternocleidomastoid and scalene muscles at their maximal mechanical advantage. Breath sounds are usually globally diminished, and wheezing may be present. While clubbing is not seen with COPD, it may accompany the development of bronchiectasis or other suppurative complications.

The chest x-ray also reflects hyperinflation. The chest has a widened AP diameter with flattened diaphragms (appreciable on lateral chest x-ray). This is also manifest as an increase in the depth of the retrosternal air space. This space is abnormal when the distance from the sternum to the most anterior part of the ascending aorta is greater than 2.5 cm. Hyperlucency of the lungs, attenuation of the pulmonary vasculature, and

narrowing of the cardiac shadow are also seen. Compression of the trachea ("saber sheath trachea") can be seen as a result of surrounding overinflation.

Nicklaus et al. defined radiographic criteria as the most supportive of the diagnosis of COPD. These include attenuation of the pulmonary vessels, flattening of the diaphragms in the AP and lateral films, an irregular radiolucent parenchymal pattern, and increased depth of the retrosternal airspace.

The cardiac examination may reveal signs of right-sided heart failure caused by cor pulmonale. These include jugular venous distension, hepatojugular reflux, lower extremity edema, a loud, fixed, and split S2.

Pulmonary hypertension should be suspected if signs of right-sided heart failure are found. The pulmonary arteries are enlarged when the diameter exceeds 16 mm on the right and 20 mm on the left on an inspiratory chest x-ray.

The electrocardiogram reflects strain on the right ventricle resulting from pulmonary hypertension. These include P-pulmonale, right ventricular hypertrophy, right axis deviation, and a right bundle branch block.

QUESTION 4   The chest x-ray is now available and reveals an increased AP diameter, flattening of the diaphragms, and an increased retrosternal air space. The lung fields have heterogeneous density. The electrocardiogram has a right axis deviation and right bundle branch block. Laboratory evaluation revealed a WBC count of 14,000 without a left shift and a serum $[HCO_3]$ of 34 mEq/L. An arterial blood gas on 2 L of oxygen by nasal cannula was pH 7.29/ Pao_2 53 mm Hg/ $Paco_2$ of 70 mm Hg. The patient's internist tells you that his baseline blood gas is pH 7.34/$Paco_2$ 60 mm Hg/Pao_2 of 61 mm Hg with a $[HCO_3]$ of 33 mEq/L. What is your impression of these laboratory values?

This patient has developed the typical acid-base abnormality associated with COPD. The primary problem is ventilatory insufficiency and retention of CO_2. This leads to a respiratory acidosis. Retention of $[HCO_3]$ is the metabolic compensatory response. Acutely, the serum $[HCO_3]$ rises by 0.1 mEq/L for each mm Hg rise in the P_{CO_2} from baseline. In chronic respiratory acidosis the serum $[HCO_3]$ rises by 0.4 mEq/L for each mm Hg rise in the P_{CO_2} from baseline. Therefore, the pH remains close to the normal range although an acidosis persists.

In our patient there appears to be an acute process. The retention of CO_2 has led to a significant acidosis without HCO_3 retention to buffer the change of pH. The small change in $[HCO_3]$ seen acutely is the reason that the pH is lower.

Hypoxemia and hypercapnia are well tolerated in COPD and may fluctuate by 5 to 10 mm Hg without consequence. In patients with chronic respiratory acidosis, buffering maintains the pH in a near-normal range. Therefore, the best marker for assessing severity of illness is pH.

Immediate goals of oxygenation are modest. Acutely, the goal of Pa_{O_2} is 55 to 60 mm Hg. Raising the arterial Pa_{O_2} in an acutely ill patient with obstructive lung disease may lead to further CO_2 retention in part caused by development of more severe ventilation—perfusion mismatching. High levels of CO_2 may lead to depression of the patient's mental status and further hypoventilation. Additionally, overoxygenation will offset the mechanisms of HCO_3 retention. Should this occur, the patient is placed at major risk of significant acidosis superimposed on the compensatory respiratory alkalosis. When the patient returns to breathing lower concentrations of oxygen, he can develop more significant respiratory acidosis because the underlying buffering system (renal retention of bicarbonate) has been removed. Therefore, adequate oxygenation should be approached from below with small amounts of supplemental oxygen. Underoxygenation may be life threatening. Allowing a patient to remain hypoxemic increases right ventricular afterload and may impair reversal of the primary problem (bronchospasm, cardiac ischemia, respiratory muscle fatigue, etc.).

QUESTION 5 What is the role of cigarette smoking as an etiology of COPD? What are the important aspects of alpha-1 antitrypsin deficiency?

Smoking is the leading risk factor for the development of COPD. The risk of COPD in smokers is 30 times greater than non-smokers. Smoking is responsible for 80% to 90% of deaths related to COPD. A dose response relationship exists between smoking and development of airways obstruction. Cessation of smoking leads to improvement of lung function and a decline in the rate of deterioration. Additional factors that diminish lung function are air pollution, environmental exposures, passive smoking, and an ill-defined genetic predisposition to aggressive lung destruction.

Alpha-1 antitrypsin deficiency (A1AT) demonstrates codominant inheritance with early onset lower lobe bullous disease. A1AT is an antiprotease that functions to inactivate elastase elaborated by neutrophils. When deficient, the protease/antiprotease balance shifts toward increased protease activity. The most common symptom is progressive dyspnea. Smoking plays an additive role by recruiting neutrophils to the lung, inactivating A1AT enzyme activity, and opposing elastin resynthesis. The threshold level above which lung disease does *not* occur is 11 µmol/L.

QUESTION 6 At this point you suspect that the patient has COPD. The morning after admission, the patient's attending physician brings the patient's most recent pulmonary function results to the floor. They are as follows:

	DATA	% PREDICTED
FVC	2.79	70%
$FEV_{1.0}$	0.87	32%
$FEV_{1.0}/FVC$	31.2	—
DL/VA	2.05	47%
TLC	6.51	103%
FRC	5.15	155%
RV	3.53	155%

FVC = forced vital capacity; $FEV_{1.0}$ = forced expiratory volume in one second; DL/VA = diffusion capacity corrected for alveolar ventilation; TLC = total lung capacity; FRC = flunctional residual capacity; RV = residual volume.

What is your interpretation of these pulmonary function tests?

The above pulmonary function tests demonstrate the cardinal findings in a patient with COPD. A reduction of the $FEV_{1.0}$ may be seen in restrictive and obstructive lung disease. However, reduction of the $FEV_{1.0}$/FVC ratio is the hallmark of obstructive disease. In cases of restrictive lung disease, the $FEV_{1.0}$/FVC ratio remains normal.

Hyperinflation is also evident in analysis of the lung volumes. The residual volume is the amount of air left in the lung after maximal forced expiration. In COPD, airway closure results in increased air trapping distal to the site of airway collapse increasing the total lung capacity, functional residual capacity, and residual volume.

The patient also has a diffusion abnormality (DL/VA 47%). The combination of hyperinflation with a diffusion abnormality points toward emphysema. In this disease, diffusion is reduced as a result of loss of lung surface area from parenchymal destruction.

QUESTION 7 You are also informed that the patient had undergone an exercise desaturation test. On room air the patient was only able to walk 3' 15" with desaturation to 84% after 2' 30". After application of I L of oxygen by nasal cannula, he was able to ambulate 4' 30" without desaturation. Therefore, he was placed on continuous nasal cannula oxygen at home at I L. What are the qualifications and benefits of oxygen therapy in COPD?

A patient should be placed on continuous oxygen therapy when he meets either of the following criteria: (1) Pao_2 less than 55 mm Hg on room air or (2) Pao_2 between 55 and 59 mm Hg in the presence of lower extremity edema, polycythemia, or cor pulmonale. It is necessary to reevaluate each patient 3 months after institution of oxygen therapy because aggressive standard therapy with bronchodilators and corticosteroids can improve oxygenation and obviate supplemental needs. It is common to see an elevation of the $Paco_2$ from baseline levels after beginning oxygen therapy. As long as this stabilizes, it is well tolerated.

For patients with cor pulmonale oxygen improves prognosis and decreases right ventricular afterload caused by pulmonary artery dilatation. In the American Nocturnal Oxygen Therapy Trial, continuous 24-hour therapy decreased pulmonary hypertension and decreased right heart strain. In addition, therapy has been shown to ameliorate polycythemia, improve neuropsychiatric function, and subjective quality of life and longevity.

QUESTION 8 What are the most important tenets of therapy for an exacerbation of chronic obstructive lung disease?

Bronchodilators are a major treatment modality. Beta-agonists (albuterol) cause smooth muscle relaxation and bronchodilatation. Beta-agonists should be used as the major treatment for acute bronchospasm and can be given consecutively. When the patient is more comfortable, the duration between treatments can be lengthened. Inhaled anticholinergic agents should also be used. These agents block parasympathetic-mediated bronchoconstriction. Ipratropium bromide is the anticholinergic agent of choice. In an acute exacerbation a good strategy is to alternate treatments with these agents every 1 to 2 hours. A moderate level of bronchodilatation may also occur after infusion of magnesium. While the onset and offset of action are rapid (2 to 20 minutes), this may be enough to allow administration of more potent therapy.

Systemic corticosteroids are also a major treatment modality. The effect of corticosteroids does not occur until 6 to 8 hours after administration.

Therefore, steroids counteract the late broncho-spastic response related to airway inflammation. Steroids can be administered in either the oral or intravenous form with equal efficacy. Intrave-nously, solumedrol (0.5 to 2 mg/kg q8h) is the agent of choice, whereas orally, prednisone (1 mg/kg) may be given. Typically, high-dose therapy is begun acutely and tapered gradually over the next 7 to 10 days as the patient's dyspnea improves. For some patients the taper period may extend into long-term maintenance therapy at as low a dose as tolerated.

After acute therapy, an important consider-ation is in which unit to admit the patient. Admission of the acutely ill COPD patient to the intensive care unit avoids underestimation of the degree of physiologic compromise. Close moni-toring and observation allow rapid therapy of any secondary cardiopulmonary embarrassment. In-dications for admission to the intensive care unit include acute respiratory acidosis, altered mental status, new infiltrates on chest x-ray, more severe hypoxemia, if the cause for the acute problem is unknown or if clinical evaluation is concerning. Clearly sedatives should be withheld. Intubation and mechanical ventilation should be held as a treatment of last resort for patients with obstruc-tive lung disease.

When a patient demonstrates increased spu-tum production or a change in the character of the sputum, antibiotics are indicated. Because the most common organisms in this population are *S. pneumoniae* and *H. influenzae,* antibiotic therapy should be targeted at these organisms.

The use of theophylline is controversial for acute exacerbations of COPD and chronic therapy. Use of theophylline is limited by its narrow thera-peutic range. Adverse effects include tachycardia, arrhythmias (multifocal atrial tachycardia), sei-zure, nausea, vomiting, and agitation. There are also many drug interactions. Theophylline levels are elevated by concomitant use of quinolone and macrolide antibiotics, allopurinol, oral con-traceptive pills, and cimetidine. Theophylline me-tabolism is increased by phenytoin, rifampin, and barbiturates. Currently, a prudent approach to use

ACUTE EXACERBATIONS OF COPD: TEN COMMANDMENTS

* Thou shalt not unwisely admit thy patient to the floor.
* Thou shalt not overoxygenate thy patient.
* Thou shalt not underoxygenate thy patient.
* Thou shalt not undertreat with bronchodilators and corticosteroids.
* Thou shalt not unwisely sedate thy patient.
* Thou shalt not intubate thy patient unwisely.
* Thou shalt not allow thy patient to become alkalemic.
* Thou shalt not make thy intubated patient struggle to breathe.
* Thou shalt not prolong weaning unnecessarily.
* Thou shalt not starve thy patient.

From Pierson DJ: Approach to the patient with acute-on-chronic ventilatory failure: "10 commandments" for the clinician. In Pierson DJ, Kocmorek RM, eds: Foundations of respiratory care, New York, 1992, Churchill Livingstone.

of theophylline is to continue treatment in pa-tients who derive clear benefit and to maintain serum levels in the low range. Theophylline should not be used therapeutically in acute exac-erbations of COPD.

When heart failure is discovered, appropriate specific therapy is warranted. In particular, ad-ministration of oxygen may produce pulmonary artery dilatation and reduce right ventricular af-terload.

It is important not to underestimate the impor-tance of adequate nutrition. Provision of adequate calories, above baseline needs, is associated with enhanced respiratory muscle strength. Since the metabolic product of carbohydrates is carbon dioxide, diets with high carbohydrate content may place stress on the respiratory system. There-fore, protein and lipids should make up the predominance of calories.

All patients should receive yearly influenza vaccination as well as the 23-valent pneumococ-cal vaccination every 10 years.

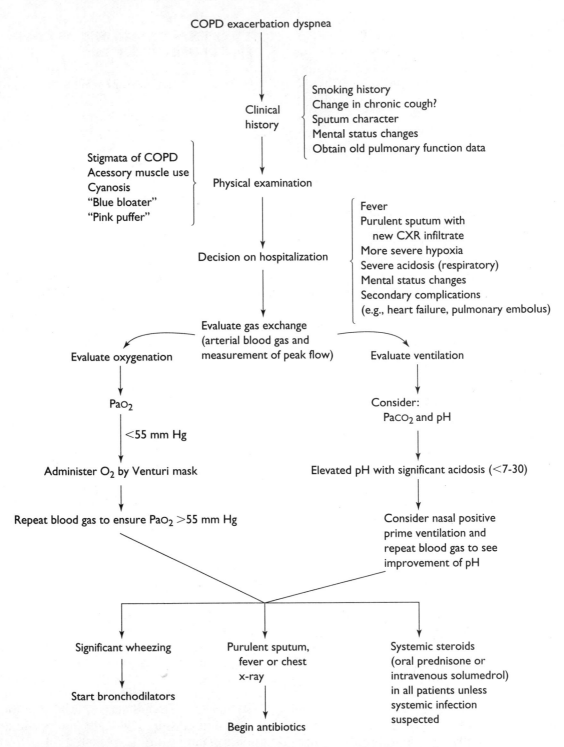

COPD exacerbation dyspnea

Clinical history

Smoking history
Change in chronic cough?
Sputum character
Mental status changes
Obtain old pulmonary function data

Stigmata of COPD
Acessory muscle use
Cyanosis
"Blue bloater"
"Pink puffer"

Physical examination

Decision on hospitalization

Fever
Purulent sputum with
    new CXR infiltrate
More severe hypoxia
Severe acidosis (respiratory)
Mental status changes
Secondary complications
(e.g., heart failure, pulmonary embolus)

Evaluate gas exchange
(arterial blood gas and
measurement of peak flow)

Evaluate oxygenation

Evaluate ventilation

PaO_2

Consider:
$PaCO_2$ and pH

<55 mm Hg

Administer O_2 by Venturi mask

Elevated pH with significant acidosis (<7-30)

Repeat blood gas to ensure PaO_2 >55 mm Hg

Consider nasal positive
prime ventilation and
repeat blood gas to see
improvement of pH

Significant wheezing

Purulent sputum,
fever or chest
x-ray

Systemic steroids
(oral prednisone or
intravenous solumedrol)
in all patients unless
systemic infection
suspected

Start bronchodilators

Begin antibiotics

11-12-1 Diagnostic approach to chronic obstructive pulmonary disease.

The box on p. 719 summarizes some of the important concepts concerning the acute therapy of an exacerbation of chronic obstructive lung disease.

CASE FOLLOW-UP The patient was admitted to the intensive care unit. He received 60 mg prednisone orally as well as alternating albuterol and atrovent by med-nebulizer every 2 hours. The steroid dose was tapered over the next 6 days. Med-nebulizer treatments were replaced by an albuterol-metered dose inhaler. The patient's exercise tolerance improved so that he was ambulating in the halls without dyspnea. He is to see you in the outpatient clinic 1 week after discharge.

• •

BIBLIOGRAPHY

Bone RC, Dantzker DR, George RB, et al: *Pulmonary and critical care medicine*, Part G, St Louis, 1994, Mosby.

Fraser RG, Pare JA, Pare PD, et al: *Diagnosis of diseases of the chest*, vol 1, Philadelphia, 1990, WB Saunders.

George RB, Light RW, Matthay MA, Matthay RA: *Chest medicine: essentials of pulmonary and critical care medicine*, ed 2, Baltimore, 1990, Williams & Wilkins.

RHEUMATOLOGY

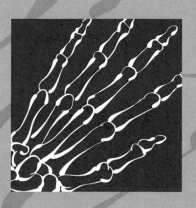

CALVIN BROWN
SECTION EDITOR

CASE

Charlotte Harris

A 42-year-old man came to the emergency room complaining of a swollen, painful right ankle. For the week before presentation he had experienced generalized achiness. His symptoms first started in his right shoulder, then moved to his knees, and then to his left wrist before localizing to the right ankle. None of these joints became swollen. He did feel feverish, but did not take his temperature until the day of presentation when it was 100.5°F. There was no history of trauma. He has smoked 1 pack of cigarettes/day for the last 23 years, drinks 12 beers/week, and is sexually active with more than one partner.

QUESTION 1 What are the key elements concerning the evaluation of joint complaints?

The evaluation of joint complaints is important chiefly because it may be the initial presenting element of a systemic disease and because now, as opposed to the past, there are many effective treatments available for the rheumatic diseases. Because joint pain can be a manifestation of a systemic disease, a full history and physical examination should be carried out. The physical examination is important because local soft tissue conditions may cause tenderness or swelling and be confused with synovitis. Examination includes inspection for the presence of erythema, palpation for bony or synovial irregularity as well as heat, comparison to other unaffected joints or the examiner's own normal joints and range of motion. The presence of crepitus suggests friction between moving joint components. Ballotment of the patella supports the presence of excessive synovial fluid. Palpation of the joint should be performed from multiple directions to reduce the possibility of pain coming from a focal area of bony or tendon tenderness.

QUESTION 2 For the patient presented, what is the differential diagnosis of a monoarticular arthritis?

The most commonly seen causes of a monarticular arthritis are infectious arthritis, crystalline induced arthritis, and monarticular presentations of inflammatory arthritis such as rheumatoid arthritis or rheumatic fever. In the case of infectious arthritis, microorganisms (bacteria, fungi, viruses) reach the joint through hematogenous spread. There is a predilection for previously damaged joints (i.e., sites of previous trauma, infection, arthritis, or sites of prosthetic joint implants). Inquiry about other sites as a source of bacteremia is important including cellulitis, recent dental work, urinary symptoms, symptoms of pharyngitis or otitis, etc., should all be made. The presence of infectious arthritis is considered a rheumatologic emergency and requires rapid institution of antibiotics and joint space drainage. Tuberculous arthritis may be found in immunocompromised individuals including the elderly, alcoholics, diabetics, and the malnourished.

Generally, calcium pyrophosphate deposition disease (Pseudogout) occurs in people who are older than our patient. Crystals are rhomboid and weakly positively birefringent. Radiography can reveal meniscal calcification of the infected joint. Alternatively, gout could also present in a man in his forties. The classic presentation of gout is the acute development of severe pain, erythema, and swelling of the great toe; however, other joints can be involved. Crystal analysis reveals negatively birefringent crystals that are intracellular and extracellular. Uric acid crystals are the product of purine metabolism. Risk factors include increased dietary intake of purines (red meats), overproduction of urate from cellular breakdown (tumor lysis, crush injury, carcinomatosis), altered metabolism (Lesch-Nyhan syndrome and HGPRT deficiency), decreased renal excretion, acidosis, thiazide diuretics, lead poisoning, and alcohol abuse. Cystic bony lesions may develop and be visible on x-ray.

The acute gouty episode may be accompanied by systemic complaints including fever, malaise, and leukocytosis. In chronic tophaceous gout, collections of white chalky material may be seen subcutaneously or extrude through the skin. Involvement more commonly involves the Achilles tendon, first metacarpophalangeal joint, elbow, and pinna of the ear. Treatment includes NSAIDs, colchicine, and intraarticular steroid injection.

An inflammatory arthritis that can present in a migratory polyarthritic manner is rheumatic fever. This is an inflammatory process that is thought to be autoimmune in etiology. Certain Group-A beta-hemolytic streptococci have an M-protein molecule or antigens on the cell wall with epitopes that share antigenic elements present in the heart. Therefore, a cross-reactive antibody can be produced that initiates an inflammatory process in the heart, joint, skin, or central nervous system. This can cause manifestations of cardites, erythema marginatum, Syndeham's chorea, or arthritis. The minor Jones criteria include arthralgia, fever, elevated ESR or CRP, prolonged PR interval on EKG, previous rheumatic fever, and preexisting rheumatic heart disease. Diagnosis is supported by the presence of two major criteria or one major and two minor criteria.

Because of the previous streptococcal infection there should be elevation of antistreptolysin O (greater than 200 to 250 Todd units), anti-DNAase or antihyaluronidase. One should also attempt to confirm the presence of infection with direct pharyngeal culture. The development of rheumatic fever is more often seen with exudative pharyngitis, longer persistence of streptococcal carriage in the pharynx, and higher ASO titers.

The most common symptoms include arthritis in 75% of patients, carditis is seen in 40% to 50%, chorea in 15%, and skin involvement in 10% of patients. Joint involvement is migratory and located in large joints and may be mild to debilitating with severe inflammation. *Jaccouds arthritis* is seen in cases of post-rheumatic fever arthropathy and is not an arthritis but the periarticular fibrosis resultant to repetitive bouts of joint inflammation.

Heart involvement can be manifest as a murmur, cardiomegaly, conduction disturbances, valve disease, and pericarditis. This is the most important symptom as it is the only manifestation of rheumatic fever that may be lethal. A diastolic murmur, known as the *Carey-Coombs murmur,* and tachycardia while sleeping are unusual associations. Valvular damage most commonly involves the mitral valve followed in order by the aortic, tricuspid, and pulmonic valves.

Sydenham's chorea, otherwise known as "St. Vitus' dance" is characterized by rapid purposeless movements, involving the face and extremities, jerky speech, and a "bag of worms" tongue due to muscle fasciculations. Characteristically, the tongue retracts involuntarily when protruded.

Subcutaneous skin nodules are seen overlying the spinous processes of the vertebrae, wrists, and occiput. These nodules do not involve the overlying skin. Erythema marginatum begins as a focal erythematous lesion that enlarges with a circinate or serpiginous border. When raised it may be known as erythema annulare. The lesion may be evanescent and may be seen to change in front of the examiner's eyes. Rheumatic fever can recur with significantly immunogenic streptococcal infection with the same serotype streptococcus.

A sexual history may yield important information. Reiter's syndrome is associated with the presence of HLA-B27 in approximately 90% of patients. Rheumatoid factor is absent and classifies this syndrome as a seronegative arthropathy. It is a reactive arthritis that may follow a diarrheal illness or sexually transmitted disease. Infection with *Chlamydia trachomatis, Salmonella, Shigella,* and *Yersisnia enterocolitica* can precede the arthritis. The triad of arthritis, conjunctivitis, and urethritis is classically described. Additional findings may include iritis, circinate balanitis, keratoderma blennorrhagicum, and buccal ulceration. Points where tendons insert into bone can become inflamed, and this is known as an *enthesopathy*. Another characteristic site of enthesopathy is inflammation at the insertion of the Achilles tendon which has been called "lover's heel." Twenty percent of patients will develop sacroiliitis. Synovial fluid is noninflammatory with elevated complement levels. Long-term sequelae can be seen in the originally affected organ systems including blindness, destructive joint disease, and urethral strictures. Up to 80% of patients will have evidence of disease at 5 years. Symptomatic palliation includes NSAIDs and sulfasalazine for severe disease refractory to NSAIDs.

Psoriatic arthritis is another seronegative arthropathy characterized by the presence of enthesopathy (Fig. 12-1-1). It is usually accompanied by characteristic psoriasiform skin lesions, nail changes including transverse ridging, pitting, onycholysis and hyperkeratosis, uveitis, and sacroiliitis. There is a strong genetic pattern of inheritance as well as HLA association with HLA-B27 being the most common (seen in 20%) along with B13, Bw17, and Cw6. However, about 50% of patients are HLA-B27 negative.

Patterns of arthritis include distal interphalangeal joint involvement associated with nail changes, symmetric polyarthritis, asymmetric oligoarthritis, psoriatic spondylitis and, arthritis mutilans (5% of cases). Radiographically, the pencil-in-cup deformity is seen. There is erosion of the middle phalanx with splaying of the base of the distal phalanx.

Dissemination of a genital gonococcal infection can lead to a monoarticular arthritis. It may present as a migratory arthralgia that then settles into one inflamed joint. The joint appears edematous, swollen, and erythematous and is tender to flexion/extension. Aspiration of synovial fluid yields suppurative material from which the organism may be cultured. As with any other septic arthritis, prompt antibiotic therapy is essential to therapy.

Hematologic abnormalities can also lead to joint symptoms. Coagulopathies or use of anticoagulants can lead to hemarthrosis and present as a monarticular process. Hemoglobinopathies can be associated with a single painful joint that may be difficult to distinguish from an inflammatory monarthritis.

Less common causes of monoarticular arthritis include: ischemic bone necrosis (avascular necrosis), pauci-articular juvenile arthritis, Charcot's arthropathy, reflex sympathetic dystrophy, and pigmented villonodular synovitis.

Rheumatoid arthritis and osteoarthritis usually present with involvement of multiple joints, but can present in a knee with an inflammatory component that can make it difficult to distinguish from acute monarticular arthritis. A comprehensive discussion of these diseases is included in Rheumatology Cases 2 and 3.

A diagnostic algorithm for monoarticular arthritis is shown in Fig. 12-1-2.

QUESTION 3 His medical history is significant for an appendectomy at age 10 and infectious mononucleosis at age 18. He takes no medications and has no known allergies to medications. He is married and is a salesman for a local radio station. Examination of our patient reveals right Achilles tendinitis and a swollen, warm, and tender right ankle. Other joints are normal. Aspiration of fluid from the right ankle yields 5 ml of yellowish fluid with a low viscosity. There are no crystals in the fluid, and gram stain is negative. There are 35,000 WBC/ml. What is the correct interpretation of the synovial fluid?

Synovial fluid is necessary to separate arthritis into the normal, inflammatory, infectious, and noninflammatory categories. Categorization is based chiefly on number of leukocytes, differential cell count, culture, glucose, and other parameters. Normal fluid has less than 200 WBC/μl with less than 25% PMNs, negative culture, and a glucose level approximately that of the serum.

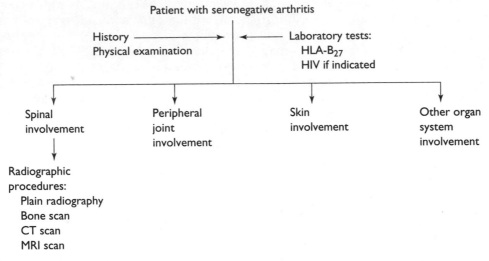

12-1-1 Diagnostic algorithm for seronegative arthritis.
(From Greene HL, Johnson WP, Maricic MJ: *Decision making in medicine*, St Louis, 1993, Mosby.)

TABLE 12-1-1   Synovial Fluid Analysis

	Normal	**Noninflamm.**	**Inflamm.**	**Septic**
WBC count	<200	200-2000	2000-100000	>100000
% PMN's	<25%	<25%	25-50%	>50%
Glucose (simultaneous drawn sample)	Approx. serum glucose	Approx. serum glucose	<50 mg less than serum	>50 mg less than serum
Culture	Negative	Negative	Negative	Positive
Color	Colorless	Yellow	Yellow	Variable
Viscosity	High	High	Low	Variable
Clarity	Transparent	Transparent	Translucent	Opaque

(Berkow R, Fletcher AJ, editors: *The Merck Manual,* ed 15, 1987, as modified from Gatter RA, and McCarty DJ: Synovianalysis, *Rheumatism* 20:2-6, 1964.)

Inflammatory fluid contains between 200 and 2000 WBC/µl with a differential cell count similar to serum. Inflammatory fluid contains between 2000 and 100,000 WBC/µl with greater than 50% PMNs, negative culture, and glucose level within 50 mg/dl of the serum glucose. Culture of these fluid types is negative. Suppurative fluid appears opaque with greater than 100,000 WBC/µl with greater than 75% PMNs and glucose level greater than 50 mg/dl below the serum level. Culture of

suppurative fluid is often positive. A summary of the characteristics of each type of fluid is in Table 12-1-1.

QUESTION 4 Further history is that he has recently separated from his wife and has had symptoms of urethral discharge for one week. Gram stain of urethral fluid reveals gram negative cocci. How does this new history impact on the preceding differential diagnosis?

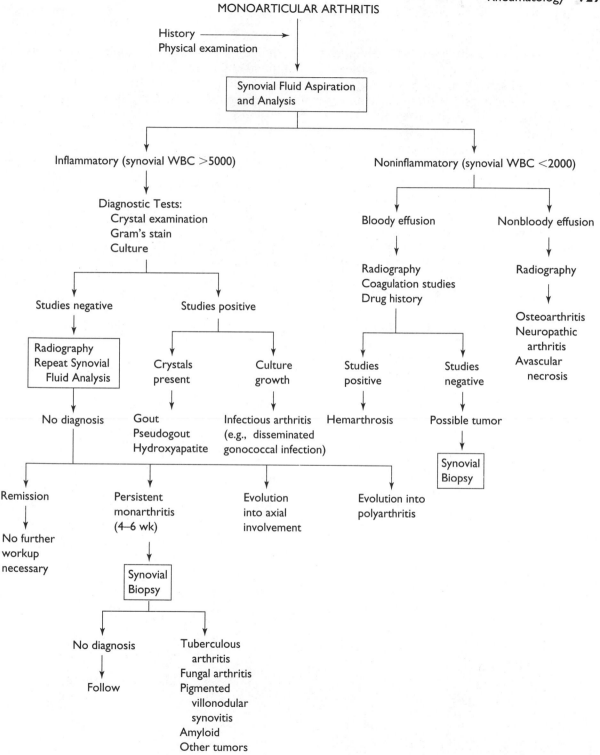

12-1-2 Diagnostic algorithm for monoarticular arthritis.
(From Greene HL, Johnson WP, Maricic MJ: *Decision making in medicine,* St Louis, 1993, Mosby.)

A history of polyarthralgias that are migratory and then settle into one joint is typical of disseminated gonococcal infection. The early stage of the disease includes constitutional symptoms, polyarthralgia, migratory tenosynovitis, and vesiculopustular eruption with only minimal joint effusion. Later the joint symptoms will localize with more pronounced synovial edema. Blood cultures are positive in only about 10% of cases, and synovial fluid cultures are positive in between 25% to 50% of cases. It is rare for both the blood and synovial fluid culture to be positive concurrently. The initial focus of infection may be silent but should be cultured empirically. The dermatitis consists of a maculopapular or a vesicular lesion. These lesions are usually asymptomatic, number less than 20 to 25, and may appear on the periphery of the extremities. The organism can be cultured from the skin lesions. The synovial fluid leukocyte count is generally lower than that seen in other bacterial infections, ranging between 50,000 and 100,000 WBC/ml.

Generally patients with gonococcal arthritis respond rapidly to antibiotics, improving within 24 to 48 hours. The response is so impressive that a therapeutic response can be used to confirm the diagnosis.

BIBLIOGRAPHY

Berkow R, Fletcher AJ, eds: *The Merck Manual*, ed 15, 1987, as modified from Gatter RA, McCarty DJ: Synovianalysis, *Rheumatism* 20:2-6, 1964.

Forbes CD, Jackson WF: *A colour atlas and text of clinical medicine*, St Louis, 1993, Mosby.

Goldenberg DL, Reed JI: Bacterial arthritis, *N Engl J Med* 312:764-771, 1985.

McCarthy DJ: Gout without hyperuricemia, *JAMA* 271:302, 1994.

Rompalo AM, Hook EW, Roberts PL: The acute arthritis—dermatitis syndrome, *Arch Intern Med* 147:281, 1987.

Wilson JD, Braunwald E: *Harrison's principles of internal medicine*, ed 12, •••.

Yu TF: Diversity of clinical features in gouty arthritis, *Semin Arthritis Rheum*, 13:360, 1984.

C A S E

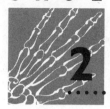

2 Charlotte Harris

A 60-year-old woman came to the office with a chief complaint of knee, ankle, and shoulder pain. She first had joint pain 20 years ago when her right shoulder hurt. She was diagnosed with bursitis and responded well to a steroid injection. She did well until 10 years later when knee pain developed, and she had her knee aspirated by an orthopedic surgeon. The knee responded to steroid injection, but she subsequently developed pain in her ankles, shoulders, and her right hip. She has had pain without swelling in her wrists, metacarpophalangeal, and proximal interphalangeal joints. She has morning stiffness that lasts 6 hours. She has had no back pain. Her primary doctor placed her on prednisone for 7 weeks, and although it helped, she stopped it because she was afraid of side effects.

Her medical history includes a hiatal hernia seen at endoscopy and a cesarean section. She has been on Darvocet and has no known allergies. She quit smoking 10 years ago and does not drink alcohol. She works as a social worker. Her family history is positive for diabetes and melanoma, but negative for arthritis.

QUESTION I Given her complaints of joint pain, what other historic features would help in forming a differential diagnosis?

The patient should be questioned about the presence of Raynaud's phenomena, dysphagia, gastroesophageal reflux, tightening on the skin of the hands and face, decreased digital flexibility, and shortness of breath. These symptoms may suggest the presence of scleroderma.

Patients with systemic lupus erythematosus (SLE) may exhibit a photosensitive rash in a malar distribution, scarring discoid skin lesions, alopecia, psychiatric disturbances, pleuritic or atypical chest pain, and oral aphthous ulcers.

Back pain, pitting changes of the nails, and typical psoriasiform skin lesions may accompany psoriatic arthritis.

A travel history to the northeast and north-central United States, a known tick bite, and classic annular skin lesions may be seen in cases of Lyme disease. A history of sarcoidosis is also important.

A history of joint trauma should be sought. Patients who have occupations that include repetitive joint trauma or movement, use of only one extremity, exposure to vibration, working in a cramped position or with a limited range of motion may lead to joint pain. Symptoms of infection should also be assessed by the interviewer.

QUESTION 2 What is the differential diagnosis of a chronic polyarthritis with regard to the expected findings associated with each disease?

Arthralgia and arthritis are two of the most common presenting features of SLE. At onset 77% of patients will have arthralgia, and 56% of patients will complain of arthritis. The arthritis can often be intermittent and is usually not destructive. The joints most frequently involved include the hands, knees, and wrists.

Extraarticular features of SLE are very common at presentation and increase in frequency as the disease progresses. At presentation, 57% will have skin disease, 23% will have pleurisy, 20% will have pericarditis, 33% will have Raynaud's phenomena, and 24% will have some manifestation of CNS disease. In our patient it would be quite unusual for SLE to be present for 10 years without extraarticular manifestations. Laboratory findings should confirm the diagnosis of SLE. Nearly all patients with SLE will have a positive antinuclear antibody (ANA). With a negative ANA there is less than a 0.14% probability of having SLE. Forty percent of SLE patients will have positive double-stranded DNA antibodies. Thirty percent of patients will have antibodies to the Smith antigen, and 23% will have U1RNP antibodies.

Scleroderma is another disease that must be considered in this differential diagnosis. Scleroderma can be categorized as either limited or diffuse. Limited disease indicates involvement of the face and skin distal to the elbows. The diffuse type refers to skin involvement proximal to the elbows. This is a condition characterized by diffuse inflammation involving the skin, gut, heart, and lung with resultant fibrosis and deposition of collagen in the dermis and viscera. A minority of patients will develop congestive heart failure and close to one third will develop fibrotic lung disease. Often these visceral manifestations occur in the first few years of disease.

Joint involvement may frequently begin as polyarticular disease involving the small joints of the hands. Eighty-five percent of patients with diffuse scleroderma have Raynaud's phenomena as an early manifestation. Diffuse bilateral swelling of the fingers is another early manifestation. As diffuse disease progresses, there is a high incidence of esophageal dysmotility (75%). In addition to inflammatory arthritis, patients with diffuse scleroderma often have tenosynovial disease. This presents with coarse leathery friction rubs that are appreciated during motion of the extensor and flexor tendons adjacent to the fingers, wrist, knees, and ankles.

The laboratory tests that are useful in the diagnosis of scleroderma include ANA, anticentromere antibody and antitopoisomerase I antibody. The ANA is positive in 95% of scleroderma patients. Forty percent of patients with diffuse scleroderma will have positive antitopoisomerase I antibodies. The absence of these components

makes scleroderma an unlikely diagnosis in this patient.

Psoriatic arthritis has different subtypes. These include a pauci-articular subset that involves less than four joints; another subset very similar to rheumatoid arthritis; disease limited to the distal interphalangeal joints; spondylitis; and a particularly destructive type called arthritis mutilans. Genetic factors are important in this disease, but, interestingly, the genetic markers seen in isolated psoriasis are different from those seen in cases of psoritic arthritis. The presence of HLA-B27 correlates with the spondylitic form of psoritic arthritis. Other HLA associations include HLA-B38, B, CW1, CW2, DRW4, and DRW7.

One must examine the skin, scalp, perianal, and umbilical regions to find the typical skin changes of psoriasis. Age of onset is typically between 30 and 50 years with males affected equally to females. While patients with psoriatic arthritis may develop arthritis first, skin involvement usually occurs within 7 years.

Sarcoidosis causes a number of joint manifestations. Nearly 25% of patients with sarcoidosis will present with extrathoracic inflammation. About 15% will have frank arthritis. Knees and other joints may become involved in an additive pattern. Spondylitis does not occur. Periarticular swelling may be more prominent than joint swelling itself. Pauci-articular disease is the most common pattern. Heel pain and tenosynovitis may be associated.

Lyme arthritis is typically monoarticular or pauciarticular. The knee is the joint most often involved. Erythema chronicum migrans is the primary lesion seen at the site of the tick bite. Often symptoms stem from joint and periarticular structures. These initial symptoms usually resolve in several months, but recur in about 60% of patients. Transient episodes of mono- or pauci-articular symptoms can flare, especially in large joints. Ten percent will develop chronic arthritis. The diagnosis can be confirmed by serologic tests and extraarticular manifestations, which include a typical skin rash, neurologic problems, and cardiac conduction abnormalities.

Rheumatoid arthritis (RA) is generally additive. Generally it is a symmetric disease typically beginning in multiple small joints. Onset of disease is insidious, developing over several weeks to months. Fatigue is a prominent syndrome, in addition to morning stiffness. Morning stiffness lasting more than an hour in duration is significant and suggests an inflammatory arthropathy. The rheumatoid factor will be positive in 85% of cases. Definite RA is 2 to 3 times more common in women than men. HLA-DR4 is present in 65% to 80% of patients with RA and is associated with more severe disease.

Physical examination will show soft tissue swelling of the joints early on. With progression of disease, laxity of ligaments and characteristic deformities will develop. These include swan neck, boutonniere deformities, subluxation, and ulnar deviation of the fingers. An important sequela of ligament, bone, and joint disease is vertebral body instability. Of particularly critical importance is the cervical spine. Subluxation of the atlanto-axial joint, which can result from minor trauma or neck hyperextension as in opening the airway, can lead to spinal cord injury or transsection with tragic results.

A diagnostic algorithm for polyarticular arthritis is shown in Fig. 12-2-1.

QUESTION 3 In our patient high rheumatoid factor and erosive changes on joint radiographs confirmed the diagnosis of RA. What are the systemic manifestations of RA?

Besides involvement of the joints, rheumatoid arthritis is a systemic disease. There are multiple pleuropulmonary manifestations of RA. Pleural disease may include development of a pleural effusion. Even though women are more often afflicted with RA, men more frequently develop pleurisy. Pleural involvement is usually insignificant; however, fibrothorax necessitating decortication occurs rarely. One should be careful to rule out tuberculosis, empyema, and malignancy before settling on RA as the diagnosis. Another pulmonary manifestation is interstitial fibrosis, which impairs gas exchange and produces restric-

tive lung disease. Again, this complication is more common in men.

Analogous to subcutaneous rheumatoid nodules are intraparenchymal necrobiotic nodules. These lesions characteristically cavitate. Caplan described a syndrome in coal miners with RA who developed round lung densities that enlarge rapidly and may cavitate. The lesion consists of layers of necrotic collagen and dust. Besides coal workers, this can also be seen in RA patients who work as sandblasters, potters, and boiler scalers. This is a disease separate from interstitial fibrosis seen in coal worker's pneumoconiosis. Both the necrobiotic nodules and the nodules seen in Caplan's syndrome are more common in men.

Skin involvement includes the development of subcutaneous nodules. These commonly develop in areas of pressure including elbows, sacrum, and occiput. A leukocytoclastic vasculitis can develop as evidenced by splinter-shaped lesions under the nail bed or on the digital pulp. In the malleolar areas, larger areas of vasculitis can develop leading to skin sloughing. A more severe vasculitis, rheumatoid vasculitis, is associated with fever, depressed complement, and systemic symptoms. This lesion may be confused with polyarteritis nodosa.

Cardiac disease includes pericarditis. The spectrum of involvement reaches from mild inflammation to development of pericardial effusion and acute tamponade. However, cases are usually mild with chest pain, dyspnea, and peripheral edema. The physician should be vigilant for the development of jugular venous distension, peripheral edema, clear lungs, and hemodynamic instability.

Mononeuritis multiplex is a neuropathy involving different nerves in a patchy distribution. Biopsy reveals the presence of vasculitis of the vasonervorum. Synovial proliferation can also lead to nerve compression syndromes such as carpal tunnel syndrome.

Hematologic complications include a hypochromic, microcytic anemia. Felty's syndrome is the combination of splenomegaly and neutropenia. Ophthalmologic complications include epi-

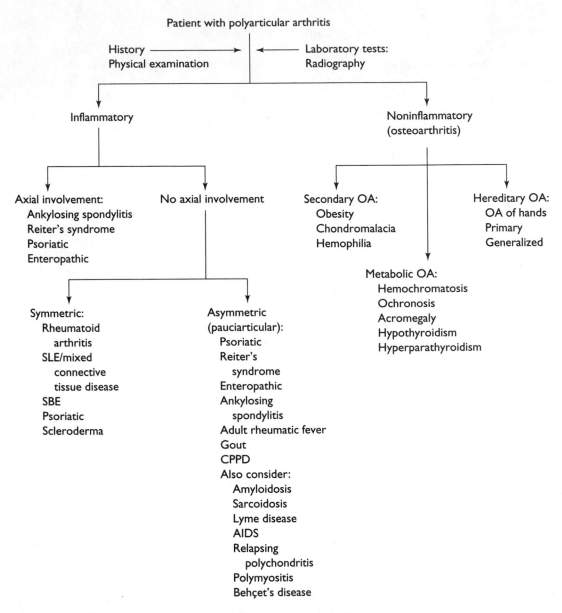

Patient with polyarticular arthritis

History ──────────────→ ←────── Laboratory tests:
Physical examination   Radiography

Inflammatory

Noninflammatory
(osteoarthritis)

Axial involvement:
  Ankylosing spondylitis
  Reiter's syndrome
  Psoriatic
  Enteropathic

No axial involvement

Secondary OA:
  Obesity
  Chondromalacia
  Hemophilia

Hereditary OA:
  OA of hands
  Primary
  Generalized

Metabolic OA:
  Hemochromatosis
  Ochronosis
  Acromegaly
  Hypothyroidism
  Hyperparathyroidism

Symmetric:
  Rheumatoid
    arthritis
  SLE/mixed
    connective
    tissue disease
  SBE
  Psoriatic
  Scleroderma

Asymmetric
(pauciarticular):
  Psoriatic
  Reiter's
    syndrome
  Enteropathic
  Ankylosing
    spondylitis
  Adult rheumatic fever
  Gout
  CPPD
  Also consider:
    Amyloidosis
    Sarcoidosis
    Lyme disease
    AIDS
    Relapsing
      polychondritis
    Polymyositis
    Behçet's disease

12-2-1   Diagnostic algorithm for polyarticular arthritis.
(From Greene HL, Johnson WP, Maricic MJ: *Decision making in medicine,* St Louis, 1993, Mosby.)

scleritis, scleromalacia perforans, and Sjögren's syndrome.

QUESTION 4   In that the diagnosis of RA is secure, what is the accepted treatment approach for this disease?

Salicylates may be used as initial treatment. Doses required are usually greater than those taken for analgesia. A serum level of 20 to 30 mg/dl is necessary and translates to 3 to 6 grams of aspirin a day. Enteric-coated preparations are preferable to help avoid gastric irritation. Patients should be made aware of how to recognize melena or hematochezia and be encouraged to use stool guaiac cards at home periodically.

Newer, nonsteroidal agents are an alternative to salicylates. Relative contraindications include peptic ulcer disease, asthma, congestive heart failure, and renal insufficiency. Nonsteroidal agents are usually no more effective, but may be better tolerated than salicylates.

Additional agents include gold salts. These agents should be added when symptom relief is not fully afforded by aspirin with/without NSAI agents. Gold arrests active inflammation, can produce disease remission, and may decrease the rate of bony erosion. Gold is contraindicated in renal or hepatic dysfunction and in the presence of blood dyscrasias. Important adverse effects include proteinuria, agranulocytosis, thrombocytopenic purpura, aplastic anemia, pruritis and skin rash, and stomatitis. Before the patient starts therapy a urinalysis, CBC, and platelet count are necessary. Through the first month of therapy, these tests should be repeated before each injection. If the drug is continued chronically, these lab tests should be performed at definite intervals to avoid serious adverse reactions.

If mild toxic reactions occur, the drug should be withheld for two weeks and may be restarted gradually. Severe skin reactions may necessitate use of topical corticosteroids. A severe gold reaction can be treated with the gold chelator dimercaprol.

D-penicillamine is an alternative to gold therapy if toxicity is encountered. The dose is slowly increased until a clinical response is seen and then maintained at that level. The CBC, platelet count, and urinalysis should be monitored. Proteinuria, nephrosis, myasthenia, pemphigus, Goodpasture's syndrome, polymyositis, and a lupus-like syndrome (antihistone antibody positive) may develop.

Methotrexate is a drug that has been widely used to treat rheumatoid arthritis. Its most serious side effects are pulmonary and hepatic toxicity. Neutropenia and thrombocytopenia can also occur. There have been a few cases of lymphoma developing while on methotrexate.

The antimalarial agent hydroxychloroquine (Plaquinil) is another second-line agent. Side effects include dermatitis and myopathy. Irreversible retinal deterioration may develop. Therefore, periodic eye examination is necessary. This drug should be discontinued after 3 to 6 months if no clinical response is seen.

Corticosteroids are used as short-term agents to treat inflammation. It is important to use the lowest effective dose. Steroids will not arrest the progressive joint destruction. Complications include a rebound effect after discontinuation, immunosuppression, osteoporosis, glucose intolerance, hypertension, and gastrointestinal bleeding.

Intraarticular joint injection is useful when the number of joints affected is small. Long-acting agents such as triamcinolone hexacetonide and prednisolone tertiary-butylacetate are preferred. Local inflammation may flare transiently because of the crystalline state of the agent.

Steroid-sparing agents include azathioprine and cyclophosphamide. However, these agents risk development of immunosuppression, hepatic and renal disease, and lower the threshold for development of secondary malignancy with long-term use.

BIBLIOGRAPHY

Harris ED: Rheumatoid arthritis: pathophysiology and supplications for therapy, *N Engl J Med* 322:1277, 1990.

Incus T, Callahan LF: Early mortality in RA predicted by poor clinical states, *Bull Rheum Dis* 41:4, 1992.

MacKenzie AH: Differential diagnosis of rheumatoid arthritis, *Am J Med* 85(Suppl 4):2, 1985.

C A S E

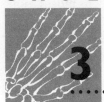

3

Charlotte Harris
···········

A 68-year-old obese woman came to the office with a chief complaint of right knee pain and swelling for the past 4 weeks. She describes 3 to 4 hours of morning stiffness such that it is difficult to walk. One year before presentation, she had pain with mild swelling in the 5th PIP joint of her right hand. No other joints have been symptomatic recently. She took aspirin as needed for these symptoms, and they gradually resolved. She cannot recall a history of trauma.

Two months before presentation she was hospitalized for streptococcal pharyngitis that required intravenous penicillin. She denies a recent history of fever, skin rash, or dental work. She has a monogamous heterosexual relationship with her husband. She has been taking Ibuprofen 400 mg bid with only partial symptomatic improvement.

She has no known allergies, does not smoke, drink alcohol, or use illegal drugs. She lives with her husband and works as a nurse's aide. She was born in the Virgin Islands and came to the United States in 1986. Her grandmother had arthritis, but the details of her illness are not known.

Review of systems is negative for chest pain, shortness of breath, abdominal pain, history of peptic ulcer disease, Raynaud's phenomena, photosensitive rash, sicca syndrome, or alopecia.

QUESTION 1 How would you characterize this type of arthritis? What would be the first test of choice to evaluate this problem?

This is a chronic monoarticular arthritis. Furthermore, the patient's obese stature may contrib-

ute to the symptoms. There is a family history of joint disease that remains unspecified because of lack of knowledge on the part of the patient. Nevertheless, this should be kept in mind as different etiologic factors are evaluated. Another confounding factor is that the patient has been taking Ibuprofen for the last 10 to 14 days. This may obscure a pure presentation of the underlying syndrome.

She does have a history of another joint being involved one year ago, but it is difficult to connect these two episodes with the prolonged time course and lack of known unifying diagnosis.

The first investigational test is arthrocentesis. It is important to perform this test under specific guidelines. Crystal analysis should be performed early as the crystals can deteriorate as the sample sits idle. In the emergency room setting this may require a phone call to the lab to make certain that the gram stain and crystal analysis is carried out immediately. The needle should be inserted into the joint through an area of normal skin so that the needle remains sterile and no infectious agents are introduced into the joint space. When pus is withdrawn, the joint should be drained as much as possible.

A diagnostic algorithm for monarticular arthritis is shown in Fig. 12-3-1 on p. 739.

QUESTION 2 On physical examination vital signs are T 98.4°F, BP 110/70 mm Hg , P 88 bpm, and RR 14/min. General physical examination is unremarkable. Musculoskeletal examination reveals normal muscle strength. All joints are normal except the right knee, which had full range of motion but a large, moderately warm effusion. There is no overlying erythema. The joint is only painful at the extremes of range of motion. Twenty milliliters of clear yellow-tinged fluid of low viscosity were drained from the right knee. No crystals were seen, and gram stain was negative. Analysis included: WBC count was 100 with 10% polymorphonuclear leukocytes and 90% lymphocytes with 31 RBC/ml. Based on the recovery of this synovial fluid, what is the differential diagnosis of this problem?

The synovial fluid profile is consistent with a non-inflammatory process. Clear fluid is not indicative of an inflammatory or septic joint disease. A full explanation of the interpretation of synovial fluid is included in Rheumatology Case 1.

In this case the differential diagnosis must include acute infection. Even though the fluid is not consistent with a septic process, this diagnosis is a rheumatologic emergency and must be ruled out definitively. The physician should rank disease in a differential diagnosis based on likelihood, but should never leave off an emergent disorder that may require immediate therapy. An example is a patient in a similar situation who mistakenly took or was too embarrassed to admit that she used antibiotics from another family member or friend. The fluid should be gram stained quickly and cultured for infectious agents. An acute bacterial process or chronic infection such as tuberculous or fungal arthritis should be considered. Generally acute infection will have synovial WBC counts in the 50,000-100,000 range with a predominance of polymorphonuclear cells. One exception is the joint effusion produced by *Neisseria gonorrhea* infection (see Rheumatology Case 1). In this condition the inflammatory response is much milder with leucocyte counts in the 15,000 to 30,000 range.

Traumatic problems also present as a monoarticular process with near normal synovial fluid leucocyte counts but may be hemorrhagic. Removal of blood and/or clots is an important reason to carry out arthrocentesis. The appropriate history is necessary to confirm the diagnosis. The physical examination may reveal lacerations, swelling, erythema, warmth, patellar dislocation, or bony fracture. For this reason, plain radiographs of the affected joint are important.

Neuropathic arthropathy (Charcot-joint) is caused by loss of sensory function with chronic trauma on ambulation. Associated conditions include diabetes mellitus, tabes dorsalis, syringomyelia, leprosy, peripheral neuropathy, hereditary neuropathies (Charcot-Marie-Tooth disease, hereditary sensory neuropathy), use of analgesics, amyloid neuropathy, and nerve root compression syndromes. The joint fluid is usually normal, and the distribution is usually monoarticular.

Hypertrophic pulmonary osteoarthropathy (HPO) is a condition of reactive periostitis that usually affects the proximal portions of the long bones (i.e., fibula or ulna). The most important association is with neoplasm of the lung. The lesion may precede, be concurrent, or show up after the development of the tumor. The lesion may also resolve with treatment of the neoplasm and may be categorized as a paraneoplastic syndrome. In some cases, lung neoplasms may be found at an early enough stage to afford cure.

Behçet's disease includes joint disease along with gastrointestinal and CNS vasculitis, recurrent oral and genital aphthous ulcers, migratory thrombophlebitis, iridocyclitis of the anterior chamber, or involvement of the posterior chamber including choroiditis and uveitis. The arthritis is usually self-limited and nondestructive and usually involves the knee or a large joint.

Another disease that must be considered is acute rheumatic fever as the patient provides a history of a recent streptococcal infection. A full discussion of acute rheumatic fever is included in Rheumatology Case 1.

Ehlers-Danlos syndrome is characterized by a disorder of connective tissue and collagen. The connective tissue is hypermotile and fragile. Sickle cell disease is associated with the development of avascular necrosis of bone. This is also usually monoarticular with a noninflammatory joint effusion. Amyloidosis, apart from periph-

738 Diagnostic Strategies for Internal Medicine

eral neuropathy, causes an arthropathy that mimics RA.

Additional diagnoses that may have a noninflammatory-inflammatory synovial fluid include the joint manifestations of SLE, RA, and progressive systems sclerosis (scleroderma). These diseases are covered more fully in Rheumatology Case 2.

Arthritis as an extraarticular manifestation of inflammatory bowel disease, Crohn's disease or ulcerative colitis, is another syndrome that may involve a large joint and the lower extremities. Flares and quiescence of arthritis are usually concurrent to flares of colitis. Arthritis may be the first manifestation of these diseases. HLA-B27 is absent in this arthropathy. Treatment depends on treating the underlying bowel disease.

Finally, the noninflammatory nature of the synovial fluid suggests that the patient might have osteoarthritis. The distant involvement of proximal interphalangeal disease would be compatible with osteoarthritis.

QUESTION 3 Radiograph of the knee performed in the standing position was normal. What are the physical and radiographic findings, epidemiology, and pathophysiology of osteoarthritis?

Heberdeen's and/or Bouchard's nodes on the distal and proximal intraphalangeal joints are noninfestations of osteoarthritis (OA). Stiffness is evident on examination, and areas of tenderness may be focal to palpation. Crepitus, or a crunching sound, may be appreciated on passively moving the joint. Joint pain is usually exacerbated by movement and relieved with rest. Advanced findings include bony enlargement, presence of osteophytes, joint deformation, and subluxation.

Radiographic analysis has shown to be insensitive, with characteristic findings appearing later than clinical disease. Arthroscopy demonstrates pathology earlier and more definitively.

OA can involve individuals beginning in the fourth to fifth decade with incidence of about 5%, but is generally more prevalent in the elderly population. Women are twice as likely to develop OA compared with men; black women have twice the risk compared with white women.

The pathophysiology of OA is complex. The cascade of events that lead to joint damage are triggered by a change in the microenvironment of the chondrocyte. This may be due to trauma, infection, or congenital disease. Cartilage cells divide very slowly so that the response to injury is prolonged. The second step is the decreased production of proteoglycans, the substance that provides the structural framework of the cartilage. This leads to stiffening of the cartilage, development of microfractures, and subchondral bone production. Osteochondrophytes develop around the joint, bony pseudocysts develop, and the cartilage is further damaged. The articular surface loses surface area, undergoes pitting, becomes coarse, ulcerates and stimulates further proliferation of joint components that crowd normal structures and lead to deterioration of function.

Radiologically, this leads to a narrowed joint space, increased density of subchondral bone, osteochondrophytes (spurs), and pseudocyst involvement.

QUESTION 4 What is the correct approach to treatment for osteoarthritis?

The major goal of therapy is the preservation of joint integrity and function. Thus, a program of rehabilitation at an accredited location and exercise are the mainstay of joint preservation. Symptoms of pain and swelling are managed by aspirin, nonsteroidal antiinflammatory agents, or simple analgesics. Muscle relaxants can be used as an adjunct to decrease joint stress.

CASE SUMMARY Her ESR was 8 mm/hr, ASO was negative. Synovial fluid culture and gram stain were negative. One month later she returned to the office. She had 50% improvement in her symptoms on Naproxen 500 mg bid. Repeat aspiration was again negative for crystals, and MRI demonstrated tricompartmental changes of osteoarthritis.

• •

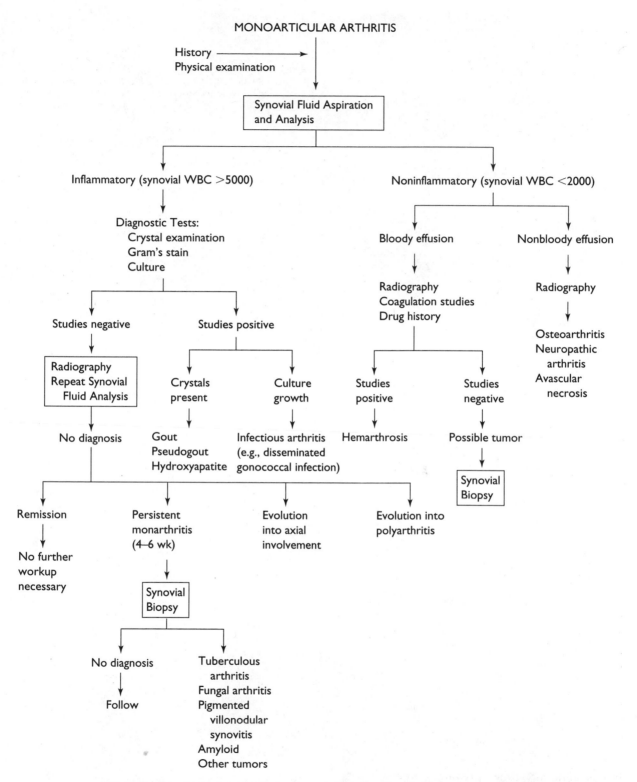

12-3-1 Diagnostic algorithm for monoarticular arthritis.
(From Greene HL, Johnson WP, Maricic MJ: *Decision making in medicine,* St Louis, 1993, Mosby.)

BIBLIOGRAPHY

Bradley JD, Brandt KD, Katz BP: Comparison of an anti-inflammatory dose of ibuprofen, and analgesic dose of ibuprofen and acetaminophen in the treatment of patients with osteoarthritis of the knee, *N Engl J Med* 325:87, 1991.

Clang RW, Falconer JW, Streberg SD: A randomized, controlled study of arthroscopic surgery versus closed needle lavage for patients with osteoarthritis of the knee, *Arthritis Rheum* 36:289, 1993.

CASE

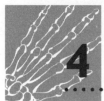

4 Winston Sequiera

A 20-year-old woman comes to the emergency room because of a low-grade fever, joint pains for 2 days, and a rash she first noticed that morning. She also had symptoms suggesting an upper respiratory tract infection and complained of a headache for which she self-medicated with enteric-coated aspirin.

In the emergency room she looks very anxious but does not appear to be ill. Her blood pressure is normal, she has no meningeal signs, and her abdomen is mildly tender. Except for a skin eruption, the rest of the examination is normal. The rash is mainly over the lower extremities and buttocks with an occasional lesion over the upper torso and limbs. The lesions are mostly discrete, palpable purpura, and nonpruritic, though a few lesions tend to coalesce and others are beginning to fade. Her CBC including platelets is normal.

She denies drug use or contact with hepatitis. Her boyfriend who accompanied her was questioned separately. He denied the use of drugs, but did admit to more than one sexual partner; he did not have urethral symptoms.

QUESTION I What is the name of this rash, and what are the possible diagnoses?

It is important to differentiate this rash from a purpura related to thrombocytopenia, which is not palpable and may be associated with ecchymosis. The CBC including the platelet count in this patient was normal. She has what is commonly referred to as nonthrombocytopenic palpable purpura. The differential diagnosis is large and includes a drug reaction to aspirin, penicillin, or sulfa drugs. Infections including hepatitis B or

C, Neisserial organisms, and endocarditis are all possibilities. She does not have the classic pustular rash on a red base or acute tenosynovitis supportive of disseminated gonoccocal infection. Blood, cervical, rectal, and throat cultures are done, and aspirin and other NSAIDs should be discontinued in order to focus on the diagnosis.

Cryoglobulinemia needs to be considered in the differential diagnosis. Cryoglobulins are immunoglobulins that precipitate in the cold with resolution during warming. There are three types of cryoglobulinemia: type 1: monoclonal immunoglobulin (e.g., macroglobulinemia); type 2: monoclonal antibody usually IgM against a polyclonal IgG; type 3: mixed polyclonal immunoglobulins. Lymphoproliferative diseases are associated with types 1 and 2, cryoglobulinemia and collagen vascular diseases with type 3. Neurologic and renal disease are associated with both types 2 and 3.

Henoch-Schönlein purpura may present with a similar rash. It is most frequently a disease of childhood with more than 75% of patients presenting before the age of 7. The rash is frequently accompanied by abdominal pain and a microscopic hematuria. There may be ocular, cardiac, or CNS involvement, but the prognosis depends upon the extent of the renal disease. In most instances the renal involvement is self-limiting, but 1% to 2% of patients may progress to end-stage renal failure and accounts for nearly 15% of patients in a pediatric dialysis program. The diagnosis is made by demonstrating IgA deposition in the vessel wall on a skin biopsy. A skin biopsy should be taken from a fresh lesion ideally less than 24-hours old.

Cryoglobulins were not detected in the patient's serum. The patient did not improve after 7 days of antibiotics. New lesions appeared, and she continued to have joint pains. Her attending physician considered the diagnosis of a collagen vascular disease and started her on low-dose prednisone and discharged her.

QUESTION 2 Her liver enzymes are normal, and a hepatitis screen is negative. She felt the same 2 days later. A new crop of lesions have appeared, and the patient is getting more anxious. Her urine has 3 to 5 white cells with 10 to 20 RBCs per high power field and no casts. In the patient's biopsy, postcapillary venules were involved with fibrinoid degeneration and infiltration with neutrophils, perivascular hemorrhage, and cellular fragments. Immunofluorescence staining was predominantly IgM with no IgG, IgA, or C3, the most common finding in nonthrombocytopenic purpura not associated with HS. The rheumatology workup is back with a rheumatoid factor (RF) of 70 (normal <40) and antinuclear antibody (ANA) of 1:320; C3 and C4 normal. Does this patient have rheumatoid arthritis, systemic lupus erythematosus (SLE), or Sjogren's syndrome as a cause of her symptoms?

Because of white cell debris noted on biopsy, another name for this lesion is a leukocytoclastic vasculitis. Leukocytoclastic vasculitis can be a presenting feature of many of the collagen vascular diseases. The American College of Rheumatolgy criteria require at least 6 weeks of symptoms before a diagnosis of rheumatoid arthritis can be made. Similarly, while one cannot totally exclude SLE, it is important to be aware that a positive ANA or RF can be found in a variety of conditions including TB, sarcoid, thyroiditis, and liver disease.

QUESTION 3 Two weeks later she is seen in the office, and the lesions have progressed. She is reexamined particularly for lymph node, spleen, or hepatic enlargement. Hairy cell leukemias and lymphomas have been associated with this type of skin rash. The examination was normal. The rash now becomes more nodular. The physician begins

HYPERSENSITIVITY VASCULITIS

DRUGS
- Sulfa agents
- Penicillin
- NSAIDs
- Cocaine
- Phenylpropanolamine

INFECTIONS
Viral
- Hepatitis B or C
- Parvovirus
- HIV
- Flu vaccine

Bacterial
- Gonococcemia
- Meningococcemia
- Streptococcal infection
- Lyme disease
- Endocarditis

COLLAGEN VASCULAR
- RA
- SLE
- Sjogren's syndrome
- Wegener's granulomatosis
- PAN

MALIGNANCIES
- Hairy cell leukemia
- Lymphoma

MISCELLANEOUS
- Henoch-Shönlein purpura
- Cryoglobulinemia
- Hypocomplementemic vasculitis

therapy with dapsone (50 mg), and the rash begins to improve. How does this change in the rash impact upon the differential diagnosis?

In retrospect this patient probably has idiopathic chronic leukocytoclastic (hypersensitivity) vasculitis. A more complete list of the differential diagnosis of this entity is seen in the box. The diagnosis is made by exclusion of other possible forms of cutaneous vasculitis and the associations that have been mentioned above. In the vast majority of these patients no identifiable cause can be found.

Other conditions that may resemble or be associated with necrotizing vasculitis are as follows. Nodular vasculitis was previously considered to be associated with tuberculosis. Lesions tend to occur on the lateral and posterior aspects of the leg. Cutaneous granulomatous vasculitis has very similar characteristics and is a variation of necrotizing vasculitis. The rash is nodular, though in a small percentage of patients, it may present as a plaque. The patients tend to be slightly older than the patient described, and it may be associated with rheumatoid arthritis most frequently, but has been described with sarcoidosis, chronic inflammatory bowel disease, and other forms of systemic granulomatous vasculitis. When the disease occurs with lymphoproliferative disorders, the prognosis is poor.

Other forms of cutaneous vasculitis include urticarial vasculitis and livedoreticularis. In urticarial vasculitis, the skin lesions are urticarial with immune complex deposition and low complement levels. It is frequently associated with SLE. Livedoreticularis, as the name suggests, is a rash with a reticulate pattern and is most commonly observed on the lower extremities. It may be asymtomatic associated with cutaneous periarteritis nodosa (PAN) or with the antiphospholipid syndromes.

PAN is a rare disease with an incidence between 0.2 to 1.8 per 100,000. The presentation may be quite nonspecific with fever and weight loss. The kidney is involved 70% of the time. Hypertension is a frequent association. Unexplained neuropathy may be indicative of vasculitis. Acute abdominal pain or gangrene with perforation of the gall bladder may be presenting features of PAN. The lab is usually nonspecific with anemia and hypoalbuminemia. Low complement levels are present in only 25% of patients. Biopsy of the skin lesions or affected organs or "beading" on angiogram help confirm the diagnosis. Cutaneous PAN is a benign disease, and unless accompanied by evidence of systemic involvement, does not require aggressive therapy.

Kawasaki disease, also referred to as mucocutaneous lymph node syndrome, is a disease of children. It appears to affect Asians most frequently but has been described in all ethnic groups. Patients may demonstrate fever, conjunctivitis, strawberry tongue, cervical lymphadenopathy, and an exfoliative erythematous rash with desquamation of the hands and feet. A major complication of this disease is coronary arteritis; the incidence of which appears to increase with the use of steroids. Steroids therefore are relatively contraindicated in this disease, which is treated with high doses of aspirin and more recently with intravenous gammaglobulin.

QUESTION 4 What are the major vasculitides that demonstrate granulomatous inflammation?

Systemic vasculitis may be classified depending upon the vessel size involved or upon histology. Table 12-4-1 divides the common vasculitidis based on the formation of granuloma.

The granulomatous vasculitis syndromes include classic Wegener's and allergic granulomatous vasculitis of Churg-Strauss. In Wegener's granulomatosis the patients usually present with chronic sinusitis, pulmonary hemorrhage or pauciimmune complex glomerular nephritis. A biopsy of the involved tissue (i.e., the sinuses or lungs) may be necessary. Inflammation of the vessel wall with granulomas and necrosis confirm the diagnosis. Because there is often a paucity of tissue involvement from the sinuses, the biopsy results are often equivocal. An open biopsy of the lung rather than a transbronchial biopsy is more likely to be diagnostic. More recently antineutrophilic cytoplasmic antibodies (ANCA) have been helpful in the diagnosis of Wegener's. Using immunofluorescence there are two patterns, c-ANCA and p-ANCA. The c-ANCA antibody is directed against proteinase 3 as the antigen with a specificity for Wegener's approaching 90%. The perinuclear staining in p-ANCA corresponds to myeloperoxidase in about 10% of patients and is

TABLE 12-4-1   **Classification of Vasculitis**

	Granulomatous	Nongranulomatous
Large arteritis	Giant cell arteritis Takayasu's arteritis	Ankylosing spondylitis Reiter's syndrome Relapsing polychondritis Cogan's syndrome
Medium and small arteritis	Allergic granulomatosis GANS Wegener's granulomatosis Lymphomatoid granulomatosis	Classical idiopathic PAN Overlap Berger's disease Kawasaki disease
Postcapillary venulitis		Hypersensitivity vasculitis

associated with microangiitis. An ANA is the most frequent cause of p-ANCA that is myeloperoxidase negative on ELISA. It has also been described with infection, chronic inflammatory bowel disease, idiopathic glomerular nephritis, and Goodpasture's syndrome.

Allergic granulomatosis of Churg-Strauss resembles Wegener's and often presents as a pneumonitis with changing radiographic densities. A history of asthma with eosinophilia, antedating the diagnosis at times by years, subcutaneous nodules, and leucocytoclastic vasculitis are common features of the disease. Abdominal symptoms with ischemia of the bowel and gall bladder may occur. The kidney is involved less frequently than in PAN. Eosinophilic infiltration of the prostate and lower urinary tract is an unusual but unique feature of this disease and may lead to urinary obstruction.

Giant cell arteritis usually presents with headaches, jaw claudication, and sudden onset of irreversible blindness may occur. A rare complication recently described is an aneurysm of the thoracic aorta, with or without aortic valvular involvement. Tenderness over the temporal artery is helpful in the diagnosis, and an elevated erythrocyte sedimentation rate (ESR) and a temporal artery biopsy will confirm the diagnosis. The mainstay of treatment is corticosteroids starting with 60 mg of prednisone and reducing the dose when the ESR normalizes. Prednisone is reduced to the lowest possible dose to keep the ESR normal. At least 2 years of treatment is required.

Takayasu's vasculitis or pulseless disease, though most often reported in young Asian women, is observed in all races. Rarely it may present with skin lesions described in the patient. More commonly the patient may first visit the physician because of hypertension, vertigo or syncope, and on occassion because of symptoms of ischemic heart disease. Steroids may be tried along with vasodilator and low-dose ASA. Prognosis depends on the vessel involved and the accessibility of the vessel to surgical correction.

QUESTION 5   What is the appropriate therapy for cutaneous vasculitis?

Treatment of cutaneous vasculitis without evidence of systemic involvement, hypersensitivity vasculitis in this case, is usually conservative. When associated with collagen vascular diseases without organ involvement, the patients may be observed, treated with dapsone (25 to 100 mg/day) or low-dose prednisone (7.5 mg/day). Treatment of the underlying infection or withdrawal of the offending drug usually results in regression of the rash. In a large group of patients, however, the underlying cause cannot be determined, and there is a tendency for recurrences every few weeks to months. Fortunately, the majority of these individuals improve spontaneously. A few

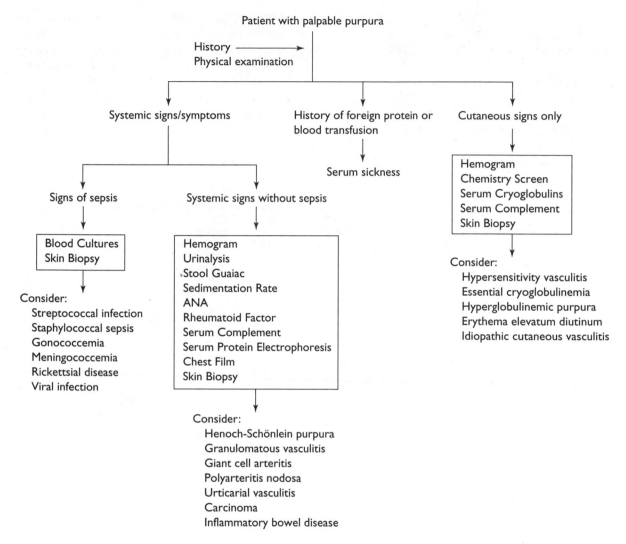

Patient with palpable purpura

History ⟶
Physical examination

Systemic signs/symptoms

History of foreign protein or blood transfusion

↓

Serum sickness

Cutaneous signs only

Hemogram
Chemistry Screen
Serum Cryoglobulins
Serum Complement
Skin Biopsy

Consider:
 Hypersensitivity vasculitis
 Essential cryoglobulinemia
 Hyperglobulinemic purpura
 Erythema elevatum diutinum
 Idiopathic cutaneous vasculitis

Signs of sepsis

Blood Cultures
Skin Biopsy

Consider:
 Streptococcal infection
 Staphylococcal sepsis
 Gonococcemia
 Meningococcemia
 Rickettsial disease
 Viral infection

Systemic signs without sepsis

Hemogram
Urinalysis
Stool Guaiac
Sedimentation Rate
ANA
Rheumatoid Factor
Serum Complement
Serum Protein Electrophoresis
Chest Film
Skin Biopsy

Consider:
 Henoch-Schönlein purpura
 Granulomatous vasculitis
 Giant cell arteritis
 Polyarteritis nodosa
 Urticarial vasculitis
 Carcinoma
 Inflammatory bowel disease

12-4-1   Approach to a patient with palpable purpura.
(From Greene HL, Johnson WP, and Maricic MJ: *Decision making in medicine*, St Louis, 1993, Mosby.)

patients, however, may have a more chronic course lasting many years, refractory to steroids and dapsone.

Cutaneous vasculitis with evidence of systemic involvement may require more aggressive treatment. Before initiating treatment, however, one should exclude conditions that may, at first glance, resemble a vasculitis (box). In patients with Wegener's and PAN the initial treatment is with coticosteroids at a dose of 1 to 2 mg/kg/day

followed by cyclophosphamide. The latter may be given IV at monthly intervals in doses of 0.5 g/m^2 or in a daily oral dose of 2 to 3 mg/kg/day. Oral therapy has shown to be very effective in Wegener's; it is used in other forms of systemic vasculitis even though no double blind studies have been performed. Pulse cyclophosphamide IV has the advantage of fewer side effects, and anecdotal reports suggest that it may be as efficacious as daily dose cyclophosphamide. Trimethoprim-

CONDITIONS THAT MAY BE MISDIAGNOSED AS VASCULITIS

VASCULAR ABNORMALITIES
- Arterial coarctation
- Dysplasias

THROMBI OR EMBOLIZATION
- Arteriosclerosis: cholesterol; emboli
- Atrial myxoma
- Endocarditis
- Anticardiolipin Ab syndrome

CONNECTIVE TISSUE DISORDER
- Ehlers-Danlos syndrome
- Pseudoxanthoma elasticum

DRUGS
- Ergot
- Cocaine

MISCELLANEOUS
- Kohlmeir-Degos disease
- Neurofibromatosis

sulfamethoxazole may be indicated for treatment of limited Wegener's disease confined to the sinuses and upper respiratory tract. Preliminary reports suggest that methotrexate may also be useful in the treatment of Wegener's granulomatosis.

CASE FOLLOW-UP Over the next few years the rash tends to flare periodically. The rest of the examination continues to be normal, and the patient is able to carry on her usual activities. She is maintained on low-dose aspirin and procardia.

BIBLIOGRAPHY

Hoffman GS, Kerr GS, Leavitt RY, et al: Wegener's granulomatosis: an analysis of 158 patients, *Ann Intern Med* 116: 488-498, 1992.

Hoffman GS, Leavitt RY, Fleisher TA, et al: Treatment of Wegener's granulomatosis with intermittent high-dose intravenous cyclophosphamide, *Am J Med* 89:403-410, 1990.

Lie JT: Diagnostic histopathology of major systemic and pulmonary vasculitic syndromes, *Rheum Dis Clin North Am* 16(2):269-292, 1990.

Nolle B, Specks U, Ludemann J, et al: Anticytoplasmic autoantibodies: their immunodiagnostic value in Wegener's granulomatosis, *Ann Intern Med* 111:28-40, 1989.

C A S E

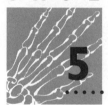

5   Winston Sequeira

A 45-year-old female lawyer presents with increasing tiredness and difficulty in getting out of a chair, climbing stairs, or even picking up an object from the floor. This is associated with severe myalgia.

The patient denied recent infections. She had been quite healthy and until a few months ago had taken no medication. About 2 or 3 months before seeing her physician, she noticed difficulty in swallowing and some abdominal discomfort and treated herself with cimetidine. She blamed all her symptoms on the stress at work. She had not noticed a change in the color of the urine. She did not smoke, drank alcohol on occasion, and had never used cocaine or heroin and was not on diuretics or laxatives. She had no family history of muscle disease.

QUESTION 1   What is your initial impression of the patient's complaints?

Easy fatigue and muscle pain are common nonspecific symptoms. It is important to be able to identify the source of the pain. In a patient with active synovitis of the shoulder it is not uncommon for the patient to complain of an ache over the deltoid and upper arm than over the glenohumeral joint. Inability to abduct the arm in such an individual is more likely to be due to the active arthritis or bursitis, but it can be difficult to exclude muscle weakness. Neuropathies are a cause of hyperesthesias and limb pain. Overuse syndromes or intense athletic activity in an untrained individual frequently result in myalgias. Viral syndromes including influenza, coxsackie, and hepatitis can occasionally present with severe arthralgias and muscle pain along with fatigue. Fibromyalgia and chronic fatigue syndrome may

also have a similar profile. Polymyalgia rheumatica would be considered in older individuals with hip and shoulder girdle pain.

QUESTION 2   She is unable to raise her head off the pillow and had III/V weakness in the proximal muscles of both the upper and the lower extremities. She had a waddling gait (grading of muscular strength is seen in the box). Her distal muscles were normal, there was no muscle wasting, and the deep tendon reflexes were present. She had no skin rash on the face, anterior chest, upper arms, or over the knuckles. The rest of the physical examination was normal. This patient had a mild normocytic normochromic anemia, normal electrolytes, and TSH. The SGOT, SGPT, and LDH were elevated as was the CPK and aldolase. The ANA was positive. What is the cause of her weakness?

This patient has demonstrable proximal muscle weakness that excludes neuropathies as a cause. It is helpful to classify the causes of proximal muscle weakness (see box). The major categories include (1) electrolyte imbalances, (2) endocrinopathies, (3) drugs, (4) metabolic, (5) collagen vascular disease, (6) muscular dystrophy, (7) neurologic dis-

. . . .

GRADING OF MUSCLE WEAKNESS

- 0 No perceptible movement
- 1 Barely perceptible movement
- 2 Unable to move against gravity
- 3 Moves against gravity but not against resistance
- 4 Moves against resistance but easily overcome
- 5 Normal strength.

. . . .

ELEVATED CPK OR PROXIMAL MUSCLE WEAKNESS: A DIFFERENTIAL DIAGNOSIS

ELECTROLYTE IMBALANCE
- Disorders of K, Na, Ca, P, Mg

ENDOCRINOPATHIES
- Hyperthyroidism or hypothyroidism
- Cushing's or Addison's disease
- Acromegaly
- Diabetic myoneuropathy

DRUGS
- Alcohol
- Steroids
- Lovastatin
- Clofibrate
- Zidovudine
- Cimetidine
- Colchicine
- Emetine
- Penicillamine

METABOLIC MUSCLE DISEASES
- Deficiencies of myophosphoralase
- Phosphofructokinases
- Acid maltase
- Carnitine
- Carnitine palmityl transferase
- Myoadenelate

COLLAGEN VASCULAR DISEASES
- Polymyositis
- Dermatomyositis,
- SLE
- Scleroderma
- RA

INFECTIONS
Viruses
- Influenza
- Hepatitis B
- Coxsackie
- HIV
- Parasites *Trichinella*
- Cysticercosis
- Toxoplasmosis

Mycobacteria
- TB
- Leprosy

NEUROLOGIC DISEASES
- Amyotrophic lateral sclerosis
- Myasthenia gravis
- Eaton-Lambert syndrome
- Landry's paralysis
- Guillain-Barré syndrome

MISCELLANEOUS
- Heat stroke
- Postexertional
- Postanesthesia

eases, and (8) infection. The most common electrolyte abnormality is hypokalemia. A history of diuretic use, laxative abuse, or the use of licorice may be useful historical points. Hypothyroidism should be considered in every individual with proximal muscle weakness because it is a frequent manifestation of this common disease. Alcohol is a cause of severe rhabdomyolysis. Chronic steroid use may be a cause of insidious muscle weakness. This patient was briefly on cimetidine, but her symptoms preceded her use of the drug, and it is unlikely that it played a part in her disease. The muscular dystrophies and enzyme deficiencies usually present in childhood. Milder forms, however, are observed in adult life. The diagnosis of polymyositis is made after excluding other causes of proximal muscle weakness. Muscle weakness toward the end of the day may be indicative of myasthenia gravis. Ptosis is a prominent feature of this disease. Tropical myositis is a deep tissue infection, usually with staphylococcus, associated with muscle necrosis and inability to move the limb because of pain. As the name suggests, it is more commonly seen in the tropics but is also found in temperate climates.

The anemia is indicative of a more chronic illness. The enzyme elevation points to a muscle disease. If the CPK was not included in the panel, it is likely that an erroneous diagnosis of liver disease may have been considered. The proximal muscle weakness with an elevated CPK and the lack of other secondary causes would make a collagen vascular disease like polymyositis a possible diagnosis.

QUESTION 3   What is the tourniquet test, and how do the results impact on the diagnosis of myositis?

A tourniquet test may be used to exclude some of the enzyme deficiencies. Baseline lactate and ammonia levels are drawn. A blood pressure cuff is applied at 20 mm Hg above the systolic blood pressure. The patient is then asked to squeeze a ball for 90 seconds. The cuff is released, and samples are drawn after 1, 5, and 10 minutes. Normally, the lactate and ammonia levels should be 3 to 4 times the baseline. In the myophosphoralase deficiencies the lactate level does not increase, and the ammonia may show a slower return to baseline. Abnormalities should be confirmed with a biopsy and special histochemical stains.

QUESTION 4   An EMG was done on the patient. Insertional irritability with low amplitude polyphasic spikes was seen and thought to be indicative of a myositis. What is the next step in the diagnostic plan?

A muscle biopsy should be done to confirm the diagnosis. Because the EMG may distort the muscle histology, it is wise to do the EMG on one side and the biopsy on the other. Tissue should be obtained from the contralateral deltoid or quadriceps. The biopsy should not be obtained from the weakest or the strongest muscle, as the results may be misleading. In the former, the muscle tissue may be replaced by fat or fibrous tissue and, in the latter, may appear normal. The specimens must be handled with care, spread across a piece of cardboard without stretching or wrinkling, and lightly moistened with saline. A frozen section should be processed for muscle enzymes and

histochemistry to exclude enzymatic defects, dystrophies, and metabolic diseases. If the disease is patchy, a larger specimen or two fragments of muscle from adjacent areas is more likely to provide a diagnosis. The needle muscle biopsy has the advantage of being a quick procedure with no scar and can be done repeatedly to follow the course of the disease. The major drawback is distortion, requiring a neuropathologist experienced in reading such specimens. This makes an open biopsy the procedure of choice for the initial biopsy.

QUESTION 5   What are the histologic features seen in dermatomyositis, polymyositis, and inclusion body myositis?

The inflammation in the interstitial and perivascular areas is indicative of an inflammatory muscle disease like dermatomyositis. In polymyositis the inflammation is within the myofibrils. Associated myofibril degeneration with phagocytosis and muscle regeneration are added features of polymyositis and dermatomyositis. Inclusion body myositis is characterized by variation in fiber size, angulation, and eosinophilic inclusions with vacuoles containing basophilic granules. On EM these vacuoles contain membranous whorls and tubular filaments.

QUESTION 6   What are the clinical features of autoimmune myositis?

Polymyositis is an autoimmune inflammatory muscle disease of unknown etiology. It is a relatively rare disease with 2 to 10 new cases per year/million people. It is more common in women with the ratio of 4:1 and associated with other collagen vascular diseases. Like other autoimmune diseases it is more frequent in African-Americans. The diagnosis is made if the patient has three of the four following features: (1) proximal muscle weakness, (2) elevated CPK, (3) an EMG compatible with myositis, and (4) inflammation on the muscle biopsy.

Dermatomyositis is the addition of a violaceous

heliotrope rash around the eyes often associated with scaly plaques over the knuckles referred to as Gottron's papules. The onset may be acute or insidious with the patient only seeking medical advice when significantly disabled. Involvement of the neck flexors makes it difficult for the patient to raise the head off the pillow. Dysphagia and dysphonia are characteristics of pharyngeal muscle weakness predisposing patients to the development of aspiration pneumonia. The weak intercostal muscles may contribute to ventilatory failure. Interstitial lung disease may precede the myositis but is generally diagnosed later. A strong correlation with the Jo-1 antibody and interstitial lung disease in polymyositis exists. Fever, weight loss, and arthritis may be present in all forms of myositis but is commonly described with polymyositis. The arthritis is generally nondeforming and nonerosive, but on occasion ulnar deviation may be evident. Cardiomyopathy leading to congestive heart failure or more commonly arrhythymias or conduction abnormalities may be observed. The elevated MB fraction found in polymyositis may not necessarily be indicative of cardiac involvement or ischemia. Calcinosis, more common in childhood dermatomyositis, tends to be linear and along the muscle fascicles. Vasculitis leading to bowel infarcts may be associated with dermatomyositis usually in children.

Patients with dermatomyositis should be screened for malignancy because there is evidence that the incidence may be higher in these patients even if one corrects for age. There is debate over the intensity with which this search should be carried out. Most rheumatologists believe that a compulsive physical examination coupled with the standard methods used to screen for malignancies in the general population is quite adequate. Bohan and Peter's classification has been modified recently to include inclusion body myositis (box). This involves older men with distal muscle involvement.

The cause of polymyositis or dermatomyositis is not known, but environmental factors, possibly viruses, in a genetically susceptible host is felt to play a part. Jo-1 is a histidyl t-RNA synthetase. It

CLASSIFICATION OF INFLAMMATORY MUSCLE DISEASE

- 1. Polymyositis
- 2. Dermatomyositis
- 3. Polymyositis/dermatomyositis associated with malignancy
- 4. Childhood polymyositis dermatomyositis
- 5. Associated with other collagen vascular diseases
- 6. Inclusion body myositis
- 7. Granulomatous myositis

(Modified from Bohan A and Peter JB: Polymyositis dermatomyositis, N Engl J Med 292:344-347, 1975.)

is speculated that Jo-1 and other synthetases might form immunogenetic complexes with t-RNA like structures on picornaviruses. The complimentary viral and host structures might lead to antisynthetases by antiidiotype mechanisms. In dermatomyositis the disease appears to be humorally mediated with evidence of immune complexes, complement activation, vascular damage, and muscle necrosis. In contrast, cell-mediated cytotoxicity appears to play a role in polymyositis. Elevated IL-1B, IL-2, and IL-2 receptors are associated with active inflammation. An MRI may be able to detect active inflammation as opposed to weakness due to muscles that are atrophic or replaced by fat. Using an MR spectroscope and P_{31}, one can determine the ratio of inorganic phosphorous and phosphokinase that is elevated in active muscle disease along with reduction of intracellular ATP. These are still research tools, however, and usually not used in day-to-day practice.

QUESTION 7 What autoantibodies are associated with polymyositis or dermatomyositis?

A number of autoantibodies have been described in patients with polymyositis and dermatomyositis. The most common of these is the

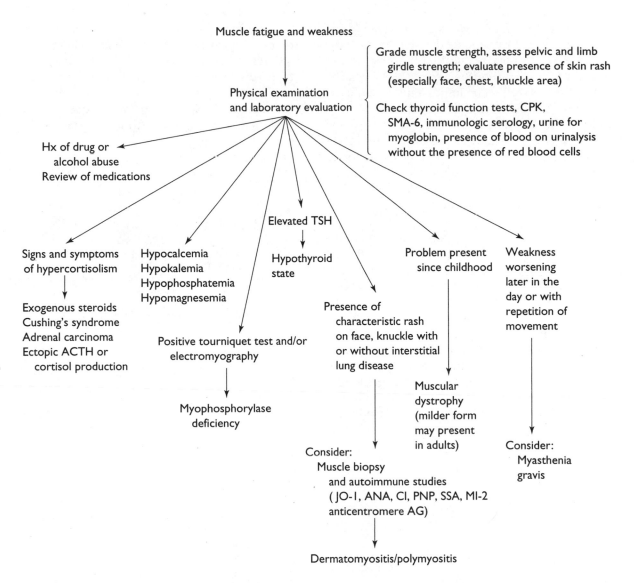

12-5-1   Diagnostic algorithm for muscle fatigue and weakness.

antinuclear antibody observed in nearly 70% of patients. The others include antibodies to U_1RNP, SSA, and the anticentromere (noted in less than 10% of patients). Anti-Jo-1 antibody is associated with interstitial lung disease and is the most common of the anticytoplasmic aminacyl t-RNA synthetases, identified in 20% of patients. These antibodies have been observed when the antinuclear antibodies are negative. Signal recogni-

tion antibodies (anti-SRP) are associated with cardiac disease and poor response to therapy. About 10% of patients may have anti-Mi-2, and this antibody tends to identify patients with muscle disease and features of scleroderma or dermatomyositis.

QUESTION 8   What is the traditional treatment regimen for polymyositis and dermatomyositis?

Treatment is usually with steroids in doses of 1 to 2 mgm/kg. Most patients do well on this dose and begin to feel better within a couple of weeks but may take a few months. Serial CPKs should be monitored, as well as the improvement in muscle strength. Steroids may nonspecifically reduce CPKs, as in muscular dystrophies, without actual remission in the disease. Therefore, it is important to note a parallel reponse between a reduction in CPKs and increased muscle strength. If muscle strength is not improving, the patient should be reassessed, and the history and the biopsy should be reviewed.

Azathioprine (2 to 4 mg/kg) or weekly methotrexate (0.1 to 0.3 mg/kg) may be used. The latter may be given orally, intravenously, or intramuscularly. As any muscle injury may increase the CPK level, intramuscular injections should be avoided. Cyclosporine and, more recently, IV gammaglobulin, have been used in refractory cases. Cyclophosphamide, effective in the treatment of other autoimmune diseases, does not appear to be that effective in the management of polymyositis or dermatomyositis. Plasmapheresis has been tried but not found to be of use in this disease.

The long-term survival rate is worse for patients with cancer-related myositis. Patients with dermatomyositis, myositis with other connective tissue diseases, do better with a 5-year survival rate of 80%. Patients with anti-SRP have the worst prognosis with a survival rate of 30%. There is residual disability in one third of survivors. Only a small number of patients with inclusion body myositis respond to treatment.

BIBLIOGRAPHY

Bohan A, Peter JB: Polymyositis dermatomyositis, *N Engl J Med* 292:344-347, 1975.

Hochberg MC, Feldman D, Steven MB: Adult onset polymyositis/dermatomyositis analysis of clinical and laboratory features and survival in 76 patients with a review of the literature, *Semin Arthritis Rheum* 15:168-178, 1986.

Plotz PH, Dalakas M, Leff RL, et al: Current concepts in idiopathic inflammatory myopathies: polymyositis dermatomyositis and related disorders, *Ann Intern Med* 111:143-157, 1989.

Targoff IN, Johnson AE, Miller EW: Antibody to signal recognition particle in polymyositis, *Semin Arthritis Rheum* 33:1367-1310, 1990.

CASE

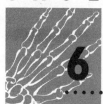

6
Paul R. Delbusto
. . . .

A 32-year-old man comes to your office with back pain. He states that his lower back has been increasingly painful over the last 4 months. The symptoms are worse in the morning and after naps. His symptoms seem to "work themselves out" over 2 to 3 hours. Approximately 2 weeks ago he developed the onset of bilateral heel pain. The pain is worse with weight bearing, and he has been unable to stand for prolonged periods of time. This has interfered with his work as a trader where he is required to be on his feet all day. He has taken acetaminophen with codeine without relief. He has lost 4 lbs over the past 4 months but denies any fever or chills.

His medical history is significant for testicular cancer 4 years ago. He required an orchiectomy but no radiation.

Physical examination reveals a temperature of 98.8°F. There is no skin disease. Conjunctiva are nonerythematous. There are no oral ulcers. A heart murmur is not present. Abdominal examination is benign. The back examination revealed no spinal tenderness. The patient is not able to touch his toes on forward flexion. Hip range of motion is normal. There is tenderness over the buttocks around both sciatic notches. There is pain on palpation of the medial aspect of both heels. The testicular examination reveals an orchiectomy without other abnormalities. Lymphadenopathy was not present.

QUESTION I What is the differential diagnosis, and what bedside test should be performed?

Back pain is the most common reason for patients to seek medical attention. The most common causes of back pain are mechanical.

Mechanical low back pain is defined as pain secondary to overuse of a normal anatomic structure (i.e., muscle strain) or pain secondary to trauma or deformity of an anatomic structure (i.e., herniated disc). Most episodes of back pain are self-limited. Ninety percent of mechanical causes of back pain last less than 8 weeks.

In this patient, there are historic clues to suggest that a mechanical cause of back pain may not be present. First, the patient's back pain has persisted over 4 months. This duration of back pain must be taken seriously as most episodes of back pain spontaneously remit. Second, the patient has had a 4-lb weight loss that suggests systemic disease. Fevers and chills may be other clues to systemic disease but are not present in this case. Third, the character of the back pain implies inflammatory disease. Mechanical back pain tends to worsen as the day progresses. Many patients are asymptomatic before any of the day's activity. In this patient, stiffness and pain worsening upon awakening and improving as the day progresses suggests an inflammatory nature of the pain. Fourth, bilateral heel pain does not accompany mechanical causes of back pain. The tenderness of the medial aspects of both heels is caused from plantar fasciitis. Plantar fasciitis and the other enthesopathies often accompany the inflammatory back diseases. Enthesopathies are sites of inflammation at insertion of ligaments and tendons onto bone. Other examples of enthesopathies include costochondritis and achilles tendonitis. The plantar fascia, when symptomatic, presents as heel pain worse upon first weight bearing. Symptoms often improve as the day progresses.

The bedside test to help identify the inflammatory back disorders (or spondyloarthropathies) is the Schoeber test. The Schoeber test identifies decreased expansion of the lumbar vertebrae on flexion of the back. A 10-cm line is made on the spine with the patient upright from the level of the iliac crests superiorly. The patient is then asked to fully flex the back by bending over and touching his or her toes. The line is then remeasured. A normal back should expand the line to measure over a total of 15 cm. A measurement of less than 15 cm implies limited lumbar expansion and consideration of the diagnosis of a spondyloarthropathy.

Physical examination in patients with back pain may help identify catastrophic causes of back pain. Neurologic deficits may suggest spinal cord compression or cauda equina syndrome. Abdominal examination may reveal an aortic aneurysm. Physical examination may also ellicit neighboring causes of back pain such as hip disease or trochanteric bursitis. Pain on palpation of the buttocks at the sciatic notches in this patient suggests sacroiliitis from the spondyloarthropathies. Sacroiliac tenderness and detection of sacroiliitis by physical examination, however, are often unreliable.

The history of testicular cancer in this patient raises the possibility of metastatic cancer as a cause of this patient's pain. Metastatic bone lesions or retroperitoneal involvement by tumor may present as back pain. Back pain caused from malignancy is often worse with recumbency, and patients may report they have been sleeping in a chair for relief of pain. Again, this patient's plantar fasciitis would not be seen in metastatic testicular cancer, and therefore metastatic testicular cancer is lower on our differential diagnosis.

The patient's poor response to acetaminophen with codeine is not unusual in the spondyloarthropathies. The spondyloarthropathies tend to respond better to the nonsteroidal antiinflammatory agents than to simple analgesia since inflammation is the basis for the pain in these conditions.

QUESTION 2 Which diagnostic tests are recommended to help make the diagnosis of inflammatory back pain in this patient?

A complete blood count and chemistry panel may help identify systemic inflammatory disease. Patients with inflammatory arthritis may have a normocytic, normochromic anemia (anemia of chronic disease). The albumin may be depressed, and the globulin fraction elevated on the chemistry panel reflecting inflammation. The sedimentation rate, a nonspecific measure of inflammation, is commonly elevated in the inflammatory back diseases and is often a good clue that a nonmechanical cause of back pain is present.

The best test in this patient and for the spondyloarthropathies is plain sacroiliac radiographs. Sacroiliitis may be identified and represents inflammatory chondritis and osteitis of the adjacent subchondral bone. HLA-B27 testing is neither necessary nor cost effective in this patient as plain radiography confirmed bilateral sacroiliitis. HLA-B27 typing may occasionally be useful for the diagnosis of the spondyloarthropathies in patients who have a clinical history somewhat suggestive of inflammatory back disease and negative sacroiliac radiographs. Bone scan, CT scan (computed tomography), and most recently MRI (magnetic resonance imaging) have been used to identify sacroiliitis in patients with negative plain sacroiliac radiographs (Fig. 12-6-1).

QUESTION 3 You place the patient on indomethacin 50 mg tid. The patient returns 3 months later and complains of a 10-lb weight loss and bloody diarrhea. He has 5 to 6 episodes of bright red loose stools per day. He has felt weak and his appetite has been poor. His back and heel pain have improved on indomethacin. Physical examination reveals diffuse abdominal tenderness and bright red blood on rectal examination. What is the rheumatologic diagnosis, and what diagnostic test do you recommend?

The spondyloarthropathies consist of ankylosing spondylitis, Reiter's syndrome, psoriasis, and inflammatory bowel disease. Reiter's syndrome classically is characterized by a triad of arthritis, urethritis, and conjunctivitis. Reiter's syndrome develops in the setting of postdysenteric or

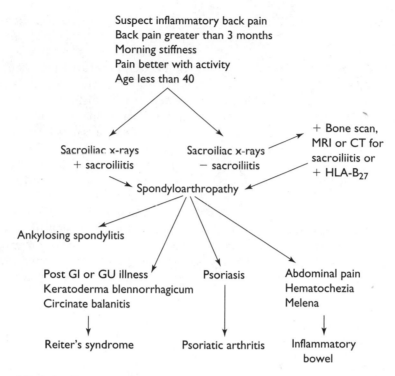

Suspect inflammatory back pain
Back pain greater than 3 months
Morning stiffness
Pain better with activity
Age less than 40

Sacroiliac x-rays
+ sacroiliitis

Sacroiliac x-rays
− sacroiliitis

+ Bone scan,
MRI or CT for
sacroiliitis or
+ HLA-B$_{27}$

Spondyloarthropathy

Ankylosing spondylitis

Post GI or GU illness
Keratoderma blennorrhagicum
Circinate balanitis

Psoriasis

Abdominal pain
Hematochezia
Melena

Reiter's syndrome

Psoriatic arthritis

Inflammatory
bowel

12-6-1   Diagnostic algorithm for the patient with inflammatory back pain.

postvenereal illness. The characteristic rashes of keratoderma blennorrhagicum and circinate balanitis may be present. Psoriatic spondyloarthropathy is characterized by psoriatic plaques. The skin involvement may be subtle and should be searched for carefully. The cleft of the buttock, hair line, and penis are not unusually involved. Inflammatory bowel disease consists of ulcerative colitis and Crohn's disease. Both ulcerative colitis and Crohn's disease have an associated spondyloarthropathy. Diarrhea and/or hematochezia with or without abdominal pain are common presentations for these diseases. A diagnosis of ankylosing spondylitis may be made when specific features of Reiter's syndrome, psoriasis, or inflammatory bowel disease are absent.

Although this patient may have been diagnosed with ankylosing spondylitis at the onset, the patient has now developed symptoms of inflammatory bowel disease. The gastrointestinal symptoms of inflammatory bowel disease may develop after the spondyloarthropathy. Ulcerative colitis is more likely than Crohn's disease to possess this property.

Inflammatory bowel disease has two distinct arthritic syndromes: the spondyloarthropathy and peripheral arthritis. Peripheral arthritis characteristically involves large joints, and the lower extremity is more commonly involved than the upper extremity. Activity of the bowel disease correlates directly to the activity of the peripheral arthritis. Therefore, control of the bowel disease often results in control of the peripheral arthritis. Conversely, the activity of the spondyloarthropathy is independent of the bowel activity. In this case, the symptoms of the spondyloarthropathy were controlled, yet the patient developed active bowel disease.

Indomethacin as a possible cause of gastrointestinal bleeding cannot be understated. Peptic ulcer disease, esophagitis, and small bowel erosions have been described in patients who use nonsteroidal antiinflammatory drugs. However, this patient has hematochezia, which suggests lower intestinal tract bleeding.

Bilateral symmetrical sacroiliitis is more commonly seen in ankylosing spondylitis and inflammatory bowel disease. Asymmetrical sacroiliitis is a feature mostly seen in Reiter's syndrome and psoriasis. In this patient, bilateral sacroiliitis and hematochezia with abdominal pain suggest ulcerative colitis spondyloarthropathy. Therefore, the study of choice at this point would be colonoscopy.

QUESTION 4   The colonoscopy in this patient was consistent with ulcerative colitis, and the diagnosis of ulcerative colitis spondyloarthropathy was made. What is the appropriate therapy for this disease process?

Treatment of ulcerative colitis spondyloarthropathy consists of medications and physical therapy. Physical therapy in these patients may prevent progressive deformity and disability. The patient should walk erect, perform back extension exercises regularly, and sleep on a firm mattress. Nonsteroidal antiinflammatory drugs can limit the pain and stiffness that the spondyloarthropathies may cause. Though all nonsteroidal antiinflammatory agents may have clinical efficacy in the spondyloarthropathies, indomethacin continues to be the favored agent by most rheumatologists. Nonsteroidal antiinflammatory drugs may vary with respect to toxicity and efficacy among individuals, but controlled data comparing agents are lacking.

In some individuals with inflammatory bowel disease, nonsteroidal antiinflammatory drugs may exacerbate the bowel symptoms. When patients fail or are unable to take these medications, second-line agents are offered. Sulfasalazine is the best studied of the second-line drugs. Sulfasalazine however is more efficacious in the treatment of the peripheral arthritis rather than the spondyloarthropathy. There is little role of chronic corticosteroid administration in the treatment of the spondyloarthropathies.

Corticosteroids may be necessary to control the bowel symptoms in selected patients but will have little effect on the axial arthritis. Judicious use of intraarticular corticosteroid or enthesopathy injections are often effective. Rarely, other immunosuppressive drugs such as methotrexate or azathioprine have been used to treat progressive disease not controlled by other agents. Removal of the colon in ulcerative colitis does not improve the symptoms of the spondyloarthropathy.

BIBLIOGRAPHY

Borenstein DG, Wiesel SW: *Low back pain: medical diagnosis and comprehensive management,* Philadelphia, 1989, WB Saunders.

Brooks PM: Nonsteroidal anti-inflammatory drugs-differences and similarities, *N Engl J Med* 324:1716-1724, 1991.

Brown MD: The source of low back pain, *Semin Arthritis Rheum* 18 (Suppl 2):67-72, 1989.

Dixon A Stj: Progress and problems in back pain research, *Rheumatol Rehabil* 12:165-175, 1973.

Furey JG: Plantar fasciitis. The painful heel syndrome, *J Bone Joint Surg* 57A:672-673, 1975.

Gabriel SE, Jackkimainen L, Bombardier C: Risk for serious gastrointestinal implications related to the use of nonsteroidal anti-inflammatory drugs: A meta-analysis, *Ann Intern Med* 115:787-796, 1991.

Hadler NM: Regional back pain, *N Engl J Med* 315:1090-1092, 1986.

Nachemson A: The lumbar spine: an orthopaedic challenge, *Spine* 1:59-71, 1976.

Weiner SR, Clark J, Taggart NA, Utsinger PD: Rheumatic manifestations of inflammatory bowel disease, *Semin Arthritis Rheum* 20:353-366, 1991.

CASE

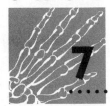

7

Paul R. Delbusto

. . . .

A 38-year-old woman comes to your office with a 2-week history of painless swelling of both hands including her fingers. She denies any symptoms of Raynaud's phenomena, arthritis, weakness, rash, alopecia, fever, chills, or weight loss.

Her medical history is significant for Grave's disease at age 26. She received radioactive iodine and is currently on thyroid replacement. She does not smoke or drink alcohol. There is no family history of arthritis, but her mother had "knobs on the knuckles" of both hands.

Physical examination is significant for a blood pressure of 112/74 mm Hg and a temperature of 99°F. Both hands and fingers are edematous and pitting diffusely. Obvious synovitis is not present. The systemic examination is completely normal.

QUESTION 1 What is the differential diagnosis, and which laboratory investigations would be helpful at this time?

Painless swelling of the hands is a nonspecific early presentation of several rheumatic conditions. Rheumatoid arthritis (RA), systemic lupus erythematosus (SLE) scleroderma, amyloid, and pseudogout may present this way. Edematous hands is the most common presentation of overlap syndromes. Remitting seronegative symmetrical synovitis with pitting edema (RS3PE) is a condition seen in elderly men. Thyroid acropachy can occur years after hyperthyroidism with clinical findings of painless swelling of the fingers, exophthalmos, clubbing, pretibial, myxedema, and periostitis. Carpal tunnel syndrome secondary to median nerve compression can sometimes

accompany edematous hands, but in this case neurologic symptoms are absent.

A complete blood count, chemistry panel, and urinalysis would be helpful to identify systemic disease and other organ involvement. A serum and urine protein electrophoresis may identify a monoclonal protein from amyloid. A rheumatoid factor (RF) and antinuclear antibody (ANA) may assist in determining which autoimmune illness may be responsible for these symptoms. Thyroid function tests should be obtained to exclude thyroid disease in this patient who has a history of Grave's disease. Radiographs of the hands may reveal evidence of chondrocalcinosis from pseudogout. The "knobs on the knuckles" of her mother's hands were most likely Heberden's and Bouchard's nodes from osteoarthritic involvement of the distal and proximal interphalangeal joints, respectively. Her mother's disease has no relationship to her current illness.

QUESTION 2 The patient returns upon your request in 2 weeks. She states that in addition to having swollen hands her fingertips turn white and then blue upon exposure to cold. The laboratory results from last visit include a normal blood count, chemistry panel, and urinalysis. The RF was negative, and the ANA was positive at 1:2560 with a nucleolar pattern. Chemically, her thyroid was compensated. Discuss how your differential diagnosis now changes with the new clinical information and which clinical investigations would now be helpful in determining the diagnosis.

The patient has developed Raynaud's phenomenon characterized by the change in color of her fingertips upon exposure to cold temperature. Raynaud's phenomenon may be present in rheumatoid arthritis, SLE, scleroderma, overlap conditions, as well as other rheumatic conditions. The differential diagnosis of Raynaud's phenomenon includes structural vasculopathies, malignancies, as well as other vasospastic disorders. Raynaud's phenonomenon may occur without an underlying medical disorder (primary Raynaud's phenomenon). The presence of Raynaud's phenomenon in this patient does not allow us to narrow the differential diagnosis.

The absence of other organ involvement identified by the normal blood count, chemistry, and urinalysis does not allow us to identify a specific autoimmune process. However, it is not unusual for organ involvement to evolve over time in rheumatic conditions. For example, if this patient developed thrombocytopenia, malar rash, and urinary sediment, a diagnosis of SLE would be likely.

RF was not present in this patient but may be present in all diagnoses being considered. In fact, 25% of patients with RA may be seronegative for RF. Though ANAs may be seen in RA, SLE, scleroderma, and overlap syndromes, the nucleolar pattern in high titer is suggestive of scleroderma. Specific scleroderma antibodies such as anticentromere antibody and antibody to SCL-70 (topoisomerase) can now be ordered to help confirm the diagnosis.

You place the patient on nifedipine for symptoms related to Raynaud's phenomenon and ask the patient to return.

The patient returns 3 months later and now has developed headache, arthralgias, dyspnea, and heartburn. Physical examination reveals a blood pressure of 240/130 mm Hg. There was evidence of papilledema and retinal hemorrhages on funduscopic examination. The patient is in congestive heart failure. Her hands and wrists developed thickened, bound-down skin. There are flexion contractures at the proximal interphalangeal joints. You also notice that the patient's skin disease has extended to her trunk and face. You send the patient to the emergency room.

Laboratory data in the emergency room reveals a hemoglobin of 9 g/dl and a platelet count of 200,000/ml. The reticulocyte count is 18%, and microangiopathic hemolytic anemia is present on the peripheral smear. Her serum creatinine is 3.2. Urinalysis reveals 5 to 10 red blood cells and 1+ protein. Outpatient labs from your office return and are negative for anticentromere and SCL-70 antibodies.

QUESTION 3 Do you now doubt the diagnosis of scleroderma? If so, what is the rheumatologic diagnosis, and what complication has she now suffered? What is the treatment of choice for this complication?

The patient has scleroderma characterized by Raynaud's phenomenon, arthralgias, skin involvement, esophageal disease, and now renal crisis.

There are two main subtypes of systemic scleroderma: diffuse and limited. Diffuse disease differs from limited scleroderma in many ways. In limited scleroderma, skin involvement is limited to skin distal to the elbow or knee. In diffuse scleroderma, skin involvement is seen proximal to the knee or elbow, as well as distal. In diffuse disease the skin involvement progresses rapidly, but in limited scleroderma skin disease is slower to advance. In addition, the internal organ involvement in diffuse scleroderma occurs more rapidly and carries a worse prognosis. Diffuse scleroderma has a 10-year mortality of more than 50%, whereas limited scleroderma has a 10-year mortality of less than 50%. Raynaud's phenomenon is usually present for many years before the development of skin involvement in limited scleroderma. In diffuse scleroderma, Raynaud's phenomenon frequently occurs after development of skin disease. Pulmonary scleroderma in the form of pulmonary fibrosis is more common in diffuse scleroderma, whereas pulmonary hypertension is more frequent in limited scleroderma. Renal crisis is almost exclusively seen in diffuse scleroderma. Anticentromere antibodies are found in 4% to 98% of limited scleroderma patients. Antibodies

DIFFUSE VERSUS LIMITED SCLERODERMA

DIFFUSE SCLERODERMA
* Skin involvement proximal and distal
* Rapid organ involvement
* Raynaud's phenomenon after skin involvement
* Pulmonary fibrosis in 70%
* Renal crisis common
* Antibody to SCL-70 (topoisomerase)
* 10-year survival <50%
* Raynaud's phenomenon 90%
* Finger swelling 95%
* Tendon friction rubs 70%
* Arthralgias 98%
* Proximal weakness 80%
* Calcinosis 20%
* Telangiectasias 60%
* Esophageal dysmotility 80%
* Small bowel involvement 40%
* Myocardiopathy 15%
* ANA 90%
* Sicca 15%

LIMITED SCLERODERMA
* Skin involvement distal only
* Slow onset of organ involvement
* Raynaud's phenomenon before skin involvement
* Pulmonary hypertension in 25%
* Renal crisis uncommon
* Antibody to centromere
* 10-year survival >50%
* Raynaud's phenomenon 99%
* Finger swelling 90%
* Tendon friction rubs 5%
* Arthralgias 90%
* Proximal weakness 60%
* Calcinosis 40%
* Telangiectasias 90%
* Esophageal dysmotility 90%
* Small bowel involvement 60%
* Myocardiopathy 10%
* ANA 90%
* Sicca 15%

to SCL-70 are present in 25% to 75% of diffuse scleroderma patients. Other clinical manifestations of scleroderma include tendon friction rubs, muscle weakness, calcinosis, telangiectasias, small bowel involvement, cardiomyopathy, and sicca syndrome. Tendon friction rubs, when present, suggest diffuse scleroderma in almost all cases (see box).

Our patient has diffuse scleroderma characterized by proximal and distal skin involvement and renal crisis. The presence of skin involvement before Raynaud's phenomenon also suggests diffuse scleroderma. Absence of scleroderma-specific antibodies does not exclude this clinical diagnosis. This patient has suffered one of the most dreaded complications of scleroderma, which is renal crisis. Renal crisis in scleroderma usually presents with hypertensive crisis. Our patient has funduscopic changes, as well as heart failure. Renal insufficiency has developed. Renal crisis in scleroderma is renin-mediated, and therefore angiotensin-converting enzyme inhibitors are the treatment of choice. Since the development of angiotensin-converting enzyme inhibitors, pulmonary disease is now the most frequent cause of death in scleroderma patients.

Nifedipine did not prevent the development of renal crisis in this patient but may have worsened the esophageal symptoms. Calcium blockers decrease gastroesophageal sphincter tone and may have uncovered occult esophageal disease. Therefore calcium blockers should be used with caution in scleroderma patients.

QUESTION 4 Retrospectively, how would you evaluate the initial differential diagnosis with respect to specific elements in this patient's full presentation, and what is the final diagnosis?

It is now easy in retrospect to differentiate scleroderma from the other possibilities in our differential diagnosis (Fig. 12-7-1). RA has skin manifestations, but they are usually the result of vasculitis or ulcers. RA does not frequently involve the kidney except from drug toxicity. NSAIDS (nonsteroidal antiinflammatory drugs),

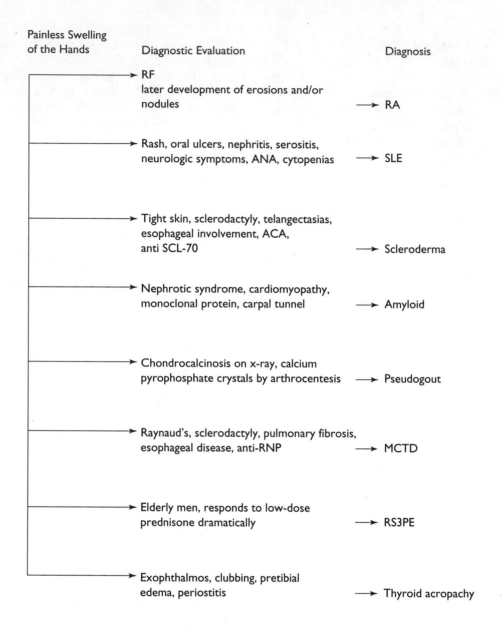

Painless Swelling
of the Hands   Diagnostic Evaluation   Diagnosis

RF
later development of erosions and/or
nodules   ⟶ RA

Rash, oral ulcers, nephritis, serositis,
neurologic symptoms, ANA, cytopenias   ⟶ SLE

Tight skin, sclerodactyly, telangectasias,
esophageal involvement, ACA,
anti SCL-70   ⟶ Scleroderma

Nephrotic syndrome, cardiomyopathy,
monoclonal protein, carpal tunnel   ⟶ Amyloid

Chondrocalcinosis on x-ray, calcium
pyrophosphate crystals by arthrocentesis   ⟶ Pseudogout

Raynaud's, sclerodactyly, pulmonary fibrosis,
esophageal disease, anti-RNP   ⟶ MCTD

Elderly men, responds to low-dose
prednisone dramatically   ⟶ RS3PE

Exophthalmos, clubbing, pretibial
edema, periostitis   ⟶ Thyroid acropachy

ANA - antinuclear antibody
ACA - anticentromere antibody
RF - rheumatoid factor
RS3PE - remitting seronegative symmetrical synovitis
              with pitting edema

12-7-1   Differential diagnosis of painless swelling of the hands.

gold, and penicillamine may cause renal abnormalities.

SLE can cause skin abnormalities and renal disease. The common skin manifestations include the malar and discoid rash, photosensitivity, oral ulcers, vasculitic lesions, and others. Tightened, thick skin is not a manifestation of SLE. Nephritis is a common renal manifestation of SLE. SLE frequently has serosal, neurologic, and hematologic abnormalitics.

Amyloid can rarely mimic the skin disease of scleroderma. Other features of amyloid such as nephrotic syndrome, carpal tunnel syndrome, or cardiomyopathy are not present in this patient. Pseudogout does not have internal organ involvement and is a diagnosis made by identifying calcium pyrophosphate crystals by arthrocentesis. Skin tightening, Raynaud's phenomenon, ar-thralgias, esophageal disease, and renal crisis in this patient represent a constellation of symptoms seen in scleroderma.

BIBLIOGRAPHY

Cardelli MB, Kleinsmith DM: Raynaud's phenomenon and diseases, *Med Clin North Am* 73:1127-1141, 1989.

Kinsella RA, Black DK: Thyroid acropachy, *Med Clin North Am* 52:393, 1968.

McCarty DJ, O'Duffy JD, Pearson L, Hunter JB: Remitting seronegative symmetrical synovitis with pitting edema (RS3PE) syndrome, *JAMA* 2545:3763-276, 1985.

Seibold JR: Systemic sclerosis. In Klippel JH, Dieppe PA, eds: *Rheumatology,* St Louis, 1994, Mosby.

Steen VD, Costantino JP, Shapiro AP, et al: Outcome of renal crisis in systemic sclerosis: relation to angiotensin converting enzyme (ACE) inhibitors, *Ann Intern Med* 113:352-357, 1990.

INDEX